fifteenth edition

Rypins' Medical Boards Review

volume **I**
Basic Sciences

Rypins' Medical Boards Review

fifteenth edition

Edited by

Edward D. Frohlich, M.D.

Vice President for Academic Affairs,
Alton Ochsner Medical Foundation;
Staff Member, Ochsner Clinic;
Professor of Medicine and Physiology,
Louisiana State University School of Medicine;
Adjunct Professor of Pharmacology and
Clinical Professor of Medicine,
Tulane University School of Medicine
New Orleans, Louisiana

With the Collaboration of a Review Panel

J. B. LIPPINCOTT COMPANY • Philadelphia

Grand Rapids • New York • St. Louis • San Francisco
London • Sydney • Tokyo

Acquisitions Editor: Charles McCormick
Sponsoring Editor: Delois Patterson
Project Editor: Linda J. Stewart
Indexer: Ruth Elwell
Design Coordinator: Doug Smock
Cover Designer: Mark A. James
Production Manager: Carol A. Florence
Production Coordinator: Pamela Milcos
Compositor: Bi-Comp, Inc.
Printer/Binder: Murray Printing Company

Fifteenth Edition

Library of Congress Cataloging-in-Publication Data

Rypins, Harold, 1892–1939.
  Rypins' medical boards review.

  Rev. ed. of: Rypins' medical licensure examinations.
14th ed./edited by Edward D. Frohlich, with the
collaboration of a review panel. c1985.
  Includes index.
  Contents: v. 1. Basic sciences—v. 2. Clinical
sciences.
  1. Medicine—Handbooks, manuals, etc. 2. Medicine—
Examinations, questions, etc. 3. Medical sciences—
Examinations, questions, etc. I. Frohlich, Edward D.,
[Date]. II. Rypins, Harold, 1892–1939. Medical
licensure examinations. III. Title. IV. Title:
Medical boards review. [DNLM: 1. Licensure, Medical.
2. Medicine—examination questions. W18 R995m]
R834.5.R96   1989   610.76   89-7952
  ISBN 0-397-50906-5 (v. 1)
  ISBN 0-397-50907-3 (v. 2)

Editorial Review Panel

Preface

Publication of the 15th edition of *Rypins' Medical Boards Review* provides the opportunity to take stock of our past performance, the present perception of the value of the volume to our readers, and our future role in medical education and the overall learning process. Clearly, our past performance is nothing short of an outstanding success. This is attested by 56 years of confidence by medical students and physicians desiring a comprehensive review prior to their sitting for licensure examinations. Over these years, if imitation is the sincerest form of flattery, many volumes have entered and left the bookstalls, but *Rypins'* continues to endure and to merit the confidence of its readers. As further evidence of the esteem in which this textbook is held I have received many letters and telephone calls from Europe, Africa, Asia, and Latin America asking when the next edition is scheduled for publication and what will be new in the forthcoming edition.

Initially, this textbook was prepared for physicians planning to take state board medical licensure examinations. It consisted of short treatises or summaries in nine major areas of medicine, each followed by typical essay-type questions from past examinations. This format remained rather constant over the first 14 editions. Multiple-choice questions and their answers were included in the 13th edition to help students prepare for the more recently introduced national board type of examination.

Most experts, teachers, students, and specialists in preparing examinations would agree that all examinations have their faults. Nevertheless, licensing examinations remain the only means available for objectively testing the knowledge and competence of individuals to practice the art and science of medicine. Coincidentally, the examinations and their scope and objectives have become more sophisticated and expanded with the introduction of additional types, from the qualifying examination to national board examinations and the several examinations that test the knowledge of practicing physicians worldwide. Each state jealously (and justifiably so) guards its right to determine which physicians should be granted the privilege of practicing medicine within its borders; as a result, more than 50 jurisdictions have in the past prepared their own medical licensure examination. These examinations have varied so widely in kind, quality, and rate of failure of prospective practitioners that some states have refused to accept the licenses of others, placing serious obstacles in the way of the interstate movement of physicians.

To resolve some of these difficulties, the Federation of State Medical Boards of the United States, after some years of study and research, developed a clinically oriented, reliable examination, the Federation Licensing Examination, which is offered to any state board for use as its own licensing examination. It is prepared by a committee of the federation in collaboration with the National Board of Medical Examiners (NBME). Known by the acronym FLEX (Federation Licensing Examination), this examination is given in all participating states of the United States twice a year on the same three days, in June and December.

By far the largest number of graduates from American medical schools take another series of examinations, not identical to the FLEX, that is offered in three parts by the NBME: The first is given after completion of the first two preclinical years in medical school; the second part, which focuses on clinical medicine, is taken after the second two years; and the third, taken after at least six months of the first postgraduate training year, is an objective test of general clinical competence. The U.S. Congress is constantly revising health manpower legislation that may affect medical licensure. The use by all states of these high-quality examinations, either under state board auspices or by a nationally constituted medical licensure examination, may help forestall legislation of a single federal licensing examination for graduates of American medical schools.

Nevertheless, the use of federal licensing examinations seems to be unavoidable because of the need to determine the adequacy of the knowledge of graduate physicians from foreign medical schools who are applying for a license to practice medicine in the United States. Over the years a number of types of examinations have been developed for foreign medical graduates. The first of these was the Educational Commission for Foreign Medical Graduates (ECFMG), a one-day test, in English, that consisted of 300 well-chosen NBME multiple-choice questions. Five of every six questions came from the traditional clinical fields and one of every six from the basic medical sciences. Also included in the ECFMG examination was a one-hour test designed to assess the graduate's understanding of the English language.

A second type of test, the Visa Qualifying Examination (VQE), was introduced under mandate by an Act of Congress in 1976. This law required that all foreign medical graduates who are accepted for graduate training in the United States pass the VQE before a visa might be issued to enter the United States. This examination was taken in three parts: the first in the basic sciences, the second in the clinical sciences, and the third in clinical and patient problems. Indeed, passing the VQE was declared equivalent to passing parts I and II of the standard NBME examination.

The VQE, however, was abandoned in favor of a revised format, the Foreign Medical Graduate Examination in the Medical Sciences (FMGEMS) and ECFMG English test. This examination takes place in two half-day sessions. The preclinical areas of medical inquiry are comprehensively reviewed on the first day, and the second day includes an English language test and an examination of clinical knowledge. Refer to Chapter 1 for further discussion, including appropriate reference to the source for obtaining specific details and for an application to sit for these examinations.

Another area of medical licensure, of relatively recent importance, is the requirement for relicensure by state medical boards or by certain subspecialty organizations. In summary, therefore, a variety of examinations have been designed to determine medical knowledge and competence. These have undergone a tremendous evolution and growth in sophistication and number and in the demands they place on the fundamental knowledge of the professional physician.

This brings us to the present 15th edition of *Rypins' Medical Boards Review,* which has dramatically changed with respect to the 14th edition. In this edition we see a new title that reflects this evolution in medical (licensure) examinations to the present national, state, and specialty board examinations as well as the FMGEMS. We have also decided to make this textbook available in two volumes, one for the basic preclinical sciences and the other for the clinical sciences. This should provide the reader with a less "weighty" tome while reading, a greater ease in keeping up-to-date from one edition to the next, and a means for utilizing more directly the supplementary *Rypins' Questions and Answers for Medical Boards Review* for the 14th edition, which deals with the basic preclinical sciences.

Several additional innovations are provided in this new edition. These include the introduction of key words highlighted in bold italics within the substance of each chapter. These key words provide the reader with a valuable notation of terms critical to the topic under study.

Certainly the most valuable innovations are the participation of six new contributors on our Review Panel (three new authors contributed to Volume I, and three new authors contributed to Volume II). Each individual has had considerable teaching experience as well as broad recognition by his peers for expressing with clarity the chapter topic. Thus we warmly welcome Drs. Robert Roskowski, Jr., Ronald B. Luftig, Margaret A. Reilly and John C. McGiff, who have extensively revised and remarkably updated the material in the Biochemistry, Microbiology and Immunology, and Pharmacology chapters in the fundamental preclinical sciences volume.

We also welcome Drs. Ronald C. Elkins and Martin L. Pernoll, who have provided extensively revised chapters in Surgery and in Obstetrics and Gynecology in the clinical sciences volume. With the untimely death of my dear friend and colleague Dr. Solomon Papper, I elected to assume authorship responsibilities for the Internal Medicine chapter. I invited my friend and colleague at the Ochsner Clinic, Dr. George A. Pankey, to coauthor this chapter with me. He has broad experience in clinical teaching and in the study of infectious diseases and is well recognized for his earlier work in national testing programs.

These new contributors to the ''Rypins' family'' join our earlier mainstays and experienced ''heavies'' of the editorial review panel. Each of the contributors is widely recognized as an academic leader of the first order. All have been selected because of their ability to express and teach highly complex material in a simple and yet straightforward manner.

Each of these world-class teachers has drastically revised and updated his past material. The reader will find new material on molecular and cellular biology and immunology presented in a crystal-clear manner; this is integrated with the material of other chapters dealing with disease mechanisms, patient evaluation, management, and treatment. Note also the new tables, figures and pedagogic text material.

Thus we see a very dramatic and broadly revised 15th edition—a textbook markedly restructured in physical organization, contributors, and, most importantly, in content and scientific material. We are all very pleased with this new and exciting edition.

We hope that this textbook will continue to be of value to all who are concerned with medical examinations—those who prepare the examination, those who must prepare and qualify for medical licensure, and those already licensed who are required to sit for relicensure examination. In addition, this textbook may be of value to the medical educator planning for courses in continuing medical education, to the medical student who is interested in reviewing material for specific course examinations, and to the practicing physician interested in gaining a quick resume of the present state of knowledge in some area of medical pedagogy. This has been the text's aim for over half a century: to present, in a clear and concise manner, the most comprehensive and up-to-date knowledge of the various fields of medicine and to make the accompanying questions as pertinent and clinically oriented as possible. With respect to the questions that are appended to each chapter, it is suggested that the reader should not only review the rhetorical questions, but also consider carefully the multiple-choice questions. As indicated, these multiple-choice questions follow the style and format of the questions devised by the NBME, FLEX, and FMGEMS examinations. The questions in each chapter are followed by an answer key.

And what of the future of *Rypins'*? Well, this all depends on you, the readers. We always value your comments, suggestions, and needs. We sincerely hope that this textbook continues to merit your confidence and support.

It is appropriate and gratifying to express to those who are so close to me personally and professionally my deep appreciation for being able to put forth this new edition. I am truly grateful to my colleagues at the Ochsner Clinic and at the Alton Ochsner Medical Foundation for the opportunity, the time, and the ambience to pursue and complete this academic challenge. Over the years, I have always valued the support and constant loyalty of an office staff that is a great source of personal satisfaction and appreciation. Midway in the preparation of this edition my longstanding assistant, Elizabeth Murray, achieved the distinction of a well-earned promotion to her retirement years. And, I am indeed fortunate that her position has been filled by two equally competent and dedicated assistants, Barbara Buetow and Melissa Chiasson. To each of these people I express my deep gratitude and appreciation. Clearly, my expression of appreciation is also in order to the publishing staff of J. B. Lippincott.

But, most of all, I again and always wish to express my deep love and inexpressible thanks to my wife, Sherry, and to my children, Margie, Bruce, and Lara. Only they know of their love and patience, their unselfish understanding of the time, effort, and commitment that is required to bring this idea and textbook to fruition. Without their support and encouragement it would have been impossible to organize, review, and get this material published within the schedule planned. It has been said that "Medicine is a jealous mistress"; jealousy has been no part of my family's relationship with me and endeavors such as this attest to their love and support. Indeed, it has been that loving understanding that has made this, and whatever else I do, worthwhile, possible, and personally rewarding and hence a labor of love.

Edward D. Frohlich, M.D.

Preface to the First Edition

This book is an expression of the writer's conviction that the average American medical graduate of today is well prepared for the practice of his profession and that consequently there is little basis for the obvious dread with which he approaches the ordeal of the licensing examination. It is based on fifteen years' experience as Secretary of the New York State Board of Medical Examiners, during which period he has had intimate contact not only with medical schools and boards of medical examiners throughout the country, but also with large numbers of candidates for the licensing examination.

After a critical survey of many thousands of questions actually used throughout the whole United States, a selection of typical questions has been made, and these immediately follow the review presented in each of the nine major medical subjects. By placing these questions at the end of the chapters the thought processes of the student are stimulated and his best interests more fully served than in the older forms of questions and answers.

It is the proper function of the state to submit to examination all candidates for the right to practice medicine, and the state medical licensing examination can, and in some instances does, serve as a valuable check upon the work of the medical schools. There should be, however, closer co-operation between licensing boards and medical schools. Medical faculties should recognize more clearly the function and intention of the licensing boards, and licensing boards should be more clearly aware of the progress which is being made in medical schools. It is evident that the examining boards are slowly realizing that medical schools are in better position than themselves to test the student's academic or encyclopedic knowledge of such subjects as anatomy, chemistry, and bacteriology; that such testing may be safely left in the hands of medical faculties; and that examining boards should limit themselves to inquiring into the ability of the medical graduate to apply such knowledge clinically.

As for the graduate's attitude toward the state licensing examination, his fear arises from failure to understand the point of view of the state examiners as well as from an ability to muster in due proportion the vast amount of material presented to him during his medical course.

Careful study of licensing examinations throughout the United States indicates a general agreement among examiners regarding the material essential for the candidate. It is this ground, and only this ground, that the present volume aims to cover.

Every effort has been made to treat as concisely as possible those portions of the medical curriculum generally selected for use by the various examining boards. Repetition and overlapping have been avoided. Where a subject such as rabies, for example, has been covered in the chapter on Preventive Medicine, it is not repeated under the consideration of the Filtrable Viruses in Bacteriology. The arrangement of the material emphasizes the relations of the whole and its parts. It is taken for granted that the student has been adequately trained in the medical sciences and there is no attempt to teach him anything new. The object is, not to cram his mind, rather, to assist him in selecting and rearranging his material intelligently and practically.

Deliberate omission has been made of nearly all technical procedures, such as physical diagnosis, blood-counting and blood-chemistry, basal metabolism, x-ray, or surgical technic. Technical procedures cannot be taught in books and the ability to employ them properly should be assumed in the modern graduate. For similar reasons there is no separate section on materia medica or prescription-writing. References to the use of therapeutic agents are included in the consideration of the disease for which they are indicated.

To the authors in the various fields of medicine from whose books and articles he has freely drawn, the author desires to express his appreciative thanks. His gratitude to Miss E. Marion Pilpel, Miss Florence S. Muffson, and particularly to his wife, Senta Jonas Rypins, for invaluable secretarial assistance, he is most happy to acknowledge.

HAROLD RYPINS
Albany, N.Y.

Contents

fifteenth edition

Rypins' Medical Boards Review

Medical Qualifying Examinations

Edward D. Frohlich, M.D.
Vice President for Academic Affairs, Alton
Ochsner Medical Foundation; Staff Member,
Division of Hypertensive Diseases, Ochsner Clinic;
Professor of Medicine and of Physiology, Louisiana
State University School of Medicine; Adjunct
Professor of Pharmacology and Clinical Professor
of Medicine, Tulane University School of Medicine,
New Orleans, Louisiana

The testing of professional competence before certifying for public responsibilities is an age-old practice. In China, for example, candidates for public service were required to submit to special examinations at least 3,000 years ago, and the tests were said to be not unlike those employed today. In the United States the practice developed slowly, first as a kind of contribution by the profession itself to public welfare; later as a responsibility of the state. In New York State the problem arose in the early 19th century as far as the practice of medicine is concerned. At that time, the Legislature found that attempts to control the practice of "physic and surgery" in unorganized fashion had been most unsatisfactory, since charlatans and quacks abounded, and passed "an act to incorporate Medical Societies for the purpose of regulating the practice of Physic and Surgery in this state." This law provided for the establishment of a medical society in each county and gave to the practicing physicians themselves, thus legally organized, the power to grant licenses to qualified applicants and to regulate the practice of medicine in their counties.

Methods of testing varied. In general, tests were clinical and practical, limited to questions or discussions concerning the diagnosis and the treatment of diseases, for the candidates were chiefly those who had received their training as apprentices to practicing physicians. Not until nearly midcentury did the number of physicians who had had their education and training in medical schools predominate. Soon thereafter the states themselves assumed responsibilities for licensure and, consequently, for establishing formal testing procedures. With this development, Boards of Examiners, or similar bodies, were appointed to examine officially all applicants for fitness to practice the medical profession. Today, all 50 states, as well as the District of Columbia and the Commonwealth of Puerto Rico, have official medical licensing agencies.

The usual means of measuring knowledge is the formal written examination, and it has an important place in all educational programs. "Examination," the late President Eliot of Harvard once stated, "is the most difficult of the educational arts and its influence on both students and teachers may be very great." Indeed, intelligently and thoughtfully prepared examinations can be made a most valuable educational exercise in any course of study. They not only force the student to review and stimulate him to keep up with his work, but they also may serve to test the quality of teaching if the examination is well designed and the results are interpreted carefully.

How effective are formal written examinations in testing professional competence? Perhaps not as effective as they are in an educational program. Nevertheless, they are the only practical means of assessing the competence of large numbers of applicants for professional licensure. Although this practice is not ideal and does not test for such essential attributes as ethical and moral standards, carefully designed tests do play a definite role in separating the qualified practitioner from the unqualified and, in doing so, protect the public from the charlatan and the incompetent.

Examinations for licensure, however, have not always kept pace with the remarkable advances in medical knowledge and the resultant changes in methods of training for the practice of medicine. For this reason, many of the examination methods employed in former years have become inadequate. Thus, the purpose of the licensing examination is not so much to test the candidate's general knowledge in such individual subjects as anatomy, pathology, medicine, and surgery as to determine his or her ability to apply this knowledge to the diagnosis and treatment of disease and to determine the candidate's general fitness to practice the art and the science of medicine. In the past, unfortunately, most licensing examinations failed miserably in this last category.

The existence of separate licensing boards in all the states, the District of Columbia and the Commonwealth of Puerto Rico, each setting its own type of qualifying examination for licensure, has led to great variation in the kind and quality of the examinations. This has worked against unity of procedures and standards and has made difficult the movement of physicians from one licensing jurisdiction to another. However, as will be described in more detail later, through the efforts of the Federation of State Medical Boards of the United States, a high quality examination—the Federation Licensing Examination (FLEX)—prepared by a special Federation committee for administration twice a year, has been offered to any state medical board that wishes to use the examination as its own licensing test. A measure of its success is shown by the fact that it has been used by nearly all states since 1973. The prerequisites for licensure still varies from one state to another; and it would be well for any physician interested in licensure in any specific state to write directly to the State Board of Medical

Licensure of that state for specific requirements and information.

Another confusing element in the licensing procedure has been added by the establishment in a number of states of separate boards of examiners in the basic sciences. These tests are designed to be given to candidates for admission to all branches of the healing professions, not only medicine but such other areas as chiropractic and neuropathy. In these jurisdictions certification by the basic science boards is required before admission to the specific professional examination is granted.

In most instances the members of these boards are teachers of such subjects as general chemistry, physics, biology, and anatomy. The tests therefore are not specifically prepared for physicians who have had intensive training in the basic medical sciences that form an integral part of medical education. The purpose of this examination is to determine whether the candidate has had adequate training in the fundamental sciences considered essential for admission to the licensing examination of the particular healing art the applicant wishes to practice. At best these tests are elementary when compared with the comprehensive training in the basic medical sciences given in schools of medicine. The consequent repetition, in part at least, of an examination in basic sciences by the medical licensing boards in these states has complicated still further the licensing of physicians. Fortunately, the number of these basic science boards is diminishing, and the time appears not far off when they will be done away with.

Thus, with all their defects and deficiencies, examinations are essential to the licensing procedure. They form not only an essential part of any well-planned program of education but are also, when well constructed, the only generally satisfactory method thus far devised for determining the professional competence and fitness to practice for a large number of candidates. They constitute a dependable measure of coordinated thinking as well as a test of knowledge not to be gained in any other way. Examinations are therefore here to stay, and the objective of all boards of medical licensure must be to administer examinations that are as fair, comprehensive and valid tests of fundamental knowledge and clinical competence as it is possible to make.

TYPES OF EXAMINATIONS

Essay Examination

Until rather recently many state boards of medical examiners employed the so-called essay examination, but it is no longer generally used in licensing tests. In this test a limited number of questions is asked, and the candidate answers each one in a short composition or dissertation. The essay examination emphasizes description, definition, explanation and discussion. Symptoms, signs, abnormalities in function, pathologic changes, etiology, and the diagnosis and treatment of disease conditions are described, and discussed by the candidate, sometimes at considerable length.

The advantages of the essay test are that it gives the candidate an opportunity to consider thoughtfully each of a limited number of problems posed, to reveal his ability to organize his answer, to demonstrate his skill at description and to present evidence of his general scholarship, his writing ability, penmanship, spelling, composition and neatness of execution. All of these qualities are desirable accomplishments, but not all of them are the particular attributes that define a physician's overall competence to practice medicine.

Among the disadvantages are the relatively long time it takes to grade essay answers, the difficulty the examiner has of being uniformly fair in grading answers to the same question on different papers and the frequent quandary the examiner finds himself in when, because of poor penmanship or a lack of knowledge of English on the part of the candidate, he cannot interpret an answer. The grading of essay examinations is therefore slow, subject to considerable subjective variation in evaluation of answers, and occupies an excessive amount of an examiner's time.

Finally, in view of the continued rapid expansion of medical knowledge in every field, it is now recognized that a limited number of essay questions does not permit as adequate testing of the candidate's general knowledge as is desired. Occasionally, therefore, oral or practical tests have been used to supplement the written test. With the additional information that such tests provide, the examining boards feel more secure in certifying a candidate for licensure. The great difficulty with this type of individual test, however, is that it cannot be given within a reasonable time, nor can adequate numbers of examiners be provided when great numbers of candidates must be examined. At present, if given at all, these individual tests are limited to those states where the number of candidates is small.

Multiple-Choice Examination

In recent years more and more State Boards of Examiners have been turning to the objective or multiple choice examination. In this type of test each question is so prepared that the candidate is faced with a problem, the correct answer to which is included in the question and must be selected and indicated on the answer sheet by making a mark in the appropriate place. The characteristic feature of these tests is that the candidate answers the questions by blackening, with a special pencil on the answer sheet, the space he believes to indicate the correct answer. Although this is considered a written examination, no actual writing of sentences is required. This kind of test has two important advantages: A great many more questions covering a much wider range of subjects can be asked in a given time than is possible in the essay examination; and the answers can be graded more objectively and with greater speed and accuracy than in any other type of examination. Thus, the number of questions that can be asked in an allotted period can be increased from 8 or 10, or at most 12, in an essay test to 100, 150, or even more, in the objective test, thereby effectively broadening the scope of the examination.

At first the objective or multiple-choice examination met with considerable disapproval on the candidate's part because the technique was so new and different, and on the examiner's part because the construction of valid, unambiguous, and reliable questions proved to be so difficult (far more difficult, in fact, than the preparation of essay questions). But with the passage of time the objective examination has come into its own as a valid, comprehensive and dependable test of a candidate's knowledge and, when applied effectively, of his competence and ability. Moreover, this type of examination seems to be the most searching, valid, and comprehensive type of test to administer to large groups of candidates.

Many different forms of objective, multiple-choice questions have been devised to test not only medical knowledge but those subtler qualities of discrimination, judgment and reasoning. Certain types of questions may test an individual's recognition of the similarity or dissimilarity of diseases, drugs, physiologic or pathologic processes. Other questions test judgment as to cause and effect or the lack of causal relationships. Case histories or patient problems are used to simulate the experience of a physician confronted with a diagnostic problem; a series of questions then tests the individual's understanding of related aspects of the case, such as associated laboratory findings, treatment, complications, and prognosis. In this type of examination each question has only one correct response among a number of possible choices—most often one correct response out of five choices, although the ratio may be somewhat less or considerably more.

Ambiguity of questions is exceedingly rare due to the intensive review process by the examination committees before they are used. The preparation of objective or multiple choice examinations is extremely difficult, for the work of the examiners, instead of consisting of the time-consuming and usually tiresome reading and grading of essay-type answers, shifts to the preparation of the many questions included in the tests. Because generally the objective is to construct questions with only one correct answer, the preparation of an examination is best done by a group, usually an examination construction committee. The members of each group or committee should be skilled in one basic or clinical science discipline. Usually each member prepares questions in advance of a committee meeting, at which each question will be subjected to a critical review. Doubtful items are revised, modified, or discarded and new items may be developed. All items not approved unanimously are discarded. An examination prepared in this way, which is the method used by the National Board of Medical Examiners, contains only material that has been thoroughly worked over and agreed upon as appropriate, free from ambiguity and representative not only of important aspects of the subject but also of high standards of education.

SCORING OF MULTIPLE-CHOICE EXAMINATIONS

When objective multiple-choice examinations are used, the examinations are usually scored by electronic machines. To the casual observer, this machine scoring may look like a highly mysterious business. The answer sheets are loaded into the machine, a button is pressed, and the machine reads the sheets, matches the answers against an answer key, and punches the examinee's score into the automated machine data card. A manual check is also made to avoid the possibility of any technical error. Furthermore, these machines are not robots making their own decisions; they perform only in the way that they are programmed to perform. The responsible examiners determine whether an individual should pass or fail.

A grade of 75 has been established as the passing score for the examinations of the National Board. But it does not follow that it is necessary to respond correctly to 75% of the items in order to obtain this grade. Indeed, the scoring procedure is such that usually a score of about 50% to 60% of the questions answered correctly results in a passing grade

of 75. In arriving at the passing score, the distribution curve of all those taking an examination is given consideration.

Examinations of the multiple-choice type have certain advantages over the time-honored essay tests. Although essay tests may probe more deeply into a limited number of subjects, multiple-choice examinations sample a much greater breadth of medical knowledge. Because the answer sheets can be scored by machine, the grading can be accomplished rapidly, accurately and impartially. With this type of examination it becomes possible to determine the level of difficulty of each test and to maintain comparability of examination scores from test to test and from year to year for any single subject. Moreover, of even greater long range significance is the facility with which the total test and the individual questions can be subjected to thorough and rapid statistical analysis, thus providing a sound basis for comparative studies and the continuing improvement in the quality of the test itself.

NATIONAL BOARD OF MEDICAL EXAMINERS

In the years following the issuance of the Flexner Report on the medical schools of the nation [Flexner A: Medical Education in the United States and Canada, bulletin no. 4. New York, Carnegie Foundation for the Advancement of Teaching, 1910] it became evident that not only medical school programs, but also the licensing examinations of the various states, needed upgrading. One physician who took seriously the licensing examination matter was Dr. W. L. Rodman of Philadelphia, who, in 1915, founded the National Board of Medical Examiners. This Board, a voluntary and unofficial examining agency, was organized "to prepare and to administer qualifying examinations of such high quality that legal agencies governing the practice of medicine within each state" could, at their discretion, "grant a license without further examination to those candidates" who had passed the National Board examinations and had become Diplomates of the Board. The membership of the National Board of Medical Examiners has grown in strength and importance over the years and now includes representatives from the faculties of leading American medical schools and from the Association of American Medical Colleges, the American Medical Association, the Federation of State Medical Boards of the United States, the American Hospital Association, and various Federal medical services.

The National Board, however, is in no sense a licensing agency, and the last interest this board could have would be the responsibility of licensing physicians on a national basis. It is the function of each individual state to determine who shall practice within its borders and to set the standards of medical practice in accordance with its own rules and regulations. As its name implies, the National Board is an examining board, and currently all but a few states are willing to issue licenses to practice medicine within their borders to holders of the National Board Diploma; a few states do so with minor additional requirements. In a majority of states the National Board Diploma is accepted for full licensure. In New York State, for example, in 1973 approximately 37% of all physicians licensed were licensed on the basis of their National Board qualifications. It goes without saying that the candidate preparing for licensure in a specific state should communicate directly with that state's Board of Medical Examiners to learn the requirements of that state.

Eligibility to take the National Board examinations is currently limited to candidates who are regularly enrolled as students in, or are graduates of, any approved medical school in the United States or Canada. Graduates of foreign medical schools are not admitted, although, before they may serve as interns or residents in any United States hospital, they must take and pass a special qualifying examination. The special testing procedures that are required of all foreign medical graduates will be discussed later.

The examination of the National Board of Medical Examiners has from the outset been given in three parts, Part I in the basic medical sciences, Part II in the clinical sciences, and Part III as a practical examination involving clinical and patient problems. Over the years, however, the examinations have not been static but have been changed in form and content to keep abreast of medical progress and changes in medical education. The examinations are prepared by special committees, one for each major basic science and clinical science field. These commitees are selected with great care, and their members (usually six per committee) come from medical school faculties and the staffs of teaching hospitals all over the United States and Canada. Thus, the preparation of the examinations has been in the hands of leaders in the medical profession throughout the country, and the examinations themselves have reflected the progress and change occurring in the various fields of medicine and in science generally.

From carefully prepared essay tests in the various basic and clinical sciences the Board some years ago turned to the more efficient and valid objective or multiple-choice tests in the different subjects. The Board also decided to change from the Part III practical examinations given at the bedside in hospital centers throughout the country to a new, unique objective test of clinical competence that is taken by all candidates. This has resulted in more universally uniform and valid testing of a physician's fitness to practice, effectively eliminating the lack of uniformity that characterized the bedside examinations carried out in many different centers. The National Board has not only kept constantly abreast of progress in medicine and medical education but has actually been a leader in bringing about progressive change, especially in the quality of examination procedures.

Today the Part I and Part II examinations are set up and scored as total comprehensive objective tests in the basic sciences and clinical sciences, respectively. The format of each part is changed since it is no longer subject oriented, that is, separated into sections specifically labeled Anatomy, Pathology, Medicine, Surgery, and so forth. Subject labels are therefore missing, and in each part questions from the different fields are intermixed or scrambled so that the subject origin of any individual question is not immediately apparent, although it is known in the National Board office. Therefore, if necessary, individual subject grades can be extracted.

Part I is a 2-day written test that includes questions in anatomy, biochemistry, microbiology, pathology, pharmacology, physiology, and a recently added discipline, behavioral sciences. Each subject contributes to the examination a large number of questions designed to test not only knowledge of the subject itself but also "the subtler qualities of discrimination, judgment, and reasoning." Questions in such fields as molecular biology, cell biology, and genetics are included, as are questions to test the "candidate's recognition of the similarity or dissimilarity of diseases, drugs, and physiologic, behavioral, or pathologic processes." Problems are presented in narrative, tabular, or graphic form, followed by questions designed to assess the candidate's knowledge and comprehension of the situation described.

Part II is also a 2-day written test that includes questions in internal medicine, obstetrics and gynecology, pediatrics, preventive medicine and public health, psychiatry, and surgery. The questions, like those in Part I, cover a broad spectrum of knowledge in each of the clinical fields. In addition to individual questions, clinical problems are presented in the form of case histories, charts, roentgenograms, photographs of gross and microscopic pathologic specimens, laboratory data, and the like, and the candidate must answer questions concerning the interpretation of the data presented and their relation to the clinical problems. The questions are "designed to explore the extent of the candidate's knowledge of clinical situations and to test his ability to bring information from many different clinical and basic science areas to bear upon these situations."

The examinations of both Part I and Part II are scored as a whole, certification being given on the basis of performance on the entire part, without reference to disciplinary breakdown. The grade for the part is derived from the total number of questions answered correctly, rather than from an average of the grades in the component basic science or clinical science subjects. A candidate who fails will be required to repeat the entire part. Nevertheless, as noted above, in spite of the interdisciplinary character of the examinations, all of the traditional disciplines are represented in the test, and separate grades for each subject can be extracted and reported separately to students, to state examining boards, or to those medical schools that request them for their own educational and academic purposes.

This type of interdisciplinary examination and the method of scoring the entire test as a unit have definite advantages, especially in view of the changing character of the curricula in modern medical schools. The old type of rigid, almost standardized, curriculum, with its emphasis on specific subjects and specified numbers of hours in each, has been replaced by a more liberal, open-ended kind of curriculum, permitting emphasis in one or more fields and corresponding deemphasis in others. The result has been rather wide variations in the totality of education in different medical schools. Thus, the scoring of these tests as a whole permits accommodation to this variability in the curricula of different schools. Within the total score, weakness in one subject that has received relatively little emphasis in a given school may be balanced by strength in other subjects.

The rationale for this type of comprehensive examination as replacement for the traditional department-oriented examination in the basic sciences and the clinical sciences is given in the National Board Examiner:

The student, as he confronts these examinations, must abandon the idea of "thinking like a physiologist" in answering a quesiton labeled "physiology" or "thinking like a surgeon" in answering a question labeled "surgery." The one question may have been written by a biochemist or a pharmacologist; the other question may have been written by an internist or a pediatrician. The pattern of these examinations will direct the student to thinking more broadly of the basic sciences in Part I and to thinking of patients and their problems in Part II.

Until a few years ago the Part I examination could not be taken until the work of the second year in medical school had been completed, and the Part II test was given only to the student who had completed the major part of the fourth year. Now a student, if he feels he is ready, may be admitted to any regularly scheduled Part I or Part II examination during any year of his medical course without prerequisite completion of specified courses or chronologic periods of study. Thus, emphasis is placed upon the acquisition of knowledge and competence rather than the completion of predetermined periods.

A candidate is eligible for Part III after he has passed Parts I and II, has received the M.D. degree from an approved medical school in the United States or Canada, and, subsequent to the receipt of the M.D. degree, has served at least 6 months in an approved hospital internship or residency. Under certain circumstances, consideration may be given to other types of graduate training provided they meet with the approval of the National Board. After passing the Part III examination the candidate will receive his Diploma as of the date of the satisfactory completion of his internship or residency. If a candidate has completed his approved hospital training prior to completion of Part III, he will receive certification as of the date of the successful completion of Part III.

The Part III examination, as noted above, is an objective test of general clinical competence. It occupies 1 full day and is divided into two sections, the first of which is a multiple-choice examination that relates to the interpretation of clinical data presented primarily in pictorial form such as pictures of patients, gross and microscopic lesions, electrocardiograms, charts, and graphs. The second section, entitled Patient Management Problems, utilizes a programmed-testing technique (answer by erasure to uncover information or results of actions) designed to measure the candidate's clinical judgment in the management of patients. This technique simulates clinical situations in which the physician is faced with the problems of management presented in a sequential programmed pattern. A set of some four to six problems is related to each of a series of patients. In the scoring of this section, candidates are given credit for correct choices; they are penalized for errors of commission (selection of procedures that are unnecessary or are contraindicated) and for errors of omission (failure to select indicated procedures).

All parts of the National Board examinations are given in a great many centers, usually in medical schools, in nearly every large city in the United States, as well as in a few cities in Canada, in Puerto Rico, and in the Canal Zone. In some cities, such as New York, Chicago, and Baltimore, the examination may be given in more than one center.

The examinations of the National Board have become recognized as the most comprehensive test of knowledge of the medical sciences and their clinical application produced in this country. Approaching them in comprehensiveness and quality are the examinations, developed in close association with the National Board by a committee of the Federation of State Medical Boards of the United States, given twice a year under the auspices of the Federation in any state wishing to use them. These are known as the Federation Licensing Examinations or by the acronym FLEX. More will be said about these examinations later.

For years the National Board examinations have served as an index of the medical education of the period and have strongly influenced higher educational standards in each of the medical sciences. The Diploma of the National Board is accepted by 47 state licensing authorities, the District of Columbia, and the Commonwealth of Puerto Rico in lieu of the examination usually required for licensure and is recognized in the American Medical Directory by the letters DNB following the name of the physician holding National Board certification.

The National Board of Medical Examiners has been a leader in developing new and more reliable techniques of testing, not only for knowledge in all medical fields but also for clinical competence and fitness to practice. In recent years, too, a number of medical schools, several specialty certifying boards, professional medical societies organized to encourage their members to keep abreast of progress in medicine and other professional qualifying agencies have called upon the National Board's professional staff for advice or for the actual preparation of tests to be employed in evaluating medical

knowledge, effectiveness of teaching, and professional competence in some medical fields. In all cases, advantage has been taken of the validity and effectiveness of the objective, multiple-choice type of examination, a technique the National Board has played an important role in bringing to its present state of perfection and discriminatory effectiveness.

FEDERATION LICENSING EXAMINATION (FLEX)

There have been several important developments in the field of medical qualifying examinations in recent years. The first significant achievement in the development of qualifying examinations was the introduction, in 1968, of the first Federation Licensing Examination (FLEX), prepared under the direction of the Examination Institute Committee of the Federation of State Medical Boards of the United States, Inc. Beginning in 1957, the Federation's Examination Institute Committee had held annual conferences designed to study examination procedures in the various states with the end in view of improving their quality and keeping them abreast of the continuing progress in medical education. As a result, there is general agreement to justify the continuation of this committee on a permanent basis.

At the present time this committee is charged: to provide state medical boards with high quality, uniform, and valid examinations for purposes of evaluating clinical competence and qualification for licensure; to place licensure in a definite relation to modern medical education by updating state board examination procedures and providing flexibility; to establish uniform levels of examinations among the states; to create a rational basis for interstate endorsement; and to provide a basis for the management of the foreign medical graduate problem.

Following publication of their first complete report, in 1961, the Examination Institute Committee continued to hold special conferences and symposia at each annual Federation meeting, and to press forward in its efforts to develop an examination of high quality that would be acceptable to the various state medical boards. At first, it was believed that the Federation itself could set up an examination center, staffed by a medical director and a specialist in examination construction and preparation, that would be in competition with other examination centers, particularly the National Board of Medical Examiners, which had been functioning for more than 50 years. Since the cost was found to be prohibitive, the Examination Institute Committee consulted with the staff of the National Board of Medical Examiners, and the Federation Licensing Examination came into being. Thus, in 1967, the Federation of State Medical Boards gave the new examination its unanimous approval at its annual meeting; and in June, 1968, candidates for licensure in six states took the first FLEX examinations. Since then, all but two states have accepted the FLEX examination as their own official licensing examination.

The FLEX is a uniform, valid, and reliable licensing examination, planned and prepared by FLEX Test Committees composed of Federation members and designed for use by any state medical licensing board. It is a 3-day examination given simultaneously by participating medical boards in the name of their own states twice a year, in June and December.

The arrangement with the National Board calls for making pools of already tested and validated objective questions in the six major basic medical science disciplines and the six major clinical fields available to the Test Committees composed of Federation members who represent the state medical boards that have decided to use the FLEX examination. From this collection of questions two subcommittees—one for the basic sciences and one for the clinical sciences—prepare the licensing examinations in these two fields. A third subcommittee selects the questions or problems to be given in the test of clinical competence.

This latter test is relatively new in licensing examinations in spite of the fact that such competence is the most essential requirement of a physician. A few state boards had attempted to solve the problem by requiring oral or practical tests in addition to the standard written tests, but for those boards that had a large number of applicants for licensure, individual tests of this kind were out of the question. The National Board of Medical Examiners had developed an ideal and unique practical test that had been used for some years with great success. This, the Federation's FLEX Committee (now called the FLEX Board) felt, met every need, and it was decided to add this practical test to those in the basic and clinical sciences. However, because of the many changes in the curricula of medical schools in this country, it was held that individual tests in anatomy, physiology, surgery, etc., were becoming outmoded. A comprehensive interdisciplinary examination that covered all basic medical science fields in one test and the clinical sciences in another was established. Questions in all of the important

areas would be included in these tests; they would be "scrambled" without regard to discipline, but with all fields adequately represented. It was decided that about 90 questions each in anatomy, biochemistry, microbiology, pathology, pharmacology, and physiology would be mixed together in the basic sciences test, and about the same number of questions each in internal medicine, obstetrics and gynecology, pediatrics, preventive medicine and public health, psychiatry, and surgery would be mixed together in the clinical sciences test.

In each examination, the origin of the individual questions is known in the central office. Therefore, in spite of the scrambled character of the questions in the actual examination, it is possible to extract specific grades in each individual subject if these are needed. The FLEX Board felt, however, that each basic science and clinical science examination should be considered as a unit, with a single grade to be given for each entire test.

The examination in the basic sciences, given on the first day, is divided into three sections, A, B, and C, each lasting about 2½ hours, in which time some 180 questions must be answered, making a total of approximately 540 questions for the day. The clinical sciences examination, given on the second day, is presented in the same way.

On the third day the examination designed to test clinical competence is given. This test is divided into two sections that resemble in all details the two sections of Part III of the National Board examination. In the first section clinical material is presented in the form of pictures of patients or specimens, roentgenograms, electrocardiograms, and graphic or tabulated material about which searching questions are asked. In the second section a distinctive technique described as programmed testing is employed, the object being to assess the candidate's judgment in the sequential management of patients in a manner similar to that which he would experience in relation to his own patients as he studied their disease processes or injuries, evaluated his findings and planned his treatment. A single overall grade is given to this entire part.

Because there will be many physicians who graduated from several to many years before appearing for this examination, the FLEX Board decided to provide, in addition to a single grade for each of the three parts (and of course, separate grades in each of the basic and clinical science subjects for those boards that might want them) a single overall grade for the entire examination, a grade that would give greater weight to the clinical, rather than the basic science, portion of the test. This is the so-called FLEX weight average. This average is developed by emphasizing the importance of the clinical parts of the examination, inasmuch as a weight of 1 is given to the basic sciences grade, a weight of 2 to the clinical sciences grade, and a weight of 3 to the clinical competence grade. How this weighted average is to be used will depend on the decision of each state medical board giving the FLEX examination. The FLEX Board recommends that a weighted average of 75 be the accepted passing grade.

Thus, there are now two important medical examinations for graduates of American and Canadian medical schools, those given by the National Board of Medical Examiners and those given under the auspices of the Federation of State Medical Boards of the United States. These two examinations do not conflict since their purposes are not exactly the same. The National Board examinations are designed to test the knowledge of students as they are learning medicine in medical schools today; these tests are focused on the student of today and the physician of tomorrow. The FLEX examination is designed to assess fundamental knowledge and, more especially, the clinical competence of the physician of today. A dual examination system has thus emerged, each examination important in its own right, each with a different objective and each aimed at its own clearly defined target.

EDUCATIONAL COUNCIL FOR FOREIGN MEDICAL GRADUATES (ECFMG) CERTIFICATION

The second significant achievement in the development of qualifying examinations was brought about as a result of the problems created by the ever increasing numbers of foreign-educated physicians, particularly from non-English-speaking countries, who were coming to the United States for further education and training, many of whom decided to remain in this country to practice. After a study by a committee representing the American Hospital Association, the American Medical Association, the Association of American Medical Colleges and the Federation of State Medical Boards of the United States, with the unofficial cooperation of the U.S. Department of State, the Educational Council for Foreign Medical Graduates (ECFMG) was created. The purpose of the Council is to develop and administer an evaluation procedure or qualifying

examination that will effectively ascertain the fitness of foreign medical graduates to serve as interns and residents in hospitals in the United States or to come to the United States to otherwise practice medicine. Also included for those who come from countries where English is not the spoken language is a 1-hour examination designed to assess comprehension of English vocabulary and language structure (the ECFMG English test).

It was only natural that the Council should turn to the National Board of Medical Examiners for advice and help. The result was that the examinations, given twice each year, were, and continue to be, prepared and scored by the National Board. Indeed, so close became the association between these two organizations because of this relationship, that the home office of the Council, formerly in Evanston, Illinois, was moved to Philadelphia, Pennsylvania, where it is now located. This is the same city in which the home office of the National Board is located.

The Council on Medical Education of the American Medical Association has adopted rules providing that no approved hospital in the United States can now employ as interns or residents any foreign-educated physicians who do not hold the ECFMG Certificate unless they already have a valid state license. In spite of some criticism (most of it unwarranted) of the Council as well as its sponsoring agencies in the first few years, the Council, after giving more than 315,000 examinations in 48 centers in the United States and Canada and in over 105 foreign countries, has fully justified its existence. Indeed, at the present time practically every state that will accept foreign-educated physicians for licensure requires that all these applicants be certified before being admitted to the licensing examination in that state.

The Council semiannually issues an information booklet and application* in which are set forth the requirements for certification, and several pages are devoted to describing the examination itself. Please refer to the following discussion on the Foreign Medical Graduate Examination in the Medical Sciences (FMGEMS) for further details.

---

* Copies of the booklet detailing information on the Foreign Medical Graduate Examination in the Medical Sciences (FMGEMS) and the ECFMG English test can be obtained by writing to the Educational Commission for Foreign Medical Graduates, 3624 Market Street, Philadelphia, Pennsylvania 19104–2685.

FOREIGN MEDICAL GRADUATE EXAMINATION IN THE MEDICAL SCIENCES (FMGEMS)

Until 1976, all foreign medical graduates desiring to undergo postgraduate medical training in the United States were required to take the ECFMG examination. This comprehensive clinical examination permitted certification by the ECFMG for acceptance into an accredited graduate medical education training program in the United States. In 1976, the United States Congress enacted amendments to the Immigration and Naturalization Act (INA) that required all foreign medical graduates who desire entrance into the United States for postgraduate training (or to practice medicine) to pass a new Visa Qualifying Examination (VQE). If this examination, a 2-day comprehensive test of preclinical (basic) and clinical knowledge, was passed, a certificate was issued by the ECFMG. This document was required to obtain the necessary visa to enter the United States. Thus, a passing grade on the VQE was deemed equivalent to passing Parts I and II of the National Board Examinations, provided the candidate also demonstrated competence in oral and written English. In 1977 (and in subsequent years) there was an extremely high rate of failure of the basic sciences (day 1) of the VQE in comparison to the ECFMG examination (that had much fewer questions in the basic sciences area).

The VQE examination is no longer given; it has been supplanted by the Foreign Medical Graduate Examination in the Medical Sciences (FMGEMS). In addition, all candidates from foreign medical schools must also pass the ECFMG English test. Passage of both examinations is therefore required for ECFMG certification.

A word of definition of a "foreign medical graduate" (FMG) is necessary before discussing the FMGEMS test. An FMG is any physician whose medical degree of qualification was conferred by any medical school located outside the United States, Canada and Puerto Rico. That medical school, however, must be listed in the *World Directory of Medical Schools,* published by the World Health Organization. Citizens of the United States who have completed their medical education in schools outside of the United States, Canada, and Puerto Rico are defined as "foreign medical graduates" (FMGs). Alternatively, foreign nationals who have graduated from United States, Canadian, or Puerto Rican medical schools are not FMGs.

Thus, the ECFMG certification provides assurance to all directors of training programs of the Ac-creditation Council for Graduate Medical Education (ACGME) that the FMG applicant has fulfilled the minimum standards for medical knowledge and mastery of the English language necessary to enter their programs. This ECFMG certification is also prerequisite for licensure to practice medicine in most states of the United States. (Some states may require that the candidate also pass the FLEX examination.)

English Language Examinations

Two English language examinations are approved by the ECFMG. The *ECFMG English test* is administered twice yearly (in January and July) in the morning of the second day (prior to the clinical science test) of the FMGEMS. The ECFMG states that examinees who take the clinical science component of the FMGEMS examination must also take the ECFMG English test that same day even if they have passed the English test at previous examinations. The only other English test that is acceptable to the ECFMG is an international or special administration of the *Test of English as a Foreign Language (TOEFL).* The ECFMG emphasizes that this testing is with the provision that applicants have previously taken an ECFMG English test. There are a number of important requirements concerning these English tests as well as details concerning the medical science examination and the registration procedures. The applicant for all examinations of this nature, therefore, should not assume that the information concerning any of the examinations described in this textbook is the final word. It is strongly recommended that the applicant communicate directly with the testing agencies. (The ECFMG address is listed by footnote on p. 9.)

Medical Science Examination

As indicated above, the examination is formulated by the ECFMG and the NBME and is given twice yearly, in January and in July, as two half-day sessions on 2 successive days. The questions on the first day relate to preclinical (basic) sciences and on the second day to the clinical sciences. The overall examination consists of approximately 950 test items constructed in a multiple-choice format. The preclinical science questions, about 500 items in number, are derived from the areas of anatomy, biochemistry, behavioral sciences, microbiology, pathology, pharmacology, and physiology. The second-day examination in the clinical sciences is preceded by the English test, which is followed by 450 question items drawn in approximately equal numbers from the disciplines of internal medicine, obstetrics and gynecology, pediatrics, preventive medicine and public health, psychiatry, and surgery. As indicated above, this new 2-day examination replaces the VQE and ECFMG examinations.

FIVE POINTS TO REMEMBER

In order for the candidate to maximize chances for passing these examinations, a few commonsense strategies or guidelines should be kept in mind.

First, it is imperative to thoroughly prepare for the examination. Know well the types of questions to be presented, the pedagogic areas of particular weakness, and devote more preparatory study time to these weak areas. Do not use too much time restudying areas in which there is a feeling of great confidence and do not leave unexplored those areas in which there is less confidence. Finally, be well rested before the test, and if possible, avoid traveling to the city of testing just that morning or late the evening before.

Second, know well the format of the examination and the instructions before becoming immersed in the challenge at hand. This information can be obtained from many published texts and brochures or directly from the testing service (e.g., FMGEMS and ECFMG's English Test from 3624 Market Street, Philadelphia, Pennsylvania 19104–2685 U.S.A.; cable: EDCOUNCIL; telephone: (215) 396–5900). In addition, the many available texts and self-assessment types of examinations are valuable for practice.

Third, know well the overall time allotted for the examination and its components and the scope of the test to be faced. These may be learned by a rapid review of the examination itself. Then, proceed with the test at a careful, deliberate, and steady pace without spending inordinate time on any single question. For example, certain questions such as the "one best answer" (questions 1 to 3 of "Examples of Questions" below) probably should be allotted 1 to 1½ minutes each. The "matching" type of questions (numbers 4 to 18) should be allotted similar time. The multiple "true-false" type should be given about 1½ minutes. Thus, each question of the five-component questions should be allotted approximately 20 seconds. With respect to the "recall" type of question, there is great need for logical judgment, for the candidate to infer an answer from the presentation of the data, and to discard illogical answers from the multiplicity of the choices. Further, the candidate should be aware that those questions containing the word "always" or "never" are unlikely to be wise choices; questions with words such as "may" and "could" are wiser selections.

Fourth, it follows that if a question is particularly disturbing, the candidate should note appropriately the question (put a mark on the question sheet) and return to this point later. Don't compromise yourself by so concentrating on a likely "loser" that several "winners" are eliminated because of inadequate time. One way to save this time on a particular "stickler" is to play your initial choice; your chances of a correct answer are always best with your first impression. If there is no initial choice, reread the question.

Fifth, allow adequate time to review answers, to return to the questions that were unanswered and "flagged" for later attention, and check every nth (e.g., 20th) question to make certain that the answers are appropriate and that you did not inadvertently skip a question in the booklet or answer on the sheet (this can happen easily under these stressful circumstances). There is nothing magical about these five points. They are simple and just make common sense. If the candidate prepared himself well and follows the preceding commonsense points, the chances are he will not return for a second go-round.

EXAMPLES OF QUESTIONS

The following questions are presented as a guide to the physician preparing for examinations in the basic and clinical sciences. They offer the variety of types of multiple-choice questions that have been devised to provide objectivity in testing a large area of subject material that demands depth in knowledge and comprehension.

Objective—Multiple Choice Type

COMPLETION TYPE

The so-called completion type item is the most common. Items of this type usually are placed together at the beginning of the test, as follows, with these directions:

Directions. Each of the following questions or incomplete statements is followed by five suggested answers or completions. Select the one that is best in each case and blacken the corresponding space on the answer sheet.

The following item illustrates this type, although obviously this question is rather easy.

Question 1:

To which one of the following systems of the body does the heart belong?

(a) The digestive system
(b) The central nervous system
(c) The circulatory system
(d) The endocrine system
(e) The musculoskeletal system

The correct answer, of course, is (c). To make this question somewhat more difficult and avoid naming the correct system among the choice, the circulatory system can be omitted and an alternative choice, "None of the above," substituted for it. Then the question will appear as:

Question 2:

To which of the following systems of the body does the heart belong?

(a) The digestive system
(b) The central nervous system
(c) The endocrine system
(d) The musculoskeletal system
(e) None of the above

The fifth choice (e), now becomes the correct response. In this manner the candidate is made to think of the various systems of the body and must know the right answer without its being suggested to him as one of the possibilities. In these examinations the choice "None of the above" will appear and sometimes will be a correct and sometimes an incorrect response.

Another variant of the completion type of item is in the negative form, where all but one of the choices are applicable, and the candidate is asked to mark the one that does not apply. The following is an example:

Question 3:

All of the following are associated with prerenal azotemia EXCEPT:

(a) Shock
(b) Dehydration
(c) Pernicious vomiting
(d) Gastrointestinal hemorrhage
(e) Multiple myeloma

The correct answer is (e).

ASSOCIATION AND RELATEDNESS ITEMS

Items of a somewhat different nature may be used effectively, as, for example, in determining the candidate's knowledge of the action and the use of closely related drugs or the distinguishing features of similar diseases. There follow specific directions for items of this type with a group of items taken from a pharmacology test and another group from a medicine test. As illustrated in this group of items, the candidate must have well-organized information about a number of related drugs and is required to demonstrate considerable understanding of the differential use of these drugs.

Directions. *Each group of questions below consists of five lettered headings followed by a list of numbered words or phrases. For each numbered word or phrase, select the one heading that is related most closely to it.*

Question 4–9:

(a) Quinidine
(b) Theophylline
(c) Amyl nitrite
(d) Glyceryl trinitrate
(e) Papaverine

4. Relaxes smooth muscle of the arterial system; causes fall in arterial pressure; commonly administered in tablets sublingually *Answer:* (d).
5. An opium alkaloid; direct vasodilator action; used in instances of coronary occlusion and peripheral vascular disease *Answer:* (e)
6. Commonly effective in relieving symptoms of bronchial asthma *Answer:* (b)
7. The best for quick treatment of cyanide poisoning *Answer:* (c)
8. Increases the contractile force of the heart and is diuretic *Answer:* (b)
9. May be used in auricular fibrillation *Answer:* (a)

Questions 10–17:

(a) Coarctation of the aorta
(b) Patent ductus arteriosus
(c) Tetralogy of Fallot
(d) Aortic vascular ring
(e) Tricuspid atresia

10. Benefitted by systemic pulmonary artery anastomosis *Answer:* (c)
11. Most common type of congenital cyanotic heart disease *Answer:* (c)

12. Corrected surgically by resection and end-to-end anastomosis *Answer:* (a)
13. Possible cause of dysphagia in infants and children *Answer:* (d)
14. Wide pulse pressure *Answer:* (b)
15. Associated frequently with atrial septal defects *Answer:* (e)
16. A continuous murmur *Answer:* (b)
17. Hypertension in the arms and hypotension in the legs *Answer:* (a)

A further elaboration of association and relatedness items is considerably more searching and calls for a discriminatory understanding of a number of similar but distinguishable factors. For example, the following question reveals considerable information about the candidate's knowledge of the causes of hypoglycemia and the related functional disturbances: four of the five situations in the numbered list below are common to one of the three functional disturbances designated by letters. The candidate is instructed to select one situation that is the exception and the functional disturbance common to the remaining four.

Question 18:

(a) Clinically significant hypoglycemia
(b) Clinically significant hyperglycemia
(c) Clinically significant glycosuria

(1) Overdose of insulin
(2) Functional tumor of islet cells
(3) Renal glycosuria
(4) Hypopituitarism
(5) von Gierke's disease

If the candidate selects (a) and (3), the correct answer, he demonstrates that he knows that (1), (2), (4) and (5) may produce clinically significant hypoglycemia; that (3) does not; and that no combination of four of the five conditions is associated with hyperglycemia or glycosuria. In other words, the possession of both positive and negative information is probed. Specific directions for handling this form of discriminatory question read as follows:

Directions. *There are two responses to be made to each of the following questions. There are three lettered categories; four of the five numbered items are related in some way to one of these categories. (1) On the answer sheet blacken the space under the letter of the category in which these four items belong. (2) Then blacken the space under the number of the item that does not belong in the same category with the other four.*

Items of this type may be used to determine knowledge of disease symptomatology, laboratory findings, or therapeutic procedures, as shown by the following:

Questions 19–21:

19. (a) Multiple neurofibromatosis (von Recklinghausen's disease)
    (b) Hemangioblastomas of the central nervous system
    (c) Multiple sclerosis

    (1) Neurofibromas of the skin
    (2) Meningeal fibromas
    (3) Congenital angiomas of the eye
    (4) Lipomas of subcutaneous tissue
    (5) Cystic disease of the pancreas

Answer: 1. (a)
        2. (5)

20. (a) Contraindications to saddle-block anesthesia
    (b) Contraindications to continuous caudal analgesia
    (c) Contraindications to local anesthesia

    (1) Deformity of the sacrum
    (2) Cutaneous infections
    (3) Perforated dura
    (4) Decreased perineal resistance
    (5) Prodromal labor

Answer: 1. (b)
        2. (4)

21. (a) Eosinophilia of diagnostic significance
    (b) Plasmacytosis of diagnostic significance
    (c) Lymphocytosis of diagnostic significance

    (1) Trichinosis
    (2) Multiple myeloma
    (3) Löffler's syndrome
    (4) Hodgkin's disease
    (5) Schistosomiasis

Answer: 1. (a)
        2. (2)

Another variant of the association and relatedness type of question is demonstrated by the following example from a test in public health and preventive medicine:

Directions. *Each set of lettered headings below is followed by a list of words or phrases. For each word or phrase blacken the space on the answer sheet under*

A if the word or the phrase is associated with (a) *only*

B if the word or the phrase is associated with (b) *only*

C if the word or the phrase is associated with *both* (a) and (b)

D if the word or the phrase is associated with *neither* (a) *nor* (b)

Questions 22–26:

(a) Maternal hygiene program
(b) School health program
(c) Both
(d) Neither

22. Periodic physical examination *Answer:* C—(a & b)
23. Audiometer test *Answer:* B
24. Nutritional guidance *Answer:* C—(a & b)
25. Serologic test for syphilis *Answer:* A
26. Immunization against rubella *Answer:* B

QUANTITATIVE VALUES AND COMPARISONS

In general, questions in this category will call for an understanding of quantitative values rather than rote memory of the quantities themselves. The test committees have agreed that these examinations should contain a minimum of questions calling for the memorizing of absolute quantitative amounts. Actual figures will be found only where the details of the information are considered to be of such importance that they should be a part of the working knowledge that a practicing physician should have in mind without recourse to a reference book. Knowledge of the comparative significance of quantitative values may be called for by items such as the following:

Directions. *The following paired statements describe two entities that are to be compared in a quantitative sense. On the answer sheet blacken the space under*

A if (a) is *greater than* (b)
B if (b) is *greater than* (a)
C if the two are *equal or very nearly equal*

Questions 27–31:

27. (a) The usual therapeutic dose of epinephrine
    (b) The usual therapeutic dose of ephedrine *Answer:* B
28. (a) The inflammability of nitrous oxide-ether mixtures *Answer:* A

(b) The inflammability of chloroform-air mixtures

29. (a) The susceptibility of premature infants to rickets *Answer:* A
    (b) The susceptibility of full-term infants to rickets
30. (a) Life expectancy with glioblastoma of the occipital lobe
    (b) Life expectancy with glioblastoma of the frontal lobe *Answer:* C
31. (a) The amount of glycogen in the cells of Henle's loop in a diabetic *Answer:* A
    (b) The amount of glycogen in the cells of Henle's loop in a nondiabetic

Directions. *Each of the following pairs of phrases describes conditions or quantities that may or may not be related. On the answer sheet blacken the space under*

A if increase in the first is accompanied by increase in the second or if decrease in the first is accompanied by decrease in the second

B if increase in the first is accompanied by decrease in the second or if decrease in the first is accompanied by increase in the second

C of changes in the second are independent of changes in the first

Questions 32–34:

32. (1) Urine volume
    (2) Urine specific gravity *Answer:* B
33. (1) Plasma protein concentration
    (2) Colloid osmotic pressure of plasma *Answer:* A
34. (1) Cerebrospinal fluid pressure
    (2) Intraocular pressure *Answer:* C

CAUSE AND EFFECT

A type of item that is especially applicable to some of the more elusive aspects of medicine and calls for an understanding of cause and effect is illustrated in the following type of questions:

Directions. *Each of the following sentences consists of two main parts: a statement and a reason for that statement. On the answer sheet blacken the space under*

A if the statement and the proposed reason are *both true* and are *related* as cause and effect

B if the statement and the proposed reason are *both true* but are *not related* as cause and effect

C if the statement is *true* but the proposed reason is *false*

D if the statement is false but the proposed reason is *an accepted fact or principle*

E if the statement and the proposed reason are *both false*

Directions Summarized:

A = True True and related
B = True True and NOT related
C = True False
D = False True
E = False False

In situations that may be presented by this type of item, the right answer may sometimes be arrived at through good reasoning from an appreciation of the basic principles involved. The sample items are as follows:

Questions 35–39:

35. Herpes simplex usually is regarded as an autogenous infection BECAUSE patients given fever therapy frequently develop herpes. *Answer:* A

36. Cow's milk is preferable to breast milk in infant feeding BECAUSE cow's milk has a higher content of calcium. *Answer:* D

37. The corpus luteum of menstruation becomes the corpus luteum of pregnancy BECAUSE progesterone inhibits the activity of the anterior portion of the pituitary gland. *Answer:* B

38. The sinoauricular node serves as the pacemaker BECAUSE after its removal the heart fails to beat. *Answer:* C

39. A higher titer of antibody against the H antigen of the typhoid bacillus is a good index of immunity to typhoid BECAUSE any antibody to an organism can protect against disease caused by that organism. *Answer:* E

Question 40:

A modification of the true-false type of question that calls for careful thought and discrimination is the "multiple true-false" variety. In this question a list of numbered items follows a statement for which several possible answers are given and the candidate is required to select the appropriate response from a list of answers designated by letters:

40. Live virus is used in immunization against:
1. Influenza
2. Poliomyelitis
3. Cholera
4. Smallpox

Answers:
A. Only 1, 2 and 3 are correct
B. Only 1 and 3 are correct
C. Only 2 and 4 are correct
D. Only 4 is correct
E. All are correct

STRUCTURE AND FUNCTIONS

Diagrams, charts, electrocardiograms, roentgenograms, or photomicrographs may be used to elicit knowledge of structure, function, the course of a clinical situation or a statistical tabulation. Questions then may be asked in relation to designated elements of the same.

CASE HISTORIES

The most characteristic situation that confronts the practicing physician can be simulated by a clinical case history derived from a patient experience, which is followed by a series of questions concerning diagnosis, signs and symptoms, laboratory determinations. treatment, and prognosis. In answering these questions, much depends on arriving at the proper diagnosis, for, if an incorrect diagnosis is made, related symptoms, laboratory data, and treatment also will be wrong. These case history questions are set up purposely to place such emphasis on the correct diagnosis comparable with the experience of actual practice.

Directions. *This section of the test consists of several case histories, each followed by a series of questions. Study each history, select the best answer to each question following it, and blacken the space under the corresponding letter on the answer sheet.*

The patient is a 21-year-old white man with a complaint of malaise, cough, and fever. The present illness had its onset 10 days prior to admission with malaise and a nonproductive cough, followed in 24 hours by a temperature varying from 100°F to 101°F that persisted up to the time of admission. On about the fourth day of illness the cough became more severe, producing scant amounts of white viscid sputum. Three days prior to admission, paroxysms of coughing began, followed sometimes by vomiting. Chilly sensations were noted but no frank shaking chills. Anterior parasternal pain on coughing has been present since the fifth day of illness.

On physical examination the temperature is 101°F; the pulse rate 110 beats per minute; the respiratory rate 32 per minute; and the blood pressure 108 mmHg systolic, 60 mmHg diastolic. The patient is well developed and well nourished, appears to be acutely but not chronically ill, and is dyspneic but not cyanotic.

Positive physical findings are limited to the chest and are as follows:

Vocal and tactile fremitus and resonance are within normal limits. In the left axilla a few fine rales are heard, and the bronchial quality of the sounds is increased, although the intensity is normal.

Blood findings are reported as follows:

White blood count, 3400 (polymorphonuclears 30%, lymphocytes 62%, monocytes 5%, eosinophils 3%).

Roentgenogram of the chest reveals an increase in the density of the perihilar markings with ill-defined areas of patchy, soft, increased radiodensity at both bases and in the left upper lung field.

Questions 41–45:

41. Which one of the following is the most likely diagnosis?
    (a) Tuberculosis
    (b) Pneumococcal pneumonia
    (c) Primary atypical pneumonia *Answer:* (c)
    (d) Coccidioidomycosis
    (e) Bronchopneumonia
42. Which one of the following is the most likely additional physical finding?
    (a) Splenomegaly
    (b) Signs of meningeal irritation
    (c) Pleural friction rub
    (d) Frequent changes in distribution of chest findings *Answer:* (d)
    (e) Signs of frank lobar consolidation
43. Which one of the following laboratory findings is consistent with the diagnosis?
    (a) Elevation and further increase of cold agglutinins *Answer:* (a)
    (b) Positive blood culture
    (c) Marked leukocytosis with the beginning of recovery
    (d) Positive sputum examination
    (e) Positive skin test
44. Which one of the following is the therapy that should be given?
    (a) Bed rest and streptomycin
    (b) Bed rest and penicillin
    (c) Streptomycin and paraaminosalicylic acid
    (d) Bed rest and Aureomycin *Answer:* (d)
    (e) Psychotherapy and physical rehabilitation
45. Which one of the following is the probable outcome of this disease in this patient if untreated?
    (a) The fever will subside spontaneously by crisis
    (b) Recovery will be gradual, with relapse not unexpected. *Answer:* (b)
    (c) Empyema will develop
    (d) Residual fibrosis will appear with healing
    (e) Lung cavitation will not be unexpected

Objective examinations permit a large number of questions to be asked, for 150 to 180 in each subject can be answered in a 2½-hour period. Because the answer sheets are scorable by machine, the grading can be accomplished rapidly, accurately, and impartially. It is completely unbiased and percentile, since the human element is not a factor. Of long-range significance is the facility with which the total test and individual questions can be subjected to thorough and rapid statistical analyses, thus providing a sound basis for comparative studies of medical school teaching and for continuing improvement in the quality of the test itself. Furthermore, multiple-choice written examinations have certain advantages of real benefit to the candidate, to the medical school and, ultimately, to state boards of medical examiners.

Review Questions

Following are examples of review questions. In those relating to the basic sciences in particular, an attempt has been made, in most of them at least, not merely to call for information based on recollection of past study but rather to relate the questions to practical clinical or patient problems. These questions are rhetorical in nature and would require an essay-type answer. The reviewer is presented these questions primarily as an overall suggestion of important areas for study and review.

QUESTIONS IN THE BASIC SCIENCES

Describe or diagram the conduction pathways of the heart. Indicate the sites of pathology or disturbances in the presence of:

(a) Paroxysmal tachycardia
(b) Adams-Stokes syndrome
(c) Heart block after myocardial infarction

Diagram the anatomy encountered in doing a tracheotomy.

What neurologic structures are found at the cerebellopontine angle, both within and outside of the brain, where pathology might be reflected in clinical symptoms?

A patient has sustained fractures of the lower left ribs posteriorly. What subjacent structures might be injured? What studies should be performed to determine the extent of the injury?

Diagram a cross section of the spinal cord at the level of L2, indicating major tracts. Indicate the blood supply to the cord at this level.

Name five congenital defects that may be detected at birth and give their embryologic derivation.

Diagram the abdominal aorta with its major branches. Indicate site of occlusion for Leriche syndrome.

Describe the embryologic development of the pituitary gland. Diagram its relationship to surrounding structures.

Diagram the relationship of the pancreas to the duodenum with its duct system. Describe its embryology.

Diagram the tracheobronchial tree, showing the major lung segments. Where will a foreign body aspirated into the tracheobronchial tree most frequently lodge?

Discuss the role of progesterone in pregnancy.

What is intermittent claudication? What is its cause?

What is meant by the specific dynamic action (SDA) of food? What is the significance of SDA in prescribing a diet for an obese patient?

Describe briefly the functions of the hypothalamus.

Define *each* of the following:

(a) Conditioned reflex
(b) Jaundice
(c) Orthopnea
(d) Emphysema
(e) Tidal air
(f) Heartburn

Name and discuss the factors responsible for the tonic activity of the respiratory center.

Explain why pulmonary edema develops first in dependent parts of the lungs.

Discuss the role of bile in fat digestion.

What is the origin of bilirubin found in the serum?

In a patient with jaundice and a mild anemia, what five *biochemical* determinations would, in your opinion, be most effective in the differential diagnosis? Explain your choices.

Define a vitamin.

Under what circumstances can hypervitaminosis develop? List the clinical and biochemical manifestations of any hypervitaminosis.

The following proteins may be found in human serum. Define four of the six listed below, list the methods by which they may be detected and explain their clinical significance:

(a) Cryoglobulin
(b) Myeloma protein
(c) Siderophilin (transferrin)
(d) Macroglobulin
(e) Cold agglutinin
(f) Haptoglobin

Define a *buffer system*. Give an example of a buffer system important in clinical medicine and explain the operation of the system in:

(a) Metabolic acidosis
(b) Respiratory alkalosis

What are the clinical manifestations of hypokalemia? What electrocardiographic changes are frequently associated with hypokalemia? List three clinical states in which hypokalemia is a common finding.

Define four of the following:

(a) Methemoglobin
(b) Thyroglobulin
(c) Respiratory quotient
(d) Pasteur effect
(e) Nitrogen balance
(f) Intrinsic factor

In advising a community hospital that is about to establish a clinical diagnostic radioisotope laboratory, what radioactive chemical compounds would you recommend? List the compounds (*not* just elements) and give at least *one* use for *each*.

Name three microorganisms sensitive to penicillin and three resistant to penicillin as it is administered in clinical practice.

Define the terms *anamnestic response* and *booster effect*. How are these principles applied to artificial immunization?

List three infections in which disease is caused primarily by the toxin of the infecting microorganism.

Name a vaccine in which the immunizing principle is a modified toxin.

Describe two laboratory tests for the diagnosis of syphilis. How may these tests be modified by antiluetic therapy?

Name two microorganisms that may induce cavitating disease of the lung. Describe briefly the morphology and the staining characteristics of each.

What streptococcus is associated with "streptococcal" sore throat? What distinguishes this microorganism on blood agar culture? What are three possible sequelae of untreated streptococcal pharyngitis?

Name three bacteria that are frequently associated with meningitis. For each of the three types of meningitis, list an antimicrobial drug that is effective in its treatment.

What is the etiologic significance of a pneumococcus in the throat culture of an adult patient with pharyngitis? In the sputum of a patient with pneumonia? In the nasopharynx of a child with otitis media?

List three cultural or biochemical characteristics of pneumococcus.

What is Sabin's vaccine? Are its antigenic constituents living or dead? Name one constituent of the vaccine in addition to those that are intended for immunization. Does the vaccine prevent infection?

Classify the etiologic agent of "Asiatic influenza."

Which antimicrobial agents are effective in the treatment of uncomplicated influenza?

What is the most frequent cause of death in influenza?

Name two microorganisms frequently implicated in the fatal termination of influenza.

Describe three characteristics by which viruses differ from bacteria.

Identify three diseases caused by rickettsia.

What are selective media? Give the name of one such medium and its purpose. Of what value is penicillinase in diagnostic bacteriology?

Name two diseases that may be prevented or modified by the parenteral injection of antibody.

Name two diseases in which antibody must be used for optimal treatment.

What is the significance of:

(a) An elevated serum ASO (antistreptolysin O) titer
(b) An elevated serum heterophile antibody titer
(c) An elevated cold agglutinin titer in the serum

Compare infectious hepatitis and serum hepatitis with respect to:

(a) Etiologic agent
(b) Epidemiology
(c) Incubation period

Indicate for *each* of the following organisms whether it is sensitive or resistant *in vitro* to penicillin and tetracycline:

Streptococcus pyogenes
Neisseria gonorrhoeae
Neisseria meningitidis
Klebsiella pneumoniae
Hemophilus influenzae
Brucella abortus

Name three vaccines that contain living and three that contain dead infectious agents, listing also the microorganisms they contain. How would you test for the efficacy of immunization with any one of these agents (without exposing your patient to disease)?

List three gram-positive and three gram-negative bacteria. For *each* organism listed, give a brief description of its morphology.

Cite two laboratory characteristics of the staphylococci that are most commonly pathogenic for humans. What is the drug of choice for treating most staphylococcal infections acquired outside the hospital?

Name three diseases in humans caused by spirochetes. What are the names of the etiologic agents of these diseases?

Briefly discuss the most common gross pathology of an adenocarcinoma of the right hemicolon and contrast it with that most often seen in the descending colon. Correlate these gross findings with the usual initial symptom complex of each.

Which of the following is the most frequent site of carcinoma of the colon:

(a) The cecum
(b) The splenic flexure
(c) The sigmoid
(d) The rectum

Which of the following figures most nearly represents the percentage of carcinoma of the colon and the rectum that are detectable by digital rectal examination:

(a) 10%
(b) 2%
(c) 20%
(d) 50%

A 55-year-old woman is admitted to the hospital with complaints of tiredness, weakness, progressive enlargement of the abdomen and continuous mild generalized abdominal discomfort for "some time." No further reliable history is obtainable. Physical examination reveals a middle-aged woman with obvious recent wasting. The blood pressure is 130/80 mmHg; pulse 80 beats per minute and regular; temperature 97°F. The *only* other significant physical finding is an enlarged, tense abdomen exhibiting shifting dullness and fluid wave. (A routine urinalysis has revealed no significant abnormality, nor has an electrocardiogram.)

In the absence of other significant physical findings, what two conditions would you consider most probable in your provisional diagnosis?

What one simple and practical procedure, utilizing the clinical laboratory, would best aid in the differential diagnosis between the two?

Indicate the characteristic clinical laboratory findings elicited by this procedure for *each* of the two conditions that you have mentioned.

Very briefly discuss cancer of the lip under the following headings:

(a) Sex incidence
(b) Location
(c) Gross pathology
(d) Microscopic pathology
(e) Spread
(f) Prognosis.

In cases of pernicious anemia, name:

(a) The fundamental defect involved in the pathogenesis
(b) Three laboratory findings indispensable to a diagnosis of pernicious anemia
(c) Three accessory laboratory findings that confirm the diagnosis

The following phrases are descriptive of characteristics of certain neoplasms. In *each* case name a neoplasm to which the phrase might correctly pertain:

(a) A tumor that has a high mortality but rarely, if ever, metastasizes
(b) A serotonin-secreting tumor that may produce spells of flushing of the skin
(c) An invasive tumor of the skin that rarely, if ever, metastasizes
(d) A neoplasm that may be mistaken for eczema
(e) A malignant neoplasm originating from the placenta
(f) A neoplasm associated with intermittent episodes of hypertension

A man, age 55 years, has had a recent myocardial infarction. Anticoagulant therapy is ordered.

What drug should be used for rapid anticoagulant effect, and what laboratory procedure should be used to check the result?

What drug should be used for long-term anticoagulant effect, and what laboratory test should be used for its control? Give the normal values for this test and the range of values optimal for the patient receiving anticoagulant therapy.

Discuss briefly the pathology of bronchogenic carcinoma, indicating usual sites of primary origin, histologic types and method of spread.

List five common sites of metastasis of bronchogenic carcinoma, arranging them in order of frequency.

Following overindulgence in food and alcohol, a man, age 30, develops sudden severe epigastric pain with moderate rigidity and tenderness of the upper abdomen. There are nausea, vomiting, cyanosis, abdominal distention, rapid pulse and shock.

Indicate two conditions that should be considered and laboratory findings that would aid in the differential diagnosis.

Describe clinical features that should suggest that a skin lesion is a malignant melanoma.

Describe briefly the histopathology of malignant melanoma.

Indicate method of spread and prognosis.

Name three diseases that can be transmitted by blood or blood products from donor to recipient.

What precautions should be taken to prevent such transmission?

QUESTIONS IN THE CLINICAL SCIENCES

A patient is admitted to a hospital unconscious immediately following an automobile accident. The neurologic examination is normal. Consciousness is not regained. Two hours later respirations are irregular, the left pupil is a little dilated and the right arm is tonic. In another hour the right side of the face begins to twitch. The right arm is spastic, and the left pupil is fully dilated. Respirations are very irregular and slow. (Consider unmentioned phenomena to be normal.)

Write the letters *a* and *b* on your answer paper. After *each* letter write the *number* preceding the word or the expression that best completes the statement.

(a) At this time the diagnosis is:
  1. Depressed skull fracture
  2. Intracranial hematoma
  3. Subdural hematoma
  4. Epidural hematoma
(b) The immediate procedure should be:
  1. Lumbar puncture
  2. Neurologic consultation
  3. Electroencephalogram
  4. Angiogram
  5. Temporal trephine

Outline the procedure to be followed in the evaluation of a severe injury of the pelvis.

What basic information must you have to order and manage intelligently a patient's fluid intake for the few days following a major abdominal surgical procedure during which oral fluids cannot be taken in adequate amounts?

Following a cholecystectomy for gallstones but with no previous history of jaundice, a patient drains bile from the incision. This drainage gradually becomes less and finally ceases after 2 weeks. Concomitantly, the patient becomes jaundiced and develops periodic attacks of chills and fever. The stools become somewhat lighter in color but are not clay colored.

What conditions would you consider in the differential diagnosis?

What laboratory tests or diagnostic procedures, if any, would definitely confirm your diagnosis?

Should this patient be operated upon?

If operation is indicated, when should it be performed?

List the procedures you might employ if necessary to arrive at the diagnosis of a lesion of the lung that has been noted on an anteroposterior chest x-ray film.

What means would you use to manage the problem presented by the elderly frail, weak individual who has great difficulty in getting rid of copious mucoid tracheobronchial secretions in the immediate postoperative period?

A 65-year-old man with chronic bronchitis and emphysema has a combined abdominal-perineal resection of the rectum and the sigmoid colon for carcinoma. During the immediate postoperative period he is being treated with an indwelling urethral catheter and an indwelling nasogastric tube. By the fourth postoperative day the patient's temperature has gradually risen since operation to 103°F by rectum.

What significance, if any, is the amount of fever?

What should be done in an attempt to explain it?

Peptic ulcers of the duodenum are treated surgically by a variety of procedures. Indicate the rational basis for the treatment of his lesion by:

(a) Vagotomy with pyloroplasty
(b) Subtotal gastric resection
(c) Gastroenterostomy

Outline your management of a patient presenting himself with a history of painless hematuria lasting for 1 day, 1 week ago.

Given a patient with severe hypertension, list some of the changes in the fundus of the eye that you would likely encounter in doing an ophthalmoscopic examination.

A 55-year-old woman with atrial fibrillation due to rheumatic heart disease experiences a sudden severe pain in the left leg. When she is seen at the hospital 4 hours later the pain is still present. The leg is cooler than the right from the knee down, and the skin is blanched. The toes can be moved, but sensation in the lower leg is decreased. Pulsation can be felt over the left common femoral artery at the level of Poupart's ligament on the left, but none below this level.

What is the clinical diagnosis?

At what specific point is the lesion most likely located?

What recommendations for management do you make?

A 32-year-old white man is found to have hypertension of 190 mmHg systolic and 100 mmHg diastolic on routine examination. What are the possible causes of this, and what clinical and laboratory findings would help in identifying these causes?

A 28-year-old Puerto Rican woman, the mother of children 6 and 8 years of age, complains of weakness, slight fever, anorexia and hemoptysis. How should this situation be managed from the diagnostic and therapeutic standpoints? What is the most likely diagnosis, and what are the implications with respect to this patient's family?

Discuss the management of *each* of the following clinical situations:

(a) Congestive failure in a child with acute rheumatic pancarditis
(b) Paroxysmal ventricular tachycardia
(c) Premature ventricular beats in a patient with acute myocardial infarction

A 3-year-old child has a generalized convulsive seizure and is rushed to you in the emergency room of a hospital. Tabulate the common causes and give the clinical and laboratory findings of *each* cause mentioned.

Indicate briefly the clinical significance of *each* of the following:

(a) Bence Jones protein in the urine
(b) A positive heterophil agglutination test
(c) A high blood alkaline phosphatase
(d) A high blood acid phosphatase
(e) A positive porphobilinogen in the urine

A moderately obese middle-aged woman presents herself complaining of recurrent belching and a sense of a lump and burning in the substernal area. These symptoms occur especially when she stoops over or after a heavy meal, and when she goes to bed at night. Discuss differential diagnosis and treatment.

Outline the clinical and laboratory differential diagnosis of hematuria in an elderly male.

A middle-aged female patient with rheumatoid arthritis has been under long-term treatment with steroids. She now requires operation for acute appendicitis. What are the implications of the prior steroid therapy in such a situation, and how would you manage the medical aspects of the case?

Tabulate briefly the major indications and contraindications for use of each of the following:

(a) Oral hypoglycemic agents
(b) Nitrogen mustard
(c) Parenteral iron preparations
(d) Intravenous aminophylline
(e) Intravenous ACTH

A young adult man has anorexia, vomiting and mild nausea for a few days and then notes dark urine and light stool. Discuss clinical and laboratory differential diagnosis and therapy.

Name one subjective complaint and one objective indication for estrogenic hormone in the management of the woman after her menopause.

A 9-year-old girl experiences prolonged vaginal bleeding. Examination reveals breast and vulvar development and a 6 cm by 9 cm tumor in the pelvis. What would you suspect?

What two complaints warrant a suspicion of gonococcal infection in the female? Indicate two procedures, either of which would confirm the diagnosis.

A 60-year-old nulliparous woman, 9 years postmenopausal, reports serous to bloody vaginal discharge on several occasions in the past month.

Indicate two probabilities.

How would you establish the diagnosis?

What two possibly predisposing factors would you consider when suspecting vaginitis is due to *Monilia?*

What would confirm that diagnosis?

What treatment would you prescribe?

A patient, gravida I, with uterus approximately term size, states that she cannot be more than 30 weeks pregnant. What three possibilities would you consider?

The child survived delivery by section when profuse antepartum bleeding was due to placenta previa. Name three possible causes if menstruation fails to occur by the sixth month postpartum.

What two observations noted during labor warrant a suspicion that defibrination of maternal blood may occur?

How can you determine if this is occurring?

If undetected, what could be the result?

Name three laboratory procedures that might be indicated repeatedly during the prenatal care of a normal patient.

Name three disadvantages inherent in "deep" general anesthesia for delivery at term.

List the activities of the U.S. Public Health Service.

What health hazards may be encountered in a boys' summer camp?

What voluntary agencies are active in the field of cardiovascular disease, and what are some of their activities?

What immunizations should be recommended for travelers to the Middle East and Africa?

What is meant by *each* of the following terms:

(a) Crude death rate
(b) Standardized death rate
(c) Infant mortality rate
(d) Birth rate

What services are offered by local health departments to the practicing physician?

Discuss health hazards in industry, and outline methods of preventing them.

Discuss health facilities provided by unions.

Anatomy

J. Robert Troyer, Ph.D.
The John Franklin Huber Professor and Chairman
of Anatomy, Temple University School of Medicine
Philadelphia, Pennsylvania

Neal E. Pratt, P.T., Ph.D.
Professor of Orthopedic Surgery and
Anatomy, Hahnemann University
Philadelphia, Pennsylvania

Human anatomy is the study of the structure of the human body. This study is often subdivided into (1) *gross anatomy,* the study of structure as seen with the unaided eye, (2) *microscopic anatomy (histology),* the study of structure as seen with the aid of a microscope; (3) *cytology,* the study of the structure of cells; (4) *embryology,* the study of the origin, growth and development of an organism from inception until birth; and (5) *neuroanatomy,* the structure of the nervous system.

The human body is organized into cells, tissues, organs, and organ systems. *Cells* are the smallest units of structure of the body that have, or had, the ability to carry on all of the vital functions of the body. *Tissues* are groups of cells and intercellular material that are specialized for the performance of specific functions. Each *organ* consists of certain arrangements of tissues that join in performing a specific bodily function or functions. An *organ system* is a group of organs that perform related functions. The major organ systems of the body are the integumentary, skeletal, muscular, nervous, circulatory (cardiovascular and lymphatic), respiratory, digestive, endocrine, urinary, and reproductive systems.

In the following review of human anatomy we will first discuss cell structure; this will be followed by a regional review of the back, upper extremity, lower extremity, head and neck, thorax, abdomen, and pelvis and perineum. The gross and micro-scopic anatomy, neuroanatomy, and embryology of the organ systems will be discussed as each region is reviewed.

CELL STRUCTURE

The cells of the body are composed of *protoplasm,* which is organized into two major components: the nucleus and the cytoplasm. The cytoplasm is separated from its surrounding environment by a plasma membrane and from the nucleus by a nuclear membrane (envelope).

NUCLEUS

Most cells possess one nucleus that in the interphase (nondividing) state consists of chromatin, one or more nucleoli, nucleoplasm and an investing nuclear membrane. Some cells (*e.g.*, red blood cells) have no nuclei, whereas quite a few cells have more than one nucleus (*e.g.*, parietal cells of stomach, hepatocytes, osteoclasts).

Chromatin. Chromatin particles in the nucleus are the threads of deoxyribose nucleic acid (DNA) and proteins of the *chromosomes.* The DNA double helix of 20-A diameter that represents the genes of the chromosomes is coiled or folded back upon itself in forming each chromatin fibrillar thread of 100-A diameter. Chromatin material occurs in two forms: (1) *heterochromatin,* consisting of tightly coiled and condensed threads of DNA and protein, and (2) *euchromatin,* comprised of less-coiled, lighter staining, and more dispersed threads. The heterochromatin seems to represent the more inactive metabolic state, whereas euchromatin is more active in the synthesis of ribonucleic acid (RNA). Although the ratio of euchromatin to heterochromatin is different in various cells of the body, the chromatin content and chromosomal number are constant for somatic and sex cells. Somatic cells contain 46 chromosomes consisting of 22 pairs of autosomes and one pair of sex chromosomes (XX in females and XY in males). Sex cells contain 23 chromosomes made up of one half of each pair of chromosomes.

Nucleolus. One nucleolus, or several nucleoli, are present in each cell. Most of each nucleolus is protein, 5% to 10% is RNA and a small amount is DNA. The protein and RNA often appear as a meandering thick thread of ribonucleoprotein called a *nucleolonema.* The nucleolonema appears as fibrillar (pars fibrosa) and granular (pars granulosa) portions of the nucleolus. A chromosomal portion of intranucleolar chromatin (nucleolar organizer) contains the genes from which ribosomal RNA (rRNA) is transcribed and synthesized. The newly formed rRNA is packaged with proteins into ribosomal subunits; these pass from the pars fibrosa and pars granulosa before being transferred to the cytoplasm where they are assembled into ribosomes.

Nucleoplasm. Nucleoplasm is an amorphous substance consisting of proteins, ions, and metabolites. Chromatin and nucleoli seem to be suspended in this substance.

Nuclear Membrane (Envelope). The nuclear membrane consists of two parallel unit membranes that are separated by a perinuclear space of about 200 A to 400 A. The *unit membrane* also is a component of the plasma membrane, Golgi apparatus, lysosomes, mitochondria, coated vesicles, and secretion granules. With the electron microscope the basic unit membrane is seen as an 80-A thick complex of an electron light area sandwiched between two electron dense areas. The dense areas seem to represent the membrane proteins and the polar ends of the phospholipid bilayers that make up the membrane. The *outer* unit membrane of the nuclear envelope is continuous with the endoplasmic reticulum. The *inner* unit membrane of the nuclear envelope is attached to the chromosomes by a fibrous network of three polypeptides called the nuclear lamina. Circular openings (nuclear pores), which are covered by thin membranes, occur at in-

tervals throughout the nuclear envelope. The nuclear pores are important passageways for the transfer of substances between the cytoplasm and the nucleus.

CYTOPLASM

The cytoplasm contains dynamic "living" structural components of the cell (organelles) and "nonliving" metabolites or products of the cell (inclusions). The organelles include the plasma membrane, ribosomes, endoplasmic reticulum, Golgi apparatus, lysosomes, mitochondria, centrioles (centrosome), fibrils, filaments, microtubules, peroxisomes, and coated vesicles. Inclusions include stored glycogen, lipid, and protein and secretion granules.

Plasma Membrane. The plasma membrane is a unit membrane 80 A thick consisting of a fluid bilayer in which there are membrane proteins. The lipid component consists of phospholipids, cholesterol, and glycolipids. The phospholipid molecules have their hydrophilic glycerol-phosphate heads oriented toward either the outer or the inner surface of the plasma membrane; the fatty acid tails of this double layer of phospholipid molecules meet in the center of the plasma membrane to form an intermediate hydrophobic zone. Cholesterol molecules stabilize the membrane, whereas glycolipids are located in the outer portion of the wall and seem to serve in cellular communication. Some membrane proteins extend through the plasma membrane (transmembrane proteins) and help to transport specific molecules into and out of the cell. Other membrane proteins extend only from the internal or external surface (*e.g.,* glycoproteins) of the membrane; these may serve as enzymes, attachment sites of the cytoskeleton or receptor sites. The membrane proteins can move around in the plasma membrane. A glycocalyx coats the outer surface of the cell. It consists of the carbohydrate components of glycolipids and glycoproteins of the membrane and also of glycoproteins and proteoglycans that have been absorbed on the cell surface.

Ribosomes. Ribosomes (rRNA plus protein) occur as free ribosomes or as the granular component of the *rough endoplasmic reticulum* (RER). Generally, the free ribosomes are involved in the synthesis of structural proteins and enzymes that stay in the cell; the RER is necessary for the *synthesis of proteins* that are secreted from the cell and for producing lysosomal enzymes used in cellular digestion.

Endoplasmic Reticulum. The endoplasmic reticulum is a membranous network of tubules and flattened sacs that are often continuous with the outer layer of the nuclear membrane. That endoplasmic reticulum that does not have attached ribosomes is called *smooth endoplasmic reticulum* (SER); that with ribosomes is RER. SER is involved in steroid production in the adrenals and gonads, excitation–contraction mechanisms of muscle, absorption of fats in the intestine, and in cholesterol and lipid metabolism and drug detoxification in the liver.

Golgi Apparatus (Golgi Complex). One or more Golgi apparatus usually is found near the nucleus. Each consists of stacks of flattened smooth-surfaced saccules composed of unit membrane. The Golgi apparatus has an immature (forming, cis) face where new stacks are added, and a maturing (trans) face where secretory vesicles seem to bud off. Protein and sugar molecules manufactured in the RER pass to the forming face through transfer vesicles. In the Golgi apparatus the protein is condensed; sugars may be added to it and the product is packaged into secretory vesicles. The Golgi apparatus also is involved in cell membrane and lysosome production.

Lysosomes. Lysosomes are unit membrane–bound vesicles of digestive (hydrolyzing) enzymes. In the digestion of worn out parts of the cell, primary lysosomes fuse with autophagic vacuoles containing the dead part. In digesting endocytized (phagocytized, pinocytized) material, primary lysosomes fuse with the internalized membrane-bound substance forming a secondary lysosome. If the material is not completely digested, a membrane-bound residual body remains.

Mitochondria. Mitochondria are filamentous or granular structures that are comprised of a double unit membrane. The inner membrane, separated from the outer membrane by a 60-A to 100-A wide space, is thrown into many transverse folds (cristae) or tubules, which project into the fluid matrix in the interior of the mitochondrion. The inner surface of the cristae is studded with many "elementary particles." Mitochondria are the sites where phosphate bond energy in the form of adenosine triphosphate (ATP) is produced. In this process, pyruvate passes through the mitochondrial membranes and into the matrix where it is converted to acetyl-coenzyme A (acetyl-CoA). Under the influence of the enzymes of the citric acid cycle in the matrix, the acetyl-CoAs are transformed into CO_2 and electrons (NADH and $FADH_2$). These electrons are then passed along an electron transport system of enzymes on the inner mitochondrial membrane and its cristae. In this process the energy that is made available is used in forming ATP by adding inorganic phosphate to adenosine diphosphate (ADP). A coupling factor (enzyme) needed in this final step of oxidative phosphorylation is located in the elementary particles of the inner membrane.

Centrosome (Cell Center). The centrosome is located near the nucleus and consists of two *centrioles* surrounded by homogenous cytoplasm. The centrioles are cylindrical ($0.15~\mu$m $\times$ 0.3 to 0.5 μm) and lie perpendicular to each other. The wall of each centriole consists of nine parallel units, each of which is made up of three fused microtubules. Basal bodies, located at the base of cilia or flagella, are similar in structure to centrioles. Centrioles seem to be nucleation centers for microtubule formation; this is apparent in the formation of the spindle during cell division.

Microtubules. Microtubules are straight or wavy cylinders whose walls are made up of rows of tubulin. Microtubules function in maintaining cell shape, in intracellular transport, and in cell movement. Cilia and flagella are motile processes that extend from the free surfaces of many different cells. They consist of a core of microtubules, the axoneme, which is arranged as two central microtubules surrounded by nine peripheral doublets, each of which share a common wall of two or three protofilaments. Dynein arms possessing ATPase activity, extend from one doublet toward an adjacent doublet. It is believed that motion of cilia and flagella is the result of doublets sliding within the axoneme as the dynein arms of one doublet walk along the adjacent doublet.

Filaments and Fibrils. Filaments are slender threads of protein molecules. Filaments less than 80 A in diameter are microfilaments, which are part of the cytoskeleton and are involved in cell contraction. Filaments between 80 A and 120 A in diameter are intermediate filaments (tonofilaments), which also lend skeletal support. Bundles of filaments comprise fibrils. Thus, myofibrils of skeletal muscle are comprised of small myofilaments (actin and myosin). Actin filaments also make up the core of microvilli, which project from the free surface of absorptive cells. The actin filaments of the microvilli intermingle with the filaments of the terminal web at the base of the microvilli.

Peroxisomes. Peroxisomes are small membrane bound vesicles containing several oxidative enzymes involved in the production of hydrogen peroxide.

Coated Vesicles. The membranes of coated vesicles are coated on their cytoplasmic surface by several proteins (*e.g.,* clathrin). Coated vesicles are involved in intracellular transport, packaging of secretory material, or are specialized for the receptor-mediated endocytosis of macromolecules from the extracellular fluid. In the latter process the macromolecules are internalized when the coated plasma membrane to which it binds is pinched off as a coated vesicle. Cholesterol is internalized by this method. Coated vesicles join to form endosomes, before they fuse with lysosomes.

Inclusions. Glycogen, lipid droplets, and pigments (*e.g.,* lipofuscin, melanin, carotene) are stored in many of the cells of the body. Secretion granules are membrane-bound vesicles containing a protein or protein–carbohydrate secretory product.

Intercellular Junctions. Cells demonstrate variable degrees of cohesion and attachment. These junctions are particularly pronounced in epithelial and muscle tissues. *Tight junctions* (zonulae occludentes) form bands around the apical wall of epithelial cells. Since the outer leaflets of adjacent cell membranes fuse in a series of ridges in this type of junction, there is a relatively tight seal that prevents passage of materials from the lumen between the cells. The *zonula adherens* is a band that forms just deep to the tight junction. Microfilaments of the terminal web insert into a dense plaque on the cytoplasmic surface of the zonula membrane. This junction retains a 20-nm intercellular space. *Desmosomes* (maculae adherentes) are small spot junctions that are similar in structure to the zonula adherens, except that tonofilaments insert into the attachment plaque and there may be dense material in the intermediate space. The *gap junction* (nexus) is characterized as being a 2-nm apposition of membranes that is bridged by connexons that permit cells to communicate with each other.

PROTEIN SYNTHESES

The mechanisms for protein synthesis are important since structural proteins comprise most of the important structures of the body, and since most of the chemical reactions in the body are catalyzed by enzymes which are proteins. The general sequence of events in protein synthesis is the (1) activation of genes, (2) transcription of DNA to form messenger RNA (mRNA), (3) recognition of amino acids by their specific transfer RNA (tRNA) molecules, and (4) translation of the mRNA by the tRNA at the ribosomes (rRNA).

Activation of Genes. *Structural genes* (cistrons) are specific segments of the DNA molecule that provide coded messages essential for the assembly of certain amino acids in the production of specific structural proteins or enzymes. In order for different genes to exist, the double helix of DNA that comprises the chromosomes must possess structures whose variation in sequencing permits different proteins to be formed. These components of DNA are sequences of **nucleotides.** Each nucleotide is assembled so that one deoxyribose sugar unit and one unit of phosphoric acid provide part of the DNA strand while a nitrogenous base forms a side chain that pairs with the base of a nucleotide in the adjacent DNA strand of the double helix. The only four nitrogenous bases that exist in DNA are two purines, adenine (A) and guanine (G), and two pyrimidines, cytosine (C) and thymine (T). When the bases pair, adenine bonds only with thymine, and cytosine only with guanine. The sequence of the bases (*i.e.,* the sequence of genetic code letters A, T, C, and G) along a single strand of DNA determines which amino acids will be put together to form a particular protein. A sequence of three nitrogenous bases (codon) codes for each amino acid. Several codons in sequence form each cistron. Thus, the **genetic code** for protein synthesis is found in the nitrogenous base sequence of DNA.

Although each somatic cell contains all of the genes for that individual, relatively few genes are activated at any one time. A gene is activated only when a specific mRNA molecule is to be transcribed from the DNA. In this activation process, it appears that a specific gene regulatory protein acts as the activator by binding to the DNA and facilitating the binding of RNA polymerase to a promoter segment of the DNA. The latter binding promotes transcription of a specific mRNA when the specific RNA polymerase recognizes a starting point and moves down the gene to its termination signal. The affinity of the specific gene regulatory protein for the DNA may be increased or decreased by inducer and inhibitory ligands, respectively.

Transcription of Messenger RNA. Messenger RNA has a structure similar to a single strand of DNA, except that ribose sugar takes the place of deoxyribose and thymine is replaced by uracil. When genes are activated, the DNA strands of the helix separate in the region of the involved cistron and the exposed nitrogenous bases serve as templates for the synthesis of a mRNA molecule. In this process adenine of the DNA pairs with uracil of the developing mRNA molecule, the thymine of DNA pairs with adenine of RNA, the guanine of

DNA pairs with cytosine of RNA, and the cytosine of DNA pairs with guanine of RNA. The newly formed mRNA separates from the DNA strand, passes into the cytoplasm and becomes associated with tRNA.

Recognition and Transport of Amino Acids by Transfer RNA. Transfer RNA molecules are multipolar structures that are produced in the nucleus. Each tRNA molecule passes into the cytoplasm, where one of its poles recognizes and binds a specific amino acid. Another pole of each tRNA molecule contains a triplet of nitrogenous bases that is able to ''read'' the complementary codon of a mRNA molecule. A third pole recognizes ribosomes.

Translation of the Messenger RNA Message. Ribosomal RNA and tRNA play roles in translating the mRNA message. The small subunit of the ribosome attaches to a start codon on the mRNA molecule and then travels down the molecule from codon to codon. At each codon the appropriate tRNA that ''reads'' the codon attaches to the mRNA and deposits its amino acid. As each amino acid is assembled into a new protein molecule, the tRNAs are released and another ribosome may read the mRNA. When each ribosome reaches a stop codon, the translation is terminated. If the protein that is produced is a structural protein, the ribosomes used are free ribosomes. If the protein is to be a secretion product, the protein molecule passes through the ribosome, into the lumen of the rough (granular) endoplasmic reticulum, and through transfer vesicles to the region of the Golgi apparatus, where it is concentrated and packaged into secretory granules (storage vacuoles). When these membrane-bound granules fuse with the plasma membrane, the secretory product is elaborated by exocytosis. In some cells the concentration step is eliminated and the product is transferred directly to the plasma membrane from the endoplasmic reticulum and Golgi region.

CELL DIVISION

Somatic cells divide by the mitotic process of cell division, whereas sex cells divide by meiosis. Prior to both of these types of division the stem cell undergoes an interphase stage wherein the DNA is replicated during the S (synthesis) phase. In this replication process, the DNA strands separate (replication fork) when the bonds between nitrogenous bases are broken, and free nucleotides attach to their complementary bases. Thus, two new helices are formed of which one DNA strand in each helix

has served as the template for the new chromatid. If mitosis occurs, the cell will divide into two daughter cells, each with 46 chromosomes. In meiosis two divisions (meiosis I and II) take place with no further replication of the DNA, thus producing four cells, each with the haploid (23) number of chromosomes.

Mitosis. After interphase the cell enters the *prophase* stage, where the chromosomal strands become coiled as they shorten and thicken. The two chromatids of each chromosome are joined by a centromere, the chromosomes are suspended in a spindle of microtubules that bridges between the two centrioles, and the nucleolus and nuclear envelope disappear. During *metaphase* the chromosomes align on a metaphase (equatorial) plate. In *anaphase* the chromosomes separate in the region of the centromeres, and each chromatid is pulled toward opposite poles of the cell. During *telophase* a cleavage furrow in the plasma membrane continues to separate the cytoplasm into two daughter cells while the nucleoli and nuclear envelope reappear.

Meiosis. In the first meiotic division (MI) cells undergo a lengthy prophase, and the homologous chromosomes come together in a synapsis. This configuration is called a tetrad of four chromatids. In metaphase these synapsed pairs line up on the equator, but they separate during anaphase and telophase so that the two new daughter cells will have only 23 chromosomes, each of which is represented by two chromatids. Thus, MI is a reduction division. In the second meiotic division (MII), the centromeres separate during metaphase so that each of the new daughter cells receive 23 chromatids, each of which becomes a new chromosome. The result of meiosis is the production of four sex cells from one stem cell, with each of the four cells having the haploid (23) number of chromosomes.

THE BACK AND THE HISTOLOGY OF BASIC TISSUES

Vertebral Column

INDIVIDUAL VERTEBRAE

Typical Vertebra. The component parts of the vertebral column are basically similar in construction. The two major portions are the anterior *body* and the posterior *vertebral* or *neural arch.* The body is in the form of a flattened cylinder that serves as the major weight bearing portion of the vertebra. The vertebral arch consists of a series of continuous projections and prominences that form (together with the posterior aspect of the body) the vertebral foramen. The paired *pedicles* project posteriorly from the posterolateral aspect of the upper half of each body, and the *laminae* project posteromedially (to join in the midline) from the posterior extents of the pedicles. The *transverse processes* extend laterally from the arch; the *single spinous* process is directed posteriorly in the midline. The pairs of superior and inferior articular processes arise from the vertebral arch at about the junction of the pedicle and lamina. Each articular process contains an articular facet.

Regional Variation. The size of the vertebral bodies steadily increases from above downward to accommodate the increasing superincumbent weight. The delicate cervical vertebrae are distinguished by a bifid spine, foramina in the transverse processes that transmit the vertebral arteries, and prominent upward flares of the superolateral aspects of the body. Thoracic vertebrae have articular facets or costal fovea (with which the ribs form synovial joints) on the posterolateral aspects of the bodies and the anterior aspects of the tips of the transverse processes, and very long spinous processes that are directed inferiorly so that they overlap the next lower vertebra. Lumbar vertebrae have very large heavy bodies and short strong spinous processes that are directed posteriorly. Their laminae are about half as high (superoinferiorly) as their bodies, and hence an interlaminar space exists between lumbar vertebrae.

CONNECTIONS BETWEEN ADJACENT VERTEBRAE

Joints. The vertebral arches are connected by the *intervertebral* or *zygapophyseal articulations.* These are synovial joints between the superior articular facets of the vertebra below and the inferior articular facets of the vertebra above. A thin joint capsule permits a limited amount of gliding motion between the articular surfaces. The orientation or plane of the joint space is a major determinant of the direction of motion that occurs between adjacent vertebrae.

The bodies are united (and separated) by a fibrocartilaginous *intervertebral disk.* This is a cartilaginous joint and as such permits limited motion. The disk is composed of a gelatinous core (*nucleus pulposus*) which is surrounded by a strong distensible envelope (*anulus fibrosus*) and separated from each vertebral body by a hyaline cartilage plate. Thus, the disk has all the physical properties of a closed fluid–elastic system, that is, any pressure is delivered equally and undiminished to all parts of the container, which in this case are the anulus fibrosus and the cartilaginous plates.

Ligaments. The ligaments of the vertebral column can be grouped into those that interconnect adjacent vertebrae and those that extend virtually the entire length of the vertebral column. The segmental ligaments include the ligamentum flavum, which connects the laminae, and the interspinous, supraspinous, and intertransverse ligaments, whose locations are self-explanatory. Two ligaments extend from the atlas to the sacrum. The anterior longitudinal ligament reinforces the anterior and anterolateral aspects of the vertebral bodies and intervertebral disks. The posterior longitudinal ligament attaches to the posterior aspects of the bodies and disks and is therefore within the vertebral canal. This ligament supports the posterior aspect of the disk in the midline but adds little support posterolaterally.

These ligaments are strong and tight and act to support the vertebral column as well as restrict motion. Spinal extension is limited by only the anterior longitudinal ligament while the rest of the above-named ligaments limit flexion. Side-bending is limited by the intertransverse ligaments.

VERTEBRAL COLUMN AS A WHOLE

Normal and Abnormal Curves. The anteroposterior curves of the vertebral column are compensatory adjustments that attempt to position the superincumbent weight above the next lower segment of support. Normally each junctional area (lumbosacral, thoracolumbar, cervicothoracic, occipitocervical) is directly above the center of gravity of the body as a whole, and as a result little or no muscular activity is necessary to hold the spine upright during quiet standing. These curves are such that the lumbar and cervical regions present posterior concavities while the thoracic and sacral regions present posterior convexities. No lateral curvature normally exists. An exaggerated lumbar curve is called *lordosis;* an exaggerated thoracic curve, *kyphosis.* Any lateral curve is *scoliosis.*

Motion of Vertebral Column. Motion of the vertebral column as a whole is the sum of the variable amount of motion that occurs between adjacent vertebrae. Although the intervertebral disk is easily distorted in any direction, and thus permits motion in any direction, its thickness does regulate the extent of motion. In addition, motion is limited by the tension of the vertebral column ligaments. The direction of motion is limited to a large degree by the orientation of the plane of the zygapophyseal joint. In the cervical region the disks are relatively thick, and although the joint spaces are oriented between the coronal and horizontal planes, they are closer to the horizontal plane. As a result, flexion, extension, lateral bending, and rotation are permitted. Flexion and extension are especially free between the occipital bone and the atlas, and rotation is very free between the atlas and axis. The rigidity imposed by the rib cage and the thin intervertebral disks greatly limits motion in the thoracic region. Lumbar disks are very thick, and the joint planes range from a sagittal orientation superiorly to a coronal orientation between L5 and S1. Although flexion and extension are quite free (especially between L5 and S1) rotation and lateral bending are limited.

Integrity of the Vertebral Column. The static support of the normally aligned vertebral column is provided primarily by the ligaments discussed above. As soon as motion occurs, the muscles become important in controlling the overall posture, but the relationship between adjacent vertebrae is still maintained by the ligaments. Bony support is a factor at only certain areas. The *thoracic region* is, of course, greatly reinforced by the thoracic cage; as a result vertebral dislocations seldom occur there. At other levels the only possible bony support is derived from the articular facets that form the zygapophyseal joints. The amount of this support, though, is dependent upon the orientation of the joint space. In the *cervical region* these joint spaces are nearly horizontal. As a result there is no bony block preventing one vertebra from sliding forward with respect to an adjoining vertebra. It follows that cervical dislocation can occur with only soft tissue damage (no fracture). On the other hand, the planes of the *lumbar* zygapophyseal joints are vertically oriented (the upper ones in the sagittal plane and the lower ones in the coronal plane), and the inferior articular facets overlap the superior articular facets of the next lower vertebra. Any tendency toward dislocation is resisted by interlocking of the articular surfaces, and fracture usually accompanies dislocation.

The stability of the lower lumbar region (especially the *lumbosacral junction*) is particularly dependent on bony support. The body of L5 is sitting on the anteriorly inclined superior aspect of the sacrum, and there is a natural tendency for this vertebra to slide (dislocate) anteriorly. This tendency is resisted by the zygapophyseal joints between L5 and the sacrum. Occasionally there is bony discontinuity of the lamina between the superior and inferior articular facets, a condition called *spondylolysis.* This means that the bony support normally provided by the zygapophyseal joint is lost, and anterior sliding of the L5 body is predisposed. Ante-

rior dislocation of the vertebral body is referred to as *spondylolisthesis.*

INTERVERTEBRAL FORAMEN

Normal Anatomy of the Intervertebral Foramen. The basic boundaries of this foramen are the same throughout the vertebral column. The superior and inferior aspects are the pedicles of the respective vertebrae. The anterior boundary consists of the intervertebral disk and portions of the adjacent vertebral bodies. Posteriorly the superior and inferior articular facets form the zygapophyseal joint. Although the specific anatomy of the foramen differs somewhat from region to region, pathology most commonly involves the more mobile cervical and lumbar regions; this description is limited to those areas.

Pathology Involving the Intervertebral Foramen. In the *cervical region* the foramen is small, the intervertebral disk forms most of the anterior wall, and the relatively large spinal nerve practically fills the opening. Protrusion or rupture of the disk into the foramen will impinge on the nerve in the foramen; that is, rupture of the disk between cervical vertebrae 5 and 6 will involve spinal nerve C6. In addition, the size of the cervical intervertebral foramen can be reduced by inflammation of the zygapophyseal joint (arthritis) and by bony projections from the vertebral bodies. These bony spurs usually result from disk degeneration, which in turn causes irritation to *Luschka's joints* on the posterolateral aspects of the vertebral bodies. In the *lumbar region* the disk forms the lower half of the anterior wall of the foramen, and the upper vertebral body, the upper half. The opening is very large, and the relatively small spinal nerve exits in the upper part of the foramen opposite the vertebral body. Rupture of the disk at this level typically does not affect the spinal nerve in the same foramen but rather the spinal nerve that is descending in the anterolateral aspect of the vertebral canal (across the posterolateral aspect of the disk) to exit from the next lower intervertebral foramen. Thus, a rupture of the disk between lumbar vertebrae 4 and 5 will usually impinge on spinal nerve L5.

MICROSCOPIC STRUCTURE OF THE CONNECTIVE AND SUPPORTIVE TISSUES

The adult connective and supportive tissues are connective tissue proper, cartilage, and bone. *Connective tissue proper* is further classified into loose irregular (areolar) connective tissue and dense regular and irregular connective tissues. These tissues contain cells and a preponderance of intercellular fibers and ground substance.

Loose Irregular Connective Tissue.   Loose connective tissue is found in the superficial and deep fascia and as the stroma of most organs. It is generally considered as the packing material of the body. Loose connective tissue contains most of the cell types and all of the fiber types found in the other connective tissues. The most common cell types are the fibroblast, macrophage, adipose cell, mast cell, plasma cell, and wandering cells from the blood. *Fibroblasts* contain the organelles that permit them to produce all of the fiber types and the intercellular material (see Table 2-2 immediately before the anatomy review questions). In their production of these proteinaceous substances, mRNA, rRNA, and tRNA are produced in the nucleus and pass to the cytoplasm. Amino acids that have been taken into the fibroblast attach to specific tRNA and are translated on the mRNA in the region of the ribosomes of the RER. The polypeptides produced pass through the cisternae of the RER to the region of the Golgi complex where they are packaged into membrane-bound procollagen macromolecules that attach to the cell surface before discharge from the fibroblast. Outside the cell, the procollagen molecules are cleaved of their registration peptides forming tropocollagen, which is assembled into *collagen* (for a summary of most secretory cells of the body and their secretion, see Table 2-2). The Golgi complex also is responsible for adding the carbohydrate components to the glycosaminoglycans (GAGs) (mucopolysaccharides) of the ground substance. *Macrophages* are part of the reticuloendothelial system (mononuclear phagocyte system). They possess large lysosomes containing digestive enzymes, which are necessary for the digestion of phagocytized materials. *Mast cells* occur mostly along blood vessels and contain granules that represent the heparin and histamine produced by these cells. *Plasma cells* are part of the immune system in that they produce circulating antibodies. They are extremely basophilic because of their extensive RER. *Adipose cells* are found in varying quantities. When they predominate, the tissue is called adipose tissue.

Collagenous, reticular, and elastic fibers are irregularly distributed in loose connective tissue. Collagenous fibers are usually found in bundles of fibers and provide strength to the tissue. Each fiber is made up of fibrils, which are composed of staggered monomers of tropocollagen giving a 640-A periodicity to most normal collagen in the body. Many different types of collagen are identified on the basis of their molecular structure. Of the five most common types, collagen type I is the most abundant, being found in dermis, bone, dentin, tendons, organ capsules, fascia, and sclera. Type II is located in hyaline and elastic cartilage. Type III probably is the collagenous component of reticular fibers. Type IV is found in basal laminas. Type V is a component of placental basement membranes. Reticular fibers are smaller, more delicate fibers that form the basic framework of reticular connective tissue. Elastic fibers branch and provide elasticity and suppleness to connective tissue.

Ground substance is the gelatinous material that fills most of the space between the cells and fibers. It is composed of acid mucopolysaccharides (GAGs) and structural glycoproteins, and its properties are important in determining the permeability and consistency of the connective tissue.

Dense Connective Tissue.   Dense irregular connective tissue is found in the dermis, periosteum, perichondrium, and capsules of some organs. All of the fiber types are present, but collagenous fibers predominate. Dense regular connective tissue occurs as aponeuroses, ligaments, and tendons. In most ligaments and tendons collagenous fibers are most prevalent and are oriented parallel to each other; fibroblasts are the only cell type present. In the ligamenta flava, elastic fibers dominate and they are considered elastic ligaments.

Cartilage.   Cartilage is composed of *chondrocytes* embedded in an intercellular matrix, consisting of fibers and an amorphous firm ground substance. Three types of cartilage (hyaline, elastic, and fibrous) are distinguished on the basis of the amount of ground substance and the relative abundance of collagenous and elastic fibers.

Hyaline cartilage is found as costal cartilages, articular cartilages, and cartilages of the nose, larynx, trachea, and bronchi. The intercellular matrix consists primarily of collagenous fibers and a ground substance rich in chondromucoprotein, a copolymer of a protein and chondroitin sulfates. The gel like firmness of cartilage depends on the electrostatic bonds between collagen and the GAGs and the binding of water to the GAGs. The GAGs are composed of chondroitin and keratan sulfates covalently linked to core proteins, which are bound to hyaluronic acid molecules. Chondrocytes occupy lacunae. During the growth period of the cartilage these cells existed as chondroblasts, and they produced the intercellular matrix. All types of cartilage grow interstitially by the mitoses of cells in the center of the cartilage mass; most types also grow appositionally by the formation of chondroblasts from undifferentiated cells in the cellular layer of the perichondrium. Unlike the fibrous layer of the perichondrium, the cellular layer and the cartilage are avascular so they receive nutriments and oxygen through diffusion from blood vessels in the fibrous layer of the perichondrium. Articular cartilages receive nutriments by diffusion from blood vessels in the marrow and from the synovial fluid. With old age, there is a decrease of acid mucopolysaccharides, an increase in noncollagenous proteins, and calcification may occur because of degenerative changes in the cartilage cells.

Elastic cartilage is found in the pinna of the ear, auditory tube and epiglottic, corniculate and cuneiform cartilages of the larynx. Elastic fibers predominate and thus provide greater flexibility. Calcification of this type of cartilage is rare.

Fibrous cartilage occurs in the anchorage of tendons and ligaments, in intervertebral disks, in the symphysis pubis, and in some interarticular disks and ligaments. Chondrocytes occur singly or in rows between large bundles of collagenous fibers. Compared with hyaline cartilage, only small amounts of hyaline matrix surround the chondrocytes of fibrous cartilage.

Bone. Bone tissue consists of *osteocytes* and an intercellular matrix that contains organic and inorganic components. The organic matrix consists of dense collagenous fibers and an osseomucoid substance containing chondroitin sulfate. The inorganic component is responsible for the rigidity of bone and is composed chiefly of calcium phosphate and calcium carbonate with small amounts of magnesium, fluoride, hydroxide, and sulfate. Electron microscopic studies show that these minerals are deposited in an orderly fashion on the surface of the collagenous fibrils in their interband areas. In the basic organization of bone tissue, osteocytes lie in lacunae and extend protoplasmic processes into small canaliculi in the intercellular matrix. The protoplasmic processes of adjacent osteocytes are in contact with one another and gap junctions are present. The matrix is organized into adjacent layers or lamellae. The number and arrangement of lamellae differ between compact and cancellous bone.

Compact bone contains haversian systems (osteons), interstitial lamellae and circumferential lamellae. *Haversian systems* consist of extensively branching haversian canals that are oriented chiefly longitudinally in long bones. Each canal contains blood vessels and osteogenic cells and is surrounded by 8 to 15 concentric lamellae and osteocytes. The collagenous fibers in adjacent lamellae run at right angles to each other and spiral around the canal. Nutriments from blood vessels in the haversian canals pass through canaliculi and lacunae to reach all osteocytes in the system. Interstitial lamellae occur between haversian systems and represent the remains of parts of haversian and circumferential lamellae. Outer and inner circumferential lamellae occur under the periosteum and endosteum respectively. Volkmann's canals enter through the outer circumferential lamellae and carry blood vessels and nerves which are continuous with those of the haversian canals and the periosteum. Sharpey's fibers are coarse perforating fibers that anchor the periosteum to the outer circumferential lamellae.

Bones are supplied by a loop of blood vessels that enter from the periosteal region, penetrate the cortical bone, and enter the medulla before returning to the periphery of the bone. Long bones are specifically supplied by arteries which pass to the marrow through diaphyseal, metaphyseal, and epiphyseal arteries. In the marrow cavity, some arteries end in sinusoids, and others branch and enter the haversian canals where they supply fenestrated capillaries. The marrow sinusoids drain to veins that leave through nutrient canals. The capillaries of the haversian canals drain to veins that pass centrifugally to the periosteum and adjacent muscles.

Bone undergoes extensive remodeling, and haversian systems may break down or be resorbed in order that calcium can be made available to other parts of the body. Bone resorption occurs by osteocytic osteolysis or by osteoclastic activity. In *osteocytic osteolysis,* osteocytes resorb bone that lies immediately around the lacunae. In *osteoclastic activity,* large multinucleated osteoclasts arise from osteoprogenitor cells and abut against an osseous surface. Here, their extensive ruffled surfaces and proteolytic enzyme secretions seem to be involved in the resorption of more extensive portions of bone. Osteoclasts are components of the mononuclear phagocyte system. In this way, portions of old haversian systems are resorbed, or longitudinal depressions are formed on the periosteal and endosteal surfaces of the bone. If new haversian systems are to be laid down in the gutters or tubes that remain after the resorptive process is complete, osteoblasts differentiate from the osteogenic cells of the enlarged haversian canal or periosteum and begin to lay down a lamella at the periphery of the space. Successive new concentric lamellae are laid down inside this initial lamella.

Cancellous bone differs from compact bone in that the lamellae are organized into trabeculae or spicules. Few haversian systems are present, and most osteocytes are generally closer to the blood supply than in compact bone.

BONE DEVELOPMENT

Development of Vertebrae and Ribs. At the end of the second postfertilization week, the primitive streak gives rise to cells that migrate laterally between the ectoderm and entoderm, forming the intraembryonic mesoderm. At approximately the same time the notochord arises from a cranial midline migration from the primitive node. As development progresses, the intraembryonic mesoderm adjacent to the notochord thickens into longitudinal masses called the paraxial mesoderm. From the 21st to 30th days, the paraxial mesoderm differentiates into 42 to 44 paired segments called somites. This craniocaudal development of somites gives rise to four occipital, eight cervical, twelve thoracic, five lumbar, five sacral, and eight to ten coccygeal somites. Each somite further differentiates so that three distinct cellular regions are apparent. The ventromedial region, sclerotome, eventually gives rise to supportive skeletal structures (e.g., vertebrae and ribs); the dorsomedial part, myotome, forms the skeletal muscles; and the dorsolateral portion, dermatome, gives rise to the dermis of the skin and subcutaneous tissue.

During the fourth week the sclerotomic mesenchymal mass of each somite begins to migrate toward the midline to become aggregated about the notochord. In this migration, cells of the caudal half of each somite shift caudally to meet the cranially migrating cranial half of the adjacent sclerotome. From each of these joined masses, mesenchymal processes grow dorsally around the neural tube to form the neural arches of the vertebrae, and also give rise to rib primordia. Since a vertebra develops from parts of two pairs of adjacent sclerotomes the original intersegmental arteries will come to pass across the middle of the vertebral bodies. The segmental spinal nerves to the myotomes will come to lie at the level of the intervertebral disks and the myotomes. The notochord degenerates in the region of the vertebral bodies but persists in the center of the intervertebral disk as the nucleus pulposus. In the cervical region, the migration of sclerotome accounts for the formation of seven cervical vertebrae from eight somites. This is due to the cranial half of the first sclerotome becoming part of the occipital bone while the caudal half of the eighth sclerotome becomes part of the first thoracic vertebra. Thus, the first cervical nerve passes between the occipital bone and first cervical vertebra while the eighth cervical nerve emerges between the seventh cervical and first thoracic vertebrae.

At 7 weeks separate *chondrification centers* develop in the bodies and the lateral half of each neural arch, and these subsequently fuse together. Later, *ossification centers* develop in the vertebral bodies, in each half of the neural arch and in each rib. These remain as separate centers throughout fetal life. The rib primordia give rise to ribs in the thoracic region, transverse processes in the lumbar region, parts of the transverse processes in the cervical region, and the alae of the sacrum. Excessive growth of the rib primordia can lead to cervical and lumbar ribs. In spondylolisthesis there is usually a defect in the formation of the pedicles due to nonunion of ossification centers. In this condition the spine, laminae, and inferior articular processes of the affected lower lumbar vertebra stay in place, while the body migrates anteriorly with respect to the vertebra below it. In spina bifida conditions there is failure of the neural arches to unite properly in the formation of the spinous process.

The Microscopic Development of Bone. There are two basic patterns of bone formation: intramembranous and endochondral. In both of these types of bone formation, the process of forming bone tissue and the histologic structure of the bone formed are identical. The major difference between these two types of development is the environment within which bone tissue is laid down.

Intramembranous bone formation occurs in flat bones of the skull and face. In this type of development mesenchymal cells differentiate into osteoblasts in a region where mesenchymal cells have produced a fine-fibered vascular membrane. The osteoblasts lay down lamellae of collagenous fibers and ground substance in the form of a meshwork of trabeculae within the membrane. Some osteoblasts become entrapped as osteocytes in this osteoid tissue. When organic *osteoid tissue* becomes impregnated with inorganic salts, it is called *osseous tissue.* Some intertrabecular spaces become marrow cavities when their mesenchyme differentiates into reticular connective tissue and blood-forming cells. Others become haversian canals as concentric lamellae are formed. At the periphery of the entire developing bone (e.g., outer and inner surfaces of skull bones) the bone becomes quite compact in its development. This is accomplished by a mesenchymal condensation around the bone that differentiates into a periosteum, the inner cells of which become osteoblasts and lay down compact bone.

Thus, the bone takes on an appearance of outer and inner tables of compact bone, between which is the diploe of spongy trabecular bone. Osteoclasts are associated with bone resorption, which takes place chiefly on the inner surfaces of the tables and trabeculae. The membranous junction between two developing flat bones is eventually ossified as a suture.

Endochondral bone formation is characterized by a cartilage model of the bone preceding bone histogenesis. In the formation of the cartilage model of a long bone, the oldest cartilage is found in the center of the shaft (diaphyseal) region. Cells in this region hypertrophy, produce phosphatase and bring about calcification of the surrounding cartilaginous matrix. The result of this calcification is inhibition of diffusion of nutrient materials to the chondrocytes, and they die or they may become osteoprogenitor cells. While the cartilage in the center of the shaft is calcifying, the chondrogenic layer of the perichondrium is becoming vascularized. In this new environment, the undifferentiated mesenchymal cells of the chondrogenic layer start to differentiate into osteoblasts, which lay down a bony collar around the shaft of the cartilage model. The perichondrium is now a periosteum. Osteogenic tissue, containing osteoprogenitor cells and blood vessels from this osteogenic layer of the periosteum, pass between the trabeculae of the bony collar and penetrate into the degenerating calcified cartilage. This periosteal bud of tissue is instrumental in resorption of some of the smaller calcified cartilage spicules between lacunae, and in the laying down of bone on remnants of the calcified cartilage. The center of the shaft now consists of osteogenic tissue and bony trabeculae that contain remnant cores of calcified cartilage. This area in the diaphysis is called the primary ossification center.

Since the newer cartilage lies toward the epiphyses, the *metaphyses* (epiphyseal plates, physes) demonstrate the following developmental gradient as the diaphysis is approached: (1) a layer of tissue where cells are not dividing (zone of resting cartilage); (2) a layer where chondrocytes are dividing mitotically and interstitially in an axial orientation (zone of multiplication); (3) a layer where cells are enlarging (zone of cellular hypertrophy and maturation); and (4) a layer where the intercellular material is calcifying and cells are dying (zone of calcification). The shaft grows in length by the multiplication of cartilage cells at the zones of multiplication in each metaphyseal region and by osseous tissue being laid down on the remnants of calcified cartilage in the zone of calcification. This process also brings about an increase in length of the primary marrow cavity. An increase in width of the marrow cavity takes place by resorption of bone on the inner surface of the periosteal bony collar. Since this resorption is not as rapid as the appositional laying down of bone on the outer surface of the bony collar, the compact bone of the shaft increases in width.

Secondary ossification centers develop later in fetal life, or after birth, in the epiphyses. These are usually characterized by hypertrophy of chondrocytes and calcification of cartilage in the centers of the epiphyses where the older cartilage cells exist. Vascular and osteogenic buds of tissue enter the area from the metaphyseal region. A thin layer of dense bone is laid down on the surfaces of the epiphyses where a periosteum is present. On articular surfaces, no periosteum or perichondrium exists, and hyaline cartilage is retained as a covering to the underlying epiphyseal bone.

Muscles of the Back

SUPERFICIAL MUSCLES OF THE BACK

The superficial muscles of the back are found superficial to the thoracolumbar fascia. They represent most of the *extrinsic muscles of the shoulder* in that they interconnect the axial and appendicular portions of the skeleton, specifically extending from the vertebral column or rib cage to the scapula, clavicle, or humerus. Functionally, they are concerned with motion of the shoulder girdle and humerus. Innervation is supplied mainly by branches of the brachial plexus. The *trapezius* is innervated by the accessory (11th cranial) nerve and controls the position of the shoulder statically as well as during virtually any motion, especially when the arm is abducted or flexed. The *latissimus dorsi* is the major extendor of the humerus and shoulder depressor (the "crutch-walking" muscle), and is innervated by the thoracodorsal nerve. A plane of three muscles underlying the trapezius connects the vertebral column and scapula. The *levator scapulae* and the *rhomboid major* and minor are innervated by the dorsal scapular nerve and direct branches of the cervical plexus. The *serratus anterior* extends from the medial border of the scapula to the anterolateral thoracic wall. It functions to hold the ventral surface of the scapula against the thorax and, working with the trapezius, is important in shoulder abduction and flexion. The long thoracic nerve innervates this muscle.

DEEP MUSCLES OF THE BACK

The deep muscles of the back, or the *erector spinae,* are deep to the thoracolumbar fascia and occupy the vertically oriented furrow formed between the spinous processes of the vertebrae and the angles of the ribs. These muscles extend from the occipital bone to the sacrum, and although they can be divided anatomically into many specific parts the entire mass functions as a unit. They are innervated segmentally by branches of the dorsal rami of spinal nerves. Bilateral contraction of these muscles produces extension of the vertebral column; unilateral contraction causes side-bending and rotation.

MICROSCOPIC STRUCTURE OF MUSCLE TISSUE

There are three types of muscle tissue: smooth, skeletal, and cardiac. All three types are comprised of muscle cells (fibers) that contain myofibrils possessing contractile filaments of actin and myosin.

Smooth Muscle. Smooth muscle cells are spindle shaped and are organized chiefly into sheets or bands of smooth muscle tissue. This tissue is found in blood vessels and other tubular visceral structures. Smooth muscle cells contain both actin and myosin filaments, but the actin filaments predominate. The filaments are not organized into patterns that give cross striations as in cardiac and skeletal muscle. Filaments course obliquely in the cells and attach to the plasma membrane. Electron microscopy shows the plasma membrane as a "typical" trilaminar membrane. In specific regions where smooth muscle cells appose each other, leaving only narrow 20-A intercellular gaps, specialized zones of contact occur, which are known as nexuses or "gap" junctions. These junctions probably facilitate the transmission of impulses for contraction. In other intercellular regions a glycoprotein coat and a small amount of collagenous and reticular fibers are found.

Skeletal Muscle. Skeletal muscle fibers are characterized by their peripherally located nuclei and their striated myofibrils. The cross striations are due to the organization and distribution of actin and myosin filaments. These striations are organized within each muscle fiber into fundamental contractile units called *sarcomeres,* which are joined end to end at the Z lines (Fig. 2-1). The striations in a sarcomere consist of an A band bordered toward the Z lines by I bands. The midregion of the A band contains a variable light H band that is bisected by an M line. The light I band contains actin filaments that insert into the Z line. These filaments interdigi-

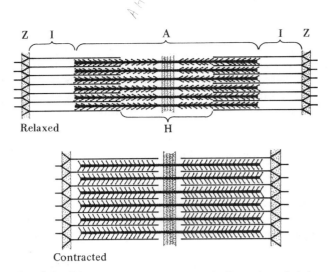

Fig. 2-1. Diagram of a sarcomere in the relaxed state *(top)* and contracted state *(bottom)*. During contraction the thin actin filaments of the I band are pulled into the A band by the myosin heads of the thick myosin filaments, thus reducing the length of the I bands and H zones. (Cormack DH: Ham's Histology, 9th ed, p 393. Philadelphia, JB Lippincott, 1987. Courtesy of E. Schultz and C. P. Leblond)

tate and are cross bridged in the A band with myosin filaments, forming a hexagonal pattern of one myosin filament surrounded by six actin filaments. In the contraction of a muscle fiber a chemical reaction takes place in the region of the cross bridges, causing the actin filaments of the I band to move deeper into the A band, thus resulting in a shortening of the I bands.

Each skeletal muscle fiber is invested with a sarcolemma (plasmalemma) that extends into the fiber as numerous small transverse T tubules. These tubules ring the myofibrils at the A-I junction and are bordered on each side by terminal cisternae of the sarcoplasmic (endoplasmic) reticulum. This arrangement of one T tubule with two terminal cisternae is called a triad. In excitation–contraction coupling, acetylcholine released from the motor end-plate causes depolarization of the muscle membrane, which is propagated to the T tubule–sarcoplasmic reticulum junction. This brings about release of calcium from the terminal cisternae of the sarcoplasmic reticulum, catalyzing the chemical reaction between the actin and myosin filaments in the region of the cross bridges. In this process, calcium attaches to the TnC subunit of troponin, resulting in movement of tropomyosin and uncovering of the active sites for the attachment of actin to the cross-bridging heads of myosin. Due to this attachment, ATP in the myosin head hydrolyzes, producing energy, Pi and ADP, which results in a bending of the myosin head and a pulling of the actin filament into the A band. The actin–myosin bridges detach when myosin binds a new ATP molecule and when calcium returns to the terminal cisternae at the conclusion of neural stimulation.

Cardiac Muscle. Cardiac muscle contains striations and myofibrils that are similar to those of skeletal muscle. It differs from skeletal muscle in several major ways. Cardiac muscle fibers branch and contain centrally located nuclei and large numbers of mitochondria. Individual cardiac muscle cells are attached to each other at their ends by *intercalated disks.* These disks contain several types of membrane junctional complexes, the most important of which is the gap junction. This junction electrically couples one cell to its neighbor so that electrical depolarization is propagated through the heart by cell-to-cell contacts rather than by nerve innervation to each cell. The sarcoplasmic reticulum–T tubule system is arranged differently in cardiac muscle than in skeletal muscle. In cardiac muscle each T tubule enters at the Z line and forms a diad with only one terminal cisterna of sarcoplasmic reticulum.

DEVELOPMENT OF SKELETAL MUSCLES

Histogenesis of Skeletal Muscle. Skeletal muscle cells develop from mesenchyme that arises from the myotomes of somites or from the mesoderm of branchial arches. Stellate mesenchymal cells differentiate into elongate multinucleate myotubes containing peripherally located myofibrils and centrally located nuclei. Later in development, myofibrils will increase in size and number and the nuclei will migrate peripherally. In the limited regeneration of muscle, new fibers may be formed from satellite cells that lie between the skeletal muscle cell and its basement membrane.

Morphogenesis of the Skeletal Musculature. Myotomes divide into dorsal epaxial and ventral hypaxial condensations of mesenchyme. Dorsal and ventral rami develop from the segmental spinal nerves and innervate the epaxial and hypaxial portions, respectively. The epaxial masses give rise to the deep muscles of the back. The hypaxial masses develop into anterior and lateral body wall muscles of the cervical and thoracolumbar regions. Muscles of the extremities and those that attach the limbs to the trunk may arise from local somatic lateral mesoderm but are innervated by the ventral rami of spinal nerves. Subsequent migrations of segmental myoblasts, trailing their respective nerves, lead to the formation of complex nerve fiber plexuses from successive spinal cord levels. In addition to migration, five other basic processes occur in the establishment of muscles: (1) fusions of portions of successive myotomes (*e.g.,* erector spinae), (2) change from the original cephalocaudal direction of the fibers (*e.g.,* transversus abdominus), (3) longitudinal splitting of a myotomic mass to form more than one muscle (*e.g.,* rhomboideus major and minor), (4) tangential splitting (*e.g.,* intercostals), and (5) degeneration of parts or all of a myotome with conversion of the degenerated part to connective tissue (*e.g.,* serratus posterior inferior and superior).

Spinal Cord and Spinal Nerves

GROSS ANATOMY OF SPINAL CORD AND SPINAL NERVES

Basic Organization. The nervous system is composed of the central and peripheral nervous systems. The *central nervous system (CNS)* is enclosed within the cranial vault and vertebral canal and consists respectively of the brain and spinal cord. The *peripheral nervous system* is outside the bony encasement and is composed of peripheral nerves, which are branches of or continuations of the cranial and spinal nerves. The *autonomic nervous system* is anatomically a portion of both the central and peripheral nervous systems. The usual definition of this system is an anatomical one that includes the motor side of the system controlling blood vessels, glands and viscera, and thus can be called the general visceral efferent system.

The spinal cord is a long cylindrical structure whose hollow core is called the *central canal* and is a portion of the *ventricular system.* The central canal is surrounded by the gray matter (cell bodies and terminal arborizations), which is in turn surrounded by the white matter (long ascending and descending cell processes). The cord is segmented, each segment corresponding to a specific portion of the body wall (including extremities) that it innervates. The diameter of the cord decreases from top to bottom with the exceptions of the low cervical and the lumbosacral regions whose enlargements reflect the upper and lower extremities, respectively. The spinal cord terminates inferiorly at the inferior aspect of the first lumbar vertebra. This termination is in the form of an inverted cone and is thus called the *conus medullaris.* Vertical lines of nerve rootlets attach to the anterolateral and posterolateral aspects of the cord. The rootlets from a single segment converge and form *anterior* and *posterior roots.* The two roots join in the intervertebral foramen to form the *spinal*

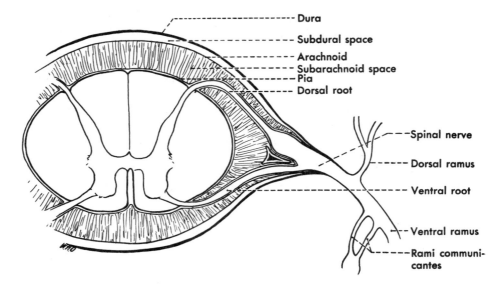

Fig. 2-2. Cross-sectional diagram of the spinal cord, nerve roots, and meninges. (Hollinshead WH: Anatomy For Surgeons, Vol 3, 3rd ed, p 175. Philadelphia, JB Lippincott, 1982)

nerve (Fig. 2-2). After exiting from the intervertebral foramen, the spinal nerve divides into *ventral* and *dorsal rami* whose muscular and cutaneous branches supply the body wall structures.

Both the brain and spinal cord are surrounded by three membranes that have both trophic and protective functions (see Fig. 2-2). For the most part the *meninges* of brain and cord are similar. The differences are outlined later in this chapter. The innermost, the *pia mater,* is a thin membrane that conforms very closely to the contours of the spinal cord and is firmly attached to the neural tissue. The vessels that supply the central nervous system are found in this membrane. The *denticulate ligament* is a series of pial extensions that project laterally and attach to the outermost covering, the *dura mater.* These ligaments serve to stabilize the spinal cord. The intermediate *arachnoid* is a thin filmy membrane attached to the pia by numerous trabeculae. The area between the arachnoid and pia is the *subarachnoid space,* which is filled with cerebrospinal fluid. This fluid holds the arachnoid tightly against the outer dura mater; since the arachnoid and dura are not firmly attached, the *subdural space* is in reality only a potential space. Together the pia and arachnoid are the soft coverings of the spinal cord called the *leptomeninges.* The dura mater is a strong thin membrane, the *pachymeninx.* It is separated from the bones and ligaments of the vertebral canal by the *epidural space* in which the epidural fat and *internal venous plexus* are found. The dura, as well as the pia and arachnoid, extends laterally at the

level of each spinal nerve and becomes continuous with the connective tissue coverings of the nerves. Inferiorly the dural sac terminates at the second sacral vertebra. Since the arachnoid is so closely held against the inner aspect of the dura, the dural sac and subarachnoid space are co-extensive.

Relationship of Spinal Cord to Vertebral Column. The spinal cord extends from the foramen magnum to the lower border of the first lumbar vertebra. This means that only the very uppermost cervical cord segments are opposite the vertebra of the same name. Upper thoracic cord segments are one vertebral level higher than their correspondingly named vertebra, while the lumbar, sacral, and coccygeal cord segments lie opposite the last two thoracic and first lumbar vertebrae. Since each spinal nerve exits through its original intervertebral foramen, only the highest cervical spinal nerves are horizontally oriented, while each next lower spinal nerve is more obliquely oriented as it travels farther to its intervertebral foramen. As a result of this incongruity between spinal cord and vertebral column, the symptoms resulting from a spinal cord lesion do not usually correspond to the vertebral level of the lesion. For example, a lesion at vertebral level T12 could logically be accompanied by symptoms that correspond to cord segments L3 and below. The *cauda equina* is composed of dorsal and ventral roots; these structures are the only neural elements in the subarachnoid space between the end of the spinal cord and the end of the dural sac. This area is the region of choice for spinal tap as there is minimal risk to neural structures when a needle is inserted into the subarachnoid space. In addition, the interlaminar space between lumbar vertebrae allows easy access.

MICROSCOPIC STRUCTURE OF SPINAL NERVES AND THE SPINAL CORD

Spinal Nerves. The basic cell type of nerve tissue is the *neuron*. Each neuron consists of a nerve cell body (perikaryon) and one or more nerve processes (fibers). The cell body of a typical neuron contains a nucleus, Nissl material of rough endoplasmic reticulum, free ribosomes, Golgi apparatus, mitochondria, neurotubules, neurofilaments, and pigment inclusions. The cell processes of neurons occur as *axons* and *dendrites.* Dendrites contain most of the components of the cell body except the nucleus and Golgi apparatus, whereas axons contain the major structures found in dendrites except for the Nissl material. At the synaptic ends of axons, the presynaptic process contains vesicles from which are elaborated excitatory or inhibitory substances. The functional dendrites of some neurons, such as the sensory pseudounipolar neurons of spinal nerves, are structurally the same as axons. Unmyelinated fibers in peripheral nerves lie in grooves on the surface of neurolemma (Schwann) cells and are incompletely invested by the plasmalemma of these cells. Myelinated peripheral neurons are invested by numerous "jellyroll" layers of Schwann cell plasma membrane that constitute a myelin sheath. The Schwann cell cytoplasm and nucleus lie peripheral to the myelin sheath. There are many Schwann cells along each myelinated fiber. In the junctional areas between adjacent Schwann cells there is a lack of myelin. These junctional areas along the myelinated process constitute the nodes of Ranvier.

Spinal nerves have an outer epineurial connective tissue investment and an inner more cellular perineurial covering that extends internally to surround nerve bundles. The cells of the perineurium form an epithelioid sheath wherein the cells are joined by occluding junctions and the layers of cells are separated by basal lamina material. This perineurial layer seems to be an effective barrier against material entering or leaving the nerve. A loose endoneurial connective tissue separates nerve processes and lies next to the basement membranes of the Schwann cells.

Spinal nerves contain the processes of neurons whose cell bodies are located in sensory dorsal root ganglia (pseudounipolar neurons), sympathetic ganglia (multipolar neurons), and in the gray matter of the spinal cord (multipolar neurons). Each spinal nerve contains myelinated and unmyelinated fibers that are invested by Schwann cells. In the ganglia, each cell body is surrounded by supportive satellite cells.

Spinal nerves contain neurons representing four functional components: (1) general somatic efferent (GSE) fibers to skeletal muscles, (2) general visceral efferent (GVE) fibers to smooth and cardiac muscle and glands, (3) general somatic afferent (GSA) fibers from the skin, muscle and tendon spindles, and joints, and (4) general visceral afferent (GVA) fibers from viscera.

Spinal Cord. The spinal cord consists of a central canal lined with ependymal cells and bounded by central gray matter and peripheral white matter. The H-shaped gray matter has anterior, posterior, and lateral horns. It consists of groups of nerve cell bodies (nuclei, cell columns), axons, dendrites, and glial cells that form a meshwork called *neuropil.* An architectural lamination permits classification of the gray matter into nine Rexed's layers.

Glial cells are the supportive cells of the CNS. They consist of ependymal cells, astrocytes, oligodendroglia, and microglia. Protoplasmic astrocytes are found mostly in the gray matter, and fibrous astrocytes are located mostly in the white matter. Astrocytes provide structural support for nerve tissue and may help to isolate groups of nerve endings from each other. Oligodendroglia invest nerve fibers to form the myelin of the CNS. One oligodendrocyte may envelope several fibers. Microglia, unlike the other glia, arise from mesodermally derived monocytes and are components of the mononuclear phagocyte system.

The *anterior horn of gray matter* contains the cell bodies of alpha and gamma motor neurons whose axons innervate extrafusal and intrafusal skeletal muscle fibers, respectively. These nerve cell bodies constitute the GSE cell column and are grouped into nuclei that supply axons to specific regions; for example, those most medial in the anterior horn go to the more axial musculature while those most lateral innervate the extremities and the lateral muscles of the trunk. The alpha motor neurons are in Rexed's layer IX, the gamma motor neurons are in layer VII, and mostly commissural neurons occupy layer VIII. Damage to alpha motor neurons results in a *lower motor neuron (LMN) syndrome* of flaccid paralysis, rapid and relatively extensive muscle atrophy, atonia, and loss of deep and superficial reflexes. If only some GSE neurons to a muscle are damaged then pareses, hypotonia, and hyporeflexia result. Preganglionic sympathetic neurons at thoracic and L1 and L2 levels are located in the intermediolateral cell column. This GVE cell column is in Rexed's layer VII. Preganglionic parasympathetic cell bodies are scattered in layer VII of cord levels S2–S4. Axons of preganglionic autonomics leave the cord by the ventral root and become part of the spinal nerve. Sympathetic preganglionics leave the nerve via the white rami communicantes and enter the sympathetic chain ganglia or become components of splanchnic nerves. They will synapse with postganglionic sympathetic neurons in the sympathetic chain or prevertebral ganglia. Unmyelinated postganglionic axons reentering the spinal nerve constitute the gray rami communicantes. Sacral parasympathetic preganglionics form pelvic nerves, which terminate on ganglia near, or in, the organs innervated.

The *posterior horn of gray matter* consists of several nuclear groups that constitute the GSA cell column. Most prominent of these nuclei are the posteromarginal nucleus of Rexed's layer I, substantia gelatinosa in layer II, the nucleus proprius mostly in layer IV, and nucleus dorsalis of Clarke in layer VII. These nuclei are "nuclei of termination" for incoming somatic afferents in the dorsal roots, and they are involved in processing sensory information. Pain and temperature first-order afferent neurons terminate on second-order neuron cell bodies in the posteromarginal nucleus, nucleus proprius, and deeper layers of the posterior horn. Axons of these second-order neurons transmit impulses contralaterally through the anterior white commissure and ascend in the lateral funiculus as the lateral spinothalamic tract. This tract synapses on third-order neurons in the ventral posterolateral (VPL) nucleus of the thalamus. Axons of VPL cells pass to the postcentral gyrus (areas 3, 1, 2; primary somesthetic area) of the parietal lobe and to an area of parietal cortex immediately above the lateral fissure (somatic sensory area II). Sensory information from intrafusal fibers of neuromuscular spindles and tendon spindles is transmitted via IA and IB myelinated first-order neurons, respectively. These synapse on cells of the nucleus dorsalis (Clarke) at cord levels C8 to L3. Axons of these second-order neurons pass ipsilaterally to the cerebellum as the posterior spinocerebellar tract. IA and IB neurons entering the cervical cord above C8 ascend in the posterior white column to the medulla where they synapse on the accessory cuneate nucleus. Cuneocerebellar and posterior spinocerebellar fibers pass through the inferior cerebellar peduncle to reach the anterior lobe and paravermal areas of the cerebellum. Incoming fibers for crude (light) touch synapse in cells of the posterior horn. Most of the axons of these second-order neurons cross in the anterior white commissure and ascend in the anterior funiculus as the anterior spinothalamic tract. This tract synapses in the VPL nucleus of the thalamus and the impulses are probably relayed to the postcentral gyrus. Visceral sensation (GVA) is probably received by nuclei of termination in the lateral portion of the posterior horn. Its transmission to higher centers is probably through multisynaptic ascending paths in the funiculus proprius lying adjacent to the gray matter. Collaterals from incoming neurons of the dorsal root enter the gray matter and synapse on internuncials and alpha motor neurons for reflex purposes. Those coming from spindle receptors and ending directly on alpha motor neurons are part of the monosynaptic stretch (myotatic) reflex. Terminals of association neurons interconnecting different segmental levels, as well as terminals of descending axons from suprasegmental levels, end on internuncials that synapse with gamma and alpha motor neurons.

The *white matter* is organized into posterior, lateral and white funiculi. Each funiculus contains both ascending and descending pathways (Fig. 2-3). In the posterior funiculus (posterior white column) the most prominent pathway is that concerned with two-point touch, vibratory and joint senses, and stereognosis. Spindle information by way of IA fibers from neuromuscular spindles and IB fibers from Golgi tendon organs also are transmitted in the posterior white column. Axons of these pathways in the posterior white column arise from cell bodies in the dorsal root ganglia, enter the cord in the medial bundle of the dorsal root, and ascend to the medulla where they synapse on second-order neurons in the nuclei gracilis and cuneatus (see Fig. 2-22). Those axons entering dorsal roots below the T6 level constitute fasciculus gracilis and terminate in nucleus gracilis; those at and above T6 are in fasciculus cuneatus and terminate in nucleus cuneatus. Axons of the second-order neurons from the nuclei gracilis and cuneatus cross the midline as internal arcuate fibers and ascend as the medial lemniscus to the VPL nucleus of the thalamus where they synapse with third-order neurons whose axons go to the postcentral gyrus.

The most clinically prominent tracts of the lateral funiculus are the posterior spinocerebellar tract, the lateral spinothalamic tract, the lateral corticospinal tract, and the lateral reticulospinal tract (see Fig. 2-3). The posterior spinocerebellar tract is peripherally located beneath the posterolateral fasciculus at

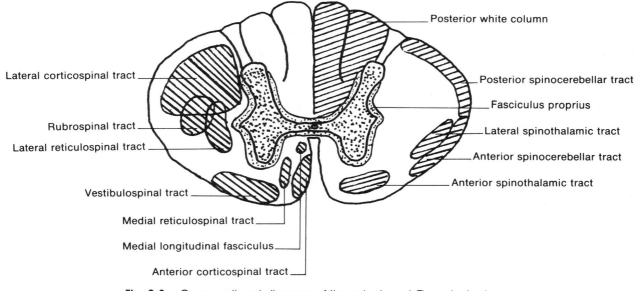

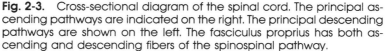

Fig. 2-3. Cross-sectional diagram of the spinal cord. The principal ascending pathways are indicated on the right. The principal descending pathways are shown on the left. The fasciculus proprius has both ascending and descending fibers of the spinospinal pathway.

all levels of the spinal cord above L4. It conveys spindle information to the cerebellum. The lateral spinothalamic tract (see Fig. 2-21) is located ventrolaterally in the lateral funiculus and just deep to the anterior spinocerebellar tract. As previously mentioned, it represents the axons of second-order neurons of the pain and temperature pathway. The lateral corticospinal tract (see Fig. 2-3) is located just medial to the posterior spinocerebellar tract, mostly in the dorsal half of the lateral funiculus. This tract arises from pyramidal cells in the precentral gyrus and premotor area (areas 4 and 6) and postcentral (areas 3, 1, 2) gyrus (see Figs. 2-20, 2-23). From these gyri, axons descend in the brain stem, cross in the pyramidal decussation and descend in the contralateral lateral funiculus before terminating on internuncial neurons, which, in turn, synapse on alpha and gamma motor neurons. The lateral corticospinal tract constitutes the upper motor neurons of the pyramidal motor system. It is involved primarily in fine voluntary movements involving chiefly the more distal phylogenetically "newer" musculature, and it is facilitory to the antagonists of the antigravity muscles. The lateral reticulospinal tract arises from large cells (nucleus gigantocellularis) in the medial reticular formation of the medulla. Axons from these cells descend ipsilaterally in the lateral funiculus and are somewhat interspersed with axons of the lateral corticospinal tract.

Stimulation of cells of the lateral reticulospinal tract inhibits alpha and gamma neurons innervating antigravity muscles (*i.e.*, extensors of the lower extremity and flexors of the upper extremity). Damage to these two tracts in the lateral funiculus results in the ***upper motor neuron (UMN) syndrome.*** This syndrome is discussed later in the section on somatic motor control mechanisms. Other pathways are found in the lateral funiculus. These are the rubrospinal pathway from the red nucleus, descending central autonomics from the hypothalamus, the spinotectal pathway to the superior colliculus of the mesencephalon, spinoreticular fibers to the brain stem reticular formation and interconnections between the spinal cord and inferior olivary nucleus.

In the anterior funiculus, the anterior spinothalamic tract, anterior corticospinal tract, lateral vestibulospinal tract, medial reticulospinal tract, and medial longitudinal fasciculus (MLF) are most prominent (see Fig. 2-3). The anterior spinothalamic tract is located just anterior to the ventral horn. Its origin, destination, and crude touch role were described previously. The anterior corticospinal tract has a similar origin and path to that of the lateral corticospinal tract, but it differs in that it is located near the anterior median fissure, it usually descends only to upper thoracic levels, and its axons have not crossed in the pyramidal decussation. These axons will cross, however, at the level where they terminate on internuncials that synapse with gamma and alpha motor neurons, supplying muscles of the upper extremity and neck. The vestibulospinal tract is interspersed with the anterior spinothalamic tract. It arises from cells in the lateral vestibular nucleus and descends ipsilaterally to end on internuncials that synapse with gamma and alpha motor neurons supplying antigravity muscles. Stimulation of this pathway results in facilitation of extensors of the lower extremity and of flexors of the upper extremity. The medial reticulospinal tract arises from nuclei in the medial portion of the pontine reticular formation. It descends ipsilaterally, lies lateral to the anterior corticospinal tract in the anterior funiculus and is involved in facilitation of antigravity muscles. The MLF lies in the most dorsal portion of the anterior funiculus next to the anterior median fissure. This composite tract contains axons arising from the mesencephalic tectum (tectospinal tract), vestibular nuclei (medial vestibulospinal tract), and the reticular formation of the brain stem (medial reticulospinal tract). Thus, unlike descending fibers of the lateral funiculus, which are facilitory to the antagonists of antigravity muscles and inhibitory to antigravity muscles, the descending fibers of the anterior funiculus are facilitory to antigravity muscles.

The spinal cord is supplied by descending branches from vertebral arteries and from radicular branches of segmental arteries. From these vessels paired posterior spinal arteries arise that descend dorsal to the posterior funiculus, while a single midline anterior spinal artery arises from the paired anterior spinal arterial branches of the vertebral. An arterial vasocorona plexus, lying in the pia adjacent to the lateral funiculus, interconnects the anterior and posterior radicular branches. The posterior spinal arteries supply the posterior funiculus, dorsal part of the dorsal horn of gray matter, and the posterolateral fasciculus (Lissauer). Sulcal branches of the anterior spinal artery supply all other parts of the spinal cord except the most peripheral portion of the lateral funiculus supplied by the arterial vasocorona. Spinal veins have a distribution that is generally similar to arteries. Sulcal and posterior veins empty into anteromedial, anterolateral, posteromedial, and posterolateral veins. These drain, in turn, to radicular veins that enter the epidural venous plexus.

Destruction of the posterior white column ipsilaterally results in astereognosis and in a loss of two-point touch and vibratory sense on the same side below the lesion. Damage to the lateral funiculus results in (1) a loss of pain and temperature con-tralaterally starting one segment below the lesion and extends caudally; (2) spastic paralysis, exaggerated deep reflexes, loss of superficial reflexes, and loss of fine distal motor activity ipsilaterally below the lesion; and (3) a Horner's syndrome of ptosis, pupillary constriction, and blanched and dry facial skin ipsilaterally if the lesion is above the upper thoracic intermediolateral cell column level.

DEVELOPMENT OF THE SPINAL CORD AND SPINAL NERVES

The CNS appears early in the third embryonic week of development as a thickened neural (medullary) plate of ectoderm. This plate is elongate, wider cephalically than caudally, and is located rostral to the primitive node of Hensen. It is continuous laterally with ectoderm that will give rise to the epidermis of the skin. With further development the lateral edges of the plate elevate to form neural folds that close the neural groove into a *neural tube*. The closure begins at the fourth somite and progresses cephalically and caudally, with the anterior and posterior neuropores closing by the 25th day. Ectoderm arising at the junction of neural ectoderm with general surface ectoderm becomes segmentally arranged as the *neural crest* material lying dorsolateral to the neural tube. The cephalic enlargement of the neural tube differentiates into the brain and gives rise to motor components of cranial nerves. The caudal part becomes the spinal cord and also gives rise to the ventral roots of spinal nerves. Neural crest gives rise to sensory neurons comprising the dorsal root ganglia and sensory cranial nerve ganglia, postganglionic autonomic ganglia of cranial and spinal nerves, Schwann cells, satellite cells, parenchyma of the adrenal medulla, pigment cells, and cartilage cells in the head region.

Histogenesis of the Spinal Cord. The early neural tube consists of a neuroepithelium that differentiates into neuroblasts and spongioblasts (glioblasts). *Neuroblasts* differentiate into neurons whose cell bodies are localized into a mantle layer and whose axons contribute to a more peripheral marginal layer. Some of these axons ascend or descend in the marginal layer and become the association fibers of the tracts of the white matter. Others leave the white matter and become motor (efferent) nerve fibers of the ventral roots and spinal nerves. *Spongioblasts* lining the central canal differentiate into ependymal cells while others migrate into the marginal and mantle layers and become astrocytes and oligodendroglia.

The lateral walls of the neural tube are separated into dorsal alar plates and ventral basal plates by a longitudinally running sulcus limitans. The thin roof plate is obliterated in the fusions accompanying the formation of the posterior median septum; the floor plate remains as the anterior white and gray commissures. The mantle layer of the alar plate develops into the posterior horn of gray matter that contains the nuclei of termination for GSA and GVA neurons. Neurons of the posterior horn are internuncial, commissural and association neurons. The mantle layer of the basal plate becomes the anterior horn and lateral horn of gray matter. Neuroblasts of the anterior horn give rise to gamma and alpha GSE neurons whose axons leave the cord in the ventral root and innervate intrafusal and extrafusal skeletal muscle fibers, respectively. Neuroblasts of the lateral horn give rise to preganglionic sympathetic neurons of the intermediolateral cell column at thoracic and L1–L2 levels. Preganglionic parasympathetic neurons arise in a similar position at S2–S4 levels.

Histogenesis of Spinal Nerves. GSA and GVA neurons arise from neural crest material, and their cell bodies are located in dorsal root ganglia. Axons of the sensory cells terminate in the posterior horn or, as in the case of the GSA discriminatory touch pathway, ascend in the posterior white column as the fasciculus gracilis and fasciculus cuneatus. GSE and preganglionic visceral efferent axons in spinal nerves arise from neuroblasts of the mantle layer as previously described. Postganglionic autonomic neurons differentiate from neural crest. Their cell bodies are aggregated into sympathetic and parasympathetic ganglia. Postganglionic axons are unmyelinated; those that traverse the spinal nerve enter it through the gray communicating rami. The myelin of all myelinated fibers in spinal nerves develop from neural crest material by the wrapping of differentiating Schwann cells around axons.

Nerve Degeneration and Regeneration. Injury to a nerve fiber leads to degeneration of the axon and myelin in the entire portion distal to the lesion (Wallerian or secondary degeneration) and also for a distance of one to two internodes in the proximal stump of the fiber (retrograde or primary degeneration). If injured neurons are components of ascending sensory pathways in the CNS, the sensory loss will be reflected as an anesthesia, hypesthesia, astereognosis, hypalgesia, or analgesia below the lesion. The degeneration, however, will be primarily in the entire distal stump above the lesion. Damage to the sensory levels (*e.g.*, dorsal roots) of reflexes can lead to hypotonia or atonia and hy-poreflexia or areflexia at the level of the lesion. When injured neurons are components of descending motor pathways then the loss may be expressed as paresis, paralysis of movement or atrophy. Both the motor functional deficit and degeneration of the distal stump are below the lesion.

In degeneration of myelinated peripheral nerves, myelin in the distal stump and in the region of damage will retract from the nodes, break up into segments and will be phagocytized by Schwann cells. Most myelin has degenerated by 3 weeks after the injury, but some may remain for up to 3 months. The axon of the distal stump swells, fragments, and is phagocytized by the Schwann cells. Schwann cells of the distal stump, and for one to two internodes in the proximal stump, increase in size, divide and form longitudinal bands. These bands of Büngner move into the center of the nerve fiber as the myelin and axon degenerate, thus leaving a neurolemmal tubular space between the Schwann cells and their basement membrane. If the damage to the neuron is near the cell body, the whole neuron will degenerate. If the injury is farther away, the cell will not die but the cell body will swell, chromatolysis occurs, and the nucleus moves eccentrically to a position opposite the axon hillock. Chromatolysis is due to dispersion of RER and ribosomes and is not accompanied by loss of RNA.

In regeneration of the peripheral nerve, Nissl material starts to reappear around the nucleus in the third week, the nucleus returns to its original position, and turgescence subsides. Schwann cells bridge the area of the cut, and the swelling axon tip splits into fine fibers that enter neurolemmal tubes. Of the new fibers that enter each tube, the one that is usually first to reach the nerve ending will be moved deeply into gutters on the surface of the Schwann cells while the others degenerate. If the regenerating neuron is to become myelinated, the Schwann cells will wrap it with their plasmalemma. If it is to remain unmyelinated, it will be incompletely invested in the Schwann cell gutters.

Degeneration and regeneration processes of the CNS are similar to those in peripheral nerves, but regeneration is seldom as complete or successful. Since Schwann cells are absent, oligodendroglia perform similar functions but have more limited capacities. Vascular and neuroglial elements respond more to trauma. Microglia and astrocytes proliferate and extend into the cut area and compete with poor neurolemmal tube formation in the damaged area. Thus, regenerating fibers in the CNS pass into poor neurolemmal tubes if they are not first blocked by extensive scar tissue formation.

UPPER LIMB

BONES AND JOINTS OF THE UPPER LIMB

The bones of the upper limb include the clavicle and scapula (which form the shoulder [pectoral] girdle), the humerus of the arm, the radius and ulna of the forearm, and the carpals, metacarpals, and phalanges of the hand.

Clavical and Sternoclavicular and Acromioclavicular Articulations. The clavicle, through its articulations, is the only bony connection between the upper limb and the axial skeleton. As such, it keeps the limb away from the body, thereby enabling a large range of motion. Proximally directed force through the upper limb frequently causes clavicular fracture. These fractures are usually in the middle third of the bone because of its doubly curved shape; they are also easily diagnosed by palpation because of the clavicle's completely subcutaneous location.

The medial end of the clavicle articulates with the superolateral aspect of the manubrium at the *sternoclavicular joint.* The bones are separated by an intra-articular disk, and thus two synovial cavities exist. The bones are held in position by the articular capsule and sternoclavicular, interclavicular, and costoclavicular ligaments.

The lateral end of the clavicle articulates with the acromion at the *acromioclavicular joint.* The synovial space is enclosed by a capsule, but the major supports for this joint are the coracoclavicular ligaments (conoid and trapezoid ligaments), which extend between the clavicle and the coracoid process.

Humerus. The humerus articulates with the scapula proximally and with the radius and ulna distally. The head forms a nearly hemispheric articular surface covered with articular cartilage. A constricted anatomic neck marks the attachment of the capsule of the shoulder joint. Lateral to the head is the greater tubercle. The lesser tubercle lies anteriorly below the head and receives the subscapularis. Between these tubercles is the intertubercular groove lodging the tendon of the long head of the biceps. Immediately below the tubercles is the tapering surgical neck, so named because of the frequency of fracture in that area. The spiral groove curves around the posterolateral aspect of the midshaft of the humerus, passing inferior to the laterally placed deltoid tuberosity.

The lower end of the humerus presents the *trochlea* medially and the rounded *capitulum* laterally. The trochlea articulates with the trochlear notch of the ulna and the capitulum with the radial head.

Above the trochlea anteriorly the coronoid fossa receives the coronoid process of the ulna when the elbow is flexed. Above the trochlea posteriorly the olecranon fossa is occupied by the olecranon process of the ulna when the elbow is extended. The lateral epicondyle is smaller than the medial.

Shoulder Joint. The shoulder joint (Fig. 2-4) is a loose ball and socket joint formed by the articulation of the *head of the humerus* with the *glenoid fossa* of the scapula. In this joint maximal mobility is available at the expense of stability. The very loose articular capsule is redundant inferiorly when the joint is in the anatomic position. The glenoid cavity is deepened to a small degree by the glenoid labrum, a dense fibrocartilaginous wedge that attaches to the periphery of the glenoid fossa. The capsule extends from the rim of the glenoid fossa and the labrum to the anatomic neck of the humerus. It is reinforced anteriorly by the variable glenohumeral ligaments and by the coracohumeral ligament. The tendon of the long head of the biceps brachii ascends through the intertubercular groove and then passes across the superior aspect of the humeral head (between the fibrous and synovial portions of the capsule) to attach to the supraglenoid tubercle.

The major supports of this joint are the muscles of the *rotator* (musculotendinous) *cuff:* the subscapularis, supraspinatus, infraspinatus, and teres minor. The tendons of these muscles blend with the anterior, superior, and posterior aspects of the fibrous capsule and thus support the joint in those

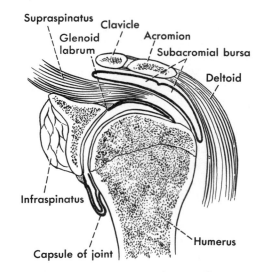

Fig. 2-4. Frontal section through the shoulder and suprahumeral space. (Hollinshead WH: Anatomy For Surgeons, Vol 3, 3rd ed, p 316. Philadelphia, JB Lippincott, 1982)

areas. The inferior aspect of the joint capsule, however, is virtually unsupported in an area through which the humeral head may pass in an anterior dislocation of the shoulder.

Motion at the shoulder joint is very free and occurs around an infinite number of axes. Although shoulder joint motion is a major factor in allowing the hand to assume innumerable locations and positions, proper function of the entire shoulder complex is absolutely necessary. Scapular motion as well as motion of the clavicle accompanies virtually every positional change of the upper limb. A loss of scapular, sternoclavicular, acromioclavicular, or glenohumeral range of motion can reduce the range of the entire upper limb. Scapular motion is controlled primarily by the trapezius and serratus anterior muscles. The motions listed below refer strictly to the shoulder joint, and the muscles indicated are the prime movers at that joint:

Flexion: anterior deltoid, pectoralis major, (especially the clavicular portion) coracobrachialis
Extension: latissimus dorsi, posterior deltoid, teres major
Abduction: middle deltoid, supraspinatus
Adduction: latissimus dorsi, pectoralis major (sternal portion)
Medial rotation: pectoralis major, latissimus dorsi, teres major, anterior deltoid, subscapularis
Lateral rotation: posterior deltoid, teres minor, infraspinatus

Suprahumeral Space. This is not a space in any sense but rather an area that is packed with structures of various types. The suprahumeral space (see Fig. 2-4) is between the head of the humerus and the arch formed by the acromion, coracoid, and the intervening coracoacromial ligament. The major structures within this space are the superior portion of the capsule of the shoulder joint, the tendon along with part of the supraspinatus muscle, the subdeltoid (subacromial) bursa, and the tendon of the long head of the biceps brachii muscle. Humeral motion accompanies virtually every motion of the upper limb, so the structures in this space are compressed between the head of the humerus and the coracoacromial arch. This compression is especially necessary during flexion and abduction. Inflammation of any of these tissues results in loss of range of motion of the shoulder area.

Radius, Ulna, and Their Articulations. The radius is the lateral bone of the forearm. It has a small head proximally that is cylindrical in shape, and an expanded distal extremity, which is the major forearm contribution to the wrist joint. The ulnar notch is on the medial aspect of the expanded distal portion, and the lateral palpable radial styloid is the most distal bony prominence of the forearm. The dorsal radial tubercle (of Lister) is the most prominent ridge on the posterior aspect of the distal radius. The radial (bicipital) tuberosity is on the ventral proximal aspect of the radius.

The ulna is large proximally but narrows distally into the small round (but flat distally) head with the ulnar styloid extending past the head medially. The proximal portion has the deep ventrally directed trochlear notch. The distal lip of the notch is the coronoid process; the proximal portion is the olecranon process and forms the point of the elbow. The lateral aspect of the proximal ulna is indented to form the radial notch.

The ulna and radius are united through synovial joints both proximally and distally, with the interosseous membrane interconnecting the two shafts between these synovial joints. The *proximal joint* is between the radial head and the radial notch of the ulna; the *distal joint* is between the ulnar head and the ulnar notch of the radius. The proximal joint is stabilized primarily by the annular ligament of the radius, which attaches to the edges of the radial notch of the ulna and surrounds the head of the radius. The distal joint is reinforced primarily by an intra-articular disk that extends from the distal medial radius to the ulnar styloid. The proximal joint shares an articular capsule with the elbow joint; the distal joint shares one with the wrist.

Pronation and *supination* occur between the two bones of the forearm at the proximal and distal radioulnar joints. When the hand is supinated the two bones are parallel. When the hand is pronated the radius is wrapped around the ulna. Pronation is produced primarily by the pronator teres and pronator quadratus; supination by the biceps brachii and the supinator.

Elbow Joint. The elbow joint is formed between the trochlea of the humerus and the trochlear notch of the ulna medially, and between the capitulum of the humerus and the head of the radius laterally. The motion permitted at this joint—flexion and extension—is essentially determined by that part of the joint between the humerus and ulna. A common joint capsule encloses both the two portions of the elbow joint in addition to the proximal radioulnar joint. The capsule is thickened medially to form the ulnar collateral ligament and laterally to form the radial collateral ligament. The major flexors at the elbow are the brachialis, biceps brachii, and brachioradialis. The major extensor is the triceps brachii.

Bones of the Hand.   The bones of the hand include the 8 carpal bones, 5 metacarpals and 14 phalanges. The bones of the carpus are arranged in two rows. From lateral to medial, the proximal row consists of the *scaphoid,* the *lunate,* the *triquetrum,* and the *pisiform* bones. The distal row is composed of the *trapezium,* the *trapezoid,* the *capitate,* and the *hamate* bones. Each of the digits is composed of three phalanges except the thumb, which has only two. The phalanges are named by their position, that is, proximal, middle, and distal.

Wrist Joint and Joints of the Hand.   The proximal articular surface of the wrist or *radiocarpal joint* is formed by the distal aspect of the radius and the medially placed intra-articular disk. This disk interconnects the ulnar styloid and the distomedial aspect of the radius. The distal articular surface is formed primarily by the scaphoid and lunate, with a small contribution from the triquetrum. The wrist joint has its own synovial cavity, which is separated from the distal radioulnar joint by the articular disk. The *midcarpal articulation,* which also has a separate joint cavity, is found between the two rows of carpal bones. The capsules of both joints are reinforced by collateral as well as dorsal and palmar ligaments. The motions that occur in the area of the wrist are contributed to by movement at both the radiocarpal and midcarpal joints. These motions and their major motors are:

Flexion: flexor carpi radialis, flexor carpi ulnaris
Extension: extensor carpi radialis longus, extensor carpi radialis brevis, extensor carpi ulnaris
Abduction or radial deviation: extensor carpi radialis longus, flexor carpi radialis, abductor pollicis longus
Adduction or ulnar deviation: flexor carpi ulnaris, extensor carpi ulnaris

The *carpometacarpal (CM) articulations* of the four medial digits allow essentially no motion, even though they are synovial joints. The CM joint of the thumb is between the base of the first metacarpal and the trapezium. The shapes of these joint surfaces permit flexion, extension, abduction, adduction and, hence, circumduction. Rotation of the thumb is essential to opposition. Rotation occurs primarily at this joint and is provided by the action of the opponens pollicis.

The *metacarpophalangeal (MP) joints* are synovial in type and permit flexion, extension, abduction, adduction, and circumduction. Abduction and adduction are free only in extension as the collateral ligaments become taut in flexion and thereby virtually eliminate any side-to-side movement. Abduc-

tion and adduction are very limited at the MP joint of the thumb. The *interphalangeal (IP) joints* are all synovial articulations that permit only flexion and extension.

The muscles producing motion in the hand are:

MP flexion (not thumb): lumbricals, dorsal and ventral interossei, flexor digitorum profundus, flexor digitorum superficialis
MP extension (not thumb): extensor digitorum
Digital abduction: dorsal interossei
Digital adduction: ventral interossei
Proximal IP (PIP) extension: lumbricals, dorsal, and ventral interossei
Distal IP (DIP) extension: lumbrical, dorsal, and ventral interossei
Proximal IP flexion: flexor digitorum superficialis, flexor digitorum profundus
Distal IP flexion: flexor digitorum profundus
NOTE: The combination of MP flexion and IP extention produces a functional position that is used in many activities requiring infinite control and gradation. These motions are the combined functions of the lumbricals and the interossei muscles.
Thumb flexion: flexor pollicis longus and brevis
Thumb extension: extensor pollicis longus and brevis
Thumb abduction: abductor pollicis longus and brevis
Thumb adduction: adductor pollicis
Opposition of the thumb: opponens pollicis, abductor pollicis brevis, and flexor pollicis brevis

COMPARTMENTATION OF THE UPPER LIMB

Arm.   The arm is divided into anterior and posterior compartments by the medial and lateral intermuscular septa, which extend from the investing brachial fascia to the humerus. The muscles in the anterior compartment are the biceps brachii, brachialis, and coracobrachialis. These muscles are innervated by the musculocutaneous nerve and produce flexion at the elbow and supination of the forearm. Only the triceps brachii is found in the posterior compartment. This elbow extensor is innervated by the radial nerve.

Cubital Fossa.   The cubital fossa is the depression anterior to the elbow and proximal part of the forearm. This fossa is bounded laterally by the brachioradialis muscle, medially by the pronator teres muscle, and proximally by a line interconnecting the medial and lateral epicondyles of the humerus. The tendon of the biceps brachii muscle disappears into this fossa as it passes toward the radial tuberosity; the bicipital aponeurosis extends medially from the biceps tendon to the investing fascia of the forearm. This aponeurosis separates the superficially positioned median cubital vein from the deeper structures that pass through the fossa. The deeper structures are the brachial artery, which passes medially to the biceps tendon, and the median nerve, which is medial to the brachial artery.

Forearm. The forearm is separated into anterior and posterior compartments by the medial and lateral intermuscular septa, which extend from the antebrachial fascia to the ulna and radius, respectively, and by the interosseous membrane, which interconnects the radius and ulna. The muscles in the anterior compartment originate from the medial humeral epicondyle and the ventral aspects of the radius and ulna, and they function to pronate the forearm and flex the wrist and fingers. The pronator teres, flexor carpi radialis, palmaris longus, flexor digitorum superficialis, flexor pollicis longus, pronator quadratus, and the lateral half of the flexor digitorum profundus (to digits 2 and 3) are innervated by the median nerve. The flexor carpi ulnaris and medial half of the flexor digitorum profundus (to digits 4 and 5) are innervated by the ulnar nerve. The muscles in the posterior compartment originate from the lateral humeral epicondyle and the dorsal

aspects of the radius and ulna. These muscles, all innervated by the radial nerve, function to supinate the forearm and extend the wrist and digits at the MP joints. These posterior muscles are the brachioradialis, extensor carpi radialis longus, extensor carpi radialis brevis, extensor digitorum, extensor digiti minimi, extensor carpi ulnaris, supinator, abductor pollicis longus, extensor pollicis brevis, extensor pollicis longus, and extensor indicis.

Carpal Tunnel. The carpal tunnel (Fig. 2-5) interconnects the anterior compartment of the forearm and the palm of the hand. It is a fibro-osseous canal, formed posteriorly and on both sides by the carpal bones and ventrally by the deep part of the flexor retinaculum (transverse carpal ligament). The structures that pass through this tunnel (canal) include the tendons of the flexor digitorium superficialis, flexor digitorum profundus, and flexor pollicis longus muscles, the synovial sheaths of those tendons, and the median nerve. Any of these structures, particularly the median nerve, can be compressed within the canal (carpal tunnel syndrome). The ulnar nerve and artery, tendon of the palmaris longus muscle, and palmar branch of the median nerve also cross the ventral aspect of the wrist but pass superficial to the deep part of the flexor retinaculum.

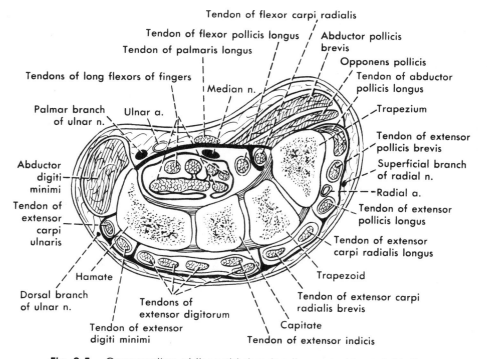

Fig. 2-5. Cross section at the wrist showing the carpal tunnel. (Hollinshead WH: Anatomy For Surgeons, Vol 3, 3rd ed, p 471. Philadelphia, JB Lippincott, 1982)

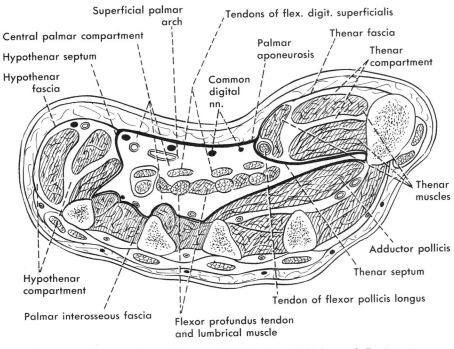

Fig. 2-6.   Cross section of the hand. (Hollinshead WH, Rosse C: Textbook of Anatomy, 4th ed, p 236. Philadelphia, JB Lippincott, 1985)

Hand.   The ventral aspect of the hand is separated into thenar, hypothenar, and central compartments (Fig. 2-6). The antebrachial fascia continues into the hand and attaches along the first and fifth metacarpals. In the central region of the palm this fascia is greatly thickened to form the ***palmar aponeurosis.*** From the lateral border of this aponeurosis the thenar intermuscular septum extends into the palm and attaches to the first metacarpal. This septum together with the investing fascia around the lateral aspect of the palm delimits the ***thenar compartment,*** which contains the abductor pollicis brevis, flexor pollicis brevis, and opponens pollicis muscles. These muscles are innervated by the recurrent or thenar branch of the median nerve. The hypothenar intermuscular septum extends between the medial extent of the palmar aponeurosis and the fifth metacarpal and combines with the investing fascia on the medial aspect of the palm to form the ***hypothenar compartment.*** This compartment contains the abductor digiti minimi, flexor digiti minimi brevis, and opponens digiti minimi, all of which are innervated by the deep branch of the ulnar nerve. The ***central compartment*** is deep to the palmar aponeurosis in the center of the palm. It is bounded by the aponeurosis, the thenar and hypothenar intermuscular septa and a layer of fascia, the adductor interosseous or palmar interosseous fascia, that ex-

tends between the first and fifth metacarpals deep in the palm. Only the four small lumbrical muscles are found in this compartment. The two lateral lumbricals are innervated by the median nerve; the two medial ones, by the ulnar nerve. The long flexor tendons to the digits pass through this compartment. This compartment also contains the superficial palmar arterial arch, which is between the palmar aponeurosis and the long flexor tendons. The cutaneous branches of the median and ulnar nerves are distributed with the branches of the superficial arterial arch. The ***adductor interosseous compartment*** is essentially between the metacarpals. It is bounded dorsally by the dorsal interosseous fascia and ventrally by the adductor interosseous fascia. This space contains the dorsal and ventral interossei along with the adductor pollicis, all of which are innervated by the deep branch of the ulnar nerve.

Bursae and Spaces.   The ***radial*** and ***ulnar bursae*** are synovial tendon sheaths that surround the long flexor tendons of the digits. They both start proximal to the wrist, pass through the carpal tunnel with the tendons and extend either partially or completely through the palm and into the fingers. The radial bursa is associated only with the tendon of the flexor pollicis longus. The ulnar bursa surrounds all four tendons of both the flexor digitorum superficialis and profundus muscles. That part of this bursa associated with the little finger usually extends through the palm and into the digit while the others terminate at midpalmar levels. Thus, the synovial portions of the digital tendon sheaths of the index, middle, and ring fingers are not continuous with the ulnar bursa, *per se.*

A pair of potential spaces (really fascial planes) exists at the approximate level of the adductor interosseous fascia, that is, in the plane just deep to the long digital flexor tendons in the central compartment. This plane is divided into a medial ***midpalmar space*** and a lateral ***thenar space*** by a septum that extends from the palmar aponeurosis to the third metacarpal. As indicated above, these are only potential spaces but can become actual spaces when filled with blood or inflammatory material.

NERVES OF THE UPPER LIMB

Brachial Plexus. Most of the muscles of the upper limb are supplied by branches of the brachial plexus (Fig. 2-7). The plexus is formed by the ventral rami of spinal nerves C5, 6, 7, 8, and T1. Ventral rami of C5 and 6 unite to form the ***superior trunk,*** C7 continues as the ***middle trunk,*** and the ***inferior trunk*** is formed by the union of C8 and T1. Each of the three trunks split into anterior and posterior divisions. This separation into divisions determines the basic innervation pattern for the extremity; that is, the nerves formed from the anterior divisions innervate the muscles in the anterior compartments, and those from posterior divisions innervate posterior compartment muscles. The ***lateral cord*** is formed from the anterior divisions of the

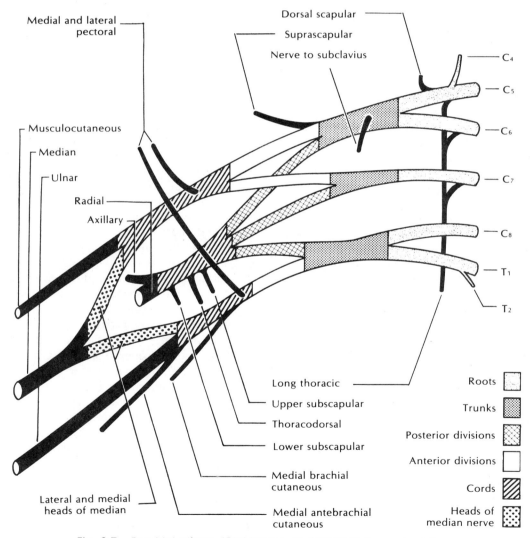

Fig. 2-7. Brachial plexus. (Christensen JB, Telford IR: Synopsis of Gross Anatomy, 5th ed, p 64. Philadelphia, JB Lippincott, 1988)

superior and middle trunks, and the anterior division of the inferior trunk continues as the *medial cord.* The posterior divisions of all three trunks unite to form the *posterior cord.* The cords of the plexus receive their names from their relationships with the second part of the axillary artery. The terminal peripheral nerves are formed in the axilla from the cords. The *median nerve* (C6–T1) is formed by contributions from both the medial and lateral cords. The remainder of the medial cord forms the *ulnar nerve* (C7–T1), and the termination of the lateral cord is the *musculocutaneous nerve* (C5, 6). The posterior cord gives rise to the *radial* (C5–8) and *axillary nerves* (C5, 6).

Branches from the plexus proper are called *collateral branches,* and they supply most of the extrinsic and intrinsic muscles of the shoulder. (Extrinsic muscles extend from the axial skeleton to the scapula, clavicle or humerus; intrinsic muscles connect the scapula or clavicle with the humerus.) The branches from the ventral rami are the *dorsal scapular nerve* (C5), which supplies both rhomboids and part of the levator scapulae, and the *long thoracic nerve* (C5–7) to the serratus anterior. Two branches arise from the superior trunk: the *nerve to the subclavius* (C5) and the *suprascapular nerve* (C5, 6), which innervates the supraspinatus and infraspinatus muscles. The *medial* (C8, T1) and *lateral* (C5–7) *pectoral nerves* branch from the medial and lateral cords, respectively. The medial pectoral nerve innervates the pectoralis major and minor; the lateral, only the major. The three *subscapular nerves* branch from the posterior cord. The *upper* and *lower subscapular nerves* (C5, 6) innervate the subscapularis and teres major muscles. The *thoracodorsal nerve* (middle subscapular) (C6–8) innervates the latissimus dorsi muscle.

Median Nerve. The median nerve passes through the arm in the medial neurovascular bundle, which is located where the medial intermuscular septum joins the brachial fascia. In the distal part of the arm it inclines laterally and passes through the cubital fossa just medial to the brachial artery. The median nerve enters the forearm by passing through the pronator teres muscle and descends in the forearm between the superficial and deep grounds of muscles. At the wrist the median nerve (see Fig. 2-5) is between the tendons of the flexor carpi radialis and the palmaris longus. It enters the hand by going through the carpal tunnel. Just distal to the deep part of the flexor retinaculum (transverse carpal ligament) the nerve branches into the *thenar* (recurrent) and *digital* (common and proper) *branches.* The thenar branch innervates the

muscles in the thenar compartment. The digital branches supply the skin on the ventral aspect of the lateral three and a half digits and some of the corresponding part of the palm. The lateral midpalmar skin is supplied by the *palmar branch* of the median nerve. This branch arises proximal to the wrist and does not pass through the carpal tunnel.

Musculocutaneous Nerve. From its origin in the axilla this nerve inclines laterally, going first through the coracobrachialis muscle and then between the biceps brachii and the brachialis. It enters the subcutaneous tissue in the distal lateral arm, after which it continues into the forearm as the *lateral antebrachial cutaneous.* It supplies the skin of the lateral aspect of the forearm.

Ulnar Nerve. The ulnar nerve passes through the proximal half of the arm in the medial neurovascular bundle. It inclines posteriorly in the distal half of the arm, enters the posterior compartment and then passes behind the medial epicondyle of the humerus to enter the forearm. The nerve passes through the forearm under cover of the flexor carpi ulnaris, and at the wrist it is deep to the tendon of the same muscle (see Fig. 2-5). It enters the hand by passing superficial to the deep part of the flexor retinaculum and lateral to the pisiform. Just distal to the pisiform it divides into *deep* and *superficial branches.* The superficial branch splits into common and proper digital nerves, which innervate the palmar skin of the medial one and a half digits and the corresponding part of the palm. The deep branch passes through the hypothenar compartment and then sweeps laterally across the palm deep to the long flexor tendons. It innervates the interossei as it crosses the palm and terminates in the adductor pollicis. The ulnar nerve also innervates the dorsal skin of the medial one and a half digits. This is accomplished by the *dorsal cutaneous branch,* which arises proximal to the wrist.

Radial Nerve. The radial nerve descends in the posterior compartment of the arm by curving obliquely around the posterior aspect of the midshaft of the humerus in the spiral groove. In the distal third of the arm it enters the anterior compartment by piercing the lateral intermuscular septum and is positioned between the brachioradialis and the brachialis muscles. Just proximal to the elbow and deep to the brachioradialis it divides into *superficial* and *deep branches.* The superficial branch descends in the forearm under cover of the brachioradialis. It enters the subcutaneous tissue in the distal forearm and is cutaneous to the dorsal surface of the lateral three and a half digits and corresponding part of the dorsal hand. The deep branch enters the posterior compartment of the forearm by wrapping around the neck of the radius in the substance of the supinator muscle. It then branches into its many muscular branches and continues through the forearm as the *posterior interosseous nerve,* which terminates at the level of the wrist.

Axillary Nerve. The axillary nerve passes anteroinferior to the shoulder joint (where it is occasionally stretched in an anterior shoulder dislocation) and then horizontally around the posterior aspect of the surgical neck of the humerus. It then enters the under surface of the deltoid muscle.

PERIPHERAL NERVE LESIONS IN THE UPPER LIMB

Radial Nerve. When the radial nerve is interrupted in the axilla, the following symptoms are apparent:

1. Extension of the elbow and wrist are lost, and wrist drop results.
2. Extension of the thumb is lost; abduction is weakened.
3. Extension of the MP joints of the index, middle, ring, and little fingers is lost.
4. Grasp is weakened, due to inability to extend and stabilize the wrist.
5. Supination of the forearm is weakened.
6. Radial and ulnar deviation of the wrist are weakened.
7. Sensation is lost on the dorsolateral aspects of the hand, arm and the dorsal aspect of the forearm.

A radial nerve lesion at the level of the elbow would differ from that above primarily in that elbow extension would be unaffected; the severity of the other motor symptoms would depend upon the exact level of the involvement. Sensory loss would be limited to the dorsolateral hand.

Median Nerve. Paralysis of the median nerve at the wrist (as it passes through the carpal tunnel, resulting in a carpal tunnel syndrome) produces the following problems:

1. Flexion of the thumb is weakened.
2. Opposition of the thumb is lost, resulting in a derotated and adducted thumb (simian hand).
3. Flexion of the MP joints of the middle and index fingers is weakened, resulting in a slight clawing of these fingers.
4. Sensation is lost on the palmar surface of the lateral three and a half fingers and the corresponding portion of the distal palm.

Paralysis of the median nerve proximal to the elbow or in the axilla causes additional difficulties:

5. Flexion of the IP joints of the index and middle fingers is lost, resulting in an extension deformity, especially of the index finger.
6. Flexion of the PIP joints of the little and ring fingers is lost, resulting in slight clawing of those two fingers. (The combination of 5 and 6 produces a benediction attitude of the hand.)
7. Flexion of the IP joint of the thumb is lost.
8. Pronation of the forearm is lost.
9. Flexion of the wrist is weakened.
10. Sensation is lost on the palmar surface of the lateral three and a half fingers and the entire lateral palm.

Ulnar Nerve. Paralysis of the ulnar nerve at the wrist results in these difficulties:

1. Abduction and adduction of the fingers are lost.
2. Flexion of the MP joints and extension of the IP joints are weakened in the index and middle fingers and virtually lost in the ring and little fingers. As a result, clawing is severe in the little and ring fingers, and moderate in the middle and index fingers.
3. Adduction of the thumb is virtually lost.
4. Opposition of the little finger is lost.
5. Opposition of the thumb is somewhat difficult.
6. Palmar sensation of the medial one and a half digits and the corresponding portion of the palm is lost.

Paralysis of the ulnar nerve proximal to the elbow results in these additional problems:

7. Flexion of the DIP joints of the little and ring fingers is lost.
8. Flexion of the wrist is weakened and is accompanied by radial deviation.
9. Sensation of the dorsal aspects of the medial one and a half digits and corresponding portions of the hand is lost.

Combined Median–Ulnar Nerves. Interruption of both the median and ulnar nerves at the wrist results in:

1. Flexion of the MP joints and extension of the IP joints is lost; there is severe clawing of all four fingers.
2. Digital abduction and adduction are lost.
3. Thumb and little finger opposition are lost, hence a simian hand.
4. Sensation on the entire ventral surface of the hand is lost.

Blockage or lesion of the median and ulnar nerves proximal to the elbow causes the following additional difficulties:

5. Flexion of all joints distal to the elbow is lost.
6. Pronation of the forearm is lost.

Axillary Nerve. Paralysis of the axillary nerve as it leaves the posterior cord results in:

1. Virtual loss of useful shoulder joint abduction. Only a few degrees of abduction remain.
2. Weakened shoulder flexion.
3. Loss of sensation on the proximal lateral arm.

Musculocutaneous Nerve. Paralysis of the musculocutaneous nerve at its origin results in:

1. Very weakened elbow flexion
2. Weakened supination of the forearm
3. Loss of sensation on the lateral forearm.

BLOOD SUPPLY OF THE UPPER LIMB

Arteries. The blood supply of the upper limb is provided by the *subclavian artery,* which becomes the *axillary artery* as it crosses the first rib (Fig. 2-8). The first part of the axillary artery extends from the first rib to the pectoralis minor muscle, the second part is deep to the muscle, and the third part extends between the pectoralis minor and the lower border of the teres major muscle. The superior thoracic artery to the upper chest wall branches from the first part of the artery. There are two branches of the second part: the thoracoacromial trunk, which supplies the acromial, deltoid, pectoral, and clavicular regions, and the lateral thoracic branch, which descends along the anterolateral chest wall. The branches of the third part of the artery are the subscapular artery, which bifurcates into the circumflex scapular and thoraco-dorsal arteries, and the anterior and posterior humeral circumflex arteries, which arise at the level of the surgical neck of the humerus. The circumflex scapular artery forms potential anastomoses posterior to the scapula with branches of the subclavian artery. The posterior humeral circumflex artery accompanies the axillary nerve as it passes around the posterior aspect of the proximal humerus.

The *brachial artery* is the continuation of the axillary artery that passes through the arm in the medial neurovascular bundle. It then inclines laterally in the distal half of the arm and crosses the elbow by passing through the cubital fossa. In the cubital fossa it is medial to the tendon of the biceps brachii muscle and lateral to the median nerve (between these two structures), and it is separated from the more superficial median cubital vein by the bicipital aponeurosis. It divides into the radial and ulnar arteries just opposite the radial head. Its largest branch is the deep brachial artery, which arises in the axilla and spirals around the humerus with the radial nerve. *? profunda brachii*

The *ulnar artery* passes through the medial aspect of the forearm deep to the flexor carpi ulnaris muscle, and at the wrist it is just lateral to that muscle's tendon. It enters the hand by passing superficial to the deep part of the flexor retinaculum and lateral to the pisiform. Its largest branch is the common interosseous artery, which arises high in the forearm and divides into the anterior and posterior interosseous arteries.

The *radial artery* descends through the lateral part of the forearm under cover of the brachioradialis muscle. At the level of the radial styloid it inclines dorsally and enters the dorsum of the hand by passing through the *anatomic snuff box.* (The anatomic snuff box is bordered by the tendons of the abductor pollicis longus and extensor pollicis brevis laterally and the tendon of the extensor pollicis longus medially.) At the wrist a radial pulse can be obtained somewhat proximally, just lateral to the tendon of the flexor carpi radialis.

The course of the ulnar artery in the hand is similar to that of the ulnar nerve in that it has a superficial and a deep branch. The superficial branch gives rise to the *superficial palmar arch*. This arch is at the level of the palmar border of the extended thumb between the palmar aponeurosis and the long flexor tendons. The arch is completed by the superficial palmar branch of the radial artery, which branches proximal to the wrist and passes superficially through the thenar muscles. The arch has common digital branches to the fingers and a proper digital branch to the thumb. The radial artery passes through the snuff box and then between (passing dorsal to ventral) the first and second metacarpals. This course brings it into the deep part of the lateral palm where it gives rise to the *deep palmar arterial arch*. This arch, completed by the deep branch of the ulnar artery, accompanies the deep ulnar nerve. The position of this arch is proximal to the superficial arch and deep to the long flexor tendons. The palmar metacarpal branches of the deep arch communicate with branches of the superficial arch and the dorsal carpal arterial network.

Veins. The veins of the upper extremity consist of two sets: the *deep* and the *superficial.* The deep veins accompany the arteries and communicate frequently with the superficial veins, which are in the subcutaneous tissue.

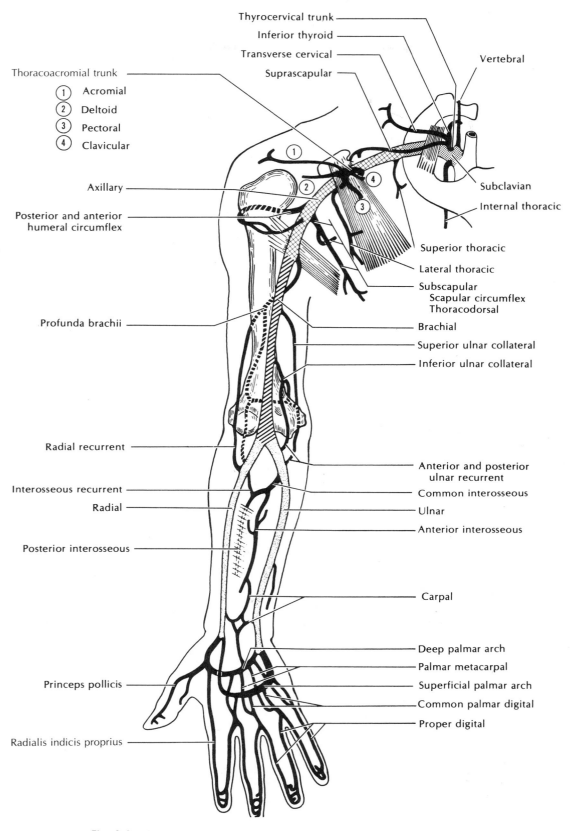

Fig. 2-8. Summary of arterial supply of the upper extremity. (Christensen JB, Telford IR: Synopsis of Gross Anatomy, 5th ed, p 86. Philadelphia, JB Lippincott, 1988)

Thyrocervical trunk
Inferior thyroid
Transverse cervical
Suprascapular
Vertebral

Thoracoacromial trunk
(1) Acromial
(2) Deltoid
(3) Pectoral
(4) Clavicular

Axillary

Posterior and anterior humeral circumflex

Subclavian
Internal thoracic

Superior thoracic
Lateral thoracic
Subscapular
Scapular circumflex
Thoracodorsal

Profunda brachii

Brachial
Superior ulnar collateral
Inferior ulnar collateral

Radial recurrent

Anterior and posterior ulnar recurrent
Common interosseous
Ulnar
Anterior interosseous

Interosseous recurrent
Radial

Posterior interosseous

Carpal

Deep palmar arch
Palmar metacarpal
Superficial palmar arch
Common palmar digital
Proper digital

Princeps pollicis

Radialis indicis proprius

The superficial veins are the basilic, cephalic, and median cubital. The **basilic vein** arises on the ulnar side of the back of the hand and extends along the ulnar side of the forearm to the elbow. It crosses the anteromedial aspect of the elbow, pierces the brachial fascia, and empties into the brachial vein.

The **cephalic vein** begins at the radial side of the dorsal venous network and continues proximally through the lateral forearm and arm. At the shoulder it passes through the deltopectoral groove (separating the deltoid and pectoralis major muscles), after which it empties into the axillary vein.

The **median cubital vein** interconnects the cephalic and basilic systems superficial to the cubital fossa.

LOWER LIMB

BONES AND JOINTS OF THE LOWER LIMB

Pelvis. The pelvis is composed of the two hip bones (os coxae) and the sacrum. The three bones are united at the two sacroiliac joints and the single symphysis pubis, thus forming the pelvic ring.

The **os coxae** is made up of three bones that fuse early in life: the pubis, ischium, and ilium. The **pubis** is anteromedially located. It consists of a body (which forms the symphysis with the body of the opposite side) and posterolaterally directed superior and inferior rami. The superior pubic ramus unites with the ilium; the inferior, with the ischium. The palpable pubic tubercle springs from the anterior aspect of the body. The **ischium** is the posteroinferior portion of the hip bone. It has a heavy body, a palpable ischial tuberosity, and an ischial spine. The tuberosity is the inferiormost aspect of the hip bone and the point of origin of the hamstring muscles. The ischial spine projects posteromedially above the tuberosity and is palpable via rectal or vaginal examination. The **ilium** is the superiormost part of the os coxae, and its body is united with both the ischium and the pubis. The flattened and superiorly located iliac wing has a thickened crest that terminates anteriorly and posteriorly in the anterior and posterior superior iliac spines. The gluteal muscles attach to the lateral aspect of the iliac wing, and the iliacus muscle attaches medially. The posteromedial aspect of the iliac body presents the surface that articulates with the sacrum.

Inferiorly, portions of the pubis and ischium surround the obturator foramen. Superior to the obturator foramen and on the lateral aspect of the os coxae, the three component bones form the socket of the hip joint, the acetabulum. Posteriorly and inferiorly, the area between the ischial tuberosity and ischial spine is the lesser sciatic notch; the area between the ischial spine and the posterior inferior iliac spine is greater sciatic notch.

The bones of the pelvis are involved in the formation of the walls of both the pelvic and abdominal cavities. The **pelvic inlet** separates the true pelvis below from the false pelvis (part of the abdominal cavity) above. The inlet is formed posteriorly by the sacral promontory, laterally by the arcuate line of the ilium and the iliopectineal line, and anteriorly by the superior aspects of the pubic bodies and symphysis.

Although there are many variations in pelvic architecture, the following classification has received general acceptance. Also, it must be stressed that although the following discussion considers four categories of pelvic shape, in reality most pelves are mixtures of the various types. The **gynecoid pelvis** is regarded as the characteristic female pelvis. It is distinguished by an oval inlet with the transverse diameter exceeding the anteroposterior diameter. This pelvis is shallow with straight walls. The ischial spines are not prominent, and the subpubic arch is wide. It also has the appearance of being flattened from top to bottom, making it shorter and wider than the male pelvis. The **android pelvis** (male) has a heart-shaped inlet, is longer and heavier, and the angle of the subpubic arch is more acute. The **anthropoid pelvis** has an oval inlet with the long axis along the anteroposterior diameter. The **platypelloid pelvis** has a flattened oval inlet, which is caused by marked reduction in the anteroposterior diameter.

Femur. The femur is the largest and longest bone in the body. Proximally, the superomedially directed head is separated from the shaft by the neck, which joins the shaft at the trochanteric region. The head is slightly more than half of a sphere and is covered with articular cartilage, except in the region of the fovea. The angle between the neck and shaft is about 90 degrees in the female and greater than that in the male. The palpable greater trochanter is located superolaterally at this junctional area; the lesser is inferomedially. The long shaft inclines medially from above downward. The distal end of the femur has two separate condyles, both of which are covered by articular cartilage. The articular surface comes together anteriorly to form a groove for the patella. An intercondylar fossa separates the condyles inferiorly and posteriorly. Each condyle is expanded superiorly to form an epicondyle.

Hip Joint. The **acetabulum** is a deep socket with the horseshoe-shaped articular surface oriented so

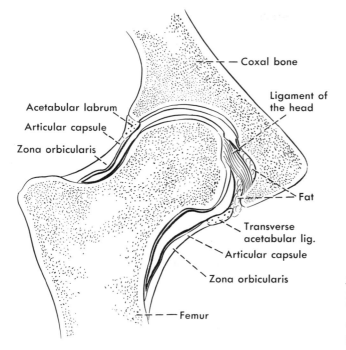

Fig. 2-9. A frontal section through the hip joint. (Hollinshead WH, Rosse C: Textbook of Anatomy, 4th ed, p 395. Philadelphia, JB Lippincott, 1985)

that its open end is directed inferiorly (Fig. 2-9). Therefore the articular surface is incomplete centrally and inferiorly. The head of the femur also has an area that is not covered by articular cartilage, the centrally located fovea. The two bony surfaces are quite congruent. The head of the femur is actually gripped by the fibrocartilaginous **acetabular labrum,** which, in addition to deepening the socket, also reduces its diameter and thereby holds the femur in place. That part of the labrum that bridges the gap inferiorly between the two limbs of the horseshoe-shaped acetabulum is the transverse acetabular ligament.

The **capsule** of the hip joint extends from the labrum and corresponding part of the os coxae across the joint and well down the femoral neck. Anteriorly it extends over the entire length of the neck and attaches to the area of the intertrochanteric line. Posteriorly it extends about two thirds of the way distally so that there is an extracapsular portion of the neck posteriorly. It is important to note that only the fibrous portion of the capsule is attached to the femur as just indicated. The synovial layer reflects on itself at these attachments and passes proximally along the neck to attach at the border of the articular surface of the head of the femur. Most of the blood vessels supplying the head and neck of

the femur pass proximally along the neck of the femur deep to the synovial layer of the capsule. They are firmly held against the bone and vulnerable to laceration when the femoral neck is fractured. Again, it is important to note that the entire anterior aspect of the neck is intracapsular, but only the medial two thirds is intracapsular posteriorly.

A major amount of support of the hip joint is provided by three extracapsular ligaments that blend with the fibrous portion of the joint capsule. The **iliofemoral ligament** (Y ligament of Bigelow) extends from the anterior aspect of the body of the ilium across the front of the hip joint to the lower part of the intertrochanteric line. This ligament becomes taut as the hip is extended and is a major stabilizing force of the hip joint. The **ischiofemoral ligament** curves around the superior aspect of the joint. As the ligament tightens during hip extension, it forces the head of the femur into the acetabulum. The **pubofemoral ligament** crosses the joint inferiorly. The fovea of the head of the femur and the nonarticular portion of the acetabulum are connected by the ligament of the head of the femur (ligamentum teres), an intra-articular ligament that conveys a small blood vessel to the head of the femur and offers virtually no joint support.

Although the number of potential motions that can occur at the hip joint is infinite, it is convenient to describe those that correspond to the cardinal planes of the body. These motions and their major motors are:

Flexion: psoas, iliacus, rectus femoris
Extension: biceps femoris, semitendinosus, semimembranosus, posterior portion of the adductor magnus, gluteus maximus
Abduction: gluteus medius, gluteus minimus
Adduction: adductor magnus, adductor longus, adductor brevis, adductor minimus, gracilis
Lateral rotation: gluteus maximus, obturator internus and externus, gemelli, quadratus femoris
Medial rotation: gluteus medius and gluteus minimus, tensor fasciae latae

It should be noted that, based on the position of the hip (flexion or extension), certain adductors may rotate the thigh either medially or laterally.

Tibia and Fibula. The *tibia* is the weight bearing bone of the leg and therefore is the major bone in the formation of both the ankle and knee joints. Superiorly it is expanded to form the flat tibial plateau, which is composed of the medial and lateral tibial condyles. These condyles are separated by the intercondylar area, which contains the intercondylar eminence. The anterior border of the shaft is subcutaneous throughout its length with an obvious protrusion superiorly where it begins as the tibial tuberosity. Inferiorly the tibia is expanded to form the articular surface for the ankle joint with the medialmost aspect extending distally as the medial malleolus.

The *fibula* is the lateral bone of the leg whose most apparent function is that of providing muscle attachments. This thin bone articulates with the tibia both proximally and distally. The interosseous membrane connects the two bones throughout most of their lengths. The inferior extent of the fibula is the lateral malleolus.

Knee Joint. The knee joint is formed between the rounded femoral condyles and the relatively flat tibial condyles (tibial plateau). The length of the articular surface (front to back) of the femoral condyles greatly exceeds that of the tibial condyles; as a result, most knee motion is a gliding of the femoral condyles on the tibial condyles. There is, however, some rocking motion between the two bones during the last few degrees of extension.

The poor congruency between the two sets of articular surfaces produces a dead space. This dead space is filled in part by the wedge-shaped disks or *menisci.* Each of these is somewhat C shaped and sits on the periphery of each tibial condyle and attaches centrally to the intercondylar area of the tibia. In addition to deepening the socket and increasing the congruency, the menisci absorb shock that is transmitted from femur to tibia and protect the capsule by keeping it from being pinched between the two bones. The lateral meniscus is almost a complete circle so that its central attachments are very close together. It is also loosely attached to the capsule, continuous with the meniscofemoral ligament and connected to the popliteus muscle. Thus, the lateral meniscus is relatively movable; presumably this is why it is seldom injured. The medial meniscus is relatively immovable and therefore very frequently injured as it is caught between the medial tibial and femoral condyles. It is immovable both because it is C shaped (and thus has wide central attachments) and it is attached firmly to the capsule and the medial collateral ligament.

The fibrous and synovial portions of the *joint capsule* do not correspond to one another. The fibrous portion encloses the entire joint area and is made up of the quadriceps tendon, patella, and patellar ligament anteriorly, the patella retinacula anteromedially and anterolaterally, and the iliotibial tract (band) laterally. Medially the tibial collateral ligament blends with the fibrous capsule. The synovial lining encloses the articular surfaces, but the intercondylar area is outside the joint space (but within the fibrous capsule). The volume of the joint space is largest when the knee is slightly flexed (approximately 15 degrees), and thus patients whose knees are effused will usually be most comfortable with their knees in that position.

The major ligamentous support of the knee is provided by the **collateral** and **cruciate ligaments.** The *lateral* (fibular) *collateral ligament* extends between the lateral femoral epicondyle and the head of the fibula and restricts medial displacement of the leg on the thigh. This ropelike structure is easily palpable and separated from the joint capsule. The *medial* (tibial) *collateral ligament* is a strong broad band, which connects the medial femoral epicondyle and the medial tibial condyle; it restricts lateral displacement of the leg on the thigh. It is palpable as a thickening in the joint space medially. The collateral ligaments are taut when the knee is extended but loosen somewhat when the knee is flexed, thus permitting rotation in that position. The cruciate ligaments occupy the intercondylar area and give the knee anteroposterior stabilization. From its anterior tibial attachment, the *anterior cruciate ligament* passes posteriorly, superiorly, and laterally to attach to the medial aspect of the lateral femoral condyle. It protects against posterior dislocation of the femur on the tibia. The *posterior cruciate* extends from its posterior tibial attachment anteriorly, superiorly, and medially to attach to the lateral aspect of the medial femoral condyle. It protects against anterior dislocation of the femur on the tibia. Although the cruciate ligaments are most taut in full flexion (posterior) and extension (anterior), portions of both are tense throughout the range of motion. And even though all of these ligaments are strong and reinforce the knee joint, the major stabilization of this joint is provided by the muscles (mainly quadriceps and hamstrings) that cross the joint.

The motions that occur at the knee and the major muscles that cause them are:

Extension: quadriceps femoris
Flexion: biceps femoris, semitendinosus, semimembranosus, gastrocnemius
Medial rotation: semimembranosus, semitendinosus, sartorius, popliteus
Lateral rotation: biceps femoris

Bones of the Foot. The bones of the foot are the *tarsals, metatarsals,* and *phalanges.* The seven tarsal bones are arranged in two rows with one bone between the rows. Proximally the talus sits on the calcaneus, and distally the bones (medial to lateral) are the medial, intermediate, and lateral cuneiforms and the cuboid. The navicular is essentially between the cuneiforms and the talus. The talus is the highest bone in the foot and it receives all of the superincumbent weight from the leg. The metatarsals and phalanges are similar in number and position to the metacarpals and phalanges of the hand.

The bones of the foot are arranged to provide flexibility and stability, that is, they must perform the weightbearing function while providing for a soft landing and forceful takeoff. These requirements are met by the presence of several *arches* that are arranged so that weight hits the floor at the calcaneal tuberosity posteriorly and at the heads of the metatarsals anteriorly. The most important arch is the medial longitudinal arch, which consists of the calcaneus, talus, navicular, three cuneiforms, and the three medial metatarsals. The lateral longitudinal arch is made up of the calcaneus, cuboid, and two lateral metatarsals. A transverse arch exists at the level of the distal row of tarsals and bases of the metatarsals. The major static support of these arches (primarily the medial longitudinal arch) is provided by ligaments, which are the very important plantar calcaneonavicular (spring) ligament, the long plantar ligament, and the ligament-like plantar aponeurosis. Dynamic support is added by the intrinsic muscles of the foot. Three extrinsic muscles of the foot, the tibialis anterior and posterior and the peroneus longus, may provide additional dynamic support.

Ankle Joint. The ankle joint is formed superiorly by the tibia and fibula and inferiorly by the trochlea of the talus. The *trochlea* is a cylindrically shaped process with its long axis oriented from side to side and its articular surface located on both its rounded upper aspect and flat ends. The tibia articulates with the superior aspect and medial end (via the medial malleous) of the talus; the lateral malleolus, with the lateral end. The talus glides around in the mortise formed by the tibia and fibula. The anterior aspect of the trochlea is wider than the posterior. As a result, in dorsiflexion the widest portion of the trochlea is wedged between the malleoli (good bony stability). In plantar flexion this support is lost. Thus, most sprains occur when the ankle is plantar flexed. The distal tibia and fibula are lashed together by anterior and posterior tibiofibular ligaments. The major ligaments supporting the ankle joint are the medial (deltoid) and lateral collateral ligaments. The deltoid ligament is a broad band that connects the medial malleolus with the talus, navicular, and calcaneus. The lateral collateral ligament is composed of three distinct bands: the anterior and posterior talofibular ligaments and the calca-

neofibular ligament. The anterior talofibular ligament is the most commonly injured ligament, accompanying the frequent plantar flexion-inversion sprain of the ankle.

The motions of the ankle and their major motors are:

Plantar flexion: gastrocnemius, soleus, tibialis posterior
Dorsiflexion: tibialis anterior

Subtalar and Transverse Tarsal Joints. Although the motions of the foot (other than toe motion) are the sum totals of the individual amounts of motion that occur at each intertarsal joint, there are two areas (called functional joints) where most of this motion does occur. These functional joints are the subtalar and transverse tarsal (midtarsal) joints. The motions of the foot are *inversion,* which is a combination of adduction and supination, and *eversion,* which is a combination of abduction and pronation. The subtalar joint is under the talus between the talus and the calcaneus. The two sets of articular surfaces that form this joint are separated by a strong interosseous ligament. The orientation of these joint spaces is an inclined plane that is directed anteriorly, medially, and inferiorly. The transverse tarsal joint consists of two joints that extend transversely across the foot. The medial articulation is between the talus and the navicular, the lateral between the calcaneus and the cuboid.

The motors of these foot motions are:

Inversion: tibialis anterior, tibialis posterior, flexor hallucis longus, flexor digitorum longus
Eversion: peroneus longus and brevis

COMPARTMENTATION OF THE LOWER LIMB

Hip Region. Although there are no compartments *per se* around the hip, the muscles in this region can be placed in logical groups. The *gluteal muscles* are the lateral and posterolateral muscles of the hip. The gluteus maximus is innervated by the inferior gluteal nerve, and the gluteus medius and minimus and the tensor fascia lata are supplied by the superior gluteal nerve. Deep to the gluteus maximus there is a group of muscles called the short external rotators of the thigh. These muscles are innervated by direct branches of the lumbosacral plexus and consist of the piriformis, obturator internus, superior and inferior gemelli, and the quadratus femoris. Anteriorly, the iliopsoas (iliacus and psoas major muscles) extends from the abdominal cavity into the proximal thigh. This major hip flexor is supplied by direct branches of the lumbar plexus.

Thigh. The investing fascia of the thigh is the fascia lata. It is dramatically thickened laterally as the iliotibial tract or band. Two intermuscular septa extend from this investing fascia to attach to the femur. Thus, these medial and lateral intermuscular septa separate the thigh into anterior and posterior compartments. The anterior compartment is actually anterolateral and the posterior compartment posteromedial. The muscles in the *anterior compartment* are innervated by the femoral nerve and consist of the sartorius and the four components of the quadriceps femoris—the rectus femoris, vastus medialis, vastus intermedius, and vastus lateralis. The posterior compartment has two groups of muscles—the medial femoral or adductors and the posterior femoral or hamstrings. The *medial femoral muscles* are mostly innervated by the obturator nerve and consist of the adductor longus, adductor brevis, adductor magnus, pectineus, gracilis, and obturator externus. The *hamstrings* are primarily innervated by the tibial portion of the sciatic nerve and consist of the biceps femoris, semitendinosus, and semimembranosus.

Femoral Triangle. The femoral triangle is not a compartment *per se,* but it contains important structures. The triangle is defined by the inguinal ligament above, the sartorius muscle laterally, and the medial border of the adductor longus muscle medially. The floor is formed by the adductor longus, pectineus, and iliopsoas muscles. The superficial and deep inguinal lymph nodes are found respectively superficially and deep to the investing fascia in this area. In addition to receiving superficial lymphatics from the lower extremity, the superficial nodes drain the lower abdominal wall, buttock, perineum, and lower portion of the anal canal and vagina. From lateral to medial the following structures descend through the triangle: the femoral nerve, the femoral artery, and the femoral vein. The femoral artery is midway between the anterior superior spine of the ilium and the pubic tubercle. The femoral sheath is an extension of transversalis fascia that forms a sleeve around the femoral vessels as they enter the thigh. The area just medial to the vein is within the sheath and is called the femoral canal, and it is the usual path of a femoral hernia. After leaving the triangle, the femoral vessels pass through the thigh just deep to the sartorius muscle, an area called the *adductor* (subsartorial) *canal.*

Popliteal Fossa. The popliteal fossa is a deep diamond-shaped area behind the knee. It is bounded superomedially by the tendons of the semitendinosus and semimembranosus muscles, superolaterally by the tendon of the biceps femoris, and inferiorly by the heads of the gastrocnemius muscle. Its floor is the posterior (supracondylar) portion of the distal femur. The popliteal vessels pass vertically through this fossa with the artery closest to the bone and thereby vulnerable to laceration when this part of the femur is fractured. The tibial nerve passes through the middle of this fossa superficially, and the common peroneal nerve follows the tendon of the biceps femoris muscle. This space is packed with loose connective tissue.

Leg. The leg has anterior, lateral, and posterior compartments. The major partition consists of the subcutaneous tibia, the interosseous membrane, the fibula, and the posterior intermuscular septum, which separates the posteromedially situated posterior compartment from an anterolateral region. This anterolateral area is subdivided into anterior and lateral compartments by the anterior intermuscular septum. The *anterior compartment* contains the tibialis anterior, extensor hallucis longus, extensor digitorum longus, and peroneus tertius muscles, all of which are innervated by the deep peroneal nerve. These muscles dorsiflex the ankle, invert the foot, and extend the toes. The *lateral compartment* muscles are primarily everters of the foot. The two muscles in this compartment— the peroneus longus and brevis—are innervated by the superficial peroneal nerve. All *posterior compartment* muscles are innervated by the tibial nerve and function to plantar flex the ankle, invert the foot, and flex the toes. The posterior compartment muscles are the gastrocnemius, soleus, and plantaris superficially, and the deep group consisting of the flexor hallucis longus, flexor digitorum longus, tibialis posterior, and popliteus.

Foot. The organization of the foot is similar to that of the hand, but the compartmentation is less complete in the foot. There is a definitive compartment associated with the small toe and a deep one more or less between the metatarsals. However, fascial separations complete the formation of neither a central compartment nor one associated with the great toe.

For the most part the muscles of the foot are similar to those of the hand but are usually described in layers rather than in compartments. All of the plantar muscles are innervated by either the medial or lateral plantar nerves, both branches of the tibial nerve. The *superficial layer* consists of the adductor hallucis (medial plantar), flexor digitorum brevis (medial plantar), and abductor digiti minimi (lateral plantar). The *intermediate layer* is limited to the central area of the foot and is formed by the tendon(s) of the flexor digitorum longus and related muscles, that is, the quadratus plantae (lateral plantar) and lumbricals (medial and lateral plantar nerves). The *deep layer* consists of the flexor hallucis brevis (medial plantar), adductor hallucis (lateral plantar), and flexor digiti minimi (lateral plantar). A fourth layer is usually described; it consists of both the plantar and dorsal interossei, all of which are supplied by the lateral plantar nerve. The foot differs from the hand also in that it has dorsal intrinsic muscles. These muscles, the extensor hallucis brevis and extensor digitorum brevis, extend the toes and are innervated by the deep peroneal nerve.

NERVES OF THE LOWER LIMB

Lumbosacral Plexus. Branches of the lumbosacral plexus (Fig. 2-10) supply most of the lower extremity. The *lumbar plexus* is formed in the sub-

stance of the psoas major muscle from the ventral rami of L1 through L4. All of L1 and part of L2 give rise to cutaneous nerves that supply the lower abdominal wall, the anterior part of the perineum and the proximal portion of the lower limb. The rest of the plexus forms major nerves of the lower extremity. The *sacral plexus* (L4 through S4) is formed in the pelvis on the ventral aspect of the piriformis muscle. The combined contribution of L4 and L5 is the lumbosacral trunk, which enters the pelvis by passing just lateral to the sacral promontory.

Femoral Nerve. The femoral nerve (L2–4) emerges from the lateral aspect of the psoas major muscle and enters the thigh by passing deep to the inguinal ligament. Upon entering the femoral triangle, it immediately branches into its many muscular branches. Its terminal branch, the cutaneous saphenous nerve, continues through the thigh in the ad-

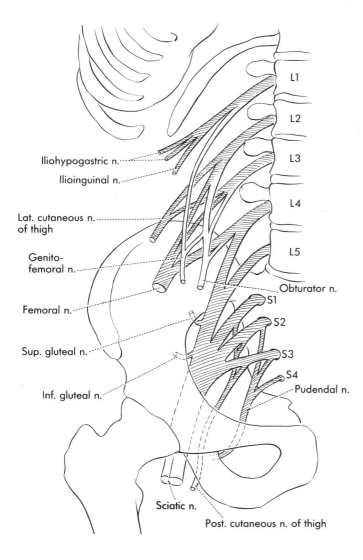

Fig. 2-10. Diagram of the lumbosacral plexus. (Hollinshead WH, Rosse C: Textbook of Anatomy, 4th ed, p 338. Philadelphia, JB Lippincott, 1985. After a figure from Sections of Neurology and the Section of Physiology, Mayo Clinic and Mayo Foundation: Clinical Examinations in Neurology, 2nd ed. Philadelphia, WB Saunders, 1963)

ductor canal. It enters the subcutaneous tissue in the distal thigh and supplies the skin on the medial aspect of the leg and foot.

Obturator Nerve. This nerve (L2–4) emerges from the medial aspect of the psoas major muscle just above the pelvic brim. It then enters the pelvic cavity and passes anteriorly and ventrally toward the obturator canal, through which it enters the medial aspect of the thigh. It ends there by dividing into its terminal muscular and cutaneous branches. The cutaneous branches of this nerve supply the medial thigh and knee.

Gluteal Nerves. The superior gluteal nerve (L4–S1) arises in the pelvis but immediately exits by passing above the piriformis muscle and through the greater sciatic notch. It passes anteriorly between the gluteus medius and minimus muscles (supplying both) and terminates by supplying the tensor fasciae latae muscle. The inferior gluteal nerve (L5–S2) also arises in the pelvis and exits immediately by passing below the piriformis and through the greater sciatic notch directly into the substance of the gluteus maximus muscle.

Sciatic Nerve. The sciatic nerve is the largest nerve in the body. It consists of the tibial and common peroneal nerves, which are enclosed in a common connective tissue sheath. The sacral plexus essentially terminates as the sciatic nerve. This nerve leaves the pelvis by passing below the piriformis (usually) and through the greater sciatic notch. It descends through the middle of the posterior thigh between the medial and lateral hamstring muscles. It typically divides into the common peroneal and tibial nerves in the distal thigh as it enters the popliteal fossa.

The **common peroneal nerve** passes superficially through the popliteal fossa just medial to the biceps femoris muscle and its tendon. It passes superficial to the lateral femoral condyle and then wraps around the lateral aspect of the neck of the fibula. The nerve divides into its terminal branches, the superficial and deep peroneal nerves, as it passes the neck of the fibula. The **superficial peroneal nerve** enters the lateral compartment of the leg where it descends to innervate the skin on the dorsum of the foot. The **deep peroneal nerve** passes through the lateral compartment into the anterior compartment. It descends through this compartment and enters the dorsum of the foot where it supplies the extensor digitorum brevis and the extensor hallucis brevis muscles. It has a very small cutaneous distribution to the web space between the great and second toes.

The **tibial nerve** descends superficially through the center of the popliteal fossa. It enters the posterior compartment of the leg by passing between, and then deep to, the two heads of the gastrocnemius muscle. It descends through the leg between the superficial and deep groups of muscles and enters the foot by passing behind the medial malleolus. As it enters the foot, it divides into the **medial** and **lateral plantar nerves**. The medial plantar nerve is homologous with the median nerve of the hand. It passes into the medial aspect of the foot and divides into muscular branches and cutaneous branches (plantar digital nerves) that supply the skin on the plantar surface of the medial three and a half toes and corresponding part of the ball of the foot. The lateral plantar nerve is similar in course and distribution to the ulnar nerve in the hand. It passes diagonally across the plantar aspect of the foot by going between the flexor digitorum brevis and quadratus plantae muscles. It then terminates by dividing into superficial and deep branches. The superficial branch has muscular branches and is cutaneous to the plantar aspect of the lateral one and one half toes and corresponding part of the sole in that area. The deep branch dives deeply and passes medially across the foot deep to long flexor tendons and terminates by supplying the adductor hallucis.

PERIPHERAL NERVE LESIONS IN THE LOWER LIMB

The lower limb is used almost exclusively as a means of locomotion. The muscles are concerned with both weight bearing and forward propulsion of the entire body. Therefore, in analyzing peripheral nerve lesions, it is only reasonable to evaluate the disturbances in the normal gait pattern that are caused by nerve damage.

Superior Gluteal Nerve. The abductors of the hip maintain the coronal balance during the stance phase of gait; that is, when an individual is standing on one foot, the hip abductors on the weight-bearing side prevent dropping of the pelvis to the opposite side (hip adduction). A patient with a superior gluteal nerve injury will exhibit a positive **Trendelenburg sign** during the stance phase of gait or when asked to stand on one foot; that is, his pelvis will drop to the non-weightbearing side, and he will shift his trunk laterally to the weight-bearing side in order to bring the center of gravity over the supporting limb.

Inferior Gluteal Nerve. At heel-strike there is a tendency for the trunk to bend forward, that is, hip flexion. This is counteracted by the gluteus maximus. If this nerve is totally severed, the patient will compensate by throwing the trunk backward at heel-strike, thus preventing the line of gravity from moving anterior to the hip joint.

Femoral Nerve. At heel-strike and continuing through most of the stance phase, the quadriceps muscles maintain knee extension and thus support the body weight. With a loss of quadriceps function the patient must lock the knee and keep the line of gravity well in front of the joint. As a result this patient will whip his leg into extension by forceful thigh flexion followed by a rapid halt of this flexion (by way of the gluteus maximus), which snaps the knee into extension by pendulum action. As soon as the knee is extended he plants the heel on the floor, extends his hip (to hold the knee extension), and flexes his trunk (to get the line of gravity ahead of the knee joint). He then *vaults* over a rigidly extended knee.

Deep Peroneal Nerve. During gait the anterior compartment muscles of the leg shorten the length of the limb during the swing phase by dorsiflexing the ankle; they also prevent plantar flexion (footslap) at heel-strike. When a patient with a deep peroneal nerve lesion (total paralysis) takes a step, he must lift his leg high so the plantar flexed foot can clear the ground *(steppage gait).* There is no heel-strike because the ball of the foot hits the ground before the heel. If there is partial paralysis of the deep peroneal nerve (the tibialis anterior is weakened), the foot can be dorsiflexed during the swing phase, but at heel-strike the weakened muscle cannot prevent plantar flexion and the ball of the foot hits the ground with a *slap.*

Tibial Nerve. The forward momentum for locomotion is provided by the foot pushing down and back against the ground (plantar flexion). This function is lost with a tibial nerve lesion. The result is a noticeable lag in forward momentum at the point of push-off.

BLOOD SUPPLY OF THE LOWER LIMB

Arteries. Most of the lower extremity is supplied by the *femoral artery* (Fig. 2-11). The gluteal region receives the *superior* and *inferior gluteal arteries* from the internal iliac, and the *obturator artery* (also a branch of the internal iliac) supplies a portion of the medial thigh. The femoral artery is the continuation of the external iliac artery, which enters the thigh by passing deep to the inguinal ligament. It descends through the femoral triangle and adductor canal. As it enters the popliteal fossa by passing through the adductor hiatus, its name changes to the popliteal artery. A femoral pulse is taken about midway between the anterior superior spine of the

ilium and the pubic tubercle. The largest branch of the femoral is the *deep femoral artery,* which arises in the femoral triangle and descends just medial to the femur. The *medial and lateral circumflex arteries* arise from the deep femoral soon after it arises. The deep femoral also has perforating branches that pass into the posterior compartment of the thigh.

The *popliteal artery* passes through the deepest portion of the popliteal fossa, where it has several genicular branches. When a popliteal pulse is taken the artery must be compressed against the femur. This is done with the knee flexed to remove the tension on the fascia covering the fossa. The artery terminates by dividing into the anterior and posterior tibial arteries as it enters the posterior compartment of the leg.

The *anterior tibial artery* immediately enters the anterior compartment of the leg by passing above the superior margin of the interosseous membrane. It descends through the anterior compartment and enters the foot by crossing the anterior aspect of the ankle; there it becomes the *dorsalis pedis artery*. On the dorsum of the foot—where the dorsalis pedis pulse is best taken—the artery is between the tendons of the extensor hallucis longus and the extensor digitorum longus. The dorsalis pedis artery terminates into branches, most of which supply the dorsum of the foot. One of these branches, the deep plantar branch, passes into the plantar aspect of the foot by going between the first and second metatarsals and there helps form the *plantar arterial arch.*

The *posterior tibial artery* descends through the deep portion of the posterior compartment of the leg, inclining medially as it descends. It enters the foot behind the medial malleolus where a posterior tibial pulse can be taken. It terminates as it passes around the medial malleolus by dividing into *medial and lateral plantar arteries.* It has a large peroneal branch high in the posterior compartment, the *peroneal artery,* which descends in the lateral part of the posterior compartment and terminates around the ankle.

The medial and lateral plantar arteries correspond in course and distribution to the medial and lateral plantar nerves. There is only one arterial arch in the foot, which corresponds to the deep arch of the hand, and is formed by the deep branch of the lateral plantar artery and the deep plantar branch of the dorsalis pedis artery.

Veins. The veins of the lower extremity consist of deep and superficial veins. The deep veins correspond rather closely to the pattern of the arteries. The two saphenous veins are the main superficial veins. The *greater saphenous vein* begins on the dor-

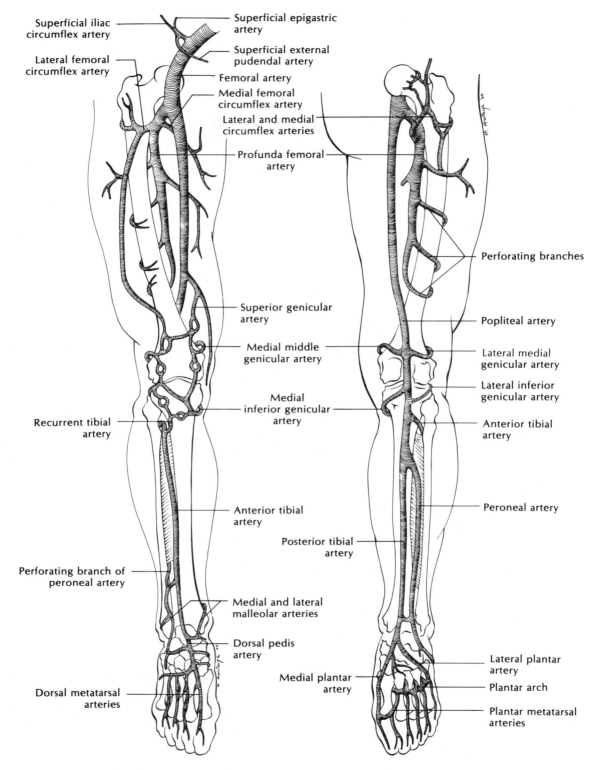

Fig. 2-11. Arteries of the lower limb. (Christensen JB, Telford IR: Synopsis of Gross Anatomy, 5th ed, p 278. Philadelphia, JB Lippincott, 1988)

somedial aspect of the foot and ascends along the anteromedial aspect of the leg and thigh. It terminates by passing through the saphenous opening of the fascia lata and emptying into the femoral vein just distal to the inguinal ligament. The greater saphenous vein passes just anterior to the medial malleolus, where it is commonly secured for venous cutdown. The *lesser saphenous vein* begins as a network on the dorsolateral aspect of the foot. It ascends behind the lateral malleolus and through the middle of the calf, and it terminates by emptying into the popliteal vein in the popliteal fossa.

HEAD AND NECK

SUPERFICIAL STRUCTURES OF THE HEAD AND NECK

Major Surface Landmarks and Regions. The anterolateral aspect of the neck is divided into anterior and posterior triangles by the prominent sternocleidomastoid muscle. The *anterior triangle* is in front of this muscle and extends to the inferior margin of the mandible and to the midline. Behind the sternocleidomastoid the *posterior triangle* is also delimited by the superior border of the trapezius muscle and the middle third of the clavicle. The face can be divided into several areas that include the orbit, nose, forehead, temporal region, maxillary region, and mandibular region. It is convenient to start with the well-defined orbit, which is protected and delimited by the prominent supraorbital and infraorbital margins, which meet laterally. Extending posteriorly at the level of the infraorbital margin, the zygomatic arch separates the temporal region above from the mandibular or lower jaw region below. The mandibular region extends inferiorly and then anteromedially to join the same region of the opposite side. The maxillary or upper jaw region is inferior to the infraorbital margin and lateral to the nose. The posterior part of the head is the occipital region.

Microscopic Structure of the Skin and Scalp. The skin consists of an outer *epidermis* of stratified squamous keratinized epithelium and an underlying *dermis* of dense irregularly arranged fibroelastic connective tissue. Beneath the dermis is a *subcutaneous layer* of loose connective tissue. The epidermis varies in structure and thickness, depending on the region of the body. On the palmar surface of the hand and on the soles of the feet the epidermis consists of four layers. These are, from the dermis to the surface, the stratum germinativum, stratum granulosum, stratum lucidum, and stratum corneum.

The stratum germinativum is further divisible into a stratum basale and stratum spinosum. Epidermal cells in both of these layers are capable of mitoses. Cells of the stratum spinosum (prickle cells) are joined at numerous desmosomes (macula adherens) where many tonofilaments converge toward the plasma membrane. Desmosomes are dense bodies where plasma membranes of adjacent cells appear thickened because of a dense layer on their cytoplasmic surfaces. A thin intermediate lamina occurs in the intercellular space at a desmosome. Tonofilaments will give rise to the fibrous protein keratin. Melanin granules are found in the deeper cells of the stratum germinativum in caucasians and in more of the deeper layers in colored races. Melanin is produced in melanocytes, which arise from neural crest. The melanin granules are distributed to the epidermal cells. The color of the skin is dependent on the amount of melanin, carotene, and the vascularity of the skin.

The stratum granulosum represents cells that are older and further differentiated in the keratinization process than those of the deeper layers. Keratohyalin granules predominate and will give rise to the interfilamentous amorphous matrix that will be prevalent in the stratum corneum. Membrane-coating granules in the granulosal cells provide the intercellular "sealing" cement between cells of the stratum corneum. The stratum lucidum contains flattened translucent cells, with orderly arrays of tonofilaments, that have lost their nuclei. Cells of the stratum corneum also have lost their organelles and contain soft keratin, which consists of tightly packed filaments embedded in an amorphous matrix.

The dermis is divisible into papillary and reticular layers. The papillary layer is immediately underneath the epidermis and contains dense fine collagenous fibers, blood vessels and free and encapsulated (*e.g.,* Meissner's tactile corpuscles) nerve endings. The reticular layer contains coarser bundles of collagenous fibers. Smooth muscle can be found in this layer in the nipple and scrotum. Hair follicles, sebaceous glands, and the ducts of sweat glands are located in the reticular layer. The secretory portions of simple tubular sweat glands, the roots of hairs, and pacinian corpuscles (deep pressure receptors) are constituents of the subcutaneous layer. Extensive accumulations of fat in this layer determine it as the panniculus adiposus.

Secretory portions of sweat glands consist of a high cuboidal epithelium invested by contractile myoepithelial cells. Since no part of the cell is lost in the secretory process, it is classified as a merocrine type of secretion. The ducts are stratified cuboidal, except for the intraepidermal portion, which is lined by the epidermal epithelium.

Sebaceous glands have short ducts that empty into hair follicles, except for those in the labia minora and glans penis where they open directly to the surface. The secretory portion of the sebaceous gland is stratified cuboidal; the lumen is generally filled with rounded cells containing numerous fat droplets. The secretion of sebum involves the holocrine discharge of sebaceous cells. New cells proliferate and differentiate from more basal regions of the gland.

Hairs are most prevalent in the scalp and are lacking in such areas as the palms of the hands and soles of the feet. Each hair consists of a root and a shaft. The root is enclosed by a tubular hair follicle that consists of inner and outer epithelial root sheaths, both derived from epidermis, and an outer connective tissue root sheath that corresponds to the dermis. At its lower end the follicle and root expand into a hair bulb, which is indented by a connective tissue hair papilla. The hair, consisting of an inner medulla, a cortex, and outer cuticle, grows upward from the differentiation of matrix cells in the hair bulb. Pigment in the cortical layer and air in the cortex and medulla determine the color of the hair. Arrectores pilorum of smooth muscle run in the obtuse angle between the follicle and epidermis, and they attach to the follicle deep to the sebaceous glands. Contraction causes erection of the hair and dimpling of the skin (goose flesh) at the smooth muscle attachment in the dermis. In the scalp and face, skeletal muscles are found in the superficial fascia.

Organization of the Blood Vessels to the Head and Neck. The common carotid arteries are the major arteries to the head and neck. The external carotid supplies most of the head and neck structures outside the cranial cavity; the internal carotid supplies the cranial cavity and orbit. On the right the vessel is one of the main terminal branches of the brachiocephalic trunk, while on the left it is a direct branch from the arch of the aorta. In a plane deep to the sternocleidomastoid muscle each artery extends along a line that passes behind the sternoclavicular joint and through the midpoint between the angle of the mandible and the mastoid process. It terminates by dividing into the internal and external carotids between the levels of the hyoid bone and the thyroid cartilage prominence (laryngeal prominence or Adam's Apple), where the carotid body and sinus can be palpated. The *internal carotid* has no branches and passes directly toward the carotid canal through which it enters the cranial cavity.

The *external carotid* artery ascends to the neck of the mandible where it divides into its terminal branches: the *maxillary artery,* which passes deep to the neck of the mandible into the infratemporal fossa, and the *superficial temporal artery,* which ascends into the temporal region to supply that region and the anterior part of the scalp. Six other branches commonly arise from the external carotid artery. The *superior thyroid artery* supplies primarily the thyroid gland and larynx. The *lingual artery* passes deeply toward the tongue. The *facial artery* crosses the inferior margin of the mandible just anterior to the angle (where a facial pulse can be taken). From this point the facial artery follows a tortuous course obliquely across the face toward the angle between the nose and medial aspect of the eye. It supplies the superficial structures of the face as it winds superficial and deep to them. The *ascending pharyngeal artery* supplies the pharyngeal and palatal regions. The *occipital* and *posterior auricular branches* supply primarily the superficial regions designated by their names.

The *jugular system of veins* drains most of the head and neck. The main vessel is the internal jugular vein, which begins at the base of the skull where it receives most of the venous blood from the cranial cavity. It descends through the neck in company with the carotid arteries, receiving multiple tributaries from outside the cranial cavity, and terminates by joining the subclavian vein to form the brachiocephalic vein.

Cutaneous Nerves. The cutaneous innervation is easily defined if the head and neck are divided into three areas (Fig. 2-12). The first includes the entire face and the anterior part of the scalp, extending posteriorly to a line across the top of the head that connects the two external auditory meatuses (interauricular line). The skin of this area is innervated by the three divisions of the fifth cranial (trigeminal) nerve. The ophthalmic nerve innervates the bridge of the nose, upper eyelid and cornea, forehead, and scalp. The maxillary division covers the lateral aspect of the nose, cheek, and anterior temporal region. The mandibular innervation corresponds to the area overlying the mandible and the posterior temporal region. The second area includes the medial aspect of the posterior neck and the corresponding part of the occipital region, which extends anteriorly to the interauricular line. This area is supplied by cutaneous branches of the dorsal rami of cervical spinal nerves. The third area includes the anterolateral neck, posterior triangle

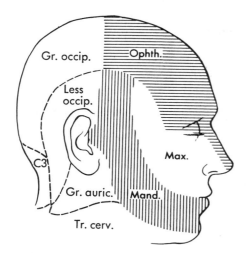

Fig. 2-12. Approximate cutaneous distribution of the three divisions of the fifth nerve and of cervical nerves to the face and scalp. (Hollinshead WH: Anatomy For Surgeons, Vol 1, 3rd ed, p 317. Philadelphia, JB Lippincott, 1982)

and shoulder pad region, and the skin surrounding the ear posteriorly. This third area is innervated by the cutaneous branches of the cervical plexuses (lesser occipital, great auricular, transverse cervical, and supraclavicular nerves).

Facial Muscles. The muscles of facial expression are found essentially in the subcutaneous tissue of the face, neck (platysma), and scalp (epicranius). They function to move the skin and regulate the shape of the openings on the face. Many muscles are associated with the muscle surrounding the mouth (orbicularis oris) and those surrounding the eyes (orbicularis oculi). The buccinator muscle is deeply located in the cheek and represents the only muscle in that area. All of these muscles are innervated by the seventh cranial (facial) nerve.

Parotid Gland. The largest of the salivary glands is located anteroinferior to the ear and extends inferiorly to the level of the angle of the mandible. It has a deep portion that extends posterior and then medial to the ramus of the mandible. The main trunk of the facial nerve enters the posterior aspect of the gland and divides into its main divisions within the substance of the gland. The parotid duct passes anteriorly around the masseter muscle and empties into the oral cavity just opposite the second upper molar.

Microscopic Structure of Major Salivary Glands. The parenchyma of the parotid gland consists of *serous acini* and ducts. The acini are grouped into lobules and lobes by connective tissue septa. Pyramid-shaped cells with apical accumula-

tions of zymogen granules and basal concentrations of RER line the small lumina of the serous acini. Myoepithelial cells lie between the acinar cells and the basal lamina. The serous secretion of the acinar cells passes into *intercalated ducts,* which empty into *striated ducts.* Both of these ducts are intralobular ducts. Intercalated ducts have small lumina and are lined by simple cuboidal epithelium. Striated (salivary) ducts are larger and are lined by a simple columnar epithelium whose cells have extensive infoldings of the plasma membrane on their basal surfaces. These basal striations with their interposed mitochondria are like those in cells of the distal convoluted tubules of the kidney and perform similar functions in the reabsorption of sodium and water from the luminal fluid. After reabsorption, the secretion in the striated ducts passes successively to interlobular, interlobar, and the main excretory (Stensen's) ducts. The simple columnar epithelial lining of the ducts gets taller as the main duct is approached. Stensen's duct is lined by pseudostratified columnar epithelium that contains some goblet cells. At the opening of the duct into the oral cavity, the epithelium becomes stratified squamous nonkeratinized epithelium.

The submandibular gland is a mixed seromucous gland whose acini are preponderantly serous. *Mucous alveoli* are frequently capped by *serous demilunes* or have serous cells lining their terminal portions. The secretion from serous demilunes passes between mucous cells to reach the lumen. Mucous cells contain basally flattened nuclei, RER, and apical membrane-bound mucigen droplets. The ducts of the submandibular gland are microscopically similar to those of the parotid, but salivary ducts are longer and more numerous. The main duct (Wharton's) opens into the mouth beneath the tongue.

The sublingual gland is a mixed gland, but the mucous alveoli predominate. Salivary ducts and intercalated ducts are few in number. The main excretory ducts open into the mouth at the side of the frenulum and, like the main ducts of the parotid and submandibular gland, are lined by pseudostratified columnar epithelium.

FASCIAL PLANES AND COMPARTMENTS OF THE NECK

Fascial Planes. The *superficial layer* (investing layer) of cervical fascia encircles the neck and encloses the sternocleidomastoid and trapezius muscles (Fig. 2-13). The *prevertebral fascia* surrounds the vertebral column and its associated muscles,

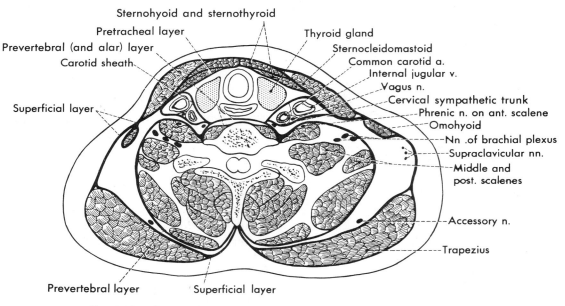

Sternohyoid and sternothyroid
Pretracheal layer
Prevertebral (and alar) layer
Carotid sheath
Superficial layer
Thyroid gland
Sternocleidomastoid
Common carotid a.
Internal jugular v.
Vagus n.
Cervical sympathetic trunk
Phrenic n. on ant. scalene
Omohyoid
Nn. of brachial plexus
Supraclavicular nn.
Middle and post. scalenes
Accessory n.
Trapezius

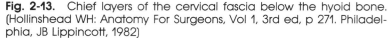

Prevertebral layer   Superficial layer

Fig. 2-13. Chief layers of the cervical fascia below the hyoid bone. (Hollinshead WH: Anatomy For Surgeons, Vol 1, 3rd ed, p 271. Philadelphia, JB Lippincott, 1982)

that is, the longus capitis and colli, the scalenes, and the deep muscles of the back in the cervical region. The visceral structures of the neck are enclosed in a sleeve of fascia called the *pretracheal fascia* anteriorly and laterally and the *buccopharyngeal fascia* (between the pharynx or esophagus and the vertebral column) posteriorly. The infrahyoid muscles have their own fascia, which is between the investing and pretracheal layers of cervical fascia. In the lateral part of the neck and deep to the plane of the sternocleidomastoid muscle, the several layers of cervical fascia meet and contribute to the formation of the vertically oriented *carotid sheath.*

Anterior Triangle. Many surgical approaches to the viscera of the neck are made through this area, which is bounded by the midline, inferior margin of the mandible and the sternocleidomastoid muscle. The part of the anterior triangle above the digastric muscle is the submandibular triangle, and the area below the digastric is sometimes divided into the carotid triangle above the omohyoid muscle and muscular triangle below. The carotid sheath structures—the vagus nerve, the carotid artery, and the internal jugular vein—pass vertically through this area, located deep to the sternocleidomastoid muscle. The cervical sympathetic chain is deep in the triangle on the anterolateral aspects of the cervical vertebrae. The lateral lobes of the thyroid gland are immediately adjacent to the lateral aspects of the

trachea and lower larynx, while the isthmus of the thyroid crosses the midline in front of the upper rings of the trachea. The parathyroids are related to the posterior surface of the upper and lower aspects of the lateral lobes of the thyroid. The esophagus lies behind the trachea and larynx.

The submandibular triangle contains the submandibular gland, the facial artery and vein, the mylohyoid vessels and nerves, and the hypoglossal nerve.

Posterior Triangle. The posterior triangle is bounded by the superior border of the trapezius, the posterior border of the sternocleidomastoid, and the middle third of the clavicle. This area is easily visualized by asking the patient to hunch his shoulder anteriorly and turn his head to the opposite side. Several major structures supplying the upper limb are accessible through this triangle.

The cutaneous branches of the cervical plexus enter the subcutaneous tissue after curving around the posterior middle third of the sternocleidomastoid muscle. The accessory nerve emerges from beneath the middle of the posterior border of the sternocleidomastoid, passes obliquely across the triangle and dives deep to the superior border of the trapezius about 3 cm above its clavicular attachment. The inferior belly of the omohyoid muscle crosses the inferior aspect of the triangle a few centimeters above the clavicle.

The floor of the posterior triangle is muscular,

consisting of the splenius capitis and cervicis, levator scapulae, and the scalene muscles. The anterior and middle scalene muscles attach inferiorly on the first rib. These two muscles, together with a small portion of the first rib, form a narrow triangle (*scalene triangle* or scalene groove) through which the roots (ventral rami) of the brachial plexus and the subclavian artery enter the posterior triangle. Any of these structures can be compressed as they pass through this narrow opening. This neurovascular compression can be caused by muscle hypertrophy, the occurrence of a cervical rib, and so forth. Since the posterior border of the anterior scalene muscle corresponds to the lower part of the posterior border of the sternocleidomastoid muscle, the scalene groove is readily palpable. Therefore, the roots of the plexus are palpable as hard cords, and the subclavian pulse can be taken by compressing the subclavian artery against the first rib. In addition, the inferior deep cervical lymph nodes are associated with the anterior scalene. These *anterior scalene nodes*—the final sentinel nodes for the thoracic duct on the left and the right lymphatic duct on the right—are palpated in the same area.

Although only a portion of the *subclavian artery* is in the posterior triangle, it is included here. This artery is divided into three parts on the basis of its relationship to the anterior scalene muscle (see Fig. 2-8). The first part arises from the arch of the aorta on the left and the brachiocephalic trunk on the right. It passes superolaterally to the medial margin of the anterior scalene. The branches of the first part are the *vertebral artery,* which ascends deep to the anterior scalene to enter the transverse foramen of C6; the *thyrocervical trunk,* which has suprascapular, transverse cervical, and inferior thyroid branches; and the *internal thoracic artery,* which descends deep to the costal cartilages just lateral to the sternum. The second part of the subclavian lies posterior to the anterior scalene. Its only branch is the *costocervical trunk,* which gives rise to the deep cervical and highest intercostal arteries. The third part extends from the lateral border of the anterior scalene to the first rib. The *dorsal scapular artery* may arise from this part.

VISCERAL STRUCTURES OF THE NECK

Larynx.   The larynx (Fig. 2-14) is a tubular organ composed of nine cartilages that are connected by elastic membranes and synovial joints. It is lined by a mucosa that covers the vocal cords and is innervated by branches of the vagus nerve. The cartilages of the larynx are (1) epiglottis, (2) thyroid (Adam's apple), (3) cricoid, (4) two arytenoids, (5) two corniculates, and (6) two cuneiforms.

The larynx is that portion of the airway between the pharynx and the trachea. It is anterior to cervical vertebrae 4 through 6, and related anteriorly to the infrahyoid muscles and laterally to the inferior constrictor muscle of the pharynx and the lobes of the thyroid gland.

The vocal apparatus *(glottis)* consists of the true vocal folds and the opening *(rima glottidis)* between the folds. The area above the true folds, extending to the laryngeal additis (entrance), is the *vestibule* or *supraglottic portion.* The false vocal folds are above the true folds, and the area extending laterally between the true and false folds is the *ventricle.* The vocal fold (true vocal cord) contains the thin cranial edge of the conus elasticus. This free edge is the so-called vocal cord. The *vocal fold* is divided into anterior *intramembranous* and posterior *intracartilaginous portions.* The intramembranous portion stretches between the thyroid and arytenoid cartilages and is capable of tension change and vibration. The intracartilaginous portion is formed by the arytenoid cartilage. The numerous intrinsic muscles moving the laryngeal cartilages lie deep to the thyroid cartilage except the cricothyroid, which alone is innervated by the external branch of the superior laryngeal nerve, and which functions to tense the vocal cords. The others are innervated by the inferior (recurrent) branch of the

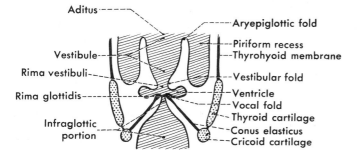

Aditus

Vestibule

Rima vestibuli

Rima glottidis

Infraglottic portion

Aryepiglottic fold

Piriform recess
Thyrohyoid membrane

Vestibular fold

Ventricle
Vocal fold
Thyroid cartilage
Conus elasticus
Cricoid cartilage

Fig. 2-14. Cavity of the larynx and its subdivisions in a frontal section. (Hollinshead WH: Anatomy For Surgeons, Vol 1, 3rd ed, p 420. Philadelphia, JB Lippincott, 1982)

vagus. These include the posterior cricoarytenoid, which abducts the vocal cords; the transverse arytenoid and lateral cricoarytenoid, which adduct the vocal cords; and the thyroarytenoid and vocalis muscles, which relax the vocal cords. The internal branch of the superior laryngeal nerve is sensory to the supraglottic portion of the larynx and the adjacent part of the pharynx. The recurrent laryngeal nerve innervates the infraglottic mucosa of the larynx. The blood supply is provided by the superior and inferior thyroid arteries.

Pharynx. The pharynx extends from the base of the skull to the beginning of the esophagus. Posteriorly it is in contact with the upper six cervical vertebrae; laterally it is related to the internal and the common carotid arteries, the internal jugular vein, the sympathetic trunk, and the last four cranial nerves. Anteriorly it communicates with the nasal cavity and the oral cavity; inferiorly it communicates with the larynx and esophagus.

That portion of the pharynx above the soft palate is the *nasopharynx.* The auditory (eustachian) tube opens on the lateral wall of the nasopharynx. The projecting cartilage of the auditory tube produces a marked elevation (the torus tubarius) around the opening, and the pharyngeal recess is the fossa behind the posterior lip of the torus. The pharyngeal tonsil ("adenoid") is found on the posterior wall of the nasopharynx. The *oropharynx* is posterior to the oral cavity, and it is limited above by the soft palate and below by the superior aspect of the epiglottis. The oral pharynx communicates with the oral cavity through the *fauces* (throat), which is below the soft palate and above the root of the tongue. Laterally the fauces are bounded by two mucosal-covered muscular columns (pillars of the fauces): anteriorly the palatoglossal fold and posteriorly the palatopharyngeal fold. The lateral area between the folds is the tonsillar fossa, which contains the palatine tonsil. The *laryngopharynx* extends from the superior edge of the epiglottis inferiorly to the lower border of the cricoid cartilage, essentially surrounding the larynx laterally and posteriorly. The vertical groove between the lateral aspect of the larynx and the pharyngeal wall is the piriform recess.

The *muscles of the pharynx* are the three constrictors and the stylopharyngeus, the latter passing downward between the superior and the middle constrictors. The constrictors overlap each other from below upward and surround the pharynx, and all three are inserted into a fibrous raphe in the posterior midline. Between muscles and mucous membrane is the pharyngobasilar fascia, which is especially strong above where it is attached to the

basilar process of the occipital bone and the petrous portion of the temporal bone. The inferior constrictor arises from the cricoid cartilage and the oblique line of the thyroid cartilage and encircles the pharynx. The middle constrictor arises from the greater and the lesser horns of the hyoid bone. The superior constrictor arises from the lower end and the hamulus of the medial pterygoid plate, the pterygomandibular ligament and the posterior end of the mylohyoid line on the inner surface of the mandible. The constrictor muscles are innervated by the tenth cranial nerve and the stylopharyngeus by the ninth cranial nerve. The ninth cranial nerve is also a major sensory nerve innervating the pharyngeal mucosa. As a result, the sensory limb of the gag reflex is the ninth cranial nerve and the motor limb the tenth cranial nerve.

Microscopic Structure of the Thyroid and Parathyroid Glands. The thyroid gland is invested by a thin capsule of connective tissue that projects into its substance and divides it imperfectly into lobes and lobules. The parenchyma consists of *follicles* that are closed epithelial sacs lined by simple cuboidal or simple columnar epithelium, the cells being low when the gland is underactive and taller when the gland is overactive. Follicles vary from $50\ \mu$ to $500\ \mu$ in diameter, and the size of each follicle is somewhat dependent on the degree of distention by the stored colloid in the lumen of the follicle. In the production of thyroxine and triiodothyronine the follicular cells receive iodide and amino acids from extensively distributed fenestrated capillaries lying adjacent to the basement membrane. Through the mechanisms of a basally located RER and apically oriented Golgi apparatus, a glycoproteinaceous thyroglobulin is produced. This substance is discharged at the apical end of the cell into the follicular lumen where it is stored along with nucleoproteins and proteolytic enzymes as colloid. Under the influence of thyroid-stimulating hormone (TSH), portions of thyroglobulin are taken into the apex of the follicular cell by pinocytosis, and the droplets are hydrolyzed by lysosomal activity into thyroxine and triiodothyronine. These substances are then secreted from the basal aspect of the cell into the surrounding capillaries. *Parafollicular cells* located between follicle cells and the basement membrane, and also found between follicles, differ structurally from follicle cells by being larger and lighter staining. They produce calcitonin.

A connective tissue capsule separates parathyroid glands from the thyroid gland. Fine connective tissue septa penetrate the parathyroid glands and divide the parenchyma into irregular cords of chief (principal cells) and oxyphil cells. *Chief cells* produce parathyroid hormone and are found in two functional states as light and dark chief cells. Dark chief cells contain membrane-bound argyrophilic secretory granules, a relatively large Golgi complex, and large filamentous mitochondria. Light cells have a smaller Golgi complex and few secretory granules. Oxyphilic cells are very acidophilic, are engorged with mitochondria and have a small nucleus, and do not appear until the end of the first decade of life. Their function is unknown.

Microscopic Structure of the Larynx and Trachea. As previously mentioned, the tubular larynx is composed of nine cartilages connected by elastic membranes and intrinsic skeletal muscles. It is lined with a mucosa whose folds form the true and false vocal folds. The mucosa of the *true vocal folds* covers the vocal ligament (free margin of the conus elasticus) and vocalis muscle. The lining epithelium of the true vocal fold and of most of the epiglottis is stratified squamous nonkeratinized epithelium. Some taste buds may be found in the epiglottic epithelium. The rest of the lining is pseudostratified ciliated columnar epithelium that contains goblet cells and is underlain by a lamina propria containing mixed seromucous glands. Inhaled particulate matter is entrapped in the sticky mucous secretion, which is transported to the pharynx by ciliary movement in the more fluid serous medium. There are no glands in the true vocal folds, but the surface is kept moist by the secretions that arise from numerous glands lining the ventricles. Lymphatic tissue in the ventricles may constitute the laryngeal tonsil. The thyroid, cricoid, and most of the arytenoid cartilages are hyaline cartilage. The epiglottis, cuneiform, corniculate, and tips of the arytenoid cartilages are elastic cartilage.

The trachea is a tubular structure whose wall, from the luminal surface outward, consists of a mucosa, submucosa, and adventitia. The mucosa is similar to that of most of the larynx in that it is comprised of a pseudostratified ciliated columnar epithelium with goblet cells, the most prominent basement membrane in the body, and a lamina propria that contains many longitudinally directed elastic fibers. The indistinct submucosa contains seromucous glands that also extend between the C- and Y-shaped hyaline cartilage rings in the adventitial layer. The open interval of the C-shaped cartilages faces the esophagus and is bridged with fibroelastic tissue and a trachealis smooth muscle that runs circularly, attaching at the inner surface of each cartilage end.

Microscopic Structure of the Pharynx. The wall of the pharynx consists of a mucosa, muscularis, and fibrosa. A submucosal layer exists only in the superior lateral region and near the junction with the esophagus. The epithelium of the nasopharynx is pseudostratified ciliated columnar epithelium with goblet cells; that of the oropharynx and laryngopharynx is stratified squamous nonkeratinized epithelium. The lamina propria contains many elastic fibers that constitute a dense elastic layer immediately adjacent to the muscularis. Mucous glands are found beneath the stratified squamous epithelium, whereas mixed glands occupy the lamina propria under the pseudostratified ciliated columnar epithelium. Aggregations of lymphatic nodules in the posterior nasopharyngeal mucosa constitute the pharyngeal tonsils (adenoids). The superior, middle, and inferior constrictor muscles and the stylopharyngeus and salpingopharyngeus muscles constitute the skeletal muscle of the muscularis layer. The fibrosa layer is a tough fibroelastic layer that attaches the pharynx to surrounding structures.

TEMPORAL AND INFRATEMPORAL REGIONS

Osteology. The *temporal fossa* is superficial to those areas of the frontal, parietal, and squamous portions of the temporal and greater wing of the sphenoid bones that are bounded superiorly and posteriorly by the temporal lines. It extends inferiorly to the zygomatic arch and anteriorly to the frontal process of the zygomatic bone.

The *infratemporal fossa* is deep to the ramus of the mandible and the zygomatic arch. It is limited above by the infratemporal crest of the sphenoid, medially by the lateral pterygoid plate, anteriorly by the maxilla, and inferiorly by the alveolar border of the maxilla. The infratemporal fossa is continuous medially with the pterygopalatine fossa via the pterygomaxillary fissure. It communicates with the middle cranial fossa by openings in its roof: the foramen ovale and foramen spinosum. Connections with the orbit are established through the inferior orbital fissure.

Temporomandibular Joint. The temporomandibular articulation is formed between the anterior portion of the mandibular fossa and the articular tubercle of the temporal bone above and the condyle of the mandible below. The articular surfaces are covered by fibrocartilage and are separated by an articular disk. The strong joint capsule is reinforced by the sphenomandibular and stylomandibular ligaments. The condyle moves like a hinge on the articular disk while the disk glides forward toward the articular eminence. Consequently, when the mandible is depressed as in opening the mouth, the mandibular condyle slides anteriorly and inferiorly and thus out of the mandibular fossa.

Muscles of Mastication. The muscles of mastication are the masseter, temporalis, and the medial and lateral pterygoids. They are found both in the temporal and infratemporal fossae and superficial to the ramus of the mandible.

The *masseter* extends from the zygomatic arch to the outer surface of the ramus of the mandible, and it is an elevator of the mandible. The *temporalis* muscle arises from the temporal fossa of the skull and inserts on the borders and the inner surface of the coronoid process. It elevates and retracts the mandible. The *medial pterygoid* arises from the inner surface of the lateral pterygoid plate and inserts on the angle and the inner surface of the ramus of the mandible. The *lateral pterygoid* arises from the zygomatic surface of the greater wing of the sphenoid and the outer surface of the lateral pterygoid plate. It inserts in the depression in front of the neck of the mandible and the articular disk. Both pterygoid muscles (especially the lateral) cause deviation of the mandible to the opposite side and are thereby responsible for the grinding action of chewing. In addition, the medial pterygoid is an elevator and the lateral pterygoid is a protruder of the mandible. Mandibular depression is produced by the lateral pterygoid and floor of the mouth muscles. All muscles of mastication are innervated by the mandibular division of the trigeminal nerve.

Contents of the Infratemporal Fossa. In addition to the pterygoid muscles, the infratemporal fossa contains the proximal portion of the maxillary artery, the mandibular division of the trigeminal nerve, and the pterygoid plexus of veins.

The *maxillary artery* is the larger of the two terminal branches of the external carotid. It arises in the substance of the parotid gland and enters the infratemporal fossa by passing deep to the ramus of the mandible. It passes obliquely through the fossa (either deep or superficial to the lateral pterygoid muscle) on its course to the pterygopalatine fossa via the pterygomaxillary fissure. While in the infratemporal fossa it gives off the anterior tympanic, deep auricular, middle meningeal, inferior alveolar, pterygoid, masseteric, buccal, and deep temporal branches. The *middle meningeal artery* enters the middle cranial fossa through the foramen spinosum and is the major arterial supply to the cranial dura mater.

The *mandibular nerve* enters the infratemporal fossa through the foramen ovale. The main trunk of

this nerve is short (1 cm) so that it branches high in the fossa. It has muscular branches to the muscles of mastication, and the mylohyoid, tensor tympani, and tensor veli palatini. Its sensory branches are the buccal nerve to the cheek, the auriculotemporal nerve to the posterior temporal region, the lingual nerve to the oral cavity, and the inferior alveolar nerve to the mandibular dentition and the skin covering the chin.

Parasympathetics are distributed in certain branches of this nerve. The otic ganglion is located medial to the main trunk of the nerve. The preganglionic input to this ganglion is from the lesser petrosal nerve, whose fibers exit the brainstem in cranial nerve IX. (Between cranial nerve IX and the lesser petrosal these fibers pass through the tympanic nerve and the tympanic plexus.) The postganglionic fibers from the otic ganglion are distributed with the auriculotemporal branch to the parotid gland. The chorda tympani branch of the seventh cranial nerve enters the infratemporal fossa through the petrotympanic fissure and joins the lingual nerve high in the fossa. The lingual nerve transports these preganglionic fibers to the submandibular ganglion (located in the submandibular triangle) where they synapse and are then distributed to the submandibular, sublingual, and lingual glands.

The *pterygoid plexus of veins* surrounds the pterygoid muscles. It receives blood from the face, nasal cavity, orbit, palate, cranial cavity, pharynx, and infratemporal fossa. It drains into the maxillary vein, which joins the superficial temporal vein to form the retromandibular vein.

PTERYGOPALATINE FOSSA

Osteology. The pterygopalatine fossa is between the maxilla in front and the pterygoid portion of the sphenoid behind. Medially it is bounded by the perpendicular plate of the palatine bone. It communicates laterally with the infratemporal fossa by the pterygomaxillary fissure, medially with the nasal cavity by the sphenopalatine foramen, inferiorly with the oral cavity by the palatine canal and the greater and lesser palatine foramina, posterosuperiorly with the middle cranial fossa by the foramen rotundum, anterosuperiorly with the orbit by the inferior orbital fissure, and posteromedially with the pharynx by the pharyngeal canal. The pterygoid canal is a canal through the pterygoid portion of the sphenoid that opens onto the posterior wall of the pterygopalatine fossa.

Contents of the Pterygopalatine Fossa. This fossa contains the terminal portion of the maxillary artery, the maxillary division of the trigeminal nerve, and the *pterygopalatine parasympathetic ganglion.* The preganglionic parasympathetic fibers that synapse in this ganglion exit the brain stem in the facial nerve. From the facial nerve the course of these fibers is in the greater petrosal nerve, which passes into the middle cranial fossa by the hiatus of the facial canal and then out of the fossa by a small foramen in the region of the foramen lacerum. The greater petrosal nerve then joins the deep petrosal nerve (which contains postganglionic sympathetic fibers), and together they pass through the pterygoid canal as the nerve of the pterygoid canal. This nerve terminates in the ganglion, the parasympathetics synapsing, and sympathetics merely passing through. Both fiber types are then distributed with branches of the maxillary nerve. The parasympathetic secretomotor fibers are thus distributed to the mucosa of the nasal cavity, palate, pharynx, and paranasal sinuses and to the lacrimal gland. The course of these fibers to the lacrimal gland is circuitous; they pass sequentially in the infraorbital nerve, its zygomatic branch, a communicating branch between the zygomatic and lacrimal nerves, and the lacrimal nerve to the gland.

The *maxillary nerve* continues as the infraorbital nerve, which passes into the floor of the orbit and eventually terminates on the face by the infraorbital foramen. The branches of the maxillary nerve and the proximal portion of the infraorbital nerve are the palatine (greater and lesser) to the palate, the nasopalatine and lateral nasal branches to the nasal cavity, the pharyngeal nerve to the nasopharynx, the zygomatic nerve to the skin of the zygomatic region of the face, and the superior alveolar nerves to the maxillary sinus and dentition.

The branches of the **pterygopalatine artery** are the posterior superior alveolar to the maxillary sinus and maxillary dentition, the infraorbital artery, the descending palatine artery to the palate, the pharyngeal artery, and the sphenopalatine artery to the nasal cavity.

ORAL CAVITY

The mouth or oral cavity consists of a vestibule and the mouth proper. The vestibule of the mouth lies between the lips and cheeks externally and the gums and teeth internally. It receives the parotid duct opposite the second upper molar tooth.

The *mouth proper* is bounded laterally and in front by the alveolar arches and the teeth; behind, it communicates with the pharynx through the fauces. It is roofed by the hard and the soft palates. The floor is composed of the tongue and the reflection of its mucous membrane to the gum lining the inner aspect of the mandible; the midline reflection is elevated into a fold called the frenulum linguae. On each side of this fold is the caruncula sublingualis containing the openings of the submandibular (Wharton's) ducts. Behind these are the openings of the ducts of the sublingual glands.

Lips and Cheeks. The lips are muscular folds covered externally by skin and internally by mucosa (mucous membrane). The upper lip extends to the nasolabial sulcus and contains a vertical midline groove, the philtrum. The mentolabial sulcus separates the lower lip from the skin of the chin. The lips receive their blood supply from labial branches of the facial artery. Their sensory nerve supply is by infraorbital branches of the trigeminal nerve to the upper lip and mental branches to the lower lip; the facial nerve supplies the orbicularis oris muscle. Microscopically the cutaneous surface consists of a thin skin, which possesses hairs, and sweat and sebaceous glands. The vestibular surface consists of stratified squamous nonkeratinized epithelium, lamina propria, and a submucosa rich in mucous and mixed seromucous labial glands. The orbicularis oris muscle lies between the dermis and submucosal layers. The red area of the lip lies in the free margin of the lip at the junction between skin and mucosa. It is covered by nonkeratinized epithelium containing deeply indenting vascular papillae. No glands are present, and the epithelium is kept moist by licking of the lips.

The cheeks are similar in structure to the lips. Thick submucosal fibers tightly bind the mucosa to the buccinator muscle, thus reducing the chance of chewing on mucosal folds. Mixed buccal glands occupy the submucosa.

Tongue. The tongue is a muscular organ whose bilateral muscle masses are separated in the midline by a fibrous septum. Extrinsic muscles interconnect the tongue and the hyoid bone (hyoglossus), styloid process (styloglossus), mandible (genioglossus), and palate (palatoglossus). Portions of the genioglossus function in protrusion of the tongue; the styloglossus and palatoglossus elevate the tongue; the hyoglossus depresses the sides; and the styloglossus and other portions of the genioglossus serve in retraction of the tongue. Intrinsic muscles are oriented in vertical, longitudinal, and transverse bundles and function to control the shape of the tongue. Both intrinsic and extrinsic muscles, with the exception of the palatoglossus (which is innervated by the vagus nerve), are innervated by the hypoglossal (12th) nerve. At its root the tongue is connected to the pharynx, palate, and epiglottis; the glossoepiglottic folds attach the root to the epiglottis and bound the vallecula.

The tongue is divisible into an anterior two thirds and a posterior one third by a V-shaped sulcus terminalis on the dorsum of the tongue. The apex of the V points posteriorly and ends in the foramen cecum, which marks the site of the embryonic thyroid diverticulum.

The mucosa over the anterior two thirds is characterized by filiform and fungiform papillae. *Filiform papillae* are the most numerous and uniformly distributed. They have a slender vascular core of connective tissue and are covered by a hyalinized, but not fully keratinized, epithelium. *Fungiform papillae* are knoblike projections that are larger and more scattered than the filiform papillae. Their epithelium is stratified squamous nonkeratinized and contains taste buds. *Vallate papillae* are the largest and least numerous of the papillae. They are oriented parallel to the sulcus terminalis and are 9 to 12 in number. Each papilla is surrounded by a trench into which underlying serous glands of von Ebner empty. The sides of the papillae and trench contain many *taste buds,* which extend intraepithelially from the basement membrane to the surface. Taste buds contain spindle-shaped neuroepithelial cells that receive sensory nerve endings. Anterior lingual glands are located near the tip of the tongue and are mixed seromucous glands.

The mucosa over the root of the tongue is stratified squamous nonkeratinized epithelium overlying connective tissue, lymphatic nodules, and mucous glands. Aggregations of lymphatic nodules around single crypts constitute lingual tonsils.

The tongue and floor of the mouth receive their blood supply from branches of the lingual artery. Branches of the lingual vein drain the tongue. The fifth, seventh, ninth, tenth, and twelfth cranial nerves supply the tongue. The hypoglossal nerve (twelfth) supplies SE fibers to the skeletal muscles. Temperature, pain, and touch receptors are supplied in the anterior two thirds of the tongue by GSA fibers of the lingual nerve from the mandibular branch of the trigeminal nerve (fifth), while GVA fibers of the glossopharyngeal (ninth) nerve subserve the same function in the posterior one third of the tongue. Taste buds in the anterior two thirds are supplied by special visceral afferent (SVA) fibers of the facial nerve (seventh) by the chorda tympani and lingual nerves. Taste buds of the vallate papillae are supplied by SVA fibers of the glossopharyngeal nerve. Taste buds and general sensations near the epiglottis are supplied by the superior laryngeal branch of the vagus nerve.

Teeth. Teeth, gums, and alveolar bone provide a wall between the vestibule and the mouth proper. There are 20 deciduous teeth and 32 permanent teeth equally distributed between the upper and lower jaws. Each tooth consists of a free crown, a root buried in an alveolus (socket) of the jaw, and a neck between the crown and root at the gum margin. Dental pulp of connective tissue, vessels, and nerves occupies a pulp chamber in the crown and root. The root is suspended in the alveolar bone by a periodontal membrane. The wall of the tooth consists of enamel, dentin, and cementum. *Enamel* is the hardest structure in the body, and it covers the crown. It consists of radially arranged rodlike enamel prisms that were elaborated by ameloblasts before the tooth erupted. Ameloblasts developed from the enamel organ, which differentiated from a dental ledge of oral ectoderm. Each of the enamel prisms is invested by a prism sheath, which is rich in organic matter. Adjacent prism sheaths are cemented together by interprismatic substance. *Dentin* lines the pulp chamber and lies internal to enamel in the crown and internal to cementum in the root. Dentin consists of a meshwork of collagen fibers oriented parallel to the surface of the tooth, and a calcified ground substance composed of GAGs and mineral salts. This dentin matrix is permeated by radially arranged dentinal tubules containing dentinal fibers (of Tomes), which are processes of odontoblasts lining the pulp chamber. These cells are necessary for the production of the dentin matrix. *Cementum* is like a bony covering of the dentin; it is more acellular and avascular than bone, but collagen lamellation and bone cells (cementocytes) are present. Cementocytes and odontoblasts arise from mesenchyme.

The sensory nerves to the maxillary teeth are branches of the maxillary division of the fifth nerve. The posterior superior alveolar nerve supplies the molars, the middle superior alveolar innervates the bicuspids, and the anterior superior alveolar supplies the canine and incisor teeth. These branches and palatine branches of the maxillary nerve also supply the gums. The lower teeth are supplied by the inferior alveolar nerve from the mandibular branch of the trigeminal nerve. Blood supply is by way of the superior alveolar branches of the maxillary artery and the inferior alveolar artery.

Palate, Isthmus of the Fauces, and Palatine Tonsil. The palate forms the roof of the mouth and consists of hard and soft portions. The *hard palate* is formed by the palatine processes of the maxillae and the horizontal portions of the palatine bones. An incisive canal penetrates it anteromedially, and greater and lesser palatine foramina lie posterolaterally. The bony palate is covered inferiorly by a mucoperiosteum that is much like that of the gums in that it consists of a stratified squamous epithelium that contains a cornified layer. An accumulation of fat is found anteriorly in the submucosa; mucous glands are plentiful in the submucosa of the posterior two thirds of the hard palate. Transverse corrugations of the mucosa in the anterior region and a median raphe also are characteristic features.

The *soft palate* is a muscular organ that extends posteriorly from the hard palate. It is lined on the nasopharyngeal side by pseudostratified cillated columnar epithelium and on the oral side and free margin by stratified squamous nonkeratinized epithelium. The submucosa contains mucous glands on the oral side and mixed glands on the nasal side. Most of the skeletal muscles of the soft palate insert into either the palatine aponeurosis, which is continuous with the pharyngobasilar fascia, or are continuous with their opposite partner in the midline. The lowest or most anterior layer of muscle is the palatoglossal muscle. As indicated previously, this muscle and the mucosa covering it constitute the anterior pillar of the fauces (glossopalatine arch). The most posterior layer of muscle is formed by the palatopharyngeus muscle, which with its mucosa constitutes the posterior pillar of the fauces (palatopharyngeal arch). The uvular muscles extend from the hard palate to the tip of the uvula.

The levator veli palatini and the tensor veli palatini are the major muscles of the palate. The tensor veli palatini arises from the scaphoid fossa at the root of the pterygoid plate; its tendon passes around the hamulus and spreads just above the glossopalatine muscle and attaches to the palatine aponeurosis. The levator veli palatini arises from the under surface of the petrous bone behind the tensor and spreads out in the soft palate above the tensor. These two muscles elevate the soft palate.

All of the muscles of the soft palate except the tensor are supplied by the vagus nerve; the tensor veli palatini is supplied by the mandibular division of the fifth cranial nerve. The principal artery of the hard palate is the greater palatine branch of the maxillary artery. It enters through the greater palatine foramen and runs forward toward the incisive canal where it anastomoses with branches of the sphenopalatine artery. The soft palate is supplied by the lesser palatine artery, ascending palatine branches of the facial artery, and branches of the ascending pharyngeal artery. Palatine veins are tributaries to the pterygoid plexus.

The isthmus of the fauces is the communication between the oral cavity proper and the oral pharynx. It is bounded above by the soft palate, below by the tongue, and laterally by the glossopalatine arch.

The palatine tonsil is located between the anterior and posterior pillars. It bulges into this depression and is covered by a mucosal fold of the anterior pillar; there is a depressed supratonsillar fossa above the tonsil. The free surface of the tonsil, lined by stratified squamous nonkeratinized epithelium, dips into the underlying lymphatic nodular aggregation as 10 to 20 branching primary and secondary crypts. Lymphocytes from the underlying diffuse and nodular lymphatic tissue often heavily infiltrate the epithelium. The tonsils produce lymphocytes; the presence of plasma cells indicates that tonsils are involved in antigen-antibody reactions. The presence of many neutrophils is characteristic of tonsillar inflammation. Each tonsil is partially invested basally by a connective tissue capsule that sends septa around the aggregations of nodules that invest each crypt. Some mucous glands and the superior pharyngeal constrictor and styloglossus muscles lie peripheral to the capsule. Efferent lymphatic vessels penetrate the pharyngeal wall and pass to superior deep cervical nodes, especially the jugulodigastric node. The arterial supply to the palatine tonsil is by the ascending palatine branch of the facial artery, tonsillar branch of the facial artery, palatine branch of the ascending pharyngeal artery, dorsal lingual branch of the lingual artery, and descending palatine branch of the maxillary artery. The nerves innervating the tonsil are branches of the maxillary division of the trigeminal nerve and the glossopharyngeal nerve.

NASAL CAVITY AND PARANASAL SINUSES

Nasal Cavity.   The nasal cavity (Fig. 2-15) extends from the base of the anterior cranial fossa to the roof of the mouth (palate) and is divided into right and left sides by the *nasal septum.* The septum is formed by the perpendicular plate of the ethmoid, the vomer, and the septal cartilage. The nasal cavity is related superiorly to the anterior cranial fossa; laterally to the ethmoid air cells, maxillary sinus, and orbit; inferiorly to the oral cavity; and posterosuperiorly to the sphenoid sinus. It opens anteriorly on the face by way of the vestibule and nares and is

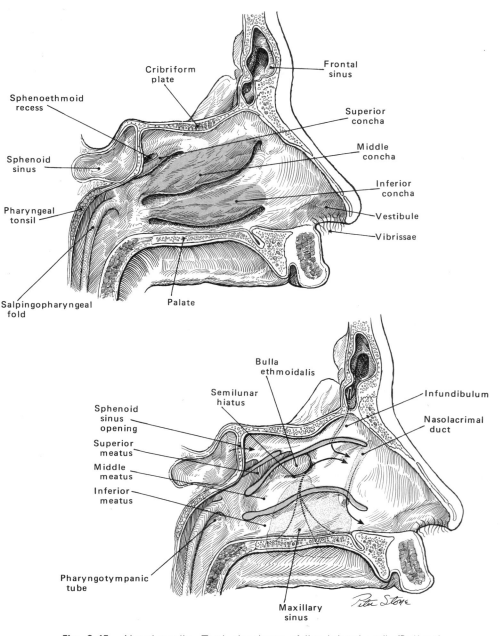

Fig. 2-15. Nasal cavity. *(Top)*, structures of the lateral wall. *(Bottom)*, drainage pathways of the paranasal sinuses and the nasolacrimal duct, with conchae removed. (Christensen JB, Telford IR: Synopsis of Gross Anatomy, 5th ed, p 395. Philadelphia, JB Lippincott, 1988)

continuous posteriorly by the choanae with the na-sopharynx. The superior, middle, and inferior *con-chae* divide the cavity into superior, middle, and inferior *meatuses.* The area posterosuperior to the superior concha is the sphenoethmoidal recess.

Most of the nasal cavity is lined by a mucoperios-teum consisting of a pseudostratified ciliated colum-nar epithelium, seromucous glands, and an exten-

sive blood supply. The venous plexuses of the conchae and septum can become engorged with blood, thus restricting the nasal passage by swelling of the mucosa. The rostral direction of the arterial blood flow in the mucosa aids in warming the air. The superior portion of the nasal cavity constitutes the *olfactory mucosa* whose pseudostratified colum-nar olfactory epithelium consists of modified bipolar neuroepithelial cells and basal and supporting cells. Nonmotile cilia of the bipolar cells are considered to be the olfactory receptor mechanism of the functional dendrite, and its axon passes to the olfactory bulb. Serous glands of Bowman empty to the olfactory surface where their secretion washes the cilia and prepares them to respond to new stimuli.

The GSA fibers to the mucosa of the nasal cavity are from the anterior and posterior ethmoidal nerves (ophthalmic V), and the lateral nasal and nasopalatine nerves (maxillary V). The olfactory epithelium in the upper part of the nasal cavity is innervated by SVA fibers from the olfactory (first cranial) nerve. All parasympathetic (GVE) fibers are from the pterygopalatine ganglion and distributed by branches of the maxillary division of the trigeminal nerve. The blood supply to the nasal cavity is provided by three arteries: the maxillary, ophthalmic, and facial arteries. The anterosuperior portions of the lateral wall and septum are supplied by the anterior and posterior ethmoidal branches of the ophthalmic artery. Most of the lateral wall (posteroinferior portion) is supplied by the lateral nasal branches of the maxillary artery, and the same area of the septum is supplied by the sphenopalatine branch of the maxillary. The area around the external nares is supplied by the superior labial branches of the facial artery.

Paranasal Sinuses. The *maxillary sinus* is related to the orbit above, the nasal cavity medially, the posterior maxillary teeth inferiorly, the infratemporal fossa posterolaterally, and the cheek anterolaterally. The sinus empties into the middle meatus by way of the hiatus semilunaris and is best drained when lying on the opposite side. Since the opening is well above the inferior extent of the sinus, the top of the head should be lower than the lower jaw for complete drainage to be accomplished.

The *frontal sinus* is in the frontal bone deep to the superciliary ridge. It is related anteriorly to the forehead, posteriorly to the anterior cranial fossa, and inferiorly to the orbit, ethmoid air cells, and the nasal cavity. It empties into the middle meatus and is best drained in the upright position.

The *ethmoid air cells* are interposed between the upper portion of the nasal cavity and the orbit. They are related superiorly to the anterior cranial fossa and inferiorly to the maxillary sinus. These sinuses drain into the superior and middle meatuses. The locations of these openings are variable, and hence the optional drainage position varies between upright and lying on the opposite side.

The *sphenoid sinus* is in the body of the sphenoid bone. It is inferior to the sella turcica, the hypophysis and the optic nerve, and bounded laterally by the cavernous sinus. The pterygoid canal is in the floor of the sinus. This sinus empties into the sphenoethmoidal recess. It drains best with the head flexed more than 90 degrees.

The mucosa of the paranasal sinuses is continuous with that of the nasal cavity but contains a thinner pseudostratified columnar epithelium and sparser glands whose mucus flows toward the nasal cavity. The secretomoter fibers to the mucosa are postganglionic parasympathetics from the pterygopalatine ganglion that are distributed primarily with branches of the maxillary nerve.

ORBITAL REGION

Osteology. The orbital cavities are four-sided pyramids. The roof of each is formed by the orbital plate of the frontal bone and the lesser wing of the sphenoid. The floor is formed by the orbital surface of the maxilla, the orbital process of the zygoma, and the orbital process of the palatine bone. The medial wall is formed by the nasal process of the maxilla, the lacrimal, the ethmoid, and the sphenoid bones. The lateral wall is formed by the orbital process of the zygomatic bone and the greater wing of the sphenoid. The orbit is related superiorly to the frontal sinus and anterior cranial fossa; medially to the nasal cavity, ethmoid air cells, and sphenoid sinus; inferiorly to the maxillary sinus; and laterally to the temporal fossa and the middle cranial fossa. The orbit communicates with the cranial cavity by way of the superior orbital fissure and the optic canal, with the infratemporal and pterygopalatine fossae by way of the inferior orbital fissure, and with the sphenoid sinuses and nasal cavity by way of the anterior and posterior ethmoidal foramina.

Contents of the Orbit. The contents of the orbit are enclosed in a tough, conically shaped layer of fascia, the *periorbita*. The periorbita is only loosely attached to the walls of the orbit (in reality it is the periosteum of these bones), and it is continuous at the apex of the orbit through the optic canal and the superior orbital fissure with the periosteal layer of cranial dura. The meningeal layer of cranial dura forms a tubular sleeve around the optic nerve; this layer blends with the sclera of the eyeball. As the arachnoid and pia also follow the optic nerve to the eyeball, the subarachnoid space surrounds the optic nerve and extends the same distance. Within the confines of the periorbita the extraocular structures are embedded in fat.

The *extraocular eye muscles* control the movements of the eyeball and the upper eyelid. The inferior oblique, levator palpebrae, and the superior, medial, and inferior rectus muscles are all innervated by the oculomotor (third) nerve. The lateral rectus is supplied by the abducens (sixth) nerve and the superior oblique by the trochlear (fourth) nerve.

The *optic nerve* enters the orbit through the optic canal and passes through the center of the orbital cone toward the eyeball. The *oculomotor, trochlear, ophthalmic,* and *abducens nerves* enter by way of the superior orbital fissure. The oculomotor nerve has two divisions: the superior supplies the superior rectus and levator palpebrae muscles, and the inferior provides the motor root (preganglionic parasympathetics) to the ciliary ganglion and innervates the medial and inferior rectus muscles and the inferior oblique. The trochlear nerve is very small and passes superomedially to the superior oblique muscle. The ophthalmic nerve divides into the lacrimal nerve, which supplies the lacrimal gland; the frontal nerve, which terminates as the supratrochlear and supraorbital nerves; and the nasociliary nerve, which has ethmoidal and infratrochlear branches. The abducens nerve passes through the lateral part of the orbit to the lateral rectus.

The *ciliary ganglion* is a parasympathetic ganglion located in the posterior third of the orbit just lateral to the optic nerve. Preganglionic fibers reach this ganglion through the motor root of the oculomotor nerve and after synapsing reach the eyeball by way of the short ciliary nerves. These fibers innervate the *sphincter pupillae* and the *ciliary muscle.* Sensory (GSA) fibers to the eyeball are provided by the nasociliary branch of the ophthalmic nerve. These fibers reach the bulb via the long ciliary nerves, which are branches of the nasociliary. In addition, the nasociliary nerve provides a sensory root to the ciliary ganglion through which sensory fibers reach the bulb by way of the ganglion and the short ciliary nerves. Sympathetic fibers reach the bulb through either long or short ciliary nerves as well as with various arteries. The *sympathetics* innervate the *dilator pupillae* muscle and the *superior tarsal muscle.*

The *ophthalmic artery* arises from the internal carotid artery as the latter passes the optic nerve. The ophthalmic artery then enters the orbit by passing inferior to the optic nerve and through the optic canal. The *central artery of the retina* enters the optic nerve about halfway along the orbital course of the nerve. It travels to the retina within the substance of the nerve (with the central vein of the retina) and is therefore surrounded by the subarach-noid space and is vulnerable to any pressure changes in that system. Other major branches of the ophthalmic artery are the ciliary branches to the eyeball, the lacrimal artery, and the ethmoidals. The superior and inferior ophthalmic veins drain primarily into the cavernous sinus, although there are communications with the pterygoid plexus and the veins of the face.

Eyelid. The upper and lower eyelids are movable folds that are separated by a palpebral fissure at their free margins. Each lid is covered by thin skin that is modified posteriorly into a mucous membrane called the palpebral conjunctiva. The palpebral conjunctiva consists of a lamina propria and stratified epithelium whose surface cells fluctuate in various regions between squamous and columnar. The palpebral conjunctiva is continuous with the bulbar conjunctiva at the fornix. The lamina propria of the palpebral conjunctiva is firmly attached to the *tarsal plate* of dense connective tissue that contains the sebaceous tarsal (meibomian) glands. The tarsal glands open onto the free border of the lid. In the upper lid the superior tarsal muscle and tendinous slips of the levator palpebrae superioris attach to the tarsal plate. Ptosis of the eye can occur in (1) Horner's syndrome, in which there is damage to the sympathetic innervation of the involuntary superior tarsal muscle; or (2) oculomotor nerve damage, in which the innervation to the skeletal superior levator palpebrae muscle is compromised. The tarsal plate is attached laterally to the zygomatic bone and medially to the frontal process of the maxilla by lateral and medial palpebral ligaments. Anterior to the tarsal plate is the palpebral portion of the orbiculus oculi muscle. A subcutaneous tissue, which seldom contains fat, lies between the skin and the orbicularis oculi muscle. Cilia (eyelashes) are large hairs arranged in two or three irregular rows on the free margins of the eyelids. Large sebaceous glands (Zeis) and large spiral sweat glands (Moll) are closely associated with the cilia.

Lacrimal Apparatus. The lacrimal apparatus consists of the lacrimal gland, lacrimal ducts, lacrimal sac, and the nasolacrimal duct. The lacrimal gland is situated near the front of the lateral roof of the orbit. Its main ducts open onto the upper lateral half of the conjunctival fornix. Microscopically this gland resembles the parotid in that it is comprised of serous acini. Tears from the lacrimal gland move across the eyeball to the medial angle of the eye where they enter the lacrimal canaliculi. The canaliculi arise on the medial margins of the upper and lower lids at the lacrimal puncta on the lacrimal papillae. The lacrimal ducts carry the lacrimal secretion medially to the lacrimal sac, which is an upward expansion of the nasolacrimal duct. The nasolacrimal duct is lined by columnar epithelium and passes downward, backward, and slightly laterally to enter the nasal cavity at the inferior meatus.

Eyeball. The eyeball consists of three layers: (1) an outer fibrous tunic composed of the sclera and cornea; (2) a vascular coat (uvea) of choroid, ciliary body, and iris; and (3) the retina formed of pigment and sensory (nervous) layers (Fig. 2-16). The anterior chamber lies between the cornea anteriorly and the iris and pupil posteriorly; the posterior chamber lies between the iris anteriorly and the ciliary processes, zonular fibers, and lens posteriorly. Both chambers possess aqueous humor, which is produced in the region of the ciliary processes and exits through the uveal meshwork and canal of Schlemm at the lateral iris angle of the anterior chamber. The canal of Schlemm drains into the anterior ciliary veins. The vitreous body occupies the space between the lens and the retina.

In embryonic development the optic nerve and retina developed as an evagination of the diencephalon, the pigment layer of the retina arising from the outer layer, and the nervous layer arising from the inner layer of the optic cup formed by indentation of the optic vesicle. The lens developed from a lens vesicle that took origin from a thickened lens placode of general surface ectoderm. The outer epithelium of the cornea also developed from surface ectoderm. The other investing tunics of the eyeball developed from head mesenchyme, while the extrinsic eye muscles arose from head (eye) somites.

The *cornea* constitutes the anterior one sixth of the eye. Its front free surface is lined with stratified squamous nonkeratinized epithelium, and its posterior surface is lined with endothelium that is continuous with the spaces of the uveal meshwork. Underlying the endothelium is a prominent basement membrane called Descemet's membrane; below the anterior epithelium is a thin connective tissue membrane (Bowman's membrane). Between both membranes is the substantia propria comprising the bulk of the cornea. This layer consists of many lamellae of collagenous fibrils held together by a glycoprotein ground substance. The collagen fibrils of adjacent layers run perpendicular to each other and may interweave from layer to layer.

The *sclera* forms the posterior five sixths of the fibrous tunic and is composed of dense fibrous connective tissue. Although continuous with the cornea, it is delimited from the cornea by internal and external scleral sulci. Nerve fibers of the optic nerve perforate it posteromedially at the optic disc, forming the lamina cribrosa. Extrinsic eye muscles insert into the sclera, and the loose outer scleral layer is continuous with the loose tissue of Tenon's space investing the eyeball. Ciliary vessels and

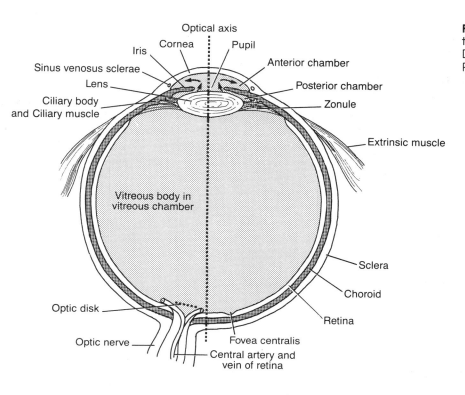

Fig. 2-16. Diagram of a horizontal section of the eye. (Cormack DH: Ham's Histology, 9th ed, p 680. Philadelphia, JB Lippincott, 1987)

nerves perforate the sclera around the entrance of the optic nerve; other emissaria, which transmit venae vorticosae from the choroid layer, occur midway between the sclerocorneal junction and the optic nerve.

The *choroid* layer consists of vascular loose connective tissue; it is separated externally from the sclera by a potential perichoroidal space and firmly attached internally to the pigment layer of the retina. The vessel and capillary layers of the choroid are the most prominent layers. The capillary layer supplies the outer layers of the retina and is the only portion of the choroid not continued forward into the ciliary body.

The *ciliary body* is bounded posteriorly at the ora serrata by the retina and choroid; laterally by the sclera; medially by the posterior chamber, vitreous body, and lens; and anteriorly by the iris. The posterior two thirds of the ciliary body is smooth on its inner surface, whereas the anterior one third bears radially arranged *ciliary processes.* The forward continuation of the choroid forms the ciliary muscle layer, vessel layer, and lamina vitrea. The forward continuation of the retina gives rise to the outer pigment and inner ciliary epithelial layers and to the internal limiting membrane. The smooth muscle of the ciliary body is oriented in meridional, radial, and circular directions. Its action is to relax the tension on the suspensory zonular ligaments, thus allowing the lens to become more convex due to its elasticity. It is supplied by parasympathetic fibers of the oculomotor nerve. Preganglionic fibers arise in the Edinger–Westphal complex of the mesencephalon, course through the oculomotor nerve and short motor root of the ciliary ganglion, and synapse with postganglionic cell bodies in the ciliary ganglion. Myelinated postganglionic nerves traverse the 12 short ciliary nerves and choroid layer to reach the ciliary body.

The vascular layer is thick in the ciliary processes, contains fenestrated capillaries, and is covered by the pigment and ciliary epithelia. The ciliary epithelium, over the summits of the processes, is modified by basal infoldings of the plasmalemma for transport. This epithelium is involved in aqueous humour formation. Occluding junctions between ciliary epithelial cells may be a major site of a blood–aqueous barrier.

The *iris* is attached peripherally to the anterior end of the ciliary body. The anterior surface of the iris demonstrates an inner pupillary zone separated from an outer ciliary zone by a collarette (iris frill). The iris is lined anteriorly by a discontinuous layer of fibroblasts and melanocytes, and posteriorly by

pigment epithelium. Underlying the anterior surface layer is an anterior border layer formed principally of chromatophores; deep to this is a vascular stromal layer containing the sphincter pupillae muscle. These layers are an anterior continuation of the uvea. The vascular stroma is bordered posteriorly by the pigment epithelium and the more deeply lying dilator pupillae muscle; these two layers are a forward continuation of the retina. The color of the iris depends on the thickness of the anterior border layer and on the pigmentation of its cells. If the layer is thick and heavily pigmented, the eyes are seen as brown; if the layer is small and little pigment is present, the light passes through the vascular stroma and is reflected off of the pigment epithelium as blue. The arterial supply to the iris is by way of long ciliary and anterior ciliary arteries from the ophthalmic division of the internal carotid arteries. These vessels form a major arterial circle in the vessel layer of the attached margin of the iris. Radial branches from this circle pass toward the pupillary margin, forming a minor arterial circle. The sphincter pupillae and dilator pupillae muscles arise from the pigment epithelium and thus are of neural ectodermal origin. The sphincter pupillae is innervated by parasympathetic fibers of the oculomotor nerve by a pathway that is similar to that for the ciliary muscle. The dilator pupillae muscle is supplied by postganglionic sympathetic fibers that arise from cell bodies in the superior cervical ganglion, follow the internal carotid artery to the cavernous plexus, pass through the nasociliary and its long ciliary branch, and traverse the choroid to reach the iris. The preganglionic sympathetic neurons arise in the intermediolateral cell column of T1 and T2 spinal cord segments, and their axons traverse the ventral roots, white communicating rami, and sympathetic trunk to attain the superior cervical ganglion.

The *retina* is divisible into ten layers: (1) pigment epithelium, (2) layer of rod and cone outer and inner segments, (3) external limiting membrane, (4) outer nuclear layer, (5) outer plexiform layer, (6) inner nuclear layer, (7) inner plexiform layer, (8) ganglion cell layer, (9) nerve fiber layer, and (10) internal limiting membrane. The simple cuboidal cells of the pigment epithelium have melanin-containing cytoplasmic processes that interdigitate with the rod and cone outer segments. Layers 2 to 5 contain the *rod* and *cone* receptors of the light pathway. The outer segments of rods and cones contain numerous stacked membranous discs derived from the plasma membrane and containing visual pigments. The outer discs of the rods differ from cones in that they lose their plasma membrane continuity and are discharged from the cell. Pigment cells phagocytize these extruded discs and also supply vitamin A to the receptor cells. The outer segment of cones and rods is connected to the inner segment by a connecting stalk containing a cilium. The inner segment contains the protein-producing endoplasmic reticulum and Golgi complex necessary for the replacement of rod discs and the nurturing of cone discs. The cell bodies and nuclei of rods and cones constitute the outer nuclear layer. The axons (pedicles) of these cells pass into the outer plexiform layer where they synapse with dendrites of bipolar cells and processes of horizontal cells. *Bipolar cells* are the second-order neuron in the visual pathway. Their nuclei are in the inner nuclear layer, and their axons synapse with dendrites of the third-order neuron ganglion cells in the inner plexiform layer. The cell bodies of midget and diffuse *ganglion cells* constitute the ganglion cell layer, and their axons form the nerve fiber layer. By these arrangements of cells one cone may synapse with one bipolar cell, which in turn synapses with one midget ganglion cell, or several rods or cones may synapse with one bipolar cell, which synapses with a diffuse ganglion cell. Horizontal interconnections are accomplished between rods and cones by horizontal cells and between ganglion cells by amacrine cells. The outer and inner limiting membranes are formed by the ends of processes of supporting Müller's cells whose nuclei, like those of bipolar, horizontal, and amacrine cells, are located in the inner nuclear layer.

All of the retinal layers external to the inner nuclear layer receive nourishment from choroid capillaries. The rest of the retina is supplied by capillaries derived from branches of the central retinal artery of the optic nerve. The retinal arteries enter at the optic disc and branch into superior and inferior nasal and superior and inferior temporal arteries, the larger branches of which run in the nerve fiber layer. The veins accompany the arteries. Diagnostically the arteries are bright red; the veins are wine colored. The arterial "reflex" from the bloodstream is broader and brighter than the venous "reflex." Choroidal vessels are pinker, flatter and more bandlike than the retinal vessels.

In examination of the fundus of the eyeball, a macula lutea is seen in the visual axis about 2½ disc diameters to the temporal side of the optic disc. It is a darker oval area in the reddish retinal field. It is devoid of vessels, and in its center is a depressed area, the fovea centralis. The *fovea* is a site for acute central vision where cones predominate and most retinal layers have been "moved aside" for more immediate access of light rays to the cones.

The *lens* is a biconvex body whose posterior surface has a greater convexity. It consists of a capsule, anterior epithelium, and lens substance. The capsule consists of basal and reticular laminae ensheathing the lens into which zonular fibers insert. The anterior epithelium contains simple cuboidal cells that become elongate at the equator of the lens where they give rise to new lens fibers. The lens substance consists of prismatic lens fibers that are meridionally arranged, with older fibers more centrally located than the newer ones. Desmosome junctions are present between the newer cells; sutures mark the junction of fibers in the central part of the lens.

EAR

Temporal Bone. The temporal bone houses the middle ear cavity, contains a network of interconnected canals that form the internal ear, and participates in the formation of various cranial and extracranial fossae. It is composed of squamous, mastoid, petrous, and tympanic parts. The *squamous portion* forms part of the mastoid process, external auditory meatus, and the mandibular fossa and has the zygomatic process, which forms part of the zygomatic arch. It helps define the middle cranial fossa. The *mastoid portion* forms most of the mastoid process and part of the wall of the posterior cranial fossa. The *tympanic part* forms most of the external auditory meatus and all of the styloid process. The *petrous portion* projects anteromedially toward the dorsum sellae where it ends. Its petrous ridge separates the anterior face from the posterior face. The anterior face forms the posterior portion of the floor of the middle cranial cavity. The posterior face is the anterolateral aspect of the posterior cranial fossa and contains the opening of the internal auditory meatus.

External Ear. The external ear is composed of the external cartilaginous portion, the pinna or auricle, and the external auditory meatus. The external auditory meatus is about 3 cm in length, connects the auricle and the middle ear cavity, and consists of a lateral cartilaginous and a medial osseous portion. In the infant the osseous meatus is merely a bony ring; in the adult it is about 2 cm long. It is narrowest at the isthmus about 0.5 cm from the tympanic membrane. The entire external auditory meatus is S shaped. The convexity of the outer cartilaginous portion is directed upward and posteriorly while that of the inner osseous portion is directed downward and anteriorly.

Middle Ear.   The middle ear, or tympanic cavity, is generally shaped like a flat cigar box. Its long axis parallels the tympanic membrane so that it is obliquely oriented, sloping medially from above downward and from behind forward. The cavity is divided into three regions: the middle ear cavity proper at the level of the tympanic membrane; the attic, or epitympanum, above the membrane; and the hypotympanum below the membrane. The cavity communicates posterolaterally with the mastoid air cells by way of the attic and mastoid antrum, and anteromedially with the nasopharynx by way of the auditory tube.

The *lateral wall* is formed primarily by the tympanic membrane. This membrane is angularly concave with its apex—the umbo—directed medially. It is composed of a fibrous stratum covered laterally by skin and medially by mucous membrane. The greater part of the periphery of the membrane is a thickened fibrocartilaginous ring that attaches to the bony tympanic sulcus. Superiorly the sulcus and fibrous stratum are deficient, and thus the membrane is lax (pars flaccida). The rest of the membrane is called the pars tensa.

The *medial wall* of the middle ear cavity separates that cavity from the inner ear. Prominent on that wall are (1) the promontory, which corresponds to the first turn of the cochlea; (2) the oval window, which contains the foot plate of the stapes and lies a little above and behind the promontory; (3) the round window below the oval window; and (4) the pyramid containing the stapedius muscle.

The roof is the *tegmen tympani,* a thin portion of the petrous temporal bone, which forms part of the floor of the middle cranial fossa. The *floor* of the middle ear is formed by the roof of the jugular foramen. The *anterior wall* is formed below by the roof of the carotid canal; above it is deficient where the auditory tube opens into the tympanic cavity. The *posterior wall* is formed inferiorly by the descending portion of the facial canal; superiorly the attic is in communication with the mastoid antrum.

The *ossicles* of the middle ear are the malleus, incus, and stapes. The manubrium of the malleus attaches to the umbo of the tympanic membrane, the foot plate of the stapes fits into the oval window, and the incus interconnects the stapes and malleus.

The *chorda tympani* nerve branches from the facial nerve and passes between the incus and malleus. The *tympanic plexus* is located on the promontory. It contains sympathetics (by way of the caroticotympanic branch of the internal carotid plexus), and sensory and parasympathetic fibers (both by way of the tympanic branch of the glossopharyngeal nerve).

The *auditory (eustachian) tube* is about 3.8 cm to 4 cm in length, extending from the tympanum obliquely forward, downward and inward. Its first third is bony; the pharyngeal two thirds are cartilaginous.

The air cells of the mastoid process communicate with the middle ear by means of the antrum and the attic. Up to the age of 5 years there is usually only one cell, the antrum, after which the mastoid consists of a large number of cells communicating with one another and the antrum. This area is lined with a continuation of the mucous membrane of the tympanum.

Inner Ear or Labyrinth.   The inner ear is contained in the petrous portion of the temporal bone and consists of an osseous labyrinth containing a membranous labyrinth. Between the bony and membranous labyrinth is perilymph. Within the membranous labyrinth is endolymph.

The *osseous labyrinth* is a series of cavities in bone consisting of a central vestibule off of which are three semicircular canals posterolaterally and the cochlea anteromedially. The vestibule is separated from the laterally situated middle ear cavity by a bony wall containing the fenestra ovalis. This oval window is closed by the foot plate of the stapes. In the posteromedial wall of the vestibule is the opening of the vestibular aqueduct, which extends to the posterior wall of the petrous portion of the temporal bone. The three *semicircular canals* are oriented at right angles to each other. The anterior (superior) and posterior canals are vertically oriented; the lateral (horizontal) canal is horizontally positioned. The positioning of the semicircular canals is such that the anterior canal of one osseous labyrinth runs parallel to the posterior canal of the other side. The anterior canal runs transverse to the long axis of the petrous bone. Its anterior limb is dilated into an ampulla just before its entrance into the vestibule; the posterior limb joins the anterior limb of the posterior canal to enter the vestibule as a crus commune. The posterior canal runs parallel to the posterior wall of the petrous bone, and its posterior limb enters the vestibule just beyond the ampulla. Both limbs of the lateral canal enter the vestibule, and an ampulla is located on the anterior limb. The *cochlea* is conical, has two and one half turns, and its apex is directed forward, outward, and downward. Mesenchymal epithelium lines the periosteum of the osseous labyrinth.

The *membranous labyrinth* consists of an interconnected series of fibrous sacs lined by simple squamous epithelium. The epithelium is derived from an otic vesicle that developed from an otic placode of general surface ectoderm. With the exception of the vestibule, the membranous labyrinth conforms generally to the contour of the osseous labyrinth. The larger membranous portion in the upper posterior part of the vestibule is the utricle; that in front of the utricle is the saccule. The utricle receives the openings of the membranous semicircular canals. The saccule communicates with the membranous cochlear duct by the ductus reuniens. An utriculosaccular duct interconnects the utricle and saccule and continues backward through the vestibular aqueduct as the endolymphatic duct. The latter duct terminates as an endolymphatic sac under the dura lining the posterior surface of the petrous portion of the temporal bone. There are six neuroepithelial receptor areas in each labyrinth: (1) macula utriculi, (2) macula sacculi, (3–5) one crista ampullaris in each ampulla, and (6) organ of Corti in the cochlear duct. The organ of Corti is supplied by the cochlear division of the eighth nerve; the maculae and cristae are innervated by the vestibular division.

The *cristae ampullares* are thickened ridges of epithelium and connective tissue placed transversely to the long axis of each semicircular canal. The epithelium of each crista consists of sustentacular cells and two configurations (types I and II) of neuroepithelial cells called *hair cells*. Each hair cell contains one kinocilium and many stereocilia that project into an overlying gelatinous mass called the cupula. In the horizontal canals the kinocilia are on the utricular side of the hair cells; in the superior (anterior) and posterior canals the kinocilia are located away from the utricle. Displacement of the stereocilia toward the kinocilia increases the rate of discharge from the hair cells, while movement in the opposite direction decreases the rate of discharge in the vestibular nerve. Thus, movement of *endolymph* toward the utricle in the ampullary end of the horizontal semicircular canal causes an increased rate of discharge in that crista. Thus, when an individual is first rotated while the lateral canals are in a horizontal position, the endolymph flow in the horizontal canal on the side of direction of rotation would be essentially ampullopetal, resulting in increased rate of discharge, while the endolymph in the other horizontal canal is ampullofugal, and there is a decreased rate of discharge. In postrotation the opposite occurs. If the head is positioned so that the horizontal canals are vertically oriented, and warm water is added to one ear, then convection currents

produce an ampullopetal flow in that ear resulting in a rate of discharge that exceeds that from the unstimulated ear. The use of cold water produces an opposite direction of endolymph flow; thus, the results are opposite to those for warm water. Both the type I and type II hair cells are innervated by the dendritic terminals of bipolar cells of the vestibular ganglion. Some cells receive efferent neurons. The vestibular ganglion lies in the upper part of the outer end of the internal auditory meatus. Axons from the vestibular ganglion pass medially in the internal auditory canal as the vestibular portion of the vestibulocochlear nerve and enter the brain stem at the pons-medulla junction.

The *maculae* are similar to the cristae in that they are local thickenings of the membrane, they contain hair cells and sustentacular cells, and their hair cells penetrate a gelatinous membrane. The macular gelatinous membrane contains calcium carbonate crystals called otoliths (otoconia) and is called the otolithic membrane. The hair cells in various regions of the macula utriculi have their kinocilia placed on different sides so that the macula can detect linear acceleration and the position of the head in respect to gravitational forces. The macula of the saccule also is involved with equilibratory action.

The *organ of Corti* is located on the basilar membrane of the membranous cochlear duct. The *cochlear duct* (scala media) is filled with endolymph, runs throughout most of the cochlea, and is separated from the upper scala vestibuli by the vestibular membrane and from the lower scala tympani by the basilar membrane. The basilar membrane is suspended between the centrally located osseous spiral lamina of the modiolus and the peripherally located periosteal thickening called the spiral ligament. On the lateral wall of the cochlear duct is the stria vascularis. It is highly vascular, is lined with pseudostratified columnar epithelium and is involved in endolymph production. The organ of Corti is an arrangement of supportive and hair cells on the upper border of the basilar membrane. The neuroepithelial hair cells are arranged into inner and outer hair cells by their relationship to an inner tunnel (of Corti) formed by inner and outer pillar cells. The hair cells are supported by outer and inner phalangeal cells whose phalangeal processes form a firm reticular lamina at the peripheral surfaces of the hair cells. The microvillous hairs of the hair cells are in contact with the overlying gelatinous tectorial membrane, thus establishing a mechanism wherein movement of the basilar membrane will cause stimulation of hair cells by bending of the microvilli.

This mechanical stimulus is transduced into electrical energy by the hair cells and transmitted to the terminal dendritic endings of the special somatic afferent (SSA) cells of the spiral cochlear ganglion. Axons of these bipolar nerve cells pass into the axis of the modiolus, course upward into the internal acoustic meatus, become the cochlear portion of the vestibulocochlear nerve, and synapse in the dorsal and ventral cochlear nuclei at the pons-medulla junction of the brain stem.

The blood supply of the labyrinth is by way of the internal auditory (labyrinthine) and stylomastoid arteries. The stylomastoid is a branch of the posterior auricular. The internal auditory arises from the basilar artery, or in common with the anterior inferior cerebellar artery, and traverses the internal acoustic meatus before branching into cochlear and vestibular branches. The veins accompany the arteries and drain as internal auditory veins into the superior petrosal or transverse sinuses.

PITUITARY GLAND

The pituitary gland, or hypophysis, (Fig. 2-17) is located in the sella turcica of the body of the sphenoid bone. It is attached to the hypothalamus by its pituitary stalk, which penetrates the diaphragma sellae, a dural covering to the sella turcica. The hypophysis is in relation laterally to the internal carotid artery and the other contents of the cavernous sinus; it is bounded rostrally and superiorly by the optic chiasma. It is composed of an adenohypophysis and a neurohypophysis. The gland is about 1.5 cm in its greatest diameter and about 1 cm in its rostrocaudal extent.

The *adenohypophysis* consists of a pars tuberalis, which forms an anterolateral cuff to the infundibulum, a *pars distalis* (anterior lobe), which produces most adenohypophyseal hormones, and a pars intermedia, which is interposed between the pars distalis anteriorly and the pars nervosa posteriorly.

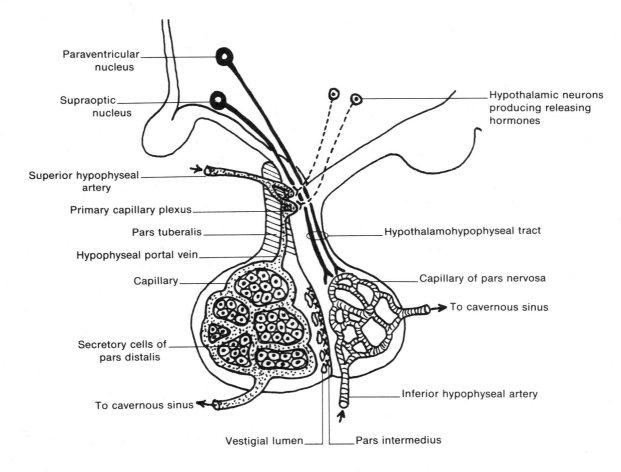

Fig. 2-17. Diagram of the pituitary gland, its vascularity, and the hypothalamo-hypophyseal pathways.

The parenchyma of the pars distalis is comprised of cords of cells that are closely apposed to fenestrated sinusoidal capillaries. The latter receive venous trunks originating from capillary loops (primary capillary plexus) that extend into the pars tuberalis and infundibular stalk; this vascular arrangement constitutes the hypophyseal portal system. The capillary loops are supplied by superior hypophyseal arteries, which arise from the internal carotid and posterior communicating arteries. The cell cords of the pars distalis are comprised of chromophils and chromophobes. Chromophobes are considered to be degranulated chromophils. Chromophils are divisible by the staining reaction of their secretion granules into various types of **basophils** and **acidophils** which produce the hormones of the pars distalis (Table 2-1). The release of these hormones into the adjacent capillaries is controlled by releasing and inhibiting hormones produced in hypothalamic neurons, and secreted into the portal system in the infundibular stalk. The pars intermedia and pars tuberalis consist mainly of basophils.

The **neurohypophysis** consists of the infundibular stalk and pars nervosa, and by some definitions includes the median eminence and secretory neurons of the hypothalamus. The secretory cells of the neurohypophysis are hypothalamic neurons. Cell bodies in the supraoptic and paraventricular nuclei of the hypothalamus give rise to unmyelinated axons that help make up the **hypothalamohypophyseal tract** of the infundibular stalk before termination in adjacent fenestrated capillaries in the pars nervosa. Glial supportive cells of the pars nervosa are called pituicytes. The hormones produced and transported in the neurons (Table 2-1), their binding protein (neurophysin), and ATP constitute a neurosecretory material that may accumulate in the axons and their endings as Herring bodies before discharge into the capillaries. Secretory neurons from other hypothalamic nuclei (*e.g.*, preoptic, arcuate, dorsomedial) send axons to the infundibular stalk where they empty their releasing or inhibitory hormones into the primary capillary plexus of the portal system. The neurohypophysis is supplied by inferior hypophyseal arteries from the internal carotid. The veins of the hypophysis are the lateral hypophyseal veins, which drain to the cavernous and intercavernous sinuses.

DEVELOPMENT OF THE HEAD AND NECK

Development and Fate of the Branchial Arches. During the third and fourth weeks of development the embryo develops head and tail folds that result in the incorporation of the dorsal portions of the primitive yolk sac entoderm as foregut, midgut, and hindgut. The rostral portion of the *foregut* (primitive pharynx) develops five lateral pairs of *pharyngeal pouches;* these and the floor of the pharynx give rise to the tongue, pharynx, thyroid gland, parathyroid glands, and thymus gland. The more caudal portions of the foregut will develop into the esophagus, stomach, part of the duodenum, and the liver and pancreas.

While the pharyngeal pouches are forming internally, five pairs of branchial (pharyngeal) arches appear externally. These are numbered 1, 2, 3, 4, and 6. They are separated by branchial (pharyngeal)

TABLE 2-1. Hormones of the Pituitary Gland

HORMONES	CELLS OF ORIGIN	RELEASING AND INHIBITING HORMONES
Pars distalis		
Growth hormone (GH)	Acidophils	Growth hormone–releasing factor (GRF)
		Somatostatin (growth-inhibiting hormone, GIH)
Prolactin (PRL)	Acidophils	Prolactin-releasing factor (PRF)
		Prolactin-inhibiting factor (PIF)
Thyroid-stimulating hormone (TSH)	Basophils	Thyrotropin-releasing hormone (TRH)
Follicle-stimulating hormone (FSH)	Basophils	Gonadotropin-releasing hormone (GnRH)
Luteinizing hormone (LH)	Basophils	Gonadotropin-releasing hormone (GnRH)
Adrenocorticotropic hormone (ACTH)	Basophils	Corticotropin-releasing factor (CRF)
Pars intermedia		
Melanocyte-stimulating hormone (MSH)	Basophils	MSH-releasing factor (MRF)
		MSH-inhibiting factor (MIF)
Pars nervosa		
Oxytocin	Paraventricular neurons	
Antidiuretic hormone (ADH, vasopressin)	Supraoptic and paraventricular neurons	

grooves, which are aligned with the pharyngeal pouches to form branchial (pharyngeal) membranes consisting of outer ectodermal and inner entodermal layers. Each groove is numbered according to the arch that lies rostral to it. Each branchial arch is comprised of an outer ectodermal layer and an inner entodermal lining with a vertical bar of mesoderm and a cranial nerve interposed between the two layers.

The first arch is divisible into mandibular and maxillary arches. The surface ectoderm of these arches will become the epidermis of the upper and lower jaws, the epithelium of most of the oral cavity, the parenchyma of the major salivary glands, and the enamel of the teeth. The mandibular and maxillary divisions of the trigeminal nerve course in these arches and supply the skin of the face with sensory nerves (GSA) and the muscles of mastication with motor (SVE) nerves. The muscles developing from the mandibular arch are the temporalis, masseter, medial and lateral pterygoids, mylohyoid, anterior belly of the digastric, tensor veli palatini, and tensor tympani. Mesenchyme and neural crest of the mandibular arch develop into a transitory Meckel's cartilage before forming a mandible, malleus and incus; mesenchyme of the maxillary arch forms the maxilla. The first branchial groove gives rise to the external acoustic meatus. The first branchial membrane develops into the tympanic membrane, and the first pharyngeal pouch presages part of the auditory (eustachian) tube and middle ear cavity.

The second (hyoid) arch grows back over arches 3 to 6 and will fuse with them, obliterating branchial grooves 3 to 6 and a transitory cervical sinus that was formed in this caudal growth. Improper obliteration of the cervical sinus can result in a cervical cyst. Cervical (branchial) fistulas may remain if communications are retained externally or internally through the branchial membranes. Since the ectoderm of the second arch gives rise to the epidermis of much of the neck, the openings of external branchial fistulas occur in the neck along the anterior margin of the sternocleidomastoid muscle. Internal fistulas most often occur into the second pouch. Since the tonsil develops in the region of the second pouch, internal fistulas of the second pouch open into the tonsillar region. Mesenchyme of the second arch gives rise to the muscles of facial expression, the stapedius, posterior belly of the digastric and stylohyoid muscles. It, along with neural crest, also gives rise to the stapes, styloid process, stylohyoid ligament, and lesser cornua of the hyoid bone. The facial nerve runs in the second arch and supplies SVE neurons to the muscles developing from this arch.

The third pharyngeal arch gives rise to the stylopharyngeus muscle supplied by the glossopharyngeal nerve and to the body and greater cornua of the hyoid bone. The entoderm of the dorsal part of the third pharyngeal pouch gives rise to parathyroid III, which will develop further into the parenchyma of the inferior parathyroid gland. The ventral part of the third pharyngeal pouch becomes the thymus gland.

The fourth and sixth arches give rise to the laryngeal cartilages and the pharyngeal, palatal, and laryngeal muscles. All of these, except the tensor palatini and stylopharyngeus, are innervated by the vagus (and accessory?) nerve, with the superior laryngeal branch supplying the fourth arch and the recurrent laryngeal branch passing through the sixth arch. The dorsal part of the fourth pharyngeal pouch gives rise to the superior parathyroid gland; the fate of the ventral part is not certain. The fifth (sixth) pharyngeal pouch gives rise to the ultimobranchial body, which is implicated in the formation of the calcitonin-producing parafollicular cells of the thyroid gland.

Aortic arches arise from the aortic bulb and enter each branchial arch, where they run chiefly caudal to the cranial nerve of each arch. The first two aortic arches in the mandibular and hyoid arches disappear (see Fig. 2-27). The third aortic arch becomes a part of the internal carotid and common carotid arteries. The right fourth arch becomes part of the right subclavian artery, and the left fourth arch becomes the arch of the aorta. The proximal portions of both sixth aortic arches become parts of the pulmonary arteries; the left distal part becomes the ductus arteriosus. Since the recurrent laryngeal is caudal to the sixth aortic arch, retention of the ductus arteriosus as the ligamentum arteriosum accounts for the left recurrent laryngeal looping around the arch of the aorta caudal to the ligament, whereas the right loops higher around the subclavian artery.

The tongue develops from elevations in the floor of the primitive pharynx and by forward migration of developing muscle from occipital somites. The body of the tongue arises from two lateral swellings and a median tuberculum impar in the floor of the mandibular arch. The root of the tongue develops from a copula of mesenchyme of the second, third, and fourth arches. The epiglottic swelling also comes from mesenchyme of the fourth arch. The muscles of the tongue develop from occipital somites and are innervated by SE fibers of the hypoglossal nerve. Since the oral membrane, demarcating the ectodermally lined stomodeum from the entodermal primitive pharynx, existed just in front of the fauces, most of the epithelium of the body of the tongue arose from ectoderm while the root and foramen cecum area developed from entoderm. Thus, general sensation of the anterior two thirds of the tongue is supplied by branches of the trigeminal nerve, whereas the posterior one third is innervated by the glossopharyngeal nerve. The thyroid gland develops as an evagination from the floor of the pharynx at the level of the first pharyngeal pouch. It migrates caudally to the region of the larynx, leaving the foramen cecum as the site of original evagination and often leaving thyroglossal duct cysts along its migratory course. Thyroglossal duct cysts can be found in the root of the tongue and in or behind the hyoid bone.

Development of the Face, Nasal Cavity, and Oral Cavity. By the sixth week of embryonic development a frontal prominence overhangs the cephalic end of the stomodeum. It is bounded laterally by nasal pits surrounded by horseshoe-shaped elevations. The medial portion of the horseshoe-shaped elevation is the *nasomedial process;* the lateral portion is the *nasolateral process.* The nasolateral process is delimited from the maxillary process by the naso-optic (nasolacrimal) furrow. The developing oral cavity is bounded inferiorly by distal fusion of the mandibular processes of the first branchial arch. As the maxillary processes become more prominent they fuse with the nasomedial processes and push them toward the midline; this displaces the frontal prominence upward and leads to fusion of the nasomedial processes in the midline. The fused nasomedial processes (intermaxillary segment) give rise to the medial part of the upper lip and distal nose, incisor teeth and associated upper jaw, and the primary palate (median palatine process). The *maxillary process* gives rise to the rest of the upper lip, teeth, and jaw and the palatine shelves forming the secondary palate. The lower lips, jaw, and teeth are formed from the *mandibular processes.* The nasolacrimal duct is formed at the point of obliteration of the naso-optic furrow by fusion of the nasolateral and maxillary processes. Inability of these processes to fuse leads to an oblique facial cleft. The nasolateral processes give rise to the alae of the nose.

The *nasal pits* become deeper and break through the bucconasal membrane into the primitive oral cavity. Toward the end of the second embryonic month the *palatine shelves* (lateral palatine processes) of the maxillary processes grow medially and fuse with the primary palate, rostrally, and with each other and with the inferiorly growing nasal septum caudally. The lateral palatine processes thus give rise to a secondary palate, which separates the nasal cavity above from the definitive oral cavity below. The caudal free borders of the palatine shelves project as the soft palate into the pharynx, dividing it into an upper nasopharynx and lower oropharynx. Incomplete degeneration of the bucconasal membrane can lead to choanal atresia. Failure of the palatine shelves to fuse in the midline, or to fuse with the primary palate, produce cleft palate. Such clefts can be divided into three groups: (1) those occurring between the palatine shelves and the primary palate (anterior, primary palate types); (2) those occurring posterior to the incisive foramen at the point of fusion of the palatine shelves with each other (posterior, secondary palate types); and (3) those involving defects in both the anterior and posterior palate (complete unilateral or bilateral types). The anterior and complete types may be associated with cleft lip if the nasomedial and maxillary processes fail to merge (fuse). Median cleft of the upper lip and jaw is due to the lack of fusion of the nasomedial processes with each other.

Development of the Hypophysis. The hypophysis arises from two sources: Rathke's pouch and the infundibulum. Rathke's pouch arises as an evagination of stomodeal ectoderm that pinches off from the stomodeum and migrates toward the diencephalon where it becomes adherent to the rostral surface of the infundibulum. The infundibulum develops as an outgrowth of neural ectoderm from the hypothalamus of the diencephalon. The infundibulum gives rise to the neurohypophysis; Rathke's pouch develops into the adenohypophysis.

CENTRAL NERVOUS SYSTEM AND CRANIAL NERVES

The structure and localization of the spinal cord and spinal nerves were covered previously in the section on the back.

Cranial Cavity. The cranial cavity (Fig. 2-18) is formed by a roof (calvaria) and a floor. The calvaria is formed by the single frontal and occipital bones, the paired parietal bones, and portions of the greater wings of the sphenoid, and the squamous parts of the temporal bones. The parietal bones are united by the sagittal suture and with the frontal bone at the coronal suture. Posteriorly the occipital and parietal bones are united at the lambdoidal suture.

The floor of the cranial cavity is divisible into

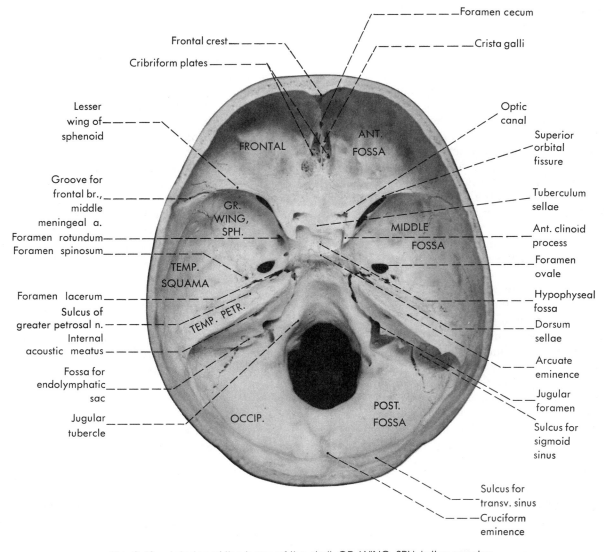

Foramen cecum

Crista galli

Frontal crest

Cribriform plates

Lesser wing of sphenoid

Optic canal

Superior orbital fissure

FRONTAL

ANT. FOSSA

Groove for frontal br., middle meningeal a.

GR. WING, SPH.

Tuberculum sellae

Foramen rotundum

Ant. clinoid process

Foramen spinosum

MIDDLE FOSSA

Foramen ovale

TEMP. SQUAMA

Foramen lacerum

Hypophyseal fossa

Sulcus of greater petrosal n.

TEMP. PETR.

Dorsum sellae

Internal acoustic meatus

Arcuate eminence

Fossa for endolymphatic sac

Jugular foramen

Jugular tubercle

OCCIP.

POST. FOSSA

Sulcus for sigmoid sinus

Sulcus for transv. sinus

Cruciform eminence

Fig. 2-18. Interior of the base of the skull. GR. WING, SPH. is the greater wing of the sphenoid; TEMP. SQUAMA and TEMP. PETR. are the squamous and petrous portions of the temporal bone; and OCCIP. is the occipital bone. (Hollinshead WH: Anatomy For Surgeons, Vol 1, 3rd ed, p 57. Philadelphia, JB Lippincott, 1982)

three cranial fossae: anterior, middle, and posterior. The **anterior cranial fossa** is formed medially by the cribiform plate of the ethmoid and the crista galli, and laterally by the orbital plate of the frontal bone. Posteriorly both the body of the sphenoid and its lesser wing participate in the formation of this fossa, which is related anteromedially to the frontal sinus and inferiorly to the nasal cavity, ethmoid sinuses, and the orbit. The multiple openings in the cribiform plate transmit the rootlets of the olfactory nerve; the foramen cecum anterior to the crista galli may transmit an emissary vein between the nasal cavity and the superior sagittal sinus. The anterior

cranial fossa houses the frontal lobes of the brain and the olfactory bulbs and tracts.

The **middle cranial fossa** has a central and two lateral portions. The **central part** is formed by the body of the sphenoid and consists of the sella turcica posteriorly and the chiasmatic groove anteriorly; it houses the hypophysis (pituitary) and optic chiasm. This part of the fossa is related inferiorly (and anteriorly) to the sphenoid sinus and laterally to the cavernous sinus. The optic canals convey the optic nerves open into the orbits.

The **lateral part of the middle cranial fossa** houses the temporal lobe of the brain and is formed by the greater wing of the sphenoid and parts of both the squamous and petrous portions of the temporal bone. This part of the fossa is related inferiorly to the infratemporal fossa and middle ear cavity, laterally to the temporal fossa, anteriorly to the orbit, and medially to the sphenoid sinus. There are a number of openings in this fossa. The superior orbital fissure (containing the ophthalmic division of the trigeminal, oculomotor, trochlear, and abducens nerves, and the ophthalmic veins) opens into the orbit; the foramen rotundum (containing the maxillary division of the trigeminal nerve) opens into the pterygopalatine fossa; the foramen ovale (containing the mandibular division of the trigeminal nerve) and the foramen spinosum transmitting the middle meningeal artery) open into the infratemporal fossa. The foramen lacerum is an irregularly shaped opening at the apex of the petrous pyramid; in life, this opening is filled by fibrous tissue and is the floor of the carotid canal and thus nothing passes through the opening.

The *posterior cranial fossa* is formed by the posterior aspect of the body of the sphenoid, a portion of the petrous portion of the temporal bone, and the occipital bone. Anteriorly in the midline the inclined plane formed by the sphenoid and the basilar portion of the occipital bone is occupied by the brain stem; the midbrain is surrounded by the notch of the tentorium cerebelli. The cerebellum occupies the rest of the posterior fossa. The foramen magnum, the large single opening in this fossa, transmits the spinal cord–brain stem junction and its meningeal coverings, the accessory nerve, the vertebral and the anterior and posterior spinal arteries, and the communication between the dural venous sinuses and the internal vertebral venous plexus. The hypoglossal canal transmits the hypoglossal nerve, and the jugular foramen contains the glossopharyngeal, vagus, and accessory nerves, and the continuity between the dural venous sinuses and the internal jugular vein. The internal acoustic meatus is an opening on the posterior face of the petrous pyramid, which transmits the facial and vestibulocochlear nerves and the labyrinthine artery.

Gross Brain Topography. The brain consists of three basic parts, the cerebral hemispheres (telencephalon), the brain stem, and the cerebellum. The cerebral hemispheres and cerebellum cover much of the superior and lateral surface of the brain stem. From the cerebral hemispheres to the spinal cord the brain stem consists of (1) the diencephalon, (2) the mesencephalon, (3) the metencephalon (pons), and (4) the myelencephalon (medulla). In relation to the skull the frontal and temporal lobes of the cerebral hemispheres lie in the anterior and middle cranial fossae, respectively; the cerebellar hemispheres are in the posterior cranial fossa. The diencephalon, mesencephalon, and pons rest on the superior surface and clivus of the body of the sphenoid bone, while the medulla occupies a groove on the basilar part of the occipital bone extending from the sphenoid to the foramen magnum. The brain is invested by dura, arachnoid, and pia mater.

The *dura* serves as the periosteum of the skull and also reflects between the cerebral hemispheres in the longitudinal cerebral fissure as the falx cerebri. The falx is continuous posterioriy with another dural reflection, the tentorium cerebelli, lying in the transverse cerebral fissure between the occipital lobe of the telencephalon above and the cerebellum below. Important venous sinuses are found in the dura. The superior sagittal sinus in the attached margin of the falx cerebri drains to the transverse sinuses at the periphery of the tentorium cerebelli. These in turn drain to the internal jugular veins via the sigmoid sinuses. An inferior sagittal sinus in the free margin of the falx cerebri and the great vein of Galen from the brain drain to the straight sinus running in the junction of the falx and tentorium. The straight sinus drains to the transverse sinus. An anterior group of sinuses includes the cavernous, intercavernous, superior and inferior petrosal sinuses and basilar plexus.

The *arachnoid* does not project into the sulci of the telencephalon, and it is separated from the pia by a subarachnoid space. This space is enlarged into subarachnoid cisterna at the cerebellum–medulla junction (cisterna magna), between the cerebral peduncles (interpeduncular cistern), superior and lateral to the midbrain (cisterna ambiens), and at several other areas. Arachnoid granulations, projecting nto the superior sagittal sinus, serve as a mechanism for the flow of cerebrospinal fluid from the subarachnoid space into the venous system. The *pia* is vascular, and the underlying glial membrane blends with the walls of pial blood vessels as they penetrate the brain substance. Tight junctions of the nonfenestrated brain capillaries provide the chief component of the *blood–brain barrier.*

The *cerebral hemispheres* are interconnected by a corpus callosum and an anterior commissure of commissural fibers and by the lamina terminalis, which lies rostral to the third ventricle. Each cerebral hemisphere consists of an outer gray *cortex* (pallium), underlying white matter, a deeply located nuclear mass called the *basal ganglia,* and a lateral ventricle. The cortex and its underlying white matter are thrown into a fairly consistent localization of gyri and sulci that make it possible to define frontal, parietal, temporal, occipital, insular, and limbic lobes. The more rostral *frontal lobe* is separated from the parietal lobe by the central sulcus (of Rolando). In the frontal lobe the precentral gyrus (motor area) borders the central sulcus, and is demarcated from the more rostral superior, middle, and inferior frontal gyri by the precentral sulcus (see Fig. 2-20). On the basal surface the frontal lobe is comprised of an olfactory bulb and tract lying between the gyrus rectus and the orbital gyri. The *parietal lobe* consists of the more rostral postcentral gyrus (somesthetic area) and the posteriorly located superior and inferior parietal gyri. On the medial aspect the parietal and occipital lobes are divisible by the parieto-occipital sulcus; laterally the boundary is less precise. The lateral fissure (sulcus) helps to form an inferior boundary to the frontal and parietal lobes. It terminates caudally where the inferior parietal gyrus caps it as the supramarginal gyrus. The rest of the inferior parietal gyrus abuts against the posterior extent of the superior temporal sulcus and is called the angular gyrus.

The lateral surface of the *occipital lobe* consists of lateral occipital gyri. The medial surface is divided by the calcarine fissure into a cuneus above and a lingual gyrus below. That portion of the cortex immediately bordering the calcarine fissure is the striate (visual) cortex. The lateral surface of the *temporal lobe* is comprised of superior, middle, and inferior temporal gyri. The transverse temporal gyri (of Heschl) lie medial to the superior temporal gyrus in the floor of the lateral fissure. It is the primary receptive area for hearing. The insula lies deep in the lateral fissure and constitutes a cortical cover to the lenticular nucleus. On the basal surface of the temporal lobe the occipitotemporal gyrus and parahippocampal gyri lie medial to the inferior temporal gyri. The more medial parahippocampal gyrus ends rostrally as the uncus, is bounded laterally by the collateral fissure and medially by the hippocampal fissure, and is continuous around the caudal end (splenium) of the corpus callosum with the cingulate gyrus. The rostral part of the parahippocampal gyrus, the uncus, and the lateral olfactory stria and gyrus (which project from the olfactory trigone and tract), comprise the primary olfactory receptive area. The *limbic lobe* includes the subcallosal, cingulate, and parahippocampal gyri, as well as the dentate gyrus and hippocampus, which lie deep to the hippocampal fissure.

The *diencephalon* contains the third ventricle and is divisible into four parts: the roof or epithalamus, the dorsolaterally located thalamus, the floor and ventromedially oriented hypothalamus, and the ventrolateral subthalamus. The diencephalon is bounded above by the transverse cerebral fissure. While this fissure extends caudally between the occipital lobe and cerebellum and is occupied by the tentorium cerebelli, rostrally it lies between the corpus callosum and fornix above and the epithalamus (tela choroidea, pineal body, habenula) and thalamus below. It extends laterally and ventrally as the choroid fissures adjacent to the choroid plexuses of the lateral and third ventricles, respectively. Rostrally, the transverse cerebral fissure ends blindly behind the interventricular foramen (of Monro) where the choroid plexus of the third ventricle is continuous with that of the lateral ventricle. The diencephalon is bounded laterally by the internal capsule and the cerebral peduncles. Basally the surface shows anteroposteriorly the optic chiasm, infundibular stalk and pituitary gland, and mammillary bodies.

The *mesencephalon* lies between the diencephalon and pons. Its dorsal surface consists of two superior colliculi, two inferior colliculi, the brachia of these colliculi, which connect to the lateral and medial geniculate nuclei of the diencephalon, respectively, and the emerging trochlear (fourth) nerve. Ventrally the mesencephalon demonstrates cerebral peduncles, interpeduncular fossa, and emerging oculomotor (third) nerves. An iter (cerebral aqueduct of Sylvius) connects the third ventricle of the diencephalon with the fourth ventricle in the pons.

The *pons* is bounded dorsally by the attached cerebellum. The lateral surface is made up of the middle cerebellar peduncle with its emerging root of the trigeminal (fifth) nerve. Ventrally the basis pontis forms a bridge between the middle cerebellar peduncles. On the superior aspect the superior medullary velum, superior cerebellar peduncles, and cerebellum form the roof of the fourth ventricle. The tegmentum forms the floor of the ventricle and demonstrates a facial colliculus in the medial eminence located medial to the sulcus limitans.

The *cerebellum* overlies the posterior surface of the pons and upper medulla. It consists of a midline vermis and two lateral hemispheres. The surface of the cerebellum has elevations called folia, which are separated by sulci. On the superior surface a primary fissure separates an anterior lobe (paleocerebellum) from the posterior lobe (neocerebellum). On the inferior surface a posterolateral fissure demarcates the posterior lobe from the flocculonodular lobe (archicerebellum). There is another phylogenetic division of the cerebellum into a vermis (archicerebellum), paravermis (paleocerebellum), and lateral hemispheres (neocerebellum). The cerebellum is attached to the brain stem by paired inferior, middle, and superior cerebellar peduncles—which basically connect the cerebellum to the medulla, pons, and mesencephalon, respectively. The substance of the cerebellum consists of a cortex of gray matter, a medullary core called the arbor vitae, and four pairs of deep nuclei. Afferent neurons to the cerebellum enter primarily by way of the inferior and middle cerebellar peduncles and ascend in the arbor vitae to synapse on cells of the granular layer of the cortex. Axons of granular cells ascend to the molecular layer where they run parallel to the folia and synapse with dendrites of Purkinje cells, which send axons to the deep nuclei. Of these Purkinje axons, those from the neocerebellum synapse on cells of the dentate nuclei, those from the paleocerebellum synapse in the emboliform and globose nuclei, and those from the archicerebellun synapse in the fastigial nuclei. Axons from cells in the dentate, emboliform, and globose nuclei project to the thalamus and red nucleus by way of the superior cerebellar peduncles, while those from the fastigial nuclei pass by way of the inferior cerebellar peduncle (juxtarestiform body) to terminate in vestibular nuclei.

The upper part of the *medulla* (open medulla) contains a portion of the fourth ventricle. A tela choroidea of pia and ependyma form the roof of this part of the fourth ventricle. The floor is divisible into a medial eminence and a more lateral vestibular area. At the junction of the pons and medulla the fourth ventricle is open laterally to the subarachnoid space through the foramen of Luschka. A midline opening, the foramen of Magendie, is located at the caudalmost tip of the tela choroidea. The dorsal surface of the more inferior closed part of the medulla represents an enlarged upward continuation of the fasciculus cuneatus and fasciculus gracilis of the spinal cord. These areas are referred to as the tuberculum cuneatum and tuberculum gracilis (clava). They lie caudal and lateral to the fourth ventricle.

The ventral surface of the medulla, from the midline laterally, consists of pyramids and pyramidal decussation, preolivary sulcus, olivary eminence, and postolivary sulcus. The abducens (sixth) nerve exits at the pons–medulla junction in line with the hypoglossal (twelfth) nerve rootlets, which emerge from the preolivary sulcus. The glossopharyngeal (ninth), cranial accessory (eleventh), and vagus (tenth) nerves exit from the postolivary sulcus. The facial (seventh) and vestibulocochlear (eighth) nerves emerge below the lateral recess of the fourth ventricle at the pons–medulla junction. They are in close anatomic relationship to the inferior cerebellar peduncle (restiform body), which courses anterior to the lateral recess in passing from the medulla to the cerebellum.

Blood Supply to the Brain. The brain is supplied by the vertebral and internal carotid arteries. The *vertebral arteries* enter the foramen magnum and give off posterior inferior cerebellar and anterior and posterior spinal arteries. The *vertebral arteries* unite at the pons–medulla junction to form the basilar artery. The basilar artery runs in the basilar sulcus of the pons and terminates at the level of the mesencephalon by branching into posterior cerebral arteries. The basilar gives off the anterior inferior cerebellar, labyrinthine, paramedian, short and long circumferential and superior cerebellar arteries. Branches of the vertebral and basilar arteries supply the cerebellum, mesencephalon, pons, medulla, medial portion of the occipital lobe, and part of the temporal lobe and diencephalon.

The *internal carotid artery* courses through the cavernous sinus and emerges from the sinus medial to the anterior clinoid process. It gives off the ophthalmic artery to the eye; the posterior communicating artery to the posterior cerebral artery; and the anterior choroidal artery, which supplies the optic tract, choroid plexus of the lateral ventricle, basal ganglia, posterior part of the internal capsule, and the hippocampus. Lateral to the optic chiasm the internal carotid bifurcates into the middle cerebral and anterior cerebral arteries. The anterior cerebral arteries, connected by an anterior communicating artery, supply the medial surface of the frontal and parietal lobes. The middle cerebral artery passes into the lateral fissure and supplies the insula, lateral surface of the cerebral hemisphere, and part of the inferior surface of the temporal lobe. Basal ganglia and part of the internal capsule are supplied by the lenticulostriate branches of the middle cerebral artery. The internal carotid and vertebral arterial supplies are interconnected, forming the *circle of Willis,* which consists of the anterior communicating, anterior cerebral, posterior communicating, and posterior cerebral arteries. Central branches from the circle of Willis supply the basilar portion of the brain stem and basal ganglia and give rise to the hypophyseal portal arterial system of the adenohypophysis.

Lesions resulting in vascular deficiency of the anterior cerebral artery result in contralateral UMN paralysis or paresis of the leg and foot and loss of two-point touch and vibratory sense in the leg and foot region. Compromise of the posterior cerebral artery leads to contralateral homonymous hemianopsia and may damage portions of the thalamus. Middle cerebral artery damage can give UMN and sensory losses to the contralateral upper extremity trunk and face. It may also result in aphasia, agnosia, and apraxia. Posterior inferior cerebellar artery occlusion can result in Horner's syndrome, a contralateral loss of pain and temperature on the extremities and trunk, an ipsilateral loss of pain and temperature on the face, and a loss of functions mediated by way of the glossopharyngeal and vagus nerves.

Superficial and deep cerebral veins drain to the dural venous sinuses. The great cerebral vein (Galen) receives the internal cerebral veins and drains to the straight sinus. Superior, middle, and inferior superficial veins drain to the superior sagittal or basal sinuses. The midbrain, pons, and medulla drain by small veins into the sinuses at the base of the brain. The cerebellum is drained by superior and inferior cerebellar veins into adjacent dural venous sinuses.

Circulation of Cerebrospinal Fluid. Cerebrospinal fluid is formed by the choroid plexuses of the lateral, third, and fourth ventricles. Cerebrospinal fluid passes from the lateral ventricle through the interventricular foramen (of Monro) to the third ventricle and thence through the iter into the fourth ventricle. It exits through the foramina of Luschka and Magendie into the subarachnoid space (cisterna magna) and diffuses into the superior longitudinal sinus through the arachnoid granulations. Internal hydrocephalus may result from blockage of the ventricular pathway and most commonly occurs in the iter. Hydrocephalus resulting from blockage of the foramina of Luschka and Magendie affects all of the ventricles.

Development of the Brain. By the fourth week of embryonic development the neural tube of the cephalic region appears as three vesicles: the prosencephalon, mesencephalon, and rhombencephalon. The prosencephalon enlarges into two lateral telencephalic hemispheres and a midline diencephalon by the fifth week. The mesencephalon does not subdivide further, but the rhombencephalon differentiates into a more cephalic metencephalon and a caudal myelencephalon. With the extensive growth of the brain at this period the brain flexes in its confined space. The cephalic flexure occurs between the mesencephalon and metencephalon, the pontine flexure at the metencephalon–myelencephalon junction, and the cervical flexure at the junction of the myelencephalon and spinal cord. The metencephalon develops into the pons and cerebellum; the myelencephalon differentiates into the medulla.

In later development, the telencephalic hemispheres enlarge greatly, flex into C-shaped structures and fuse with the lateral wall of the diencephalon at a point that will be occupied later by the posterior limb of the internal capsule. The pontine flexure will become more pronounced and a metencephalic rhombic lip of alar plate material will grow dorsally and develop into the cerebellum. The mantle layers of both the cerebral hemispheres and cerebellum give rise to deep nuclei and migrate peripherally to form the cortical gray material. The deep nuclei of the cerebral hemispheres are the basal ganglia consisting of amygdaloid, caudate, lenticular (putamen and globus pallidus), and claustrum nuclear complexes.

In the brain stem, the differentiation of mantle and marginal layers does not result in as distinct a layering of gray and white matter as in the cerebral hemispheres, cerebellum, and spinal cord. Individual nuclei and fiber tracts are identifiable, but in many areas nuclei and fibers are interspersed and constitute a *reticular formation.* In addition to this major organizational difference between the spinal cord and brain stem, the structure of the latter also differs from the cord as a result of (1) the expansion and thinning out of the roof plate in those areas that develop ventricles, (2) the development of phylogenetically newer structures, (3) the acquisition of cell columns for three new functional components of cranial nerves, and (4) the specialization and lack of segmentation that leads to cranial nerves that do not all have the same functional components.

The *cell columns* of the brain stem develop from the mantle layer. Those developing from the basal plate are nuclei of origin for motor (efferent) neurons whose axons leave the brain stem in cranial nerves. Those developing from the alar plate are nuclei of termination on which incoming sensory (afferent) axons will synapse; these nuclei of termination represent cell bodies of association and internuncial neurons. Seven functional components are formed, but no cranial nerve contains all seven. These functional components are (1) SE to skeletal muscles of occipital and eye somite origin, (2) SVE to skeletal muscles of branchial arch origin, (3) GVE to postganglionic parasympathetic ganglia, (4) GVA receiving sensory neurons from visceral structures, (5) SVA receiving neurons from taste and olfactory receptors, (6) GSA from exteroceptive neurons, and (7) SSA receiving neurons from the eye and ear.

The cell columns of the brain stem are more discontinuous in their cephalocaudal extent than those of the spinal cord, and their localization corresponds generally to the emergence of the cranial nerves. A notable exception to this is the GSA cell column, which continues upward from the dorsal horn of the spinal cord (as the spinal and chief nuclei of cranial nerve V) to the midpons level, receiving trigeminal nerve fibers throughout its extent. There are no cell columns for the olfactory and optic nerves. Thus, the cell columns are limited to the mesencephalon, pons, and medulla. The cross-sectional localization of brain stem cell columns differs markedly from those of the spinal cord. Most of this difference is due to the development of the ventricles. It is recalled that in the spinal cord the gray matter is oriented vertically into a dorsal horn (alar plate) and ventral horn (basal plate) lying lateral to the central canal. With the expansion of the central canal into the ventricles of the brain, the roof plate becomes stretched out as the tela choroidea (ependyma plus pia), and the alar plate is displaced lateral to the basal plate. Consequently in the pons and medulla the nuclei of termination transmitting sensory input are located lateral to the nuclei of origin for motor output. The basic sequential localization from the midline laterally is SE, SVE, GVE, GVA, SVA, GSA, SSA. All of the nuclei of these columns in the pons and medulla lie in the floor of the fourth ventricle or near the central canal, with the exception of the SVE column, which migrates ventrolaterally into the reticular formation.

In the phylogenetic development of the brain stem, the older systems dealing with crude sensibilities and gross axial movements are retained centrally, while the phylogenetically newer structures dealing with discriminatory sensation and with the regulation of finer and more discrete movements are added more ventrolaterally.

The complex topography of the diencephalon and telencephalon and their interrelationships are better appreciated through an understanding of their development. As the ventricles of the diencephalon and telencephalon form, the roof plate of each becomes attenuated as the tela choroidea. Vascularized portions of this pia and ependyma extend into the ventricles as the choroid plexuses of the third and lateral ventricles. These choroid plexuses are continuous with each other at the interventricular foramen. The diencephalon may arise entirely from the alar plate; the optic nerve and retina develop as an evagination of the diencephalon.

The lamina terminalis arises as the most rostral wall of the telencephalon. As the telencephalic hemispheres grow tremendously in size, they grow forward, then backward, circumscribing a C-shaped growth pattern terminating at the temporal pole. The forward growth leaves the lamina terminalis displaced posterior to the frontal pole; the anterior commissure and corpus callosum develop in the lamina terminalis.

The C-shaped growth pattern is reflected in the formation of the anterior horn, body, and inferior horn of the lateral ventricle. The caudate nucleus follows this path with its head in the ventral–lateral floor of the anterior horn and its tail extending into the dorsal–lateral wall of the inferior horn of the lateral ventricle. The caudate nucleus ends near the amygdaloid nucleus located just rostral to the inferior horn of the lateral ventricle. The caudate nucleus grows around the lenticular nucleus, which is anchored at its point of fusion with the diencephalon. The internal capsule develops in this point of fusion. The insular cortex, anchored to the lenticular nucleus, is overgrown by the extensive peripheral growth of the C-shaped hemisphere. The C-shaped growth is also reflected by the fornix. This structure is a fiber pathway that extends from the hippocampal formation in the temporal lobe to the mammillary bodies in the hypothalamus; it forms the anterior boundary of the interventricular foramen in its route.

Internal Topography of the Brain Stem. The brain stem is an upward continuation of the spinal cord. As each of the higher brain stem and cortical centers was added to the nervous system in its phylogenetic development, connections between each of the levels were established, older centers at each level were retained, and many parts were traversed by tracts interconnecting the cerebral cortex with the spinal cord. In addition to these pathways and centers, central connections with cranial nerves also can be localized at the various brain stem levels.

Medulla. The lower part of the closed medulla is similar to the spinal cord in that it has a central canal, fasciculus gracilis, fasciculus cuneatus, lateral and anterior spinothalamic tracts, posterior and anterior spinocerebellar tracts, lateral reticulospinal tracts, and anterior corticospinal tracts in essentially the same locations as in the spinal cord. The substantia gelatinosa and posterolateral fasciculus continue upward as the spinal nucleus and tract of cranial nerve V, respectively. The major difference between the low medulla and spinal cord is that the lateral corticospinal tract is just forming by the decussation of fibers from the *pyramids* of the medulla. At this and higher levels there will be more of an admixture of gray matter and fibers in that area that corresponds to the gray matter of the spinal cord.

At higher regions of the closed medulla the ascending axons of the posterior funiculus synapse on cell bodies in the nucleus gracilis and nucleus cuneatus. Since these nuclei are displaced at higher levels by the expanding fourth ventricle, axons from these nuclei arch ventrally around the central canal as the internal arcuate fibers and decussate to form the *medial lemniscus.* This bundle of ascending fibers represents the axons of second-order neurons for the stereognosis—two-point touch pathway that will traverse the medulla, pons, and mesencephalon before synapsing in the ventral posterior lateral nucleus of the thalamus. In the medial lemniscus, fibers carrying impulses from sacral levels are localized just above the pyramid, while fibers representing cervical levels are located more dorsally just below the MLF.

The inferior olivary nucleus occupies the ventral part of the medulla lateral to the medial lemniscus and pyramids. The vestibulospinal tract runs dorsal to this nucleus. The spinothalamic and spinocerebellar tracts lie along the lateral margin of the medulla in the postolivary sulcus region.

The *hypoglossal nucleus* (SE) extends throughout most of the medulla and lies dorsal to the MLF. Lateral to it is the dorsal motor nucleus (GVE) of the vagus. Axons from the hypoglossal nucleus pass ventrally and exit in the preolivary sulcus. Axons from the *dorsal motor nucleus* course laterally and exit from the postolivary sulcus. GVA and SVA fibers, which enter the brain stem in the vagus nerve and at higher levels in the glossopharyngeal and facial nerves, descend in the fasciculus solitarius and terminate on the cells of the *nucleus solitarius* and dorsal sensory nucleus of the vagus lying adjacent to the fasciculus. In the closed medulla the fasciculus and nucleus solitarius lie dorsal to the dorsal motor nucleus of cranial nerve X, and at open-medulla levels they lie lateral to the motor nuclei.

In the open medulla the hypoglossal and vagal nuclei form prominences in the floor of the fourth ventricle medial to the sulcus limitans. The sensory nuclei, that is, the nucleus solitarius (GVA and SVA), vestibular nuclei (SSA), and spinal nucleus of cranial nerve V (GSA), lie lateral to the sulcus limitans. At high-medulla levels the *vestibular nuclei* (SSA) lie dorsomedial to the spinal nucleus and form a vestibular area in the floor of the fourth ventricle lateral to the sulcus limitans. At the level of the lateral recess, *cochlear nuclei* (SSA) form the most lateral prominence in the floor of the fourth ventricle. The *nucleus ambiguus* (SVE) is located in the reticular formation halfway between the spinal nucleus of cranial nerve V and the inferior olivary nucleus. Axons from this nucleus loop dorsomedially before exiting laterally in the vagus, accessory, and glossopharyngeal nerves. Lateral to the spinal tract of cranial nerve V is the *inferior cerebellar peduncle.* It consists of the posterior spinocerebellar tract, olivocerebellar fibers from the contralateral inferior olivary nucleus, cuneocerebellar fibers from the accessory cuneate nucleus, and some other ascending and reticular connections. The reticular formation is divisible into medial and lateral groups of nuclei. The lateral groups are sensory in that they receive ascending sensory information. The lateral small-celled area is associated with respiratory responses and is where the pressor center is located. The medial gigantocellular nucleus gives rise to the lateral reticulospinal tract and is inhibitory to antigravity muscles. This and adjacent medial nuclei constitute centers involved in respiratory and depressor circulatory responses. An ascending reticular activating system of multisynaptic connections arises primarily from the medial nuclei of the reticular formation.

Pons. The pons is divisible into a dorsal tegmentum and a ventral phylogenetically newer basis pontis. The *tegmentum* is an upward continuation of the medulla. It differs from the medulla in that the inferior olivary nucleus disappears and a central tegmental tract and superior olivary nucleus are located in its place; the medial lemniscus is oriented horizontally in the basal part of the tegmentum; the spinothalamic tracts are located at the lateral tip of the medial lemniscus; the corticospinal tracts are in the basis pontis and not in pyramids; cell columns and pathways relating to cranial nerves V to VIII are present.

At the pons–medulla junction the inferior cerebellar peduncle passes ventral to the lateral recess of the fourth ventricle before entering the cerebellum. At this location dorsal and ventral cochlear nuclei lie dorsolaterally and ventrally, the spinal tract and nucleus of cranial nerve V are medial, and the vestibular nuclei are dorsomedial to the inferior cerebellar peduncle. The cochlear nuclei receive axons of the bipolar neurons of the spiral cochlear ganglion. Axons from the cochlear nuclei pass medially through the tegmentum to ascend contralaterally and ipsilaterally just lateral to the spinothalamic tracts as the lateral lemniscus. Some of the axons of this pathway synapse in the superior olivary nucleus and nucleus of the lateral lemniscus before terminating in the inferior colliculus. The superior olivary nucleus lies dorsal to the spinothalamic tracts in the ventrolateral tegmentum. The vestibular nuclei receive axons from bipolar neurons of the vestibular ganglion and from the cerebellum. They send axons to the cerebellum, to the center for lateral gaze, to the oculomotor nuclei and spinal cord via the MLF, and into the spinal cord as the lateral vestibulospinal tract.

The *basis pontis* contains the corticospinal (pyramidal) tract, corticobulbar (corticonuclear) fibers to cranial nerve motor nuclei, and corticopontine fibers that terminate on pontine nuclei. Axons of the pontine nuclei cross the midline and pass laterally and dorsally into the cerebellum as the *middle cerebellar peduncle.*

In lower pontine levels the *facial* (SVE) *nucleus* occupies the ventrolateral tegmentum. Axons from this nucleus course dorsomedially and superiorly and loop around the *abducens nucleus* before passing ventrolaterally and inferiorly to exit at the pons–medulla junction. The loop (internal genu) of the facial nerve and the adjacent abducens nucleus form an abducens (facial) colliculus in the floor of the fourth ventricle. Axons from the abducens (SE) nucleus pass ventrally and inferiorly to exit at the pons–medulla junction. A parabducens group of cell bodies representing a center for lateral gaze lies inferior to the MLF in the paramedian pontine reticular formation (PPRF). Superior and inferior salivatory nuclei, containing the cell bodies of parasympathetic preganglionic nerves of the facial and glossopharyngeal nerves respectively, occupy the tegmentum but are not sharply localized.

At mid-pons levels, the trigeminal nerve penetrates the middle cerebellar peduncle and runs to the lateral tegmentum. GSA fibers of this nerve, whose cell bodies are located in the trigeminal ganglion, terminate in the *principal (chief, main) sensory nucleus* and *spinal nucleus of cranial nerve V* (Fig. 2-19). The principal sensory nucleus is the upward continuation of the spinal nucleus and receives touch fibers. Axons from this nucleus cross and ascend in the ventral secondary tract of cranial nerve V, running adjacent to the medial lemniscus, and terminate in the ventral posterior medial (VPM) nucleus of the thalamus. Some axons from the principal sensory nucleus ascend uncrossed to the VPM nucleus as the dorsal secondary tract of cranial nerve V running lateral to the MLF. Some entering touch fibers of the trigeminal nerve bifurcate and send descending branches to the upper part of the spinal nucleus of cranial nerve V. Pain fibers enter in the trigeminal nerve, descend as the spinal tract of cranial nerve V and terminate on cell bodies in

the caudal portion of the spinal nucleus of cranial nerve V. Axons from the spinal nucleus of cranial nerve V cross the midline and ascend in the ventral secondary tract of cranial nerve V. The *motor* (SVE) *nucleus of cranial nerve V* lies medial to the chief sensory nucleus of cranial nerve V. Its axons emerge from the pons in the motor root (portio minor) of the trigeminal nerve. A *mesencephalic nucleus of cranial nerve V* of unipolar neurons extends into the mesencephalon from midpons levels. It lies next to the lateral portion of the central gray material and represents the first-order neurons of a proprioceptive pathway of the fifth nerve. Thus, these cells are unique in that they are sensory ganglion cells that did not end up in ganglia but were retained in the brain stem during development of the neural tube.

At upper pons levels, the fourth ventricle narrows as the isthmus region of the pons–mesencephalon junction is approached. The superior medullary velum and *superior cerebellar peduncles* form the roof and lateral walls of the ventricles. In the region of the isthmus, the superior cerebellar peduncles move ventrally into the tegmentum. The fibers of these peduncles will decussate in the tegmentum of the mesencephalon and will ascend to the red nucleus and ventral lateral nucleus of the thalamus.

The reticular formation of the pons is an upward continuation of that in the medulla. The caudal and oral pontine reticular nuclei give rise to the pontine (medial) reticulospinal tract, which is facilitory to antigravity muscles. The main ascending pathway of the reticular formation is the central tegmental tract.

Mesencephalon. The mesencephalon is divided at the level of the cerebral aqueduct into a dorsal *tectum* and into two ventral *cerebral peduncles.* The tectum consists of two superior colliculi and two inferior colliculi. Each cerebral peduncle is subdivided into a dorsal tegmentum and a ventral crus cerebri by the substantia nigra.

At the inferior colliculus level axons of the lateral lemniscus terminate in the *inferior colliculus.* Fibers from this relay nucleus of the hearing pathway pass laterally into the brachium of the inferior colliculus and synapse on cells of the medial geniculate body which, in turn, send axons to the transverse temporal gyri (of Heschl). The mesencephalic nucleus and root and the nucleus pigmentosus (locus ceruleus) lie ventral to the inferior colliculi in the lateral extent of the central gray. In the dorsomedial limits of the tegmentum the *trochlear nucleus* nestles in the dorsal surface of the MLF. Below the

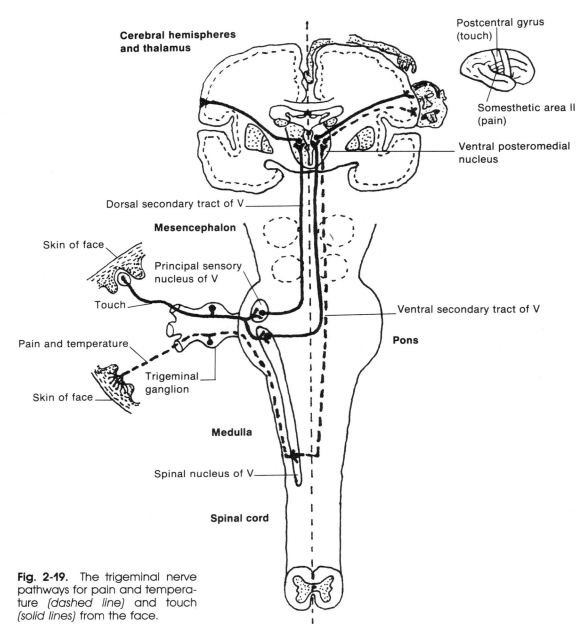

Fig. 2-19. The trigeminal nerve pathways for pain and temperature *(dashed line)* and touch *(solid lines)* from the face.

MLF fibers of the superior cerebellar peduncle decussate before passing upward toward the red nucleus; the medial lemniscus, secondary tracts of cranial nerve V and spinothalamics lie ventral and lateral to this decussation. Axons from the trochlear nucleus course dorsally in the central gray, decussate in the superior medullary velum and exit below the inferior colliculi. The crus cerebri contains the corticopontine, corticobulbar, and corticospinal pathways. Corticobulbar and corticospinal fibers occupy the middle third of the crus.

The most significant features of the superior colliculus levels are the superior colliculi, oculomotor nuclear complex and nerves, and the red nucleus. The **superior colliculus** receives optic fibers from the optic tract and occipital cortex by way of the brachium of the superior colliculus. The superior colliculus is involved in aligning the fovea on a visual target (fixation reflex). The oculomotor nuclear complex consists of the **oculomotor** (SE) and **Edinger–Westphal** (GVE) **nuclei,** which are located medial to the MLF. The oculomotor nerve passes ventrally to exit medial to the crus cerebri in the interpeduncular fossa. SE axons innervate the medial rectus, superior and inferior recti, and inferior oblique muscles. Preganglionic parasympathetic axons from the Edinger–Westphal nucleus run to the ciliary ganglion where they synapse on postganglionic neurons that innervate the sphincter pupillae and ciliary muscles. The *red nucleus* lies in the ventromedial tegmentum and is surrounded by dentatothalamic axons of the superior cerebellar peduncle that are going to the ventral lateral nucleus of the thalamus. Some axons of the superior cerebellar peduncle synapse on cells of the red nucleus. The red nucleus also receives corticorubral fibers. Major efferent paths from the red nucleus are the rubroreticular and the rubrospinal tracts.

The *pretectal area* at the junction with the diencephalon is considered part of the mesencephalon. Features of this area are the pretectal nuclei, posterior commissure, and subcommissural organ. Pretectal nuclei lie rostral to the superior colliculi, receive optic tract axons by way of the brachium of the superior colliculi and send crossed and uncrossed axons to the Edinger– Westphal nucleus. The pretectal nuclei constitute the association limb of the pupillary light reflex. The crossing fibers of this reflex either pass through the posterior commissure or decussate in the central gray below the cerebral aqueduct. The posterior commissure lies dorsal to the cerebral aqueduct at the level where it joins the third ventricle. The subcommissural organ is modified ependyma located beneath the posterior commissure. The columnar ciliated cells of this organ may secrete aldosterone and may serve as a volume receptor.

The *reticular formation* consists of many nuclei whose cells release a variety of neurotransmitters. A median (raphe) group of nuclei contains serotonergic neurons. A medial group, which includes the cells of origin of the medial reticulospinal (nucleus pontis oralis and caudalis) and lateral reticulospinal (nucleus gigantocellularis) tracts, produces serotonin and possibly substance P. A lateral group of nuclei (*e.g.*, locus ceruleus) constitutes a norepinephrine and epinephrine system. A dopaminergic system of neurons includes cells of the substantia nigra.

Diencephalon. The diencephalon consists of an epithalamus, thalamus, hypothalamus, and subthalamus. The *epithalamus* is in the roof of the third ventricle and is composed of the tela choroidea, striae medullares, habenular trigones, and pineal gland. The stria medullaris conveys fibers from the septal and preoptic area to the habenular nuclei. Axons from the habenular nuclei pass to the mesencephalon through the fasciculus retroflexus.

The *thalamus* is bounded laterally by the posterior limb of the internal capsule and medially by the third ventricle. It extends anteroposteriorly from the interventricular foramen to the pretectal area, and it lies above the hypothalamus and subthalamus. The thalamus is separated into medial, lateral, and anterior nuclear groups by the internal medullary lamina. The medial group nuclei are the midline and dorsomedial nuclei. The midline nuclei make connections with the hypothalamus. The dorsomedial nucleus receives afferents from the amygdaloid nucleus, hypothalamus, and temporal cortex and sends axons to the prefrontal cortex. Intralaminar nuclei receive spinothalamic fibers and reticulothalamics from the reticular activating system. The centromedian nucleus is an intralaminar nucleus that receives fibers from the motor cortex (area 4) and globus pallidus and sends axons to the putamen. The lateral group of thalamic nuclei are divisible into a ventral tier and a dorsal tier. The ventral tier consists of the ventral anterior, ventral lateral, and ventral posterior (VPL and VPM) nuclei. All of these ventral tier nuclei are relay nuclei. The VPL nucleus receives the medial lemniscus and spinothalamics. The VPM receives secondary ascending trigeminal pathways. Axons from both nuclei pass into the posterior limb of the internal capsule and terminate in the great somesthetic area (postcentral gyrus, area 3, 1, 2), those from VPM terminating closer to the more ventral portion of the postcentral gyrus than those from the VPL. Some axons conveying nociceptive information from the VPL and VPM nuclei terminate in somatic sensory area II located in the parietal lobe above the lateral fissure. The ventral lateral nucleus receives dentatothalamic fibers and pallidothalamic fibers and sends axons to the precentral gyrus (motor cortex). The latter fibers arise from cells in the medial aspect of the globus pallidus and pass through the fasciculus lenticulans to reach the prerubral field. From here they loop laterally over the zone incerta to enter the thalamus via the thalamic fasciculus. The ventral anterior nucleus receives pallidothalamic fibers by this same pathway and projects axons to the premotor cortex. The dorsal tier nuclei are the lateral dorsal, lateral posterior, and pulvinar. These nuclei are association nuclei and have interconnections with the parietal cortex. The pulvinar receives fibers from the metathalamus (medial and lateral geniculate bodies) and sends axons to the parastriate (area 18) and peristriate (area 19) areas in the occipital cortex and also to the inferior parietal cortex. The anterior nucleus of the thalamus relays mammillothalamic impulses from the mammillary bodies to the cingulate gyrus.

The *subthalamus* lies ventral to the thalamus between the hypothalamus and posterior limb of the internal capsule. It consists of the subthalamic nucleus, zona incerta, fasciculus lenticularis, prerubral field (of Forel), and the fasciculus thalamicus. The subthalamic nucleus lies on the internal capsule and substantia nigra and is separated form the zona incerta above by the fasciculus lenticularis. It has interconnections with the globus pallidus. Lesions of this nucleus produce hemiballism contralaterally.

The *hypothalamus* consists of groups of nuclei in the floor of the third ventricle. The nuclei are divided into medial and lateral groups by the fornix as it passes through the hypothalamus on its way to the mammillary body. The lateral group includes the lateral and tuberal nuclei. The medial group is subdivided anatomically into three groups: (1) anterior group, which includes the preoptic, anterior, supraoptic, and paraventricular nuclei; (2) middle group, containing the dorsomedial and ventromedial nuclei; and (3) posterior group of posterior and mammillary nuclei.

The hypothalamic nuclei can also be grouped on the basis of their functional connections into autonomic, neuroendocrine and olfactory groups. The anteromedial hypothalamic group of nuclei generally are concerned with parasympathetic regulation, whereas the posterolateral group is more involved in sympathetic regulation. Both nuclear groups receive ascending GVA, GSA, and SVA (taste) input from the reticular formation and send out descending central autonomics to preganglionic neurons by way of reticulospinal and reticuloreticular pathways. These regions also receive olfactory input from the amygdaloid and septal areas and have interconnections with the thalamus, prefrontal cortex, and limbic lobe.

The neuroendocrine nuclei are the supraoptic and paraventricular group, which produce posterior pituitary hormones, and a hypophysiotrophic group, which produce adenohypophyseal releasing and inhibiting factors. These nuclei and their manner of secretion have been discussed previously.

The mammillary, preoptic, and lateral hypothalamic nuclei receive input from the olfactory cortex. These nuclei have reciprocal connections with the limbic lobe and also project to other hypothalamic and brain stem nuclei.

Telencephalon (Cerebral Hemispheres). The *primary receptive areas* of each cerebral hemisphere (Fig. 2-20) are the postcentral gyrus (areas 3, 1, 2) for two-point touch, joint sense, and vibratory sense; the striate cortex (17) for vision; the transverse temporal gyri (41 and 42) for hearing; the base of the postcentral gyrus (43) for taste and the peri-

amygdaloid region (34) for smell. The gyri adjacent to these areas constitute the *unisensory association areas* where sensory information is recognized as that perceived before (gnosis). These unisensory areas are the adjacent postcentral gyrus (5), superior parietal gyrus (7), and supramarginal gyrus (40) for areas 3, 1, 2; the peristriate (19) and parastriate cortex (18) for area 17; the adjacent superior temporal gyrus (42 and 22) for 41 and 42; areas 5 and 40 for area 43; and the parahippocampal gyrus (42 and 22) for area 34. The angular gyrus (39) and adjacent areas 19 and 22 constitute *multisensory association areas* where one can recognize an object through perception of one sense and can recall what the other sensations would be for that object (*e.g.*, seeing and recognizing a chicken and recalling what it would feel, taste, sound, and smell like). This multisensory area of the parietotemporal cortex is an area for language and the formulation of complex motor activities, especially in the dominant hemisphere (usually the left). Thus, damage to the angular gyrus on the left side may result in receptive aphasia and apraxia. Lesions of unisensory areas in the dominant hemisphere result in agnosia (*e.g.*, visual agnosia, astereognosis). Lesions of the right posterior and inferior parietal lobe may lead to extinction and denial of ones contralateral body parts or environment.

Fibers from the parietal-temporal-occipital cortex by way of the arcuate, superior longitudinal and inferior occipitofrontal fasciculi connect with the prefrontal, premotor, and motor cortex of the frontal lobe. The *prefrontal cortex* is for initiative, judgment, and creativity. Broca's area in the inferior frontal gyrus of the dominant hemisphere is the motor speech area. Lesions of this area result in expressive aphasias. The frontal eye fields (8) and Exner's writing center (8) are located in the posterior part of the middle frontal gyrus. Destructive lesions of the former lead to transient conjugate gaze to the side of the lesion, whereas lesions of the latter result in a writing apraxia. The *motor cortex* (area 4) in the precentral gyrus and the *premotor cortex* (6 and 8) in front of area 4 control motor activity, especially of the contralateral extremities.

The cerebral cortex receives and projects fibers from and to lower centers by way of the *internal capsule.* The anterior limb of the internal capsule between the head of the caudate and lenticular nucleus contains connections with the prefrontal cortex. The posterior limb of the internal capsule between the thalamus and lenticular nucleus contain corticospinal fibers from the frontal lobe and re-

A

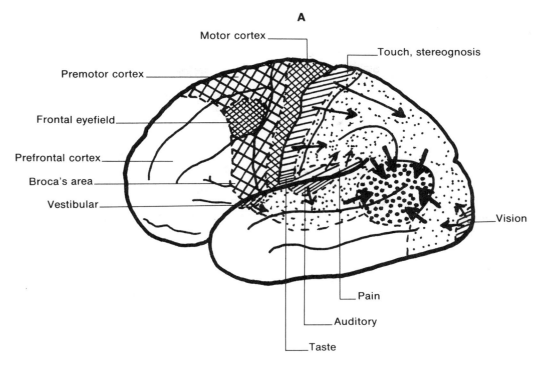

Motor cortex

Touch, stereognosis

Premotor cortex

Frontal eyefield

Prefrontal cortex

Broca's area

Vestibular

Vision

Pain

Auditory

Taste

B

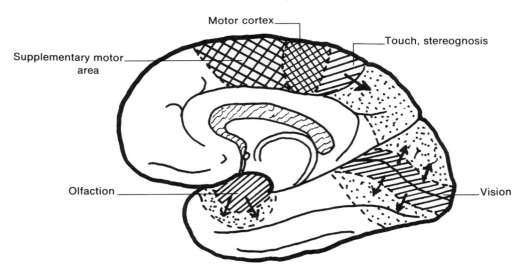

Motor cortex

Touch, stereognosis

Supplementary motor area

Olfaction

Vision

Fig. 2-20. Functional areas of the cerebral cortex as shown in lateral view *(A)* and in medial view *(B)*. The primary receptive areas are shown in diagonal lines. The unisensory association areas are shown in small dots. The multisensory association area is shown in large dots. The motor areas are cross hatched.

ceive projections to the parietal and temporal lobes. The genu of the internal capsule at the level of the interventricular foramen transports corticobulbar fibers. Sublenticular fibers of the internal capsule are auditory and optic radiations. Retrolenticular fibers are also optic radiations.

Summary of Cranial Nerves. The *first (olfactory) nerve* is comprised of the central processes of bipolar olfactory cells (SVA) whose cell bodies are located in the olfactory epithelium on the upper part of the nasal septum and the lateral nasal wall. These unmyelinated fibers (fila olfactoria) pass into the anterior cranial fossa through the lamina cribrosa of the ethmoid bone and enter the olfactory bulb. After synapse with the mitral cells of the bulb the impulses travel in the olfactory tract to the lateral olfactory stria and terminate in the pyriform lobe. The pyriform lobe is the cortical receptive area for olfaction; it consists of the lateral olfactory stria, the uncus (periamygdaloid area) and the anterior part of the parahippocampal gyrus.

The *second (optic) nerve* is formed by the central processes of the retinal ganglion cells (SSA), which converge at the optic papilla. After piercing the sclera, the optic nerve passes through the orbital fat, traverses the optic canal, and joins with its opposite fellow to form the optic chiasma. The visual pathway from retina to occipital cortex consists of four orders of neurons. The first-order neurons are the rods and cones. The second-order neurons are bipolar cells, and the third-order neurons are ganglion cells. Axons of the ganglion cells comprise the optic nerve, chiasm, and tract and terminate in the lateral geniculate body. Those axons from the nasal half of the retina decussate in the optic chiasm; those from the temporal half of the retina remain uncrossed. Thus the optic tract consists of axons from the temporal half of the ipsilateral eye and the nasal half of the contralateral eye. The fourth-order neurons are located in the lateral geniculate nucleus. Axons of these cells pass into the sublenticular and retrolenticular portion of the internal capsule, loop over the roof of the inferior horn of the lateral ventricle, and course posteriorly as the optic radiations to the striate cortex (area 17) located above and below the calcarine fissure in the occipital lobe. This pathway is also referred to as the *geniculocalcarine tract*. The pathway from the upper retina projects to the cuneus while that from the lower retina projects to the lingual gyrus below the calcarine fissure.

Lesions in the visual pathway give rise to deficits in the visual fields and some loss of visual reflexes. Since light rays from specific portions of the visual field project to opposite parts of the retinal fields, lesions in the nasal retinal field will result in loss of vision in the temporal visual field while damage to the upper retinal field will demonstrate blindness in the lower visual field. In recalling the topographic distribution of fibers in the pathway, it is readily apparent that (1) lesions in front of the chiasma lead to blindness (anopsia), or partial blindness, on the side of the damaged optic nerve or retina; (2) midline lesions of the optic chiasm result in bitemporal heteronymous hemianopsia; and (3) lesions of the pathway posterior to the chiasm give homonymous

hemianopsias (or quadrantic anopsias) to the side opposite to that of the lesion. Because of the topography of optic radiations and terminations in the striate cortex, lesions in the rostral portion of the temporal lobe or below the calcarine fissure can give upper quadrantic anopsias to the opposite side.

When light is shone into one eye, the ipsilateral pupil will constrict (direct response) and the contralateral pupil will constrict (consensual response). The afferent limb of this pupillary light reflex consists of rods and cones → bipolar cells → ganglion cells whose axons pass through the brachium of the superior colliculus to the pretectal area. The association limb is comprised of neurons of the pretectal nucleus that send axons ipsilaterally, and contralaterally (by way of the posterior commissure or central gray) to the Edinger–Westphal nucleus. The efferent limb of the pupillary light reflex involves innervation of the sphincter pupillae muscles by a pathway involving the preganglionic neurons of both Edinger–Westphal nuclei and oculomotor nerves, and the postganglionic neurons of both ciliary ganglia. Section of one optic nerve results in blindness in that eye and loss of direct and consensual pupillary light response when light is shone into the blind eye. When light is shown into the other eye the direct and consensual responses are intact. Damage to an oculomotor nerve results in loss of pupillary constriction in that eye regardless of which eye is stimulated.

When a person focuses on a near object after focusing on a far object three responses take place: (1) convergence of the eyes by contraction of the medial recti muscles, (2) pupillary constriction by contraction of the sphincter pupillae muscles, and (3) rounding of the lens due to constriction of the ciliary muscle. This reflex is referred to as the near reflex (accommodation–convergence–pupillary reflex). There are two notable distinctions between this reflex and the pupillary light reflex: (1) the pathway involves cortical connections, and (2) the efferent limb involves both SE and GVE parasympathetic components. The afferent limb involves rods and cones → bipolar cells → ganglion cells → lateral geniculate nucleus → area 17. The association limb consists of connections from area 17 → area 18 (parastriate) → area 19 (peristriate) and its corticomesencephalic axons to the oculomotor complex. The efferent limb involves the oculomotor and Edinger–Westphal nuclei, the oculomotor nerves, and the ciliary ganglia and nerves.

In the reflexes involving the turning of the head and eyes in response to visual impulses, there are cortical connections that project to a center for convergence in the midbrain tegmentum, the rostral interstitial nucleus of the MLF for vertical gaze in the midbrain and diencephalon, and in the paramedian pontine reticular formation for lateral gaze. The lateral conjugate gaze center and pathways will be discussed further in the section on the abducens nerve. The association limb for reflex turning of the head probably relays through the superior colliculus and tectospinal tract to anterior horn cells and spinal accessory neurons in the cervical cord.

The *third (oculomotor) nerve* contains both SE and GVE parasympathetic fibers. These fibers arise from the oculomotor (SE) and Edinger–Westphal (GVE) nuclei of the midbrain run ventrally through the tegmentum, and emerge on the medial aspect of the cerebral peduncles. The third nerve traverses the cavernous sinus and enters the orbital cavity through the superior orbital fissure. Preganglionic neurons terminate on postganglionic cells of the ciliary ganglion. Axons of the postganglionic cells run as short ciliary nerves and innervate the sphincter pupillae and ciliary muscles. SE fibers supply the levator palpebrae superioris, the superior, inferior, and medial recti, and the inferior oblique muscles.

Damage to the oculomotor nerve results in several characteristic symptoms. Ptosis (drooping of the upper eyelid) occurs as a result of denervation of the levator palpebrae superioris; the pupil is dilated, since the dilator pupillae is unopposed by the sphincter pupillae; and the direct and consensual responses of the pupillary light reflex are lost. The ciliary muscle is paralyzed and accommodation is impaired. Denervation of the extrinsic muscles results in external strabismus due to unopposed action of the lateral rectus and superior oblique muscles.

The *fourth (trochlear) nerve* arises from the trochlear nucleus (SE) at the inferior colliculus levels. Axons of these cells pass dorsally around the cerebral aqueduct, decussate with fibers of the opposite side, and emerge as the fourth nerve at the superior medullary velum. The fourth nerve passes ventrally around the brain stem, traverses the cisterna basalis and the cavernous sinus, and enters the orbit through the superior orbital fissure. It supplies the superior oblique muscle, which intorts the eye when abducted, and depresses the eye when adducted.

The *fifth (trigeminal) nerve* contains both general somatic afferent fibers and special visceral efferent fibers. The motor fibers arise from the motor nucleus of cranial nerve V in the pons and emerge laterally from the middle cerebral peduncle in the motor root of the trigeminal nerve. The motor root passes beneath the trigeminal ganglion, exits the skull through the foramen ovale, and joins sensory fibers to form the mandibular nerve. Motor branches of the mandibular nerve innervate the muscles of mastication and tensor tympani and tensor veli palatini muscles. Sensory pseudounipolar neurons have their cell bodies located in the trigeminal ganglion. They distribute their functional dendrites over the ophthalmic, maxillary, and mandibular nerves and send axons to the pons as the sensory root of cranial nerve V. Upon entering the pons, the fibers from pain and temperature receptors descend as the spinal tract of cranial nerve V to terminate in its spinal nucleus. Touch fibers end in the principal sensory nucleus and in the upper part of the spinal nucleus of the fifth nerve. Crossed secondary fibers for pain, temperature, and touch ascend as the *ventral secondary tract of the fifth nerve* to the VPM nucleus. Some touch fibers ascend ipsilaterally in the *dorsal secondary tract* to the VPM nucleus. Third-order neurons of the VPM nucleus send axons to the postcentral gyrus.

The cell bodies of proprioceptive fibers are located in the mesencephalic nucleus of cranial nerve V. The location of pathways to the cerebral cortex and cerebellum from this nucleus has not been completely established.

The *ophthalmic nerve* passes from the trigeminal (semilunar) ganglion in the wall of the cavernous sinus through the superior orbital fissure. In the superior orbital fissure it breaks up into three terminal branches: (1) the frontal nerve with supraorbital, frontal, and supratrochlear branches; (2) the lacrimal nerve; and (3) the nasociliary nerve.

The *maxillary nerve* arises from the anterior border of the trigeminal ganglion, traverses the wall of the cavernous sinus, and passes into the pterygopalatine fossa through the foramen rotundum. From the pterygopalatine fossa the nerve enters the orbit through the inferior orbital fissure and becomes the infraorbital nerve. This nerve passes into the infraorbital canal, where it gives off superior alveolar nerves, and emerges at the infraorbital foramen to supply the face through inferior palpebral, external nasal, and superior labial branches. Major branches in the pterygopalatine fossa are (1) zygomatic nerve, which supplies the skin of the side of the forehead and cheek, and communicates postganglionic parasympathetic fibers from the pterygopalatine ganglion to the lacrimal nerve, and (2) pterygopalatine nerves, which supply the posterior superior nasal cavity, nasopharynx, palate, orbit, and posterior upper teeth. A middle meningeal nerve arises from the maxillary nerve near its origin and passes with the middle meningeal artery to the dura mater.

The *mandibular division* supplies the muscles of mastication and is sensory to the lower teeth, gums, mandible, tongue, lower lip, lower part of the face, and the skin of the auricula and temporal region. Just outside the foramen ovale it gives off a meningeal branch, which enters the skull through the foramen spinosum, and a medial pterygoid nerve supplying the medial pterygoid muscle and otic ganglion. Beyond these branches, the mandibular nerve divides into anterior and posterior divisions. The anterior division gives off motor branches to the temporalis, masseter, and lateral pterygoid muscles and gives off a sensory buccal branch to the mucous membrane and skin of the cheek. The posterior division is mainly sensory and has several major branches: (1) the auriculotemporal whose roots encircle the middle meningeal artery and carry sensory fibers to the temporal and ear regions as well as postganglionic parasympathetic fibers to the parotid gland from the otic ganglion; (2) the inferior alveolar supplying the mylohyoid muscle, lower teeth, lower lip, and chin; and (3) the lingual nerve supplying the mucosa of the anterior two thirds of the tongue with GSA exteroceptive fibers of the fifth nerve and with SVA taste fibers of the facial nerve, the latter entering the lingual nerve by way of the chorda tympani nerve.

Lesions of the trigeminal nerve result in exteroceptive deficits of pain, temperature, and touch in the areas supplied by the damaged components. Lesions of the ophthalmic division result in loss of the afferent limb of the corneal blink reflex. Damage to one ophthalmic nerve produces loss of the direct and consensual blink. If the efferent limb, mediated by the facial nerve, were damaged and the ophthalmic was intact then stimulation of the cornea would result in blink of only that eye that had an intact seventh nerve. Lesion to the mandibular nerves could result in deviation of the jaw to the affected side upon opening of the jaws due to the unopposed action of the contralateral external pterygoid muscle.

The *sixth (abducens) nerve* leaves the brain at the posterior border of the pons, traverses the cavernous sinus, enters the orbit through the superior orbital fissure, and innervates the ipsilateral lateral rectus muscle. This nerve arises from SE cell bodies in the floor of the fourth ventricle at the facial colliculus level of the pons. The abducens nucleus receives afferents from the ipsilateral *lateral gaze center* (parabducens nucleus, PPRF) located near the abducens nucleus below the MLF. Some axons from the abducens nucleus cross the midline and ascend in the contralateral medial longitudinal fasciculus to reach cells of the oculomotor nucleus that innervate the contralateral medial rectus muscle. Thus, stimulation of neurons in the PPRF results in conjugate deviation of the eyes to the side stimulated, since the ipsilateral abducens and lateral rectus, and contralateral oculomotor and medial rectus are activated. The abducens and oculomotor nuclei also are supplied by fibers that course through the MLF from vestibular nuclei and superior colliculi.

Section of the abducens nerve may lead to medial deviation (strabismus) of the affected eye since the medial rectus is unopposed. There is diplopia and inability to turn the eye laterally. Lesion of the abducens nucleus area often involves both the abducens and lateral gaze center. In this type of lesion there is inability for both eyes to look laterally toward the side of the lesion, and there is a tendency for persistent conjugate deviation toward the opposite side.

The *seventh (facial) nerve* contains GSA, SVA (taste), GVA, SVE, and GVE functional components. GSA fibers arise from receptors in a small area near the external ear, pass to pseudounipolar cell bodies in the geniculate ganglion, and course into the pons at the pons–medulla junction to terminate in the spinal nucleus of cranial nerve V. SVA fibers arise from taste buds in the anterior two thirds of the tongue and traverse the lingual nerve and chorda tympani to reach the geniculate ganglion. Axons of these cells enter the pons and descend in the fasciculus solitarius to end in the upper part of the solitary (gustatory) nucleus. GVAs arise from the submandibular, sublingual, lacrimal, nasal, and minor salivary glands. Their cell bodies are in the geniculate ganglion, and their axons terminate in the nucleus solitarius. GVE preganglionic parasympathetic neurons arise in the superior salivatory nucleus of the pons and are distributed (1) to the pterygopalatine ganglion by way of the greater petrosal nerve, and (2) to the submandibular ganglion by way of the chorda tympani and lingual nerves. Postganglionic fibers from the pterygopalatine ganglion supply the lacrimal gland and the small glands of the pharynx, palate, paranasal sinuses, and nasal cavity. Postganglionics leaving the submandibular ganglion supply the submandibular, sublingual, and minor oral salivary glands. SVE neurons arise in the facial motor nucleus, form an internal genu around the abducens nucleus, emerge in the facial nerve at the pons–medulla junction and are distributed through numerous branches to the muscles of facial expression, the stapedius muscle, posterior belly of the digastric muscle, and stylohyoid muscle.

The facial nerve leaves the pons as two roots: (1) the motor root, and (2) the nervus intermedius. The latter nerve contains taste and parasympathetic fibers. Both roots enter the internal acoustic meatus with the vestibulocochlear nerve. At the fundus of the meatus, the facial nerve enters the facial canal in the petrous portion of the temporal bone. Near the tympanic cavity it bends (external genu) posteriorly above the oval window and descends to exit at the stylomastoid foramen. The geniculate ganglion is located at the bend, and the greater superficial petrosal nerve branches from this region. The nerve to the stapedius muscle and chorda tympani arise from the nerve while it is in the facial canal. The chorda tympani courses through the bone, enters the posterior wall of the tympanum, and passes deep to the mucous membrane and medial to the tympanic membrane and manubrium of the malleus. It exits anteriorly from the tympanum, emerges from the skull, and joins the lingual nerve. That portion of the facial nerve exiting from the stylomastoid foramen divides into posterior auricular, digastric, stylohyoid, temporal, zygomatic, buccal, mandibular, and cervical branches.

Lesions of the facial nerve (such as in Bell's palsy) result in weakness to all of the facial muscles ipsilateral to the lesion. This is distinct from lesions of the UMNs (corticobulbar tract), which bilaterally innervate that part of the facial nucleus supplying the upper facial muscles but only contralaterally supply cells to the lower face. Thus, in UMN lesions there is weakness to the contralateral lower face. Peripheral nerve lesions also may result in (1) loss of taste in the anterior two thirds of the tongue, (2) impaired lacrimation, and (3) hyperacusis due to loss of the dampening effect of the stapedius muscle.

The *eighth (vestibulocochlear) nerve* is a SSA nerve arising from receptors for hearing in the cochlear duct and arising from the maculae and cristae of the vestibular apparatus. It is comprised of the processes of bipolar cells whose cell bodies lie in the spiral cochlear ganglion and vestibular ganglion. Axons of these cells run in the internal acoustic meatus and enter the pons at the pons–medulla junction.

Cochlear fibers synapse in the dorsal and ventral cochlear nuclei. From these nuclei axons pass bilaterally, synapsing in the superior olivary nucleus, nucleus of the lateral lemniscus, and inferior colliculus. From the inferior colliculus axons pass to the medial geniculate nucleus where impulses are relayed to the transverse temporal gyrus (of Heschl). Lesions of one nerve result in deafness to that ear. Unilateral lesions of the central pathway lead only to a diminution in hearing due to the bilateral representation.

Entering *vestibular fibers* may pass directly to the flocculonodular lobe of the cerebellum or synapse on vestibular nuclei. The vestibular pathway to consciousness is not known. There are reflex connections from vestibular nuclei to the spinal cord (by way of the MLF and vestibulospinal tract), to the center for lateral conjugate gaze and to motor nuclei of the brain stem reticular formation. Some of these connections are better appreciated when the pathways involving reflex activities that accompany angular rotation of the head are considered. When the head is inclined 30 degrees forward and is first rotated to the right the endolymph of both horizontal semicircular canals does not move initially as fast as the cristae ampullares. This gives a relative displacement of endolymph to the left, although endolymph is actually moving to the right. After rotation the cristae stop moving, but there is continued brief movement of endolymph to the right in the direction of rotation. Since stimulation of cristae of the horizontal canal toward the utricle results in depolarization of the hair cells, an imbalance occurs during rotation and postrotation between the two canals. In postrotation to the right the left vestibular nerve is stimulated while the right vestibular nerve is being inhibited. This results in rapid alternating eye movements (nystagmus). The pathway for the slow component of nystagmus to the right in postrotation to the right involves the left vestibular nerve, left vestibular nuclei, right lateral gaze center, right abducens nucleus and nerve, left MLF, and oculomotor nucleus and nerve. In this pathway axons from vestibular nuclei may ascend in the MLF to reach the oculomotor nucleus and cross to the opposite abducens nucleus, or they may go to the opposite lateral gaze center, which in turn, makes connections with the abducens and oculomotor nuclei. Accompanying past-pointing and a tendency to fall to the right are mediated through connections of the left vestibular nucleus with the cerebellum and through connections of the left vestibulospinal tract with anterior horn cells of antigravity muscles, thus causing a thrust to the right. Nausea, increased salivation, and vomiting are mediated through connections of the vestibular nuclei with such motor nuclei as the dorsal motor nucleus of cranial nerve X, the nucleus ambiguus, the salivatory nuclei, and other reticular nuclei.

The *ninth (glossopharyngeal) nerve* contains

GSA, SVA (taste), GVA, SVE, and GVE functional components. GSA fibers arise from skin receptors in the posterior part of the external auditory meatus and auricula. These fibers are distributed in the auricular branch of the vagus. They pass to the glossopharyngeal near the jugular foramen and the pseudounipolar cell bodies of these GSA neurons are located in the superior ganglion in the jugular foramen. Axons of these cells enter the upper medulla, in the postolivary sulcus, and synapse on cells of the spinal nucleus of cranial nerve V.

SVA fibers arise from taste buds in the posterior one third of the tongue. They pass through lingual branches and their cell bodies are in the inferior ganglion. Axons terminate in the solitary (gustatory) nucleus. GVA fibers arise in the mucosa and glands of the posterior tongue, fauces, and pharynx. Their cell bodies are located in the inferior ganglion, and their axons terminate in the solitary nucleus. The carotid sinus nerve of the glossopharyngeal conveys GVA fibers from the carotid sinus to the nucleus solitarius. Axons from this nucleus course to the dorsal motor nucleus of cranial nerve X, where they synapse on neurons whose fibers pass into the vagus nerve and constitute the efferent limb of the carotid sinus reflex.

SVE fibers arise in the nucleus ambiguus and pass through the glossopharyngeal nerve to innervate the stylopharyngeus. GVE preganglionic parasympathetics have their cell bodies in the inferior salivatory nucleus. Axons of these neurons pass into the tympanic nerve. This nerve arises from the inferior ganglion, courses through the temporal bone, runs on the promontory, and helps to form the tympanic plexus in the middle ear cavity. The preganglionics leave the plexus in the lesser superficial petrosal nerve and synapse on postganglionics in the otic ganglion. Postganglionic axons run in the auriculotemporal branch of the trigeminal nerve and are distributed to the parotid gland.

In the gag reflex, the afferent limb is by way of GVA fibers from the oropharynx to the association limb in nucleus solitarius. Axons of the latter nucleus are both crossed and uncrossed to the hypoglossal nucleus for tongue movements and to the nucleus ambiguus for pharynx, larynx, and soft palate movements. Lesions of the glossopharyngeal can result in some loss of taste in the posterior third of the tongue and in a loss of the gag reflex when the affected side is stimulated.

The *tenth (vagus) nerve* contains the same five functional components as do the facial and glossopharyngeal nerves. The small GSA component travels from the external ear in the auricular branch of the vagus and has its cell bodies located in the superior (jugular) ganglion lying in the posterior part of the jugular foramen. Axons from this ganglion enter the medulla in the postolivary sulcus and end in the spinal nucleus of cranial nerve V. The SVA fibers arise from taste buds in the region of the epiglottis. SVA cell bodies are in the inferior (nodose) ganglion, located inferior to the jugular foramen, and their axons terminate in the gustatory part of the nucleus solitarius. GVA fibers arise in the mucosa and walls of the intestine (as far as the splenic flexure), the stomach, esophagus, pharynx, larynx, trachea, lungs, heart, carotid body, and kidney. Their cell bodies are located in the inferior ganglion, and their axons terminate in the nucleus solitarius.

SVE nerves arise from the nucleus ambiguus and are distributed to the skeletal muscles of the pharynx, soft palate, larynx, and esophagus. Pharyngeal branches supply the pharyngeal plexus that gives branches to the pharyngeal constrictor muscles and all of the palatine muscles except the tensor veli palatini. The external branch of the superior laryngeal nerve supplies the cricothyroideus and part of the inferior pharyngeal constrictor muscles. The internal branch of the superior laryngeal supplies sensory and parasympathetic secretomotor fibers to the larynx and epiglottis. All of the laryngeal muscles, except the cricothyroideus, are supplied by the recurrent (inferior) laryngeal nerve. The right recurrent arises in the root of the neck and arches under the subclavian. The left recurrent arises in the upper thorax, loops around the arch of the aorta just below the ligamentum arteriosum, and ascends to the larynx.

The GVE fibers arise from the dorsal motor nucleus of cranial nerve X. These preganglionics are distributed through numerous branches of the vagus to terminal parasympathetic ganglia in or on the heart, larynx, trachea, lungs, and digestive system from the pharynx to the splenic flexure. The terminal ganglia of most of the gastrointestinal tract are the myenteric and submucosal nerve ganglia and plexi. Postganglionic axons from terminal ganglia supply smooth and cardiac muscle and glands.

The peripheral branches of the vagus nerve are extensive. In the jugular fossa, the vagus gives off auricular and meningeal nerves. In the neck it gives off pharyngeal, superior laryngeal, right recurrent laryngeal, and the superior cardiac nerves. In the thorax the vagus gives off the left recurrent, inferior cardiac, anterior and posterior bronchial, and esophageal nerves. The right and left vagus form an esophageal plexus around the esophagus from which most of the left vagus enters the abdomen as the anterior vagus; most of the right contributes to the posterior vagus. Vagal branches in the abdomen are the gastric, hepatic, and celiac.

A unilateral lesion of the vagus nerve or its nuclei produces paresis of the ipsilateral vocal cord, resulting in abnormal phonation and hoarseness. In addition, the affected side of the soft palate is lower than the normal side. Upon phonation, the uvula points toward the normal side. Lesions of the vagus also demonstrate abnormal gag and swallowing reflexes since the vagus constitutes the efferent limbs of those reflexes.

The *eleventh (accessory) nerve* consists of two parts, a cranial and a spinal part. The cranial part arises in the nucleus ambiguus (SVE), exits from the postolivary sulcus of the medulla, passes through the jugular foramen, and merges with the vagus near the inferior vagal ganglion. The spinal part arises from anterior horn cells of the upper five cervical segments. Axons of these cells pass laterally through the lateral funiculus, ascend between the dentate ligament and the dorsal roots, and pass as a nerve trunk through the foramen magnum into the cranial cavity. This nerve trunk communicates with the cranial part of the accessory and the vagus and exists from the jugular foramen to distribute fibers to the sternocleidomastoid and trapezius muscles.

Lesions of the spinal accessory produce weakness in shoulder shrugging on the affected side, and the arm cannot be raised above the vertical plane because of paresis of the trapezius. In addition, there may be weakness in rotating the head and face to the opposite side.

The *twelfth (hypoglossal) nerve* is an SE nerve that arises from the hypoglossal nucleus and emerges from the preolivary sulcus of the medulla. It passes through the hypoglossal canal, loops ventrally and anteriorly above the hyoid bone, and innervates the tongue musculature.

Unilateral lesions of the hypoglossal nerve or nucleus result in deviation of the tongue to the affected side upon protrusion. This is due to the action of the unopposed genioglossus of the normal side. There may be fasciculations and wasting on the affected side. Since corticobulbar fibers are crossed, damage to these fibers causes the tongue to deviate away from the lesion upon protrusion.

Major Ascending and Descending Pathways. The following outline is a summary of some of the major clinically significant ascending and descending pathways that course through the spinal cord. Lesions of the ascending pathways produce loss of

sensation ipsilaterally if the lesion occurs below the decussation, and contralaterally if the lesion is above the crossing second-order neuron.

Ascending Pathways of the Spinal Cord

1. *Pain and temperature pathway* (Fig. 2-21)
   Neuron I: Cell bodies in dorsal root ganglion and axon in dorsal root.
   Neuron II: Cell bodies in the posteromarginal nucleus and nucleus proprius. Axons cross to the opposite side in the anterior white commissure and ascend as the lateral spinothalamic tract.
   Neuron III: Cell bodies in the VPL nucleus of the thalamus. Axons ascend in the posterior limb of the internal capsule to the postcentral gyrus and to a region of the parietal lobe bordering the lateral fissure (somesthetic area II).

2. *Two-point touch, stereognosis, vibratory sense pathway* (Fig. 2-22)
   Neuron I: Cell bodies in dorsal root ganglion. Axons of dorsal root ascend in the posterior white column. Those entering below T6 ascend in the fasciculus gracilis; those entering above T6 ascend in fasciculus cuneatus.
   Neuron II: Cell bodies in nucleus gracilis and cuneatus. Axons cross and ascend as the medial lemniscus.
   Neuron III: Cell bodies in the VPL nucleus of the thalamus. Axons to the postcentral gyrus by way of the posterior limb of the internal capsule.

3. *Crude (light) touch pathway* (see Fig. 2-21)
   Neuron I: Cell bodies in the dorsal root ganglion. Axons of the dorsal root enter the dorsal horn.
   Neuron II: Cell bodies in the dorsal horn. Axons are mostly crossed and ascend as the anterior spinothalamic tract.
   Neuron III: In the VPL nucleus of the thalamus; send axons to the postcentral gyrus.

4. *Posterior spinocerebellar and cuneocerebellar pathways*
   Neuron I: Dendrites arise in neuromuscular spindles and Golgi tendon organs as IA and IB fibers respectively. Cell bodies in the dorsal root ganglia. Axons enter via dorsal roots; those below L3 and above C8 ascend in the posterior white column. The rest will enter the nucleus dorsalis near the level of entry.
   Neuron II: Cell bodies in the nucleus dorsalis

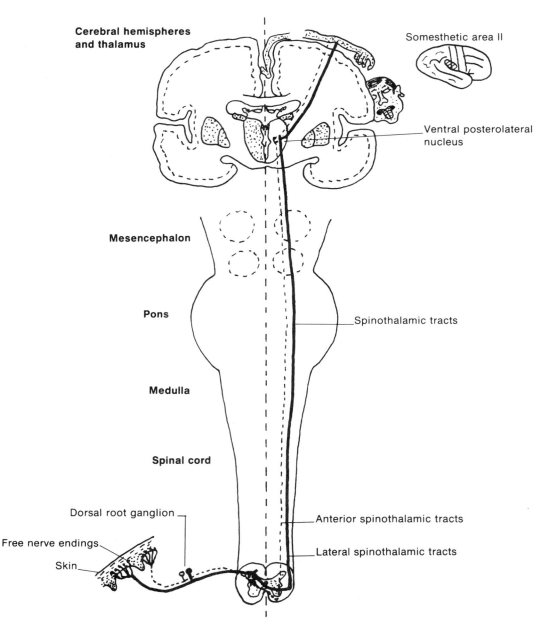

Fig. 2-21. Lateral spinothalamic tract *(solid lines)* for pain and temperature and anterior spinothalamic tract *(dashed lines)* for light touch.

(Clarke's column) receive first-order neurons from below the C8 cord level. Axons of these cells ascend ipsilaterally as the posterior spinocerebellar tract to the cerebellum. Cell bodies in the accessory cuneate nucleus receive ascending first-order neurons from levels above C8. Axons from this nucleus form the cuneocerebellar tract, which becomes part of the inferior cerebellar peduncle.

Ascending Pathways Arising at Brain Stem Levels

1. *Pain and temperature pathway* (see Fig. 2-19)
   Neuron I: Dendrites in the maxillary, mandibular, and ophthalmic division of the trigeminal nerve. Cell bodies in the trigeminal ganglion. Axons enter the pons and descend to the low medulla as the spinal tract of cranial nerve V. Some first-order neurons from the posterior ear region are part of the facial,

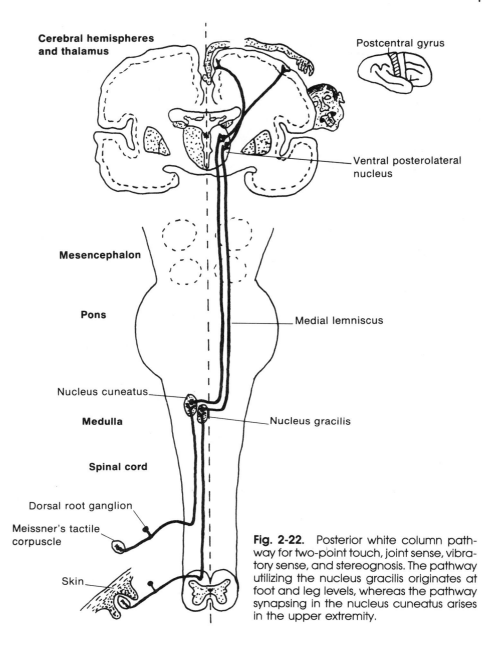

Cerebral hemispheres
and thalamus

Postcentral gyrus

Ventral posterolateral
nucleus

Mesencephalon

Pons

Medial lemniscus

Nucleus cuneatus

Medulla

Nucleus gracilis

Spinal cord

Dorsal root ganglion

Meissner's tactile
corpuscle

Skin

Fig. 2-22. Posterior white column pathway for two-point touch, joint sense, vibratory sense, and stereognosis. The pathway utilizing the nucleus gracilis originates at foot and leg levels, whereas the pathway synapsing in the nucleus cuneatus arises in the upper extremity.

glossopharyngeal, and vagus nerves. Their axons enter the spinal nucleus of cranial nerve V.

Neuron II: Cell bodies in the spinal nucleus of cranial nerve V. Axons cross and ascend as the ventral ascending secondary tract of cranial nerve V.

Neuron III: Cell bodies in the VPM nucleus. Axons to the postcentral gyrus and somesthetic area II via the posterior limb of the internal capsule.

2. *Touch pathways* (see Fig. 2-19)

Neuron I: Cell bodies in the trigeminal ganglion. Axons to the principal sensory nucleus and to the upper part of the spinal nucleus of cranial nerve V.

Neuron II: Cell bodies in the principal sensory nucleus and spinal nucleus of cranial nerve V. Axons from both nuclei cross and ascend as the ventral secondary ascending tract of cranial nerve V. Some axons from the principal sensory nucleus of cranial nerve V ascend ipsilaterally as the dorsal secondary ascending tract of cranial nerve V.

Neuron III: Cell bodies in the VPM nucleus of the thalamus; axons go to the postcentral gyrus.

3. *Hearing pathway*

Neuron I: Dendrites from the hair cells of the organ of Corti to bipolar cells in the spiral cochlear ganglion; axons to the pons–medulla junction.

Neuron II: Cell bodies in the dorsal and ventral cochlear nuclei; axons are both crossed and uncrossed and ascend as the lateral lemniscus to the inferior colliculus. There may be relays through the superior olivary nucleus, nucleus of the lateral lemniscus, and nucleus of the trapezoid body in this ascent

Neuron III: Cell bodies in the inferior colliculus. Axons pass into the brachium of the inferior colliculus.

Neuron IV: Cell bodies in the medial geniculate body. Axons pass in the sublenticular limb of the internal capsule to the transverse temporal gyri of Heschl.

4. *Visual pathway*

Neuron I: Rods and cones

Neuron II: Bipolar cells of the retina

Neuron III: Cell bodies are the ganglion cell layer of the retina. Axons course as the optic nerve, optic chiasm, and optic tract. Axons from the nasal half of the retina cross in the optic chiasm.

Neuron IV: Cell bodies in the lateral geniculate body. Axons pass in the sublenticular and retrolenticular limbs of the internal capsule and in the geniculocalcarine tract (optic radiations) to the calcarine striate cortex (area 17).

Descending Pathways of the Brain and Spinal Cord

1. Pyramidal system (see Fig. 2-23)
   a. By way of corticospinal tract
      UMN: Cell bodies are in the precentral gyrus (area 4) and in the postcentral gyrus and premotor cortex. Axons descend in the posterior limb of the internal capsule, the crus cerebri, basis pontis, and pyramids. Most cross at the pyramidal decussation and descend in the lateral corticospinal tract. They synapse on internuncials at the level of the lower motor neuron innervated.
      LMN: Cell bodies in the anterior horn of the spinal cord as alpha motor neurons to extrafusal muscle fibers and as gamma efferent

neurons to intrafusal muscle fibers. This pathway tonically facilitates the antagonists of antigravity muscles and phasically controls the distal muscles in fine movements.

   b. By way of corticobulbar pathways
      UMN: Cell bodies located near the lateral fissure in the precentral and postcentral gyri and in the premotor cortex. Axons pass through the genu and posterior limb of the internal capsule and crus cerebri. Those from frontal eye fields to the lateral gaze center (PPRF) for saccadic eye movements, to that portion of the hypoglossal nucleus that supplies the genioglossus nuclei, and to that portion of the facial motor nucleus that supplies muscles of the lower face are crossed. Those that supply the lateral gaze center for smooth pursuit movements and those that terminate on the spinal accessory nucleus are uncrossed. All other corticobulbar fibers are both crossed and uncrossed.
      LMN: Cell bodies in the SE and SVE nuclei of cranial nerves III through VII and IX through XII.

2. Major extrapyramidal tracts (see summary of tracts in Fig. 2-3)
   a. By way of vestibulospinal tract
      UMN: Cell bodies are located in the lateral vestibular nucleus. Axons of this tract are located in the anterior funiculus and end on internuncial neurons.
      LMN: Gamma and alpha motor neurons to antigravity muscles are facilitated.
   b. By way of lateral reticulospinal tract
      UMN: Cell bodies are in the gigantocellular nucleus in the reticular formation of the medulla. Axons of this tract are in the lateral funiculus.
      LMN: Gamma and alpha motor neurons to antigravity muscles are inhibited.
   c. By way of medial reticulospinal tract
      UMN: Cell bodies are in the oral and caudal pontine reticular nuclei. Axons of this tract descend in the reticular formation of the brain stem and in the anterior funiculus.
      LMN: Gamma and alpha motor neurons of antigravity muscles are facilitated.
   d. By way of rubrospinal tract
      UMN: Cell bodies are in the red nucleus. Axons cross in the ventral tegmental decussation and descend in the rubrospinal tract. This tract is located in the lateral reticular

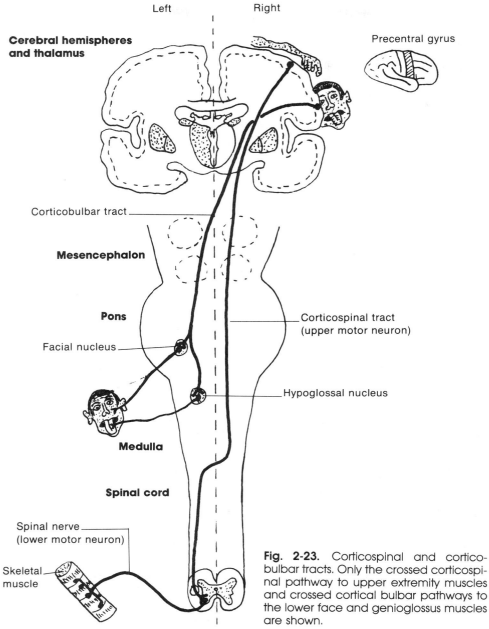

Left   Right

Cerebral hemispheres
and thalamus

Precentral gyrus

Corticobulbar tract

Mesencephalon

Pons

Facial nucleus

Corticospinal tract
(upper motor neuron)

Hypoglossal nucleus

Medulla

Spinal cord

Spinal nerve
(lower motor neuron)

Skeletal
muscle

Fig. 2-23. Corticospinal and cortico-bulbar tracts. Only the crossed corticospinal pathway to upper extremity muscles and crossed cortical bulbar pathways to the lower face and genioglossus muscles are shown.

formation of the brain stem and in the lateral funiculus of the spinal cord. Axons end on internuncials.

LMN: Gamma and alpha motor neurons probably facilitate the antagonists of antigravity muscles.

Somatic Motor Control Mechanisms. The somatic motor anterior horn cells of the spinal cord and the SE (nuclei 3, 4, 6, and 12) and SVE (nucleus ambiguus and motor nuclei of 5 and 7) neurons of the brain stem are regulated by afferent and association fibers from all levels of the CNS. Afferent and internuncial neurons innervating anterior horn cells within one level of the spinal cord constitute a segmental level of motor control. An example of this is the myotatic stretch reflex where IA fibers from the muscle spindle of a stretched muscle convey impulses monosynaptically at the level of entry of the dorsal root, with an alpha motor neuron supplying the extrafusal muscle fibers of that muscle.

Intersegmental connections of afferent and association neurons within the spinal cord constitute a mechanism for intersegmental regulation of motor activity. Such connections may involve collaterals from long ascending and descending pathways or shorter spinospinal fibers of the fasciculus proprius. An example of this is the pain withdrawal reflex wherein pain fibers are stimulated. The impulse is carried to several levels of the cord by way of the fasciculus proprius in order that motor neurons involved in the body adjustment of withdrawal can be stimulated.

Suprasegmental control pathways involve connections of the spinal cord with higher centers of the CNS. This constellation of numerous suprasegmental connections can best be appreciated if they are divided into phylogenetically older and newer systems. Such a scheme can include older antigravity and vestibular regulation, the next oldest regulation of the more stereotyped grosser movements involving the more axial musculature and the newer fine discrete movements.

Antigravity and vestibular connections involve input from muscle spindles and the vestibular apparatus. These afferents make connections through the spinocerebellar tracts and vestibular nuclei with the cerebellum; the vestibular fibers end in the flocculonodular lobe, while spindle information is conveyed to vermal and paravermal areas of the anterior and posterior lobes of the cerebellum. Cerebellar efferents, through dentatorubral fibers of the superior cerebellar peduncle, synapse in the red nucleus with cells of the rubrospinal tract, which bring about the facilitation of antagonists of the antigravity muscles. Cerebellar efferents from the flocculonodular lobe arise from the fastigial nuclei and terminate in the lateral vestibular nuclei. Axons from the lateral nucleus constitute the lateral vestibulospinal tract, which is facilitory to antigravity muscles. The medial and lateral reticulospinal tracts receive input from all levels of the CNS and are facilitory and inhibitory, respectively, to the antigravity muscles.

The regulation of *gross stereotyped movements* involves the basal ganglia and their ascending connections with the cortex and their descending connections through the reticular formation. In these circuits the premotor cortex and centromedian nucleus of the thalamus receive ascending afferent input and relay this information to the caudate and putamen. The neostriatum (putamen and caudate) also receive input from the substantia nigra. The neostriatal nuclei send axons to the globus pallidus and probably have an inhibitory effect on it. The efferent outflow from the basal ganglia (lenticular

nucleus) is from the globus pallidus to (1) the motor and premotor cortex by way of the ventral anterior and ventral lateral nuclei of the thalamus, and (2) the motor neurons of the spinal cord and brain stem by way of the subthalamus, prerubral field, red nucleus and the reticulospinal, rubrospinal, and reticuloreticular pathways. Pallidal efferents to the thalamic nuclei course through the internal capsule and then pass between the subthalamic nucleus and zona incerta in the fasciculus lenticularis to reach the prerubral field (of Forel). From the prerubral field, axons loop laterally toward the thalamus in the fasciculus thalamicus, or they descend in the reticular formation to contralateral motor nuclei. Other pallidal efferents loop around the internal capsule in the ansa lenticularis in their pathway to the thalamus.

Lesions of the basal ganglia, subthalamus, and substantia nigra are associated with disturbances in involuntary movements (dyskinesias) and in muscle tone. Lesions of the subthalamic nucleus can lead to hemiballism on the opposite side due to release of the globus pallidus from the inhibitory control of the subthalamus. Parkinsonism (paralysis agitans) is characterized by a decrease of dopamine in the substantia nigra and neostriatum (caudate and putamen). The tremor at rest and rigidity of this disorder may be due to inability of the neostriatum to inhibit the globus pallidus. Lesions producing chorea and athetosis are probably in the striatum but are not as clearly localized as the other basal ganglia disorders.

The pathways involved in the initiation and performance of a *fine coordinated movement* involve (1) input to the cortex, (2) a feedback loop between the cerebral cortex and the cerebellum, (3) corticospinal and corticobulbar pathways, and (4) alpha and gamma motor neurons of the spinal cord and brain stem. In these pathways ascending exteroceptive input is relayed through the thalamus to the primary receptive areas of the cortex (areas 3, 1, 2; 41 and 42; 43; 17). Projections from the primary receptive areas go to unisensory association areas lying adjacent to the primary receptive areas (see Fig. 2-20). The specific sensation for each receptive area is "recognized" in each unisensory association area. Projections from the unisensory association areas congregate in multisensory association areas in the junctional area of the inferior parietal gyrus (areas 39 and 40), superior temporal gyrus, and lateral occipital gyri. In this area gnosis from more than one sensation is utilized in the initiation and formulation of learned complex motor activity.

Axons from these parietal, occipital, and tempo-

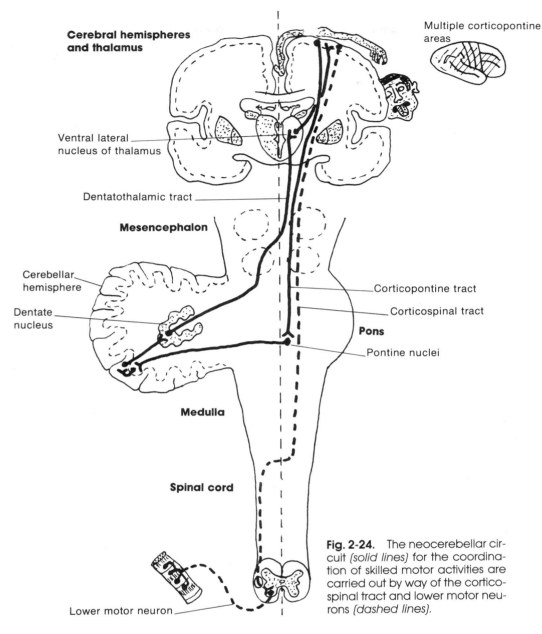

Cerebral hemispheres and thalamus

Multiple corticopontine areas

Ventral lateral nucleus of thalamus

Dentatothalamic tract

Mesencephalon

Cerebellar hemisphere

Dentate nucleus

Corticopontine tract

Corticospinal tract

Pons

Pontine nuclei

Medulla

Spinal cord

Lower motor neuron

Fig. 2-24. The neocerebellar circuit *(solid lines)* for the coordination of skilled motor activities are carried out by way of the corticospinal tract and lower motor neurons *(dashed lines)*.

ral regions, as well as axons from the prefrontal cortical center for initiative and judgment and from premotor and motor regions, descend as corticopontine pathways to pontine nuclei (Fig. 2-24). Frontopontine fibers descend through the anterior limb of the internal capsule and medial portion of the crus cerebri. The other corticopontine fibers descend in the posterior limb of the internal capsule and lateral part of the crus cerebri. After they synapse on cells of the pontine nuclei, axons of the latter cells carry impulses across the midline of the basis pontis and ascend to the cerebellar cortex in the middle cerebellar peduncle. These pontocere-

bellar fibers are mossy fibers that end in the granule cell layer. From here impulses spread through the molecular layer of the neocerebellar cortex of the posterior lobe and are transmitted to Purkinje cells. Axons of Purkinje cells pass to the dentate nucleus, where they synapse on cells whose fibers cross the midline in the decussation of the superior cerebellar peduncle and ascend to the ventral lateral nucleus of the thalamus. From the ventral lateral nucleus axons ascend to the motor cortex.

The ultimate descending pathway for fine discrete movements is by way of the corticospinal and corticobulbar tracts to anterior horn cells and brain stem

SE and SVE neurons. In this complex pathway, which involves a double crossing of fibers in the cerebral cortex–cerebellar loop and a single crossing of the corticospinal tract, the cerebellum acts as a computer coordinating the activity of numerous neurons.

Lesions of the cerebellum may demonstrate deficits in motor activity. Neocerebellar lesions produce a lateral cerebellar syndrome where the symptoms are on the same side of the body as the involved cerebellar hemisphere. This syndrome demonstrates an asynergia of voluntary skilled activity characterized by hypotonia and postural fixation defects, especially of the limbs. Some clinical signs and abnormal reflexes of neocerebellar disease are dysmetria, intention tremor, rebound phenomenon, disdiadochokinesis, explosive speech, decomposition of movement, and tendency to fall to the side of the lesion. Flocculonodular syndrome is primarily a disorder of locomotion and equilibrium. This is characterized by truncal ataxia with the patient falling, or walking on a wide base or with a drunken gait.

Lesions of various portions of the cerebral cortex lead to deficits in motor activity. Immediately after partial or complete lesions of the precentral gyrus, there is flaccid paralysis of the contralateral limbs and loss of superficial and deep reflexes, and hypotonus and exaggerated deep reflexes may occur. Involvement of the premotor area and corticoreticular fibers may lead to spastic paralysis. Lesions of Broca's area in the inferior frontal opercular and triangular areas of the dominant hemisphere may result in expressive aphasia. Sensory aphasias are more often associated with lesions of the posterior temporoparietal region. Ideomotor and ideational apraxias appear to be associated with lesions of the dominant parietal lobe in the region of the inferior parietal gyrus. Ablative lesions of the frontal eye fields in the posterior part of the middle frontal gyrus interfere with voluntary conjugate eye movements to the opposite side. Corticobulbar lesions can result in contralateral lower facial paralysis, a deviation of the tongue to the opposite side upon protrusion, and ipsilateral weakness in shoulder shrugging. Damage to the corticospinal tract in the spinal cord will give an ipsilateral UMN complex of symptoms within several weeks of the onset of the injury. This constellation of symptoms includes: (1) increased segmental muscle tone (hypertonus), especially in extensors of the lower extremity and in flexors of the upper extremity due to loss of lateral reticulospinal fibers; (2) increased deep tendon reflexes (hyperreflexia); (3) absence of or diminished superficial reflexes; (4) presence of pathologic reflexes such as the Babinski reflex; and (5) loss of fine movements. Lesions of LMNs produce flaccid paralysis or paresis, loss of deep and superficial reflexes, and denervation atrophy.

Visceral Motor Control Mechanisms. The hypothalamus is the highest subcortical center for the regulation of visceral activity. It receives ascending information from the spinal and cranial nerves by way of the reticular formation. In addition to these spinoreticular and reticuloreticular pathways, the hypothalamus receives input from the thalamus, basal ganglia, and cerebral cortex. Efferents from the hypothalamus descend to the brain stem and spinal cord and also terminate in the thalamus, cortex and hypophysis.

As previously indicated, hypothalamic nuclei are structurally divisible into medial and lateral groups by the columns of the fornix. The lateral group includes lateral and tuberal nuclei. The medial group is further subdivided into anterior, middle, and posterior groups. The anterior group includes the preoptic, anterior, supraoptic, paraventricular, and periventricular nuclei. The dorsomedial and ventromedial nuclei comprise the middle group; the posterior and mammillary nuclei make up the posterior group.

Functional classification of nuclei into autonomic and endocrine neurosecretory groups makes the hypothalamic regions easier to appreciate. An anteromedial group of nuclei are involved in parasympathetic regulation. A posterolateral group of posterior, tuberal, and lateral nuclei regulate sympathetic activity. Outflow from the hypothalamus to preganglionic parasympathetic and preganglionic sympathetic cells of the brain stem and spinal cord is by way of periventricular fibers that multisynaptically utilize the dorsal longitudinal fasciculus or the reticuloreticular and reticulospinal pathways.

The endocrine neurosecretory nuclei are the supraoptic and paraventricular and the hypophysiotrophic area of nuclei. The supraoptic and paraventricular nuclei produce antidiuretic (vasopressin) and oxytocin hormones that are secreted in the pars nervosa. The hypophysiotrophic nuclei include several hypothalamic nuclei (*e.g.*, ventromedial, arcuate, preoptic) whose axons terminate in the infundibular stalk adjacent to capillary loops of the hypophyseal portal vascular system. Releasing and inhibiting factors produced in neurons of the hypophysiotrophic area pass into these capillary loops and are transported by way of venous trunks of the pituitary stalk and capillaries of the pars distalis to the chromophobes and chromophiles of the anterior pituitary.

Visceral motor activity is influenced by descending pathways from the olfactory cortex and the limbic system. Olfactohypothalamic fibers course from the pyriform cortex to the hypothalamus. Impulses from the amygdala course in a ventral path and also in the stria terminalis to reach the hypothalamus and septal nuclei. Basal olfactory regions and the septal area are connected through the hypothalamus with the mesencephalic reticular formation by way of the medial forebrain bundle. The septal region is also in communication with the mesencephalic reticular formation through a pathway that includes the stria medullaris, habenular nucleus, habenulopeduncular tract (fasciculus retroflexus), interpeduncular nucleus, and tegmental nuclei.

The *limbic cortex* is phylogenetically "older" cortex that forms a ring around the corpus callosum and diencephalon. It includes the subcallosal area, cingulate gyrus, isthmus (retrosplenial area), parahippocampal gyrus, and hippocampal formation (hippocampus and dentate gyrus). All of these regions are connected through an association bundle called the cingulum. Axons from the hippocampal formation pass as the fimbria and fornix to the mammillary bodies and septal region. The mammillary bodies are linked to the cingulate gyrus through the mammillothalamic tract and its relay through the anterior nucleus of the thalamus. The mammillotegmental tract is a descending pathway from the mammillary bodies to the reticular formation of the brain stem.

In addition to the interconnections of the hypothalamus and amygdala with the phylogenetically older olfactory and limbic cortex, there are neocortical connections in the limbic lobe. An important circuit is that between the prefrontal cortex and the hypothalamus through a relay in the dorsomedial nucleus of the thalamus.

Lesions of the hypothalamus affect visceral activity. Damage to the lateral hypothalamic nucleus may abolish appetite and lead to weight loss, whereas lesions of the satiety center in the ventromedial nucleus may lead to obesity through excessive eating. Lesions of the supraoptic nuclei can lead to diabetes insipidus. Bilateral temporal lobe lesions involving the pyriform cortex, amygdala, and hippocampal formation may produce disturbances in emotional behavior and recent memory.

THORAX

The thorax is bounded posteriorly by the thoracic vertebrae and the ribs, laterally by the ribs and the intercostal spaces, and anteriorly by the sternum, the costal cartilages, and ribs. The sternal angle (of Louis) is formed by the junction of the manubrium and the body of the sternum. It marks the level of the second costal cartilages, the bifurcation of the trachea, and the lower aspect of the fourth thoracic vertebra.

SURFACE MARKINGS

Lungs and Pleura. The boundaries of the lungs and pleura may be mapped on the surface of the body as follows: The apex of the pleura extends about 2.5 cm above the medial third of the clavicle. Its border then passes medially behind the sternoclavicular joint, and the two pleura meet in the midline behind the sternal angle. The medial edge passes inferiorly to about the seventh costal cartilage where it inclines laterally. The medial edge of the left pleura inclines laterally at the level of the fourth costal cartilage because of the heart. This indentation of the medial edge of the pleura on the left is the cardiac notch. In the midclavicular line (below the middle of the clavicle), the lower border is at the level of the eighth rib and in the midaxillary line is at the tenth rib. Posteriorly at the scapular line (vertebral border of the scapula), the level of the pleura corresponds to the twelfth rib. The surface projection of the superior aspect of the lung corresponds to that of the pleura. The lung does not extend quite as far medially as the pleura so that the costal and mediastinal layers of parietal pleura are adjacent, thus forming the *costomediastinal recess.* The inferior border of the lung inclines laterally at the sixth costal cartilage. At the midclavicular line it is at the level of the sixth rib, at the midaxillary line the eighth rib, and at the scapular line the tenth rib. The area of pleural cavity below the inferior margin of the lung, where the parietal layers of costal and diaphragmatic pleura are adjacent, is called the *costodiaphragmatic recess.* During deep inspiration the lung descends into this recess.

The *interlobar fissures* separating the lobes of the lungs can also be reflected on the surface. The oblique fissure of the left lung divides the superior lobe from the middle lobe; that of the right lung separates the inferior lobe below from the superior and middle lobes above. The *oblique fissure* is at the level of the fourth rib posteriorly (base of the spine of the scapula), the fifth rib in the midaxillary line, and the sixth rib in the midclavicular line. A *horizontal fissure* separates the superior lobe from the middle lobe of the right lung. This fissure is at the level of the fourth costal cartilage next to the sternum, and at the level of the fifth rib in the midaxillary line where it joins the oblique fissure.

Surface Projections of the Heart. The heart may be mapped on the anterior thoracic wall by lines connecting four points. Point 1 is at the level of the second left costal cartilage, 1 cm to 2 cm lateral to the edge of the sternum. Point 2 lies 1 cm to 2 cm lateral to the edge of the sternum at the level of the third costal cartilage on the right. Point 3 is located at the level of the right sixth costal cartilage, 1 cm to 2 cm from the sternal margin. Point 4 lies 7 cm to 8 cm from the midline in the left fifth intercostal space, and marks the location of the apex of the heart. The lower (diaphragmatic) border corresponds to a line drawn from the apex through the xiphisternal articulation to point 3. The *right border* is indicated by a slightly convex line running from the right third costal cartilage to the right lower border. It is formed by the right atrium below and the superior vena cava above. The *left border* is formed by the left ventricle and the left auricular appendage. It curves from the second left costal cartilage to the apex. The *posterior surface* or base of the heart is formed largely by the left atrium and a portion of the right atrium. All of the great veins—pulmonary and venae cavae—enter this portion of the heart. Most of the *anterior* (sternocostal) *surface* of the heart is formed by the right ventricle, with smaller portions of the left ventricle, to the left and the right atrium to the right. The *inferior* or diaphragmatic *surface* is formed predominantly by the left and right ventricles.

The pulmonary and aortic orifices lie opposite the upper and lower margins of the third costal cartilage along the left margin of the sternum. The aortic valve lies behind the left side of the sternum at the level of the third interspace. The pulmonary valve is located to the left of the third chondrosternal articulation. The right atrioventricular (tricuspid) valve is in the midsternal line at the level of the fifth intercostal space. The left atrioventricular (mitral) valve lies at the left fourth sternochondral articulation.

Surface Projections of the Major Vessels. The *thoracic aorta* may be mapped on the surface of the body as follows: The ascending aorta extends from the aortic orifice on the left sternal margin to a point on the right margin of the sternum at the upper border of the second costal cartilage. The arch of the aorta curves to the left and backward, and its upper convexity lies about 2 cm below the suprasternal notch. The descending thoracic aorta extends from the left side of the lower border of the fourth thoracic vertebra to the aortic hiatus of the diaphragm located in front of the body of the twelfth thoracic vertebra. The branches arising from the aortic arch are the brachiocephalic trunk in the midline, the left common carotid a little to the left, and the left subclavian still farther to the left and on a more dorsal plane.

The right and the left brachiocephalic veins unite to form the *superior vena cava* behind the first right chondrosternal junction. Posterior to the right sternoclavicular joint the brachiocephalic artery divides and the right brachiocephalic vein begins. Posterior to the left sternoclavicular joint, the left common carotid and the left subclavian enter the neck, and the left brachiocephalic vein begins.

MEDIASTINUM

The mediastinum contains all the thoracic viscera except the lungs. It is located between the pleural cavities and between the sternum and vertebral column. It is divisible into superior, anterior, posterior, and middle regions.

Superior Mediastinum. The superior mediastinum is that part of the mediastinum located above the sternal angle. It contains the aortic arch and its branches, the superior vena cava and its tributaries, the vagus, recurrent laryngeal and phrenic nerves, trachea, esophagus, thoracic duct, left highest intercostal vein, the remains of the thymus, and some lymph nodes.

Anterior Mediastinum. The anterior mediastinum is the area in front of the pericardial cavity. It contains the thymus, internal thoracic vessels, lymph nodes, and surrounding connective tissue.

Posterior Mediastinum. The posterior cavity behind the heart and the great vessels contains the thoracic aorta, esophagus, vagus nerves, thoracic duct, azygos and hemiazygos veins, lymph nodes, and sympathetic trunks.

Middle Mediastinum. The middle mediastinum contains the heart and the pericardium.

HEART

Gross Structure of the Heart. The heart is a four-chambered organ consisting of two ventricles and two atria. An interatrial septum separates the two atria; an interventricular septum lies between the left and right ventricles. Anterior and posterior interventricular sulci on the sternocostal and diaphragmatic surfaces of the heart mark the location of the interventricular septum. The coronary sulcus encircles the heart at the atrioventricular (A-V) junction. The sulci are occupied by portions of the coronary vessels that supply the heart.

The borders of the heart were discussed previously in the section on surface markings. The *apex* of the heart is part of the left ventricle, and it points downward and to the left. It is located deep to the left fifth intercostal space about 4 cm below and 2 cm medial to the left nipple, and it is overlapped by an extension of the pleura and lungs. The *base* of the heart faces upward, to the right and toward the back. It consists mainly of the left atrium, part of the right atrium, and proximal parts of the great vessels. Its superior boundary is at the bifurcation of the pulmonary artery, and its inferior boundary is at the coronary sulcus. The left boundary of the base is at the oblique vein of the left atrium, and the right boundary is at the sulcus terminalis. The base is separated from the bodies of T5–8 vertebrae by the thoracic aorta, esophagus, and thoracic duct. The *sternocostal surface* of the heart is occupied by the right atrium, right ventricle, and a small part of the left ventricle. The *diaphragmatic surface* is comprised of the two ventricles.

The *right atrium* is larger than the left and is comprised of two parts: (1) a principal cavity (sinus venarum), and (2) an auricula. The smooth-surfaced sinus venarum is that part of the atrium between the ostia of the superior and inferior venae cavae and the right A-V opening. The superior vena cava opens into the upper and posterior part of the sinus venarum; the inferior vena cava opens into the lowest part of the sinus venarum near the interatrial septum. The coronary sinus opens between the ostium of the inferior vena cava and the A-V foramen. Rudimentary valves guard openings of the inferior vena cava and coronary sinus. The auricula is rough surfaced because of muscular ridges (musculi pectinati). It is demarcated externally from the sinus venarum by the sulcus terminalis and internally by the crista terminalis.

The dorsal wall of the right atrium consists of the interatrial septum. The fossa ovalis, representing the embryonic foramen ovale, is an oval depression in the septal wall located above the openings of the coronary sinus and inferior vena cava. It is bounded above and at its sides by the limbus fossa ovalis representing the embryonic free margin of septum secundum.

The *right ventricle* is bounded on the right by the coronary sulcus and on the left by the anterior interventricular sulcus. Its superior part, the conus arte-riosus (infundibulum), is continuous with the pulmonary trunk. Inferiorly, its wall forms the acute margin of the heart. The wall of the right ventricle is about one third the thickness of the left ventricle, but the capacity (85 ml) of both ventricles is the same. The internal surface is quite irregular because of ridges of muscle called trabeculae carneae. Some of these project from the wall of the ventricle and insert through chordae tendineae on the apices, margins, and ventricular surfaces of cusps of the right A-V valve.

The right A-V (tricuspid) valve has anterior (infundibular), posterior (marginal), and medial (septal) cusps. The anterior cusp is the largest, the posterior is the smallest. These leaflets are composed of strong fibrous tissue that is continuous at their bases with the anuli fibrosi of the fibrous skeleton separating the atria from the ventricles. The anterior papillary muscle arises from the anterior and septal walls and is attached to the anterior and posterior cusps by chordae tendineae. The septomarginal trabecula (moderator band) extends from the interventricular septum to the base of the anterior papillary muscle. The posterior papillary muscle arises from the posterior wall, and its chordae tendineae insert on the posterior and septal cusps.

The *conus arteriosus* has a smooth inner surface. It is limited from the rest of the ventricle by a ridge of muscular tissue called the crista supraventricularis. At the summit of the conus is the orifice of the pulmonary trunk. The pulmonary valve consists of three cusps: anterior, right, and left. Each cusp contains a sinus behind it and has its convexity directed toward the ventricle. Adjacent cusps attach at a common commissure. A thin marginal lunula portion of each cusp runs from each commissure to a thickened nodule in the central free margin of the cusp. When the valve is closed, the lunulae and nodules of the cusps are in contact.

The *left atrium* consists of a principal cavity (sinus venarum) and an auricula. The smooth-walled sinus venarum receives the four pulmonary veins. The interatrial septum covering the fossa ovalis of the right atrium constitutes a valve of the foramen ovale. The left auricula is longer than that of the right atrium. It curves ventrally around the base of the pulmonary trunk, and it lies over the proximal portion of the left coronary artery.

The *left ventricle* is longer, more conical and thicker than the right. It forms the apex of the heart and is separated from the right ventricle by the muscular and membranous parts of the interventricular septum. It has two openings, the left A-V (mitral), which is guarded by the mitral valve, and the aortic, which is limited by the aortic valve. The left A-V valve consists of a large anterior (aortic) and a smaller posterior cusp. Each cusp receives chordae tendineae from both the anterior and posterior papillary muscles. The aortic opening is anterior and to the right of the mitral valve. The portion of the ventricle below the aortic orifice is called the *aortic vestibule.* The aortic valve consists of three cusps, posterior, right, and left. The cusps are similar in structure to those of the pulmonary valve, but they are bigger and stronger. The right and left coronary arteries originate from the right and left aortic sinuses (of Valsalva), respectively.

The *skeleton of the heart* consists of a series of fibrous rings (anuli fibrosi) and fibrous trigones. Fibrous rings surround each A-V orifice, the aortic opening, and the pulmonary orifice. The cusps of each of the associated valves are attached to the rings. The membranous part of the interventricular septum also is continuous with the fibrous tissue of these anuli. At the junction of the A-V rings with the aortic ring a right fibrous trigone is formed. A left fibrous trigone occurs between the aortic and left A-V rings.

Microscopic Structure of the Heart. The heart wall consists of three layers: (1) an inner endocardial layer, (2) a middle myocardial layer, and (3) an outer epicardial layer. The *endocardium* consists of endothelium and a subendothelial connective tissue layer of fine collagenous and elastic fibers and some smooth muscle fibers. The endocardium of the atria is thicker than that of the ventricles. A subendocardial layer of loose connective tissue and blood vessels binds the endocardium to the myocardium. This layer in the ventricles contains the specialized muscle fibers of the conduction system.

The *myocardium* consists of spiraling bundles of cardiac muscle that take origin from the anuli fibrosi. In the atria the myocardium is a thin layer of fibers with a simple arrangement. The muscle of the ventricles is more complex and consists of several layers. The ventricular bands of muscle originate from the fibrous anulus and course in a helical manner from right to left and toward the apex. Some of the more superficial fibers can be traced in a mantle covering both ventricles. Some intermediate fibers weave from ventricle to ventricle by way of the septum. The more numerous deeper fibers pass into either of the ventricular walls and end by piercing deeply and becoming the papillary muscles. The microscopic structure of cardiac muscle was reviewed with skeletal muscle tissue in the section on the back.

The *epicardium* consists of mesothelium and an underlying connective tissue layer. A subepicardial layer of loose connective tissue containing blood vessels, nerves and fat binds the epicardium to the myocardium. The epicardium is the visceral pericardium.

The A-V valves consist of a core of dense connective tissue, which is continuous with the anuli fibrosi, and an outer layer of endocardium. The endocardium on the atrial surface of the valves is thicker than that on the ventricular side. Chordae tendineae are composed of dense regularly arranged connective tissue. The aortic and pulmonary semilunar valves resemble the atrioventricular valves, but they are much thinner.

Recent work indicates that the atrial myocytes contain granules which have been identified as one or several polypeptides called atriopeptin(s), which are responsible for a profound natriuresis.

Conduction System of the Heart. This system is composed of specialized cardiac muscle found in the sinoatrial (S-A) node and in the A-V node and bundle. The heart beat is initiated in the *S-A node (pacemaker of the heart)* located in the right atrium in the upper part of the crista terminalis just to the left of the opening of the superior vena cava. Cells of the S-A node are slender and fusiform. From the S-A node the cardiac impulse spreads throughout the atrial musculature to reach the *A-V node* lying in the subendocardium of the atrial septum directly above the opening of the coronary sinus. The A-V node has small irregularly arranged branching fibers that contain few myofibrils. Thereafter the impulse is conducted to the ventricles by passing through the specialized tissue of the A-V bundle (of His). This bundle consists of a crus commune and right and left bundle branches. The common bundle travels from the A-V node into the membranous part of the interventricular septum. It divides into right and left bundle branches that pass in the subendocardium along the muscular part of the septum and distribute to the ventricles as Purkinje tissue. *Purkinje cells* are large specialized cardiac muscle cells that usually are binucleate and contain much centrally located sarcoplasm.

The innervation of the heart is from both the parasympathetic and sympathetic divisions of the autonomic nervous system. Right and left thoracic cardiac branches from the vagus nerves arise from the recurrent laryngeal nerves and pass to the deep cardiac plexus where they synapse on postganglionic parasympathetic neurons. The vagus nerves also give rise to superior and inferior cervical cardiac nerves. The left inferior cervical cardiac nerve ends in the superficial cardiac plexus; the rest end in the deep plexus. Superior, middle, and inferior cervical cardiac nerves arising from sympathetic ganglia also descend to cardiac plexi. The left superior cervical cardiac sympathetic nerve ends in the superficial cardiac plexus; the rest end in the deep plexus. The deep cardiac plexus also receives thoracic cardiac branches from the upper five thoracic sympathetic ganglia. The coronary and pulmonary plexi and the right and left atria are supplied by branches from the superficial and deep plexi. The right vagal and sympathetic branches end chiefly in the region of the S-A node while the left branches end chiefly in the region of the A-V node.

Heart rate and force of contraction appear to be controlled mainly through the inhibitory action of the vagus nerves. Reflex slowing of the heart results from stimulation of the carotid sinus and the special pressure end organs in the carotid body. Impulses ascend in the carotid branch of the glossopharyngeal nerve to the inferior ganglion, thence to the solitary nucleus, and finally to the dorsal motor nucleus of the vagus in the medulla. Efferent cardioinhibitory impulses pass down the vagi to the cardiac plexus to synapse there with postganglionic fibers that terminate at the S-A node.

Cardiac pain impulses arise in free nerve endings, in the cardiac connective tissue and adventitia of the cardiac blood vessels. They then travel in visceral sensory fibers through the cardiac plexus, the middle and the inferior cervical cardiac and thoracic cardiac nerves, and the sympathetic chain ganglia of the neck and the upper thorax. All the pain fibers continue through the white rami communicantes of spinal nerves T1 and T5 and traverse the corresponding dorsal roots and their ganglia. Their cell bodies are located in the dorsal root ganglia, and the central fibers pass from these spinal ganglia to the dorsal horns of the upper thoracic cord segments.

Cardiac pain is referred to cutaneous areas that supply sensory impulses to the same segments of the cord that receive the cardiac sensation. Thus, they involve mainly the region of C7 through T5 and lie predominantly on the left side. The C8 and T1 segments are responsible for referred pain along the medial side of the arm and the forearm.

Blood Vessels of the Heart.   The arterial supply of the heart (Fig. 2-25) is provided by right and left coronary arteries. Venous drainage is chiefly through cardiac veins, which empty into the coronary sinus.

The *right coronary artery* originates from the right aortic sinus and courses ventrally between the pulmonary trunk and the right atrium. It descends in the right part of the A-V groove, passing onto the posteroinferior aspect of the heart. It terminates by dividing into two branches: the posterior interventricular artery, which passes toward the apex in the posterior interventricular sulcus where it anastomoses with the anterior interventricular branch of the left coronary, and a short continuation of the main trunk which anastomoses with the circumflex branch of the left coronary. Its marginal branch passes along the lower border of the right ventricle.

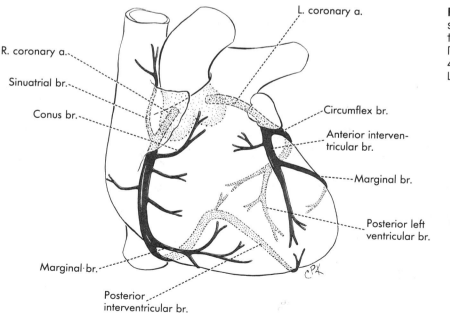

Fig. 2-25.   The coronary arteries shown from an anterior view of the heart. (Hollinshead WH, Rosse C: Textbook of Anatomy, 4th ed, p 535. Philadelphia, JB Lippincott, 1985)

The *left coronary artery,* which is usually larger than the right, originates from the left aortic sinus. It passes posterior and then to the left of the pulmonary trunk, branching into the circumflex and anterior interventricular arteries as it emerges from behind the pulmonary trunk. The circumflex artery passes to the left in the left A-V sulcus and anastomoses with the right coronary artery on the posteroinferior aspect of the heart. The anterior interventricular artery descends toward the apex in the anterior interventricular sulcus and passes onto the diaphragmatic surface where it anastomoses with the posterior interventricular branch of the right coronary.

For the most part, the *cardiac veins* accompany the coronary arteries and open into the coronary sinus, which empties into the right atrium. The remainder of the drainage occurs by means of small anterior cardiac veins that drain much of the anterior surface of the heart and terminate directly into the right atrium.

The *coronary sinus* is located in the posterior A-V groove and drains into the right atrium at the left of the mouth of the inferior vena cava. It receives three veins: (1) the great cardiac vein, which runs in the anterior interventricular groove, (2) the middle cardiac vein, located in the posterior interventricular groove; and (3) the small cardiac vein, which accompanies the marginal branch of the right coronary artery.

PERICARDIUM

The pericardium consists of two parts, an outer fibrous layer and an inner serous layer that adheres to the inner surface of the fibrous pericardium and reflects onto the outer surface of the heart.

Fibrous Pericardium. This tough connective tissue membrane surrounds the entire heart. Posteriorly and superiorly it blends with the adventitia of the great vessels. Inferiorly, it blends with the central tendon of the diaphragm. It is attached to the manubrium by a superior pericardiosternal ligament and to the xiphoid process by an inferior pericardiosternal ligament. In the area between these two ligamentous attachments, most of the anterior surface of the pericardium is separated from the thoracic wall by the lungs and pleural cavities. Only a small portion of the pericardium is intimately related to the lower left portion of the sternum and the medial ends of the fourth through the sixth costal cartilages. In this region no lungs or pleura intervene between the chest wall and fibrous pericardium. This small portion of the pericardium corresponds to the cardiac notch in the left lung and underlies the left fourth and fifth intercostal spaces. This relation permits needle entry to the pericardial cavity without traversing the pleural cavity. The fibrous pericardium is in contact posteriorly with the bronchi, esophagus, and descending thoracic aorta. The lateral outer surfaces of the fibrous pericardium are in close contact with the adjacent parietal pleura. The phrenic nerve and the pericardiocophrenic vessels descend between these two layers.

Serous Pericardium. This is a thin membrane comprised of mesothelium and an underlying connective tissue lamina. This membrane lines the pericardial cavity with a smooth glistening surface that facilitates cardiac movement. The serous pericardium, by its location, is divisible into two layers, parietal and visceral. The parietal layer lines the fibrous pericardium. At the points where the fibrous pericardium blends with the walls of the great vessels entering and leaving the heart, the parietal layer of the serous pericardium is reflected onto the vessels and then the heart muscle to form the visceral layer (epicardium) of the serous pericardium. These reflections are in the form of two tubular sheaths, one sheath for the aorta and pulmonary trunk (arterial mesocardium), and the other for the pulmonary veins and venae cavae (venous mesocardium). That portion of the pericardial cavity passing horizontally between the two tubular sheaths remains as the *transverse pericardial sinus.* The reflection of the visceral pleura over the veins forms an inverted U-shaped cul-de-sac dorsal to the heart that is referred to as the *oblique pericardial sinus.*

MAJOR VESSELS OF THE THORAX

The great vessels entering and leaving the heart are constituents of either the pulmonary or systemic vascular circuits. The pulmonary circulation is represented by the (1) pulmonary trunk originating from the right ventricle and branching into left and right pulmonary arteries, and (2) four pulmonary veins returning blood from the lungs to the left atrium. The systemic circulation is represented by the aorta, which originates from the left ventricle, and the superior and inferior venae cavae, which return blood to the right atrium. Lymphatic drainage from the thorax is by way of the thoracic duct and right lymphatic duct.

Pulmonary Trunk. This vessel arises from the infundibulum of the right ventricle and ascends obliquely and dorsally to the level of the sternal end of the second left costal cartilage where it divides into the left and right pulmonary arteries. In its course it passes in front of and then to the left of the ascending aorta. Anteriorly the pulmonary trunk is separated from the sternal end of the second left intercostal space by the left lung, pleura, and pericardium. At its origin it is related on the left to the left auricle and the left coronary artery, on the right to the right auricle and occasionally the right coronary artery.

Pulmonary Arteries. The right pulmonary artery is longer and wider than the left. It passes horizontally to the right and enters the hilus of the lung immediately below the upper lobe (eparterial) bronchus. In its course it passes dorsal to the ascending aorta, the superior vena cava, and the superior right pulmonary vein and lies ventral to the esophagus, right bronchus, and anterior pulmonary plexus. The left pulmonary artery passes laterally and posteriorly toward the root of the left lung, passing anterior to the left bronchus and the descending aorta. The ligamentum arteriosum connects the arch of the aorta above with the left pulmonary artery below. The superior left pulmonary vein lies at first ventral and then inferior to the left pulmonary artery.

Pulmonary Veins. These vessels emerge from each of the five lobes of the lung. Upon entering the lung root, however, those from the superior and middle lobes of the right lung unite. Thus, four terminal pulmonary veins course from the roots of the lungs to the left atrium. The superior right pulmonary vein passes dorsal to the superior vena cava, and the inferior right pulmonary vein passes behind the right atrium before both enter independently through the dorsal and right wall of the left atrium. The superior and inferior left pulmonary veins course anterior to the descending aorta and enter separately through the posterior wall of the left atrium near its left border. Fusion of the left pulmonary veins into a common trunk is not uncommon.

Aorta. This vessel is the main arterial trunk of the systemic circulation. It ascends from the left ventricle, arches to the left and dorsally over the root of the left lung, descends within the thorax on the left side of the vertebral column and enters the abdominal cavity through the aortic hiatus of the diaphragm. Thus, the parts of the aorta are the ascending aorta, the arch of the aorta, and the thoracic and abdominal portions of the descending aorta.

The *ascending aorta* arises from the base of the left ventricle at the caudal level of the third left costal cartilage. It passes obliquely upward to the right as far as the level of the second right costal cartilage. Initially, it is related anteriorly to the pulmonary trunk and the right auricle; more superi-

orly, it is separated from the sternum by the pericardium, variable portions of the right pleura, ventral margin of the right lung, loose areolar tissue, and the remains of the thymus. The coronary arteries arise from the ascending aorta.

The *arch of the aorta* lies in the superior mediastinum. It begins at the upper border of the second right sternocostal articulation. It curves cranially and dorsally to the left and then descends along the left side of the vertebral column to the level of the intervertebral disk between the fourth and fifth thoracic vertebrae where it continues as the descending aorta. In its course it passes at first ventral to the trachea and then to the left of this structure and the esophagus. Arising from the superior aspect of the aortic arch are three large vessels: the brachiocephalic artery (innominate), the left common carotid artery, and the left subclavian artery.

The *brachiocephalic artery* is the first branch from the arch of the aorta. It arises behind the middle of the manubrium sterni and courses obliquely upward toward the right sternoclavicular joint where it divides into the right subclavian and common carotid arteries.

The *left common carotid artery* arises from the arch of the aorta behind and immediately to the left of the brachiocephalic artery. Its thoracic portion extends up to the level of the left sternoclavicular joint. In its course it passes in front of the trachea, left recurrent laryngeal nerve, esophagus, thoracic duct, and left subclavian artery.

The *left subclavian artery* arises from the arch of the aorta about 2.5 cm distal to the left common carotid. It ascends almost vertically on the left side of the trachea to the root of the neck where it arches upward and laterally. It lies behind the left vagus nerve, left phrenic nerve, left superior cardiac sympathetic nerve, and left brachiocephalic vein. It passes in front of the left lung, pleura, esophagus, and thoracic duct.

The *thoracic portion of the descending aorta* lies in the posterior mediastinum. It extends downward from the upper border of the body of the fifth thoracic vertebra to the aortic opening in the diaphragm at the level of the twelfth thoracic vertebra. It has branches that supply the walls and viscera of the thorax. The thoracic descending aorta is related posteriorly to the left pleura and lung, the vertebral column, and the hemiazygous veins. Anteriorly, from above downward, it is related to the root of the left lung, pericardium, esophagus, and diaphragm. On its right side are the azygos vein and thoracic duct, while on the left side are the left lung and pleura.

Superior Vena Cava. The vessel returns blood to the right atrium from the upper half of the body. It arises from the junction of the right and left brachiocephalic veins at the level of the lower border of the first right costal cartilage and enters the right atrium at the level of the third right costal cartilage. The superior vena cava is related posteromedially to the trachea and anteromedially to the ascending aorta. The phrenic nerve is positioned between the superior vena cava and the parietal layer of mediastinal pleura on the right. The superior vena cava receives the *azygos vein* on its posterior surface at the level of the second costal cartilage. The azygos vein enters the thorax through the aortic hiatus in the diaphragm, passes along the right side or anterior aspect of the vertebral column, receives the hemiazygos vein at the T9 level (and possibly the accessory hemiazygos vein at the T8 level), and arches anteriorly over the root of the lung before entering the superior vena cava.

Both *brachiocephalic veins* are formed by the union of the internal jugular and subclavian veins. The right brachiocephalic vein arises dorsal to the sternal end of the clavicle and passes almost vertically downward in front of the trachea and vagus nerve and behind the sternohyoid and sternothyroid muscles and right lung and pleura. The left brachiocephalic vein is longer than the right. It courses obliquely downward and to the right from its origin deep to the medial end of the clavicle, and it joins the right brachiocephalic vein at the lower border of the right first costal cartilage. The thoracic portion of each brachiocephalic vein receives an internal thoracic and often an inferior thyroid vein. In addition, the left receives the left highest intercostal vein.

Inferior Vena Cava. This vessel returns blood to the right atrium from the caudal half of the body. It enters the thorax by piercing the diaphragm (vertebral level T8) between the middle and right leaflets of the central tendon. It ascends in a slightly anteromedial direction in the middle mediastinum and pierces the fibrous pericardium. The inferior vena cava is separated, in its extrapericardial course, from the right pleura and lung by the right phrenicopericardiac ligament. In its short intrapericardial course it is invested on its right and left sides with a reflection of the serous paricardium.

Thoracic Duct. The thoracic duct is the common trunk of all lymphatics of the body except those that drain to the right lymphatic duct from the upper right quadrant of the body. It originates in the cistena chyli of the abdomen at the second lumbar vertebra, enters the thorax through the aortic hiatus of the diaphragm, and ascends through the posterior mediastinum between the aorta and azygos vein, and posterior to the esophagus. At the level of the T5 vertebra it crosses the midline to the left side, enters the superior mediastinum and ascends between the esophagus and pleura to enter the venous system at the junction of the left subclavian and internal jugular veins.

Right Lymphatic Duct. This duct receives lymph from several lymphatic vessels: from the right side of the head and neck through the right jugular trunk; from the right upper extremity by way of the right subclavian trunk; and from the right side of the thorax, right lung, and part of the convex surface of the liver through the right bronchomediastinal trunk.

Microscopic Structure of Vessels. Blood and lymphatic vessels generally consist of three tunics: tunica intima, tunica media, and tunica adventitia. These tunics are most pronounced in the larger vessels and vary with the type and size of vessels as to their constituents. Capillary walls consists of an endothelium, basal lamina, and surrounding connective tissue. The endothelium may be continuous and contain no pores, or it may be fenestrated with pores closed by a thin membrane. Either type of endothelium contains tight intercellular junctions. Fenestrated capillaries can be found in the kidney and endocrine organs. In larger arteries and veins the three tunics are more pronounced. The *tunica intima* consists of endothelium, subendothelial connective tissue with smooth muscle, and an internal elastic membrane. In larger arteries the internal elastic membrane is fenestrated, often doubled and highly developed. The *tunica media* is more pronounced in arteries than in veins. In medium-sized (muscular, distributing) arteries it contains mostly circularly arranged smooth muscle and some elastic fibers. In large arteries (elastic, conducting) elastic lamellae predominate, but smooth muscle is present. The media of arterioles consists of several layers of circularly arranged smooth muscle. The adventitia of arteries is not as pronounced as the tunica media. It is comprised of elastic and collagenous fibers and, in larger vessels, vasa vasorum that supply the outer layers.

Veins have a poorly defined tunica media, but the *tunica adventitia* is well developed. In medium-sized veins this outer layer contains mostly collagenous fibers. In the adventitia of large veins are longitudinally running smooth muscle fibers. Venous valves are local foldings of the intima. Venules have relatively thinner walls than arteries of similar diameter.

Lymphatic vessels are microscopically similar to veins. Lymphatic capillaries appear as endothelium-lined clefts in connective tissue and have very thin walls. The thoracic duct has a thick tunica media consisting of longitudinal and circular smooth muscle bundles. Its tunica intima is prominent, but the adventitia is poorly defined.

DEVELOPMENT OF THE HEART AND MAJOR VESSELS

The heart and major vessels arise from blood islands of hemangioblastic tissue that were derived from mesoderm. The heart begins to form in the third embryonic week. An embryonic and two extraembryonic (umbilical and vitelline) vascular circuits are completed by the end of the first month of development.

Early Development of the Heart and Vascular Circuits. Two *endocardial tubes* are formed deep to the epimyocardial (myocardial mantle) thickening of splanchnic mesoderm by the coalescence of blood islands. These tubes run longitudinally and are deep to the horseshoe-shaped prospective pericardial cavity. With the lateral folding and forward growth of the embryo, the endocardial tubes are shifted ventrocaudally and fuse in the midline. The adjacent epimyocardium fuses in the midline around the fused endocardial tubes, forming a single hollow heart tube that is suspended in the primitive pericardial cavity by the dorsal mesocardium.

The coalescence of other blood islands in the embryo forms blood vessels that are in continuity with the heart tube. In the *embryonic circulation,* paired anterior and posterior cardinal veins drain the embryo cranial and caudal to the heart, respectively, and join to form the paired common cardinal veins (ducts of Cuvier); the latter veins drain into the caudal extent of the endocardial tube at the sinus venosus. Blood leaves the cranial extent of the endocardial tube and is distributed into five paired aortic arches that pass dorsally around the foregut in the branchial arches to empty into the paired dorsal aortae. Blood then circulates through branches of the aortae to capillaries that are in continuity with tributaries of the cardinal veins.

Blood vessels developing in the placenta (chorion) are linked to the embryonic circuit to form an *umbilical* (allantoic, placental) *circuit.* In this circuit umbilical arteries arise from the aorta, pass through the body stalk and go to capillaries of the placenta. Oxygenated and nutritive blood returns by the left umbilical vein to the sinus venosus. The

right umbilical vein disappears soon after it is developed.

The *vitelline circuit* involves vascular channels in the yolk sac. Vitelline (omphalomesenteric) arteries arise from the abdominal aorta and pass along the yolk stalk to capillaries in the yolk sac. Blood returns to the sinus venosus by vitelline (omphalomesenteric) veins.

After birth the umbilical arteries will remain, in part, as a portion of the internal iliac and superior vesical arteries and the lateral umbilical ligaments. The umbilical vein persists as the round ligament of the liver. Portions of the vitelline veins become the portal vein. The vitelline artery gives rise to the superior mesenteric artery.

Folding and Partitioning of the Heart. With fusion of the endocardial tubes, several dilations become apparent. These are, from cephalic to caudal, the bulbus cordis (truncus arteriosus plus the conus arteriosus), ventricle, atrium, and sinus venosus. Arteries leave the cephalic end of the bulbus cordis from a swelling called the aortic bulb (aortic sac). Veins enter at the sinus venosus. With the loss of the dorsal mesocardium, except where the veins and arteries enter and leave, the heart begins to flex into an S-shaped structure. The first flexure occurs at the junction of the bulbus cordis and ventricle. The second flexure causes the sinus venosus and atrium to shift dorsally. The adjacent bulboventricular walls disappear, and this part of the bulbus and primitive ventricle become part of a common ventricular chamber. The atrium becomes sandwiched between the pharynx dorsally and the rest of the conus and truncus ventrally, causing the atrium to bulge laterally into right and left swellings. The sinus venosus becomes shifted to the right and eventually is incorporated into the primitive right atrial swelling. The pattern of blood flow is from veins to atrium, to ventricle, to conus, to truncus, to aortic bulb, and then to aortic arches.

During the second month of development the heart is partitioned into four chambers (two atria and two ventricles), A-V valves are formed, and the conus, truncus, and aortic bulb are partitioned into ascending aorta and pulmonary trunk (Fig. 2-26).

In *partitioning of the atrium* endocardial tissue from the dorsal and ventral walls fuses into an endocardial cushion that separates the A-V communication into right and left A-V canals. While this is taking place an endocardial septum primum grows toward the endocardial cushion from the dorsal wall of the atrium. Before fusing with the cushion, an ostium primum exists temporarily between the free margin of the septum primum and the cushion. This

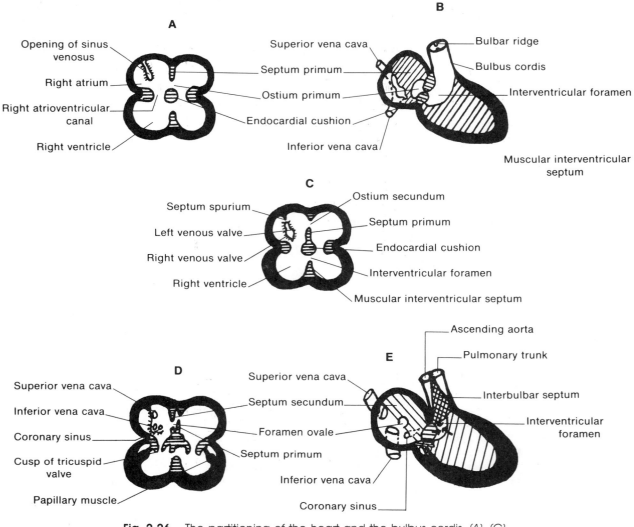

Fig. 2-26. The partitioning of the heart and the bulbus cordis. *(A), (C)* and *(D)* are frontal views. *(B)* and *(E)* are lateral views as seen from the right side. *(A)* and *(B)* represent the development in a 4-week-old embryo, and *(D)* and *(E)* represent development in a 6.5-week-old embryo.

ostium will not disappear before an ostium secundum arises from the degeneration of septum primum cephalically. In the seventh week a septum secundum grows dorsocaudally to the right of septum primum and leaves a crescentic free area covered only by septum primum. The communication from the right to the left atrium through the crescentic opening and ostium secundum is the foramen ovale. The valve of the foramen ovale is part of septum primum. The interatrial septum thus arises from septum primum and septum secundum.

The sinus venarum of the right atrium is formed by the incorporation of the sinus venosus into the right atrium so that the developing great veins enter independently. The smooth-surfaced portion of the

left atrium arises after the absorption of the common trunk of the pulmonary veins, thus leaving four pulmonary veins entering at the boundaries of this area.

In *partitioning of the ventricle* a muscular interventricular septum grows toward the endocardial cushion. Just caudal to the cushion an interventricular foramen remains for a short time before it is closed by endocardial tissue from the free margin of the interventricular septum, the endocardial cushion and the conal septum.

In *septation of the aortic bulb, truncus arteriosus, and conus arteriosus* a ridge of endocardial tissue develops on opposite walls of each of these structures. These ridges fuse in the middle of the lumen to form a bulbar (aortic, conal, truncal) septum. This septum spirals about 180 degrees as it descends from the aortic bulb into the conus, thus establishing a pulmonary trunk that intertwines with the ascending aorta. Semilunar valves develop in these vessels as localized swellings of endocardial tissue. The conal septum eventually descends to help close the interventricular septum.

In *development of A-V valves,* subendocardial and endocardial tissues project into the ventricle just below the A-V canals. These bulges of tissue are excavated from the ventricular side and invaded by muscle. Eventually all of the muscle, except that remaining as papillary muscles, disappears, and three right cusps of the right A-V valve and two cusps of the left A-V valve remain as fibrous structures.

Development of Major Arterial Vessels. Five pairs of aortic arches develop cephalocaudally in branchial arches (Fig. 2-27A,B). They bridge from the ventral aortic roots to the dorsal aortae. In comparative studies the five aortic arches represent the first, second, third, fourth, and sixth aortic arches. In humans the first, second, and distal part of the right sixth (fifth) disappear. The remaining aortic arches, ventral aortic roots, and dorsal aortae give rise to major arteries. The internal carotid arteries develop from the third aortic arches and the dorsal aortae cephalic to the third arches. The common carotids arise from the ventral aortic roots and the proximal part of the third arches. The external carotids arise in a similar position to the ventral aortic roots lying cephalic to the third arch. The right subclavian artery arises from the right fourth arch, the

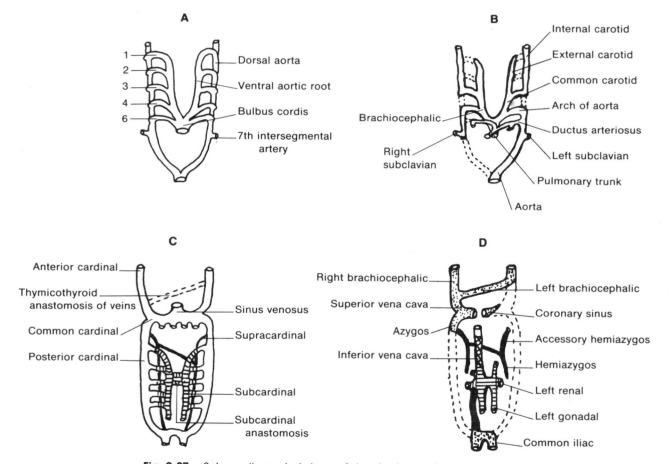

Fig. 2-27. Schematic ventral views of developing major blood vessels. *(A)* represents early aortic arch development. *(B)* shows the fate of the aortic arches. The dashed lines represent degenerating arteries. *(C)* represents early formation of the cardinal system of veins. The thymicothyroid anastomosis of veins *(dashed lines)* is a later acquisition. *(D)* shows the fate of the cardinal system of veins in the development of the superior and inferior venae cavae and the azygos system of veins.

seventh dorsal intersegmental artery, and the intervening portion of the right dorsal aorta. The left subclavian artery arises from the left seventh dorsal intersegmental artery. The arch of the aorta develops from the left fourth aortic arch and some septation of the aortic bulb. The pulmonary arteries arise from the proximal portions of the sixth arches along with some new vascular buds. The ductus arteriosus, linking the pulmonary trunk with the aorta, is the distal portion of the left sixth arch. The brachiocephalic artery originates from the right ventral aortic root between the fourth and sixth arches. The right dorsal aorta caudal to the right seventh dorsal intersegmental arteries disappears down to the embryonic low thoracic region where the paired dorsal aortae had fused into one midline vessel. The dorsal aortae between the third and fourth arches degenerates.

Development of Major Venous Channels.   The superior and inferior caval systems and the portal vein arise from early embryonic vessels (Fig. 2-27C,D).

The *superior vena cava* forms from the right common cardinal vein and a caudal portion of the right anterior cardinal vein up to the entrance of the left brachiocephalic (innominate) vein. The latter vessel arises from a thymicothyroid anastomosis of veins. The right brachiocephalic develops from the right anterior cardinal vein between this anastomotic venous attachment and the right seventh intersegmental vein (right subclavian). The left common cardinal vein and part of the left horn of the sinus venosus become the coronary sinus that drains the heart wall into the right atrium.

The *inferior vena cava,* from heart to common iliacs, arises from (1) a small portion of the right vitelline vein, (2) a new vessel in the mesenteric fold of the degenerating mesonephros, (3) the right subcardinal vein, and (4) a sacrocardinal vein joining the caudal extent of the posterior cardinal veins. The subcardinals and their anastomosis, which developed to drain the mesonephros, also give rise to the renal, gonadal, and suprarenal veins.

The *azygos venous system* arises mostly from the supracardinal veins and their anastomosis. The most cephalic portion of the azygos vein is derived from the right posterior cardinal vein.

The *portal and hepatic veins* arise from the vitelline (omphalomesenteric) veins and their anastomoses.

Fetal Circulation.   The circulation of the blood in the embryo results in the shunting of well-oxygenated blood from the placenta to the brain and the heart while relatively desaturated blood is supplied to the less essential structures.

Blood returns from the placenta by way of the umbilical vein, is shunted in the ductus venosus through the liver to the inferior vena cava and thence to the right atrium. There is relatively little mixing of oxygenated and deoxygenated blood in the right atrium because the valve overlying the orifice of the inferior vena cava directs the flow of oxygenated blood from that vessel through the foramen ovale into the left atrium, while the deoxygenated stream from the superior vena cava is directed through the tricuspid valve into the right ventricle. From the left atrium the oxygenated blood and a small amount of deoxygenated blood from the lungs passes into the left ventricle and thence into the ascending aorta from which it is supplied to the brain and the heart through the vertebral, the carotid and the coronary arteries.

Because the lungs of the fetus are inactive, most of the deoxygenated blood from the right ventricle is shunted by way of the ductus arteriosus from the pulmonary trunk into the descending aorta. This blood supplies the abdominal viscera and the inferior extremities and is carried to the placenta, for oxygenation, through the umbilical arteries arising from the aorta.

Circulatory Changes at Birth.   When respiration begins, the lungs expand, resulting in increased blood flow through the pulmonary arteries and a pressure change in the left atrium. This pressure change brings the septum primum and the septum secundum together and causes functional closure of the foramen ovale. Simultaneously, active contraction of the muscular wall of the ductus arteriosus results in its functional closure. Several months later it will become ligamentous as the ligamentum arteriosum. The ductus venosus functionally closes and becomes the ligamentum venosum. The fate of the umbilical arteries and veins was described previously in the section on extraembryonic circuits.

CONGENITAL ABNORMALITIES OF THE HEART AND GREAT VESSELS

The complicated sequence of development of changes in the heart and the major arteries accounts for the many congenital abnormalities that alone or in combination may affect these structures.

Septal defects include patent foramen ovale (incidence of about 10%) and other atrial or ventricular septal defects. An ostium secundum (foramen ovale) defect lies in the interatrial wall and is relatively easy to close surgically. An ostium primum defect lies directly above the A-V boundary and is often associated with a defect in the membranous part of the interventricular septum and in the A-V valves. A high interatrial septal defect may result, which is an improper shifting and incorporation of the sinus venosus into the right atrium.

Interventricular septal defects usually involve the membranous part of the interventricular septum and are due to improper formation of the conal septum. Rarely the septal defect is so large that the ventricles form a single cavity, giving a trilocular heart (cor triloculare biatriatum).

Congenital pulmonary stenosis may involve the trunk of the pulmonary artery and its valve or the infundibulum of the right ventricle. If this is combined with an interventricular septal defect, the compensatory hypertrophy of the right ventricle develops sufficiently high pressure to shunt blood through the defect into the left side of the heart; this mixing of blood results in the child's being cyanosed at birth.

Fallot's tetralogy is the most common congenital abnormality causing cyanosis. It is comprised of pulmonary stenosis, right ventricular hypertrophy, a septal defect and an overriding aorta, the orifice of which lies cranial to the septal defect and receives blood from both ventricles.

Transposition of the great vessels is due to improper spiraling of the bulbar septum in the formation of the great vessels. This results in either complete transposition, where the aorta is from the right ventricle and the pulmonary trunk is from the left ventricle, or in incomplete transposition where both vessels are reversed but both exit from the right ventricle.

Aortic stenosis is due to either bulbar septum displacement or localized improper growth in supravalvular, valvular, and subvalvular regions of the aorta.

Patent ductus arteriosus is a relatively common developmental abnormality. If not corrected it causes progressive work hypertrophy of the right heart and pulmonary hypertension.

Aortic coarctation may be due to abnormal retention of the fetal isthmus or to incorporation of smooth muscle from the ductus into the wall of the aorta. The constriction may occur from the level of the left subclavian artery to the ductus arteriosus, the latter being widely patent and maintaining the circulation to the lower part of the body. In other cases the coarctation may involve only a short segment near the ligamentum arteriosum, and the circulation to the lower limb is maintained by collateral arteries around the scapula that anastomose with the intercostal arteries.

Dextrorotation of the heart is the most spectacular of the abnormalities. The heart and its emerging vessels lie as a mirror image to the normal anatomy.

It may be associated with reversal of all the intra-abdominal organs.

Abnormal development of the aortic arches may result in the arch of the aorta lying on the right or actually being double. Rarely an abnormal right subclavian artery arises from the dorsal aorta and passes behind the esophagus and thus causes difficulty in swallowing (dysphagia lusoria). Double aorta is due to retention of the right dorsal aorta between the seventh dorsal intersegmental artery and the point of fusion of the aortae. If this portion remains and the right fourth aortic arch disappears, then the right subclavian arises from the aorta.

TRACHEA AND LUNGS

Gross Structure of the Trachea and Lungs. The trachea extends from the cricoid cartilage (vertebral level C6) to the level of the upper border of T5, where it bifurcates into left and right bronchi. It is related posteriorly to the esophagus and anteriorly to the thyroid gland and vessels, the sternohyoid and sternothyroid muscles, the thymus, the manubrium sterni, the major arteries and veins, and the deep cardiac plexus.

The right bronchus is both shorter and wider and diverges from the midline less than the left bronchus. Each bronchus enters the hilus of the lung at the mediastinal surface along with the pulmonary and bronchial arteries and veins, lymphatic vessels and lymph nodes, and autonomic nerve fibers. The right bronchus divides into three lobar bronchi: the superior, middle, and inferior. The left bronchus divides into a superior and inferior lobe bronchus. Each of the lobar bronchi in turn subdivides to supply bronchopulmonary segments. In the right lung these segments are (1) the apical, posterior, and anterior of the superior lobe; (2) the medial and lateral of the middle lobe; and (3) the superior, medial basal, lateral basal, anterior basal, and posterior basal of the inferior lobe. In the left lung these bronchopulmonary segments are (1) the apical-posterior, anterior, superior, and inferior of the superior lobe; and (2) the superior, anteriormedial basal, lateral basal, and posterior basal of the inferior lobe. The segmental bronchi further subdivide to smaller bronchi and bronchioles in the substance of the lung.

The lungs project laterally from the mediastinum and are invested by visceral pleura, which is continuous at the hilum with the parietal pleura. The pleural cavity lies between the visceral and parietal pleura, and it surrounds the lung. The pleura is a moist serous membrane, and under normal circumstances its surfaces do not adhere to one another.

Costal, mediastinal, and diaphragmatic subdivisions of the parietal pleura are recognized.

Each lung is conical in shape and has an apex and base; three borders, the inferior, posterior, and anterior; and three surfaces, the costal, diaphragmatic (base), and mediastinal. The apex extends 2.5 cm to 4.0 cm into the root of the neck, while the base rests on the convex surface of the diaphragm. The costal surface faces the ribs. The mediastinal surface is in contact with mediastinal pleura and bears a cardiac impression in the region facing the pericardium. The posterior border is in the concavity on either side of the vertebral column. The anterior border is sharp and projects into the costomediastinal recess, except on the left in the cardiac notch region where the pericardium is not overlapped anteriorly by the lung. The inferior border is sharp and projects into the costodiaphragmatic recess. The right lung is divided into superior, middle, and inferior lobes by two interlobar fissures; the left lung is divided into superior and inferior lobes by one interlobar fissure. The surface projections of these fissures are described previously in the section on surface markings.

The *afferent and the efferent innervation* of the lung is derived from the anterior and the posterior pulmonary plexuses, which receive branches from the vagus and the thoracic sympathetic trunk. Stimulation of the vagi brings about constriction of bronchioles, while stimulation of the sympathetic fibers causes dilation. The visceral afferents transmit pain and reflex activity, and return to the CNS by way of both the vagal and sympathetic pathways.

Microscopic Structure of the Lungs. The *conducting portion* of the respiratory system includes the nasal cavity, nasopharynx, laryngopharynx, trachea, bronchi, and bronchioles down to and including the terminal bronchioles. All but the bronchioles are characterized by (1) a mucosa of pseudostratified ciliated columnar epithelium with goblet cells and an underlying connective tissue containing mixed seromucous glands, and (2) usually a cartilaginous or bony support. The *respiratory portion* consists of respiratory bronchioles, alveolar ducts, alveolar sacs, and alveoli. A respiratory bronchiole and its branches constitute a lobule. All respiratory portions contain alveoli in their walls.

The microscopic structure of the larynx and trachea was described in the section on the head and neck. The main bronchi and segmental bronchi are similar to the trachea. The smaller bronchi have cartilaginous plates instead of rings. In bronchioles the cartilage disappears, circular smooth muscle becomes more prominent, and the ciliated epithelium becomes simple columnar and simple cuboidal. Glands are no longer present in the terminal bronchioles.

Respiratory bronchioles have simple cuboidal epithelium except at those sites where alveoli are present (Fig. 2-28). Alveolar ducts are completely lined by alveolar sacs and alveoli, and their lumina are marked by spiraling bundles of smooth muscle. Alveoli are separated from each other by interalveolar septa that contain an extensive capillary net, reticular and elastic fibers, blood cells, macrophages and lymph nodes, and nodules. The alveolus is lined by an extremely attenuated simple squamous epithelium. Blood in the capillaries is separated from the air in the alveoli by nonfenestrated endothelial cells and their basal lamina and the simple squamous (*alveolar type I*) cells and their basal lamina. The basal laminae of the alveolar and endothelial epithelia are fused in the thinnest blood–air transport regions. *Great alveolar (septal, type II)* cells bulge between the squamous cells into the alveolar lumen and produce surfactant. Alveolar phagocytes (dust cells) migrate into alveolar spaces and engulf debris.

Bronchial arteries, carrying nourishment to the lungs, course along the bronchi to the respiratory bronchioles. Venous return of this blood is mainly through pulmonary veins, but some blood returns by way of the bronchial veins to the azygos system. Pulmonary arteries branch and follow the air tubes to the capillary plexi in the alveoli. Oxygenated blood is returned through pulmonary veins that travel in the interlobular connective tissue septa.

ESOPHAGUS

Gross Structure of the Esophagus. The esophagus extends from the pharynx at the C6 level to the stomach. It passes in front of the bodies of the vertebrae in the superior and posterior mediastinum and penetrates the diaphragm at the esophageal hiatus (vertebral level T10). It is supplied by the vagal nerves and sympathetic fibers that form an esophageal plexus around the esophagus. In the lower thorax, anterior and posterior vagal trunks accompany the esophagus through the diaphragm to the stomach. Parasympathetic preganglionic fibers penetrate the wall and synapse on postganglionic neurons in the myenteric (Auerbach's) and submucosal (Meissner's) plexi.

Microscopic Structure of the Esophagus. The esophagus demonstrates well the general microscopic plan of the gastrointestinal system. The wall consists of four layers: (1) mucosa, (2) submucosa,

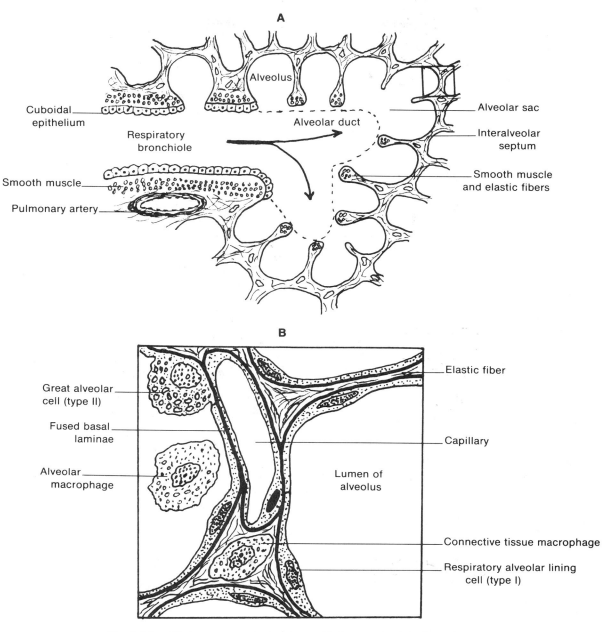

Fig. 2-28. *(A)* shows a respiratory bronchiole opening into two alveolar ducts whose lumina are outlined by the knobs of smooth muscle that border the openings into alveoli and alveolar sacs. *(B)* is an enlargement of the interalveolar septum area outlined in *(A)*. The simplest blood–air barrier consists of the cytoplasm of alveolar lining cells and endothelial cells and their fused basal laminae.

(3) muscularis externa, and (4) adventitia or serosa. The ***mucosa*** consists of stratified squamous nonkeratinized epithelium, a lamina propria with some mucous glands at the upper and lower extents of the esophagus, and a well-developed muscularis mucosae of smooth muscle. The ***submucosa*** contains some mucous glands and the autonomic submucosal nerve plexus. The ***muscularis externa*** consists of an outer longitudinal and inner circular layer of muscle with the myenteric plexus sandwiched between the two layers (Fig. 2-29). The submucosal and myenteric plexi contain post-ganglionic parasympathetic neurons and in some configurations cells of the enteric nervous system. In the upper

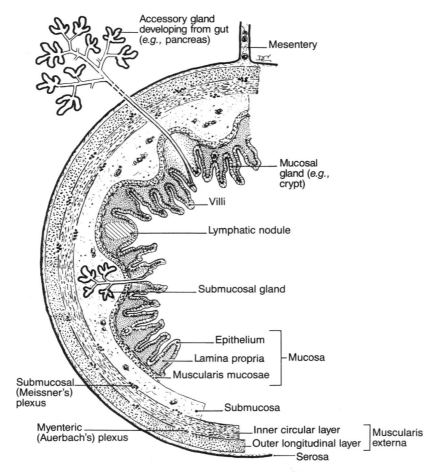

Fig. 2-29. General plan of the gastrointestinal tract. (Cormack DH: Ham's Histology, 9th ed, p 492. Philadelphia, JB Lippincott, 1987)

esophagus the muscle is skeletal; in the lower portion it is smooth muscle, and in the middle it is mixed. The *adventitia* is connective tissue that merges imperceptibly with that of the surrounding mediastinum. In the short abdominal portion of the esophagus, the outer layer is peritoneum and thus consists of mesothelium and underlying connective tissue and is called a serosa.

DEVELOPMENT OF THE TRACHEA, LUNGS, ESOPHAGUS, AND DIAPHRAGM

An *entodermal respiratory diverticulum* develops from the floor of the foregut just caudal to the last pharyngeal pouch. The larynx, trachea, and lungs develop from this diverticulum. The esophagus differentiates from the foregut caudal to this outgrowth. In the development of the larynx, the opening is constricted into a narrow T-shaped laryngotracheal orifice by underlying mesodermal ar-

ytenoid swellings. There is a transitory period when the opening is completely obliterated by an overgrowth of epithelium. Persistence of portions of this may lead to webs that obstruct the laryngeal opening.

All cartilage, muscle, and connective tissue of the larynx, trachea, and lungs arise from splanchnic mesoderm. The epithelium and glands develop from branching of the entodermal diverticulum. The main bronchi divide dichotomously through 17 generations of subdivisions by the end of the sixth month. An additional six divisions will occur by early childhood.

As the bronchial buds divide, the lung increases in size, and it bulges laterally into the embryonic coelom. The early coelom consists of a more ventral prospective pericardial cavity in continuity with a more dorsal pleural cavity, which is continuous caudally above the septum transversum with the prospective peritoneal cavity. Right and left pleuropericardial folds project from the lateral body wall and septum transversum, grow medially between the heart and lungs, and fuse with the primitive mediastinum. Thus, these folds become part of the definitive mediastinum and separate the pleural from the pericardial cavities. Pleuroperitoneal folds grow from the septum transversum at right angles to the pleuropericardial membranes. These folds invest the esophagus and, along with the septum transversum, contribute to the formation of the diaphragm. In addition the definitive diaphragm receives a major contribution of muscle in its development from the lateral body wall.

Tracheoesophageal fistulas may develop from improper separation of the respiratory diverticulum from the foregut, by malformation of the esophagotracheal septum, or by secondary fusion of the esophagus with the trachea. In the most usual circumstance the upper part of the esophagus ends blindly, while a lower portion is connected to the trachea by a narrow canal. This may result from dorsal deviation of the esophagotracheal septum in its caudal growth.

Diaphragmatic hernias can arise from improper formation of either the septum transversum, the pleuroperitoneal folds, or the muscular component from the body wall.

LYMPHATIC ORGANS OF THE THORAX

Thymus. The thymus is larger in the infant than it is in the adult. It consists of two lateral lobes invested by a connective tissue capsule that sends septa into the gland and divides it into lobules. The gland lies in the anterior part of the superior mediastinum and it extends from the fourth costal cartilage to the lower border of the thyroid gland. It lies anterior to the great vessels and fibrous pericardium. Microscopically the thymus is divisible into a central medulla and an outer cortex. The reticular cell meshwork contains lymphocytes (thymocytes) and differs from the other lymphatic tissues in that the reticular cells are derived from entoderm (of the third pharyngeal pouch). The cortex contains more lymphocytes and is less vascular than the medulla. Thymic (Hassall's) corpuscles in the medulla are concentric arrangements of flattened, and often hyalinized, cells. The corpuscles vary in size and occurrence and seem to be indicative of degeneration of reticular cells of the thymus.

Branches of the internal thoracic and thyroid arteries pass through thymic septa and enter the cortex–medulla junctional area as arterioles. Here, the arterioles give off direct branches to the medulla and also feed capillaries that loop into the cortex before draining into postcapillary venules of the medulla and cortex-medulla junction. Macromolecules cannot pass through the walls of the capillary loops, since the endothelial cells have a thick basement membrane that is bounded by reticular cells. Thus, the cortical lymphocytes seem to be protected from circulating antigens by a *blood–thymus barrier.* Large numbers of lymphocytes pass through the walls of the postcapillary venules and drain by way of thymic veins into the left brachiocephalic, inferior thyroid, and internal thoracic veins. The thymus is essential for the production of thymus-dependent (T) lymphocytes that are involved in cell-mediated immunologic responses and that also assist B-lymphocytes in humoral responses.

Lymph Nodes of the Thorax. The lymphatic nodes of the thorax are divided into parietal and visceral groups. The *parietal nodes* include the sternal, intercostal, and diaphragmatic nodes. The *sternal nodes* are located along the internal thoracic artery and receive afferents from the mammae, the deeper structures of the anterior thoracic wall, and the upper surface of the liver. Their efferents pass as a trunk to the junction of the subclavian and internal jugular veins. The *intercostal nodes* occupy the posterior parts of the intercostal spaces. They receive afferents from the posterolateral chest area. Efferents from the lower intercostal nodes carry lymph to the cisterna chyli, while the upper nodes send efferents to the thoracic duct and right lymphatic duct. *Diaphragmatic nodes* located anteriorly drain toward the sternal nodes, whereas those in the middle and posterior drain to the posterior mediastinal nodes. Superficial lymphatic vessels of the thoracic wall ramify beneath the skin and converge toward the axillary nodes. Lymphatic vessels of the mammary glands drain toward the surface along the interlobular septa and empty into a plexus located deep to the areola. This plexus also receives lymph from the areola and skin over the gland. It drains in two trunks to the axillary lymph nodes. Some drainage from the medial portion of the gland goes to the sternal nodes, while some efferents pass to interpectoral glands deep to the pectoralis major muscle, and others pass inferiorly toward abdominal nodes.

The *visceral lymph nodes* consist of anterior and posterior mediastinal and tracheobronchial nodes. The anterior mediastinal nodes are located in front of the great vessels and receive afferents from the thymus, pericardium and sternal nodes. Their efferents unite with those of the tracheobronchial nodes to form the right and left bronchomediastinal nodes.

The posterior mediastinal nodes lie behind the pericardium and along the esophagus and descending aorta. Their afferents come from the liver, esophagus and pericardium. Most efferents from these nodes go to the thoracic duct. The tracheobronchial nodes filter lymph from the trachea, bronchi, lungs, and heart.

Microscopically, lymph nodes are bean shaped, possess a hilum, and are surrounded by a capsule that sends trabeculae into a stroma of reticular tissue containing lymphocytes. Nodules of dense lymphatic tissue are located peripherally in the cortical region. If the node is in the "active" stage, the nodules contain germinal centers that consist of medium-sized lymphocytes and larger undifferentiated lymphocytes. These areas produce small lymphocytes that are pushed peripherally in the nodule and then into surrounding lymphatic sinuses. Nodes receive lymph peripherally through afferent vessels that penetrate the capsule and drain into a subcapsular sinus. This sinus drains along cortical peritrabecular sinuses to medullary sinuses (which lie between trabeculae and medullary cords of lymphatic tissue) before exiting from the lymph node at the hilum through efferent lymphatic vessels. Reticular cells and macrophages lining the sinuses perform a filtering function by phagocytizing dead cells and particulate matter and by offering antigens to the lymphocytes.

Lymph nodes also play a role in the immune response. The B-lymphocytes are found in the subcapsular cortical tissue, in germinal centers, and in medullary cords. In bacterial infections, antigens pass to the B-lymphocytes and trigger them to form blast cells in the germinal centers that proliferate and differentiate into antibody-producing lymphocytes and plasma cells. These cells pass to the medullary cords where antibodies and B-lymphocytes pass into efferent lymphatic vessels and are transported by the circulatory system to the site of infection. T-lymphocytes are located in deep cortical (paracortical) areas known as the *thymus-dependent zone*. This zone contains many postcapillary venules, whose cuboidal endothelium permits a recirculating pool of T-lymphocytes, and some B-lymphocytes, to enter the lymph node. It is thought that uncommitted lymphocytes from the thymus and bone marrow enter the lymph nodes through these venules and react with antigens from foreign cells. In this response, T-lymphocytes in the deep cortex become blast cells, proliferate, and form small long-lived memory cells and short-lived effector (killer) cells which enter the circulation.

MUSCLES, NERVES, AND VESSELS OF THE THORACIC WALL

Muscles. The major muscles are the external and internal intercostals, the subcostal, and the transversus thoracis. The *intercostal muscles* fill the intercostal spaces, the external sloping medially from above downward and the internal sloping laterally from above downward. *Subcostal muscles* are fasciculi of the internal intercostals which extend over two or more intercostal spaces near the angles of the ribs. The *transversus thoracis muscle* arises from the dorsal surface of the lower sternum and xiphoid process and extends upward and laterally to insert on the second through the sixth costal cartilages. In respiration, the intercostals apparently maintain both size and rigidity of the intercostal spaces while the entire rib cage is elevated by the scalene muscles.

Nerves. The intercostal muscles are innervated by *intercostal nerves,* which are the continuations of the ventral rami of thoracic spinal nerves. The intercostal nerves and vessels occupy the costal grooves (on the inferior aspects of the ribs), with the nerves inferior to the intercostal arteries and veins. Each intercostal nerve has two cutaneous branches: the lateral cultaneous nerve in the midaxillary line and the anterior cutaneous nerve just lateral to the sternum.

Arteries and Veins. Posterior intercostal arteries arise from the aorta and, in the upper spaces, from the costocervical trunk of the subclavian artery. They supply the deep muscles of the back, contents of the spinal canal and most of the intercostal space, and end by anastomosing with the anterior intercostal arteries, which are branches of the internal thoracic artery. The posterior intercostal veins are tributaries to the azygous system while the anterior intercostal veins empty into the internal thoracic veins. Both systems—the arterial and the venous—represent potential collateral vascular routes.

CIRCULATING BLOOD

Blood cells (formed elements) constitute 45% of the total volume of circulating blood; plasma comprises the remaining 55%. Of the 45% cell volume, erythrocytes (red blood corpuscles, RBCs) make up 44%, and the remainder is composed of leukocytes (white blood cells). The plasma, minus its blood clotting factors, is called *serum*.

Plasma acts as a medium for metabolic substances and circulating cells. Like tissue fluid, its primary components are water, inorganic salts, and a number of proteins. Albumin, the most abundant plasma protein, maintains the colloid blood pressure. Gamma globulins are also important since they include the circulating antibodies. Beta globulins transport lipids, hormones, and metal ions. Prothrombin and fibrinogen are essential components of the clotting process. Chylomicrons are microscopic particles of fat that are especially prominent in the plasma after a fatty meal.

Erythrocytes, when mature, are anucleate biconcave discs approximately 8 μm in diameter and 2-μm thick. There are about 4.8 and 5.5 million erythrocytes per cubic millimeter of blood in the normal female and normal male, respectively. Erythrocytes lack the usual complement of organelles, and they do not have the capacity for protein synthesis. Each RBC exists for about 120 days, and it lacks the mechanism to reproduce itself. About 17% of the erythrocytes possess some residual ribosomal material and, due to their stained appearance, are called *reticulocytes;* they are considered to be immature erythrocytes. The reticulocyte count provides a rough index of the rate of erythrocyte development.

Leukocytes are divisible into granular leukocytes and nongranular leukocytes. The granular leukocytes are further classified as eosinophils, basophils, and neutrophils on the basis of the affinity of their granules for different stains. The nongranular leukocytes are the lymphocytes and monocytes.

Neutrophils are about twice the size of erythrocytes and make up about 60% to 70% of the white blood cells. Their nuclei consist of three to five lobes that are interconnected by fine filaments of nuclear material. Two types of granules are present in the cytoplasm: the specific granules, which stain with neutral dyes, and nonspecific granules, which are azurophilic. Both types of granules contain hydrolytic enzymes that are used by the cell in the digestion of phagocytized materials.

Eosinophils are about the size of neutrophils, but constitute only 1% to 3% of the total leukocyte population. The nucleus is usually bilobed and the chromatin is dense. The eosinophilic granules are membrane-bound vesicles containing lysosomal enzymes.

Basophils are about the same size as the other granular leukocytes. They constitute only 0.5% of the white blood cells. The nucleus is usually S-shaped and its chromatin is less dense than that of the other granular leukocytes. The basophilic membrane-bound cytoplasmic granules contain histamine and heparin.

Lymphocytes constitute 20% to 35% of the white blood cell population. Most of the mature lymphocytes are the size of erythrocytes, but larger cells traditionally called large and medium lymphocytes are occasionally seen in circulating blood. The small lymphocyte has a relatively large round or slightly indented nucleus of dense chromatin. The nucleus is surrounded by a thin rim of cytoplasm containing a few ribosomes and some nonspecific azurophilic granules. The small lymphocytes are further designated as T- and B-lymphocytes. *T-lymphocytes* are cytotoxic cells of the cell-mediated response that "kill" foreign cells and sensitizing agents that enter the body. They also assist the *B-lymphocytes* (and their subsequent plasma cells) in their humoral antibody response to such invasive organisms as bacteria and viruses.

Monocytes range from 9 μm to 20 μm in diameter and make up 3% to 8% of the circulating leukocytes. The nucleus is oval, kidney shaped, or horseshoe shaped. The cytoplasm contains a few azurophilic granules, a Golgi complex, polyribosomes, and some glycogen; it is more abundant than that of the lymphocytes. Monocytes give rise to macrophages when they pass into connective tissues.

Platelets (thrombocytes) are small, irregular disk-shaped structures that are 1 μm to 2 μm in diameter. They are basophilic fragments of megakaryocytes containing a variety of granules. There are 250,000 to 300,000 platelets in a cubic millimeter of blood. They have a natural tendency to cling to each other and to all wettable surfaces they contact when blood is shed. Platelets contain serotonin, which helps to constrict small blood vessels during vascular injury. They also contain thromboplastin, a substance released by platelets and injured endothelial cells. Thromboplastin helps convert prothombin of the plasma to thrombin. The thrombin then converts plasma fibrinogen to fibrin which forms a network trapping blood cells and platelets. Thus, a blood clot, or thrombus, is formed.

BLOOD CELL FORMATION (HEMOPOIESIS)

The main hemopoietic tissue in the body is bone marrow. Since all of the erythrocytes, platelets, and granular leukocytes are produced in bone marrow, these blood components are called the *myeloid elements.* The specific development of these elements is referred to as myelopoiesis. Although the nongranular elements are produced in both lymphatic tissues and bone marrow, they are referred to as *lymphoid elements;* their development is termed lymphopoiesis.

The first blood cells develop in the third embryonic week from yolk sac and body stalk mesoderm. During the second month of development hemopoietic sites arise in the liver, spleen, and mesonephric kidneys. In later months of fetal development, bones are established, and the bone marrow becomes the dominant hemopoietically active tissue. *Red bone marrow* consists of a reticular fiber meshwork, which contains and supports reticular cells, myelopoietic (blood forming) cells, adipose cells, and thin-walled sinusoids. The myelopoietic cells occur in many stages. Some are relatively undifferentiated stem cells from which all myeloid elements come. Some are mature erythrocytes, granular leukocytes, and nongranular leukocytes, which are about ready to leave the bone marrow through the sinusoids and veins. The majority of cells, however, are in the numerous stages of differentiation that stem cells go through during erythropoiesis, granulopoiesis, and thrombopoiesis.

Erythropoiesis is the formation of erythrocytes from stem cells. In this process pluripotent stem cells, which have the potential to give rise to any blood cell type, differentiate into proerythroblasts. The latter cells divide into basophilic proerythroblasts, which contain free polyribosomes, a condensed nucleus, and no nucleoli. Without nucleoli the cells cannot produce ribosomes. Thus, when they divide into smaller polychromatophilic erythroblasts, their basophilia disappears and their acidophilia increases due to accumulating hemoglobin. When these cells have acquired their full amount of hemoglobin and their nuclei become very small and concentrated, they are called normoblasts (orthochromatic erythroblasts). When the nuclei are extruded they become erythrocytes. Erythropoietin, produced by the kidney, regulates proerythroblast formation. The maturation of erythrocytes is regulated by the extrinsic factor (vitamin B_{12}) and the intrinsic factor (a mucoprotein produced in the stomach).

Granulopoiesis is the formation of basophils, eosinophils, and neutrophils from stem cells that differentiate through myeloblast, promyelocyte, myelocyte and metamyelocyte stages. The myeloblast has a large nucleus with several prominent nucleoli; its cytoplasm is basophilic. When these cells acquire azurophilic granules, they are called promyelocytes. As promyelocytes mature into myelocytes, their nuclei become more dense, non-

specific azurophilic granules increase in number, and specific granules make their appearance. If the latter are neutrophilic, then the cell is a neutrophilic myelocyte; if basophilic or eosinophilic granules are present, the cell is a basophilic myelocyte or eosinophilic myelocyte. All of the cells from myeloblast through myelocyte are capable of mitosis. This ceases when the myelocyte nucleus becomes dense and more deeply indented as a metamyelocyte is formed. During maturation of the metamyelocyte into a mature granulocyte, the nucleus becomes more deeply indented and then becomes lobated or S shaped. As this takes place, certain juvenile forms of cells are detected. In neutrophil formation the horseshoe-shaped nucleus often designates the cell as a band or stab cell. Since the life span of granular leukocytes is considerably shorter (about 14 hours) than that of erythrocytes (120 days), there are more developmental forms of granular leukocytes in the marrow than there are of erythrocytes.

Thrombopoiesis is the formation of blood platelets from megakaryocytes. In this process, plasma membranes of megakaryocytes partition off cytoplasmic fragments, which are released from the cell and pass into the blood stream as platelets. The megakaryocyte may then die and is replaced by a stem cell in the marrow. Megakaryocytes are very large cells with multilobed nuclei. Blood platelets live for only about 8 to 11 days.

Lymphopoiesis is the formation of lymphocytes from a stem cell. In this process a stem cell differentiates into a large lymphocyte (lymphoblast) that further divides and matures into medium lymphocytes and then into small lymphocytes. The sites of these lymphopoietic changes are in the bone marrow and in the lymphatic tissues of the spleen, thymus, lymph nodes, tonsils, and mucous membranes of the body. The theory that the small lymphocyte is an end point of differentiation is questioned, for it appears that the small lymphocyte can be the stem cell for large lymphoblasts that produce other small lymphocytes and antibody-producing plasma cells. In the establishment of the immune system, stem cells are sent to the thymus, the mucous membrane of the gut, and return to the bone marrow. In the thymus the stem cells become T-lymphocyte precursors, which pass to other tissues and become small cytotoxic "killer" lymphocytes. Stem cells that return to the bone marrow become lymphocytes that develop into antibody-producing B-lymphocytes.

Monopoiesis is the formation of monocytes from stem cells. Monocytes seem to develop in the marrow from pluripotent stem cells. After a few days developing in the marrow, monocytes pass into the circulation for 1 or 2 days before entering the connective tissue and becoming macrophages.

MAMMARY GLAND

The mammary glands are integumentary glands located from the level of the second to sixth or seventh rib on the anterior of the thorax. In fetal development they first appear as ectodermal thickenings along a milk line extending between the upper and lower extremities. As development proceeds, 15 to 20 ectodermal invaginations branch and hollow out to give rise to the 15 to 20 lobes of the mammary gland, which are arranged in a radial fashion deep to the nipple. Thus, each lobe has a single excretory duct opening on the nipple. Each of these ducts diverges at the base of the nipple and increases in size to form an ampulla (lactiferous sinus). Deep to the ampulla the ducts branch into intralobular ducts. In the male and nonpregnant gland there are few ducts present, and the epithelium changes from stratified to simple cuboidal epithelium in proceeding from larger to smaller ducts. In the lactating gland the ducts have proliferated, and their terminal portions develop into secretory alveoli lined by a simple pyramidal epithelium invested by myoepithelial cells. The lining epithelium secretes milk proteins by the exocytosis of secretion granules (merocrine type of secretion); milk lipids in the membrane-bound lipid vacuoles are externalized by the apocrine type of secretion. The lobes of the gland are supported by a dense connective tissue sheath, between the interstices of which are large accumulations of fat. Suspensory ligaments (of Cooper) run through the gland, attaching the deep layer of the superficial fascia to the dermis. The areola is covered by a thin, delicate pigmented skin. Underlying glands (of Montgomery) open on its surface. Smooth muscle fibers also lie deep to the nipple and areola.

The nerves to the mammary gland are the intercostals (second to sixth), by way of lateral and anterior cutaneous branches. Sympathetic fibers accompany these nerves or the vessels supplying the gland. The arteries are the second and third perforating branches of the internal thoracic and the two external mammary branches of the lateral thoracic artery. Additional twigs from the intercostal arteries may enter the deep surface of the gland.

DIAPHRAGM

The diaphragm is a thin dome-shaped muscle consisting of a series of radial fibers that arise from the inner side of the thoracic outlet and insert into a central aponeurosis or tendon. On the right its dome reaches to the fifth rib; on the left, to the fifth interspace.

The diaphragm arises from three areas: (1) a small sternal part that attaches to the posterior aspect of the xiphoid process, (2) an extensive costal portion that attaches to the subcostal margin, and (3) a lumbar portion. The lumbar portion consists of the right and left crura, which arise from the anterior aspects of the lumbar vertebra and surround the aortic hiatus (T12), through which pass the aorta and thoracic duct. The esophageal hiatus (T10) is anterior to the aortic hiatus; and the opening for the inferior vena cava (T8) is more anterior and to the right. The diaphragmatic muscle is supplied by the phrenic nerves; the peripheral part of the diaphragm receives sensory fibers from the intercostal nerves. The diaphragm flattens as it contracts and thus draws the central tendon downward. This movement increases the thoracic volume and decreases the pressure within the thoracic cavity.

The phrenic nerve arises from the ventral rami of spinal nerves C3–5. It decends over the cupula of the pleura, in front of the root of the lung, and between the pericardium and pleura, to reach the diaphragm. Referred pain from the diaphragm occurs in the shoulder because both structures are innervated by sensory fibers to the C4 level of the spinal cord.

CROSS SECTIONS OF THE THORAX

The following cross sections are included to demonstrate relationships and emphasize the importance of cross-sectional anatomy in the interpretation of computerized tomographic, ultrasound (and so forth) images. The orientation of all cross sections corresponds to that used clinically in displaying the various types of cross-sectional images, for example, the reader is viewing the inferior aspect of the section with the patient's left on the right of the page.

Figure 2-30 is a section approximately through the junction of the superior and inferior parts of the mediastinum. The plane passes through the junction of thoracic vertebrae four and five, the lower aspect of the manubrium of the sternum, and includes ribs one through five. The arch of the aorta is passing posterolaterally to the left and is cut so that the origins of its three branches are apparent. From proximal to distal, these are the brachiocephalic, left common carotid, and left subclavian arteries. The fourth opening in this section is a slice through

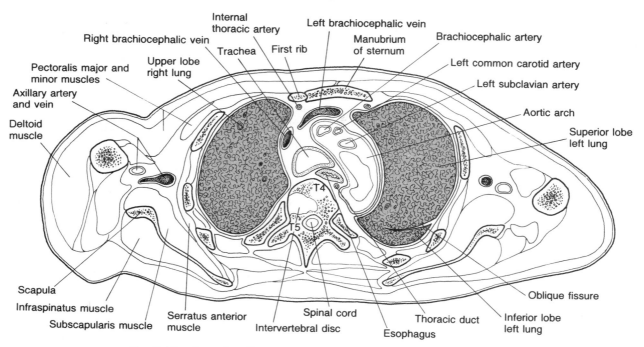

Fig. 2-30. A section through the junction of the superior and inferior parts of the mediastinum.

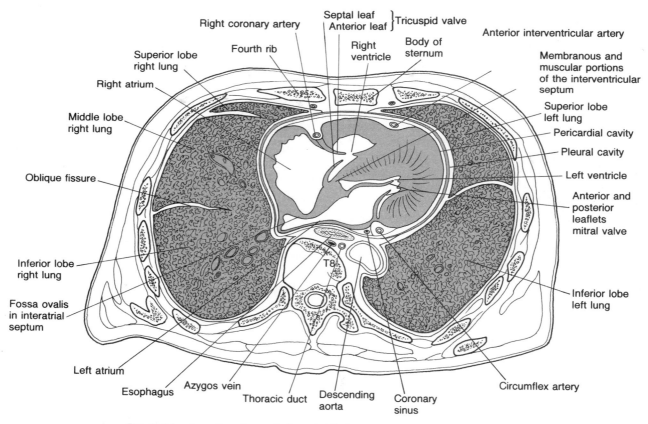

Fig. 2-31. A section through the eighth thoracic vertebra, the junction of the fourth rib with the sternum and the middle mediastinum.

a slightly abnormal arching of the aorta. The left brachiocephalic vein is passing to the right in front of the aorta, just superior to the level where it joins the right brachiocephalic vein to form the superior vena cava. The trachea, just superior to its bifurcation, is separated from the vertebral column by the esophagus, which is somewhat to the left at this level. The thoracic duct is posterolateral to the esophagus. The internal thoracic arteries are posterior to the lateral aspects of the sternum. The lungs are sectioned superior to the hilar regions. Thus, the pleural cavities are seen completely surrounding the lungs. The oblique fissure of the left lung separates the anteriorly located superior lobe from the more posteriorly positioned inferior lobe.

The plane of Figure 2-31 is through vertebra T8, the junction of the fourth rib with the sternum, and the middle mediastinum. The oblique fissure clearly separates the superior and inferior lobes of the left lung. On the right, both oblique and horizontal fissures are present so the superior, middle, and inferior lobes are partially demarcated.

The heart is sectioned so that all four chambers are visible. The posterior surface is formed almost entirely by the left atrium while the right atrium forms the right border. Note that the interatrial septum is essentially in the coronal plane. The right and left ventricles form the anterior and right borders respectively. The latter two chambers are separated by the obliquely oriented interventricular septum; both its muscular and membranous portions are visible. The tricuspid valve is anterior and somewhat to the right of the mitral valve. The coronary (A-V) sulcus houses the right coronary artery anteriorly and the coronary sinus and circumflex branch of the left coronary posteriorly. The anterior interventricular sulcus is not easily seen, but its location is marked by the anterior interventricular artery.

In the posterior mediastinum the esophagus descends directly posterior to the right atrium. The azygous vein and thoracic duct are essentially between the esophagus and vertebral column, with the azygous vein to the right of the thoracic duct. The descending portion of the thoracic aorta is anterolateral (on the left) to the vertebral bodies.

ABDOMEN

SURFACE ANATOMY

Regions.   The regions of the abdomen may be defined by two horizontal and two vertical lines. The right and left *semilunar lines* correspond to the lateral edges of the rectus abdominis muscles. The *transpyloric plane* is a horizontal line through a point halfway between the suprasternal notch and the upper border of the pubic symphysis; this plane is also midway between the xiphisternal joint and the umbilicus. The *transtubercular plane* is a lower horizontal line at the level of the top of the iliac crest. These four lines subdivide the abdomen into the following nine regions: in the center the epigastric, the umbilical, and the pubic regions; on the sides the right and the left hypochondriac, lumbar, and inguinal regions.

The abdomen may also be divided into four areas by a vertical line and a horizontal line that pass through the umbilicus. The division establishes right and left upper and lower quadrants.

The transpyloric plane is at the level of the pylorus, the body of the first lumbar vertebra, the tip of the ninth costal cartilage on each side, and the fundus of the gallbladder on the right side. The semilunar line is the lateral border of the sheath of the rectus abdominis muscle and is a slightly curved line extending from the tip of the ninth costal cartilage to the pubic tubercle. The linea alba is the vertical median line between the rectus abdominis muscles.

Stomach.   The stomach varies considerably in size and position, but its cardiac and pyloric portions are relatively fixed. The cardiac orifice is opposite the seventh costal cartilage about 2.5 cm to the left of the xiphisternal joint. The pyloric orifice is on the transpyloric plane about 1.5 cm to the right of the midline. The lesser curvature is indicated by a curved line that passes downward and to the right and connects these two points. The fundus reaches the fifth interspace in the left semilunar line. The greater curvature may extend to the level of the umbilicus or lower. The pregastric space (Traube) overlies the stomach, is semilunar in outline, and is bounded by the lower edge of the left lung, the anterior border of the spleen, the left costal margin, and the lower edge of the left lobe of the liver.

Small Intestine.   The duodenum may be mapped by four continuous lines: (1) a transverse line from the pylorus to the junction of the transpyloric and the right semilunar lines, (2) a descending line passing inferiorly to the lowest level of the subcostal margin (subcostal line at L3), (3) another transverse line passing from right to left and ending about 3.0 cm to the left of the midline, and (4) an ascending line for one to two vertebral levels that terminates at the duodenojejunal flexure. The rest of the small intestine occupies a large amount of the abdominal cavity. The coils of the jejunum are predominantly in the upper left quadrant and those of the ileum in the lower right quadrant. The ileocolic junction is slightly below and medial to the intersection of the right semilunar and transtubercular lines.

Large Intestine and Vermiform Appendix. The cecum lies in the right iliac and hypogastric regions. The middle of its lower border is located about one third (5 cm) of the distance along a line from the right anterior superior iliac spine to the umbilicus. This point (McBurney's) is where tenderness can be elicited when the appendix is inflamed. The right colic flexure is on a level just below the transpyloric plane 2.5 cm lateral to the right semilunar line. The left colic flexure lies just above the transpyloric plane 2.5 cm lateral to the left semilunar line.

Liver. The upper border of the liver corresponds to a horizontal line passing just below the nipples. The inferior border of the liver rather closely parallels the right inferior costal margin, which it leaves at the tip of the ninth costal cartilage, extending from this point across the subcostal angle to just below the left nipple.

Pancreas. The head of the pancreas occupies the curve of the duodenum and is bounded accordingly. The neck is in the midline at the transpyloric line. The body extends to the left and slightly superiorly, and the tail is in contact with the spleen.

Spleen. The spleen is situated posteriorly beneath the left ninth, tenth, and eleventh ribs. The upper pole lies about 3 cm lateral to the left of the tenth thoracic spine. The lower pole extends as far forward as the midaxillary line at the level of the eleventh rib.

Kidney. The kidneys are about 10 cm long, with about one third of their length being above the transpyloric plane, and the left kidney is about 1 cm to 1.5 cm higher. The upper pole is about 5 cm from the midline; the lower pole, 7.5 cm from the midline. Both kidneys extend above the level of the twelfth rib. The hilum is 5 cm from the middle line at the level of L1. On the dorsal aspect of the body the position of the kidneys may be indicated by a parallelogram. Two vertical lines are drawn 2.5 cm and 10 cm from the midline, and the parallelogram is completed by two horizontal lines at the levels of the tips of the spinous processes of T11 and L3.

Ureter. The location of the ureter is indicated by a line from the hilum of the kidney to the bifurcation of the common iliac artery where the ureter enters the pelvis. This vertical line is 3 cm to 4 cm lateral to the midline and is anterior to the transverse processes of the lumbar vertebrae.

ABDOMINAL WALL

Superficial Fascia. This fascia is composed of superficial and deep layers. The superficial or fatty layer *(Camper's fascia)* is continuous with the superficial fascia of adjacent areas, for example, thigh and perineum. The deep or fibrous layer *(Scarpa's fascia)* attaches to the deep fascia of the thigh but continues into the perineum as the superficial perineal fascia. Thus, fluid collecting in the superficial perineal space can extravasate into the abdominal wall (between the fibrous layer of the superficial fascia and the fascia of the external abdominal oblique muscle) but not into the thigh.

Muscles. The interval between the inferior costal margin and the superior aspect of the pelvis (pubis, inguinal ligament, iliac crest) contains four major muscles, all of which are segmentally innervated by thoracic and lumbar nerves. The external abdominal oblique, internal abdominal oblique, and transversus abdominis are lateral to the semilunar line; the rectus abdominis is medial. The most superficial muscle is the external oblique whose fibers are directed anteriorly, medially, and inferiorly. The fibers of the internal oblique are perpendicular to those of the external oblique. The transversus abdominis fibers are transversely oriented. The aponeuroses of all three muscles extend medially, and together they form the rectus sheath. The rectus abdominis is the only vertically oriented muscle, and it extends between the superomedial aspect of the pubis and the medial aspect of the inferior costal margin and the xiphoid process. Its tendinous intersections account for the "ripples" seen on the surface of the abdomen.

Inguinal Region. The inferior aspect of the abdominal wall is composed primarily of the aponeuroses of the abdominal muscles. The inferior margin of the external oblique aponeurosis forms the *inguinal ligament* as it stretches between the anterior superior iliac spine and the pubic tubercle. This tough band also is an attachment for some of the other abdominal muscles, and it participates in the formation of the inguinal canal.

The *inguinal canal* is an obliquely oriented pathway through the abdominal wall (Fig. 2-32). It stretches between the superficial (external) and deep (internal) inguinal rings and is directed inferomedially just above the inguinal ligament. The *superficial ring* is a split in the external oblique aponeurosis just superolateral to the pubic tubercle. The medial and lateral edges of the ring are called the medial (superior) and lateral (inferior) crura.

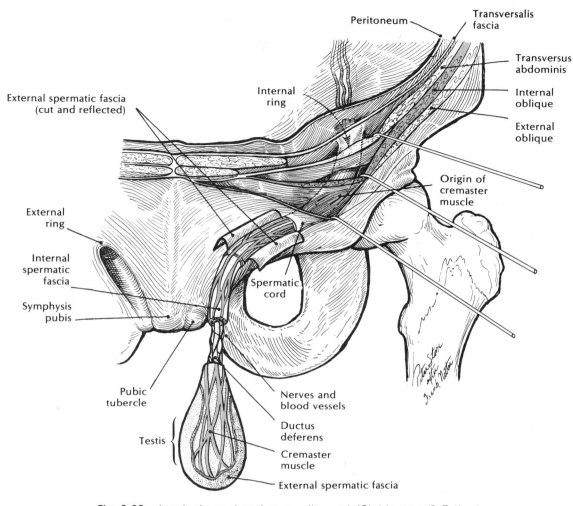

Fig. 2-32. Inguinal canal and spermatic cord. (Christensen JB, Telford IR: Synopsis of Gross Anatomy, 5th ed, p 151. Philadelphia, JB Lippincott, 1988, Langley LL, Telford IR, Christensen JB: Dynamic Anatomy and Physiology, 5th ed. New York, McGraw Hill, 1980)

The **deep ring** is the beginning of a sleeve of transversalis fascia that extends along the spermatic cord. This ring is located about halfway between the anterior superior iliac spine and the pubic tubercle.

The boundaries of the inguinal canal are as follows: (1) floor: inguinal ligament; (2) anterior wall: external oblique aponeurosis; (3) posterior wall: medially the conjoined tendon (falx inguinalis), which is composed of the arching medial attachments of the internal oblique and the transversus abdominis, and laterally the transversalis fascia; and (4) roof: conjoined tendon as it arches over the contents of the canal.

The spermatic cord consists of the vas deferens and its artery, the pampiniform plexus of veins,

lymphatics, sympathetic nerve fibers, the ilioinguinal nerve, the nerve and artery to the cremasteric muscle, and the testicular artery. Most of these structures are enclosed within the (1) **internal spermatic fascia,** which is derived from the transversalis fascia; (2) the **cremasteric muscle** and **fascia,** which are derived from the internal oblique; and (3) the **external spermatic fascia,** which is derived from the aponeurosis of the external oblique.

Inguinal hernias are either direct or indirect, based on the path of the herniating sac. The **indirect hernia** follows the course of the testis during development, that is, it passes into the canal through the internal opening and then through the canal. After exiting through the superficial ring, it usually passes into the scrotum. The neck of this type of hernia is found lateral to the inferior epigastric vessels, and the hernial sac is covered with peritoneum and the three fascial coverings of the spermatic cord. A *direct hernia* passes through Hesselbach's triangle, that is, the triangular area defined by the lateral border of the rectus abdominis, the inferior epigastric vessels, and the inguinal ligament. The neck of this type of hernial sac is medial to the inferior epigastric vessels and covered by a layer of peritoneum and transversalis fascia. Since this hernia will pass through the superficial ring, it is also covered by the external spermatic fascia.

CONTENTS OF THE ABDOMINAL CAVITY
PERITONEUM AND MESENTERIES

The peritoneum is similar to the pleura in that it consists of a parietal layer that lines the abdominopelvic cavity and a visceral layer that is reflected over organs. It is also similar in that the peritoneal cavity contains nothing other than a small amount of lubricating fluid and in reality is a potential space. It differs from the pleura in that its visceral layer reflects in varying degrees over multiple organs. Some organs—jejunum and ileum—are almost completely covered by peritoneum and attached to the posterior body wall by a mesentery and thus are said to be (completely) peritonealized. Other organs (kidneys) are essentially outside the peritoneum and covered by peritoneum on only one side. These organs are extraperitoneal or, if located on the posterior body wall, retroperitoneal. Those organs that are neither peritonealized nor extraperitoneal, but are somewhere in between, are partially peritonealized.

The *peritoneal cavity* is separated into greater and lesser peritoneal sacs. The *lesser sac* (omental bursa) is posterior to the stomach, lesser omentum, and caudate lobe of the liver. The *greater sac* is the rest of the peritoneal cavity. The two areas are connected only through the *epiploic foramen* (of Winslow), which is small. The anterior border of this foramen is the right free margin of the lesser omentum, which is formed by the hepatoduodenal ligament and contains (1) the common bile duct, (2) the portal vein, (3) the proper hepatic artery, and (4) lymphatics and nerves.

Within the peritoneal cavity there are areas where inflammatory material can accumulate and become sequestered. These areas are as follows: In the abdomen there are the subphrenic and subhepatic spaces, and the paravertebral gutters. The *subphrenic spaces* are found between the liver and the diaphragm, being separated into right and left portions by the coronary and falciform ligaments and lesser omentum. The subhepatic spaces are inferior to the visceral surface of the liver, the right being inferior to the right and caudate lobes of the liver, and the left (omental bursa) inferior to the quadrate lobe. These *subhepatic spaces* are connected through the epiploic foramen. The *paravertebral gutters* are vertically oriented and on either side of the lumbar vertebral bodies. Each is subdivided into two gutters by the ascending and descending portions of the colon. Thus, each paravertebral gutter consists of a *medial* and a *lateral paracolic gutter.* Material in the paracolic gutters tends to move superiorly into the subphrenic and subhepatic spaces. In the pelvis of both the male and female there are *pararectal fossae* on either side of the rectum. In the male the *rectovesical pouch* is found between the rectum and the bladder. In the female the uterus and broad ligament divide that area into two pouches, the *vesicouterine pouch* anteriorly and the *rectouterine pouch* (of Douglas) posteriorly.

Folds and fossae of the peritoneum occur on the lower part of the anterior abdominal wall. These consist of the single median umbilical fold, and the medial and lateral umbilical folds. The median fold overlies the remains of the urachus; the medial folds are formed by the obliterated umbilical arteries and the lateral by the inferior epigastric vessels. The *supravesical fossae* are between the median and medial folds; the *medial* and *lateral inguinal fossae* are medial and lateral respectively to the lateral fold. Indirect hernias pass through the lateral inguinal fossa while direct hernias pass through the lateral inguinal fossa while direct hernias pass through either the supravesical or medial inguinal fossa.

The specific peritoneal relationships of each organ are covered with the discussion of that organ.

Stomach. This organ extends from the cardiac opening of the esophagus to the pylorus. It consists of a fundus, a body and a pyloric portion, the latter made up of the pyloric antrum, canal, and sphincter. Its right or upper border forms the lesser curvature, to which the lesser omentum attaches. The lower and left border forms the greater curvature and gives attachment to the greater omentum and gastrolienal ligament. Posteriorly the stomach is in contact with the spleen, the splenic artery, the diaphragm, the left kidney and suprarenal, the pancreas and the transverse mesocolon; anteriorly it is in contact with the liver, the diaphragm, and the abdominal wall. The blood supply to the stomach is provided by the three main branches of the celiac trunk: the common hepatic, left gastric, and splenic arteries. Each of these main branches has branches that pass along the greater or lesser curvatures of the stomach. Venous and lymphatic drainage parallels the arterial supply. The veins are tributaries of the portal vein, and the lymphatics all eventually pass to the celiac group of aortic lymph nodes.

Small Intestine.   The *duodenum* is a C-shaped tube surrounding the head of the pancreas (Fig. 2-33). It is divided into four parts, most of which are retroperitoneal. The first part is short and ascends

slightly from the gastroduodenal junction. It is related anteriorly to the gallbladder and liver and posteriorly to the portal vein, common bile duct, gastroduodenal artery, and the inferior vena cava. The second part descends in the right medial paracolic gutter. Posteriorly it is related to the right kidney and suprarenal gland while anteriorly it is crossed by the transverse colon. The common bile duct and main pancreatic duct empty into it posteromedially. The third part passes from right to left in front of the vena cava, the body of the third lumbar vertebra

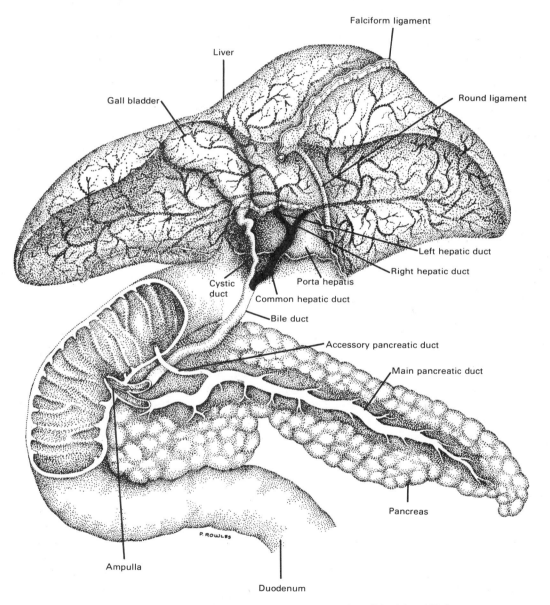

Fig. 2-33.   Duct systems of the liver, pancreas, and gallbladder. (Christensen JB, Telford IR: Synopsis of Gross Anatomy, 5th ed, p 168. Philadelphia, JB Lippincott, 1988)

and the aorta; it passes behind the superior mesenteric vessels. The fourth part is short and curves superiorly and then anteriorly at the duodenojejunal junction. It is suspended from the area of the right crus of the diaphragm by a peritoneal fold called the suspensory ligament of Treitz.

The mesenteric portion of the small intestine is divided into the proximal *jejunum* and distal *ileum.* The *mesentery* is a fan-shaped double layer of peritoneum continuous with the serosa of the jejunum and ileum and enclosing their vessels. The root of the mesentery is about 15 cm long, and its attachment to the posterior body wall extends from the duodenojejunal junction obliquely down and to the right, crossing the third part of the duodenum, the inferior vena cava, and the right ureter. The mesentery contains the intestinal and ileocolic branches of the superior mesenteric vessels as well as lymphatics and autonomics. The transition from jejunum to ileum is not abrupt, but certain differences do exist. The amount of mesenteric fat tends to increase from above downward, as does the number of arcades formed by the vessels in the mesentery. However, the blood supply to the jejunum is greater, so that its pink color is more intense than that of the ileum. The jejunum has a thicker wall as the plicae circulares are higher and more numerous.

Large Intestine.   This portion, the *colon,* extends from the ileocecal valve to the anus. It is characterized by sacculations (haustra), which are produced by three longitudinal muscle bands (taenia) that converge at the appendix. Between the sacculations are the semilunar folds, and along the free surface of the colon there are pouches containing fat (appendices epiploicae).

The *cecum* is a cul-de-sac of the colon below the entrance of the ileum. It is found in the right iliac fossa and is most often almost entirely enveloped in peritoneum. The ileocecal valve is formed by two liplike folds projecting into the medial aspect of the cecum.

The *vermiform appendix* is a blind tube that comes off the posteromedial aspect of the cecum about 2.5 cm below the ileocecal valve. It is most commonly found behind the cecum (retrocecal), although it may be in a variety of positions including hanging into the pelvis. It has a slight valve and, although variable, is usually about 10 cm in length. It has no true mesentery but is covered with a peritoneal fold and is supplied by an appendicular branch of the ileocolic artery.

The *ascending colon* is the continuation of the cecum that passes superiorly against the posterior body wall and the right kidney. Just below the right

lobe of the liver, it makes a sharp bend to the left. This bend is the right colic or hepatic flexure. The *transverse colon* extends between the hepatic and the splenic flexures and is suspended from the posterior abdominal wall by the transverse mesocolon. The attachment of the mesocolon crosses the second part of the duodenum and the pancreas, then attaches to the greater curvature of the stomach. The transverse colon is related to the liver, gallbladder and stomach anteriorly, and to the spleen superiorly. The *descending colon* extends from the splenic flexure to the left iliac fossa, passing along the lateral aspect of the left kidney and posterior body wall before becoming the *sigmoid colon.* Both the ascending and descending portions of the colon are typically partially peritonealized and therefore fixed in place, as opposed to the mobile transverse colon.

Liver.   The anterior, superior, and posterior surfaces of the liver form a dome that is related to the thoracic diaphragm. Through the diaphragm the liver is related to the lungs, pleura, heart, and pericardium. Its posteroinferior or visceral surface is related to the hepatic flexure of the colon, right kidney and suprarenal gland, gallbladder, duodenum, esophagus, and stomach. The visceral surface has an H-shaped configuration in which the center bar of the H is the *porta hepatis* where the portal vein, autonomics, and hepatic artery enter, and the common hepatic duct and lympathics exit. The limb of the H extending anteriorly on the right contains the gallbladder; posteriorly on the right is the inferior vena cava; anteriorly on the left is the ligamentum teres; and posteriorly on the left is the ligamentum venosum. That part of the liver between the two anterior limbs is the *quadrate lobe;* that portion between the two posterior limbs is the *caudate lobe.* Functionally the liver is separated into a large right lobe and a smaller left lobe, which includes the quadrate and caudate lobes.

The liver is partially enclosed within a complicated system of peritoneal folds (Fig. 2-34). The *falciform ligament* reflects from the anterior belly wall to the liver and contains the ligamentum teres in its inferior border. Anteriorly the falciform ligament reflects over the right and left lobes of the liver. On the superior and posterior aspects of the dome of the liver the two layers of this ligament initially diverge toward the sides of the liver. At the most lateral extents of these reflections, each layer turns sharply medially and posteriorly; the two layers converge toward one another in the region of the ligamentum venosum. As the two layers of the falciform ligament diverge and then converge in this pat-

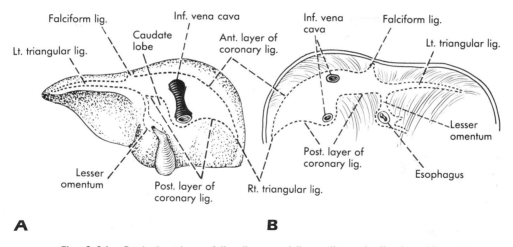

Fig. 2-34. Posterior view of the liver and its peritoneal attachments, illustrated schematically. *(A)* shows the posterior diaphragmatic and visceral surfaces, with lines of reflexion of peritoneum and ligaments indicated; *(B)* shows attachments to the diaphragm. (Hollinshead WH, Rosse C: Textbook of Anatomy, 4th ed, p 646. Philadelphia, JB Lippincott, 1985)

tern, they reflect onto the diaphragm. This crown-shaped pattern of peritoneal reflections between the posterosuperior surface of the liver and the under surface of the diaphragm is termed the *coronary ligament.* It surrounds the bare area of the liver, an area in which no peritoneum separates the liver and the diaphragm. The right and left extents of the coronary ligament are called the right and left *triangular ligaments* respectively. The lesser omentum extends from the visceral surface of the liver to the lesser curvature of the stomach. The free edge of the lesser omentum is formed as the peritoneum surrounds the portal vein, hepatic artery, and common bile duct. This free edge extends between the first part of the duodenum and the porta hepatis and forms the anterior boundary of the epiploic foramen (of Winslow), which is the entrance to the lesser omental sac.

The *portal system* includes all of the veins that drain the blood from the abdominal part of the digestive tube (except for the lower part of the rectum) and from the spleen, the pancreas, and the gallbladder. The portal vein is formed behind the neck of the pancreas by the union of the superior mesenteric and the splenic veins. It enters the porta of the liver and there, with the hepatic artery, divides into right and left lobar branches. These branches supply the liver lobules and eventually drain to the inferior vena cava by way of hepatic veins. At the porta hepatis, the hepatic artery and the common bile duct are in front of the portal vein with the artery to the left, the duct to the right.

In *portal obstruction* there are several alternate routes that blood may take to get from the portal venous system into the systemic circulation without going through the liver. These potential communications are between (1) the superior rectal veins with the middle and inferior rectal veins (which are tributaries of the internal iliac and internal pudendal respectively); (2) esophageal branches of the left gastric with esophageal tributaries of the azygous systems of veins; (3) portal tributaries in the mesenteries with body wall (retroperitoneal) tributaries of the lumbar, renal, and phrenic veins; (4) portal tributaries in the liver with tributaries to the abdominal wall veins in the falciform ligament; and (5) portal tributaries in the liver with phrenic veins across the bare area of the liver.

Gallbladder and Ducts. The *bile passages* include the gallbladder, the cystic duct, the hepatic duct, and the common bile duct (see Fig. 2-33). The gallbladder is a pear-shaped viscus lying below the liver between the right and the quadrate lobes. It has a broad fundus, a body, and a neck that narrows into the cystic duct. The body of the gallbladder is related superiorly to the liver, inferiorly to the transverse colon, and posteriorly to the duodenum or pyloric end of the stomach. The fundus of the gallbladder is at the tip of the ninth costal cartilage.

The cystic duct unites with the hepatic duct to form the common bile duct. The common bile duct and the main pancreatic duct unite just proximal to the point at which they empty into the second part of the duodenum at the major duodenal papilla. This common opening is protected by the sphincter of Oddi.

Pancreas. The pancreas (see Fig. 2-33) lies between the stomach and the posterior abdominal wall, and extends from the duodenum to the spleen. It is completely retroperitoneal. It is divided into a head, lying within the concavity of the duodenum; a neck, which is constricted posteriorly by the portal vein; a triangular body; and a tail that rests upon the spleen. The secretions of the neck, body, and tail portions of the pancreas are carried through the main pancreatic duct, through which they enter the duodenum. The accessory pancreatic duct of Santorini traverses the head of the pancreas and enters the duodenum 2 cm above the major duodenal papilla.

The main arteries supplying the pancreas are the superior and the inferior pancreaticoduodenal and the splenic, the latter running behind the upper part of the body and the tail of the pancreas.

Spleen. This organ occupies the left hypochondrium and the epigastrium under the ribs. Its parietal surface is in relation to the dome of the diaphragm. Its visceral surface is related to the stomach, left kidney, splenic flexure of the colon, and the tail of the pancreas. It is completely peritonealized and connected by peritoneal reflections to the posterior body wall in the region of the left kidney by the lienorenal ligament and to the stomach by the gastrolienal ligament. Its blood supply is provided by the splenic artery.

Kidney. The kidneys are surrounded by perirenal fat and supported by the renal fascia. They extend from the last thoracic to the third lumbar vertebrae, the right kidney being lower than the left. The kidneys are entirely retroperitoneal and are partially separated from the peritoneum by the duodenum on the right and the pancreas on the left.

The kidneys occupy the most dorsal position of all the abdominal organs. Each kidney lies against the diaphragm and the 12th rib above and against the psoas major and the quadratus lumborum below. The anterior relationships of the left kidney are the spleen, stomach, pancreas, left colic flexure, and the small intestine. The anterior surface of the right kidney is related to the liver, second part of the duodenum, and the right colic flexure.

The renal hilus is directed anteromedially and is the concave aspect of the kidney. The renal artery enters the kidney through this area, while the renal vein and ureter exit at this site. The final collecting cistern for urine is the *renal pelvis.* The pelvis occupies a large percentage of the hilus and is usually at the level of the body of L1. The pelvis narrows

rapidly to form the *ureter,* which conducts the urine to the bladder. The ureter is retroperitoneal and descend through the abdominal cavity almost vertically on the anterior aspect of the psoas major muscle. The right ureter is related anteriorly to the duodenum, the vessels to the ascending colon, the root of the mesentery, and the testicular or ovarian vessels. The left ureter is related anteriorly to the left colic vessels, testicular or ovarian vessels, and the sigmoid colon. At roentgenographic examination in which the ureters are filled with contrast medium, they are seen to cross the transverse processes of the lumbar vertebrae. As the ureters enter the pelvis, they incline medially and usually cross the termination of the common iliac arteries (or their branches). Their pelvic courses are inferomedial to the posterior aspect of the bladder. The ureters have three natural constrictions: at the junction of the renal pelvis and the ureter, where they cross the common iliac arteries, and as they pass through the wall of the bladder.

Generally, each kidney is supplied by a single large renal artery that is a direct branch from the abdominal aorta. A common variation, though, is two or three renal arteries on one or both sides.

Suprarenal Glands. The retroperitoneal suprarenal (adrenal) glands sit on the superior poles of each kidney. Both glands are related posteriorly to the diaphragm. The right suprarenal is related anteriorly to the liver and medially to the inferior vena cava. The anterior aspect of the left gland forms part of the posterior wall of the omental bursa and may be related to the splenic artery and the pancreas. Each gland receives a rich blood supply by way of branches from the renal and inferior phrenic arteries and from the aorta.

BLOOD SUPPLY OF THE ABDOMEN

The abdominal aorta (Fig. 2-35) enters the abdomen through the aortic hiatus (T12) and extends to the lower portion of the fourth lumbar vertebral body where it terminates by dividing into the large *common iliac arteries* and into its true continuation, the rudimentary *median sacral artery.* The aorta descends vertically along the anterior (or slightly to the left) aspect of the lumbar vertebral bodies.

Its branches are as follows:

Inferior phrenic. This pair of arteries arises just below the diaphragm or from the celiac trunk and distribute to the inferior surface of the diaphragm.

Celiac trunk. The highest of the unpaired vessels, it arises at L1. This artery is very short; it passes

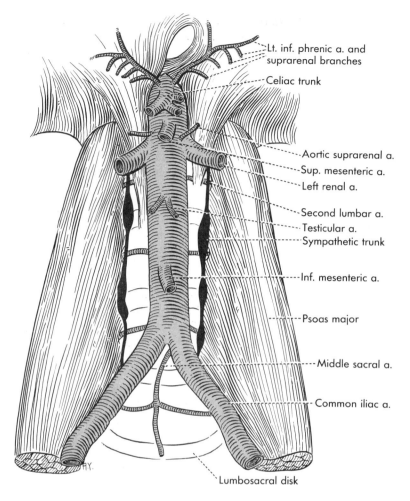

Lt. inf. phrenic a. and suprarenal branches

Celiac trunk

Aortic suprarenal a.

Sup. mesenteric a.

Left renal a.

Second lumbar a.

Testicular a.

Sympathetic trunk

Inf. mesenteric a.

Psoas major

Middle sacral a.

Common iliac a.

Lumbosacral disk

Fig. 2-35. The abdominal part of the aorta and its branches. (Hollinshead WH, Rosse C: Textbook of Anatomy, 4th ed, p 686. Philadelphia, JB Lippincott, 1985)

anteriorly behind the peritoneum and above the pancreas where it divides into its three branches: the left gastric, splenic, and common hepatic. The *left gastric* passes to the left, distributes to the lesser curvature of the stomach, and has esophageal and hepatic branches. The *splenic* passes to the left along the upper surface of the pancreas. It forms part of the floor of the lesser omental sac and supplies the pancreas and spleen and has the short gastric and left gastroepiploic branches to the greater curvature of the stomach. The *common hepatic artery* runs anterolaterally to the right toward the upper aspect of the first part of the duodenum. Its gastroduodenal branch descends behind the duodenum and has anterior and posterior superior pancreaticoduodenal, and right gastroepiploic branches. The continuation of the common hepatic after the gastroduodenal branch is the proper hepatic artery. This artery passes to the right and ascends to the porta hepatis through the lesser omentum. The right gas-

tric artery usually branches from the proper hepatic soon after its beginning; the cystic artery branches where the proper hepatic passes the cystic duct.

Middle suprarenal. These vessels are usually single, one passing directly to each suprarenal gland.

Superior mesenteric. The branches of this vessel supply the gastrointestinal tract from the middle of the duodenum through the transverse colon. One of its branches, the inferior pancreatico-duodenal artery, divides into anterior and posterior branches that form the pancreaticoduodenal arcades with the anterior and posterior superior pancreaticoduodenal arteries. The other branches are the intestinal arteries, the ileocolic artery, the right colic artery, and the middle colic artery.

Renal artery. Arising at about the level of the second lumbar vertebra, these two large arteries pass across the crura of the diaphragm and the psoas major muscles in their transverse courses to the hila of the kidneys. The right is longer than the left, and it passes posterior to the inferior vena cava.

Testicular or ovarian arteries. These small arteries arise just inferior to the renal arteries. The retroperitoneal testicular arteries descend obliquely toward the deep inguinal ring where they become part of the spermatic cord. The ureteric branches arise as the testicular arteries cross the ureters. The abdominal course of the ovarian arteries is similar to that of the testiculars. As they reach the pelvic brim, the ovarian arteries swing medially and pass through the suspensory ligament of the ovary to the ovary.

Inferior mesenteric. Arising just below the third part of the duodenum, this artery passes obliquely downward and to the left, behind the peritoneum. Its left colic, sigmoid, and superior rectal branches supply the descending colon, the sigmoid colon, and the upper portion of the rectum.

Lumbar arteries. The four lumbar arteries supply primarily the body wall and those structures within the vertebral canal.

Common iliac arteries. The large terminal branches of the aorta, the common iliacs, arise slightly to the left of the midline in front of the body of the fourth lumbar vertebra. The common iliacs divide into the internal and external iliac arteries just lateral to the sacral promotory. Each internal iliac enters the pelvis to supply pelvic and perineal structures. The external iliac passes under the inguinal ligament where it becomes the femoral artery.

Middle sacral artery. The true caudal continuation and termination of the aorta, this vessel arises from the posterior aspect of the aorta just above its bifurcation. It passes inferiorly on the ventral aspect of the lumbar vertebrae, enters the pelvis, and descends on the anterior surface of the sacrum and coccyx. It gives rise to parietal branches in its course.

NERVE SUPPLY OF THE ABDOMEN

Body Wall. The skin of the abdominal wall is innervated by the anterior and lateral cutaneous branches of intercostal nerves seven through eleven (T7–11), the subcostal nerve (T12), and the iliohypogastric branch of the first lumbar nerve. The underlying muscles of the abdominal wall are innervated segmentally by muscular branches of the same nerves.

Viscera. Autonomic innervation of the viscera of the abdominal cavity is provided by sympathetic fibers from spinal cord segments T5 through L1 or 2 and parasympathetic fibers from the vagus nerve and spinal cord segments S2 through 4. These fibers generally are distributed in periarterial plexuses that are associated with the abdominal aorta and its branches. The continuous plexus (Fig. 2-36) found on the ventral aspect of the aorta and associated with the three large unpaired arteries is divided into the celiac, superior mesenteric, and inferior mesenteric plexuses, with the intermesenteric plexus connecting the superior and inferior mesenterics and the inferior mesenteric plexus continuing inferiorly as the superior hypogastric plexus. Continuations of these plexuses follow various other branches of the aorta to their respective destinations and bear the names of the arteries, for example, the renal plexus.

The sympathetic input into the celiac and superior mesenteric plexuses is from the **greater** (T5–10), **lesser** (T10–12), and **least** (T12) **splanchnic nerves.** These nerves arise in the thorax and enter the abdomen by passing through the crura of the diaphragm.

The intermesenteric, inferior mesenteric, and superior hypogastric plexuses receive additional sympathetic fibers from the **lumbar splanchnic nerves.** The fibers in the thoracic and lumbar splanchnic nerves are preganglionic. They synapse with postganglionic fibers in ganglia associated with the aortic plexuses. The largest and most demonstrable of these is the celiac ganglion.

Vagal (parasympathetic) **fibers** supply the organs of the abdomen and the gastrointestinal tract as far distally as the splenic flexure of the large intestine. The vagus nerves enter the abdomen with the esophagus as the anterior and posterior vagal trunks. The trunks distribute on the anterior and posterior aspects of the stomach and enter the celiac plexus.

The **pelvic splanchnics** (parasympathetic fibers from spinal cord segments S2–4) provide direct retroperitoneal branches to the descending and sigmoid portions of the large intestine.

The fibers in both the vagus and pelvic splanchnic nerves are preganglionic. They synapse with postganglionic fibers either in or very near the organ innervated.

Afferent fibers from the abdominal viscera reach the CNS through both the vagus and splanchnic nerves. Those sensory fibers in the vagus are concerned with muscular and secretory reflexes. Most pain fibers are thought to be carried in the splanchnic nerves.

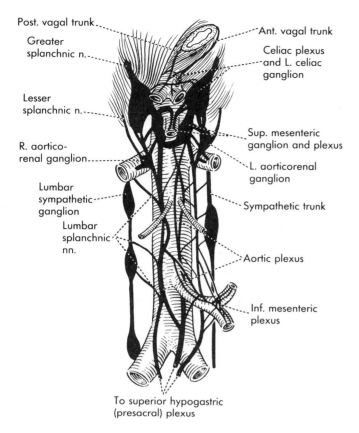

Post. vagal trunk

Greater
splanchnic n.

Lesser
splanchnic n.

R. aortico-
renal ganglion

Lumbar
sympathetic
ganglion

Lumbar
splanchnic
nn.

Ant. vagal trunk

Celiac plexus
and L. celiac
ganglion

Sup. mesenteric
ganglion and plexus

L. aorticorenal
ganglion

Sympathetic trunk

Aortic plexus

Inf. mesenteric
plexus

To superior hypogastric
(presacral) plexus

Fig. 2-36. The autonomic nerve plexuses and gan-glia associated with the aorta. (Hollinshead WH, Rosse C: Textbook of Anatomy, 4th ed, p 697. Philadelphia, JB Lippincott, 1985)

CROSS SECTIONS OF THE ABDOMEN

Figure 2-37 represents a section through the upper portion of the first lumbar vertebra. The liver occupies most of the right half of the abdomen, with the left lobe extending to the left and anterior to the stomach. The left and quadrate lobes are separated by the fissure containing the ligamentum teres, and the right lobe is most of the large portion on the right. The caudate lobe is posterior (and superior) to the porta hepatis. In the porta hepatis the portal vein is posterior to both the common hepatic duct and the proper hepatic artery, with the duct being to the right of the artery. The superior pole of the right kidney is related anteriorly to the right lobe of the liver and the right suprarenal gland. The right suprarenal gland is bounded anteriorly by the inferior vena cava, posteriorly by the right kidney, laterally by the right lobe of the liver, and medially by the right crus of the diaphragm. The celiac trunk passes anteriorly from the aorta and branches into the left gastric artery, which passes anteriorly, and the common hepatic artery, which passes to the right. The left kidney is related laterally to the spleen and anteriorly to the body and tail of the pancreas, the

left suprarenal, and the descending colon. The left suprarenal is posteromedial to the splenic vein and body of the pancreas, anteromedial to the left kidney, and lateral to the left crus of the diaphragm. The splenic vein is positioned between the pancreas anteriorly and the left suprarenal posteriorly. The splenic vein would be displaced (splenic vein sign) anteriorly by a mass in the left suprarenal and posteriorly by a pancreatic mass. The pyloric antrum of the stomach is posterior to the left lobe of the liver and anterior to the pancreas.

Figure 2-38 represents a section that passes through the intervertebral disc between lumbar vertebrae one and two. Only portions of the right and quadrate lobes of the liver are found at this level, with the gallbladder found in the groove between the two. The inferior vena cava is positioned slightly to the right of the vertebral column; the left renal vein passes to the right anterior to the aorta and posterior to the superior mesenteric artery on its way to the inferior vena cava. The portal vein is seen where it is formed, posterior to the neck of the pancreas and anterior to the uncinate process. The first and second parts of the duodenum are continuous, the second passing posteriorly from the first.

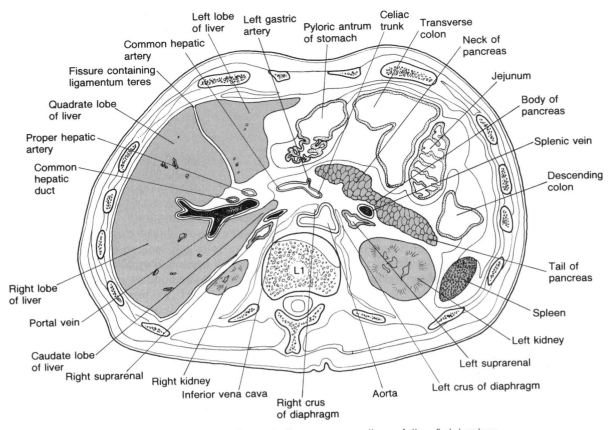

Fig. 2-37. A section through the upper portion of the first lumbar vertebra.

The head of the pancreas is related to the first and second parts of the duodenum and has the common bile duct embedded in its posterior aspect. The transverse colon passes from right to left, crossing the duodenum and the pancreas. The descending colon descends along the posterior abdominal wall, passing anterior to the left kidney.

Figure 2-39* represents a section through the third lumbar vertebra. The inferior vena cava is anterior and somewhat to the right of the vertebral column; the aorta is anterior and somewhat to the left. The third part of the duodenum passes from right to left across the vertebral column, anterior to the great vessels and posterior to the superior mesenteric artery. The hepatic flexure of the colon is related laterally to the inferior tip of the right lobe of the liver. The right kidney, which is still present at this level, is related anteriorly to the hepatic flexure of the colon and the second part of the duodenum. The ureters descend across the an-

terolateral aspects of the psoas major muscles. The superior mesenteric artery occupies the root of the mesentery.

MICROSCOPIC STRUCTURE OF ABDOMINAL ORGANS

Gastrointestinal Tract. The general histologic plan of the gastrointestinal tract consists of an inner mucosa, a submucosa, a muscularis externa, and an outer serosa (see Fig. 2-29). These were reviewed in the section on the esophagus. Different parts of the gastrointestinal tract retain the basic plan but differ as to their internal configuration of the mucosa, epithelial lining, type and extent of mucosal and submucosal glands, and by their thickness and configuration of muscle.

The *stomach* is structurally modified for the production of hydrochloric acid and pepsin and for the mixing of food with these substances. In the empty stomach the mucosa is thrown into longitudinal folds called rugae. Throughout the stomach the simple columnar lining epithelium produces mucus and indents into the mucosa as gastric pits. One or more

* The authors of this chapter wish to acknowledge the fine work of Ms. Carolyn Volpe for the five cross-sectional illustrations used in this chapter.

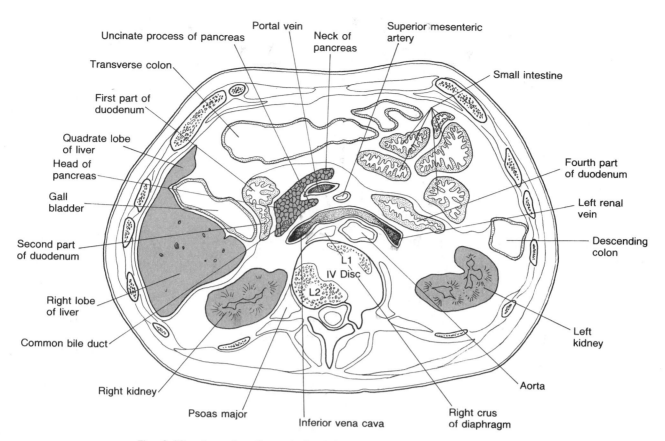

Fig. 2-38. A section through the intervertebral disc between the first and second lumbar vertebrae.

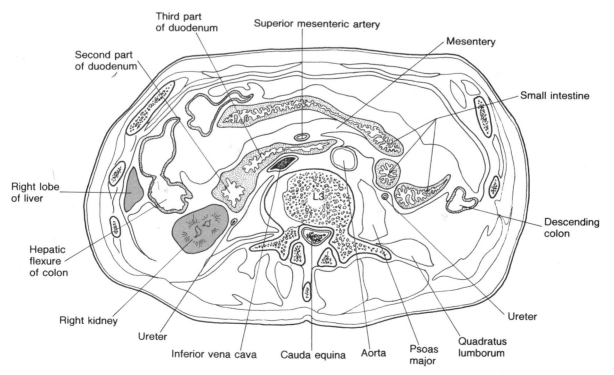

Fig. 2-39. A section through the third lumbar vertebra.

mucosal glands empty into the base of each pit. The length of glands and pits and the glandular cell types differ in the cardiac, body (fundus), and pyloric regions of the stomach. Gastric glands of the body and fundus are the most prevalent and contain the most diverse cell types. In this type of gland, chief cells are located mostly in the base (fundus), parietal cells are located in the neck and isthmus region, mucous neck cells are in the neck, and argentaffin (enteroendocrine, enterochromaffin, amine precursor uptake [and] decarboxylation [APUD]) cells are scattered. Undifferentiated columnar cells in the neck region of the gland differentiate and move upward to replace the lining epithelium, which turns over every 3 to 7 days. Other undifferentiated cells move into the glands where they differentiate into the gland cells.

Chief cells produce pepsin and are typical enzyme-secreting cells in that they contain much RER, a well-established Golgi apparatus, and membrane-bound zymogen granules. In these cells, amino acids attached to tRNA are carried to rRNA of the RER where the pepsinogen code is translated from mRNA. The protein product passes into the cisterna of the RER and is carried to transfer vesicles near the Golgi apparatus. In this region the membrane-bound pepsinogen granule is formed. The granule passes to the apical surface of the cell where the product is discharged when the membrane of the granule fuses with the plasma membrane and then opens to the lumen (exocytosis, merocrine secretion). *Parietal cells* produce HCl and seem to produce the intrinsic antipernicious anemia factor. They are rounded, or pyramidal, cells whose apices open to the lumen through an intercellular canal between adjacent chief cells. An extensive infolding of the surface membrane forms intracellular canaliculi into which microvilli project. SER and mitochondria are prevalent, and the cells are often binucleate. In the production of HCl, sodium chloride probably passes to the intracellular canaliculi where hydrogen ion, supplied by carbonic acid in the cell, is exchanged for sodium. Thus, HCl passes into the lumen of the gland while bicarbonate passes from the cell into the blood. Mucous neck cells produce mucus of a different nature than that of the surface epithelium. Argentaffin cells are sandwiched between the other gland cells and the basement membrane. Some of these produce serotonin while other types of these cells produce cholinesterase; both of these secretions are discharged into the blood stream. Other *enteroendocrine* (APUD) *cells* seem to produce a glucagonlike substance, while still others produce gastrin.

Pyloric and cardiac glands contain only cells that are similar to the neck mucous cell. In the pyloric region the gastric pits are deep, and the glands are very tortuous and appear shorter.

The muscularis externa layer of the stomach contains three layers, an outer longitudinal, a middle circular, and an inner oblique layer. The two inner layers are thickened as the pyloric sphincter muscle. The serosa is continuous at the greater curvature with the two layers of the greater omentum and at the lesser curvature with the two layers of the lesser omentum.

The *small intestine* is structurally modified for the absorption of nutritive substances. The absorptive surface is large because of (1) mucosal and submucosal folds called plicae circulares, (2) mucosal projections called villi, and (3) microvilli forming a striated border on the simple columnar lining epithelium. Mucus is secreted by goblet cells in the lining epithelium. These cells increase in number at progressively lower levels of the gastrointestinal tract where drier wastes are accumulating. *Crypts of Lieberkühn* are mucosal glands that are found throughout the intestine; they empty at the bases of the villi. Their cells replace the lining cells of the villi every 7 to 8 days and thus show mitoses and gradations of differentiation. Some of the enteroendocrine gland cells produce secretin and cholecystokinin. Argentaffin cells and Paneth's cells are present in the crypts of Lieberkühn. In the upper part of the duodenum, Brunner's glands occupy the submucosa and empty into the crypts or at the bases of villi. Their cells are similar to those in the pyloric glands and produce an alkaline glycoprotein secretion. The lower ileum contains aggregations of lymphatic nodules called Peyer's patches. These are located opposite the mesentery attachment, chiefly in the mucosa. The muscularis externa consists of inner circular and outer longitudinal smooth muscle layers. Myenteric and submucosal nerve plexi containing autonomic postganglionic cell bodies and cells of the enteric nervous system are present throughout the intestine and stomach.

The absorption of fats, carbohydrates, proteins, and water in the small intestine takes place through the simple columnar lining cells of the villi since the tight junctions (zonula occludens) of the *junctional complexes* (zonula occludens, zonula adherens, macula adherens) do not permit intercellular passage. Thus, carbohydrates, fats, and proteins must be broken down in the lumen before absorption can take place. Some of this is accomplished by pancreatic enzymes and liver bile salts. Intestinal juices produced by crypt glands and the lining epithelium are also involved in the terminal hydrolytic digestion of carbohydrates and proteins. The active sites of much of this activity seem to be in the microvillus region near the glycoprotein "fuzz" coat of the plasma membrane. Substances absorbed through the surface epithelium pass to capillaries or the central lacteal of the villi for distribution in the portal vein or thoracic duct, respectively. In fat absorption, bile salts and lipase produce micelles of fatty acids and monoglycerides which passively enter the cell. In the cytoplasm, the SER resynthesizes triglycerides and the RER produces proteins in the production of chylomicrons; these are discharged into the intercellular space, where they pass mostly to the lacteals.

The *large intestine* absorbs much water and produces mucus that lubricates the feces. No villi are present, and the crypts open directly on the surface. The lining epithelium is simple columnar with a striated border, and it contains many goblet cells. The outer longitudinal layer of the muscularis externa is thickened into three longitudinally running bands of smooth muscle (taenia coli).

The *appendix* is microscopically similar to the colon except that it is smaller, does not have taenia, and possesses a prominent ring of lymphatic nodules that occupy most of the lamina propria and the submucosa.

The *anal canal* functions to retain and eliminate wastes. The colonlike mucosa of the upper portion forms longitudinal anal columns just above the horizontally oriented anal valves. Epithelium over the anal valves is stratified squamous nonkeratinized epithelium. It becomes keratinized about 2.5 cm below the valves. The lamina propria contains large internal hemorrhoidal veins and circumanal glands. The inner circular layer of the muscularis becomes the internal anal sphincter. The outer longitudinal layer disappears and is replaced in position by skeletal muscle of the external anal sphincter.

Liver and Gallbladder.   The liver is surrounded by a tough connective tissue capsule that penetrates it at the porta to produce many septa. These septa provide support for the parenchyma and divide it into lobes and lobules. Branches of the portal vein and hepatic artery further subdivide within the septa and supply the lobules. These vessels and bile ducts constitute portal triads (portal canals, spaces) at the junction of adjacent lobules.

The *hepatic lobules* consist of a central vein from which anastomosing hepatic plates of cells, usually one cell thick, radiate toward the periphery (Fig. 2-40). Between the plates are hepatic sinusoids that connect the portal vein and hepatic artery peripher

ally with the central vein centrally. Blood drains from the central vein to sublobular veins and leaves the liver by way of the hepatic veins. The sinusoids are discontinuously lined by endothelial cells and phagocytic Kupffer cells of the reticuloendothelial system. The lining cells abut against microvilli of the hepatocytes, leaving a space (of Disse) between the base of the endothelial cell and the hepatocyte; this space is continuous with the sinusoids, thus providing for efficient interchange between blood in the sinusoid and the hepatocyte. Bile canaliculi lie between adjacent cells in the hepatic plates and are expansions of the intercellular spaces between the cells. They are separated from the rest of the intercellular space by occluding junctions; microvilli of the hepatic cells extend into the canalicular lumen. These canaliculi receive bile produced by the hepatocytes and conduct it peripherally into small ducts that open into the bile ducts of the portal triad. Bile is transported out of the liver in hepatic ducts; it then traverses the cystic duct and is stored and condensed in the gallbladder. Bile is discharged from the gallbladder through the cystic duct and common bile duct and empties at the sphincters of Oddi and Boyden into the duodenum. The epithelium lining the bile ducts grades from low cuboidal to high columnar with the increasing caliber of the ducts. *Hepatocytes* are polyhedral, with one or more large rounded nuclei. They contain a wide range of organelles that are consistent with the many and diverse functions these cells perform. The SER is involved in the synthesis of glycogen, in the inactivation and detoxification of drugs, in the synthesis of bile acids, and in the production of water-soluble bilirubin glucuronide. The RER synthesizes lipoproteins, prothrombin, albumin, and fibrinogen. Hepatocytes also store lipids, carbohydrates, and vitamins; recirculate bile acids; and can carry out gluconeogenesis. Kupffer cells, like other cells of the mononuclear phagocyte system, produce bilirubin by the breakdown of hemoglobin from phagocytized worn-out erythrocytes.

Two methods of classification of liver lobules are used other than the classic hepatic lobule mentioned above. The *portal lobule* has a portal triad at the center, with the periphery of the lobule being those adjacent portions of hepatic plates that drain into the bile duct of the portal triad. The *hepatic* (Rappaport) *acinus* is a diamond-shaped area that drains into an interlobular vein between adjacent hepatic lobules; the periphery of the acinus extends to the central veins of the two adjacent lobules.

The *gallbladder* is lined by a mucous membrane that is thrown into folds. It possesses a simple co-

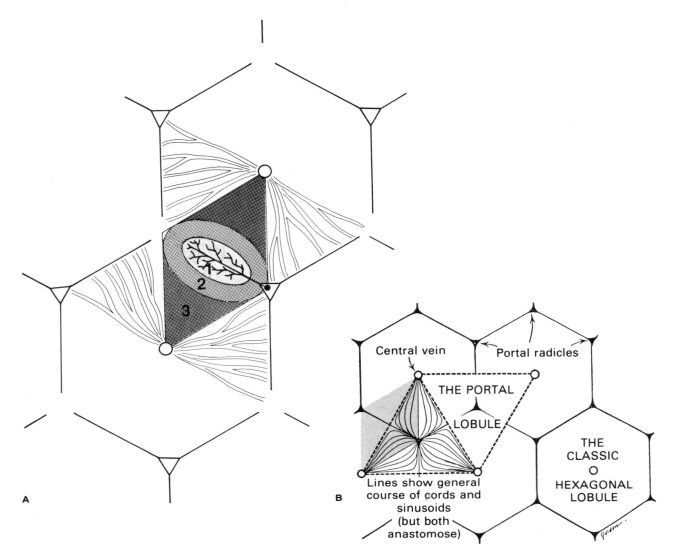

Fig. 2-40. Diagrammatic representation of *(A)* the liver acinis and *(B)* the classic lobule and portal lobule. In *(A)* the numbers indicate the distance of zones from the blood supplied by the vascular backbone extending from the portal area. In *(B)* the portal area is the center of the portal lobule, whereas the central vein is the center of the classic lobule. (Cormack DH: Ham's Histology, 9th ed, p 527. Philadelphia, JB Lippincott, 1987)

lumnar epithelium whose sodium pump transports sodium chloride through the epithelium and extensive lateral intercellular spaces to underlying capillaries; this leads to the passive reabsorption of water and the concentration of bile. A circularly arranged smooth muscle layer is present and is surrounded by a prominent connective tissue layer.

Pancreas. The pancreas is divided into lobules by connective tissue septa. The lobules are packed with serous acini consisting of enzyme-secreting pyramidal cells and centroacinar cells. The serous-secreting cells are similar in structure to other protein-secreting cells (*e.g.*, chief cells of the stomach). The cells are arranged in acini with small centroacinar cells lining the lumen. The pyramidal secretory cells are regulated by cholecystokinin, which causes secretion of proteases, nucleases, amylase, and lipase. The centroacinar and intercalated duct cells, when stimulated by secretin, produce high concentrations of sodium bicarbonate. The intercalated ducts drain acini to larger intralobular ducts, which empty successively to interlobular ducts and the main pancreatic duct (of Wirsung) or accessory duct. The larger ducts have simple columnar epithelium, goblet cells, and mucous glands; the smaller ducts are lined with simple cuboidal epithelium.

Islets of Langerhans are heavily vascularized groups of cells scattered throughout the pancreas. There are several cell types present in the islets. The most common type is the insulin-producing beta cell. Absence or malfunction of these cells leads to diabetes mellitus. Another prominent cell type of the islets is the alpha cell which produces glucagon, a hyperglycemic-glycogenolytic factor. Delta cells in the islets produce somatostatin and possibly gastrin, while PP cells may help regulate acinar cell secretion.

Spleen.   The spleen is the largest lymphoid organ in the body, and it is specialized for filtering blood. The spleen consists of white pulp (splenic nodules) and red pulp. The *white pulp* is dense lymphatic tissue; the *red pulp* is looser and consists of lymphatic splenic cords of tissue and venous sinusoids. Arterial blood enters the spleen at the hilum in the splenic artery. Branches of this artery pass in connective tissue trabeculae that radiate from the capsule at the hilar region. These are trabecular (interlobular) arteries. At the ends of the trabeculae the adventitia of the arteries takes on the character of reticular tissue and becomes infiltrated with lymphocytes forming splenic nodules (white pulp). These arteries are eccentrically located in the nodules and are called central arteries. After numerous branchings these arterioles leave the white pulp and enter the reticular connective tissue of the red pulp that surrounds the splenic nodules. In the red pulp the pulp arterioles divide into sheathed arterioles that empty into sinusoids via terminal arterial capillaries or empty first into the pulp reticulum and then filter between the lining cells of the sinusoids. Many macrophages of the reticuloendothelial (mononuclear phagocytic) system lie outside the walls of the sinusoids and phagocytize worn-out RBCs. The venous sinuses empty into pulp veins that pass to trabecular veins before blood is emptied by way of the splenic vein. In addition to the filtering of blood, the spleen controls the blood volume by storing RBCs and by periodically discharging the blood through the contraction of smooth muscle and the action of elastic fibers in the capsule and trabeculae. The spleen also produces lymphocytes, monocytes, plasma cells, and antibodies. Most of the lymphocytes that leave the spleen are from the recirculating pool of lymphocytes; relatively few new lymphocytes are formed in the spleen. The spleen is involved in both the cell-mediated and humoral

responses to antigens. In the white pulp, T-lymphocytes are located in the periarterial sheath with B-lymphocytes being located more peripherally. When B cells are activated, they move to the germinal center and give rise to plasma cells, which elaborate antibodies in the red pulp. Activated B cells also return to the general circulation by way of the red pulp sinuses. In the secondary responses to antigens by memory cells, the spleen is one of the most active organs in antibody secretion.

Suprarenal (Adrenal) Glands.   The suprarenal glands are divisible into two parts: a mesodermally derived cortex and a neural ectodermally derived medulla. A thick connective tissue capsule sends radially directed trabeculae of reticular fibers into the underlying cortex. The *cortex* consists of an outer zona glomerulosa, a middle zona fasciculata, and an inner zona reticularis. Columnar cells of the zona glomerulosa are arranged in arches. They produce mineralocorticoids (*e.g.,* aldosterone). The zona fasciculata consists of cords of cells that radiate inward from the zona glomerulosa. These cords are two cells thick, contain cuboidal cells that are often binucleate, and are separated from adjacent cords by fenestrated capillaries that radiate inward from the capsule. Fasciculata cells often contain much lipid and appear vacuolated. The zona reticularis consists of irregularly arranged cords of cells that may contain lipofuscin pigment. Fasciculata and reticularis cells are under the control of adrenocorticotropic hormone (ACTH) from the adenohypophysis; they produce glucocorticoids (*e.g.,* cortisol, corticosterone) and the sex hormone dehydroepiandrosterone. The most prominent organelle in adrenal cortical cells is an extensive SER, which is indicative of steroid-secreting cells.

The *suprarenal medulla* produces epinephrine and norepinephrine in its polyhedral basophilic cells. These cells receive terminations of preganglionic sympathetic nerve fibers, and each cell is located between a venule and a capillary. The cells exhibit the chromaffin reaction. The blood supply of the suprarenal gland is by branches of the suprarenal arteries that (1) go directly to the medulla, and (2) go indirectly to the medulla through capsular arterioles and their radiating capillary plexuses that pass between the cortical cords of cells before reaching the medulla.

Kidney, Ureter, and Bladder.   The *kidney* is divisible into an outer cortex and an inner medulla (Fig. 2-41). The *medulla* consists of renal pyramids, with the broad base of each pyramid facing the cortex, while the apex (renal papilla) opens into a minor calyx. The 10 to 16 minor calyces open into two

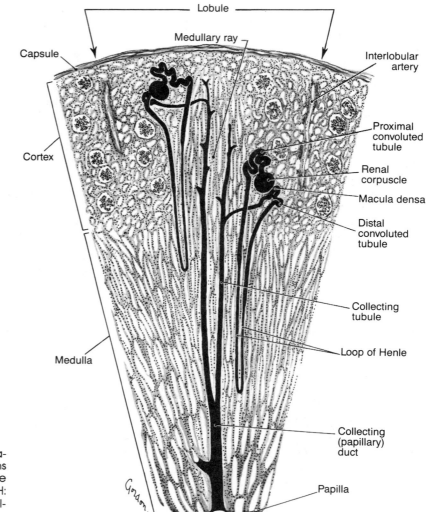

Lobule

Medullary ray

Capsule

Interlobular artery

Cortex

Proximal convoluted tubule

Renal corpuscle

Macula densa

Distal convoluted tubule

Collecting tubule

Loop of Henle

Medulla

Collecting (papillary) duct

Papilla

Fig. 2-41. Diagrammatic representation of a kidney lobule. Two nephrons emptying into collecting tubules are represented in black. (Cormack DH: Ham's Histology, 9th ed, p 569. Philadelphia, JB Lippincott, 1987)

or three major calyces, which in turn empty into the funnel-shaped renal pelvis at the hilus of the kidney. The *cortex* lies peripheral to the medulla and extends between the pyramids as renal columns. The cortex consists of medullary rays (pars radiata) and cortical labyrinths (pars convoluta). The medullary rays are parallel accumulations of collecting tubules and thick and thin limbs of the loop of Henle, which radiate toward the medulla. Each of these is surrounded by cortical labyrinth tissue of glomeruli and convoluted tubules that empty into the tubules of the medullary ray. A medullary ray and its associated cortical labyrinth constitute a lobule. A kidney lobe is a renal pyramid with its overlying cortex and renal columns.

The functional unit of the kidney is the *uriniferous tubule,* which consists of a nephron and collecting tubule. The nephron is comprised of the renal corpuscle (of glomerulus and Bowman's capsule), the proximal convoluted tubule; the thick descending limb, thin portion, and thick ascending limb of the loop of Henle; and the distal convoluted tubule (see Fig. 2-41). The glomerulus is a tuft of fenestrated capillaries fed by an afferent arteriole and drained by a smaller efferent arteriole. It is invested by podocytes of the visceral layer of Bowman's capsule. The podocytes have pedicles that interdigitate with those from adjacent podocytes and attach to a basal lamina between the podocyte and the capillary endothelium. Filtration slits 250 A wide exist between pedicles and communicate with the lumen of Bowman's capsule. At the basal lamina surface these slits are connected by a thin slit membrane. The podocytes, basal lamina and fenestrated endothelium constitute the *filtration barrier.* Mesangial phagocytic (stalk) cells in the glomerulus probably remove filtration residues from the basal lamina which is the main filter for large molecules. The parietal layer of Bowman's capsule consists of simple squamous epithelium.

The *proximal convoluted tubule* is the longest and widest portion of the nephron. It is comprised of a simple pyramidal epithelium possessing a brush border (microvilli) and indistinct lateral borders. The proximal convoluted tubule is located in the cortical labyrinth. It is continuous with, and histologically similar to, the thick descending limb of Henle's loop that courses in the medullary ray. Both the proximal and straight descending tubules resorb 85% or more of the water and sodium chloride of the glomerular filtrate. Glucose and amino acids also are resorbed by the epithelium of these tubules. The *thin portion of Henle's loop* is comprised of simple squamous epithelium. Its descending and ascending portions function similarly to the thick descending and ascending portions respectively.

The thick ascending and *distal convoluted tubules* have a low cuboidal epithelium with scattered microvilli and an extensive infolding of the basal plasma membrane. In these tubules sodium is transported out of the cells, and the filtrate becomes hypotonic and acidic. Where the distal tubule abuts against the afferent glomerular arteriole the epithelium is columnar and constitutes the macula densa. The muscle cells of the adjacent afferent glomerular arteriole are replaced by large pale juxtaglomerular cells containing granules. These cells produce renin and along with cells of the mucula densa and some interposed cells constitute the *juxtaglomerular complex.* Renin acts on its substrate, angiotensinogen, producing angiotensin I, which is converted to angiotensin II; the latter brings about increased secretion of aldosterone by the adrenal cortex. Aldosterone acts on the distal convoluted tubule to bring about reabsorption of sodium and thus reduce sodium loss in the urine.

The *collecting tubules* consist of pale, clear simple cuboidal epithelium with distinct lateral boundaries. These tubules join to form papillary ducts lined by simple columnar epithelium. Under the influence of antidiuretic hormone from the neurohypophysis, the epithelium of the collecting tubules becomes more permeable to water, and the latter is passively removed from the urine.

Arterial blood is carried to the hilar region of the kidney by the renal artery. This artery branches into interlobar branches that give rise to arcuate arteries passing along the cortex–medulla junction. Interlobular arteries arise from the arcuate arteries and

pass peripherally in the cortical labyrinths to give rise to afferent glomerular arterioles supplying the glomeruli. From the glomeruli, efferent arterioles supply the capillary plexi around the tubules. Capillaries of the medulla are supplied by arteriolae rectae from the efferent arterioles. Venous drainage is by venae rectae, interlobular, arcuate, interlobar, and renal veins that accompany the arteries.

The *ureters* are lined with transitional epithelium. External to the lamina propria is a muscularis layer consisting of inner longitudinal and outer circular smooth muscle layers. Near the bladder an additional outer longitudinal layer is added.

The *urinary bladder* is histologically similar to the lower part of the ureter in that it has a mucosa with transitional epithelium, a three-layered muscularis layer, and an outer connective tissue layer. The superficial (facet) transitional cells have a luminal plasma membrane of thick plates separated by thinner membrane. During contraction of the bladder the thick areas invaginate and form vesicles of reserve membrane.

DEVELOPMENT OF ABDOMINAL ORGANS

The development of the urogenital system will be covered in the section on the pelvis and perineum.

Development of the Digestive System. The entodermal *foregut* gives rise to the pharynx, esophagus, stomach, liver, pancreas, and part of the duodenum. The *midgut* gives rise to the rest of the small intestine, ascending colon, and proximal two thirds of the transverse colon. The *hindgut* develops into the rest of the large intestine as far as the upper part of the anal canal. The lower part of the rectum and much of the anal canal is established by the separation of the cloaca into a dorsal anorectal canal and ventral urogenital sinus by the urorectal septum. The rest of the anal canal develops from an ectodermally lined anal pit.

The *stomach* appears in the fourth embryonic week as a dilation of the foregut. As it shifts caudally from its position above the septum transversum, it rotates so that its original left surface faces anteriorly and its dorsal greater curvature extends to the left.

The *intestines* develop from cephalic and caudal limbs of a midgut loop that extends into the belly stalk. The cephalic limb extends from the upper duodenum to the yolk stalk. It gives rise to the rest of the small intestine, except the last 40 cm to 50 cm of the ileum. The caudal limb extends from the yolk stalk to the hindgut and it gives rise to the rest of the ileum, the cecum, the ascending colon, and the proximal two thirds of the transverse colon. As the loop develops it rotates counterclockwise (in an AP view) around the omphalomesenteric (vitelline) artery, the latter becoming the superior mesenteric artery (Fig. 2-42A,B). This rotation places the transverse colon above the jejunum and ileum, anterior to the duodenum, and just below the stomach. By the 10th week the abdomen enlarges, and the gut loop reenters the abdomen. The cephalic limb enters first, crowding the descending colon to the left. Partial persistence of the yolk stalk may remain as a Meckel's diverticulum attached to the ileum 40 cm to 50 cm from the ileocolic junction.

The *liver* arises in the fourth embryonic week as a ventral diverticulum of the foregut. This diverticulum grows through the ventral mesentery and into

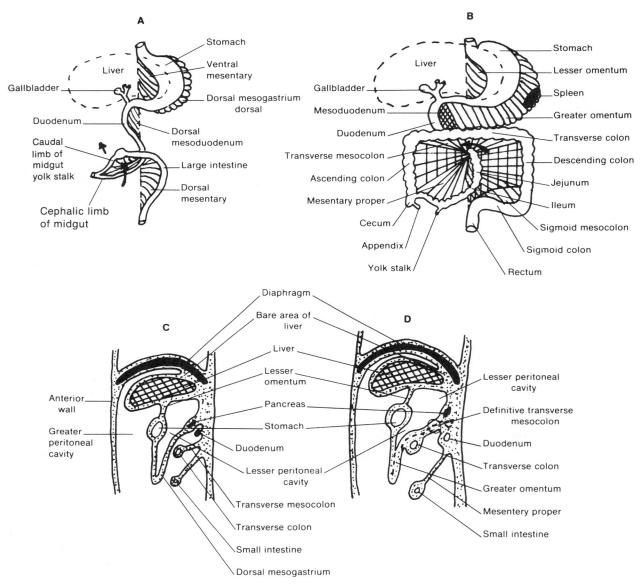

Fig. 2-42. Rotation of the gut and development of the mesenteries. *(A)*, early, and *(B)*, late, are anterior views of the rotation of the stomach and gut. The crosshatched areas of the mesentery are areas where it has become secondarily fused to the dorsal body wall. *(C)*, early, and *(D)*, late, are sagittal sections of the abdomen showing the greater and lesser peritoneal cavities, the formation of the definitive greater omentum and transverse mesocolon, and the secondarily retroperitoneal formation of the duodenum and pancreas.

the caudal face of the septum transversum. The more proximal part of the hepatic diverticulum gives rise to the common bile duct, cystic duct, gallbladder, and hepatic ducts. The more distal portions differentiate into the hepatic plates and the smaller bile ducts. Since the liver grows in the septum transversum and bulges from its caudal face, it is covered by peritoneum lining the septum transversum, except at the bare area of the liver where it abuts directly against the septum (diaphragm).

The *pancreas* forms from dorsal and ventral entodermal buds located at the level of the duodenum. The dorsal bud grows into the dorsal mesentry. The proximal portion of the ventral bud joins with the common bile duct, whereas the distal portion grows into the dorsal mesentery and fuses with the dorsal bud. The pancreatic duct (of Wirsung) develops from the ventral bud and the distal part of the dorsal primordium. The proximal portion of the dorsal bud may give rise to the accessory duct (of Santorini).

Development of the Abdominal Mesenteries and Spleen. The abdominal mesenteries develop primarily from the embryonic dorsal mesentry. The ventral mesentery may give rise to the lesser omentum and the falciform ligament, although the latter probably forms from a "shearing" of peritoneum covering the body wall. The peritoneum covering the liver reflects at the bare area of the liver to form the coronary and triangular ligaments of the liver. Much of the dorsal mesogastrium suspending the stomach fuses with the dorsal body wall to form the dorsal lining of the lesser sac. The rest of the dorsal mesogastrium fuses with the embryonic transverse mesocolon to form the definitive mesentery of the transverse colon and then drapes over the small intestine to become the greater omentum (Fig. 2-42C,D). The spleen develops from mesoderm of the dorsal mesogastrium. Most of the dorsal mesentery of the duodenum fuses with the dorsal body wall, making it and the pancreas secondarily retroperitoneal. The dorsal mesentery of the jejunum and ileum becomes the mesentery proper. The dorsal mesentery of the ascending and descending colon mostly fuses with the dorsal body wall. The dorsal mesentery of the sigmoid colon becomes the sigmoid mesocolon.

PELVIS AND PERINEUM

GROSS BOUNDARIES OF THE PELVIS AND PERINEUM

Pelvis. The osteology of the bones that form the pelvis and the basic types of pelvic architecture are discussed in the section on the lower extremity. The discussion here includes a definition of the pelvic cavity and the various planes of the pelvis.

The *pelvic cavity proper* (minor or true pelvis) is below the pelvic inlet and above the pelvic diaphragm or pelvic floor. The inlet is defined by the sacral promontory, arcuate line of the ilium, pecten pubis, and the upper aspect of the symphysis pubis. The area above this plane is the major or false pelvis and is part of the abdominal cavity. The *floor of the pelvis* is a muscular sling composed of the levator ani and coccygeus muscles. This trough-shaped sling is inclined from lateral to medial and from posterior to anterior. Its lateral attachment extends along a tendinous arch from the symphysis pubis to the ischial spine. The levator ani attaches to this arch and, after descending toward the midline, attaches to the levator ani of the opposite side along a median raphe. The coccygeus fills the gap between the ischial spine and the sacrum and coccyx. The lateral wall of the pelvic cavity consists of the obturator internus and piriformis muscles along with the corresponding portions of the hip bone.

The *plane of the pelvic inlet* is the plane that has the greatest dimensions. The distance between the sacral promontory and the uppermost aspect of the symphysis pubis is the anteroposterior diameter of the inlet or the *conjugate* vera (true conjugate). Not strictly part of the pelvic inlet but important obstetrically is the *obstetric conjugate,* the distance between the promontory and the most posterior aspect of the symphysis pubis. The *diagonal conjugate* can be measured by vaginal exam and is the distance between the promontory and the inferior aspect of the symphysis pubis. The transverse diameter of the inlet is the greatest distance between the arcuate lines.

The *plane of the pelvic outlet* is defined by the inferior aspect of the symphysis pubis, the ischiopubic rami, the ischial tuberosities, the sacrotuberous ligaments, and the tip of the sacrum. The AP diameter extends from the inferior aspect of the symphysis pubis to the tip of the sacrum. The transverse diameter of the outlet is the distance between the inner edges of the ischial tuberosities.

The *plane of the midpelvis* is the plane of least dimensions. The AP diameter of this plane extends from the inferior aspect of the symphysis to the sacrum, at the level of the ischial spines. The transverse diameter of the midpelvis is the distance between the ischial spines, which is the smallest diameter of the pelvis.

Perineum. The perineum (Fig. 2-43) is best defined as the region of the pelvic outlet below the

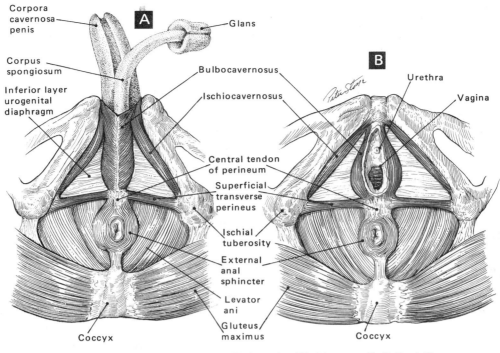

Corpora cavernosa penis
Glans
Corpus spongiosum
Inferior layer urogenital diaphragm
Bulbocavernosus
Ischiocavernosus
Urethra
Vagina
Central tendon of perineum
Superficial transverse perineus
Ischial tuberosity
External anal sphincter
Levator ani
Gluteus maximus
Coccyx
Coccyx

Fig. 2-43. Perineum: *(A)* male; *(B)* female. (Christensen JB, Telford IR: Synopsis of Gross Anatomy, 5th ed., p 203. Philadelphia, JB Lippincott, 1988)

pelvic floor. It is a diamond-shaped area that is defined by the inferior aspect of the symphysis pubic anteriorly, the ischiopubic rami anterolaterally, the ischial tuberosities laterally, the sacrotuberous ligaments posterolaterally, and the coccyx posteriorly. An imaginary line between the two ischial tuberosities separates the perineum into two triangular areas: the anterior urogenital triangle and the posterior anal triangle. The roof of the perineum is the floor of the pelvis, that is, the pelvic sling that is formed by the levator ani and coccygeus muscles.

In the ***urogenital triangle*** (Fig. 2-44) the urogenital diaphragm is a horizontal musculofascial shelf that stretches between the ischiopubic rami. It is formed by superior and inferior layers of fascia that enclose the sphincter urethrae and deep transverse perineal muscles. In the male it contains the bulbourethral glands (Cowper's glands). This diaphragm is penetrated by the membranous urethra in both sexes and the vagina in the female. The area between the superior and inferior fasciae of the urogenital diaphragm encloses the ***deep perineal space*** or pouch.

The ***superficial perineal space*** is inferior or superficial to the inferior fascia of the urogenital diaphragm. It is limited externally or superficially by

the membranous (fibrous) layer of subcutaneous tissue (Scarpa's fascia) of the abdomen, which continues into the perineum (as Colles' fascia) and attaches to the posterior edge of the urogenital diaphragm. This limiting layer also attaches to the isochiopubic ramus and the fascia later of the thigh so that urine from a ruptured urethra or blood from hemorrhage may extravasate up into the abdominal wall (but not into the thigh) from the superficial perineal space. In the male this space contains the crura of the corpora cavernosa and related ischiocavernosus muscles, the corpus spongiosum and bulb of the penis with the related bulbospongiosus muscle, and the superficial transverse perineal muscle. In the female this space contains the crura of the clitoris and related ischiocavernosus muscles, the bulbus vestibuli and related bulbospongiosus muscle, the superficial transverse perineal muscle, and the greater vestibular glands (Bartholin's glands). The urethral opening is approximately 2.5 cm posterior to the clitoris.

The ***ischiorectal fossa*** is the fat-filled, wedge-shaped area that is inferolateral to the pelvic sling and medial to the lower portions of the obturator internus muscle and the os coxae. In the region of the anal triangle, the floor of the fossa is the subcutaneous tissue and skin. The posterior recess of this

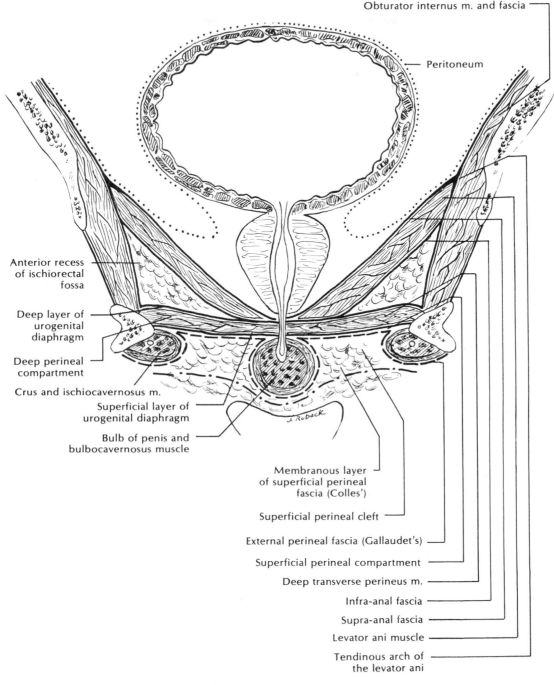

Obturator internus m. and fascia

Peritoneum

Anterior recess
of ischiorectal
fossa

Deep layer of
urogenital
diaphragm

Deep perineal
compartment

Crus and ischiocavernosus m.

Superficial layer of
urogenital diaphragm

Bulb of penis and
bulbocavernosus muscle

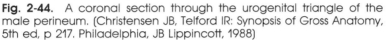

Membranous layer
of superficial perineal
fascia (Colles')

Superficial perineal cleft

External perineal fascia (Gallaudet's)

Superficial perineal compartment

Deep transverse perineus m.

Infra-anal fascia

Supra-anal fascia

Levator ani muscle

Tendinous arch of
the levator ani

Fig. 2-44. A coronal section through the urogenital triangle of the
male perineum. (Christensen JB, Telford IR: Synopsis of Gross Anatomy,
5th ed, p 217. Philadelphia, JB Lippincott, 1988)

fossa extends posterolaterally under the inferior
margin of the gluteus maximus muscle. The anterior
recess extends into the urogenital triangle above the
urogenital diaphragm. The pudendal (Alcock's) canal is a slit in the obturator internus fascia along the

lateral wall of this fossa in the anal triangle. The
internal pudendal vessels and the pudendal nerve
traverse this canal as they pass anteriorly into the
urogenital triangle. The inferior rectal arteries and
nerves branch from the parent structures in the pu-

dendal canal and pass through the ischiorectal fossa toward the rectum and anal canal.

The nerve supply to the perineum is provided primarily by the pudendal nerve (S2–4). Its branches are the inferior rectal, perineal, and posterior scrotal (labial) nerves. These branches supply all of the muscles and most of the skin of the perineum. The skin of the anterior part of the perineum is supplied by the anterior scrotal (labial) branches of the ilioinguinal nerve. Autonomics to the perineum are apparently distributed through the pudendal nerve.

VISCERA OF THE PELVIS AND PERINEUM

Gastrointestinal Tract. The *sigmoid colon* begins at the pelvic rim, descends to the left pelvic wall, traveses the pelvis from left to right, and bends upon itself to join the rectum in the midline. It is supported by the sigmoid mesocolon. The sigmoid and its mesocolon are extremely variable in length, exceeding by far the variability in other parts of the gastrointestinal system.

The *rectum* is that portion of the bowel below the midsacral region where the sigmoid mesocolon ceases. The lowest part of the infraperitoneal portion presents a dilated ampulla. Anteriorly the upper two thirds of the rectum is in contact with the coils of the ileum. In the male the lower third is related anteriorly to the trigone of the bladder, the seminal vesicles, the ductus deferens, and the prostate. In the female the lower third is in contact anteriorly with the vagina and the cervix. Posteriorly it is related to the sacrum in both sexes.

The upper third of the rectum is covered anteriorly and laterally by peritoneum; the middle third, only anteriorly; and the lower third passes below the peritoneum.

The *anal canal,* which is sometimes called the second portion of the rectum, is 2.5 cm to 3.5 cm in length. It turns dorsally, making a right angle as it passes through the pelvic floor to the anus, and is surrounded by internal and external sphincters.

The following structures can be palpated during a rectal examination in the normal male: the anorectal ring, anteriorly the prostate, posteriorly the coccyx and sacrum, and laterally the ischiorectal fossa and the ischial spines. The normal female presents the same structures with the exception of anteriorly, where the perineal body and the cervix of the uterus are palpable.

Urinary System. The pelvic portion of the *ureter* passes in front of the sacroiliac joint and medial to the internal iliac artery. In the male it passes posterior and inferior to the ductus deferens. In the female it passes inferior to the uterine artery and lateral to the cervix of the uterus. The vesical portion runs obliquely downward and medially through the bladder about 20 mm to 25 mm from its counterpart.

The empty *bladder* is posterior to the pubic symphysis and totally within the pelvic cavity below the pelvic inlet. The fully distended bladder of the adult projects well into the abdominal cavity. The bladder is extraperitoneal with its superior and posterosuperior surfaces covered with peritoneum. Laterally it is related to the levator ani and the obturator internus muscles. In the male the bladder is related superiorly to coils of small intestine and the sigmoid colon; posteriorly to the rectovesical pouch, the rectum, the seminal vesicles, and termination of the vas deferens; and inferiorly to the prostate gland. In the female it is related superiorly to coils of small intestine and the body of the uterus, posteriorly to the vagina and supravaginal portion of the cervix, and inferiorly to the pelvic fascia and the urogenital diaphragm.

The *male urethra* extends from the bladder to the glans penis, traversing (1) the prostate gland, (2) the urogenital diaphragm, and (3) the length of the corpus spongiosum. The prostatic portion contains the numerous small openings of the prostatic ducts and the crista urethralis, with the colliculus seminalis containing the openings of the ejaculatory ducts. As the urethra passes through the urogenital diaphragm, it is somewhat narrowed and is surrounded by the sphincter. In the cavernous portion the urethra is dilated at the openings of the Cowper's glands and also terminally at the fossa navicularis.

The *female urethra* is short and it passes through the urogenital diaphragm, where it is surrounded by the sphincter urethrae, and ends shortly thereafter.

Male Reproductive System. The testis and the epididymis lie in the scrotum and are separated from those of the opposite side by the scrotal septum. The epididymis lies along the posterior border of the testis. It is enlarged above to form a head and tapers to a body and small tail below. It is formed predominantly by the greatly contorted duct of the epididymis, which empties into the beginning of the ductus deferens.

The ductus deferens ascends toward the inguinal canal, which it traverses. At the internal abdominal ring it leaves the spermatic cord, passes downward and backward over the lateral surface of the bladder and medially to the ureter, penetrates the prostate gland, and opens into the prostatic portion of the urethra through the ejaculatory duct. Just before it enters the prostate, it is joined by the club-shaped seminal vesicles.

The prostate gland surrounds the urethra between the inferior surface of the bladder and the superior surface of the urogenital diaphragm. It is related anteriorly to the symphysis pubis, laterally to the levator ani muscles, inferiorly to the urogenital diaphragm, and posteriorly to the rectum.

Female Reproductive System. The *ovaries* lie against the lateral pelvic walls just below the pelvic inlet and posteroinferior to the lateral aspect of the uterine tubes. Each ovary is enclosed in a mesovarium, a posterior reflection of peritoneum from the broad ligament. The ovary is suspended from the lateral pelvic wall by the suspensory ligament of the ovary, through which the ovarian vessels, nerves, and lymphatics pass to the gland. Each ovary is connected to the uterus just below the uterine tube by the ovarian ligament.

The *uterus* consists of the fundus, body, and cervix. The cavity of the uterus is continuous superolaterally with the narrow lumen of the uterine tubes and inferiorly with the cavity of the vagina. The fundus is the superior domed portion that projects above the cavity of the body. The body is the major portion of the uterus, and the cervix is the inferior portion, part of which projects into the vagina. The uterine cavity is largest within the body. It narrows abruptly at the body–cervix junction to form the internal os. The lumen of the cervix (cervical canal) is narrow and ends inferiorly as the narrow external os, which is readily palpated during a rectal examination. The normally positioned uterus rests on the posterosuperior aspect of the bladder so that the uterovesical pouch is usually empty. The rectouterine pouch (of Douglas) separates the uterus from the rectum posteriorly. Laterally the uterus is related to the broad ligament and the ureter; the latter passing just lateral to the supravaginal portion of the cervix and inferior to the uterine artery.

The *uterine* (fallopian) *tubes* extend laterally from the superolateral aspects of the uterus. Each tube consists of a narrow-lumened isthmus, a dilated and long ampulla, and the terminal infundibulum, which is composed of numerous fingerlike fimbriae. The tubes curve posteriorly near the lateral pelvic walls where their fimbriae partially cover the ovaries. The uterine tubes are the most superior structures in the broad ligament.

The normal uterus is both anteflexed and anteverted. Anteflexion is a forward bend within the uterus itself at the level of the internal os. Anteversion is a forward bend of about 90 degrees at the junction of the uterus and the vagina. The places the uterus in approximately the horizontal plane with its anterior surface resting on the posterosuperior surface of the bladder. Malposition usually involves one of the following: (1) turning of the entire organ, retroversion (backward turning) or anteversion (forward turning); (2) bending of the body on the cervix, retroflexion (backward bending) or anteflexion (anterior bending); or (3) shifting in the position of the entire organ, retrocession, anteposition, prolapse or procidentia, the latter is the extreme degree of prolapse in which the cervix extrudes from the introitus. This results from extreme relaxation of the pelvic floor, the urogenital diaphragm, and the uterine ligaments.

The *vagina* extends from above the inferior extent of the cervix of the uterus to its external opening in the vestibule. From above downward it is inclined anteriorly as it passes through the pelvic floor and the urogenital diaphragm. The upper portion of the vagina, which surrounds the inferior part of the cervix, is divided into anterior, lateral, and posterior fornices. The vagina is related anteriorly to the base of the bladder and the urethra; posteriorly through the very thin wall of the posterior fornix, to the rectouterine pouch, rectum and anal canal; and laterally to the levator ani muscle and the ureter, which passes near the lateral fornix.

In a *vaginal examination* the urethra, bladder, and symphysis pubis are palpable anteriorly; the rectum and rectouterine pouch posteriorly; the ovary, uterine tube, and lateral pelvic wall laterally; and the cervix in the apex of the vagina.

The vestibule is surrounded by the labia minora and receives the vagina, urethra, and major and minor vestibular glands.

The *broad ligament* is a reflection of peritoneum that passes over the uterus and related structures from front to back and extends laterally to the lateral pelvic walls. As such it forms a curtain across the pelvis from side to side; the broad ligament has an anterior and a posterior layer. Lateral to the uterus the most superior structure in the broad ligament is the uterine tube; below and behind that is the ovarian ligament; and below and anterior is the round ligament. The mesovarium is the reflection of the posterior layer that suspends the ovarian ligament and ovary. That part of the broad ligament above the mesovarium that suspends the uterine tube is called the mesosalpinx. That part of the broad ligament below the mesovarium is the mesometrium. At the base of the broad ligament posteriorly, the posterior layer of mesometrium is elevated over the underlying uterosacral ligament as the rectouterine fold. The extraperitoneal connective tissue found between the layers of the broad ligament is the parametrium. The parametrium in the base of the broad ligament is thickened and forms the cardinal ligaments.

BLOOD SUPPLY TO THE PELVIS AND PERINEUM

The blood supply to the pelvic viscera and to the perineum is provided by branches of the internal iliac artery. The umbilical artery gives rise to the artery of the ductus deferens and the superior vesical artery, which supplies the bladder. The inferior vesical artery also supplies the bladder and the prostate and seminal vesicles in the male. The uterine artery (homologue to the artery of the ductus deferens) usually arises separately and passes medially to supply the uterus, uterine tube and upper part of the vagina. The vaginal artery supplies most of the vagina. The middle rectal artery supplies the middle portion of the rectum and anastomoses with the superior and inferior rectal arteries. The internal pudendal artery exits the pelvis through the greater sciatic foramen, passes around the ischial spine, and then enters the perineum through the lesser sciatic foramen. It supplies the somatic and visceral structures of the perineum. Other branches of the internal iliac artery are the superior and inferior gluteal arteries, which supply the gluteal region; the iliolumbar and lateral sacral arteries, which supply the posterior body wall; and the obturator, which passes into the medial thigh.

MICROSCOPIC STRUCTURE OF PELVIC CONTENTS

Male Reproductive System. The *testis* is ovoid and surrounded by a thick connective tissue capsule, the tunica albuginea. This capsule penetrates the testis at the mediastinum and sends radiating septula into it, dividing the testis into lobules. Within the lobules are seminiferous tubules and a loose fibrous stroma. The stroma contains interstitial cells of Leydig, which are characterized by rod-shaped crystalloids (of Reinke), much SER, and mitochondria with tubular cristae. Under the influence of luteinizing hormone (LH), also known as interstitial cell–stimulating hormone (ICSH), these cells produce testosterone; the SER and tubular cristae are characteristic of steroid-secreting cells. The seminiferous tubules consist of contorted loops that join by straight tubules with the rete testis. The convoluted portions in the viable male are lined by a germinal (seminiferous) epithelium resting on a basal lamina that is bounded by peritubular myoid cells that probably produce a peristaltic action. The seminiferous epithelium contains supportive *Sertoli cells* and *sex cells* in various stages of spermato-

genesis. The Sertoli cells are connected to each other by occluding and gap junctions. These cells support, protect, and nurture the sex cells; they also phagocytize excess cytoplasm in spermatozoan production, and, under the influence of follicle-stimulating hormone (FSH), they secrete androgen-binding protein (ABP), which serves to concentrate testosterone needed for spermatogenesis. They also secrete transferrin, inhibin, and produce lactate needed by the germ cells. The developing sex cells are located between the Sertoli cells. Spermatogonia are located next to the basal lamina in a basal (extratubular) compartment formed by the tight junctions of the Sertoli cells. The primary spermatocytes and secondary spermatocytes lie nearer the lumen in the adluminal (intratubular) compartment between Sertoli cells. Spermatids are embedded in the apices of the Sertoli cells where they transform into spermatozoa. A cross section of a tubule may show several of six stages of development. This is due to different timing in the proliferation and division of stem cells.

Spermatogonia are the only sex cells present until the time of puberty when two different types are present. These are the A or stem cell and the B or derivative cell. A cells may divide into two A cells or into two B cells. B cells grow and differentiate into primary spermatocytes. Each primary spermatocyte undergoes the reduction division of meiosis and gives rise to two secondary spermatocytes containing the haploid number (23) of chromosomes. Each secondary spermatocyte divides quickly into two spermatids. When each spermatid undergoes transformation into a spermatozoa the nucleus condenses, an acrosome vesicle is formed by the Golgi complex, the acrosome vesicle collapses as a lysosomal head cap over the nucleus, an axial filament (flagellum) grows from the proximal centriole, and mitochondria form a helix around the proximal flagellum of the middle piece. Most of the cytoplasm is cast off, leaving only a thin cytoplasmic investment to the head, neck, middle piece, and tail of the spermatozoon. In the principal piece of the tail the cytoplasm forms a fibrous sheath that does not extend into the end piece of the tail.

Sperm are transported through straight tubules, rete testis, and efferent ductules to be stored in the tail of the epididymus where they mature and become motile. At ejaculation sperm pass from the head of the epididymus into the ductus deferens, ejaculatory ducts, and urethra.

Straight seminiferous tubules and *rete testis* are lined by simple cuboidal to columnar epithelium. These empty into 10 to 15 *efferent ductules* that are lined by alternating cuboidal and tall ciliated columnar epithelium. A basal layer of rounded cells is surrounded by a lamina propria and some circular smooth muscle fibers. The cilia of the efferent ductules move spermatozoa into the *ductus epididymidis* (epididymus). This duct contains pseudostratified columnar epithelium containing long microvilli (stereocilia). This duct supplies nutritive substances to the sperm and absorbs excess fluid accompanying the sperm. The epithelium is invested by a circular smooth muscle layer.

The *vas (ductus) deferens* has a mucosa that is similar to that of the ductus epididymidis. The muscular layer is highly developed into inner longitudinal, middle circular and outer longitudinal layers. This duct is invested in the spermatic cord by the cremasteric muscle and the pampiniform plexus of veins. The ductus deferens dilates into an ampulla before terminating as the short slender ejaculatory duct, which pierces the prostate and opens into the urethra at the urethral crest. The mucosa of these structures is folded and the epithelium is not as tall as in the rest of the ductus deferens. The supporting wall of the ejaculatory duct is made up of fibrous tissue. Muscular contraction of the ductus deferens and the ductus epididymidis propel the spermatozoa to the urethra during the ejaculatory process.

The *seminal vesicle* consists of a mucosa folded into a complex system of elevations, a prominent muscularis and an adventitia. The epithelium is low pseudostratified columnar epithelium, and it secretes a viscid alkaline fluid rich in fructose.

The *prostate* is an aggregation of 30 to 50 tubulosaccular glands. The glandular epithelium is simple cuboidal to columnar, and the cells have apical secretion granules that contribute to the formation of the faintly acid secretion that is rich in citric acid and acid phosphatase. The lumina may contain lamellated prostatic concretions (corpora amylacea). The stroma between the tubules contains smooth muscle fibers.

The *male urethra* has three parts, the prostatic, membranous, and cavernous (penile) portions. The prostatic urethra is lined mostly with transitional epithelium. The membranous and penile portions are lined with pseudostratified and stratified columnar epithelium, except at the meatus where the epithelium is stratified squamous. The prostatic urethra has a crest on its posterior wall. The paired ejaculatory ducts and prostatic utricle open on this crest. The ducts of the prostatic gland open into the prostatic uretha. The membranous urethra is encircled by a sphincter of skeletal muscle fibers from the deep transverse perineal muscle. The cavernous urethra extends throughout the penis. It occupies the corpus spongiosum and receives the ducts of the bulbourethral glands and the branching mucous urethral glands (of Littre).

The *bulbourethral glands* (Cowper's) are variably tubular, alveolar, or saccular mucous glands that are enclosed in the membranous urethral sphincter. Their ducts, containing mucous areas of epithelium, open into the cavernous urethra about 2.5 cm in front of the urogenital diaphragm.

The *penis* consists of three cylinders of erectile tissue: two dorsal corpora cavernosa and one ventral corpus spongiosum. The latter terminates distally as the glans penis, and it contains the cavernous urethra. A dense fibrous tunica albuginea surrounds the cavernous bodies and separates the corpora from one another by an incomplete median (pectiniform) septum. The three corpora are enclosed in a common loose irregularly arranged connective tissue layer that underlies the investing skin. The skin folds over the glans as the prepuce. The skin of the glans adheres firmly to the erectile tissue since the loose connective tissue layer is lacking. The epithelium of the inner surface of the prepuce and that of the glans is stratified squamous and is characteristic of that lining a moist surface. It is continuous at the urethral orifice with the epithelium lining the urethra.

The *erectile tissue* of the corpora cavernosa consists of endothelium lined lacunae that are separated by fibrous trabeculae containing smooth muscle. The lacunae are large centrally but are narrow peripherally where they communicate with a venous plexus underlying the tunica albuginea. In the corpus spongiosum the arrangement is similar except for an elastic tunica albuginea, thinner trabeculae, and uniform lacunae. The corpora cavernosa are supplied by two branches of the penile artery: the dorsal artery and the deep arteries. The branches of the dorsal arteries supply capillaries of the trabeculae that drain through the lacunae to the venous plexus. The deep arteries are the chief vessels for filling the lacunae during erection. These vessels run in the cavernous bodies and give off trabecular branches that empty directly to the lacunae through helicine arteries. The latter vessels have a thick circular muscle layer and an intima with longitudinal thickened cushions. During erection the smooth muscle in the cavernous trabeculae and helicine arteries relaxes, the helicine arteries become patent, and the lacunae are engorged with more blood than can be rapidly drained by the compressed peripheral lacunae. At the end of erection, smooth muscle contraction shuts off the blood supplied by helicine arteries and forces blood into the peripheral venous plexus.

Female Reproductive System. The *ovary* is an exocrine organ secreting secondary oocytes, and it is an endocrine organ producing estrogens and progesterone. It is divided into an outer cortex and inner medulla. The cortex basically consists of a rather cellular connective tissue stroma, ovarian follicles, and a simple cuboidal surface epithelium (germinal epithelium). The medulla consists of loose connective tissue, blood vessels, lymphatics, nerves, some smooth muscle, and a few vestigial tubular structures called rete ovarii.

An *ovarian follicle* consists of a developing ovum and an investment of follicle cells and connective tissue. Follicles originate in the embryo and undergo extensive changes during the childbearing years when they are under the influence of adenohypophyseal hormones. In the embryo, primordial sex cells develop into oogonia, which differentiate into primary oocytes; the latter go through the prophase of the first meiotic division before they enter an arrested dictyotene stage. Each of these cells is surrounded by a single layer of follicle cells from the germinal epithelium. Many of these embryonic primordial follicles die, but about 70,000 survive in the cortex of the ovary until the time of puberty.

At puberty, hypothalamic nerve cells produce gonadotropin-releasing hormone (GnRH). This hormone stimulates FSH release by basophils of the anterior pituitary gland. Under the influence of FSH and other factors, ovarian follicles develop periodically. In this process, some oocytes emerge from the arrested dictyotene stage and start to complete the first meiotic division. Coincident with this, follicle cells enlarge and proliferate to form a stratified cuboidal epithelial layer around the oocyte, thus forming a primary follicle. As the follicle enlarges, spaces between follicle cells coalesce to form an antrum filled with liquor folliculi. The growing follicle is now called a secondary (vesicular) follicle. As this follicle differentiates, the follicular cells around the antrum form a stratified epithelial membrana granulosa that sits on a prominent basal lamina. This in turn is surrounded by an inner richly vascular theca interna and an outer more fibrous theca externa. The cells of the theca interna contain much SER and produce androstenedione under the influence of LH; the androstenedione is converted to estrogen by granulosa cells under the influence of FSH. The oocyte is surrounded by a protein–polysaccharide layer called the zona pellucida. Cytoplasmic processes of the oocyte and of the immediate surrounding follicle cells of the corona radiata are closely aligned in the substance of the zona pellucida. The combined oocyte, zona pellucida, and corona radiata project into the antrum of the follicle as the cumulus oophorus.

The mature vesicular follicle occupies much of the thickness of the cortex, and it causes a bulge (stigma) on the surface of the ovary. Its primary oocyte completes the first meiotic division and becomes a secondary oocyte. The secondary oocyte is relatively metabolically inactive, but it possesses more extensive protein producing mechanisms than are found in the primary oocyte. It starts its second meiotic division and reaches the metaphase stage at about the time it is ovulated from the ovary along with the zona pellucida and corona radiata of granulosa cells. Just prior to ovulation large amounts of estrogen and small amounts of progesterone are produced by the follicle, and more luteinizing hormone is produced by the adenohypophysis.

After ovulation a small amount of blood accumulates in the collapsed follicular remains, and a clot is formed in the antrum region. Under the influence of LH the granulosa and theca interna cells enlarge, accumulate lipid, and become lutein cells of a ***corpus luteum***. The granulosa lutein cells constitute the bulk of the corpus luteum and produce progesterone and estrogen. The theca lutein cells are smaller, less in number, more deeply staining, found at the periphery, and may produce estrogens. Lutein cells possess major characteristics of steroid-secreting cells in that they have relatively more SER and have mitochondria containing "tubular" lamellae rather than cristae. After clot formation the thecal connective tissue penetrates into the developing corpus luteum and replaces the blood clot in the central core.

If the ovulated secondary oocyte is fertilized and implantation takes place the corpus luteum will survive for about 6 months under the influences of human chorionic gonadotropin (HCG) from the placenta before it starts to regress. If the secondary oocyte is not fertilized the corpus luteum will last for about 14 days. When a corpus luteum degenerates the lutein cells become swollen, then pyknotic, and a hyalinized scar of connective tissue replaces the dead lutein cells. This white scar is called the corpus albicans.

Usually only one follicle reaches maturity and is involved in ovulation during each cycle. The other maturing follicles are no longer supported by the waning levels of FSH after ovulation and they degenerate. In small follicles the oocyte degenerates and the stroma invades the follicle, leaving no trace of the follicle. In larger follicles, cells of the theca interna enlarge, and the basement membrane becomes a distinct glassy membrane before coarser stromal fibers penetrate the degenerating follicle, giving it the appearance of a small corpus albicans.

The **uterine tube (oviduct, fallopian tube)** has four regions: infundibulum, ampulla, isthmus, and interstitial (intramural) portion. The wall of each of these parts consists of a mucosa, muscularis, and serosa. The mucosa of the trumpet-shaped infundibulum, and to a lesser extent that of the ampulla, is characterized by many elongate fimbriae. The epithelium of all parts of the uterine tube is simple columnar and is comprised of ciliated cells and peg-shaped secreting cells. The relative numbers of these cell types vary, depending on the estrogenic or progesteronic influences. The muscularis consists of inner circular and outer longitudinal smooth muscle layers. These layers are relatively thicker in passing from the infundibulum to the interstitial portion. The serosa is lined by mesothelium and is a continuation of the peritoneal covering of the broad ligament.

The **uterus** is comprised of a body, fundus, and cervix. The body and fundus are histologically similar, and their walls consist of three layers: perimetrium (serosa), myometrium (muscularis), and endometrium (mucosa). The perimetrium is the serosal continuation of the broad ligament. The myometrium is composed of an inner layer of longitudinal smooth muscle, a thick middle layer of circular smooth muscle and large blood vessels, and an outer layer of longitudinal and circular smooth muscle. These smooth muscle cells undergo hyperplasia and hypertrophy during pregnancy. The basic constituents of the endometrium are simple columnar epithelium that is partly ciliated; a lamina propria stroma containing mesenchymelike cells, reticular fibers, and varying amounts of leukocytes; simple tubular glands; and two sets of arteries. One set of arteries (basal arteries) supplies the glands and stroma of the deepest part of the lamina propria. The other set (coiled, spiral arteries) supplies the rest of the endometrium.

The endometrium is under the influence of ovarian progesterone and estrogen. It reflects this influence in the marked structural changes characteristic of the **menstrual cycle.** Four uterine stages of the cycle are recognized: menstrual, proliferative (follicular, estrogenic), secretory (luteal, progesteronic), and premenstrual (ischemic). The menstrual stage takes place from days 1 to 5 of the cycle. The proliferative occurs from days 5 to 14, the secretory from days 14 to 27, and the premenstrual from days 27 to 28. These are approximate times.

During the proliferative stage the endometrium grows from a height of 0.5 mm to 2 mm to 3 mm. In this process, epithelial cells of the gland remnants form a new epithelial lining and straight glands. The stroma develops from the deep (basal) layer. Spiral arteries grow into this new functional layer. In the secretory stage, under the influence of estrogen and progesterone, the endometrium grows another 2 mm in height. An increase in interstitial fluid in part of the functional layer divides it into an inner edematous spongy layer and an outer compact layer. The uterine glands grow, become corkscrew shaped, and produce a glycogen-rich mucoid secretion. Coiled arteries elongate and empty into venous sinusoids by way of capillaries. The premenstrual stage is the result of a decrease of progesterone and estrogen production by the corpus luteum. In this stage the coiled arteries kink, there is a drop in the blood supply to the functional layer, the edema decreases, and the glands begin to fragment. During the menstrual stage the functional layer becomes anemic and ischemic. Arteries and veins break down, and blood oozes into the uterine cavity through the degenerating glands and surface epithelium. The entire functional layer is sloughed off during this stage. The basal arteries are not affected, so the basal layer is retained.

The **placenta** consists of a maternal component (decidua basalis) and a fetal component (chorion frondosum). Since the embryo implants into the compacta layer of the endometrium, the **decidua basalis** is that portion of the functional layer that lies deep to the embryo. Glands and blood vessels of this layer empty into intervillous spaces. The stromal cells swell markedly, accumulate glycogen, and are called decidual cells. The **chorion frondosum** consists of a chorionic plate off of which anchoring villi arise and attach to the endometrium. Free villi extend from the anchoring villi into the intervillous spaces. In the first third of pregnancy the villi have cores of fetal connective tissue containing fetal capillaries with nucleated RBCs. This core of tissue is covered by an inner cytotrophoblastic and an outer syncytial trophoblastic epithelial layer. Later in pregnancy, the fetal vessels contain nonnucleated RBCs, the cytotrophoblast disappears, and the syncytial trophoblast is thin except for clumps of syncytial knots where the nuclei are located. An acidophilic fibrinoid material accumulates over the syncytial trophoblast in late pregnancy. The "placental barrier" in the late placenta consists of the syncytial trophoblast, the endothelium of the fetal vessels, and the intervening basal laminae of these epithelia, which are fused into one basal lamina in the thinnest portions of the barrier. In the first trimester, the cytotrophoblast and fetal connective tissue are added layers in this barrier. The cells of the cytotrophoblast produce the syncytial trophoblast and probably a GnRH. The syncytial trophoblast cells produce estrogen, progesterone, HCG, human placental lactogen (HPL) or human chorionic somatomammatropin (HCS), and human chorionic thyrotropin (HCT).

The *cervix* consists of a mucosa, muscularis, and adventitia. It does not undergo the extensive cyclic changes of the endometrium, although some changes in structure are seen in pregnancy. The portio vaginalis of the cervix projects into the vagina. The mucosa of the cervix is thrown into folds (plicae palmatae). It consists of simple columnar epithelium with some cilia, extensive forked mucus-secreting glands, and a firm stroma that is rich in collagenous and elastic fibers. The epithelium changes to stratified squamous at the portio vaginalis. During pregnancy the cervical glands become larger and secrete a mucous plug that seals the cervical canal. At the time of parturition the lamina propria becomes more edematous, looser, and cellular. The muscularis layers are similar to those in the uterine body and fundus except that there is no inner longitudinal muscular layer. The adventitia contains collagenous fibers that are continuous with surrounding structures.

The *vagina* also is comprised of a mucosa, muscularis and adventitia. The lining epithelium of the mucosa is stratified squamous nonkeratinized, but keratohyaline granules may be found in some of the cells. Under the influence of estrogen the epithelium accumulates glycogen, and many pyknotic surface cells appear. When estrogen levels are low a basal layer of cells is prominent. The lamina propria contains many elastic fibers and some large blood vessels. No glands are present. The muscularis consists of a thin inner circular layer and thicker outer longitudinal layer of smooth muscle. A sphincter of skeletal muscle is found at the lower end of the vagina.

The *hymen* has the same structure as the vaginal mucosa. It is a thin fold at the opening of the vagina into the vestibule.

The *clitoris* corresponds to the dorsal penis in the male. It has two small cavernous bodies of erectile tissue that end in a rudimentary glans clitoridis. It is covered by stratified squamous epithelium. Specialized nerve endings, such as Meissner's and pacinian corpuscles, are located in the subepithelial stroma.

The *labia minora* flank the vestibule. They have a vascularized connective tissue core that is covered by stratified squamous epithelium possessing a thin keratinized layer. Sebaceous glands, not associated with hairs, are located in the stroma.

The *labia majora* are folds of skin that cover the labia minora. The inner surface is like that of the labia minora. The outer surface is covered by skin containing hairs, sweat glands, and sebaceous glands. The interior of these folds contains much adipose tissue.

The *vestibule* is lined by partially keratinized stratified squamous epithelium. Minor vestibular glands, placed chiefly near the clitoris and opening of the urethra, secret mucus. The longer major vestibular glands are analogous to the bulbourethral glands of the male. They are located in the lateral wall of the vestibule. Their ducts open close to the attachment of the hymen.

DEVELOPMENT OF THE UROGENITAL SYSTEM

The urinary and reproductive systems take origin from the urogenital sinus and the intermediate mesoderm.

Development of the Kidney and Ureter.   Three pairs of embryonic kidneys develop in man. These are the pronephros, mesenephros, and metanephros. The pronephros and mesonephros will degenerate, but their development is essential for the establishment of the metanephros, which becomes the definitive kidney.

The *pronephros* arises at the C3–T1 vertebral levels by the dorsal proliferation of cords of cells from the intermediate mesoderm. These cords become pronephric tubules. They grow caudally and link up with the other pronephric tubules, forming a common pronephric duct that extends caudally toward the cloaca. The pronephric kidney does not function, but the pronephric duct seems to be important for the normal formation of the mesonephric kidney.

The *mesonephros* develops by the formation of mesonephric tubules from the intermediate mesoderm of the C6–L3 vertebral levels. Unlike the pronephric tubules, these tubules do not communicate with the coelom but receive a capillary glomerulus from the aorta, which is encapsulated by the proximal blind end of the tubule. The distal end of the mesonephric tubules tap into the pronephric duct and contribute to its caudal growth. This enlarged pronephric duct taps into the cloaca, and its name is changed to the mesonephric (wolffian) duct. The extensive growth of the mesonephros produces a large urogenital ridge projecting from the dorsal body wall.

The *metanephros* arises from two sources: the ureteric bud (metanephric diverticulum) and the metanephrogenic intermediate mesoderm of the L4–S1 vertebral levels. The ureteric bud arises as a tubular outgrowth from the mesonephric duct near its entrance into the cloaca. It grows toward the intermediate mesoderm where its blind end becomes capped by metanephrogenic tissue. The ureteric bud elongates as the ureter, and its blind end enlarges as the renal pelvis and undergoes a series of branchings. These branchings give rise to the major and minor calyces and the collecting tubules. The metanephrogenic condensations capping the blind ends of the collecting tubules develop into nephrons. One end of the blind nephron forms a Bowman's capsule around a glomerulus of capillaries. The other end taps into the collecting tubule.

Development of the Urinary Bladder and Urethra. The urinary bladder and urethra develop from the entoderm of the urogenital sinus and allantois. In early development the allantois is a diverticulum of the cloaca. A urorectal septum of mesoderm arises between the allantois and hindgut, grows caudally, and divides the cloaca into a dorsal rectum and ventral urogenital sinus. With this division, the mesonephric duct empties into the urogenital sinus. As the urogenital sinus and a small adjacent portion of the allantois enlarge to form the urinary bladder, portions of the mesonephric and metanephric (ureter) ducts are incorporated into the wall of the urogenital sinus. This results in the ureters entering the bladder and the mesonephric ducts entering more caudally into the less dilated portion of the urogenital sinus. This distal portion of the urogenital sinus will become the urethra of the male and the urethra, vestibule, and part of the vagina of the female.

Development of the Reproductive System. Even though the sex of the embryo is determined at fertilization, the gonads, ducts, and external genitalia pass through an indifferent stage of development in which male and female components have the same appearance. This stage lasts until about the sixth week of development.

In the *indifferent stage,* gonads form on the medial wall of the urogenital ridges. Starting in the third week, primordial sex cells migrate from the yolk sac to the urogenital ridge. By the sixth week the coelomic epithelium has proliferated, invaginated, and surrounded the primordial sex cells to form primitive gonadal (sex) cords in the underlying mesoderm of the gonad.

In the indifferent stage of genital duct formation, both mesonephric and müllerian (paramesonephric) ducts are present. The müllerian ducts arise as longitudinal invaginations of the coelomic epithelium on the lateral wall of the urogenital ridge. Cranially this duct remains open to the coelom. Caudally it opens through the dorsal wall of the urogenital sinus. In its craniocaudal course it lies at first lateral to the mesonephric duct, then passes anterior to it, and finally fuses with the opposite müllerian duct medial to the mesonephric ducts. During this fusion the urogenital ridges of the two sides are brought together to form a genital cord (septum) between the developing bladder anteriorly and the rectum posteriorly.

In the indifferent stage of the development of the external genitalia, mesoderm invades the lateral walls of the external opening of the urogenital sinus producing elevations called urogenital (urethral) folds (Fig. 2-45C). These folds unite anterior to the urogenital opening at the genital tubercle. Labioscrotal swellings develop lateral to the urogenital folds.

In the development of the *male reproductive system* the gonadal cords become testis cords that differentiate into seminiferous tubules and rete testis. The primordial sex cells become spermatogonia, whereas ingrowing coelomic epithelial cells give rise to supportive (Sertoli) cells. Leydig cells develop from mesenchyme. Efferent ductules develop from adjacent mesonephric tubules (Fig. 2-45A). The developing testis produces müllerian-inhibiting hormone (MIH) and androgens, which lead to the degeneration of the müllerian duct and to the differentiation of the mesonephric duct into the ductus epididymidis, vas (ductus) deferens, and ejaculatory duct. The seminal vesicle arises as an outgrowth of the mesonephric duct. The urogenital sinus gives rise to the urethra and the prostate, bulbourethral, and urethral glands. The genital tubercle enlarges and carries with it inferiorly a urethral plate of entoderm. This plate is transformed into the penile (cavernous) urethra after the lateral urogenital folds fuse ventrally (Fig. 2-45D). The urethral plate, urogenital folds and genital tubercle (phallus) give rise to the definitive penis. The scrotum is formed by the ventral fusion of the labioscrotal swellings. The testes descend late in gestation from their retroperitoneal abdominal location. They are "anchored" in the scrotum by the gubernaculum testis, which is derived from mesoderm of the urogenital ridge caudal to the testis. The path of descent is indicated by the inguinal canal. This follows the embryonic pathway of the processus vaginalis evaginating from the peritoneum.

In the development of the *female reproductive*

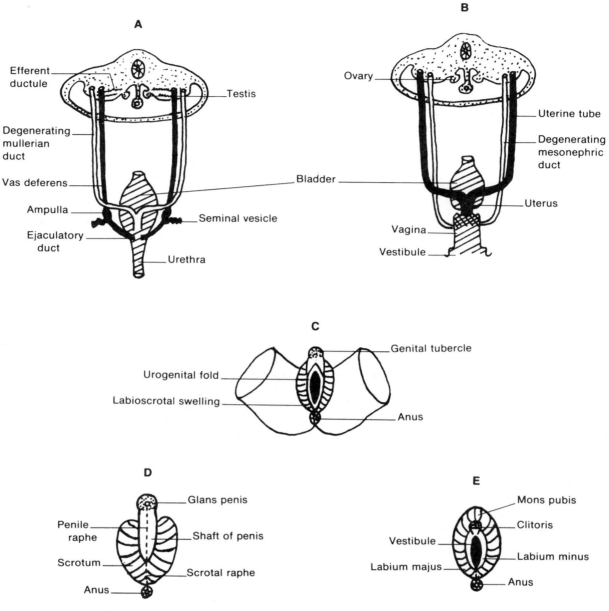

Fig. 2-45.   Development of the urogenital system. *(A)* The male reproductive ducts are shown in black developing from the mesonephric tubules (efferent ductules) and mesonephric duct; the urethra develops from the urogenital sinus (hatched). *(B)* The female reproductive ducts develop from the müllerian ducts (black) and urogenital sinus (hatched). The upper one third of the vagina (cross hatched) may develop from the müllerian ducts. *(C)* The indifferent stage of external genitalia development. *(D)* and *(E)* Male and female external genitalia, respectively, developing from the genital tubercle (stippled), urogenital folds (white), and labioscrotal swellings (hatched). The vestibule (black) is lined by entoderm of the urogenital sinus.

system the initial gonadal cords degenerate and a second series of ovarian cords develop from primordial sex cells and coelomic epithelium. This second set of cords splits into groups of follicles near the surface of the developing ovary. Each primitive ovarian follicle consists of a developing sex cell surrounded by a flattened layer of follicular cells. The sex cells complete the prophase of the first meiotic division and are in the arrested dictyotene stage by the time of birth. From the sixth month until parturition there is a tremendous rate of degeneration of primitive follicles, the number decreasing from about 6 million to about 400,000 or less.

The unfused portions of the müllerian ducts develop into the uterine tubes (Fig. 2-45B). The fused portion give rise to the uterus and part of the vagina. The genital cord remains as the broad ligament of the uterus. The proper ligament of the ovary and the round ligament of the uterus probably arise from the mesoderm of the urogenital ridge caudal to the ovary. The mesonephric duct and tubules degenerate, but some remain as the paroophoron (tubules), epoophoron (tubules and duct), and Gartner's duct (duct). Where the fused müllerian ducts empty into the urogenital sinus, some entodermal tissue forms a vaginal plate that eventually hollows out as the lower two thirds of the vagina; the upper one third is thought to arise from the müllerian ducts. The urogenital sinus caudal to the vaginal opening becomes enlarged as the vestibule.

In the female the genital tubercle remains relatively small as the clitoris (Fig. 2-45E). The urethral folds become the labia minora, and the labioscrotal swellings develop into the labia majora. The hymen probably forms from the entoderm of the vaginal plate.

Congenital Malformations of the Urogenital System. *Horseshoe kidney* is usually due to fusion of the caudal ends of the two kidneys across the midline. This probably occurs as they are approximated in their cranial migration out of the pelvis over the umbilical arteries. *Bifid ureter* is usually the result of a premature division of the ureteric bud. When this occurs it may result in double pelvis or double kidney. *Exstrophy of the bladder* is caused by failure of mesoderm to invade the area anterior to the developing bladder. This results in improper development of the anterior abdominal wall and bladder with exposure of the posterior mucosal wall to the outside. *Congenital hydrocoele* is a collection of fluid in a remnant of the processes vaginalis. In *hypospadias* the external meatus of the urethra is on the ventral surface of the penis or scrotum. This may be caused by improper closure of the urogenital folds or labioscrotal swellings and by failure of the outer ectodermal cells to grow into the glans and join the penile urethra.

Improper fusion of the müllerian ducts leads to many different abnormalities of the uterus. These range from uterus didelphys with its two bodies (bicornis) and two cervices bicollis to uterus arcuatus in which there is a minor degree of imperfect fusion in the fundus. *Double vagina* is due to incomplete canalization of the paired sinovaginal bulbs that give rise to the vaginal plate.

Pseudohermaphroditism is a condition in which the individual has either testes (male pseudohermaphrodite) or ovaries (female pseudohermaphrodite) but possesses external genitalia of the opposite sex. In *testicular feminization* the male duct system and external genitalia are not induced to develop. An immature female duct system and female external genitalia remain. In *adrenogenital syndrome* a genetic abnormality results in absence of an enzyme necessary for the production of hydrocortisone. This leads to an excess of ACTH, which causes overproduction of adrenal androgens. In females the excessive androgen causes hypertrophy of the clitoris and fusion of the labia majora, thus producing female hermaphroditism. In males the overproduction may cause precocious secondary sexual characteristics.

EARLY EMBRYOLOGY AND DEVELOPMENT OF THE PLACENTA

Fertilization. At ovulation a secondary oocyte, zona pellucida, and corona radiata of follicle cells are discharged from the ovary and drawn into the infundibulum of the uterine tube where a spermatozoan can penetrate the zona pellicuda and secondary oocyte (Fig. 2-46). In this process, acrosome enzymes aid in penetration of the corona radiata and zone pellucida, while a cytoplasmic response of the secondary oocyte gives a zonal reaction that prohibits penetration by other spermatozoa. The union of the spermatozoan and secondary oocyte in the process of fertilization brings about the following major physical consequences: (1) reactivation of the secondary oocyte, (2) completion of the second meiotic division with formation of the second polar body, (3) establishment of a zygote (fertilized ovum) with the diploid number (46) of chromosomes, and (4) establishment of the mitotic spindle for the first cleavage division.

Cleavage and Blastodermic Vesicle Formation. During cleavage a series of mitoses occur in the zygote that result in successive 2, 4, 8, and 16

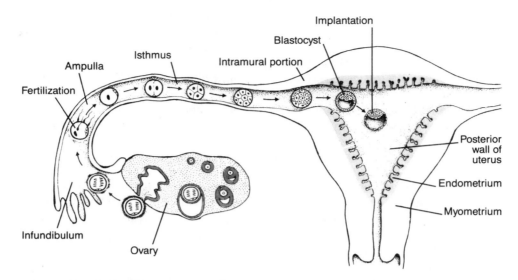

Fig. 2-46. Diagram illustrating ovulation, fertilization, cleavage, and blastocyst formation. (Cormack DH: Ham's Histology, 9th ed, p 633. Philadelphia, JB Lippincott, 1987. After Moore KL: The Developing Human. Clinically Oriented Embryology, 3rd ed. Philadelphia, WB Saunders, 1982; modified with permission)

cell stages. These divisions take place over a period of about 3 days as the developing conceptus passes down the uterine tube. At about the time the 16-cell morula reaches the uterine cavity, fluid penetrates between some of the cells and produces a cavity in the solid ball of cells. The conceptus is now called a blastodermic vesicle (blastocyst). It consists of an outer layer of cells called the trophoblast, a cavity of the blastodermic vesicle (blastocoele), and an inner cell mass. After 3 days in the uterine cavity, the zona pellucida degenerates, and the sticky trophoblastic cells adhere to the endometrium.

Establishment of Ectoderm, Entoderm, and Mesoderm. In the eighth day of development the inner cell mass cavitates to form an ectodermally lined amniotic cavity. The ectoderm of the embryonic disk will eventually give rise to the neural tube, neural crest, and epidermis. An inner entodermal layer of cells also differentiates from the inner cell mass. These cells proliferate to form the yolk sac. The dorsal portion of the yolk sac later will become incorporated into the embryo as the primitive gut. Embryonic mesoderm arises from an elongate mass of cells called the primitive streak. The mesodermal cells turn inward along the midline and move laterally, insinuating themselves between the ectoderm and entoderm. In its forward, caudal, and lateral movement, the embryonic mesoderm eventually joins the extraembryonic mesoderm that arises from the trophoblast. The notochord arises as a midline forward growth of cells from the primitive (Hensen's) node. In the third week of development, the embryonic mesoderm will have differentiated

into paraxial (somite, dorsal), intermediate, and lateral mesoderm. The paraxial mesoderm will develop further into paired somites that eventually give rise to vertebrae, ribs, skeletal muscle, and connective tissues. The intermediate mesoderm will differentiate into much of the urogenital system. The lateral mesoderm, like the extraembryonic mesoderm, splits to form a coelom. That lateral mesoderm adjacent to the ectoderm is somatic mesoderm, while that next to entoderm is splanchnic mesoderm. Somatic mesoderm later will give rise to body wall tissues. Splanchnic mesoderm further differentiates into the cardiovascular system, smooth muscle, and connective tissues in the walls of most visceral structures, mesenteries, and the spleen.

Development of the Placenta. After the attachment of the blastodermic vesicle to the uterus at about the sixth postfertilization day, the trophoblast proliferates rapidly, and the conceptus begins to implant into the compacta layer of the endometrium. It is completely embedded in the uterine stroma by the eleventh postfertilization day (see Fig. 2-46). In the rapid proliferation of cytotrophoblastic cells, fusion of the outer cells forms an outer syncytial trophoblast over the single inner layer of cytotrophoblast. The coalescence of lacunae formed in the syncytial trophoblast leads to the formation of primary stem villi. These are most extensive in the trophoblast that faces the deeper layers of the endometrium. It is in this region where most of the nutriments are being supplies to the trophoblast from invaded uterine glands and blood vessels. The primary stem villi consist of a core of cytotrophoblast surrounded by syncytial trophoblast. Later, mesoderm invades these villi, and they become secondary stem villi containing a core of connective tissue. By the end of the third week, blood vessels start to form in the secondary villi, and they are designated as tertiary villi. With the vascularization of the trophoblast it is called the chorion. That part of the chorion that is the deepest in the uterine wall becomes the chorion frondosum portion of the placenta; the rest of it loses its villi and is called the chorion laeve. An anchoring villus and its free floating villi constitute a cotyledon.

Septa of the cytotrophoblastic coating of the intervillous space project from the decidua and incompletely separate the cotyledons from each other. The functional layer of the endometrium deep to the chorion frondosum is the decidua basalis; that adjacent to the chorion laeve is the decidua capsularis; and the rest is the decidua parietalis. As the embryo enlarges the uterine cavity is obliterated, and the decidua capsularis and decidua parietalis fuse into a much compressed layer. After birth of the newborn, the decidual layers, placenta, chorion laeve, and amnion will be discharged as the afterbirth.

TABLE 2-2. Secretory Cells and Their Products*

ORGAN SYSTEM: ORGAN, TISSUE, CELLS	PRODUCT
Skeletal (Connective tissue, cartilage, bone)	
Mast cells	Heparin, histamine
Fibroblasts, chondrocytes, osteocytes	Procollagen, elastin, GAGs
Osteoclasts	Hydrolytic enzymes
Plasma cells	Antibodies
Muscular	
Smooth muscle	Elastin
Nervous	
Neurons	Neurotransmitters (e.g., epinephrine, norepinephrine, acetylcholine, GABA, dopamine, serotonin, substance P, oxytocin, ADH)
Schwann cells, oligodendroglia	Myelin*
Choroid plexus	Cerebrospinal fluid
Endocrine organs	
Pituitary gland and hypothalamus	(See Table 2-1.)
Thyroid	
Follicular cells	Thyroxine, triiodothyronine
Parafollicular cells	Calcitonin
Parathyroid Chief cells	Parathyroid hormone
Suprarenal	
Zona glomerulosa	Mineralocorticoids (e.g., aldosterone)
Zona fasciculata and zona reticularis	Glucocorticoids (e.g., cortisol) and dehydroepiandrosterone
Medulla	Norepinephrine and epinephrine
(See below for reproductive endocrine cells.)	
Digestive	
Oral Cavity	
Von Ebner's and parotid glands	Serous secretion
Submandibular and sublingual	Serous and mucous secretions
Odontoblasts	Dentin
Ameloblasts	Enamel
Esophagus	
Mucosal and submucosal glands	Mucus
Stomach	
Lining epithelium, neck mucous cells, and cardiac glands	Mucus
Chief cells	Pepsin
Parietal cells	HCl, intrinsic antipernicious anemia factor
Enteroendocrine	Gastrin, glucagon
Pyloric glands	Alkaline glycoprotein secretion
Intestines	
Goblet cells	Mucus
Brunner's glands	Alkaline glycoprotein secretion
Paneth cells	Lysozyme

(Continued)

TABLE 2-2. Secretory Cells and Their Products* (*Continued*)

ORGAN SYSTEM: ORGAN, TISSUE, CELLS	PRODUCT
Enteroendocrine cells	Secretin, cholecystokinin, glucagonlike substance, somatostatin, gastric inhibitory polypeptide, motilin, serotonin, substance P, vasoactive intestinal polypeptide
Liver	
Hepatocytes	Bile, lipoprotein, prothrombin, albumin, fibrinogen, glucose
Pancreas	
Acinar cells	Protease, nuclease, amylase, lipase
Centroacinar and intercalated duct cells	Sodium bicarbonate
Islet alpha cells	Glucagon
Beta cells	Insulin
Delta cells	Somatostatin, gastrin(?)
Respiratory	
Bowman's glands	Serous secretion
Goblet cells	Mucus
Great alveolar (type II) cells	Surfactant
Cardiovascular (blood)	
Neutrophils and eosinophils	Hydrolytic enzymes
Basophils	Heparin and histamine
Platelets and megakaryocyte precursor	Serotonin, thromboplastin
Eye	
Tarsal glands	Sebum
Lacrimal glands	Tears
Ciliary body epithelium	Aqueous humor
Ear	
Stria vascularis of cochlea, cells of crista ampullares and maculae	Endolymph
Ceruminous glands	Cerumen (ear wax)
Integumentary	
Stratum germinativum	Tonofilaments, which become keratin*
Stratum granulosum	Interfilament matrix and membrane-coating substance of stratum corneum*
Melanocytes	Melanin
Sebaceous glands	Sebum
Sweat glands	Sweat
Mammary gland	Milk proteins and lipids
Urinary (kidney)	
Juxtaglomerular cells	Renin
Reproductive	
Male	
Seminiferous epithelium	Sperm
Sertoli cells	Androgen-binding protein, transferrin, inhibin, lactate
Interstial cells of Leydig	Testosterone
Seminal vesicle	Alkaline fluid rich in fructose
Prostate gland	Acid secretion rich in citric acid and acid phosphatase
Bulbourethral and urethral glands	Mucus
Female	
Theca interna cells	Androstenedione
Membrana granulosa cells	Estrogen, progesterone
Granulosa lutein cells	Estrogen, progesterone
Theca lutein cells	Estrogen(?)
Uterine glands	Glycogen-rich mucoid secretion
Cervical glands	Mucus
Cytotrophoblast cells	GnRH, Syncytial trophoblast
Syncytial trophoblast	Estrogen, progesterone, HCG, HPL (somatomammotropin, HCS), HCT

* This list is not complete; some cell products are also parts of cells.

GAGs = glycosaminoglycans
GnRH = gonadotropin-releasing hormone
HCG = human chorionic gonadotropin

HCS = human chorionic somatomammotropin
HCT = human chorionic thyrotropin
HPL = human placental lactogen

QUESTIONS IN ANATOMY

Both essay and multiple choice questions are presented in this section. The answers to the multiple choice questions are at the end of this chapter. The answers to the essay questions are in the text.

Essay Questions

Contrast the five principal regions of the vertebral column, giving the characteristics of typical vertebrae and curvatures and the exact movements permitted in each region.

Draw the normal curves of the spine.

Describe a typical thoracic vertebra.

List the various factors that permit movement of the vertebral column. Why do lumbar dislocations usually involve fracture while cervical dislocations do not?

Why does a rupture of the disk between lumbar vertebrae 4 and 5 usually impinge on spinal nerve L5?

How do cartilage and bone differ in their vascularity and in the mode of their nutritional supply?

How do seven cervical vertebrae develop from eight pairs of cervical sclerotomes? What is the embryologic basis of spondylolisthesis? spina bifida?

Describe the major components of the growing epiphyseal disk. How does a long bone grow in length and width?

What are the major functions of the superficial muscles of the back? the deep muscles of the back? What is the innervation to these muscles?

Describe a sarcomere. Are actin and myosin found in both the A and I bands? What is the T tubular system? What are the functions of intercalated disks?

What motor functional components of nerves innervate skeletal muscle of branchial arch origin? skeletal muscle of somite origin? smooth muscle of splanchnic mesoderm origin?

Draw a cross section of the thoracic cord, indicating the principal ascending and descending tracts.

Describe the formation of a typical spinal nerve.

Describe the contents and extent of the cauda equina. What area is the region of choice for a spinal tap? Why?

Give the extent and the relationships of the spinal cord and its meninges. Into which space is an anesthetic injected through the inferior aperture of the sacral canal as in caudal analgesia?

List the functional components of a spinal nerve.

Which of these is a component of the autonomic nervous system? Where are preganglionic and postganglionic autonomic neurons located?

Name the nuclei of termination for incoming GSA fibers of spinal nerves.

Where would chromatolysis take place in hemisection of the spinal cord at the T3 level? What would be the sensory loss from this lesion? What would be the motor loss?

What is the fate of neural crest material? What cells are responsible for the formation of myelin in the CNS? in the PNS?

Describe the events of degeneration and regeneration of a peripheral nerve.

What would be the functional loss if the sulcal arteries supplying the C7 level were thrombosed? What area of the cord is supplied by the posterior spinal arteries?

Name the one bony link between the upper extremity and the axial skeleton.

What is the major support of the acromioclavicular joint?

Where is the surgical neck of the humerus?

Describe the articular capsule of the shoulder joint; its attachment.

What are the major supports of the shoulder joint?

What motions occur at the shoulder joint?

What muscles cause each of the motions at the shoulder joint?

Name the structures found in the suprahumeral space. What is the importance of the suprahumeral space?

At what joints do pronation and supination occur?

Describe the articular surfaces that form the elbow joint? What motions occur at this joint? What muscles cause the motions?

Between what bones is the wrist joint formed? What motions occur at the wrist joint? What muscles cause each of these motions?

What motions are available at the four medial carpometacarpal joints? How do the motions of the CM joint of the thumb differ from those of the other four?

List the motions that can occur at the metacarpophalangeal joints and the major motors of each.

Contraction of the muscles in the anterior compartment of the arm causes what motions? in the posterior compartment?

What nerve innervates the muscles in the anterior compartment of the arm? in the posterior compartment?

The muscles in the anterior compartment of the

forearm are innervated by what nerves? in the posterior compartment?

What motions are caused by contraction of the muscles in the anterior compartment of the forearm? in the posterior compartment?

Describe the compartmentalization of the ventral aspect of the hand. What nerve(s) innervate(s) the muscles of each compartment?

Describe the radial and ulnar bursae.

Describe the locations of the midpalmar and thenar spaces.

Describe the organization of the brachial plexus. Name the collateral branches of each part of the plexus.

Specifically define the locations of the ulnar and median nerves at the wrist.

What physical problems result following an injury to the radial nerve? musculocutaneous nerve? ulnar nerve? median nerve?

Trace the course of the brachial artery through the arm, and the radial and ulnar arteries through the forearm and hand.

Where exactly are radial and ulnar pulses taken?

Which artery terminates as the major contributor to the superficial palmar arterial arch? deep palmar arterial arch?

Describe the location and courses of the cephalic and basilic veins. Where does each empty into the deep veins?

What three bones form the os coxae? Describe the location of the acetabulum, obturator foramen, ischial spine, ischial tuberosity, greater sciatic notch, lesser sciatic notch, iliac crest with its anterior and posterior superior spines, and the pubic tubercle.

Compare the articular surfaces that form the hip joint with those that form the shoulder joint.

Compare the acetabular labrum with the glenoid labrum.

Define the extent of the articular capsule of the hip joint. What parts of the femoral neck are intracapsular and what parts are extracapsular?

Describe in general the blood supply to the femoral neck and head. What is unique about the courses of some of these vessels?

Describe the extracapsular ligaments of the hip joint. What are the functions?

What motions can occur at the hip joint? What are the muscles involved in each motion?

Describe the articular surfaces that form the knee joint.

What motions are available at the knee joint? What muscles cause these motions?

Describe the menisci. What are their functions?

Against what types of forces do the cruciate ligaments protect the knee? the collateral ligaments?

List the bones of the foot. Which of these form the medial longitudinal arch? the lateral longitudinal arch?

What ligament is the most important support of the longitudinal arches of the foot?

Describe the formation of the ankle joint.

What motions are available at the ankle joint? What muscles cause each of the motions?

What ligament is usually injured in an inversion-plantar flexion sprain?

At what joints do inversion and eversion occur primarily? These motions are produced by the contraction of what muscles?

Describe the location of the gluteal muscles; innervation; functions.

Name the muscles of the anterior compartment of the thigh; innervation; functions.

List the medial and posterior femoral muscles; innervation; functions.

Describe the femoral triangle. What structures pass through the triangle and what are their relationships?

Describe the popliteal fossa and the relationships of the structures within the triangle.

List the muscles found in each of the compartments of the leg; innervations; functions.

Describe the compartmentation of the foot. What nerves innervate the muscles in each compartment?

Fibers from which spinal cord segments are found in the lumbosacral plexus? Where is the lumbar portion of the plexus formed? the sacral portion?

Describe the courses of the medial and lateral plantar nerves and compare each with its homologous nerve in the hand.

Describe the limp that would accompany an injury of the superior gluteal, inferior gluteal, femoral, deep peroneal, and tibial nerves.

Describe the course of the femoral artery through the thigh. How does it begin? Where exactly is it located in the femoral triangle?

At what point does the femoral become the popliteal artery? Where is the artery in the popliteal fossa? How can a popliteal pulse be taken?

Describe the courses of the main arterial trunks through the leg.

Compare the arterial supply of the foot with that of the hand.

Describe the exact location of the greater saphenous vein as it crosses the ankle joint.

Which nerves leave the anterior cranial fossa?

Which structures are found in the posterior cranial fossa? What are the important foramina of this region? Name the structures passing through each foramen.

Which structures pass through the foramen magnum?

Name the structures passing from the middle cranial fossa to the orbit through: (1) the optic foramen, (2) the superior orbital fissure, (3) the foramen rotundum, (4) the foramen ovale, and (5) the foramen lacerum.

List the contents of the infratemporal fossa. Where does this fossa communicate with the cranial cavity?

Describe the important relationships of the mastoid air cells.

Describe the location and the extent of the pharynx, the parts into which it is usually divided, the structure of its walls, and the location of its various openings.

Describe the site and boundaries of the opening of the eustachian tube into the pharynx.

Describe the temporomandibular joint. In which direction does this joint usually become dislocated?

What are the structures and the spaces found just external to each part of the bony wall of the orbit? Indicate where each is related to the orbital wall.

Describe the extraocular muscles and give their nerve supply.

Describe the relationships of the palatine tonsil. Which artery is most commonly in close relation to the palatine tonsil? State the course of this artery and its relationships to the tonsil.

Give the relations of the branches of the external carotid artery? the internal carotid artery?

Describe the layers of the scalp. What are its blood and nerve supply?

Describe the meninges of the brain. In what parts of the brain are ventricles and choroid plexuses located?

Trace the pathway of the cerebrospinal fluid from its origin in the choroid plexus of the lateral ventricle to the superior sagittal sinus. What happens if the iter is occluded? At what other sites is the flow likely to be obstructed?

What are the principal fissures and lobes of the cerebrum?

Describe the internal and external topography of the medulla. Which cell columns extend into the medulla from the spinal cord?

Which cranial nerves arise from the medulla?

From what nuclei of origin in the brain stem do preganglionic parasympathetic fibers arise? Where do these fibers synapse and what organs do they supply?

Give, in general, the distribution of the vagus nerve. What are its functional components?

Give the origin, course, and distribution of the hypoglossal nerve.

What cranial nerves convey the afferent and efferent nerves (limbs) of the cough reflex? carotid sinus reflex? gag reflex? corneal blink reflex? pupillary light reflex? What are the nuclei of termination and origin of these reflexes?

What nerves supply general somatic afferent, special visceral afferent, and somatic efferent fibers to the tongue? How is the tongue mucosa modified to carry out the functions of the tongue?

If the uvula points to the right on phonation, which nerve is most likely damaged?

What is the relation of the facial nerve to the middle ear? the jugular vein? Describe the bony and the membranous labyrinths. Describe the middle ear and the mastoid. What is the anatomic basis for paralysis of only the lower contralateral face in corticobulbar lesions compared to paralysis of the whole ipsilateral side in facial nerve lesions?

Why do unilateral lesions of the auditory pathway within the CNS rarely result in deafness?

Describe the possible pathway for postrotational nystagmus starting with stimulation of the hair cells in the crista of the lateral semicircular canal.

Give the location within the central nervous system of the nuclei that directly innervate the voluntary ocular muscles. Where do afferent fibers to these nuclei originate and in which tracts do they travel to reach the nuclei? What are the necessary nerve connections for lateral conjugate gaze?

If the right fifth nerve is damaged, will the left eye blink if the right cornea is stimulated? If the right facial nerve is damaged and the fifth nerve is intact, will any eye blink if the right cornea is stimulated?

Describe the orbit and its contents.

Describe the eyeball.

Describe the normal anatomy of the fundus of the eye as seen with the ophthalmoscope. How are the arteries and the veins differentiated from each other?

What is the vascular supply of the retina? What nutritive pathway is compromised in detachment of the retina?

Describe the autonomic innervation of the eyeball and eyelid. Ptosis can occur following injury to what two nerve pathways? What are the symptoms of Horner's syndrome, and where might a lesion be located that could lead to this?

Describe the circulation of aqueous humor. In what area might blockage of the pathway lead to glaucoma?

Trace the flow of tears from their origin to their arrival in the nasal cavity. Where are the tarsal glands located and what types of glands are these?

What is the nerve pathway involved in the near reflex (accommodation, convergence, and pupillary reflex)?

Describe the optic nerve, its termination, and point of emergence from the skull.

Outline the visual pathway. Trace light rays from a point in the upper right quadrant of the visual field to the retina; then trace the impulses from the rods and cones stimulated to the specific site in the occipital cortex where the impulses would be received.

Contrast the effects of the destruction of the right optic nerve and of the left optic tract on the retina and the field of vision.

Describe the olfactory nerve, including its origin, termination, and exit from the skull.

Locate the lamina cribrosa.

Give the course and function of the pyramidal (corticospinal) tract. What is its relation to the cerebral motor cortex?

Describe the course of the medial lemniscus. Where do these fibers originate and terminate? What is the functional significance of this pathway?

Where are the primary receptive cortical areas for two-point touch, vision, hearing, and olfaction? Which relay nuclei of the diencephalon send fibers to these areas?

Where would be a likely site for a lesion that would give contralateral paralysis to the extremities and trunk and would also give paralysis of lateral gaze of the ipsilateral eye to the side of the lesion? Where would the lesion be if there was contralateral paralysis of the extremities, ipsilateral paralysis of medial gaze, ptosis, and dilated pupil?

Which functional components or pathways make up the internal capsule of the brain? Where in this structure is each component found?

Describe the paralysis resulting from a destructive lesion that involves the posterior limb of the internal capsule.

Where do the principal afferents to the cerebellum originate? Describe the course that each follows to reach its termination in the cerebellum.

What is the major output of the cerebellum? Where do the efferent pathways from the neocerebellum go? Where do the efferent pathways from the flocculonodular lobe terminate? What is the function of the cerebellum?

What is the major outflow of the lenticular nucleus? What connections are made with the subthalamic nucleus and what is the effect of this nucleus on the globus pallidus?

Which structures receive their blood supply from the internal carotid artery?

What blood vessels comprise the arterial circle of Willis?

Which major ascending and descending pathways could be compromised if there was occlusion of the anterior spinal artery where it arises from the vertebral artery?

What deficits would occur if the posterior inferior cerebral artery were occluded?

Give the position, relationships, attachments, innervation, and embryonic origin of the pituitary gland. Into what parts is the pituitary gland divided and what are the characteristics of the cells in the various parts? What is the functional significance of each of the cell types?

Describe the pathway of hypothalamic-releasing hormones from their production in the hypothalamus to their site of action on chromophils of the adenohypophysis. How does this pathway differ from the neurosecretory tracts that terminate in the neurohypophysis?

Which structures are most susceptible to injury when the pituitary gland undergoes enlargement? Where are these structures found in relation to the pituitary?

Describe the major efferent pathways of the hypothalamus. What is the relationship between the hypothalamus and autonomic nervous system? the limbic system?

What are the two main divisions of the autonomic nervous system? Discuss the origins of the two parts from the central nervous system. Where, in general, are the peripheral adrenergic and cholinergic fibers found within these two systems?

To which structures are the nerve fibers from the superior cervical ganglion distributed? What would be the results of destruction of this ganglion?

Describe the microscopic structure of the salivary glands. Where do their ducts open into the oral cavity?

Which of the major salivary glands are mixed seromucous glands? Both the pancreas and parotid can be affected in mumps. Compare the exocrine portions of these two glands. How are the cells of the striated (salivary) ducts of the parotid similar to the cells of the distal convoluted tubule of the kidney?

What are the major contents of the anterior triangle of the neck? the posterior triangle? In which triangle of the neck could you palpate the anterior scalene nodes? the roots of the brachial plexus?

Describe the carotid sheath, its contents, and its relation to the cervical sympathetic trunk.

Describe the cervical plexus and give the structures innervated by it.

Which anatomic structures are traversed in tracheotomy?

What comprises the true vocal fold? What nerves regulate the muscles of the larynx? What would be the motor and sensory loss if the superior laryngeal nerve were severed?

Give the gross and the microscopic structures of the thyroid gland and its important relations. What is its blood supply? Where may ectopic and accessory thyroids be found? Explain their location on the basis of the embryonic development of the thyroid.

Give the number, the position, and the relationships of the parathyroid glands. Describe briefly the origin and the development of these glands.

Give the position, relationships, and microscopic structure of the thymus. Explain the occasional inclusion of parathyroid tissue in the thymus. Compare the thymus gland at birth and at puberty.

If there is a complete branchial fistula at the second pharyngeal pouch and cleft, where will it open internally and externally?

Describe the development of the face. What is the embryologic basis for cleft lip? cleft palate? choanal atresia?

Outline the boundaries of the lungs and pleura on the chest wall.

Name the lobes and the fissures of each lung and explain how they can be mapped out on the chest wall.

Give the outline of the heart as projected on the surface of the anterior thoracic wall. Which structures of the heart form the boundaries described above? Which chambers lie directly beneath the anterior chest wall?

Locate the heart valves as projected into the anterior chest wall. Which of these valves lie near the surface and which are placed more deeply? If sounds from the more deeply placed valves are projected in the direction of blood flow through these valves, where would be the areas of maximum audibility for each?

What are the boundaries of the mediastinum? Give the contents of the anterior, the middle, and the posterior portions.

Give the positions and the relationships of the trachea in the thorax. At what level does it branch into the right and the left bronchi? In which of these bronchi is a foreign body most likely to lodge? Explain.

How many bronchopulmonary segments are there in each lung and lobe?

Describe the right pleural sac. Why does the lung collapse when an opening forms from the air passages of the lung into the pleural sac?

Describe the innervation of the lungs. Indicate the functional significance of the nerve fibers involved.

Describe the changes in the histology of the walls of the respiratory tract as one proceeds from the trachea to the alveoli. How far down the conducting pathways do cartilage, glands, and ciliated epithelium extend?

Describe the lining epithelium of the alveoli. What structures constitute a blood–air barrier?

Give the location and microscopic structure of the valves of the heart. What are the functions of the chordae tendineae and the papillary muscles? How are these structures arranged to subserve their functions? Compare the right and the left atrioventricular orifices and their valves. Why is one valve larger than the other?

Contrast the right and left ventricles of the heart as to structure of the walls, volume of the cavities, and valvular arrangements.

Describe the development of the interatrial septum. Where is the foramen ovale? What is the embryologic basis of the foramen ovale defect and the foramen primum defect? What embryologic structures contribute to the development of the membranous part of the interventricular septum?

Describe the arch of the aorta, including its important relationships.

Describe the fate of the five pairs of aortic arches. What is the developmental reason for a right subclavian artery arising from the arch of the aorta? How does transposition of the aorta and pulmonary artery arise?

What embryologic vessels are retained and which fail to form in the formation of double superior venae cavae? What postnatal structures arise from the left umbilical vein, vitelline veins, vitelline arteries, and umbilical arteries?

Describe the blood supply to the heart.

Describe the efferent innervation to the heart, including the location of the cell bodies of the various neurons involved.

Give the anatomic arrangements that provide for reflex slowing of the heart on stimulation of the carotid sinus.

The stellate ganglion has been removed for the relief of anginal pain. What effects other than the relief of anginal pain may result? Explain the anatomic basis for each of these additional effects.

Describe in detail the anatomic arrangement of the structures in the heart responsible for the initiation and transmission of the heart beat.

Describe in detail the anatomic modifications in the heart and the resultant changes in the circulation of the blood in a normal infant following birth. What results if these normal changes do not take place? Explain.

Describe the composition, the extent, and the attachments of the pericardial sac. Where can it be opened for drainage without going through the pleura?

Describe the diaphragm, including its origin, structure, attachments, and orifices. Give the mechanism of its action. Where is referred pain from the diaphragm commonly experienced and how is this related to its innervation?

What are the roles in inspiration of the diaphragm, abdominal muscles, intercostal muscles, and scalene muscles?

Contrast the gross and the histologic features of the esophagus and the trachea as related to the functions of each of these tubes.

What is a possible embryologic reason for tracheoesophageal fistula? for diaphragmatic hernia?

Where does the thoracic duct empty and what does it drain?

Describe the lymphatics of the thoracic cavity. What is the effect, if any, of blocking the thoracic duct at the point at which it empties into the venous system?

Describe the pathway of lymph through a lymphatic node. What is the function of the reticuloendothelial (mononuclear phagocyte) system? What is the function of a lymph node?

Compare the microscopic structure of the thymus with that of a lymph node. What is the gross relationship of the thymus to the great vessels?

Discuss the lymphatic drainage of the breast, mentioning all possible pathways and connections.

Describe the normal gross and microscopic structure of the mammary gland.

Describe the origin, the course, and the termination of the splanchnic nerves. What is the functional nature of the various fibers running in these nerves, and where are the cell bodies of these fibers located? What would be the vascular effects in the abdomen on section of the splanchnic nerves?

Divide the abdomen into nine surface regions and name them. What structures do the horizontal dividing lines represent?

Divide the abdomen into four regions.

Locate the stomach on the surface, including the cardiac orifice and the pyloric orifice.

On the surface locate the duodenum, the ileocolic junction, the cecum, and the right and left colic flexures.

On the surface outline the liver and indicate the exact location of the gallbladder.

On the surface locate the pancreas, spleen, kidneys, and ureter.

What muscles form the anterior abdominal wall?

What abdominal muscle or its aponeurosis forms the superficial inguinal ring, the deep inguinal ring, and the floor, roof, anterior and posterior walls of the inguinal canal?

Differentiate between the pathway of a direct versus an indirect inguinal hernia.

Differentiate between organs that are retroperitoneal, partially peritonealized and "completely" peritonealized. Give specific examples of each.

Describe the location of the lesser peritoneal sac.

Name the three structures in the free edge of the lesser omentum.

Describe the parts of the stomach.

What are the four parts of the duodenum?

Where are the jejunum and ileum normally located? How does the jejunum differ grossly and microscopically from the ileum?

How does the large intestine differ grossly and microscopically from the small intestine?

With what organs are the ascending, transverse and descending parts of the colon related?

With what organs is the liver related? Where is the gallbladder found with respect to the liver? With what organs is the gallbladder related?

Describe the bare area of the liver.

Describe the peritoneal relationships of the liver.

What is the relationship between the inferior vena cava and the liver?

Where are the caudate and quadrate lobes of the liver?

What organs are drained by the portal vein? What alternate pathways may blood take when the normal path for portal blood through the liver is obstructed?

Describe the bile duct system of the liver and gallbladder.

Describe the relationships of the pancreas. Into what does the main pancreatic duct empty?

Describe the peritoneal relationships of the spleen.

At what vertebral levels are the kidneys found?

What structures form the kidney bed? What structures are related to the anterior surfaces of each kidney?

Describe the course of the ureters. To what structures is each ureter related? At what locations are the ureters naturally constricted?

Describe the location and relationships of each suprarenal gland.

At what vertebral level does the aorta pass through the thoracic diaphragm? At what vertebral level does the abdominal aorta bifurcate? Where is the abdominal aorta with respect to the lumbar vertebrae?

Name the three large unpaired branches of the aorta and give the distribution of each.

What general areas are supplied by the common iliac arteries?

The sympathetic fibers that innervate the abdominal viscera originate from what spinal cord segments? Where do the synapses occur between the preganglionic and postganglionic sympathetic and parasympathetic fibers that supply the abdominal viscera?

What part of the gastrointestinal tract is supplied by the vagus nerve?

Describe the system of nerve plexuses along the ventral aspect of the aorta.

What nerves innervate the skin and muscle of the abdominal wall?

What are the major differences in character in the normal mucosa of the alimentary canal, beginning with the esophagus, and terminating at the anus? What are the associated changes in function?

Describe the stomach. Give its relations and describe the microscopic structure of gastric glands. What cells produce HCl? pepsin? mucus? serotonin?

Describe the modifications of the small intestine for the function of absorption. What structures accentuate the absorptive surface area. Locate Brunner's glands. What do they produce?

Describe the histologic structure of the vermiform appendix.

What is the microscopic structure of the liver? Describe the circulation of the blood through the liver. Explain on an anatomic basis why certain ingested poisons cause damage initially to the periphery of the liver lobules. In case of portal obstruction, what collateral venous circulation might be established?

Give the contents of the portal areas (canals, triads).

How is the mucosa of the gallbladder structurally adapted to the functions it performs?

Describe the histologic structure of the pancreas. Give the functional significance of its various structures. What are the most prominent ultrastructural characteristics of cells of the exocrine secretory units?

What is the microscopic structure of the spleen? Describe the flow of blood through the spleen. Describe the position, relationships, and peritoneal attachments of the spleen.

Describe the microscopic structure of the adrenal gland. What is the nerve and blood supply to the cortex and medulla? Locate the cell bodies of neurons that supply the medulla.

Describe the histologic structure of the kidney. What is the blood supply to the various components of the renal cortex and medulla? How are the different parts of the nephron structurally adapted to carry out their functions?

What constitutes the filtration barrier of the renal corpuscle?

What are the histologic features of the ureter and urinary bladder that permit them to readily accommodate large quantities of water?

Describe the rotation of the gut. What are the fates of the cephalic and caudal limbs of the gut loop?

How does the lesser peritoneal sac develop? What embryologic structures contribute to the formation of the greater omentum? What is the fate of the vitelline (omphalomesenteric) artery?

Locate the following structures and give their embryologic significance: (1) ligamentum arteriosum, (2) ligamentum venosum, (3) round ligament of the liver, (4) Meckel's diverticulum, and (5) lateral umbilical ligaments.

Compare the peritoneal arrangements of the various parts of the large intestine. Explain the manner in which a structure that in early development is suspended by peritoneum becomes secondarily retroperitoneal.

Describe the origin of the pancreas.

Compare the suprarenal medulla with a sympathetic ganglion as to its origin, structure, and function. Describe the development of the suprarenal gland.

How does the bare area of the liver reflect the development of the liver in the caudal face of the septum transversum? From what embryonic germ layer do the epithelium and glands of most of the digestive system arise?

Differentiate the true from the false pelvis.

Define the pelvic inlet and the pelvic outlet.

What muscles form the pelvic diaphragm? Describe their lateral attachments.

Define the AP and transverse diameters of the pelvic inlet, pelvic outlet and midpelvis.

Define the boundaries of the urogenital and anal triangles.

Describe the boundaries of the ischiorectal fossa, including its anterior and posterior recesses and its contents.

What is the pudendal canal and what are its contents?

Describe the deep perineal space. What are its contents in the male and the female?

Define the superficial perineal space. What are its contents in the male and the female?

What nerves innervate the skin of the perineum?

What structures are palpable in the male and female via rectal examination?

Define the location of the urinary bladder and name the organs to which it is related in both the male and female.

Trace the course of the urethra in both the male and female.

To what structures is the prostate gland related?

Describe the course of the ductus (vas) deferens.

Describe the location of the ovaries.

How are the ovaries related to the uterine tubes?

Define the parts of the uterus.

How is the uterus related to the vagina?

What is the normal position of the uterus? To what structures is it related?

What structures are normally palpable by a vaginal examination?

How is the broad ligament related to the uterus?

What are the mesometrium, mesovarium, mesosalpinx, parametrium, and the cardinal ligaments?

Name the visceral branches of the internal iliac artery and describe their general distributions.

Describe the origin, migration and fate of primordial sex cells in the formation of the indifferent stage of the gonad and in the formation of the testis and ovary.

Describe the histologic structure of the testis. Where and how does spermatogenesis take place?

Describe the histologic structure of the epithelium lining the rete testis, efferent ductules, ductus epididymidis, and ductus deferens.

Describe the male urethra, its parts, their characteristics and relationships. Explain on an anatomic basis where in the course of the urethra difficulty might be experienced in passing a rigid catheter.

What ducts empty into the urethra, and what is the nature of the substances being delivered to the urethra?

Describe the histologic characteristics of the pe-

nis. What structures are adapted for the function of erection? Why is the urethra not completely compressed during erection?

What is the origin of the vesicular ovarian (graafian) follicle? What is ovulation? When does it occur in relation to the menstrual cycle? When does it occur in relation to oogenesis?

Describe the development and histology of the corpus luteum.

If fertilization and implantation do not take place, when during the menstrual cycle will the corpus luteum degenerate? What is a corpus albicans?

Describe the histologic structure of the uterine (fallopian) tube. What is the function of the ciliated epithelium?

Describe the histologic structure of the uterus. State the major endometrial changes that take place during the menstrual cycle and during pregnancy. What is the effect of estrogen on the uterus? of progesterone?

Describe the mucosa of the cervix. What changes take place in the cervix during the menstrual cycle? during pregnancy?

Describe the histology of the vagina. How does its epithelium change during the menstrual cycle.

Compare the histology of the clitoris and penis.

What are the fates of the mesonephric ducts, müllerian ducts, and urogenital sinus in the male? in the female?

What is the difference in origin of the nephrons and collecting tubules?

What is the embryologic basis of double vagina? uterus didelphys? bipartite uterus?

What is the normal fate of the processus vaginalis in the male? What is hydrocoele?

What is the fate of the urethral folds and labioscrotal swellings in the male? in the female? What embryologic structures are involved in the formation of hypospadias? What causes, and what is the effect of, congenital adrenal hyperplasia?

What series of events immediately follows penetration of a secondary oocyte by a spermatozoon? Where does fertilization usually occur?

How long is the developing conceptus in the uterine tube? in the uterine cavity? On what postfertilization day does implantation occur?

Into what layers of the endometrium does the embryo implant?

Describe the development of the placenta. When are both cytotrophoblast and syncytial trophoblast present? When are nucleated red blood cells normally found?

Describe the histologic structure of the placenta.

What is the chorion frondosum? What is a cotyledon? Where are decidual cells found? What is the decidua basalis?

Describe the placental barrier. Describe the flow of blood through the placenta.

What is the fate of the primitive streak and primitive (Hensen's) node?

What is the developmental relation of the allantois to the urinary bladder?

What is the fate of the primitive yolk sac? How are the respiratory and digestive systems related to the yolk sac?

What is the fate of the neural plate?

What is the fate of the sclerotome? myotome? intermediate mesoderm?

Multiple Choice Questions

ONE-ANSWER TYPE

Select the *one* statement that most accurately completes the sentence or answers the question. Answers are at the end of this chapter.

1. In a cell with especially high energy (ATP) requirements, which of the following organelles would you expect to be most highly developed?
   (a) Rough endoplasmic reticulum
   (b) Mitochondria
   (c) Centrioles
   (d) Peroxisomes
2. Cells with large amounts of rough endoplasmic reticulum are most likely to:
   (a) Produce steroids
   (b) Line the lumen of blood vessels
   (c) Produce structural proteins that remain in the cell
   (d) Synthesize a proteinaceous secretory product
3. Regarding the nucleus:
   (a) Chromosomes in areas of euchromatin are probably less functionally active than in areas of heterochromatin.
   (b) The nucleolar membrane separates the nucleolus from the chromosomes.
   (c) The nuclear envelop consists of two membranes, and is penetrated by pores to allow passage of material between the nucleus and the cytoplasm.
   (d) Chromosomes and the nuclear envelop are most prominent during the metaphase stage of mitosis.
4. Assuming a person had received enough exposure of x-rays to the whole body to destroy

cells as they attempt to divide, which one of the following functions would survive best?
   (a) Hair growth
   (b) Red blood corpuscle production
   (c) Intestinal absorption of fat
   (d) Cardiac contraction
5. Choose the correct statement regarding the free surface specializations of epithelial cells.
   (a) Cilia contain a core of nine peripheral and two central microfilaments.
   (b) Microvilli contain a core of microfilaments.
   (c) Microvilli insert into centrioles (basal bodies).
   (d) Stereocilia contain a core of microtubules that inserts into centrioles (basal bodies).
6. Which of the following is *not* used in classifying the various types of epithelia?
   (a) The number of layers of cells
   (b) The shape of the cells at only the free surface
   (c) The terminal specialization or modification at the free surface
   (d) The relative amount of intercellular material to the cellular content
7. The specific intercellular junctional mechanism through which cells are electrically coupled is the:
   (a) Desmosome
   (b) Tight junction
   (c) Zonula adherens
   (d) Gap junction
8. Which of the following fibers or fibrils is most like collagen in its chemical composition?
   (a) Muscle fibers
   (b) Elastic fibers
   (c) Neurofibrils
   (d) Reticular fibers
9. Tendons are composed of:
   (a) Dense irregularly arranged connective tissue
   (b) Dense regularly arranged connective tissue
   (c) Large elastic fibers with fibroblasts lying between the fibers
   (d) Large collagenous fibers with fibroblasts lying in lacunae between the fibers
10. In which of the following organs would you be most likely to find elastic cartilage?
   (a) Lungs
   (b) Developing long bone
   (c) Larynx
   (d) Inner ear

11. The stiffness of cartilage is due primarily to the presence of:
    (a) Chondroitin sulfate
    (b) Collagen fibers
    (c) Hyaluronic acid
    (d) The perichondrium

12. Bone remodelling normally:
    (a) Involves removal of existing bone by osteoblasts
    (b) Involves deposition of calcified cartilage on existing trabeculae of bone
    (c) Can occur in response to mechanical stress and fluctuations in the blood calcium level
    (d) Occurs during the "growing years," but ceases by the age of 50

13. Which statement is true for muscle tissue?
    (a) Cardiac and smooth muscle cells both branch and have central nuclei.
    (b) Cardiac and smooth muscle tissue both possess gap junctions.
    (c) Skeletal muscle satellite cells lie outside the basement membrane of the muscle and are really connective tissue cells.
    (d) Cardiac and smooth muscle tissue are each more vascular than skeletal muscle tissue.

14. Neurons:
    (a) Of the central nervous system have Nissl material that extends into both dendrites and axons
    (b) Of the central nervous system are invested by myelin produced by Schwann cells
    (c) And glial cells in the gray matter of the spinal cord make up a meshwork called neuropil
    (d) Of sympathetic ganglia are unipolar or pseudounipolar

15. Which of the following is *not* produced by a neuron?
    (a) Antidiuretic hormone (ADH)
    (b) Luteinizing-releasing hormone (LHRH)
    (c) Epinephrine
    (d) Calcitonin

16. Neuromuscular spindles:
    (a) Contain both afferent and efferent nerve fibers
    (b) Contain infrafusal fibers which are usually larger than extrafusal fibers
    (c) Are located in the myenteric plexus of the intestine
    (d) Regulate the state of contraction of cardiac muscle

17. Which of the following cells is morphologically closest to the earlier "blast" stage?
    (a) Promyelocyte
    (b) Platelet
    (c) Neutrophilic metamyelocyte
    (d) Reticulocyte

18. Which of the following cell types is most numerous in a normal blood smear?
    (a) Neutrophil
    (b) Eosinophil
    (c) Lymphocyte
    (d) Monocyte

19. Myelocytes:
    (a) Have an indented nucleus
    (b) Are incapable of division
    (c) Have "specific" granules
    (d) Arise from metamyelocytes

20. In the heart:
    (a) Purkinje fibers are modified nerve fibers constituting part of the cardiac conduction system.
    (b) The endocardium of the atria is thicker than that of the ventricles.
    (c) Papillary muscles are involuntary smooth muscle tissue that insert into chordae tendinae.
    (d) The sinoatrial (S-A) node is modified connective tissue of the cardiac skeleton.

21. Afferent lymphatic vessels are found supplying:
    (a) Peyer's patches
    (b) The spleen
    (c) Lymph nodes
    (d) The thymus

22. Which one of the following does *not* transport blood through its sinusoids?
    (a) Bone marrow
    (b) Spleen
    (c) Lymph node
    (d) Liver

23. Which of the following organs is least likely to demonstrate mucus-secreting cells or glands?
    (a) Vagina
    (b) Esophagus
    (c) Cervix
    (d) Colon

24. Which of the following is a component of the mucosa (mucous membrane)?
    (a) Enteroendocrine cells of the stomach
    (b) Hair follicle
    (c) Auerbach's myenteric nerve plexus
    (d) Sweat gland

25. Which of the following is *not* correct for the small intestine?

(a) Monoglycerides and fatty acids diffuse through the absorptive cell plasma membrane.

(b) The nodules of Peyer's patches may extend into the submucosal layer.

(c) Chylomicrons are often found in the intercellular spaces between absorptive cells.

(d) The outer longitudinal layer of the muscularis externa is thickened into taenia coli.

26. In the kidney:
(a) As much as 80% of the amino acids and glucose of the ultrafiltrate are reabsorbed by the thin portion of the loop of Henle.
(b) Renin, produced by the juxtaglomerular apparatus, acts directly on arterial smooth muscle to cause vasodilation.
(c) Antidiuretic hormone causes the collecting tubules to become more permeable to water, thus concentrating the urine.
(d) Interlobular arteries arise from arcuate arteries and pass into the cortex via the medullary rays.

27. During the differentiation of a spermatozoan (spermiogenesis) the acrosome arises by accumulation of material in:
(a) Mitochondria
(b) The nucleus
(c) The Golgi complex
(d) The nuclear envelope

28. In the male reproductive system:
(a) Spermatozoa pass in order through efferent ductules, rete testis and ductus epididymidis.
(b) The ductus deferens, seminal vesicle, and prostate all have smooth muscle in their walls.
(c) The seminal vesicle is the main source of acid phosphatase in the semen.
(d) The prostate gland is a site where spermatozoa are stored and become mature.

29. In the female reproductive system:
(a) Uterine glands secrete a carbohydrate-rich substance and also are necessary for regeneration of the surface epithelium of the uterus during the menstrual cycle.
(b) The cytotrophoblast of the placenta is most prominent during the third trimester of pregnancy.
(c) Theca externa cells of ovarian follicles secrete most of the ovarian estrogen.
(d) Ovulation occurs at the time when progesterone has reached its highest level in the blood plasma.

30. Which one of the following "structure-secretory product" combinations is correct?
(a) Syncytiotrophoblast–progesterone and estrogen
(b) Acidophils of the pars distalis–follicle-stimulating hormone (FSH)
(c) Beta cells of the islets of Langerhans–glucagon
(d) Zona glomerulosa of the suprarenal gland–cortisone

31. Which of the following is characteristic of the 27th day of the menstrual cycle?
(a) Stasis of blood in the basal straight arteries of the endometrium
(b) Constriction of the coiled spiral arteries
(c) Increased proliferation of the endometrium
(d) Increased edema of the functional spongy layer of the endometrium

32. Which one of the following organs possesses all of these characteristics: has both an exocrine and endocrine organ; is under the influence of hypophyseal hormones; has cells completing the second meiotic division?
(a) Ovary
(b) Liver
(c) Testis
(d) Pancreas

33. Which one of the following organs possesses all of these characteristics: serous acini, intercalated ducts, striated ducts, no mucous alveoli?
(a) Sebaceous gland
(b) Pancreas
(c) Sublingual gland
(d) Parotid gland

34. Which one of the following organs possesses all of these characteristics: stratified squamous nonkeratinized epithelium, serous and mucous glands, skeletal muscle, special visceral afferent nerve fibers?
(a) Esophagus
(b) Tongue
(c) Vagina
(d) Anal canal

35. Three sites where substances readily pass between the vascular system and a surface lining epithelium are in the lung alveoli, renal corpuscles, and chorionic villi. Which one of the following is found in all three structures?
(a) Lining cells which secrete lipoidal or steroidal substances
(b) Macrophages

(c) Fenestrated endothelial cells

(d) Angiotensin-producing cells

36. In the ear:

(a) Endolymph fills the scala tympani and scala vestibuli.

(b) The organ of Corti contains hair cells, each of which possesses one true cilium.

(c) Bipolar neurons in the spiral cochlear ganglion each have a peripheral process that ends on hair cells, and a central process that is a component of the cochlear nerve.

(d) The stapes is located in the round window of the scala tympani.

37. In the eye:

(a) Visual pigments are located in discs of the outer segments of cells of the pigmented layer of the retina.

(b) Accommodation (focusing on a near object) involves the relaxation of ciliary smooth muscle, resulting in release of tension on the ciliary zonule and rounding of the lens.

(c) The blind spot produced by the optic disc is medial to the visual axis.

(d) The pupil gets larger in response to parasympathetic nerve stimulation.

38. Which of the following primary afferent or efferent fibers of medullary cranial nerves is paired with an *incorrect* nucleus of termination or origin?

(a) General somatic afferent (GSA) fibers of IX-nucleus solitarius

(b) Special visceral efferent (SVE) fibers of XI-nucleus ambiguus

(c) General visceral efferent (GVE) fibers of X-dorsal motor nucleus

(d) Special visceral afferent (SVA) fibers of IX-gustatory nucleus

39. After a peripheral lesion of the abducens nerve in the orbit, one might expect to find all of the following *except:*

(a) Chromatolysis in the facial colliculus of the pons

(b) Chromatolysis in the ipsilateral mesencephalic nucleus of the fifth cranial nerve

(c) Degenerating fibers in the contralateral medial longitudinal fasciculus (MLF)

(d) Paralysis of the ipsilateral lateral rectus muscle

40. Which one of the following structures is *not* supplied by direct branches of the artery with which it is matched?

(a) Spinal tract of the trigeminal nerve–posterior inferior cerebellar artery

(b) Medial lemniscus–anterior spinal artery

(c) Corticospinal tract–posterior cerebral artery

(d) Visual (striate) cortex–anterior cerebral artery

41. Bilateral injury to the facial nerves at their emergence from the pons–medulla junction could result in:

(a) Hyperacusis because of impaired stapedius muscle activity

(b) Loss of taste from the posterior one third of the tongue

(c) Loss of all flow of saliva

(d) Ptosis in both eyes

42. After a right upper motor neuron lesion of the facial nerve there is a:

(a) Loss of the sense of taste on the right anterior portion of the tongue

(b) Loss of the corneal reflex on the right side

(c) Loss of ability to wrinkle the forehead on the left side

(d) Paralysis of lower facial muscles on the left side

43. If there is a destructive lesion of the crista ampullaris in the left horizontal semicircular canal all of the following are likely to be present *except:*

(a) A tendency to fall to the left

(b) Past-pointing to the left

(c) A sense of the room rotating to the right

(d) Nystagmus with a fast component to the right

44. A tumor in the cerebellopontine angle could result in all of the following *except:*

(a) Deafness in the ipsilateral ear

(b) Lateral strabismus ipsilaterally

(c) Impaired corneal reflex

(d) Absence of normal vestibular responses

45. All of the following result in constriction of the left pupil *except:*

(a) Focusing the eye on a near object after focusing on a far object

(b) Shining light in the right eye of a normal person

(c) Shining light on only the nasal half of the retina of the right eye of a person whose optic chiasm has been totally destroyed

(d) Shining light in the right eye of a person whose left optic nerve was destroyed

46. Which of the following eye movements and reflexes would be *least* affected by bilateral destruction of the parastriate (18) and peristriate (19) areas of the cerebral cortex?

(a) Smooth eye pursuit of a moving object

(b) The near (synkinetic, accommodation-convergence) reflex
(c) The pupillary light reflex
(d) Saccadic movements occurring in the shift of gaze from one object to another

47. Destruction of which of the following would *most likely* result in a deficit of memory for recent events?
(a) Cingulate gyrus
(b) Parietal lobe
(c) Anterior–medial region of the temporal lobe
(d) Medial dorsal nucleus of the thalamus

48. The intervertebral foramen is bounded:
(a) Superiorly and inferiorly by the lamina of the involved vertebrae
(b) Posteriorly by the zygopophyseal joint
(c) Posteriorly by the posterior longitudinal ligament
(d) Anteriorly by the intervertebral disc and the anterior longitudinal ligament

49. The shoulder joint is least reinforced by muscles of the rotator cuff:
(a) Anteriorly
(b) Inferiorly
(c) Posteriorly
(d) Superiorly

50. The major origin of the superficial group of anterior forearm muscles is the:
(a) Lateral epicondyle of the humerus
(b) Proximal ventral aspects of the radius and ulna
(c) Olecranon process of the humerus
(d) Medial epicondyl of the humerus

51. Which of the following intrinsic thumb muscles is *not* found in the thenar compartment?
(a) Adductor pollicis
(b) Flexor pollicis brevis
(c) Abductor pollicis brevis
(d) Opponens pollicis

52. The muscles in the adductor–interosseous compartment of the hand are innervated by the:
(a) Median nerve
(b) Median and ulnar nerves
(c) Radial nerve
(d) Ulnar nerve

53. The anterior cruciate ligament of the knee:
(a) Is most taut when the knee is flexed
(b) Attaches to the anterior intercondylar region of the tibia
(c) Protects against posterior dislocation of the tibia on the femur

(d) Protects against anterior dislocation of the femur on the tibia

54. Palpable just medial to the patellar ligament in the interval between the femur and tibia is the:
(a) Anterior cruciate ligament
(b) Fibular collateral ligament
(c) Tendon of the popliteus muscle
(d) Medial meniscus

55. Due to bony support, the most stable position of the ankle joint is:
(a) Dorsiflexion
(b) Inversion
(c) Plantar flexion
(d) Eversion

56. The major blood supply to the posterior femoral muscles is provided by:
(a) The obturator artery
(b) The perforating branches of the deep femoral artery
(c) The medial and lateral femoral circumflex vessels
(d) The superior gluteal artery

57. On the dorsum of the foot the dorsalis pedis pulse can be taken:
(a) Medial to the tendon of the tibialis anterior muscle
(b) Between the tendons of the tibialis anterior and extensor hallucis longus muscles
(c) Between the tendons of the extensor hallucis longus and extensor digitorum longus muscles
(d) Between the tendons of the extensor digitorum longus and peroneus tertius muscles

58. The posterior tibial pulse is taken:
(a) Posterior to the medial malleolus
(b) Anterior to the medial malleolus
(c) Posterior to the lateral malleolus
(d) Between the calcaneal tendon and the lateral malleolus

59. Which of the following functions of the muscles of mastication is incorrect?
(a) Masseter: elevation of the mandible
(b) Medial pterygoid: elevation of the mandible
(c) Temporalis: retraction of the mandible
(d) Lateral pterygoid: deviation of the mandible to the same side

60. Most of the muscle of the pharyngeal wall is innervated by cranial nerve:
(a) IX
(b) X

(c) XI

(d) XII

61. The parasympathetic fibers that innervate the sphincter pupillae muscle *do not* pass through the:
    (a) Short ciliary nerves
    (b) Cranial nerve III
    (c) Long ciliary nerves
    (d) Cavernous sinus

62. Laceration of the facial nerve immediately distal to the geniculate ganglion would *least likely* cause:
    (a) An inability to close the ipsilateral eye
    (b) Loss of taste on the anterior two thirds of the tongue
    (c) Loss of lacrimation
    (d) Loss of submandibular salivation

63. The common carotid artery bifurcates:
    (a) At the level of the cricoid cartilage
    (b) Between the levels of the cricoid and thyroid cartilage
    (c) Between the levels of the thyroid cartilage prominence and the hyoid bone
    (d) Superior to the level of the hyoid bone

64. A lesion of the most superficial nerve in the posterior triangle of the neck would logically result in:
    (a) Difficulty swallowing
    (b) Difficulty breathing
    (c) Difficulty turning the head to the same side
    (d) Difficulty elevating (hunching) the shoulder

65. The pleural cavities:
    (a) Contain the lungs
    (b) Communicate across the midline
    (c) Are composed of inner parietal and outer visceral layers
    (d) Surround the lungs

66. A penetrating wound that enters the right fourth intercostal space in the midclavicular line would initially enter the:
    (a) Superior lobe of the right lung
    (b) Right lung below the oblique fissure
    (c) Inferior lobe of the right lung
    (d) Middle lobe of the right lung

67. *Not* participating in the formation of Hasselbach's triangle is the:
    (a) Falx inguinalis (conjoined tendon)
    (b) Lateral border of the rectus abdominis
    (c) Inguinal ligament
    (d) Inferior epigastric vessels

68. The inguinal ligament extends between the:
    (a) Pubic tubercle and the anterior superior iliac spine
    (b) Anterior superior and inferior iliac spines
    (c) Greater trochanter of the femur and the pubic tubercle
    (d) Ischial spine and pubic tubercle

69. The neck of an indirect hernia is found:
    (a) Medial to the pubic tubercle
    (b) Medial to the inferior epigastric vessels
    (c) Lateral to the deep inguinal ring
    (d) Lateral to the inferior epigastric vessels

70. The renal pelvis is directed:
    (a) Anteromedially
    (b) Posteromedially
    (c) Anterolaterally
    (d) Posterolaterally

71. The pelvic diaphragm slopes inferiorly from:
    (a) Anterior to posterior
    (b) Medial to lateral
    (c) Posterior to anterior
    (d) The public symphysis to the sacral promontory

72. The superficial perineal space (pouch) is continuous with the:
    (a) Subcutaneous area of the thigh
    (b) Peritoneal cavity
    (c) Ischiorectal fossa
    (d) Fascial plane in the abdominal wall between the external abdominal oblique fascia and the membraneous layer of superficial fascia

73. All of the following are true for the plasma membrane *except:*
    (a) Possesses transmembrane proteins that help to transport specific molecules into the cell
    (b) Contains glycolipids and glycoproteins
    (c) Possesses a double layer of phospholipid molecules whose fatty acid components make up an intermediate hydrophobic zone
    (d) Is coated by a glycocalyx on both its outer and inner surfaces

74. In the mitochondria:
    (a) The electron transport system of enzymes is on the inner membrane of the cristae
    (b) Pyruvate is converted to acetyl-CoA between the outer and inner membranes
    (c) Of pancreatic cells are found a preponderance of tubular cristae
    (d) The energy that is produced is used in forming ADP

75. All of the following are true statements for cytoplasmic organelles *except:*
    (a) Coated vesicles are coated with clathrin and are involved in receptor-mediated endocytosis

(b) Free ribosomes are mostly involved in the production of secretory proteins
(c) Centrioles are similar in structure to basal bodies
(d) Intermediate filaments are plentiful in epidermal cells

POSSIBLY MORE THAN ONE ANSWER

For each of the following questions answer:

(a) if only 1, 2, and 3 are correct
(b) if only 1 and 3 are correct
(c) if only 2 and 4 are correct
(d) if only 4 is correct
(e) if all are correct

1. The Golgi apparatus is involved in which of the following?
   1. Concentrating secretory products
   2. Packaging secretory products in membrane-bound vacuoles
   3. Producing thyroglobulin
   4. Adding the carbohydrate component to the glycosaminoglycans of ground substance

2. Which of the following cells characteristically contain(s) much smooth endoplasmic reticulum?
   1. Cells of the zona fasciculata of the suprarenal gland
   2. Cardiac muscle cells
   3. Granulosa lutein cells
   4. Pancreatic acinar cells

3. Which of the following cells is/are considered to be quite phagocytic?
   1. Kupffer cells
   2. Fibroblasts
   3. Macrophages
   4. Plasma cells

4. Which of the following statements is/are correct regarding epithelia?
   1. Stratified squamous epithelium lines surfaces that are subject to abrasion.
   2. Transitional epithelium is well adapted for absorptive functions.
   3. All cells of pseudostratified columnar epithelium reach the basement membrane, but not all of them reach the luminal surface.
   4. Epithelial cells usually receive nutritive substances from capillaries located in the intercellular spaces of the epithelium.

5. The basement membrane consists of:
   1. Large collagen bundles
   2. Reticular fibers
   3. The plasma membrane of basal epithelial cells
   4. A basal lamina

6. Which of the following are found within the intercellular spaces between epidermal cells?
   1. Tonofilaments
   2. Nerve fibers
   3. Meissner's tactile corpuscles
   4. Melanocytes

7. Osteons (Haversian systems) contain:
   1. Collagenous fibers that, in adjacent lamellae, run perpendicular to each other
   2. Interstitial lamellae
   3. Osteoprogenitor cells that occupy the osteon (Haversian) canal
   4. Canaliculi through which blood is transported to the osteocytes

8. Which of the following are characteristics of both hyaline cartilage and bone?
   1. Avascular tissue
   2. Cells occupy lacunae
   3. Grow by both appositional and interstitial growth
   4. The intercellular matrix contains numerous collagenous fibers and a mucoidal ground substance

9. Cardiac muscle differs from adult skeletal muscle in that cardiac muscle possesses:
   1. Intercalated discs
   2. Branching fibers
   3. Centrally located nuclei
   4. T tubules which are located at the Z line

10. During excitation–contraction coupling in skeletal muscle:
    1. Calcium is released from the cisterna of the sarcoplasmic reticulum.
    2. The interaction of actin and myosin is regulated, at least in part, by troponin and tropomyosin.
    3. A wave of membrane depolarization is carried into the depths of the muscle fiber by the T tubules.
    4. The A band shortens as a result of the interaction between thick and thin filaments.

11. Glial (neuroglial) cells are components of which of the following?
    1. Pars nervosa
    2. Pars distalis of the hypophysis
    3. Pineal gland
    4. Adrenal (suprarenal) medulla

12. A drug that interferes with mitosis would be likely to directly affect the division of:
    1. Metamyelocytes
    2. Myelocytes
    3. Normoblasts
    4. Polychromatophilic erythroblasts

13. Lymphatic nodules are found in the:
    1. Spleen

2. Lymph nodes
3. Ileum
4. Thymus

14. Which of the following statements about the respiratory system are true?
    1. Great alveolar (giant septal, pneumonocyte II) cells produce surfactant.
    2. Bronchioles possess elastic cartilage, which allows for expansion of bronchioles at inspiration.
    3. Respiratory bronchioles possess smooth muscle and alveoli.
    4. The true vocal cords (folds) and the rest of the larynx are lined by pseudostratified columnar epithelium.

15. Which of the following organs possess submucosal glands?
    1. Duodenum
    2. Fundus of the stomach
    3. Esophagus
    4. Colon

16. In which cell is/are there normally only 23 chromosomes (although there may be a normal diploid amount of DNA)?
    1. Parietal cell of the stomach
    2. Secondary spermatocyte
    3. Zygote
    4. An oocyte just after it is discharged from the ovary at ovulation

17. Which of the following statements about the liver is correct?
    1. Discontinuities in the sinusoidal epithelium permit passage of some substances between the lumen of the sinusoid and the perisinusoidal space of Disse.
    2. In the classical liver lobule bile flows toward the periphery, whereas a mixture of arterial and venous blood flows toward the center of the lobule.
    3. Hepatocytes constitute the walls of bile canaliculi.
    4. Hepatocytes possess both smooth and rough endoplasmic reticulum.

18. Following the administration of radioactive glucose, which of the following structures or substances would be labeled?
    1. The fuzz (glycocalyx) covering the free surface of the intestinal lining cell
    2. Colloid in the thyroid follicle
    3. Hyaline cartilage matrix
    4. Hepatocytes

19. Which one of the endocrine tissues listed below is correctly matched with a mechanism that is involved in the regulation of the production and/or release of the hormone produced by that tissue?
    1. Parathyroid–low levels of calcium in the blood
    2. Adrenal medulla–stimulation of preganglionic sympathetic neurons
    3. Pars distalis of hypophysis–releasing hormones that reach the pars distalis from hypothalamic neurons by way of the hypophyseal portal system
    4. Corpus luteum–placenta formation

20. Which of the following "cell–secretory product" combinations is/are correct?
    1. Plasma cell–circulating antibodies
    2. Mast cell–heparin
    3. Fibroblast–collagen precursor
    4. Enteroendocrine cell–serotonin

21. Which of the following "cell–secretory product" combinations is/are correct?
    1. Chief cell of the stomach–pepsinogen
    2. Acidophil of the pars distalis–growth hormone
    3. Zona glomerulosal cell of the adrenal gland–mineralocorticoids
    4. Parietal cell of the stomach–hydrochloric acid

22. A simple cuboidal or columnar epithelium with extensive basal infoldings of the plasma membrane is characteristically found in:
    1. Distal convoluted tubules of the kidney
    2. The lining epithelium of the small intestine
    3. Striated ducts of the parotid gland
    4. The lining epithelium of the oral cavity

23. Which of the following statements about the kidney is/are correct?
    1. The macula densa is a region of the distal tubule which is closely associated with an afferent glomerular arteriole.
    2. Collecting tubules are located in both the medulla and the cortex.
    3. Proximal convoluted tubules have an extensive microvillous (brush) border.
    4. Adjacent pedicels in the glomerulus are separated by a slit that is bridged by a very thin slit membrane.

24. Which of the following cells are correctly paired to its secretory product?
    1. Basophils of hypophysis–FSH (follicle-stimulating hormone)
    2. Oxyphil cells–parathyroid hormone
    3. Acidophils of hypophysis–prolactin (luteotropic hormone)
    4. Chromaffin cells of adrenal–aldosterone

25. Which of the following are target cells or target organs for the hormone indicated?
    1. Seminal vesicle–luteinizing hormone (LH)
    2. Prostate gland–testosterone
    3. Leydig cells–testosterone
    4. Sertoli cells–follicle-stimulating hormone (FSH)
26. Which of the following statements is/are correct for the testis?
    1. Some spermatogonia proliferate and remain as stem cells, while others differentiate into primary spermatocytes.
    2. The smooth endoplasmic reticulum of Leydig cells is essential for testosterone production.
    3. Sertoli cells help control passage of macromolecules to haploid cells.
    4. Secondary spermatocytes are usually plentiful, since they are relatively slow to divide into spermatids.
27. The luteal (secretory) phase of the menstrual cycle is characterized by:
    1. A coiling or sacculation of endometrial glands
    2. Relatively high amounts of progesterone in the blood plasma
    3. The presence of a functional corpus luteum
    4. Atresia of some ovarian follicles
28. In the membranous labyrinth of the ear:
    1. Maculae are receptors for position sense.
    2. Otoconia are components of the cristae.
    3. Efferent nerves end on some of the hair cells.
    4. Perilymph flow during head rotation produces forces on sensory hairs which cause them to fire nerve impulses.
29. Which of the following statements is/are correct for the eye?
    1. The inner nuclear layer of the retina contains the nuclei of bipolar cells, horizontal cells and amacrine cells.
    2. Aqueous humour passes, in sequence, through the posterior chamber, anterior chamber, trabecular meshwork (spaces of Fontana), canal of Schlemm, and veins.
    3. Light striking the retina (excluding the fovea centralis and the optic papilla) encounters in order: ganglion cells, bipolar cells, and rods and cones.
    4. The pathway of visual impulses in the retina is from rods and cones to bipolar cells, and from the latter to ganglion cells.
30. Bilateral destruction of the posterior white

column at spinal cord segment C5 might include a *loss* of:
    1. Two-point discrimination in both legs
    2. Vibratory sense in both hands
    3. Ability to identify objects placed in a patient's hands when the patient's hands are out of sight
    4. Appreciation of passive limb movements in the hands and feet
31. One month after ipsilateral destruction of the C3 through T3 dorsal root ganglia there would be ipsilateral:
    1. Anesthesia of the upper extremity
    2. Slight increase in deep tendon reflexes of the upper extremity
    3. Some nerve fiber degeneration in the medulla
    4. A complete dermatomal loss of sensation in only segments C6 to T1
32. Two months after complete destruction of the lateral funiculus in spinal cord segments C5 and C6 there would probably be:
    1. Ipsilateral hemiplegia
    2. Ipsilateral hypertonus at lower levels
    3. Absence of ipsilateral superficial (cutaneous) abdominal reflexes
    4. Ipsilateral exaggerated deep tendon reflexes
33. Two months after complete ipsilateral destruction of the ventral roots of the C5 through T1 spinal nerves, one would expect to find:
    1. Exaggerated myotatic (stretch) reflexes in the ipsilateral upper limb
    2. Flaccid paralysis of muscles in the ipsilateral upper limb
    3. Loss of superficial (cutaneous) abdominal reflexes
    4. Muscle atrophy in the ipsilateral upper limb
34. When an axon is damaged there is dispersal of Nissl material in the cell body (perikaryon) of the damaged neuron which is called chromatolysis. If the facial nerve was sectioned at its emergence from the brain stem, in which of the following would chromatolysis be present?
    1. Nucleus solitarius
    2. Geniculate ganglion
    3. Pterygopalatine ganglion
    4. Superior salivatory nucleus
35. A high medulla lesion involving the spinal tract and nucleus of the trigeminal nerve on one side could:

1. Produce some loss of sensation from the ipsilateral external auditory canal
2. Cause contralateral and ipsilateral loss of crude touch on the face
3. Produce some ipsilateral loss of pain on the anterior two thirds of the tongue
4. Cause a diminished jaw-jerk reflex

36. A tumor obliterating the right striate cortex above the calcarine fissure would result in:
    1. Damage to cells which receive impulses from both retinae by way of the lateral geniculate nucleus
    2. Left lower quadrantic anopsia
    3. A homonymous type of visual defect
    4. Chromatolysis of ganglion cells in the temporal half of the retina of the right eye

37. Which of the following structures are components of the hearing pathway?
    1. Superior olivary nucleus
    2. Inferior colliculus
    3. Medial geniculate body (nucleus)
    4. Lateral lemniscus

38. Destruction of the entire right tegmentum at the level of the facial colliculus would result in:
    1. Contralateral loss of pain and temperature in the trunk, extremities, and part of the face
    2. Complete contralateral loss of two-point touch in the trunk, extremities, and face
    3. Paralysis of conjugate lateral gaze to the right
    4. Positive Babinski reflex on the left

39. A lesion of the mesencephalic tegmentum, which destroys the left oculomotor nerve, left medial lemniscus, and left red nucleus and adjacent cerebellar efferents, could result in:
    1. Intention tremor in the right upper extremity
    2. Ptosis in the left eye
    3. Loss of touch on the right side of the body
    4. Loss of the consensual response in the pupillary light reflex when light is shone in the left eye

40. Which of the following "destroyed structure-signs and symptoms" combinations is/are correct?
    1. Destruction of the subthalamic nucleus–hemiballism
    2. Destruction of the left inferior parietal gyrus (area 39, angular gyrus)–apraxia
    3. Destruction of the postcentral gyrus–agnosia

4. Destruction of the supraoptic nucleus–diabetes insipidus

41. Which of the following lesions would produce the signs and symptoms indicated?
    1. A hemisection of the cord produces a contralateral loss of pain and temperature and an ipsilateral loss of two-point touch below the level of the lesion.
    2. Lesion of the vagus nerve near its emergence from the brain stem produces chromatolysis in the dorsal motor nucleus of the vagus and the nucleus ambiguus.
    3. Lesion of the hypoglossal nerve results in deviation of the tongue to the side of the lesion upon protrusion.
    4. Lesion of the inferior cerebellar peduncle causes chromatolysis in the ipsilateral nucleus dorsalis (Clarke's nucleus).

42. The location of the spinal nerve in the intervertebral foramen:
    1. Is at the level of the intervertebral disc in the cervical region
    2. Is above the level of the intervertebral disc in the lumbar region
    3. Is at the level of Luschka's joints in the lower cervical region
    4. Is at the level of the intervertebral disc in the lumbar region

43. With respect to the support provided by the ligaments of the vertebral column:
    1. The anterior longitudinal ligament resists flexion of the vertebral column.
    2. The posterior longitudinal ligament resists flexion of the vertebral canal.
    3. The interspinous ligaments resist extension of the vertebral column.
    4. The ligamenta flava resist flexion of the vertebral column.

44. With respect to the location of the ligaments of the vertebral column:
    1. The ligamenta flava interconnect the lamina of adjacent lamina.
    2. The anterior longitudinal ligament lines the anterior aspect of the vertebral column.
    3. The posterior longitudinal ligament attaches to the posterior aspects of the vertebral bodies.
    4. The anterior longitudinal ligament attaches to the pedicles of adjacent vertebrae.

45. The radial nerve:
    1. Passes posteriorly around the surgical neck of the humerus
    2. Passes ventral to the lateral aspect of the elbow joint

3. Passes medial to the biceps tendon in the cubital fossa
4. Passes around the neck of the radius

46. Which of the following is/are palpable in the anatomic snuff box?
   1. Scaphoid bone
   2. Median nerve
   3. Radial artery
   4. Pisiform bone

47. The integrity of which of the following nerves can be checked by testing the motions of the thumb?
   1. Median
   2. Ulnar
   3. Radial
   4. Musculocutaneous

48. The superficial palmar arterial arch:
   1. Is deep to the long flexor tendons
   2. Is superficial to the palmar aponeurosis
   3. Is proximal to the deep part of the flexor retinaculum
   4. Is at the same level (depth) as the common digital branches of the median nerve

49. MP flexion and IP extension of the index, middle, ring, and little fingers are produced by the
   1. Ventral interossei
   2. Lumbricals
   3. Doral interossei
   4. Flexor digitorum profundus

50. The ulnar nerve:
   1. Passes posterior to the medial epicondyle of the humerus
   2. Passes lateral to the pisiform
   3. Is deep to the flexor carpi ulnaris muscle in the forearm
   4. Passes superficial to the deep part of the flexor retinaculum

51. The median nerve:
   1. Is formed from both the medial and lateral cords of the brachial plexus
   2. Passes through the carpal tunnel
   3. Is medial to the brachial artery in the cubital fossa
   4. Is lateral to the tendon of the flexor carpi radialis muscle at the wrist

52. The musculocutaneous nerve:
   1. Passes deep to the brachialis muscle
   2. Passes through the coracobrachialis muscle
   3. Is the continuation of the medial cord of the brachial plexus
   4. Passes between the biceps and brachialis muscles

53. The capsule of the hip joint:
   1. Encloses the entire femoral neck
   2. Is reinforced by the iliofemoral, ischiofemoral, and pubofemoral ligaments
   3. Encloses the proximal two thirds of the femoral neck anteriorly
   4. Encloses the proximal two thirds of the femoral neck posteriorly

54. The transverse tarsal (midtarsal) joint is formed between the:
   1. Talus and navicular
   2. Talus and calcaneus
   3. Cuboid and calcaneus
   4. Navicular and cuboid

55. The lateral collateral ligament of the ankle extends between the lateral mallelus and the:
   1. Calcaneus
   2. Navicular
   3. Talus
   4. Cuboid

56. The femoral nerve:
   1. Passes deep to the inguinal ligament
   2. Contains fibers from spinal cord segments L2, 3, and 4.
   3. Innervates muscles which extend the knee
   4. Is medial to the femoral artery in the femoral triangle

57. The common peroneal nerve:
   1. Is the deepest structure in the popliteal fossa
   2. Passes around the neck of the fibula
   3. Innervates the major plantar flexors of the foot
   4. Is the most lateral nerve in the popliteal fossa

58. The tibial nerve:
   1. Innervates all of the intrinsic muscles of the plantar foot
   2. Enters the foot by passing behind the medial malleolus
   3. Passes through the median area of the popliteal fossa
   4. Innervates the muscles in the posterior compartment of the leg

59. The anterior cranial fossa is related to the:
   1. Orbit
   2. Nasal cavity
   3. Frontal sinus
   4. Ethmoid air cells

60. The lateral portion of the middle cranial fossa is related to the:
   1. Infratemporal fossa
   2. Middle ear cavity

3. Cavernous sinus
4. Orbit

61. The phrenic nerve:
    1. Contains fibers from spinal cord segments C3, 4, and 5
    2. Passes posterior to the root of the lung
    3. Provides the motor innervation to the skeletal muscle fibers of the respiratory diaphragm
    4. Contributes fibers to the cardiac plexus

62. The pterygopalatine fossa communicates with the:
    1. Middle cranial fossa by way of the foramen rotundum
    2. Nasal cavity by way of the sphenopalatine foramen
    3. Oral cavity by way of the palatine canal
    4. Orbit by way of the inferior orbital fissure

63. Regarding the openings of the paranasal sinuses:
    1. The anterior ethmoid air cells drain into the superior meatus of the nasal cavity.
    2. The maxillary sinus drains into the middle meatus of the nasal cavity.
    3. The frontal sinus drains into the inferior meatus of the nasal cavity.
    4. The sphenoid sinus drains into the sphenoethmoidal recess of the nasal cavity.

64. With respect to the areas or parts of the larynx:
    1. The glottis includes the true vocal folds plus the rima glottidis.
    2. The ventricle is a laterally extending pouch between the true and false folds.
    3. The vestibule and supraglottic portion are the same.
    4. The additis is the laryngeal entrance (from the pharynx).

65. Which of the following muscle-function pairs is/are correct?
    1. Cricothyroid–relaxation of vocal cords
    2. Posterior cricoarytenoid–abduction of vocal cords
    3. Lateral cricoarytenoid–abduction of vocal cords
    4. Transverse arytenoid–abduction of vocal cords

66. Relative to the heart:
    1. Its diaphragmatic surface is formed primarily by the right and left ventricles.
    2. Its posterior surface is formed predominantly by the right atrium.
    3. Its sternocostal surface is formed by portions of all four chambers of the heart.
    4. Its right border is formed by the right ventricle.

67. With respect to the relationships of the duodenum:
    1. Its first part is related posteriorly to the portal vein and common bile duct.
    2. Its second part is related medially to the head of the pancreas.
    3. Its third part is crossed anteriorly by the superior mesenteric vessels.
    4. Its third part is related posteriorly to the transverse colon.

68. The stomach is related:
    1. Posteriorly to the caudate lobe of the liver
    2. Anteriorly to the respiratory diaphragm
    3. Anteriorly to the splenic artery
    4. Posteriorly to the pancreas

69. The vermiform appendix:
    1. Usually arises from the large intestine just superior to the entrance of the ileum.
    2. Arises from the cecum at the termination of the taeniae coli
    3. Typically hangs into the (true) pelvic cavity
    4. Is usually retrocecal in position

70. The spleen
    1. Lies under ribs 9, 10, and 11 posteriorly
    2. Is related to the left kidney posteriorly
    3. Is related anteriorly to the stomach
    4. Is related to the right colic flexure

71. Pelvic splanchnic nerves:
    1. Contain preganglionic parasympathetic nerve fibers
    2. Contain fibers that innervate the gastrointestinal tract from the splenic flexure distally
    3. Contain fibers that arise from sacral spinal cord segments 2, 3, and 4.
    4. Contain the same type of efferent fibers as the lumbar splanchnic nerves

72. The portal vein is formed:
    1. Between the pancreas and the stomach
    2. By the union of the splenic and superior mesenteric veins
    3. By the junction of the superior and inferior mesenteric veins
    4. Posterior to the pancreas

73. The pudendal nerve:
    1. Arises from spinal cord segments S2, 3, and 4
    2. Passes through the pudendal canal
    3. Passes through the lesser sciatic foramen
    4. Passes through the greater sciatic foramen

74. The urogenital diaphragm:

1. Is found both anterior and posterior to the ischial tuberosities
2. Is oriented parallel to the sagittal plane
3. Is perforated by the urethra and anal canal
4. Extends between the ischiopubic rami
75. In the processes leading to protein synthesis:
    1. The genetic code is found in the nitrogenous base sequence of DNA.
    2. Messenger RNA molecules are transcribed from exposed nitrogenous bases of DNA.
    3. Both rRNA and tRNA are involved in translating the mRNA message.
    4. The tRNA places an amino acid directly into the rough endoplasmic reticulum.

ANSWERS TO MULTIPLE CHOICE QUESTIONS

Multiple Choice: One-Answer Type

1. b	12. c	23. a	34. b
2. d	13. b	24. a	35. b
3. c	14. c	25. d	36. c
4. d	15. d	26. c	37. c
5. b	16. a	27. c	38. a
6. d	17. a	28. b	39. c
7. d	18. a	29. a	40. d
8. d	19. c	30. a	41. a
9. b	20. b	31. b	42. d
10. c	21. c	32. c	43. c
11. a	22. c	33. d	44. b

45. c	53. b	61. c	69. d
46. c	54. d	62. c	70. a
47. c	55. a	63. c	71. c
48. b	56. b	64. d	72. d
49. b	57. c	65. d	73. d
50. d	58. a	66. d	74. a
51. a	59. d	67. a	75. b
52. d	60. b	68. a	

Multiple Choice: Possibly More Than One Answer

1. e	20. e	39. a	58. e
2. a	21. e	40. e	59. e
3. b	22. b	41. e	60. e
4. b	23. e	42. a	61. b
5. c	24. b	43. c	62. e
6. c	25. c	44. a	63. c
7. b	26. a	45. c	64. e
8. c	27. e	46. b	65. c
9. e	28. b	47. a	66. b
10. a	29. e	48. d	67. a
11. b	30. e	49. a	68. c
12. c	31. b	50. e	69. c
13. a	32. e	51. a	70. a
14. b	33. c	52. c	71. a
15. b	34. c	53. c	72. c
16. c	35. b	54. b	73. e
17. e	36. a	55. b	74. d
18. e	37. e	56. a	75. a
19. e	38. b	57. c	

3

Physiology

Arthur C. Guyton, M.D.
Chairman and Professor,
Department of Physiology and Biophysics,
University of Mississippi School of Medicine,
Jackson, Mississippi

Physiology is the study of function in living matter, and human physiology is specifically the study of function in the human being. This discipline attempts to answer such questions as: How do we live? How do we reproduce? How do we move about? How do we think? How do we see? And what are the basic physical and chemical principles upon which the intricate functions of the body are based?

BASIC ORGANIZATION OF THE BODY AND HOMEOSTASIS

The basic living unit of the body is the cell, of which there are about 75 trillion in the body. The cells are continually bathed in extracellular fluid, which is sometimes called the internal environment of the body. The constituents of this fluid are very exactly controlled, and, as long as they remain within normal range, each cell is capable of living as an individual unit and performing its respective tasks for the body. A very large portion of our discussion of human physiology will deal with this exact regulation of the constituents in the extracellular fluid; this is called *homeostasis,* which means simply maintenance of constant conditions in the internal environment.

FUNCTIONAL SYSTEMS OF THE BODY

The body can be divided into several major functional systems, each one of which performs a particular task in maintaining homeostasis as follows:

The ***cardiovascular system*** keeps the fluids of the internal environment continually mixed. It does this by pumping blood through the vascular system. As the blood passes through the capillaries, a large portion of its fluid diffuses back and forth into the interstitial fluid that lies between the cells.

The ***respiratory system*** provides oxygen for the body and removes carbon dioxide.

The ***gastrointestinal system*** provides the foods needed for cellular energy and for synthesis of new cellular and extracellular structures.

The ***kidneys*** provide a means for eliminating waste products left over after the chemical reactions in the cells have taken place. Most important among these are large quantities of urea, uric acid, creatinine, and nitrates. In addition to ridding the body of the unwanted end products of metabolism, the kidneys also regulate the concentrations of most of the extracellular fluid constituents including the concentrations of sodium, potassium, calcium, magnesium, chloride, bicarbonate, and phosphate ions. They also help to control the blood volume, volume of the extracellular fluid, and arterial pressure.

The ***nervous system*** directs the activity of the muscular system, thereby providing locomotion. It also controls the functions of many internal organs through the ***autonomic nervous system,*** and it allows us to be intelligent beings so that we can attain the most advantageous conditions for our survival.

The ***endocrine glands*** provide another regulatory system. Hormones secreted by these glands control many of the metabolic functions of the cells, such as growth, rate of metabolism, special cellular activities associated with reproduction, absorption and growth of bone, rate of glucose metabolism, and rate of amino acid metabolism.

The *reproductive system* provides for formation of new beings like ourselves; even this can be considered a homeostatic function, for it generates new bodies in which still trillions of more cells can exist in a well-regulated internal environment.

FUNCTION OF THE CELL

Cell Structure.   The cell is composed of two major parts: the *nucleus* and the *cytoplasm.* Surrounding the nucleus is a *nuclear membrane,* which is highly permeable, and surrounding the cytoplasm is a *cellular membrane* that is also permeable but much less so than the nuclear membrane. Both the nucleus and the cytoplasm are filled with a highly viscous fluid containing very large quantities of dissolved proteins, glucose, electrolytes, and many other substances. In addition there are many intracellular organelles, some of which we will discuss in the following paragraphs.

The most important structures of the nucleus are the 23 pairs of *chromosomes,* each of which contains several thousand *deoxyribose nucleic acids (DNAs)* that are the *genes* that regulate cellular function and reproduction.

The most conspicuous structures in the cytoplasm are the *mitochondria* and the *endoplasmic reticulum.* The mitochondria are usually elongated bodies sometimes larger than 1 micron in length and containing large quantities of oxidative and other enzymes that are responsible for supplying energy to the cells, as will be discussed below. The endoplasmic reticulum is a system of tubes and vesicles that connects with the nuclear membrane and spreads throughout the entire cytoplasm.

Energy Release in the Cell—Function of the Mitochondria.   An adequate supply of energy must always be available to energize the chemical reactions of the cells. This is provided principally by the chemical reaction of oxygen with any one of three different types of foods: glucose derived from carbohydrates, fatty acids derived from fats, and amino acids derived from proteins. On entering the cell the food molecules are split into still smaller molecules that in turn enter the mitochondria where still other enzymes remove carbon dioxide and hydrogen atoms in a process called the *citric acid cycle.* Then an oxidative enzyme system, also in the mitochondria, causes progressive oxidation of the hydrogen atoms. The end products of the reactions

in the mitochondria are water and carbon dioxide, and the energy liberated is used by the mitochondria to synthesize still another substance, *adenosine triphosphate (ATP),* a very highly reactive chemical that can diffuse throughout the cell and provide almost instantaneous energy for any cellular process that requires it.

Endoplasmic Reticulum—Synthesis of Multiple Substances in the Cell.   Most cells contain a vast network of tubes and vesicles that penetrates all portions of the cytoplasm. This network is called the endoplasmic reticulum. The membrane of the endoplasmic reticulum is an extensive manufacturing plant for multiple substances that are used inside the cell and that are excreted from some cells. These substances include proteins, carbohydrates, lipids, and structures such as lysosomes, peroxisomes, and secretory granules.

The membranes of the endoplasmic reticulum perform the synthetic processes, and many of the substances that are formed are transported in the tubules and vesicles of the endoplasmic reticulum to other parts of the cell. For the synthesis of proteins, *ribosomes* attach to the outer surface of the endoplasmic reticulum; these function in association with *messenger RNA* to synthesize many protein molecules that then enter the endoplasmic reticulum where the molecules are further modified before release for use in the cell.

Lysosomes.   An organelle found in great numbers in all cells of the body is the lysosome. This is a small spherical vesicle surrounded by a membrane and containing digestive enzymes. The enzymes are used by the cell for various digestive purposes. For instance, when bacteria or other substances are phagocytized by cells, digestive enzymes from the lysosomes digest the phagocytized particles. Also, when cells become damaged, enzymes from lysosomes can digest the damaged portions of the cells and remove these. Finally, when tissues are no longer used for their normal functions, they frequently undergo atrophy. Lysosomes in the cells cause this atrophy by digesting portions of the cellular mass.

Regulation of Protein Synthesis in the Cell by the Genes.   Proteins are the basis of almost all the functions that occur in the cells for two reasons: (1) all of the enzymes that catalyze the chemical reactions of the cells are proteins, and (2) most of the important physical structures of the cell contain structural proteins.

The genes control protein synthesis in the cell and in this way control cell function. Each gene is a double stranded helical molecule of deoxyribose nucleic acid, called DNA, and it is composed of multiple units of (a) the sugar deoxyribose, (b) phosphoric acid, and (c) four bases of different types (two purines, *adenine* and *guanine,* and two pyrimidines, *thymine* and *cytosine*). It is the sequence of bases in one of the two strands in this molecule that control the type of protein synthesized. These bases are held together in the long helical molecule by the deoxyribose and the phosphoric acid. The sequence of bases is different for each type of gene, and it is this sequence that determines the properties of each individual gene.

The Genetic Code. Each three successive bases in the strand of the DNA molecule is called a *code word* and these code words control the sequence of amino acids in a protein to be formed in the cytoplasm. One code word might be composed of adenine, thymine, and guanine, while the next code word might have a sequence of cytosine, guanine and thymine. These two code words have entirely different meanings because their bases are different. The sequence of successive code words on the DNA molecule is known as the *genetic code.*

Ribose Nucleic Acid (RNA) and Its Role in the Formation of Protein in the Cytoplasm. The deoxyribose nucleic acid molecule that makes up the gene controls the formation of a similar molecule called a *ribose nucleic acid* molecule (RNA). This molecule is composed of the sugar ribose, phosphoric acid and four different bases (the same bases as those found in DNA except that thymine is replaced by uracil). Thus, this molecule is very similar to the DNA molecule. When the DNA molecule of the gene causes formation of the RNA molecule, it transfers its code to the RNA molecule by controlling the sequence of bases in the RNA molecule. This control of RNA formation by DNA is called *transcription* because the code of the DNA is "transcribed" onto the RNA.

During the transcription process, the two strands of DNA that make up the DNA molecule pull apart from each other. One of these strands then serves as the gene and attracts to it the necessary chemicals that form the RNA molecule. The four separate bases that are part of the building blocks of the DNA molecule are mutually attractive to four complementary bases that subsequently become part of the RNA molecule (quanine attracts cytosine; cytosine attracts quinine; adenine attracts uracil; thymine attracts adenine). Thus, the code formed in the RNA molecule is a complementary code to that of the gene DNA strand. All of this takes place in the nucleus; then the synthesized RNA molecule diffuses outward from the nucleus into the cyto-

plasm where it then functions in the synthesis of a specific cell protein.

Three different types of RNA molecules are formed: (1) ribosomal RNA, (2) transfer RNA, and (3) messenger RNA. All three diffuse from the cell nucleus through the nuclear membrane into the cytoplasm, where each plays a specific role in the manufacture of protein.

Ribosomal RNA becomes a major constituent of the small particles called ribosomes. Protein molecules are then manufactured by these ribosomes.

There are 20 separate types of *transfer RNA molecules,* each one of which combines specifically with one of the 20 different amino acids and conducts this amino acid to the ribosome, where it is combined into the protein molecule.

Messenger RNA carries the genetic code that determines the sequence in which successive amino acids will be arranged in the protein molecule. Messenger RNA is a single-stranded, long molecule, having a succession of *codons* along its axis. These codons are mirror images of the code words in the gene DNA, and they also consist of three successive bases. To manufacture protein molecules, one end of the RNA strand enters the ribosome, and the entire strand then threads its way through the ribosome in a little over a minute. As it passes through, the ribosome "reads" the genetic code and causes the proper succession of amino acids to bind together by chemical bonds called peptide linkages, which will be discussed later in the chapter. Actually, the messenger RNA does not recognize the different types of amino acids but instead recognizes the different transfer RNA molecules. However, each transfer RNA molecule carries only one specific type of amino acid; one can well understand that it is that type of amino acid that will be incorporated into the protein.

To recapitulate, as the strand of messenger RNA passes through the ribosome, each one of its codons draws to it a specific transfer RNA that in turn delivers a specific amino acid. This amino acid then combines with the preceding amino acid, the sequence continuing to build until an entire protein molecule is formed. At this point a special codon appears that states the process is complete, and the protein is released into the cytoplasm or through the membrane of the endoplasmic reticulum into the interior of this reticulum. This control of amino acid sequencing by the RNA code during protein formation is called *translation.*

It is believed that there are about 100,000 different types of genes in the nucleus; thus one can well understand that a multitude of different types of proteins can also be formed in each cell. The character of each cell depends on the relative proportions of the types of proteins that are formed. In essence, then, the genes control the structure of the cell through the types of structural proteins formed, and the genes also control the functions of the cell mainly through the types of protein enzymes that are formed.

Differentiation of Cells. During the course of development of the human being from the fertilized ovum, the ovum divides again and again until trillions of cells are formed. However, the new cells gradually differentiate from each other, certain cells attaining one set of genetic characteristics while other cells attain other characteristics. This differentiation process occurs as a result of inactivation of certain of the genes and activation of others during successive stages of cellular division. This results in widely different functions in different cells.

Cellular Reproduction. Most cells of the body, with the exception of mature red blood cells, striated muscle cells, and neurons in the nervous system, are capable of reproducing other cells of their own type. Ordinarily, if sufficient nutrients are available, each cell grows larger and larger until at a certain point it automatically divides by the process of *mitosis* to form two new cells. Before mitosos occurs, all the genes in the nucleus, as well as the chromosomes carrying the genes, are themselves reproduced to create a completely new set of genes. During mitosis one set of genes enters one of the daughter cells while the other set enters the second daughter cell. Thus, not only are the physical characteristics of the two new cells alike, but they are still controlled by the same types of genes so that their functions will also be very similar. If, during the process of reproduction, one or more of the genes fails to be reproduced or becomes suppressed, then the two new cells will not be exactly alike, and the cells will become slightly differentiated from each other.

THE BODY FLUIDS

Total Body Water: Extracellular and Intracellular Fluid. Approximately 57% of the adult body is water. In the normal adult, this amounts to a *total body water* of approximately 40 liters. This can be divided into two major compartments: the *extracellular fluid,* which has a volume of about 15 liters, and the *intracellular fluid,* which has a volume of about 25 liters. The extracellular fluid is continually mixed by the circulatory system, and it is called the *internal environment* of the body. Because of this mixing, its constituents are relatively uniform in all parts of the body. Frequently, it is desirable to divide the extracellular fluid into two subcompartments: the *plasma,* which is part of the blood and amounts to approximately 3 liters, and the *interstitial fluid,* which lies between the tissue cells and amounts to approximately 12 liters.

Though the intracellular fluids are not identical in all the different cells, they are sufficiently similar so that it is usually reasonable to consider them together as one large compartment of homogeneous fluid.

Comparison of Extracellular and Intracellular Fluid. Figure 3-1 shows the concentrations of the most important substances in both the extracellular and intracellular fluids. Both of these fluids contain nutrients that are needed by the cells, including glucose, amino acids, cholesterol, phospholipids, neutral fat, oxygen, and others not illustrated in the figure. Some of the food substances are present in higher concentrations in the intracellular fluid than in the extracellular fluid because of specific concentrating abilities of the cell membranes.

A major difference between the extracellular and the intracellular fluids is in the electrolytes. Extracellular fluid contains large quantities of sodium and chloride ions but only small quantities of potassium, magnesium and phosphate ions. On the other hand,

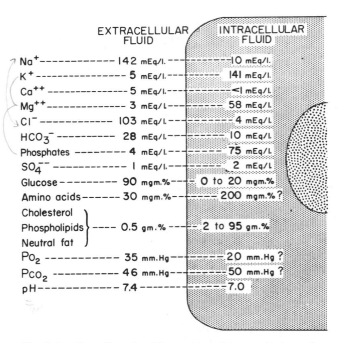

Fig. 3-1. Constituents of the extracellular and intracellular fluids. (Guyton AC: Textbook of Medical Physiology, 7th ed. Philadelphia, WB Saunders, 1986)

intracellular fluid contains very large quantities of these latter ions, potassium, magnesium, and phosphate, but very few sodium and chloride ions. Also extracellular fluid contains small quantities of calcium ions, but intracellular fluid contains almost none. These differences in the fluids cause a membrane potential to develop between the two sides of the membrane—negative on the inside and positive outside. Later in the chapter we shall see how this potential develops and the manner in which it changes during the transmission of nerve and muscle impulses.

The Fluid of the Blood. The fluid of the blood is actually a composite of about 2 liters intracellular fluid inside the blood cells and 3 liters extracellular fluid in the plasma.

The plasma is almost identical with the interstitial fluid except that it contains dissolved **plasma proteins** in a concentration of about 7% in comparison with an average protein concentration in the interstitial fluid of 2% to 3%.

EXCHANGE OF FLUID AND ELECTROLYTES THROUGH THE CELL MEMBRANE

Structure of the Cell Membrane. The cell membrane is composed basically of a lipid matrix containing mainly phospholipids, cholesterol, and triglycerides. However, it also contains many large protein molecules that protrude all the way through the membrane. Channels through the structures of the protein molecules serve as many minute pores in the membrane.

Diffusion Through the Cell Membrane. Many substances pass through the cell membrane, back and forth between the extracellular and the intracellular fluids, by the process of **diffusion.** Diffusion means simply **random motion of molecules.** That is, all molecules in liquids and gases are continually moving among each other, bouncing first one way and then another. A few substances can diffuse directly through the lipid matrix of the cell membrane. This is especially true for water molecules because these are so small and have so much energy that they can force their way between the lipid molecules. This also includes substances that are soluble in the lipid membrane, such as fats, carbon dioxide, and oxygen.

The various ions and large molecules such as glucose can enter and leave the cells only through the channels formed in the membrane by protein molecules that extend all the way through the membrane. Figure 3-2 illustrates two protein molecules protruding through the cell membrane. The one to the right is a typical membrane protein with a trans-

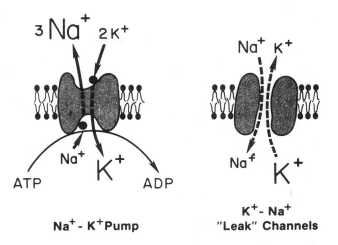

Na⁺ - K⁺ Pump   K⁺- Na⁺ "Leak" Channels

Fig. 3-2. Protein molecules protruding through the cell membrane, showing to the right an open channel and to the left a pump mechanism for pumping sodium and potassium ions. (Guyton AC: Textbook of Medical Physiology, 7th ed. Philadelphia, WB Saunders, 1986)

port channel through its molecular interstices. Depending upon various conditions of the cells, some of these channels are at times wide open and allow rapid diffusion of specific substances. However, at other times the channels are closed, and diffusion is greatly decreased. Thus, the opening and closing of these channels is a means by which movement of many substances through the cell membrane can be controlled, as we shall discuss more fully later in this chapter.

The net amount of each substance that will diffuse through the cell membrane depends not only on the permeability of the membrane for the substance but also on the relative concentrations of the substances on the two sides of the membrane. If the concentration difference is very great, the net movement of the substance will also be greatly increased from the area of high concentration toward the area of low concentration.

Facilitated Diffusion. Many substances are transported through the cell membrane by a process called facilitated diffusion, in which the substance combines chemically with a carrier in the cell membrane and is transported in combination with this carrier to the opposite side and then released. The carrier is either always or almost always one of the protein molecules that penetrates through the cell membrane; the substance is probably transported through the structure of the protein molecule itself.

The most important substance transmitted through cell membranes by the process of facilitated diffusion is glucose. Insulin greatly increases this facilitated transport of glucose.

Active Transport Through the Cell Membrane. Active transport is similar to facilitated diffusion in that the substance to be transported combines with a carrier and is released from the carrier on the opposite side of the membrane. However, active transport causes movement of the substance in only one direction. Also, it can transport the substance even when the concentration of the substance is greater on the side to which it is being transported than on the other side. To achieve those characteristics of active transport that are different from facilitated diffusion, especially the transport of substances "uphill" against a concentration gradient or against an electrical potential gradient, requires energy. This energy is supplied by the high-energy compound adenosine triphosphate (ATP) or by some other similar high-energy phosphate compound inside the cell.

The most important active transport system in the body is that for active transport of sodium out of cells and potassium into cells, which is called the sodium–potassium pump. This pump is illustrated to the left in Figure 3-2. The protein structure of the pump serves both as the carrier and as the energy transferring mechanism for moving the sodium and potassium ions between the extracellular and intracellular fluids. This pump pumps sodium out of the cells and causes the concentration of sodium inside the cells to become very low and its concentration in the extracellular fluids very high. At the same time it pumps potassium into the cells, causing the intracellular potassium concentration to build up to a very high level. It is this sodium–potassium pump that maintains most of the ionic concentration differences between the intracellular and the extracellular fluids and therefore is extremely important for function of nerve and muscle fibers, as will be described later in the chapter.

Other active transport systems include amino acid transport to the interior of cells and transport of large numbers of ions such as sodium, potassium, hydrogen, calcium, magnesium, and phosphate through the renal tubular and gastrointestinal epithelial membranes.

OSMOTIC PRESSURE AND OSMOTIC EQUILIBRIA AT THE CELL MEMBRANE

Osmosis. Water molecules pass through the cell membrane at least 100 times as easily as almost any other substance in the body fluids. Because of this, any time an excess concentration of less permeant substances occurs on either side of the membrane, water is forced by osmosis through the membrane; this can be explained as follows:

The presence of dissolved substances in a water solution reduces the concentration of water molecules in the fluid. Therefore, if such a solution is placed on one side of the cell membrane while pure water is placed on the other side, more water molecules will diffuse from the pure water, which has a high water concentration, through the membrane than from the solution which has a lower water concentration. As a result, an excess of water molecules will pass continuously from the pure water into the solution; this is osmosis.

Osmotic Pressure. If pressure is applied across a membrane through which osmosis is occurring, but with the pressure applied in the direction opposite to the osmotic flow, the osmosis can be slowed or even stopped. The amount of pressure that is required to stop the osmosis is called the osmotic pressure.

The normal concentration of osmotically active substances in the body fluids is great enough that if these fluids should be placed on one side of a cell membrane and pure water on the other side, the amount of osmotic pressure across the membrane would be approximately 5400 mm Hg, which is more than 50 times as great as the arterial blood pressure of the human being. Obviously, pure water never exists in the normal person on either side of the cell membrane, but occasionally the concentrations of the extracellular and the intracellular fluids do differ slightly. When this occurs, small amounts of osmotic pressure develop immediately across the membrane and cause water to move through the membrane, diluting the concentrated fluid and concentrating the dilute fluid until their concentrations become equal. Therefore, except for a few seconds at a time the extracellular and the intracellular fluids remain continuously in osmotic equilibrium with each other.

Isotonicity, Hypotonicity, and Hypertonicity. A solution is said to be *isotonic* if no osmotic force develops across the cell membrane when a normal cell is placed in the solution.

A solution is said to be *hypotonic* if the osmotic concentration of substances in the solution is less than their concentration in the cell. An osmotic force develops immediately when the cell is exposed to the solution, causing water to flow by osmosis into the cell; within less than a minute the cell swells until it either bursts or its fluids become diluted sufficiently to equal the concentration of the hypotonic solution.

A solution is said to be *hypertonic* when it contains a higher osmotic concentration of substances than does the cell. In this case an osmotic force develops that causes water to flow out of the cell into the solution, thereby greatly concentrating the intracellular fluid and markedly shrinking the cell.

Fluid Therapy. When fluid is administered to a patient, it is generally injected into the bloodstream or is absorbed into the blood from the gastrointestinal tract, and it immediately becomes part of the extracellular fluid. If the fluid is very hypotonic, large portions of the water in the fluid will pass by osmosis into the cells. If it is very hypertonic, it will draw large amounts of the intracellular water out of the cells, thereby shrinking the cells.

Dehydration means loss of water from the body. If pure water is lost, such as by evaporation from the respiratory tract or from the surfaces of the skin, this will concentrate both the extracellular and the intracellular fluids. However, if pure extracellular fluid, or fluid very similar to extracellular fluid, is lost from the body, as occasionally occurs in different types of kidney disease or when a person sweats profusely, the fluid loss at first will be mainly from the extracellular compartment without affecting the intracellular fluid.

EXCHANGE OF FLUIDS THROUGH THE CAPILLARY MEMBRANES

Diffusion Between the Plasma and the Interstitial Fluid. The capillaries are porous structures with several million slits or pores (the widths of which are about 8 nm) to each square centimeter of capillary surface. As the blood flows through the capillaries, very large quantities of dissolved substances diffuse in both directions through these "pores." In this way sodium, chloride, potassium, glucose, and almost all other dissolved substances in the plasma continually mix with the interstitial fluid. The rate of diffusion is so great that even cells as far as 50 microns away from the capillaries can still receive adequate quantities of nutrients.

Capillary Pressure. The blood inside the capillaries is under a considerable amount of pressure, averaging about 17 mmHg. This tends to cause fluid to leak out the pores of the capillaries into the interstitial fluid. Fortunately, however, the colloid osmotic pressure of the plasma proteins, which will be discussed below, prevents this loss of fluid and thereby helps to maintain the blood volume at a normal value essentially all of the time.

Colloid Osmotic Pressure of the Proteins. In the above discussion of osmosis and osmotic pres-

sure, it was pointed out that essentially all dissolved substances in the extracellular and the intracellular fluids cause osmotic effects at the cellular pores. However, capillary pores are far larger than cellular pores, so that only the dissolved proteins are large enough that they fail to pass to any significant extent through these pores. Since osmotic pressure is proportional to the percentage of molecules that fail to pass through the membrane, and since the total number of dissolved protein molecules is relatively small, the osmotic pressure of the plasma at the capillary membrane is only 28 mmHg, some 200 times less than the osmotic pressure that occurs at the cell membrane. Therefore, to distinguish the osmotic pressure at the capillary membrane from that at the cell membrane, the capillary osmotic pressure is called *oncotic pressure* or *colloid osmotic pressure,* because protein solutions look like colloidal solutions even though they are not. The osmotic pressure at the cell membranes is frequently called *total osmotic pressure.*

Starling's Equilibrium of the Capillaries. The capillary pressure tends to push fluid out of the capillaries, while the plasma colloid osmotic pressure tends to move fluid in. Furthermore, the pressure in the tissue spaces outside the capillaries, the *interstitial fluid pressure,* can push fluid inward if it is positive, and the protein in the interstitial fluids can cause *tissue fluid colloid osmotic pressure* on the outside of the capillaries, which tends to move fluid out of the capillaries. To determine whether or not fluid will actually move inward through the membrane or outward, one adds the inward forces and the outward forces and determines which are the greater. On the average, these two remain almost exactly equal, so that there is no net loss or gain in either blood or interstitial fluid volume. This balance between the inward and the outward forces is called Starling's *equilibrium of the capillaries,* and it can be stated mathematically as follows:

Capillary pressure + tissue fluid colloid osmotic pressure = interstitial fluid pressure + plasma colloid osmotic pressure

The normal values for these different pressures are the following:

Capillary pressure, 17 mmHg
Tissue fluid colloid osmotic pressure, 6 mmHg
Plasma colloid osmotic pressure, 28 mmHg
Interstitial fluid pressure, −5 mmHg

Note particularly that the normal interstitial fluid pressure is negative rather than positive. Putting these values into the above equation yields:

$$17 + 6 = -5 + 28$$

or

$$23 = 23$$

Thus, the forces that tend to move fluid into or out of the capillary wall are normally almost exactly balanced. (Actually, there is usually a fraction of a millimeter of mercury greater pressure tending to move fluid outward, which is what causes the formation of lymph, as we shall discuss later.)

Edema. The collection of excess interstitial fluid between the cells is known as edema. The normal negative interstitial fluid pressure keeps the cells pulled tightly together because fluid is continually pumped away from the tissues through the lymphatics. However, on occasion the interstitial fluid pressure becomes positive, which causes the interstitial fluid now to push the cells apart and cause edema. Thus, abnormalities that cause the interstitial fluid pressure to rise from its negative value into a positive range will cause edema. These include (1) *increased capillary pressure,* which can result from obstruction of a vein, excess flow of blood from the arteries into the capillaries, excess blood volume, or failure of the heart to pump blood rapidly out of the veins into the arterial system; (2) *decreased plasma colloid osmotic pressure,* which can result from failure of the liver to produce sufficient quantities of plasma proteins, loss of large quantities of proteins into the urine in certain kidney diseases, or loss of large quantities of proteins through burned areas of the skin or other denuding lesions; (3) *increased capillary permeability,* which allows excessive leakage of fluids and plasma proteins through the membranes—a number of allergic, bacterial, and toxic diseases, including especially anaphylaxis and *Clostridium nouyi* infection, cause this type of damage to the capillaries; and (4) *excessive quantities of proteins in the interstitial fluids,* which will draw fluid out of the plasma into the tissue spaces because of high tissue colloid osmotic pressure—this results most frequently from lymphatic blockage, which prevents the return of proteins from the interstitial spaces to the blood, as will be discussed in the section below.

LYMPHATIC SYSTEM

The lymphatics are a system of accessory vessels, illustrated in Figure 3-3, that accompany the blood vessels to almost all parts of the body. Minute *lymphatic capillaries,* like the blood capillaries, are found in almost all tissues; these lead into progres-

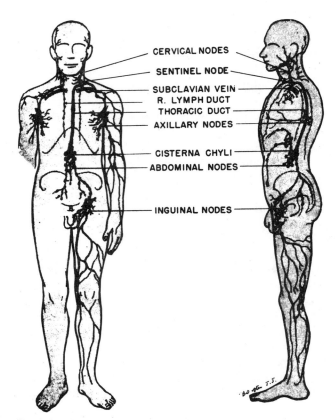

Fig. 3-3. The lymphatic system. (Guyton AC: Textbook of Medical Physiology, 7th ed. Philadelphia, WB Saunders, 1986)

sively larger lymphatic channels that finally converge mainly on the *thoracic duct,* which passes upward through the chest and empties into the venous system at the juncture of the internal jugular and subclavian veins. The lymphatic capillaries are so permeable that bacteria, various types of debris in the interstitial fluids, and large protein molecules can enter the lymph with great ease.

Lymph. Lymph is actually interstitial fluid that flows out of the interstitial spaces into the lymphatic capillaries. Therefore, its constituents are almost identical with those of the interstitial fluid. Most lymph from the peripheral tissues contains a concentration of approximately 2 g per 100 ml of protein, while that from the liver contains a concentration of about 6 g per 100 ml, and that from the intestines about 4 g per 100 ml. Since the liver produces far more lymph in proportion to its weight than any other tissue of the body, the thoracic lymph has a protein concentration of about 4 g per 100 ml.

Control of Lymph Flow. Two major factors control the rate of lymph flow: (1) the interstitial fluid pressure and (2) the rate at which the lymphatics pump. The greater the volume of fluid in the tissue spaces, the greater becomes the interstitial fluid pressure. This, in turn, promotes increased flow of fluid into the lymphatic capillaries through their large openings. Once in the lymphatic capillaries, the fluid is pumped by intermittent compression of the lymphatic vessels. The compression results either from contraction of the lymphatic walls or from external compression of the lymph vessels by contracting muscles, joint movement or any other effect that compresses the tissues. The lymphatics contain valves that allow flow to occur only away from the tissues and toward the blood stream. Therefore, during each compression cycle of a lymphatic vessel, fluid is pumped progressively along the vessel toward the circulation.

Removal of Bacteria and Debris from the Tissues by the Lymphatic System—Filtration by the Lymph Nodes. Because of the very high degree of permeability of the lymphatic capillaries, bacteria and any other type of very small particulate matter in the tissues can pass into the lymph. However, the lymph passes through a series of lymph nodes on its way to the blood. In these nodes the bacteria and other debris are filtered out, then phagocytized by macrophages in the nodes and finally digested into amino acids, glucose, fatty acids, and other small molecular substances before being released into the body fluids.

Removal of Protein From the Interstitial Fluid by the Lymphatic System. Because of their large molecular size, most proteins that leak out of the blood capillaries into the interstitial fluids cannot pass back into the blood capillaries. After these collect in the interstitial fluid and become progressively more and more concentrated, they finally flow into the lymphatic system and are returned to the bloodstream in this way. Approximately one half of all the protein in the blood leaks into the interstitial spaces each day, and were it not for its return by the lymph to the blood, a person would lose most of the plasma colloid osmotic pressure within a few hours and would no longer be able to maintain normal blood volume. Therefore, this return of protein from the interstitial spaces to the blood is probably the single most important function of the lymphatic system.

SPECIAL FLUID SYSTEMS OF THE BODY

Cerebrospinal Fluid System. The ventricles of the brain and the subarachnoid spaces around the brain are filled with *cerebrospinal fluid,* which is a special type of extracellular fluid. The brain and the spinal cord actually float in this fluid, and it cushions the nervous system against blows to the skull or the spine.

Approximately 500 ml of cerebrospinal fluid are secreted each day by the choroid plexuses in the four ventricles of the brain. This fluid then flows from the ventricular system into the subarachnoid space surrounding the cerebellum, then upward around the entire brain to be absorbed through many minute arachnoidal villi into the venous blood of the dural sinuses.

If the flow of cerebrospinal fluid is blocked at any point along its course from the choroid plexuses to the arachnoidal granulations, the fluid volume in at least part of the cerebrospinal system increases, causing *hydrocephalus,* which means simply "water in the head." The excess fluid can be inside the ventricles, in the subarachnoid space around the brain, or in both regions. Hydrocephalus can also result from excessive secretion of cerebrospinal fluid by the choroid plexus.

Ocular Fluid System. The fluid in the eyes keeps the eyeballs stretched, thereby maintaining normal dimensions between the optical elements. The fluid behind the lens is mainly a gelatinous mass called the *vitreous humor,* while the fluid lying to the side and in front of the lens is a freely flowing fluid called the *aqueous humor.* Aqueous humor is continually secreted by many ciliary processes on the surface of the ciliary body that lies inside the eye circling all the way around the lens. It then flows anteriorly through the pupillary opening and is absorbed continually into the canal of Schlemm, which lies in the sclera beneath the iridocorneal angle.

The pressure in the eyeball is regulated principally by the rate of fluid absorption into the canal of Schlemm. The pressure normally remains almost exactly 15 mmHg, but any disease that blocks normal absorption of fluid from the anterior chamber into the canal of Schlemm causes this pressure to rise. Excessive rise of pressure—to 25 mmHg to 70 mmHg—is called *glaucoma;* this can cause either slow or rapid development of blindness. The blindness results from compression of the blood vessels that supply the retina with nutrients.

Potential Fluid Spaces. A potential fluid space is one that normally contains little or no fluid but under abnormal conditions can accumulate very large quantities of fluid. These spaces include: the pleural space, the pericardial space, the peritoneal cavity, the joint spaces, and the bursae. In general, the membranes lining these spaces are very highly permeable so that the spaces communicate freely with the surrounding interstitial fluid spaces. Ordinarily, the tendency for absorption of fluid from the spaces is greater than the tendency for filtration of fluid into the spaces, and this keeps them almost completely empty except for a small amount of highly viscid fluid that lubricates the movement of the surfaces against each other. However, the same conditions that cause edema in the interstitial spaces can also cause fluid to collect in the potential spaces. These include (1) high capillary pressure, (2) low plasma colloid osmotic pressure, (3) increased capillary permeability, and (4) increased colloid osmotic pressure of the fluid in the space.

An especially important cause of large quantities of fluid in a potential space is infection. This causes large amounts of white blood cells and tissue debris to appear in the space, and these in turn occlude or partially occlude the lymphatic drainage from the space. As a result, large quantities of proteins collect, building up the colloid osmotic pressure to a point that excessive quantities of fluids are drawn by osmosis into the spaces. Such an infected fluid is called an **exudate,** while fluid that collects simply because of abnormal capillary dynamics is called a **transudate.**

KIDNEYS

FORMATION OF URINE BY THE KIDNEYS

Nephron. The functional unit of the kidney is the **nephron,** and there are approximately 2 million nephrons in the two kidneys. The functional parts of the nephron are illustrated in Figure 3-4. Each nephron is composed of a tuft of capillaries called the **glomerulus,** a capsule around the glomerulus called **Bowman's capsule,** and a series of **tubules** that lead from Bowman's capsule to the **renal pelvis.** Blood flows into each glomerulus through an **afferent arteriole** and leaves it through an **efferent arteriole,** finally flowing into a system of **peritubular capillaries** that surround the tubules.

Rate of Blood Flow Through the Kidneys. Approximately 1200 ml of blood flow through the two kidneys each minute, representing 20% to 25% of the total cardiac output.

Glomerular Filtration. The normal pressure in the glomerulus is probably about 60 mmHg, and the colloid osmotic pressure of the plasma proteins in the glomerulus averages about 32 mmHg. (This is slightly greater than the colloid osmotic pressure in other capillaries of the body because excessively large quantities of fluid are filtered through the glomerular capillaries, thereby concentrating the pro-

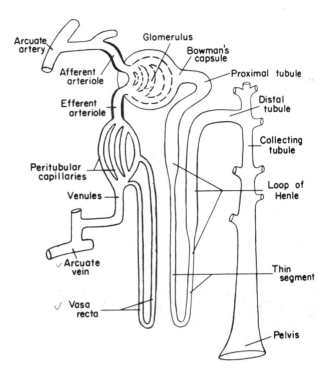

Fig. 3-4. The functional nephron. (Guyton AC: Textbook of Medical Physiology, 7th ed. Philadelphia, WB Saunders, 1986)

teins.) The pressure in Bowman's capsule on the outside of the capillaries is approximately 18 mmHg. The glomerular pressure tends to force fluid out of the capillaries, while the plasma colloid osmotic pressure and the pressure in Bowman's capsule tend to keep fluid from leaving the glomerulus. Therefore, the net force, called the **filtration pressure,** is equal to glomerular pressure minus both plasma colloid osmotic pressure and Bowman's capsule pressure. The normal filtration pressure, therefore, is 60 minus 32 minus 18, or 10 mmHg. This can be greatly altered in several ways: (1) by increasing the arterial pressure, which concomitantly increases the glomerular pressure; (2) by dilation of the afferent arterioles, which allows increased flow of blood into the glomerulus; (3) by constriction of the efferent arterioles, which impedes outflow of blood from the glomerulus; or (4) by decreasing plasma colloid osmotic pressure.

The total rate of fluid filtration from all glomeruli of both kidneys is about 125 ml per minute; this is called the **glomerular filtration rate.** This rate varies directly in proportion with the filtration pressure.

The **glomerular filtrate** is an ultrafiltrate of plasma having a composition almost identical to that of plasma except that it has almost no protein (only 0.03%).

The Renal Tubules and Tubular Reabsorption.
The renal tubular system is divided into four separate portions: (1) the proximal tubules, (2) the loops of Henle, (3) the distal tubules, and (4) the collecting ducts. As the glomerular filtrate (approximately 125 ml per minute) passes progressively down this tubular system, 124 ml are normally reabsorbed into the blood so that only 1 ml passes into the urine. About 60% is absorbed in the proximal tubules, 20% in the loops of Henle, 15% in the distal tubules, and 5% in the collecting ducts. Thus, one sees that most of the reabsorption occurs in the early portion of the tubular system.

The proximal tubules function specifically to conserve many substances that are needed by the body. For instance, all of the glucose, amino acids, acetoacetic acid, and proteins that are present in the glomerular filtrate are completely reabsorbed in the proximal tubules. Also approximately 60% of the sodium, potassium, and other electrolytes are reabsorbed. On the other hand, the proximal tubules are relatively impermeable to the waste products of the body.

In the loops of Henle a small amount of additional water and most of the remaining sodium and other electrolytes are reabsorbed, leaving about 4% of the electrolytes and 18% of the water. This ability of the loops of Henle to reabsorb most of the electrolytes plays a very important role in the ability of the kidney to dilute or to concentrate urine, as will be discussed later.

Reabsorption of fluid and dissolved substances in the distal tubules and collecting ducts is quite variable—here the kidney plays its major role in controlling concentrations of various substances in the body fluids. Thus, if the concentration of sodium is very high in the body fluids, very little sodium will be reabsorbed in the distal tubules, so that large amounts of sodium will be lost into the urine. This mechanism, as well as the control mechanisms for other electrolytes, will be discussed at greater length later.

The collecting ducts collect fluid from a large number of distal tubules and transport this fluid to the pelvis of the kidney, where it is emptied as urine. As the fluid passes through the collecting duct, about five sixths of the remainder of the fluid and small amounts of electrolytes are reabsorbed.

As the tubular fluid passes through the tubules, the usual waste products of metabolism, such as urea, creatinine, uric acid, phosphates, and sulfates, are poorly reabsorbed in comparison with water and the different electrolytes. Therefore, their concentrations become progressively greater as the tubular fluid passes from the glomerulus toward the renal pelvis. In this way, the waste products pass on into the urine and are lost.

Active Reabsorption Versus Passive Reabsorption. Reabsorption of nutrients and of many of the electrolytes from the tubules occurs by *active reabsorption,* that is, they are moved forcibly through the tubular membrane by chemical processes, as was explained earlier for cellular membranes. On the other hand, some substances such as water and urea are absorbed through the membrane only by the process of diffusion, which is called *passive reabsorption.*

The Clearance Concept. From the above discussion it can be seen that a large portion of the plasma that enters the kidneys, about one fifth of it, leaks through the glomeruli into the tubular system of the kidneys and is reabsorbed. However, during its passage through the tubules certain portions of the glomerular filtrate are entirely reabsorbed, while other portions are either not reabsorbed at all or are reabsorbed very poorly. A substance that is not reabsorbed at all never returns to the plasma and therefore is completely cleared from the plasma. For instance, creatinine is not reabsorbed at all, so that the entire 125 ml of plasma that filters into the tubules each minute is cleared of creatinine, while over 99 per cent of the water is normally reabsorbed into the blood. Therefore, it is said that the *plasma clearance* of creatinine is 125 ml per minute.

About 60 ml of plasma is cleared of urea each minute. About 1 ml is cleared of sodium, but none is cleared of glucose. Thus, the kidney acts as a "plasma clearing organ," removing those substances from the plasma that are not needed by the body while at the same time conserving those substances that are still valuable to the body.

REGULATION OF EXTRACELLULAR FLUID CONSTITUENTS AND VOLUME

Regulation of the Ratio of Interstitial Fluid Volume to Blood Volume. As has already been explained, the extracellular fluid can move with ease back and forth between the interstitial spaces and the blood. When there is excess blood volume, the capillary pressure rises above normal, causing the forces for movement of fluid out of the blood to become greater than those for moving fluid into the blood. Therefore, some of the plasma portion of the blood is automatically transferred to the interstitial spaces, until the Starling forces at the capillary membrane once again become equilibrated. Conversely, if there is too little blood volume in relation to interstitial fluid volume, then the Starling forces become overbalanced in the direction that causes fluid to move from the interstitium into the plasma. Thus, the ratio of blood volume to interstitial volume is determined by the balance of the Starling forces at the capillary membrane.

Regulation of Overall Extracellular Fluid Volume and Blood Volume.

For reasons explained above, when the extracellular fluid volume increases, the blood volume also usually increases, although this is not always true.

A long-term mechanism for control of both extracellular fluid volume and blood volume is based on the interrelationship between blood volume and arterial pressure, which we shall discuss further in a later section. Briefly, a prolonged increase in extracellular fluid volume and blood volume causes an increase in arterial pressure. The increased pressure in turn has a direct effect to increase the rate of excretion of water and electrolytes by the kidneys, which is called *pressure diuresis*. In this way, the blood volume and extracellular fluid volume are both decreased back toward the normal level. This mechanism for control of the blood volume is called the *kidney-volume–pressure control mechanism*. It is an extremely powerful mechanism that controls the extracellular and blood volumes very exactly over a period of weeks, months, and years.

For short-term control of extracellular fluid volume, two important hormonal mechanisms play an important role.

First, a 10% or greater decrease in blood volume affects the blood flow to the hypothalamus. This in turn causes the hypothalamus to secrete a hormone called *antidiuretic hormone* (or vasopressin). This hormone will be discussed at greater length in the following section. However, it has a net effect to increase the rate of water reabsorption by the tubules of the kidneys, which can cause a short-term effect to enhance both the extracellular fluid volume and blood volume.

Second, when the blood volume becomes too great and causes excessive stretch of the two atria of the heart, the atrial walls release into the blood a hormonal substance called *atrial natriuretic factor (ANF)*. This is a large polypeptide that is then carried by the blood to the kidneys where it mainly dilates the renal arterioles and increases the rate of excretion of sodium ions into the urine. When this occurs, for several reasons that will be discussed in the following section, the kidneys excrete water along with the sodium, thus decreasing both the extracellular fluid volume and the blood volume back

toward normal. Unfortunately, not enough research has yet been performed on atrial natriuretic factor to determine its overall significance in the regulation of the body fluids.

Regulation of Body Fluid Osmolality and Sodium Ion Concentration by the Antidiuretic Hormone System and by the Thirst Mechanism.

The body has two mechanisms for controlling the overall concentration of osmotically active substances in the body fluids. One of these mechanisms is the hypothalamic-pituitary *antidiuretic hormone system* and the other is the *thirst mechanism.* When the total osmotic pressure of the extracellular fluid becomes too great, this activates both of these systems, causing (1) increased thirst and therefore increased intake of water, and (2) decreased excretion of water by the kidneys because of the antidiuretic hormone, which causes greatly increased reabsorption of water in the renal tubules. Therefore, the quantity of water in the body increases, thus diluting the concentrated electrolytes. In this way, the total concentration of electrolytes is controlled within very narrow limits.

While controlling the total concentration of osmotic substances in the extracellular fluid, the same two mechanisms control the concentration of sodium. The reason for this is that between 90% and 95% of the osmotic substances in the extracellular fluid are either sodium itself or other constituents that are so closely linked to sodium that their concentrations are determined by the quantity of sodium that is available. For instance, the sum of the chloride ions and the bicarbonate ions is determined directly by the amount of sodium that is available. Therefore, the sodium ion concentration and the total concentration of all osmotically active substances in the extracellular fluids change almost exactly in parallel with each other; at the same time that the osmolality of the extracellular fluids is controlled, so also is the sodium ion concentration controlled.

Now, let us describe how the hypothalamic-pituitary antidiuretic hormone system functions and also how the thirst mechanism operates. First, a special arrangement in the kidneys affords a mechanism by which at times water can be reabsorbed more readily even than the electrolytes. To effect this, the loops of Henle of the renal tubules extend downward into the medulla of the kidney. From these tubules active reabsorption of sodium ions occurs rapidly and strongly; chloride ions are then absorbed as well to go along with the sodium, causing a very high concentration of sodium chloride in the interstitial fluids of the renal medulla. Then when the tubular fluid later passes through the collecting ducts, which also traverse the medullae, the osmotic pressure exerted by the highly concentrated medullary interstitial fluid causes rapid osmotic absorption of water from the ducts. This leaves a concentrated fluid to pass into the urine. This mechanism for concentrating the urine is called the *countercurrent mechanism.*

The second portion of the system for control of water reabsorption is the *osmoreceptor system,* which is located at the base of the brain. A high concentration of osmotic substances, especially of sodium, in the extracellular fluids causes neuronal cells in the supraoptic nucleus of the hypothalamus, called osmoreceptors, to shrink, and this excites these cells. Impulses are transmitted to the posterior pituitary gland, which in turn releases the hormone antidiuretic hormone. The antidiuretic hormone then passes by way of the blood to the kidneys where it increases the permeability of the collecting ducts, greatly increasing the rate at which water is reabsorbed osmotically. Therefore, when antidiuretic hormone is present in excess, the urine becomes highly concentrated. Without this antidiuretic hormone, the collecting ducts are almost impermeable to water; therefore, the water is lost into the urine, and the urine becomes highly dilute because of the strong reabsorption of sodium chloride by the loops of Henle.

Thus, by means of this system, excess concentration of the extracellular fluids automatically increases the secretion of antidiuretic hormone, and this causes large quantities of water to be reabsorbed, which corrects the overconcentration of the extracellular fluids. On the other hand, dilute extracellular fluid inhibits the osmoreceptor system and therefore causes excessive loss of water into the urine, again automatically readjusting the extracellular fluid concentration to normal.

Thirst is the conscious perception of need for water, and it is caused by activation of neuronal cells located in the drinking center of the anterolateral hypothalamus. Any factor that overly increases the extracellular fluid concentration, especially excess sodium, excites the thirst mechanism and makes the person seek water, thereby helping to correct the dehydration.

Regulation of Potassium Ion Concentration— Role of Aldosterone.   Aldosterone, a hormone secreted by the adrenal cortex, has effects on the renal tubules, especially the distal tubules and the collecting ducts. It increases the reabsorption of so-dium into the blood from the tubules and also increases the secretion of potassium in the opposite direction from the blood into the tubules. The increased reabsorption of sodium into the blood does not affect the blood concentrations of sodium significantly because the hypothalamic–pituitary antidiuretic hormone mechanism and the thirst mechanism discussed above still control the sodium ion concentration very exactly despite the increased sodium reabsorption from the renal tubules. On the other hand, when excess aldosterone circulates in the blood, the increased secretion of potassium into the renal tubules and subsequent excretion in the urine causes marked reduction of potassium in the extracellular fluid. Conversely, in the absence of aldosterone, the extracellular fluid potassium ion concentration increases markedly.

Now, to complete the control mechanism for potassium ion concentration: When the potassium ion concentration rises to high levels, this has a direct effect on the adrenal cortex to stimulate increased aldosterone secretion. The aldosterone then causes increased secretion of potassium into the urine and return of the potassium ion concentration back toward normal.

There is also another mechanism for regulating potassium ion concentration in the extracellular fluid that is *not* dependent upon aldosterone. This results from the fact that a high potassium ion concentration in the extracellular fluid has a direct action on the distal tubular epithelium to cause increased potassium secretion into the tubules. Therefore, at high potassium ion concentrations the tubules tend to secrete more potassium while at low extracellular potassium ion concentrations the tubules secrete less potassium. Thus, this local effect operates in parallel with the aldosterone mechanism for regulating potassium ion concentration.

Regulation of Other Extracellular Fluid Electrolytes.   Other extracellular fluid electrolytes that are regulated in similar ways include calcium, magnesium, chloride, bicarbonate, and other ions. An increase in calcium ion concentration causes decreased parathyroid hormone secretion; and this in turn causes decreased calcium reabsorption by the renal tubules and increased loss of calcium into the urine. The chloride and bicarbonate ion concentrations are adjusted by the respiratory and renal mechanisms for control of acid–base balance as will be explained in the following paragraphs.

Regulation of Acid–Base Balance.   When one speaks of acid–base balance, one actually means regulation of the *hydrogen ion concentration* in the body fluids. The hydrogen ion concentration is normally expressed in terms of pH, which is the logarithm of the reciprocal of the hydrogen ion concentration according to the following formula:

$$pH = \log\left(\frac{1}{H^+}\right)$$

Arterial blood has a normal pH of 7.4. A pH of 7.8 is considered to be highly alkaline while a pH of 7.0 is considered to be highly acidic.

Acid–Base Buffer Systems. One of the important means for regulation of the pH of the blood is the chemical acid–base buffer systems present in all the body fluids. An acid–base buffer is simply a combination of chemical substances in solution that will react chemically with either acids or alkalies, when these are added to a solution, to keep them from markedly changing the hydrogen ion concentration in the solution.

One of the major buffer systems of the body fluids is the proteins of the cells and, to a lesser extent, the proteins of the plasma and the interstitial fluids. Another buffer system that is extremely important in acid–base regulation is the bicarbonate system. This is a mixture of carbonic acid and bicarbonate ions that exists everywhere in the body fluids. The greater the carbonic acid, the lower is the pH; the greater the bicarbonate ions, the higher is the pH. The following equation, called the ***Henderson–Hasselbalch equation,*** describes this relationship:

$$pH = 6.1 + \log\frac{HCO_3^-}{CO_2}$$

The importance of the Henderson–Hasselbalch equation is twofold: First, the carbon dioxide concentration in the body fluids can be altered very rapidly by increasing or decreasing the rate of respiration. Therefore, the respiratory system can be used very effectively for short-term control of the acidity of the body fluids—that is for controlling the pH. Second, the kidneys have a powerful ability to change the bicarbonate ion concentration in the body fluids. However, this effect requires several hours to days to occur completely. Therefore, the kidneys also exert a powerful, though slowly acting, control of the acidity of the body fluids.

Respiratory Regulation of Hydrogen Ion Concentration. Rapid ventilation of the lungs decreases the concentration of carbon dioxide in the alveoli and in the pulmonary blood. When carbon dioxide leaves the blood, large portions of the carbonic acid in the body fluids immediately dissociate into water and carbon dioxide, thus reducing the concentration of carbonic acid and also of hydrogen ions. Conversely, the less the pulmonary ventilation the greater becomes the concentration of carbonic acid and the higher becomes the hydrogen ion concentration.

The hydrogen ion concentration in turn helps to control the rate and depth of pulmonary ventilation in the following manner: When the hydrogen ion concentration becomes too great, this has a direct effect on the respiratory center in the brain stem to cause an increase in the rate of pulmonary ventilation. In turn, the increased ventilation reduces the carbonic acid concentration in the body fluids and therefore returns the hydrogen ion concentration back toward normal. Conversely, if the hydrogen ion concentration becomes too low, the respiratory center becomes inhibited, pulmonary ventilation becomes reduced, and the carbonic acid concentration in the body fluids rises, thereby bringing the hydrogen ion concentration once again back near to normal. This respiratory mechanism of acid-base regulation can return the hydrogen ion concentration (and pH) about two thirds of the way back to normal within a minute or so after some foreign acid or alkali has entered the body fluids, provided the quantity is not too great.

Regulation of Hydrogen Ion Concentration by the Kidneys. When the respiratory system fails to readjust the hydrogen ion concentration to normal, the kidneys are still capable of bringing it back to normal during the ensuing 12 to 24 hours. If the kidney mechanism has plenty of time to function, it is many times as effective as either the buffers or the respiratory mechanism in readjusting the pH of the body fluids.

The kidneys readjust the hydrogen ion concentration in the following way: Hydrogen ions are continually being secreted by the tubular epithelium into the tubular fluid; these hydrogen ions represent a loss of acid from the extracellular fluids. On the other hand, bicarbonate ions are continually filtering from the blood through the glomeruli into the tubules, and this represents a loss of alkali. In acidosis, the rate of hydrogen ion secretion exceeds the rate of bicarbonate filtration because the tubular epithelial cells respond to acidosis by increased hydrogen ion secretion. This allows the body fluids to lose excess acid and therefore to correct the acidosis. On the other hand, in alkalosis, the rate of hydrogen ion secretion becomes very low, allowing excess loss of bicarbonate ion. As a result, the body fluids lose alkali and therefore become progressively more acidic, returning once again to a normal hydrogen ion concentration (and to a normal pH).

BLOOD AND IMMUNITY

BLOOD CELLS

Red Blood Cells and Their Function.   The body contains about 25 trillion red cells in an average concentration of about 4,800,000 per mm^3 of blood. The percentage of the total blood volume comprised of red blood cells is called the *hematocrit,* and this is normally about 40%.

The principal function of the red blood cells is to transport oxygen from the lungs to the tissues, but another function is to transport carbon dioxide from the tissues back to the lungs. The dynamics of these functions will be presented in the section on respiration.

Regulation of Red Blood Cell Formation.   The rate of red blood cell formation is controlled by the delivery of oxygen to the tissues. The general mechanism of this is the following: Tissue hypoxia causes the kidneys to release a hormone called erythropoietin, which then flows in the blood to the bone marrow where it stimulates erythropoiesis. In highly athletic persons, whose tissues require large amounts of oxygen, the total red cell mass in the body is often 10% to 30% above normal, and in persons residing at very high altitudes where oxygen is rare in the air the total red cell mass sometimes becomes as much as 60% to 80% above normal.

When the red blood cells are once formed, they normally have an average life span in the circulatory system of about 120 days.

Nutritive Factors Affecting Red Blood Cell Formation.   The process of red blood cell formation can be divided into two principal processes: (1) formation of the cell structure itself, and (2) formation of hemoglobin. The red cell is formed in the bone marrow by a series of divisions from the hemocytoblast. Two vitamins, vitamin B_{12} and folic acid, are necessary for normal formation of the cell structure. If either of these is missing, the cell membrane is likely to be so friable that the cells are rapidly destroyed in the circulatory system; also, the cell is likely to be too large or occasionally too small, and its shape may be globular, ovoid, or any other shape besides the normal biconcave disk. This abnormal formation of red blood cells is called *maturation failure.*

A primary nutritive factor necessary for formation of hemoglobin is iron. Iron is present in the diet in only very small quantities and even then is rather poorly absorbed from the gastrointestinal tract; therefore, many persons frequently fail to form suffi-cient quantities of hemoglobin to fill the red blood cells as they are being produced. This causes *hypochromic anemia* in which the number of cells may be normal but the amount of hemoglobin in each cell is far below normal.

White Blood Cells.   The number of white cells in the blood is normally only 1/600 the number of red blood cells, about 8000 per mm^3 of blood, but they perform the very important function of protecting or helping to protect the body from invasion by infectious agents. The white cells consist of neutrophils, eosinophils, basophils, monocytes, and platelets, all formed in the bone marrow, and lymphocytes formed in the lymph nodes.

The *neutrophils* are the most numerous of the white blood cells, representing about 60% of the total number in the blood. They are highly motile, highly phagocytic, and are attracted out of the blood into tissue areas where tissue destruction is occurring by a process called *chemotaxis,* which means attraction by the destruction products from the damaged tissues. Once in the tissue area, the neutrophils phagocytose bacteria and small amounts of dead tissue debris.

The *monocytes* are much larger cells than the neutrophils, and large numbers of them normally wander through the tissues all of the time, where they become very large and are then called *macrophages.* They can phagocytose five to ten times as many bacteria and much larger particles of tissue debris than can the neutrophils. However, they are not attracted nearly so rapidly into areas of tissue destruction as the neutrophils. In general, soon after an infection begins the concentration of neutrophils becomes very high in the infected area; then several days later the concentration of macrophages becomes very high, the macrophages replacing most of the neutrophils.

Almost all tissues of the body contain macrophages, but they are especially abundant in those tissues that are routinely exposed to bacteria, such as the lung alveoli, the sinusoids of the liver, the sinusoids of the bone marrow, the sinusoids of the lymph nodes, and the subcutaneous tissue. This extensive *monocyte-macrophage system* is frequently also called the *reticuloendothelial system.*

When tissues become infected or inflamed, breakdown products from these tissues not only cause chemotaxis of neutrophils and macrophages into the infected or inflamed tissue area, but also cause (1) rapid release of already stored white blood cells from the bone marrow, and (2) increased formation of new white blood cells.

The *eosinophils* are similar to the neutrophils except that they are less chemotactic and less phagocytic. Large numbers of eosinophils appear in the blood in allergic conditions and also when the body is invaded by certain parasites. It is possible that the eosinophils help to detoxify toxins that are released by parasites or by allergic reactions.

The *basophils* are similar to mast cells, which are found in the pericapillary tissues and secrete large quantities of heparin. Basophils, too, secrete heparin, but directly into the blood. The heparin in turn helps to prevent blood coagulation in the normal circulatory system.

The *platelets* are only fragments of cells instead of whole cells. Like heparin, they, too, are important in the blood coagulation process, as will be discussed below.

BLOOD COAGULATION

The Blood Clot. When a blood vessel ruptures, a blood clot develops within a few minutes to fill the rent and stop the bleeding—if the rupture is small enough. This process is caused by polymerization of plasma *fibrinogen* molecules into long *fibrin threads* that entrap large numbers of red blood cells, white blood cells, platelets, and plasma to form a soft gelatinous mass, the blood clot. The fibrin threads gradually contract, expressing most of the plasma from the clot, which leaves a reasonably solid barrier in the opening of the blood vessel.

Initiation of Blood Clotting. Blood clotting is caused by conversion of the plasma protein called *prothrombin* into another protein, *thrombin.* Thrombin is an enzyme that then enzymatically causes polymerization of plasma fibrinogen molecules into the fibrin threads that lead to blood clotting.

In the normal circulation, very little prothrombin is converted into thrombin each minute, so little that it is destroyed by a substance called *antithrombin* before the prothrombin can cause any blood coagulation. However, there are two principal conditions that can lead to blood clotting. These are: (1) damage to the vessel wall and (2) damage to the blood itself.

Damage to the blood vessel wall initiates a series of events called the *extrinsic pathway for prothrombin activation.* The damaged tissues in the wall of the vessel release a substance called *tissue thromboplastin.* This is mainly composed of phospholipids from the damaged tissues. The thromboplastin in turn catalyzes a series of enzymatic reactions among multiple blood plasma proteins called *blood coagulation factors.* These reactions eventually form *prothrombin activator,* which causes the pro-

thrombin to change into thrombin and thereby initiate blood coagulation.

When the blood rather than the vessel wall is damaged, another series of reactions, called the *intrinsic pathway for prothrombin activation,* occurs. The damage to the blood causes direct activation of some of the protein blood coagulation factors, and damage to the platelets of the blood causes release of *platelet thromboplastin,* which has effects similar to those of tissue thromboplastin released by torn blood vessels. The combined activation of the protein coagulation factors and release of the platelet thromboplastin leads eventually to the formation of prothrombin activator. Then, the prothrombin activator converts prothrombin to thrombin, which subsequently causes blood clotting.

Bleeding Diatheses. Several abnormalities of the blood coagulation mechanism can cause persons to become excessive bleeders. In *hemophilia* the substance called *antihemophilic factor* is absent from the plasma. This substance is required for function of the intrinsic pathway of blood coagulation; because of its absence in hemophilia, the hemophiliac person is an excessive bleeder.

The normal number of platelets in the blood is about 300,000 per mm.[3] In *thrombocytopenia* this number is greatly reduced. Platelets have the ability to attach themselves to very minute rupture points in blood vessels and thereby close these holes even without causing actual blood coagulation. In thrombocytopenia this function is lost, and as a result the person develops many minute bleeding spots over his entire body, causing petechial hemorrhages throughout all his organs and beneath the skin.

Prothrombin deficiency or *Factor VII* (another blood coagulation factor) *deficiency* frequently results from liver disease because each of these substances is a protein formed by the liver. Also, the concentration of each of them becomes reduced when vitamin K is not available to be used by the chemical systems of the liver for formation of the two substances. In deficiency of either prothrombin or Factor VII, the rate of thrombin formation is greatly reduced, thus preventing or depressing coagulation and allowing excessive bleeding.

IMMUNITY

Innate Immunity. Immunity means resistance of the body to invasion by bacteria, viruses, or other infectious agents or toxins. Each person is born with a certain amount of innate immunity that results from several special mechanisms: (1) the reticuloendothelial system and the white blood cells, which have already been discussed; (2) resistance of the intact skin to invasion by microorganisms; (3) destruction of bacterial organisms by the digestive enzymes in the stomach; and (4) substances circulating in the blood.

Adaptive Immunity—The Immune Process. In addition to the natural immunity that normally exists in all persons, a person can develop adaptive immunity to many destructive agents to which he is not naturally immune. Most destructive agents, such as bacteria, viruses, or toxins, are mostly composed of protein molecules. On entering the body, these proteins act as antigens and cause two types of immunity: one is called *humoral immunity* and the other *lymphocytic immunity.* In humoral immunity, large protein molecules called antibodies are formed, and these in turn destroy the invading agent. In the case of lymphocytic immunity, sensitized lymphocytes are formed, and these too have the capability of attacking and destroying the invading agents.

Humoral Immunity. In humoral immunity, the antigens first enter the lymphoid tissue, especially the lymph nodes. There they cause plasma cells, which are derived from lymphocytes, to produce large quantities of antibodies that are specifically reactive for the type of protein that initiated their production. Once these antibodies have been formed and released into the body fluids, which usually requires a week to several weeks, they then destroy the specific invader that had caused their formation and can also destroy any future invader of this same type.

Antibodies are large protein molecules, usually gamma globulins, that are capable of combining chemically with invading agents. The antibodies attach to the surfaces of bacteria or viruses, or they combine directly with toxins. They either destroy the invading agent or make it more susceptible to phagocytosis by the tissue macrophages or by white blood cells. Or, in the case of toxins, the antibodies can simply neutralize these by combining chemically with them.

Lymphocytic Immunity. In early fetal development of the lymph nodes, no lymphocytes are present in the nodes. Instead, the early lymphocytes are formed and processed in the liver and the thymus gland. After processing, the lymphocytes are then released into the circulating blood and eventually become entrapped in the lymph nodes. Once in these nodes, those lymphocytes processed in the liver eventually are converted into plasma cells that become part of the humoral immune process to form antibodies.

The lymphocytes that are processed in the thymus gland also end up in the lymph nodes and other lymphoid tissue of the body. However, instead of forming antibodies when the lymph node is exposed to antigens, these cells form so-called *sensitized lymphocytes,* also called *T cells* because of their earlier processing in the thymus. The T cells form chemical substances that are similar to antibodies, but these remain attached to the cell membranes of the lymphocytes. Large numbers of T cells are then released into the circulating blood, and they spread throughout the body. There are three major types of sensitized lymphocytic T cells: (1) *cytotoxic T cells* combine directly with antigens on the surfaces of invading organisms and can therefore destroy the organisms. (2) *helper T cells* function mainly in association with the plasma cells in the lymph nodes; they multiply manyfold the capability of the plasma cells to produce antibodies in response to antigens. (3) *suppressor T cells* suppress some of the immune reactions, in this way preventing the immune system from running wild and being destructive to normal tissues.

Tolerance; Autoimmune Disease. The immune process of the normal human body does not develop antibodies or sensitized lymphocytes that can destroy the body's own tissues, despite the fact that the body tissues are to a great extent like bacteria in their chemical composition. This phenomenon is called *tolerance* to the body's own proteins and tissues. This probably results mainly from destruction during fetal life of those primordial lymphocytes capable of forming antibodies or sensitized lymphocytes against the body proteins and tissues. It is likely also that special suppressor T cells also develop to help cause tolerance.

Under abnormal conditions, however, both antibodies and sensitized lymphocytes that can attack the body's own tissues do occasionally develop. This process is called *autoimmunity.* It occurs particularly in older age or after some disease causes destruction of large amounts of body tissue with release of tissue antigens into the circulating body fluids. Once the immune process has caused production of antibodies or sensitized lymphocytes that can attack the body's own tissues, these will then react against specific tissues and cause serious debility. Examples of autoimmune disease include rheumatic heart disease, rheumatoid arthritis, thyroiditis, acute glomerulonephritis, myasthenia gravis, and lupus erythematosus.

ALLERGY

There are at least three different types of allergy, two of which can occur under appropriate conditions in normal persons and one of which occurs only in persons who have a specific allergic tendency.

Allergies That Occur in Normal Persons. Two types of allergy that occur in normal persons are anaphylaxis and delayed reaction allergy.

Anaphylaxis occurs in persons who are strongly immunized against a foreign antigen. When a subsequent dose of the same foreign antigen is injected directly into the circulatory system, an immune reaction occurs in direct contact with the blood and the tissues immediately surrounding the blood vessels. This reaction causes local cellular damage. One of the effects is release of large quantities of histamine mainly from basophils, and this in turn causes extreme vascular vasodilatation and circulatory collapse. Often a person dies as a result.

Delayed-reaction allergy is caused by sensitized lymphocytes and not by antibodies. A typical example is the reaction to poison ivy. The toxin of poison ivy becomes deposited in the skin, and a small portion of it finds its way to the lymph nodes, which, over a period of several days to a week or so, form sensitized lymphocytes. These then are carried by the blood back to the original site of entry of the poison ivy toxin. Reaction of the lymphocytes with the toxin in direct association with the cells produces severe local tissue damage, which is the well-known rash and vesicles associated with poison ivy.

Allergy in the Allergic Person. Some persons, called allergic persons, tend to form a type of antibody called *reagin*. Reagins have a different protein structure from that of normal antibodies and are called IgE antibodies. Also, the reagins tend to attach themselves to basophils and mast cells throughout the tissues. When the specific antigen that reacts with the reagin (called the *allergin*) enters the tissue it combines with the reagin. This combination, occurring on the cell surface of the basophils and mast cells, causes cellular damage with release of histamine and proteolytic enzymes from the affected cells. Severe local tissue damage can result. Types of allergies of this type are hay fever, asthma, and urticaria.

TRANSFUSION; TRANSPLANTATION OF TISSUES

Successful transfusion of blood from one person to another or transplantation of tissues or organs is principally a problem of immunity; the new host may be already immune to the transfused blood or the transplanted tissues, or he may develop immunity to these after a few weeks' time, which then causes death of the cells in the transfusion or the transplant.

Transfusion Reaction. If the host is immune to transfused blood or becomes immune soon after the transfusion, a transfusion reaction is likely to result. This consists of an attack on the red blood cells by the recipient's antibodies. The antibodies attach themselves to the surfaces of the cells and make them *agglutinate* with each other, which means that the cells stick together in clumps. Occasionally the antibodies are powerful enough also to cause the cells to rupture. However, even if the cells do not rupture from this cause, the clumped cells become caught in the capillaries of the circulatory system and during the next few hours become ruptured because of progressive trauma or attack by white blood cells or by tissue macrophages. Thus, the final result in all transfusion reactions is rupture of the red cells, which is called *hemolysis,* with release of hemoglobin and other intracellular substances into the blood. Many of the intracellular components have toxic effects throughout the body, causing a febrile reaction and sometimes depressing the circulation into a shocklike state. In addition, much of the free hemoglobin in the blood filters through the glomerular membrane into the renal tubules; then water is reabsorbed from the tubules, allowing the homoglobin to become so concentrated that it precipitates. If large amounts of blood are hemolyzed, this process can block many or most of the tubules of the kidneys and causes either oliguria or anuria. As a result, a person occasionally dies a week or so later of uremia rather than as the immediate result of the transfusion reaction.

A-B-O Blood Groups. The membranes of the red blood cells in about 60% of all human beings contain one or both of two very important antigens, called *group A* or *group B agglutinogens,* that frequently cause transfusion reactions. The bloods of different persons are generally *typed,* as illustrated in Figure 3-5, on the basis of the presence or the absence of these agglutinogens in the blood cells. Thus, the four major blood groups of humans are *group A,* which contains type A agglutinogen; *group B,* which contains type B agglutinogen; *group AB,* which contains both A and B agglutinogens; and *group O,* which contains neither.

When a person does not have either A or B agglutinogens in his blood, he almost always does have antibodies that will agglutinate cells containing the missing agglutinogen. Antibodies that agglutinate the A agglutinogen are called *anti-A agglutinins,* while those that agglutinate B agglutinogen are called *anti-B agglutinins.* Thus, type A blood contains anti-B agglutinins, while type B blood contains anti-A agglutinins; type AB blood contains neither

Genotypes	Blood Groups	Agglutinogens	Agglutinins
OO	O	—	Anti-A and Anti-B
OA or AA	A	A	Anti-B
OB or BB	B	B	Anti-A
AB	AB	A and B	—

Fig. 3-5. Classification of the different blood groups, showing the presence or absence of agglutinogens in the blood cells and agglutinins in the plasma. (Guyton AC: Textbook of Medical Physiology, 7th ed. Philadelphia, WB Saunders, 1986)

of the agglutinins; and type O blood, both anti-A and anti-B agglutinins. Therefore, mixing bloods of different types will often cause agglutination of at least some of the cells and can result in a transfusion reaction.

Rh Blood Types. The blood cells of about 85% of all white persons and 95% of North American blacks also contain another antigen, called the **Rh antigen,** which exists in several different forms. Those persons who have the Rh antigen are said to be Rh positive while those who do not have any Rh antigen are said to be Rh negative.

A transfusion reaction occasionally results when Rh-positive blood is transfused into an Rh-negative person. However, this will not occur unless the Rh-negative person has been exposed previously to Rh-positive blood because, contrary to the anti-A and anti-B agglutinins, anti-Rh antibodies do not occur spontaneously in the blood. Yet, if the Rh-negative person has been exposed previously to Rh-positive blood he or she will have developed anti-Rh antibodies against the Rh factor, and a subsequent transfusion with Rh-positive blood can cause an equally severe transfusion reaction as one that occurs with the group A-B-O bloods.

The Rh factor occasionally causes a type of transfusion reaction in fetuses during pregnancy in the following way: If the mother is Rh negative, and the baby inherits the Rh-positive trait from the father, some of the Rh-positive antigens can sometimes cause the mother to develop anti-Rh antibodies; these antibodies then diffuse through the placenta into the baby and cause agglutination of the circulating red cells. This effect rarely occurs with the first Rh-positive baby but occurs much more frequently during subsequent pregnancies because immunity develops in the mother typically immediately after birth of the baby in response to antigens entering her blood from degenerating products of the placental tissues. If the mother is given antiserum against the Rh factor immediately after delivery, most instances of immunization can be prevented. But without such preventive measures, this is a cause of death in a large number of newborn or unborn children. The clinical condition, when present, is called erythroblastosis fetalis because the fetus responds with an erythroblastic reaction to form more blood cells.

Other Blood Types. In addition to the A, B, O, and Rh factors in red blood cells there are still many other protein antigens in the blood cells that occasionally cause transfusion reactions. These include the M, N, S, P, Kell, Lewis, Duffy, and Lutheran factors. However, the transfusion reactions caused by these factors are usually so mild or so rare that these factors are not considered as being important in blood transfusions, but they are all very important in forensic medicine for determining parentage of children.

Transplantation of Tissues. Almost exactly the same problems are experienced in the transplantation of tissues as in transfusion, for other cells of the body besides the red blood cells also contain antigens to which the host is either already immune or to which the host can develop immunity within a few weeks after transplantation. Especially important is another system of antigens called the HLA antigens that exist in many different forms. For this reason, successful transplantation of organs that contain living cells can usually be achieved for only a few weeks unless the recipient is treated with immunosuppressive drugs, or unless transplantation is from one identical twin to another, whose tissues contain exactly the same types of antigens. After several weeks the immune processes of the body destroy the transplant. Fortunately the use of immunosuppressive drugs now allows transplantation of kidneys, hearts and other organs. Also, procedures for "typing" the antigens in tissues have been developed so that the antigens of donor and recipient can be partially matched, thus reducing the severity of the transplant rejection reactions.

NERVE AND MUSCLE

FUNCTION OF THE NERVE FIBER

The Membrane Potential. A membrane potential occurs across the membranes of all cells. In large nerve and muscle cells this potential amounts to about 90 millivolts, with negativity inside the cell membrane and positivity outside. The development of this potential occurs as follows: Every cell membrane contains a sodium–potassium pump that pumps sodium to the outside of the cell and potassium to the inside. However, more sodium is pumped outward than potassium inward. Also, the membrane is relatively permeable to potassium, so that potassium can leak out of the cell with ease. Therefore, the net effect of this pump is principally to transport sodium outward. This active transport of sodium, which is a positively charged ion, to the outside of the membrane causes loss of positive charges from inside the membrane and gain of positive charges on the outside, thus creating negativity inside the membrane and positivity outside. The resulting membrane potential is the basis of all conduction of impulses by nerve and muscle fibers.

The Action Potential. The action potential is a sequence of changes in the electrical potential that occurs within a small fraction of a second at the membrane when a nerve or muscle membrane impulse spreads over its surface. This is caused in the following way: Any factor that makes the membrane suddenly excessively permeable—such as passing an electrical current through it, pinching the nerve fiber, pricking it with a pin, crushing it, or applying a drug such as acetylcholine—will usually cause the membrane to become very permeable to sodium ions. As a result, the positive sodium ions on the outside of the membrane now flow rapidly to the inside. Therefore, the membrane potential suddenly becomes reversed with positivity on the inside and negativity on the outside. This state is called *depolarization.*

Once depolarization has occurred, the loss of the negative potential on the inside of the membrane slows up the movement of sodium ions to the interior of the cell, and for reasons not yet understood, the membrane once more becomes almost totally impermeable to sodium ions but more permeable to potassium ions. As a result, few sodium ions are now able to pass to the inside, but large numbers of potassium ions, which are present inside the cell in high concentration, diffuse to the outside; since potassium ions are also positively charged, this once again causes loss of positive charges from the inside, reestablishing the normal negative membrane potential. This process is called *repolarization.*

The action potential can spread along a nerve or muscle fiber in the following way: Every time an action potential occurs at any given point on the membrane, the normal negative charge on the inside of the membrane is lost, which causes an electrical current to flow to the adjacent areas of the membrane and to stimulate these areas as well. As a

result, an action potential then occurs at each of these points, and the process is repeated again and again until the action potential has spread to both ends of the fiber.

In large nerve fibers, the repolarization process follows about 1/2,500 second after the depolarization process. Therefore, as many as 2,500 nerve impulses can be transmitted along a large nerve fiber per second. On the other hand, the process of repolarization is so slow in many smooth muscle fibers that not over one impulse in every few seconds can be transmitted.

The All-or-Nothing Law. A very important aspect of nerve function is that a stimulus usually causes a nerve fiber either to transmit a complete impulse (action potential) or, if the stimulus is too weak, none at all. This is called the all-or-nothing law. Furthermore, once an impulse begins, it normally travels in all directions over the fiber—either backward or forward and into all branches of the fiber—until each portion of the neuronal membrane has become depolarized.

Relationship of Nerve Metabolism to Action Potentials. It is the metabolic processes of the cell that cause active transport of sodium and potassium through the cell membrane. Therefore, if metabolism in the cell is blocked, ionic differences between the extracellular and the intracellular fluids cannot be maintained. However, nerve metabolism can be blocked for as long as several hours at a time without greatly affecting transmission of the impulse, for, once the ionic differences have been built up, impulse transmission is purely a physical phenomenon without involving the enzymatic metabolic processes of the cells. With each impulse that is transmitted, a small portion of the ions concentrated on the two sides of the membrane are lost to the opposite fluid compartment. During the ensuing few seconds or minutes, the metabolic processes of the membrane normally retransport these ions, thus restoring completely normal ionic differences. The more impulses transmitted by the nerve fiber, the greater the rate of metabolism required to maintain the appropriate ionic concentrations.

Summation of Nerve Impulses. Since nerve impulses are an all-or-nothing function, the means by which the nervous system transmits weak or strong signals is to "summate" many numbers of nerve impulses, that is, the greater the number of impulses transmitted the greater the effect at the other end of the nerve. There are two means by which summation can occur: One of these is *multiple fiber summation,* in which simultaneous impulses are transmitted over many parallel nerve fibers at the same time, and the other is *temporal summation,* in which large numbers of impulses are transmitted over the same fiber in rapid succession one after another. In either instance, the effect at the opposite end of the nerve is very much the same because the degree of reaction is dependent on the number of impulses arriving at the end of the nerve in a given period.

THE NEUROMUSCULAR JUNCTION

The neuromuscular junction is the point at which a motor nerve fiber connects with a muscle fiber. The mechanism for transmission of the impulse from a nerve fiber to a skeletal muscle fiber follows.

Release of Acetylcholine at the Neuromuscular Junction. The nerve ending, where it lies on the muscle fiber, branches like the limbs of a tree to form a broad structure with as many as 50 terminals and called the *endplate.* The nerve terminals in this endplate synthesize and store a chemical called acetylcholine. When a nerve impulse reaches the endplate, small portions of the stored acetylcholine are released into the *synaptic cleft* between the nerve terminals and the muscle membrane, and this in turn acts on the membrane of the muscle fiber to increase its permeability to sodium. Within another 1/500 second a protein enzyme called cholinesterase destroys the acetylcholine. Thus, the net result of a nerve impulse reaching the endplate is the release of a small pulse of acetylcholine that lasts just long enough to stimulate the muscle fiber.

The Endplate Potential. When the short pulse of acetylcholine increases the permeability of the muscle membrane, sodium ions immediately begin to pour to the inside of the fiber, which causes the outside of the fiber in the immediate vicinity of the endplate to become more negative and the inside more positive. This change in potential is called the endplate potential. The endplate potential in turn excites an action potential that spreads over the entire muscle fiber as described above for nerve fibers.

Occasionally the amount of acetylcholine released by the endplate is not very great, and the endplate potential is considerably less than normal. Below a certain *threshold value,* the endplate potential is not strong enough to initiate an action potential in the muscle fiber. As a result, the impulse fails to pass on into the muscle. This occurs in the disease myasthenia gravis, and it causes paralysis.

FUNCTION OF SKELETAL MUSCLE

The Basic Contractile Mechanism. In all muscle fibers there are two major types of fibrillar filaments: *actin filaments* and *myosin filaments.* In skeletal muscle fibers, these have lengths of 2.05 and 1.60 microns respectively. They are arranged linearly in the muscle fiber so that the myosin filaments alternate with the actin filaments. The ends of the myosin filaments overlap the ends of the actin filaments, and each of these then overlaps the ends of the next set of alternate filaments. This sort of arrangement continues throughout the entire length of the muscle fiber, which in some skeletal muscle is as long as half a meter. When an action potential passes over the muscle fiber membrane, the actin and myosin filaments interact with each other so that their ends slide together like pistons, thus shortening the fiber. As soon as the action potential is over, the interaction between the myosin and actin filaments disappears so that the alternate sets of filaments then slide away from each other like pistons moving backward.

Though the myosin filaments are composed entirely of myosin molecules, the actin filament is composed of long threads of actin and tropomyosin wrapped around each other in a helical manner. Also, attached periodically to the tropomyosin is a protein complex called troponin. The troponin and tropomyosin control muscle contraction, as explained in the following sections.

Initiation of Contraction: Excitation–Contraction Coupling

Transmission of an action potential over the muscle fiber membrane causes the fiber to contract a few milliseconds later, which is called *excitation-contraction coupling.* The mechanism by which this occurs is the following: Minute tubules, called *transverse tubules* or T tubules, pass transversely all the way through the muscle fiber from one side of the fiber membrane to the other side. The action potential, on reaching one of these tubules, travels to the interior of the muscle fiber along the membranes of the tubules. Thus, electrical current from the action potential is distributed to the inner substance of the muscle fiber as well as along its surface. The T tubules make physical contact inside the muscle fiber with many additional very fine tubules called *longitudinal tubules.* These are part of the endoplasmic reticulum and are collectively called the *sarcoplasmic reticulum;* they lie parallel to the myofibrils that cause muscle contraction. Also, they contain large amounts of calcium ions. When the action potential travels along the T tubules, electrical currents spread also to the longitudinal tubules and cause small amounts of calcium ions to be released from the longitudinal tubules into the fluid surrounding the myosin and actin filaments of the myofibrils.

The calcium ions then combine with the troponin complex, and in some way not understood this changes the physical relationship of the tropomyosin and actin molecules; the net result is exposure of active sites on the actin filament that attract the myosin filament, causing contraction of the muscle. Within another fraction of a second the calcium ions are actively transported back into the longitudinal tubules, which decreases the calcium ion concentration back to a very low value and thereby inactivates the myosin, allowing relaxation of the muscle.

The Ratchet Theory of Muscle Contraction. The nature of the forces that cause the actin and myosin filaments to slide along each other during the contractile process is not entirely understood. However, one theory, illustrated in Figure 3-6, is the following: Each myosin filament has approximately 200 arms, called *crossbridges*, that extend anglewise to the sides. At the end of each crossbridge is a hinged head that makes contact with one of the actin filaments. The head can attach temporarily to an active site on the actin filament, and it can also rock back and forth where it is hinged to the crossbridge. It is believed that when the head attaches to the actin filament, its molecular configuration changes, causing it to bend in a forward direction. This pulls the actin filament forward, but the forward bending also causes the head to disattach from the actin filament and to bend back to its original position. Next, it attaches to another active site farther along the actin filament. And the head bends again and pulls the actin filament still another short distance. Thus, by a process of attachment, bending, disattachment, and so forth, the actin and myosin filaments are pulled together, causing muscle contraction. The effect that initiates this contractile process is uncovering of the active sites on the actin filament, which occurs when calcium combines with the troponin complex as described above.

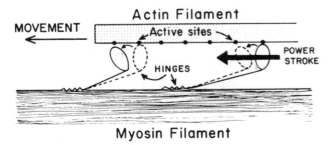

Fig. 3-6. A postulated "ratchet mechanism" for contraction of muscle. (Guyton AC: Textbook of Medical Physiology, 7th ed. Philadelphia, WB Saunders, 1986)

Energetics of Muscle Contraction. Contraction of the muscle requires energy. Each time a muscle fiber contracts, a certain amount of adenosine triphosphate, the energy-rich compound that is synthesized during the metabolism of food, is destroyed. It is believed that one molecule of adenosine triphosphate is degraded each time the head of a crossbridge bends to cause movement of the actin filament. The energy derived from this adenosine triphosphate is used to return the head back to its original "cocked" position. In this way the energy is stored in the cocked head, and it is the release of this energy that provides the force exerted by the head to pull the actin filament forward.

The more times a muscle fiber contracts and the greater the load against which the muscle contracts, the greater is the quantity of adenosine triphosphate that is degraded. When the quantity of adenosine triphosphate in the cell falls even slightly below normal, the intracellular processes for splitting and oxidizing foods go into high gear to generate new adenosine triphosphate. During extreme muscle activity, the rate of metabolism in individual muscles sometimes rises to more than 50 times the metabolic rate of the resting muscle.

Muscle Twitch and Muscle Tetanization. When a single impulse passes over the muscle fiber, the fiber contracts for a very short time, about 1/5 second in the soleus muscle, 1/15 second in the gastrocnemius muscle and 1/50 second in an ocular muscle. This single short contraction is called a *muscle twitch*. However, this twitch type of contraction normally does not occur in the body; instead, smooth and more prolonged contractions usually occur. These result from many individual muscle twitches occurring so close together, one after another, that the muscle contractions actually fuse into one long continuous contraction rather than many individual twitches. This effect is called *tetanization*.

Different Strengths of Muscle Contraction. A skeletal muscle is composed of many muscle fibers connected in parallel with each other. The strength of contraction of the entire muscle can be either very weak or very strong. To cause a weak contraction, nerve impulses are transmitted to only a few muscle fibers at a time, while to cause a very strong contraction, essentially all of the muscle fibers are contracted simultaneously. As is true in summation of nerve impulses, there are two different methods by which the strength of muscle contraction summates: (1) *multiple fiber summation,* in which many parallel muscle fibers contract simultaneously, and (2) *temporal summation,* also frequently called *wave summation,* in which successive contractions of each muscle fiber occur so close together that they add to each other.

FUNCTION OF CARDIAC AND SMOOTH MUSCLE

The basic contractile mechanism of both cardiac and smooth muscle is essentially the same as that of skeletal muscle except that in smooth muscle the actin and myosin filaments are not arranged in distinct alternate segments as is true in both skeletal and cardiac muscle. Nevertheless, an action potential traveling over the membrane causes contraction as a result of the release of calcium ions that makes the actin and myosin filaments attract each other.

Rhythmic Contraction in Cardiac and Smooth Muscle. A distinguishing characteristic of both cardiac and smooth muscle is that they can exhibit repetitive rhythmic contractions. These rhythmic contractions are caused by spontaneously occurring action potentials in the muscle fibers. Every time the membrane potential returns to the resting state, a new action potential begins because the membranes of these types of muscle are naturally very permeable to sodium ions; these ions leak into the muscle fiber, cause a change in the local membrane potential as well as membrane permeability, and the action potential. This repeats itself over and over: repolarization, depolarization, repolarization, depolarization, and so forth.

The action potential of cardiac muscle lasts about 0.3 second and of smooth muscle from as little as 0.01 second in some types of smooth muscle to more than a second in others. Also, these two types of muscle contract for more prolonged periods than the very short period that occurs in skeletal muscle, from 0.3 second to several seconds.

Tone and Plasticity of Smooth Muscle. Another important distinguishing characteristic of smooth muscle is that it can contract continuously in addition to the rhythmic contractions. The continuous contraction is called *tone.* The degree of tone can change from time to time, becoming almost none or increasing to a truly strong contraction. The intermittent rhythmic contractions are then superimposed on the basic tone. Thus, in the gastrointestinal tract, tonic contraction maintains a basal amount of pressure in the lumen of the gut, while rhythmic contractions superimposed on this cause propulsion of food along the gastrointestinal tract.

Another property of smooth muscle not evidenced by skeletal and cardiac muscle is *plasticity.* This means simply that smooth muscle can be stretched or shortened and still maintain a relatively constant amount of tension. This allows smooth muscle organs such as the urinary bladder to increase very greatly in volume without the internal pressure changing to a great extent.

HEART

RHYTHMIC EXCITATION OF THE HEART

Basic Rhythmicity of Different Types of Cardiac Muscle. Figure 3-7 illustrates the specialized conduction system of the heart called the *Purkinje system.* This system both initiates the rhythmic contraction of the heart and conducts the signal throughout the heart thus controlling heart contraction.

The natural rate of rhythmic contraction of cardiac muscle varies in different parts of the heart. The muscle fibers in the *S-A node,* a small area of special cardiac muscle located in the wall of the right atrium near the opening of the superior vena cava, have a natural rate of rhythmicity of about 72 times per minute. The natural rate of rhythmicity of atrial muscle—if it is separated from the S-A node—is 40 to 60 times per minute, and that of ventricular muscle when separated from the remainder of the heart is about 15 to 30 times per minute. It is this basic rhythmicity of cardiac muscle that causes the intermittent pumping action of the heart.

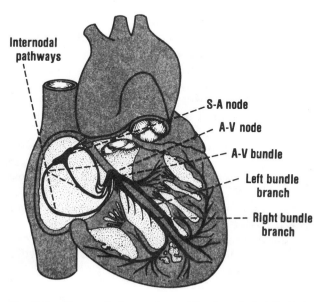

Fig. 3-7. The excitation system of the heart—the Purkinje system. (Guyton AC: Textbook of Medical Physiology, 7th ed. Philadelphia, WB Saunders, 1986)

Pacemaker Function of the S-A Node. Obviously a heart would be of less functional value if all of its parts should beat at their own natural rates of rhythm than if all parts should beat in unison. Fortunately, the portions of the heart that have naturally slow rhythmicity are excited at a faster rate by impulses coming from the S-A node. For this reason the S-A node is said to be the normal pacemaker of the heart.

The pacemaker function of the S-A node is accomplished in the following manner: Every time the muscle fibers of the S-A node contract, an impulse is transmitted to the atrial muscle and from there into the ventricular muscle. Thus, contraction of the S-A node causes contraction of the entire heart. Then, long before either the atria or the ventricles can recover enough to contract spontaneously, another excitatory impulse arrives from the S-A node. Therefore, the other parts of the heart are never allowed to contract at their natural rates of rhythm.

Conduction of the Impulse Through the Heart— The Purkinje System. Cardiac muscle fibers are arranged in a functional *syncytium*—that is, the fibers interconnect with each other so that even a single impulse in a single fiber will spread over the entire muscle mass. However, the impulse is also conducted by specifically modified cardiac muscle fibers called *Purkinje fibers* that are found in the Purkinje system. In the ventricles, these conduct the impulse at a velocity of approximately 2 m per second, which is four to six times the velocity in normal cardiac muscle. This rapid conduction allows all portions of the ventricular muscle to contract almost at the same time rather than one part contracting long ahead of another part; this in turn allows more forceful compression of the blood by the heart than would otherwise be true.

The Purkinje system begins, as illustrated in Figure 3-7, in the S-A node, located in the atrial wall near the entrance of the superior vena cava. From here, it passes through the atria by way of several internodal pathways to the *A-V node,* which lies in the posterior wall of the right atrium near the tricuspid valve. From the A-V node a large bundle of Purkinje fibers called the *A-V bundle* or the *bundle of His* passes into the ventricular septum. Then the bundle divides into *left* and *right bundle branches,* which spread respectively around the endocardial surfaces of the left and right ventricles.

The atria and the ventricles are separated from each other by fibrous tissue everywhere except where the A-V bundle passes into the ventricles. Therefore, in the normal heart the only pathway by which an impulse can travel from the atria to the ventricles is through the A-V bundle.

Another very important feature of the Purkinje system is the *junctional fibers* that occur in the A-V node. These fibers are very small and have an extremely slow velocity of impulse transmission, about one-tenth the velocity of transmission in normal cardiac muscle. This slow velocity allows a prolonged delay of the impulse so that the atria contract 0.1 to 0.2 second ahead of the ventricles. This allows the atria to pump blood into the ventricles before the ventricles begin their pumping cycle.

Heart Block. Occasionally, some pathologic condition destroys or damages the A-V bundle or A-V node so that impulses can no longer pass from the atria to the ventricles. When this happens, the atria continue to beat at the normal rate of the S-A node, while the ventricles establish their own rate of rhythm. This condition is called heart block. Usually the Purkinje fibers in the A-V bundle or in one of the bundle branches of the ventricles become the *ventricular pacemaker,* because these fibers have a higher rate of rhythm than the muscle fibers of the ventricles. The natural rate of rhythm of the ventricles after heart block can be as little as 15 beats per minute or as high as 60 beats per minute. Obviously, in heart block, the atrial contractions are not coordinated with the ventricular contractions, which prevents the ventricles from becoming as well filled before contraction as in the normal heart. This loss of atrial function impairs maximum heart pumping about 30%; however, a person with heart block can continue to live for many years because the normal heart has tremendous reserve capacity for pumping blood.

The Circus Movement—Flutter and Fibrillation. Occasionally an impulse in the heart continues all the way around the heart, and, on arriving back at the starting point, reexcites the heart muscle to cause still another impulse that again goes around the heart, this process continuing around and around the heart indefinitely. This is called a circus movement. In the normal heart it does not occur for two reasons: First, normal cardiac muscle has a very long refractory period, usually about 0.25 second, which means that the muscle fiber cannot be reexcited during this time. Second, the impulse in the normal heart travels so rapidly that it will pass over the entire heart in far less than 0.25 second, normally about 0.06 second, and therefore disappears before the heart muscle becomes reexcitable.

In the abnormal heart, however, the circus movement can occur in the following conditions: (1) Occasionally the refractory period of the cardiac muscle becomes much less than 0.25 second. (2) Sometimes the Purkinje system becomes destroyed so that the impulse takes a far longer time to travel through the ventricles because of slow conduction in the muscle fibers. (3) Occasionally either the atria or the ventricles become greatly dilated so that the length of the pathway around the heart is greatly increased; this increases the time required for the impulse to travel around the heart. (4) Often the impulse does not travel directly around the heart but instead travels in a zigzag direction, which lengthens the pathway sometimes to as much as ten times the direct distance around the heart; this obviously greatly prolongs the time for transmission of the impulse and can easily result in reexcitation of the cardiac muscle.

In the atria a regular circus movement around and around the atria causes *atrial flutter,* whereas zigzag impulses cause *atrial fibrillation.* The zigzag impulses in fibrillation also divide into multiple impulses so that there may be as many as five to ten impulses traveling in different directions at the same time. As a result, the atria remain partially contracted all the time, but they never contract rhythmically to provide any pumping action.

Flutter only very rarely occurs in the ventricles, but *ventricular fibrillation,* with many impulses of the zigzag variety spreading in all directions at once, is a very common cause of ventricular failure and death. An electric shock to the ventricles or ischemia of the ventricular muscle as a result of coronary thrombosis is a very common initiating cause of ventricular fibrillation.

THE ELECTROCARDIOGRAM

The principles of electrocardiography obviously cannot be presented in this chapter, but the normal electrocardiogram, illustrated second from the bottom in Figure 3-8, can be related to the rhythmic excitation process in the heart. The normal electrocardiogram consists of a *P wave,* which is caused by passage of the depolarization process throughout the atria; a *QRS complex of waves,* which is caused by passage of the depolarization process through the ventricles; and a *T wave,* which is caused by repolarization of the ventricles.

The PQ Interval. Normally, depolarization begins in the atria approximately 0.16 second before it begins in the ventricles. Therefore, the length of time between the beginning of the P wave and the Q wave, called the PQ interval (or PR interval when the Q wave is absent), is normally 0.16 second. Abnormally slow conduction of the impulse through the A-V bundle, as occurs when the bundle becomes ischemic following coronary thrombosis or when it becomes inflamed in the acute phase of rheumatic fever, prolongs the PQ interval sometimes to as much as 0.25 to 0.40 second. The progress of rheumatic inflammation in the heart can be assessed by following the changes in the PQ interval. As the disease becomes worse, the PQ interval often increases; as it becomes better, the PQ interval often decreases back toward normal. When the

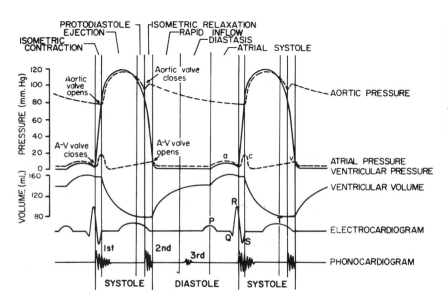

Fig. 3-8. The changes in cardiovascular pressures and ventricular volume during the cardiac cycle, and the relationships of the electrocardiogram and phonocardiogram to other events of the cycle. (Guyton AC: Textbook of Medical Physiology, 7th ed. Philadelphia, WB Saunders, 1986)

PQ interval becomes very long, conduction through the A-V bundle will eventually cease, causing heart block as explained earlier.

Abnormal QRS Waves. Since the QRS wave represents passage of the depolarization process through the ventricles, any condition that causes abnormal impulse transmission will alter the shape, the voltage, or the duration of the QRS complex. For instance, hypertrophy of one ventricle will, on the average, cause increased voltage and is likely to increase preponderantly the R or the S wave, depending on the electrocardiographic lead and the ventricle affected. Also, damage to any portion of the Purkinje system will delay transmission of the impulse through the heart and therefore will cause an abnormal shape to the QRS complex as well as prolongation of the complex.

Abnormal T Wave. The T wave represents repolarization of the ventricular muscle. Many diseases damage the ventricular muscle just enough that it becomes difficult for the muscle to reestablish normal membrane potentials after each heart beat. As a result, certain of the ventricular fibers may continue to emit electrical current far longer than usual, which causes a bizarre pattern to the T wave or sometimes even inversion of the wave. Thus, an abnormal T wave ordinarily means mild to severe damage to at least a portion of the ventricular muscle.

Elevated or Depressed S-T Segment—Current of Injury. In an occasional electrocardiogram the segment between the S and the T waves is displaced either above or below the major level of the electrocardiogram. This is caused by failure of some of the cardiac muscle fibers to repolarize between each two heart beats. As a result, between heart beats these fibers continue to emit large quantities of electrical current, called *current of injury,* that causes an elevated or depressed S-T segment. Therefore, when an elevated or depressed S-T segment is observed, one can be certain that at least some portion of the ventricular muscle has been severely damaged. This occurs very frequently following acute heart attacks.

Abnormal Rhythms. One of the most important uses of the electrocardiogram is to diagnose abnormal cardiac rhythms. For instance, in heart block the P waves are completely dissociated from the QRS and T waves. In atrial fibrillation no true P wave can be discerned at all, but in its place are many fine noise like waves continuing indefinitely in the electrocardiogram. Finally, in extrasystoles of the heart, occasional QRST waves appear in the record at points completely out of rhythm with the remaining portions of the electrocardiogram.

PUMPING ACTION OF THE HEART

Function of the Atria. The heart is actually a four chamber pump; the right side of the heart pumps blood into the pulmonary circulation, and the left side pumps blood into the systemic circulation. The atria are "primer" pumps that pump their blood into the ventricles immediately before ventricular contraction, in this way enhancing the amount of blood pumped by the ventricles. The atria are not supplied with valves to prevent back flow of blood into the veins, and their pumping force is relatively slight, but fortunately only a minute amount of force is required to move blood into the ventricles.

Even when the atria fail to pump satisfactorily, as in atrial fibrillation or in heart block, blood still flows into the ventricles because the blood in the veins simply builds up a little higher pressure and forces its way on through the atria even without the advantage of the atrial pump. For this reason persons with nonfunctional atria can nevertheless live almost normal lives as long as they do not attempt to exercise strenuously.

Mechanics of Ventricular Pumping. The ventricles are very strong pumps that are provided with inflow and outflow valves. During relaxation of the ventricles, their internal pressures are very low, which allows blood from the atria to push the *A-V valves* open and to flow into the ventricles. Then when the ventricles contract the intraventricular pressures immediately cause the A-V valves to close and the pulmonary and the aortic valves to open, and force most of the ventricular blood into the pulmonary and the systemic arterial systems. After another 0.3 second the ventricles relax, and the intraventricular pressures fall almost immediately back to zero again. In the meantime the pulmonary artery and the aorta have become distended with excess blood; a minute portion of this rushes backward toward the ventricles, catches the vanes of the outflow valves, the *pulmonary* and the *aortic valves,* and closes them. As a result, the pressures in the arteries remain high even during the period between ventricular contractions.

The period of cardiac contraction is called *systole,* and the period of relaxation is called *diastole.*

Figure 3-8 illustrates the sequential pressure changes in the heart during the cardiac cycle and their relationship to the electrocardiogram, the heart sounds, and the ventricular volume changes. Note especially that the ventricular pressure rises very high during systole, causing the aortic valve to open and blood to flow into the aorta. Then, at the end of ventricular contraction, the aortic valve closes, preventing backflow of blood from the aorta into the left ventricle. Because the aorta and large arteries are distensible, the blood pumped into the arterial system during systole is stored in these vessels and continues to flow through the systemic circulation even during diastole. At the end of diastole, the cycle begins again.

Note also in Figure 3-8 that the pressures generated in the atria are very slight, only a few millimeters of mercury, compared to those generated in the ventricles. However, these are still sufficient to fill the ventricles a fraction of a second before ventricular contraction occurs.

Finally, note that the P wave of the electrocardiogram occurs slightly before atrial contraction, the QRS waves occur at the onset of ventricular contraction, and the T wave occurs at the time of ventricular relaxation. Also, the first heart sound occurs when the inflow valves of the heart, the *semilunar valves,* close; and the second heart sound occurs when the outflow valves, the pulmonary and aortic valves, close.

Frank-Starling Law of the Heart. When increased quantities of blood flow into the heart from the veins and distend its chambers, the stretched cardiac muscle automatically contracts with increased force. This increased force in turn pumps the extra blood on through the heart into the arterial system. This is called the *Frank-Starling law of the heart,* and it obviously allows the heart to adjust its pumping capability automatically to the amount of blood that needs to be pumped. This mechanism allows the heart to pump as much as two to three times the normal amount of blood even without increasing the rate of heart beat.

Nervous Control of the Heart. The pumping action of the heart can also be altered by nervous control. Two types of nerve fibers supply the heart: *parasympathetic fibers,* which are carried in the vagus nerves, and *sympathetic fibers,* which are carried in the sympathetic nervous system. Stimulation of the sympathetic nerves increases the heart rate and also enhances the strength of the heart beat. Conversely, stimulation of the parasympathetics decreases the heart rate. In a normal person, the pumping action of the heart is regulated by both of these sets of nerves. To increase the degree of pumping action, the sympathetic nervous system is stimulated, while at the same time the normal impulses transmitted by the parasympathetic fibers are inhibited; these effects cause increased rate (up to 200 beats per minute) and strength of heart beat, which greatly enhance the overall pumping action. Conversely, during periods of rest the sympathetics become inhibited, and the parasympathetics again transmit a moderate number of impulses to the heart so that the degree of activity of the heart lessens.

This nervous control of the heart is an additional mechanism to the law of the heart to allow increased pumping action when increased quantities of cardiac output are required. For instance, in exercise these two mechanisms operate together to increase the cardiac output from the normal value of 5 liters per minute to as much as 20 to 25 liters in the normal young adult—and in well-trained athletes occasionally to as high as 35 liters per minute.

CIRCULATION

DYNAMICS OF BLOOD FLOW THROUGH THE CIRCULATION

"Circuit" Concept of the Circulation. One of the most commonly forgotten features of the circulation is that it is a complete circuit, the same blood flowing again and again through the same vessels, as illustrated in Figure 3-9. Because of this, any alteration in blood flow in any single part of the circuit alters the flow in other parts. For instance, strong constriction of the arteries in the systemic circulation might well reduce the total cardiac output, in which case the blood flow through the lungs would be decreased equally as much as the flow through the systemic circulation. Another important feature of the circuit concept is that sudden constriction of a blood vessel must always be accompanied by an opposite dilatation of another part of the circulation, because the blood volume cannot change rapidly, and blood itself is incompressible. For instance, strong constriction of the veins in the systemic circulation displaces large quantities of blood into the heart, dilating the heart and causing it to pump with increased force. This is one of the mechanisms by which the cardiac output is regulated.

Distribution of Blood in the Circulation. Approximately 80% of all the blood in the circulation is in the systemic circulatory system, approximately 10% in the lungs, and 10% in the heart. About three fourths of the blood is in the veins, about one sixth in the arteries, and one twelfth in the arterioles and the capillaries. It can be seen then that even though it is the capillary blood that supplies nutrients to the tissues and exchanges gases in the lungs, only a minute portion of the total blood volume is in the capillaries at any one time.

Blood Pressure. This is the outward force of the blood against each unit area of the vessel wall. It is

PULMONARY CIRCULATION

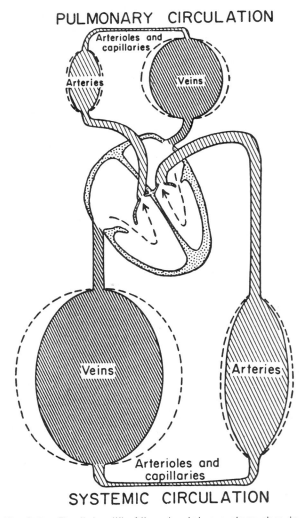

SYSTEMIC CIRCULATION

Fig. 3-9. The "circuit" of the circulatory system, showing especially the extreme distensibility of the veins. (Guyton AC: Textbook of Medical Physiology, 7th ed. Philadelphia, WB Saunders, 1986)

normally expressed in millimeters of mercury (mmHg). That is, if a vessel connected to a mercury manometer causes the mercury level to rise to a level of 100 mm, then the blood pressure is said to be 100 mmHg.

Blood Flow.   This is the rate of movement of blood along the vessels, and it is usually expressed in milliliters per minute or liters per minute.

Resistance to Blood Flow.   The viscous nature of blood causes it to flow only with difficulty through very small vessels, and the difficulty experienced by the movement of blood is called resistance to blood flow. The different factors that affect resistance are: (1) the longer the length of the vessel the greater is the resistance; (2) as the diameter of the vessel changes, the resistance changes in in-

verse proportion to the fourth power of the diameter; and (3) the resistance increases directly in proportion to the viscosity of the blood, which in turn is determined principally by the concentration of red cells in the blood.

Since changes in vessel diameter cause changes in resistance inversely proportional to the fourth power of the diameter, it is obvious that even a minute change in diameter changes the resistance tremendously. Very small vessels in the circulation have a tremendous amount of resistance, while very large vessels have so little resistance that it can be disregarded. Thus, the only portions of the circulation that offer any significant amounts of resistance are the very small arteries, the arterioles, the capillaries, and the venules, while the major arteries and the major veins normally offer almost no resistance (except where the veins are compressed by adjacent structures).

Relationship of Pressure, Flow, and Resistance.   When a blood vessel has a high pressure at one end and a low pressure at the other end, the rate of flow will be directly proportional to the difference in pressure between the two ends of the vessel, and it will be inversely proportional to the resistance to blood flow along the vessel. Thus the following formula applies:

$$\text{Blood Flow} = \frac{\text{Pressure Difference}}{\text{Resistance}}$$

SYSTEMIC CIRCULATION

Mean Pressures in the Systemic Circulation. The left ventricle normally pumps about 5 liters of blood into the aorta each minute, and the mean aortic pressure is about 100 mmHg. The resistance to blood flow through the major arteries is so slight that the mean arterial pressure even in arteries as small as 3 mm in diameter is still almost exactly 100 mmHg. Then the arteries become extremely small and lead into the arterioles where the resistance to blood flow is the greatest of any part of the systemic circulation. As a result, the mean pressure at the juncture of the arterioles and the capillaries averages only approximately 30 mmHg. The capillaries also contribute a moderate amount of resistance, causing the mean arterial pressure to fall another 20 mmHg to a level of 10 mmHg at the juncture of the capillaries and the veins. The resistance in the venous system is relatively slight, the pressure falling only 10 mmHg in the entire system. The pressure is approximately zero where the blood empties into the right atrium.

Pulsations in the Systemic Arteries. Blood is pumped by the heart in pulses, each beat of the heart normally ejecting approximately 70 ml of blood; this is called the *stroke volume output.* As a result, the arteries become greatly distended during cardiac systole, and during diastole the excess blood stored in the arterial tree "runs off" through the systemic vessels to the veins. Thus, the aortic pressure rises to its highest point during systole and falls to its lowest point at the end of diastole. The high point and the low point are called, respectively, the *systolic* and the *diastolic pressures.* In the normal adult, the systolic pressure is approximately 120 mmHg and the diastolic pressure 80 mmHg. This is usually written 120/80.

The pulsatile pressure in the aorta causes approximately equally as great pulsations in the other major arteries of the systemic circulation, but in the very small arteries and arterioles the intensity of pulsation progressively diminishes until very little occurs in the capillaries.

Regulation of Local Blood Flow by the Arterioles. In addition to having very large amounts of resistance, the arterioles are also capable of changing their resistance hundreds of times by increasing or decreasing their diameters. The arteriolar wall has an extremely strong smooth muscular coat in relation to the size of the vessel, and several different nervous and humoral stimuli can cause the arterioles to constrict so intensely that this can completely block all blood flow, while other stimuli can cause the arterioles to relax so completely that sometimes as much as 10 to 20 times normal amounts of blood are allowed to flow.

Autoregulation of Blood Flow in Each Tissue. In most tissues, blood flow in each local tissue area is autoregulated, which means that the tissue itself regulates its own blood flow. This obviously is very beneficial to the tissue because it allows the rate of delivery of oxygen and nutrients to the tissue to parallel the rate of activity.

The precise means by which autoregulation of local blood flow occurs is yet unknown. Many physiologists believe that active tissues release vasodilator substances such as adenosine, carbon dioxide, and potassium ions into the surrounding fluids and that these in turn act on the arterioles to cause them to dilate. However, other experiments indicate that this regulation might be caused very simply in the following manner: When the tissues become very active, they rapidly utilize the available oxygen in the tissue fluids. This tends to decrease the amount of oxygen available for use by the smooth muscle cells of the arteriolar walls and therefore tends to

decrease their strength of contraction. As a result, the arterioles dilate and allow adequate quantities of oxygen once more to become available to the tissues.

Nervous Regulation of Blood Flow. In essentially all areas of the body the sympathetic nerves secrete norepinephrine, and this causes vasoconstriction. Therefore, increased sympathetic stimulation causes decreased blood flow while decreased stimulation causes increased flow.

In general, nervous regulation of blood flow is concerned principally with changes in blood flow in large areas of the body at the same time. For instance, when a person becomes greatly overheated, skin vessels over the entire body become nervously dilated (vasodilation) to cause heat loss. Second, when a person exercises very strongly, the blood flow through the abdominal organs and the skin is decreased, thereby shifting the flow to the muscles. Third, when a person stands up, most of the blood vessels of the body are reflexly constricted, especially the veins. This offsets the tendency of blood to "pool" in the lower part of the body and therefore allows plenty of blood still to flow back to the heart and keep the cardiac output normal instead of falling as would otherwise occur.

Storage Function of the Veins. A reserve quantity of blood is stored in the circulatory system, especially in the veins, as illustrated in Figure 3-9, to be used in times of stress. Certain areas of the veins that store very large quantities of blood are called *blood reservoirs.* In order of importance these are (1) the sinuses of the liver, (2) the major veins of the abdomen, (3) the veins of the pulmonary system, (4) the venous sinuses of the spleen (the pulp of the spleen also stores concentrated red blood cells), and (5) the subcutaneous venous plexuses.

As much as one fourth of the total blood volume can usually be removed from a person without dire consequences because reflex nervous signals cause the veins to constrict, and blood continues to flow around the circulation almost normally.

SPECIAL AREAS OF THE SYSTEMIC CIRCULATION

Muscle Circulation. During strenuous exercise the blood flow through a muscle can increase as much as 20-fold. This increase is caused mainly by *local regulation* in the muscle itself, the increased activity of the muscle automatically causing arteriolar dilation as described above. However, the arterial blood pressure also rises, and this increases the flow as well.

Coronary Circulation. Blood flow through the myocardium obeys essentially the same principles as blood flow through the skeletal muscles. In general, coronary flow is controlled almost entirely by local regulation in the coronary vascular bed itself. The rate of blood flow parallels very closely the rate of oxygen consumption by the heart muscle, and it is believed that low oxygen concentration in the interstitial fluids of the heart muscle is in some way involved in the autoregulatory process; this was also discussed above as a possible mechanism of autoregulation throughout most of the body. Many physiologists believe that the low oxygen causes the tissues to release adenosine, and that the adenosine in turn dilates the local blood vessels.

Normal coronary blood flow is about four per cent of the resting cardiac output. When the heart works very hard, the coronary blood flow increases as much as three to four fold.

Skin Circulation. The skin circulation is specifically geared for control of body temperature. When the body temperature rises above normal, nerve signals, to be described later in this chapter, cause the blood vessels of the skin to dilate. This allows rapid flow of warm blood into the skin and therefore promotes loss of extra heat to the surroundings. Conversely, when the internal temperature of the body becomes too low, the skin vessels constrict, the skin becomes cold, and very little heat is lost.

Cerebral Circulation. The blood flow through the brain amounts to about 700 ml to 800 ml per minute, and this remains very constant under almost all physiologic conditions. In general, blood flow through the brain is controlled almost entirely by autoregulation. It is believed that autoregulation occurs in the brain mainly in response to the release of carbon dioxide from the brain tissue, the carbon dioxide dilating the blood vessels in proportion to the amount that is released. This causes the appropriate blood flow to maintain an almost exact carbon dioxide concentration at all times in the interstitial fluids of the brain. Since neuronal function is highly dependent on changes in pH, and pH in turn is highly dependent on changes in carbon dioxide, this regulatory mechanism aids in the maintenance of normal cerebral activity. Decreased blood pH or oxygen concentration will also increase brain blood flow when either of these effects is severe.

Portal Circulation. Figure 3-10 illustrates a special arrangement of the venous circulation from the gastrointestinal tract, called the portal circulation. Note that blood flows from the gastrointestinal tract and from the spleen into the portal vein and then through the liver before emptying into the systemic veins. The liver vessels offer reasonable amounts of

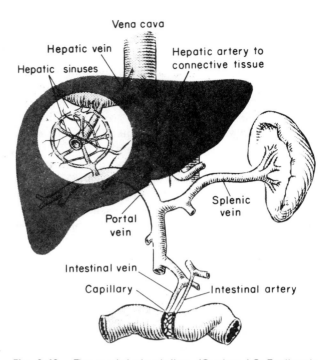

Fig. 3-10. The portal circulation. (Guyton AC: Textbook of Medical Physiology, 7th ed. Philadelphia, WB Saunders, 1986)

resistance to blood flow, which gives the portal circulatory system special characteristics of its own. Ordinarily, the portal venous pressure is about 8 mmHg because of the resistance to flow through the liver. However, in liver disease, such as *liver cirrhosis,* this resistance can increase so greatly that the portal venous pressure sometimes rises to as high as 20 or more mmHg. This causes the portal capillary pressure also to rise to a very high value, causing large quantities of fluid to leak out of the capillaries into the peritoneal cavity. Fortunately, if the blood flow through the liver becomes obstructed slowly, anastomotic channels can develop between the portal and the systemic veins. These especially occur through the esophageal veins, through the hemorrhoidal veins of the rectum and through posterior veins of the abdominal wall. Occasionally the veins of the esophagus and the hemorrhoidal veins become so enlarged that they rupture and cause serious bleeding, often causing death in the case of esophageal bleeding.

PULMONARY CIRCULATION

Pulmonary Hemodynamics. Since the circulatory system is a circuit, the same amount of blood must flow through the lungs as through the entire systemic circulation. However, the resistance to blood flow through the lungs is only about one-eighth that in the systemic circulation, and the pressures are correspondingly smaller. The pulmonary arterial systolic pressure averages 25 mmHg, and the diastolic pressure averages 8 mmHg. The mean pulmonary arterial pressure averages 15 mmHg, and the left atrial pressure averages 2 mmHg, giving a total pressure drop through the pulmonary circulation of only 13 mmHg. The pulmonary capillary pressure is approximately 7 mmHg, which is only a few millimeters greater than the left atrial pressure. This low capillary pressure is very important in keeping the alveoli dry, which will be discussed below.

Effect of Blood Flow on Pulmonary Resistance. During strenuous exercise, and in other states of physiologic stress, the cardiac output sometimes increases to as much as four to seven times normal, and in doing so the blood flow through the lungs also increases by this amount. However, the pulmonary arterial pressure rises only a moderate amount for the following reason: As the flow increases, many normally closed pulmonary capillaries open up, and those that are already open dilate more than ever. As a result, the pulmonary resistance decreases almost as much as the flow increases. Therefore, the mean pulmonary arterial pressure usually rises from 15 mmHg to only 20 to 30 mmHg when the cardiac output increases to as much as three to four times normal.

Shift of Blood From the Systemic Circulation to the Pulmonary Circulation. Approximately 10% of all the blood in the circulatory system is normally in the lungs, and about 80% is in the systemic circulation, the remainder being in the heart. Thus, there is approximately an eightfold difference in the amount of blood normally in the systemic circulation and in the lungs. However, the amounts of blood in the two circulations can change considerably when one side of the heart fails. If the right heart fails, as much as 50% of the pulmonary blood can be displaced into the systemic circulation. Conversely, if the left heart fails, then a large portion of the systemic blood can be displaced into the lungs, sometimes increasing the pulmonary blood volume to as much as 100% above normal.

Another cause of excessive shift of blood into the lungs is intense sympathetic stimulation of the circulation. This constricts mainly the systemic circulation without significantly constricting the pulmonary circulation because the sympathetic nerve supply to the pulmonary vessels is sparse. As a result, large quantities of blood are forced into the right atrium and the lungs to increase cardiac output and sometimes causing acute pulmonary edema.

Capillary Dynamics in the Lungs—the Basis of Dry Alveoli. The normal pulmonary capillary pressure is approximately 7 mmHg, while the normal colloid osmotic pressure of the plasma is 28 mmHg. Thus, the pressure tending to force fluid out of the pores of the capillaries is only 7 mmHg, while that tending to cause absorption of fluid into the capillaries is 28 mmHg. Therefore, there is a large excess of "absorption pressure" at the pulmonary membrane, which causes any fluid that enters the alveoli to be absorbed, thus keeping the alveoli dry.

Pulmonary Edema. Whenever excess blood shifts into the lungs as a result of failure of the left heart to pump adequately or as a result of excessive constriction of the systemic circulation, all of the pressures throughout the lungs, including the capillary pressure, rise very high. As long as the capillary pressure remains less than a critical level, usually about 30 mmHg, the alveoli of the lungs will remain dry, but, just as soon as the capillary pressure rises even slightly above the plasma colloid osmotic pressure, large quantities of fluid immediately begin to filter out of the capillaries into the interstitial fluid, and usually also through the alveolar membranes into the alveoli as well. This condition is ***pulmonary edema***. If the pulmonary capillary pressure rises acutely to about 50 mmHg, sufficient pulmonary edema can develop in 20 minutes to cause death, and if the pulmonary capillary pressure rises acutely to only 30 mmHg, sufficient pulmonary edema can still develop in 3 to 6 hours to cause death. However, in chronic conditions such as mitral stenosis, the pulmonary capillary pressure can remain as high as 40 mmHg for long periods of time without causing pulmonary edema, probably because very large lymphatic vessels develop in the lungs and provide extra drainage of fluid from the lung tissues.

Regulation of the Mean Systemic Arterial Pressure. Among the most important of all the control systems of the entire body are those that regulate the mean arterial pressure. The normal mean arterial pressure under resting conditions is approximately 100 mmHg, which is the force that causes blood to flow through the systemic circulation. During strenuous exercise and during other types of physiological stress, the mean pressure can rise to as high as 150 to 180 mmHg in the normal person. In hypertension, the pressure remains elevated indefinitely.

There are two basic mechanisms for regulating mean arterial pressure: (1) renal mechanisms, and (2) cardiovascular nervous reflex mechanisms.

Renal Mechanisms for Regulation of Mean Arterial Pressure. When the mean arterial pressure falls too low in the renal arteries, the kidneys cause several reactions in the circulatory system to raise the mean systemic arterial pressure. Conversely, if the mean arterial pressure rises too high in the renal arteries, the kidneys cause reverse effects on the circulation to lower the arterial pressure back to a normal level. For instance, if a person is bled a considerable amount so that his or her arterial pressure falls very low, the renal mechanisms begin immediately to bring the arterial pressure back to normal. Conversely, if excess fluids are injected into the circulatory system, elevating the arterial pressure even slightly, the renal mechanisms immediately begin to reduce the arterial pressure back toward normal once again.

Many different mechanisms have been suggested to explain the way in which the kidneys might regulate mean arterial pressure. Two of these that have received the most attention are the (renin mechanism) and the (renal-body fluid volume feedback mechanism.)

In the **renin mechanism,** the kidney secretes the enzyme renin when arterial pressure falls below normal. The renin in turn reacts with the plasma protein angiotensinogen to form a substance called angiotensin I. This in turn is converted, mainly in the capillaries of the lungs, to angiotensin II by a lung enzyme called converting enzyme. The angiotensin II then causes vasoconstriction throughout the body; this increases the total peripheral resistance and also elevates the arterial pressure back toward normal.

Angiotensin II also has two other effects that play important roles in long-term pressure regulation: (1) It has a direct effect on the kidneys to cause sodium and water retention in the body. (2) It causes increased aldosterone secretion, and this, too, causes sodium and water retention. The resulting increase in body fluid helps to raise the arterial pressure.

The most important long-term mechanism for regulation of arterial pressure is (the **renal-body fluid volume feedback mechanism.)** When the arterial pressure rises too high, the kidneys excrete greatly increased quantities of both water and salt. As a result, the extracellular fluid volume and the blood volume both decrease, and they continue to decrease until the arterial pressure falls back to that level at which the kidneys excrete normal amounts of salt and water. Conversely, when the arterial pressure falls too low, the kidneys stop excreting water and salt, and, over a period of hours to days, the person drinks enough water and eats enough salt to increase his or her blood volume, thus also returning the arterial pressure to its previous level.

This renal-body fluid volume mechanism for control of arterial pressure is slow to act, sometimes requiring several days or perhaps as long as a week or more to come to equilibrium. Therefore, it is not of major significance in acute control of arterial pressure. On the other hand, it is by far the most potent of all arterial pressure controllers for long-term control of arterial pressure. It is almost invariably involved in one way or another, either as a result of kidney damage or as a result of external factors—such as various hormones altering kidney function—in the causation of hypertension.

Regulation of Mean Arterial Pressure by Cardiovascular Nervous Reflexes. Several different nervous reflexes help to regulate the mean arterial pressure. The three most important of these are (1) the baroreceptor reflex, (2) the reflex response of arterial pressure to carbon dioxide, and (3) the reflex response of arterial pressure to cerebral ischemia.

The **baroreceptor system** operates as follows: In the walls of the carotid arteries, of the aorta, and, to a less extent of some of the other major arteries of the upper part of the body are many small stretch receptors called **baroreceptors.** When the pressure becomes excessively high in these arteries, these receptors are stimulated, and impulses are transmitted to the brain to inhibit the sympathetic nervous system. As a result, the normal sympathetic impulses throughout the body are reduced, causing the strength of the heart beat to decrease along with a simultaneous decrease in resistance in the peripheral vessels, both of which reduce the arterial pressure back toward normal. Conversely, a fall in arterial pressure decreases the number of impulses transmitted by the baroreceptors; these then no longer inhibit the sympathetic nervous system so that it becomes very active, which causes the arterial pressure to increase back toward normal.

An increase in **carbon dioxide concentration** in the blood automatically increases the mean arterial pressure by exciting the neurons of the vasomotor center in the brain stem, resulting in strong sympathetic stimulation throughout the body. This mechanism helps to ensure adequate arterial pressure during stressful conditions, since almost all types of physical stress to the body increase the basal level of metabolism and the production of carbon dioxide.

Cerebral ischemia—lack of adequate blood flow to the brain—also causes the arterial pressure to rise. In brain ischemia, the **vasomotor center** in the brain stem automatically becomes highly excited, probably because of failure of the blood to carry carbon dioxide out of the vasomotor center rapidly enough. As a result, strong sympathetic stimulation throughout the body immediately elevates the arterial pressure; this in turn increases the cerebral blood flow back toward normal and helps to relieve the ischemia.

Relative Importance of the Renal-Body Fluid Volume and Nervous Mechanisms in Regulating Mean Systemic Arterial Pressure. The renal-body fluid volume mechanism for regulating mean arterial pressure is slow to act, but it is a very powerful mechanism when it does act, having the capability of controlling the blood pressure to an extremely exact level. The cardiovascular reflexes, on the other hand, are of major importance for rapid control of arterial pressure such as (1) raising the pressure when a person stands after having been in a lying position, (2) resisting a fall in arterial pressure when a person bleeds severely, or (3) increasing the arterial pressure in times of physical stress such as during strenuous exercise. However, the cardiovascular reflexes are probably not of great importance in regulating arterial pressure from week to week, month to month or year to year because most of the nervous mechanisms eventually adapt (or "reset") to the prevailing pressure level.

HYPERTENSION

Hypertension is a disease characterized by excessively high systemic arterial pressure, and a person is usually considered to be hypertensive if the arterial pressure is greater than 140/90 mmHg. Approximately one fifth of all persons develop hypertension before death, and approximately one tenth die as a result of some secondary effect of hypertension. Yet, despite this great incidence of hypertension in the population, its cause in most cases is yet unknown. This type of hypertension is called *essential hypertension.* In the remaining cases the cause is usually renal disease or a hormonal disease that affects one of the pressure regulatory systems. The types of hypertension with known causes can be described as follows:

Renal Hypertension. Any condition that reduces the ability of the kidneys to excrete water and salt will usually cause hypertension. Such conditions include pyelonephritis, glomerulonephritis, polycystic kidney disease, amyloidosis, arteriosclerotic renal vascular disease, and many other types of renal disease.

The type of kidney debility most likely to decrease water and salt excretion is renal vascular damage, such as stenosis of the arteries to the kidneys, constriction of the afferent arterioles, or increased resistance to fluid filtration through the glomerular membrane. All of these factors decrease the ability of the kidneys to form glomerular filtrate, which in turn causes fluid and electrolyte retention and thereby increases the blood volume until the arterial pressure rises to a hypertensive level. Once the pressure has risen, normal amounts of glomerular filtrate are once again formed because of the elevated pressure, and the excretory function of the kidneys returns entirely to normal unless there is some simultaneous damage to the tubules.

The amount of increase in blood volume required to cause renal hypertension is probably less than 4 to 8 per cent, which is generally an unmeasurable quantity. However, the acute arterial pressure control mechanisms, especially the baroreceptor mechanism, oppose rapid changes in arterial pressure caused by alterations in blood volume. Therefore, an increase in blood volume that elicits hypertension will not cause the arterial pressure to rise instantaneously but instead to rise slowly over days to weeks. Even when hypertension is associated with increased blood volume, the cardiac output normally rises significantly above normal only during the onset of the hypertension. The increase in output causes excess blood flow to all the body's tissues, and the arterioles in the tissues then, as a result, automatically constrict, a process called autoregulation, thus returning the tissue blood flow back to normal. Therefore, the cardiac output returns to normal while the total peripheral resistance becomes very high.

Ischemia of the kidney can also increase the arterial pressure by causing excess formation of renin; the renin in turn causes the formation of angiotensin II in the blood. The angiotensin constricts the arterioles everywhere in the body and thereby increases the arterial pressure. This effect occurs especially in malignant hypertension, but not to a significant extent in the great majority of hypertensive patients. It also occurs in hypertension caused by unilateral renal arterial disease when the renal ischemia fails to be relieved by the high pressure.

Hormonal Hypertension. Oversecretion of certain of the hormones, especially the adrenal medullary hormones and the adrenocortical hormones, can cause hypertension. For instance, a tumor of the adrenal medulla called a *pheochromocytoma* occasionally secretes large quantities of norepinephrine and epinephrine. These two substances have almost exactly the same effect on the circulatory system as stimulation of the entire sympathetic nervous system, thereby elevating the arterial pressure. Occasionally, also, either a tumor of the adrenal cortex or hyperplastic adrenal cortices secrete excessive quantities of adrenocortical hormones. Certain of these, especially aldosterone, cause the kidneys to reabsorb large amounts of sodium and water from the tubules. The sodium and the water, in turn, lead to increased blood volume, which elevates the arterial pressure.

Essential Hypertension.   Now that we have considered the two major categories of known causes of hypertension we need to examine for a moment the possible cause of essential hypertension. Patients who develop hypertension slowly over many years virtually always have significant changes in renal function. Most important is increased renal vascular resistance, as much as several hundred per cent increase. Also, the kidneys cannot excrete adequate quantities of water and salt at normal arterial pressures, but instead require a high arterial pressure to maintain normal balance between the intake and output of water and salt. Indeed, it is highly probable that essential hypertension begins with a slowly developing increase in renal vascular resistance.

However, most research workers in the field of hypertension believe that some extraneous factor from outside the kidneys is the cause of the subsequent renal changes. For instance, a widely believed mechanism of essential hypertension is that the sympathetic nervous system is excessively active and causes hypertension by constricting the blood vessels throughout the body. It is believed that this eventually leads to the secondary changes in the kidneys that then cause the hypertension to persist. Another widely held belief is that the hypertensive person might have a genetic abnormality of the vascular smooth muscle, perhaps of the membrane of the smooth muscle cell, that causes excessive contraction of the small arterioles throughout the body, and that contraction of the arterioles in the kidneys leads to the hypertension.

REGULATION OF CARDIAC OUTPUT

The normal cardiac output in the adult is approximately 5 liters per minute, but this often increases to about four to five times this value during strenuous exercise. In general, the cardiac output is regulated in proportion to the need for blood flow through all the tissues of the body. That is, each respective tissue controls its own blood flow mainly by autoregulation, which was discussed earlier in the chapter, and the cardiac output is then regulated to supply the required blood flow. This regulation is effected in two different ways: (1) by changing the *pumping ability of the heart* and (2) by changing the rate of blood flow into the heart from the systemic vessels, which is called *venous return.*

Regulation of the Pumping Action of the Heart.   Earlier in the chapter it was pointed out that there are two major means by which the pumping action of the heart is regulated. One of these is the Frank–Starling law of the heart, and the other is nervous regulation.

In general, it can be said that, as a result of the combination of the above two mechanisms, the heart under normal physiologic conditions always pumps all the blood that flows into it without any hesitation. Therefore, in normal physiologic states it is not the pumping action of the heart that determines cardiac output, but it is the venous return to the heart that determines the output.

Regulation of Venous Return.   Venous return is regulated by three major factors: (1) the average pressure of all the blood in the systemic circulation, called the mean systemic pressure, (2) the right atrial pressure, and (3) the resistance to flow of the blood through the systemic vessels.

In the normal circulatory system, the *right atrial pressure* is *not* one of the significant factors regulating venous return because, as pointed out above, the heart normally pumps all of the blood that comes into it and therefore maintains a right atrial pressure that is essentially zero. For this reason, the other two factors, the mean systemic pressure and the resistance to blood flow through the vessels, are the major controllers of venous return.

The *mean systemic pressure* is the ''algebraic'' average of all the pressures in the systemic circulation, and this amounts to approximately 7 mmHg in the normal animal. It is this low because by far the major portion of the blood is in the veins where the pressure is low rather than in the arteries where the pressure is high. The factors that can increase the mean systemic pressure are increased blood volume and sympathetic stimulation of the blood vessels to cause constriction. Therefore, both of these increase the return of blood toward the heart. Sympathetic stimulation of the veins is particularly important because by far the major portion of the blood is stored in the veins. When the veins constrict, large quantities of blood are forced into the heart, thus distending the heart chambers and increasing the cardiac output.

When the *resistance to blood flow* decreases, blood can then flow from the systemic vessels toward the heart with greater than normal ease, thus increasing the venous return. This is one of the principal means by which venous return is regulated, for when the tissues become active, their blood vessels automatically dilate. Consequently, the venous return becomes increased, the cardiac output increases, and an adequate amount of blood flow is automatically made available to the active tissues.

Regulation of Venous Pressure. The venous pressure is regulated mainly by the same two factors that regulate cardiac output—the ability of the heart to pump blood and the venous return to the heart. Normally the heart is capable of pumping all of the blood that returns to it and therefore keeps the right atrial pressure at essentially zero. However, if the heart becomes weak, or if the venous return to the heart becomes so much greater than normal that the heart cannot pump at all, blood begins to dam up in the right atrium, and the right atrial pressure rises. This occurs to a marked extent in cardiac failure, which will be discussed below. Thus, it is the balance between pumping by the heart and venous return that determines the right atrial pressure.

The right atrial pressure in turn is a major determinant of peripheral venous pressure, because the greater the right atrial pressure, the greater must the peripheral venous pressure be to keep the blood flowing toward the heart. Ordinarily the right atrial pressure must rise to about 5 to 6 mmHg above normal before significant distention of the peripheral veins begins to occur.

The Venous Pump. In the standing position blood does not flow with ease uphill through the veins. However, the veins are provided with valves, and when the surrounding muscles intermittently contract and compress the veins, this acts as a pump to keep the blood flowing toward the heart. This mechanism is called the *venous pump.* However, if a person stands completely still so that his veins are not intermittently compressed, or if the valves in his veins have become destroyed, as occurs in varicose veins, then the venous pump is no longer effective. Under these conditions the weight of the blood in the veins makes the venous pressure in the foot of a standing person as high as 75 to 90 mmHg.

PHYSIOLOGY OF HEART FAILURE

Coronary Thrombosis and Coronary Sclerosis. The usual cause of heart failure is diminished coronary blood flow to the heart muscle, which causes ischemia of the muscle causing heart weak-ness or even destruction of portions of the heart. The most common cause of coronary insufficiency is *coronary atherosclerosis,* which occurs in virtually everyone in old age. This means, simply, fatty–fibrotic lesions of the coronary vessels, causing progressive, usually localized constriction. However, in a large number of persons another condition, *coronary thrombosis,* occurs acutely as a result of a blood clot in a coronary artery, leading to the well-known "heart attack." Both coronary atherosclerosis and coronary thrombosis normally result from *atheromata,* which means infiltration of the coronary wall with cholesterol and other fatty substances. The deposits of cholesterol form nidi for the growth of fibrous tissue and thereby cause sclerosis, or occasionally the cholesterol protrudes through the intima into the lumen of the vessel and causes a blood clot to form, thereby occluding the vessel and resulting in a heart attack.

Low Cardiac Output Failure. The immediate effect of a heart attack is usually greatly diminished pumping ability of the heart itself, which causes blood to dam up in one or both atria and the cardiac output to fall below normal. A person can live with a cardiac output as low as about one half to two thirds normal for many hours, but, if it falls permanently below this level, he usually will die.

Nervous Compensations in Heart Failure. Immediately after an acute heart attack, the fall in cardiac output and the resulting fall in systemic arterial pressure initiate intense cardiovascular reflexes that strongly excite the sympathetic nervous system. The sympathetic impulses in turn help in two ways to compensate for the diminished pumping ability of the heart: First, the strength of contraction of the nondamaged portion of the heart is increased. Second, the sympathetic impulses increase the vasomotor tone throughout the systemic circulation, which results in increased venous return of blood to the heart. As a result of these two effects, the cardiac output is often returned either to normal or almost to normal within a few minutes after a mild or even moderate heart attack, and the person will often experience nothing more than a transient period of fainting. In most severe heart attacks, however, the nervous compensations are unable to return the cardiac output to normal, but, nevertheless, do return the output part way toward normal and thereby help to prevent death of the patient.

Fluid Retention in Heart Failure. Immediately after an acute heart attack, the output of urine by the kidneys usually decreases very greatly for three reasons: (1) Sympathetic reflexes cause intense afferent arteriolar constriction in the kidneys, thereby greatly reducing the glomerular filtration rate. (2) The low cardiac output tends to reduce the arterial pressure, and this too reduces the glomerular filtration rate. (3) When the cardiac output falls very low, the kidneys secrete large amounts of renin, and large amounts of angiotensin II therefore are also formed. This in turn causes the kidneys to retain fluid by a direct effect of angiotensin on the kidneys and also indirectly by stimulating the secretion of aldosterone, which then also acts on the kidneys to reduce fluid excretion. Consequently, in severe acute cardiac failure a person may become completely anuric, while in milder degrees of acute failure, he or she usually becomes oliguric.

Obviously, the retention of fluid by the kidneys increases the total volume of extracellular fluid, most of which leaks out of the capillaries into the interstitial spaces and causes at times very serious edema. However, a small amount remains in the blood and increases the blood volume.

Value of Fluid Retention. Most physicians have long considered fluid retention in heart failure to be a detrimental factor. However, experiments in animals indicate that moderate degrees of fluid retention are beneficial to the patient because the increase in blood and interstitial fluid volumes promotes increased return of blood to the heart, primes the heart better than usual and therefore allows increased pumping. Beyond a certain degree of priming, though, the heart can become overstretched; then, further retention of fluid becomes detrimental to heart function. Also, excessive fluid retention can cause pulmonary edema and death.

Left Heart Failure Versus Right Heart Failure. Since the heart is actually two separate pumps, it is obvious that one side of the heart can fail independently of the other. More often the left heart fails because most coronary thromboses affect principally the left ventricle. However, right heart failure frequently occurs in patients who have pulmonary hypertension or in patients with certain types of congenital heart defects.

Most of the differences between left heart failure and right heart failure are obvious. Left heart failure causes excessive shift of fluid into the lungs with resulting pulmonary edema, while right heart failure causes excessive shift of blood into the systemic circulation.

In right heart failure, since only small amounts of extra blood are available in the lungs to shift into the systemic system, only a small amount of venous congestion occurs immediately in the systemic circulation. Indeed, peripheral edema does not occur

at all immediately after *acute* right heart failure but instead must await retention of fluid by the kidneys.

On the other hand, in acute left heart failure the shift of blood into the lungs from the very voluminous systemic circulation can be tremendous, and such severe pulmonary edema often occurs within a matter of minutes that it can kill the person. Yet, sometimes the pulmonary capillary pressure rises only a moderate amount immediately after the failure, not enough to cause significant edema. But during the ensuing few days, as the kidneys retain fluid, the pulmonary capillary pressure rises still higher, and severe pulmonary edema then develops, causing a respiratory death.

PHYSIOLOGY OF VALVULAR HEART DISEASE

In the past, before the availability of antibiotics, much valvular disease of the heart was caused by *rheumatic fever,* which leads to partial or total destruction of the valves. Damage occurs most frequently in the mitral valve, almost as frequently in the aortic valve, and only rarely in the tricuspid and the pulmonary valves. Sometimes the damaged vanes of the valves fail to close, which results in *regurgitation* or *insufficiency.* At other times fibrosis of the valves greatly reduces the size of the valvular opening, which is called *stenosis.* In either instance, the function of the affected ventricle is greatly compromised. Consequently, rheumatic valvular heart disease usually causes the left heart to become a very poor pump, while the right heart remains essentially normal. As discussed above, this condition often causes excessive damming of blood in the lungs, resulting in pulmonary edema and eventually a respiratory death.

A particular feature of valvular heart disease is the rapidity with which pulmonary edema sometimes occurs following exercise. In the resting state the pulmonary capillary pressure may remain slightly below the critical level at which pulmonary edema develops. But, when the person exercises, the venous return to the right heart becomes greatly increased, thus resulting in further shift of blood into the lungs, with rapid development of edema.

PHYSIOLOGY OF CONGENITAL HEART ABNORMALITIES

In many congenital heart abnormalities an abnormal opening exists somewhere between the pulmonary and the systemic arterial systems that allows much of the blood to bypass either the lungs or the systemic circulation; the condition is called a *right-to-left shunt* when the lungs are bypassed. When the blood bypasses the systemic circulation, it is called a *left-to-right shunt.*

A typical right-to-left shunt occurs in *tetralogy of Fallot* in which the principal defects are (1) an interventricular septal defect, (2) shift of the aorta to the right, its opening usually lying directly over the septal defect so that blood can flow into it from either the right or the left ventricle, (3) a greatly constricted pulmonary artery so that little blood will flow into the pulmonary system, and (4) hypertrophy of the right ventricle. In this condition the right ventricle pumps only small quantities of blood into the lungs through the constricted pulmonary artery but large quantities directly into the aorta. Thus, most of the systemic blood returning to the heart bypasses the lungs and reenters the systemic circulation without becoming aerated. The distinguishing physiologic abnormality of a right-to-left shunt, therefore, is poor aeration of the blood, and the person's skin always remains bluish, which is called *cyanotic.*

A typical left-to-right shunt is a *patent ductus arteriosus,* in which the ductus arteriosus, an important blood vessel between the aorta and the pulmonary artery in fetal life, remains patent (open) after birth of the baby. Another typical left-to-right shunt is an *interventricular septal defect.* In both of these conditions blood flows from the high pressure aorta or left ventricle into the low pressure pulmonary artery or right ventricle. As a result, the blood pumped by the left heart is forced immediately back into the pulmonary arterial system and traverses the lungs a second time and sometimes a third time before finally being pumped into the systemic circulation. Obviously, the blood that does eventually get to the systemic circulation is usually well aerated. Yet, this abnormal flow of blood around and around through the lungs markedly increases the work load of the heart, and, as a consequence, the heart is likely to fail at an early age. Also, the excess flow through the lungs often leads to progressive fibrosis of the lungs so that pulmonary debility sometimes leads to an early death.

CIRCULATORY SHOCK

Circulatory shock is a condition in which the cardiac output is so greatly reduced that tissues throughout the body begin to deteriorate for lack of adequate nutrition. Any circulatory abnormality that greatly reduces the cardiac output can cause circulatory shock. There are three major classifications of shock: (1) cardiac shock, (2) hypovolemic shock, and (3) neurogenic shock.

Cardiac Shock. This occurs most frequently in acute heart failure, in which the cardiac output often falls very low for many hours at a time. This was described above in the discussion of low cardiac output failure.

Hypovolemic Shock. This means shock resulting from greatly reduced blood volume, and this in turn can be caused by (1) blood loss, (2) plasma loss, or (3) dehydration. Obviously, hypovolemia causes shock by decreasing the venous return to the heart.

Neurogenic Shock. This is circulatory shock that results from sudden inhibition of the sympathetic nervous system throughout the body. This allows all of the systemic vessels to dilate and the blood to "pool" in the lower part of the body rather than returning to the heart. If a person with loss of sympathetic tone is kept in a standing position, this can actually kill him or her, but, if he or she is placed in a horizontal position, sufficient blood will usually still flow back to the heart to allow survival.

The Progressive Nature of Shock. One of the essential features of true circulatory shock is that it creates a vicious cycle that tends to make the shock itself worse. That is, the shock causes very poor blood flow to different tissues of the body, including the tissues of the heart and the vascular system; this causes deterioration of the heart and the vessels; the cardiac output falls still more; the tissues deteriorate more; and the vicious cycle recycles again and again. Unless the cardiovascular reflexes and other compensatory mechanisms in the body overcome this progressive tendency of shock or unless therapy is instituted, the progression continues until death.

The progressive nature of shock is often very apparent in cardiac shock, for in this condition the heart is already greatly damaged. The decreased cardiac output results in further diminished coronary blood flow that makes the heart even weaker, thus initiating a very rapid vicious cycle of cardiac deterioration. For this reason, therapy must be instituted immediately in most cases of cardiac shock to prevent death.

Irreversible Shock. Another distinguishing characteristic of shock is that, beyond a certain stage in the progressive deterioration, any amount of therapy becomes ineffective in preventing death of the patient. This is called the irreversible stage of shock. Often different types of therapy, such as blood transfusion or administration of norepinephrine, will actually return the arterial pressure to normal or above normal. Yet, after another 10 to 30 minutes the pressure begins to fall again because the cardiovascular tissues have already been damaged too much, and any amount of therapy fails to keep this from proceeding on to death. When the circulatory organs have deteriorated beyond a certain degree, even though temporary measures can return the blood pressure and cardiac output to normal for a few minutes, the tissues themselves cannot recover rapidly enough to prevent subsequent death.

CIRCULATORY ARREST

During many surgical operations, the heart arrests or fibrillates; also, since the advent of cardiac surgery, the heart is often stopped purposely. Ordinarily a person's body can stand about 3 to 4 minutes of complete circulatory arrest without any permanent damage whatsoever, but beyond 3 to 4 minutes, blood clots begin to develop in many of the peripheral vessels. With adequate preliminary anticoagulation procedures, circulatory arrest can be continued in an animal for as long as 10 to 20 minutes without serious damage to the body. Without this preliminary treatment, such extensive blood coagulation usually occurs in the vessels of the brain that permanent cerebral damage or death almost always ensues if the circulation remains arrested longer than 5 to 8 minutes.

RESPIRATORY SYSTEM

VENTILATION OF THE LUNGS

Lungs and Thoracic Cage. No muscles are attached directly to the lungs to cause them to inflate and deflate. Instead, the lungs float freely in the thoracic cage, and anytime the thoracic cage enlarges or contracts, simultaneous changes in lung volume must also occur. The space between the visceral pleura of the lungs and the parietal pleura of the thoracic cage is called the *intrapleural space*. Normally, continuous absorption of fluid by the visceral pleura keeps the space almost entirely empty except for a few milliliters of viscid material that provides lubrication for the moving lungs.

If the intrapleural space is ever opened to the atmosphere, the lungs immediately collapse because the lungs themselves are highly elastic. This elasticity results from (1) elastic fibers in the lung tissue that extend in all directions and (2) surface tension of the fluid lining the alveoli; the surface of the fluid tends to contract because of intermolecular

attraction between the water molecules. This factor is about three times as potent in causing lung collapse as are the elastic fibers.

Surface-Active Substance (Surfactant) in the Alveoli. If the alveoli were lined with pure water, the surface tension would be so great along the walls of the alveoli that they would remain collapsed all of the time. Fortunately, a substance called surface-active substance or surfactant is secreted into the fluids of the alveoli by a special type of cell in the epithelium that lines the alveoli. This substance acts to decrease the surface tension of the fluids, which allows normal expansion of the lungs. Some newborn babies fail to secrete adequate quantities of surfactant, and therefore cannot expand their lungs normally; this sometimes leads to death.

Lack of surfactant can also cause the development of pulmonary edema, because excess surface tension in the alveoli creates a powerful force to pull fluid into the alveoli from the pulmonary interstitium.

Expansion of the Lungs. The lungs can be expanded in two ways, either by increasing the length of the thoracic cavity or by increasing its thickness. The *diaphragm* is the main muscle that increases the length of the thoracic cavity; all the muscles of the thorax and the neck that pull the chest cage upward increase the thickness of the cavity, because the ribs normally hang downward but on being pulled upward extend almost straight forward.

The major muscles of expiration are the abdominal muscles. These contract around the abdominal viscera, forcing them upward against the diaphragm. Also, some of the abdominal muscles pull downward on the ribs, which reduces the anteroposterior diameter of the thorax.

Figure 3-11 illustrates increases and decreases in lung volume during a series of respiratory cycles of different intensities. At the upper part of the figure is a line that represents full expansion of the lungs. In the lower part of the figure is another line that represents the least degree of expansion of the lungs that can occur at the end of the most forceful expiration. The small excusions in this figure represent normal respiration. Some of the important features of respiratory exchange of air between the lungs and the atmosphere are described below.

Tidal Air and Minute Respiratory Volume. The amount of air taken in and expelled with each breath is called tidal air. This is normally about 500 ml. The minute respiratory volume is the sum of all the tidal air breathed during a minute. Since the normal respiratory rate is around 12 breaths per

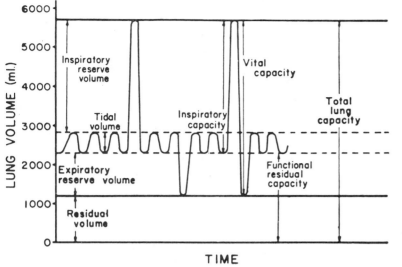

Fig. 3-11. Changes in lung volume during normal respiratory excursions and during maximal inspiration and maximal expiration. (Guyton AC: Textbook of Medical Physiology, 7th ed. Philadelphia, WB Saunders, 1986)

minute, the normal minute respiratory volume is abut 6000 ml.

Vital Capacity and Maximum Rate of Pulmonary Ventilation. The maximum amount of air that a person can expire after initially taking the deepest possible breath is called the vital capacity. In a normal male this is about 4.5 liters, and in a normal female about 3.5 liters. Thus, the vital capacity is about eight times the normal tidal air, which illustrates that there is a tremendous amount of *pulmonary reserve.* This reserve is even further enhanced by the ability of a person to breathe far more rapidly than the normal 12 breaths per minute. When a person breathes as rapidly and as deeply as he can, he can sustain for long periods a minute respiratory volume as high as 120 liters per minute and for a short time as high as 175 liters per minute. Therefore, a person can breathe about 20 to 30 times as much air per minute under stressful conditions as he breathes normally.

Dead Space and Alveolar Ventilation. Each time a person inhales air into the respiratory tract, part of the new air must be used to fill the passageways between the nose and the alveloi. Since this portion of the air does not come in contact with the pulmonary membranes that aerate the blood, it is called dead space air. The dead space of the normal respiratory system is about 150 ml. Thus, with each normal tidal volume of air, 150 ml of the 500 ml fails to reach the alveoli and therefore is not available to aerate the blood. That portion of the air that does reach the alveoli is called the alveolar ventilatory air, and it normally amounts to about 350 ml with each breath. With a normal respiratory rate of 12

per minute this amounts to an alveolar ventilation of 4.2 liters per minute.

Functional Residual Capacity. At the end of each normal expiration, approximately 2300 ml of air still remain in the lungs; this is called the functional residual capacity. And, even after the most forceful possible expiration, about 1200 ml still remain, which is called the *residual volume.* The air that remains in the lungs from breath to breath has a very important function: It keeps aerating the blood in the pulmonary capillaries even during expiration. Therefore, it prevents extensive rise and fall of blood oxygen and carbon dioxide concentrations during the respiratory cycle.

With a normal alveolar ventilatory air of only 350 ml per breath and a normal functional residual volume of 2300 ml, only about one seventh of the air in the lungs is exchanged with the atmosphere in each breath. If some foreign gas is placed in the alveoli, normal respiration will remove only half of this gas in a period of 17 seconds. Thus, it is a very false notion that the air of the lungs is completely replaced with each breath.

ALVEOLAR AIR

Concentration of the Alveolar Gases. The alveolar air normally contains major amounts of four different gases: nitrogen, oxygen, carbon dioxide, and water vapor. The relative concentrations of these are nitrogen, 74%; oxygen, 14%; carbon dioxide, 6%; and water vapor, 6%. Thus, the amount of oxygen in the alveolar air is only 14% in comparison with slightly over 20% in normal air. This difference is caused mainly by rapid absorption of oxygen from the alveoli into the blood. Also, alveolar air contains approximately 6% carbon dioxide, while normal air contains almost no carbon dioxide. This high concentration of carbon dioxide is caused by continual excretion of carbon dioxide from the blood into the alveoli.

Partial Pressures of the Alveolar Gases. In essentially all respiratory studies one expresses gas concentrations not in terms of percentage but in *partial pressures*. The partial pressure of a gas is the amount of pressure exerted by that gas alone. For instance, if a flask contains pure oxygen, and the total pressure in the flask is equal to atmospheric pressure, 760 mmHg, then the partial pressure of the oxygen is also 760 mmHg. However, if this flask contains half oxygen and half nitrogen while the total pressure is 760 mmHg, then the partial pressure of the oxygen would be 380 mmHg, and the partial pressure of nitrogen would also be 380 mmHg.

Partial pressures are used to express the concentrations of gases because it is pressure that causes the gases to move by diffusion from one part of the body to another. For instance, if the partial pressure of oxygen (P_{O_2}) is 90 mmHg in the alveoli and only 85 mmHg in the blood, then oxygen will diffuse from the alveoli into the blood. Conversely, if the pressure is greater in the blood than in the alveoli, oxygen will actually diffuse in the backward direction. Thus, the direction and the rate at which gases will diffuse depend on the pressure difference, the gases always moving from a high pressure area toward a low pressure area.

The normal partial pressures of the different gases in the alveoli are:

Oxygen, 104 mmHg
Carbon dioxide, 40 mmHg
Water vapor, 47 mmHg
Nitrogen, 569 mmHg

TRANSPORT OF OXYGEN AND CARBON DIOXIDE TO THE TISSUES

Diffusion of O_2 and CO_2 Through the Pulmonary Membrane. The normal P_{O_2} in the alveoli is approximately 104 mmHg, while the P_{O_2} of the venous blood entering the pulmonary capillaries is approximately 40 mmHg. This is a pressure difference of 64 mmHg, which causes large quantities of oxygen to diffuse through the pulmonary membrane into the blood. By the time the blood has passed through the pulmonary capillaries, it will have become almost

completely saturated with oxygen. That is, the P_{O_2} in the blood will have risen to about 100 mmHg, almost equal to that in the alveolar air.

Carbon dioxide diffuses through the pulmonary membrane in the opposite direction to the diffusion of oxygen. The pressure of carbon dioxide (P_{CO_2}) in the venous blood flowing into the lungs is approximately 45 mmHg, while the P_{CO_2} in the alveoli is 40 mmHg. This is a pressure difference of 5 mmHg that causes carbon dioxide to diffuse out of the blood into the alveoli. Carbon dioxide is far more soluble in the pulmonary membrane than is oxygen, which allows it to diffuse through the pulmonary membrane approximately 20 times as readily as oxygen. Therefore, by the time the blood has passed through the pulmonary capillaries, its P_{CO_2} will have fallen to almost exactly the P_{CO_2} in the alveoli, that is, to about 40 mmHg.

In summary, as blood passes through the pulmonary capillaries, the blood P_{O_2} and P_{CO_2} approach very nearly the alveolar P_{O_2} and P_{CO_2}.

Diffusing Capacity of the Lungs. The rate at which a gas will diffuse from the alveoli into the blood for each mmHg pressure difference is called the diffusing capacity of the lungs for that particular gas. The diffusing capacity of the lungs for oxygen when a person is at rest is approximately 22 ml per mmHg per minute. The diffusing capacity for carbon dioxide is about 20 times this value or approximately 440 ml per mmHg per minute.

Transport of Oxygen by the Blood Hemoglobin. Ninety-seven percent of all the oxygen normally carried from the lungs to the tissues is carried in chemical combination with hemoglobin in the red blood cells. Hemoglobin has the peculiar property of combining with large quantities of oxygen when the P_{O_2} is high and then releasing this when the P_{O_2} falls. Therefore, when the blood passes through the lungs, where the P_{O_2} rises to 100 mmHg, the hemoglobin picks up large quantities of oxygen. Then as it passes through the tissue capillaries, where the P_{O_2} falls to about 40 mmHg, large quantities of oxygen are released, this oxygen then diffusing to the tissue cells.

An especially important function of hemoglobin is that it releases oxygen to the tissues at a fairly constant P_{O_2}, between 20 and 50 mmHg, regardless of very wide fluctuations in the P_{O_2} in the air, for the following reason: If the oxygen in the alveolar air rises even as high as 1000 mmHg, the hemoglobin becomes 100% saturated with oxygen, which is almost exactly the same amount of oxygen as at the normal alveolar P_{O_2} of 104 mmHg, 97% saturated. Therefore, essentially the same amount of oxygen is carried by the hemoglobin to the tissues. Because of this property, hemoglobin is frequently called an *oxygen buffer.*

Diffusion of Oxygen into the Tissues. When arterial blood enters the tissue capillaries, its Po_2 is still approximately 100 mmHg. On the other hand, the tissue cells are continually using oxygen for metabolism, which keeps the Po_2 of the interstitial fluid low, about 30 to 40 mmHg. Thus, a pressure difference exists between the blood and the cells of about 60 to 70 mmHg. This immediately causes rapid diffusion of oxygen into the interstitial fluid. As the blood passes through the capillaries its Po_2 normally falls to about 40 mmHg before it enters the veins. During high metabolic activity of the tissues, this value may fall to as low as 15 to 20 mmHg.

Transport of CO_2 in the Blood. When oxygen is metabolized in the cells, large quantities of carbon dioxide are formed, causing the intracellular Pco_2 to rise to values perhaps as high as 50 mmHg. On the other hand, the Pco_2 of the arterial blood entering the tissue capillaries is only 40 mmHg. This 10 mm pressure difference makes the carbon dioxide diffuse rapidly into the blood, raising the blood Pco_2 to about 45 mmHg before the blood passes on into the veins.

The carbon dioxide in the blood, like oxygen, is also carried mainly in combination with various chemical substances. The largest proportion combines with water inside the red blood cells to form carbonic acid. This reaction is catalyzed by a protein enzyme in the red cells called carbonic anhydrase. Most of the carbonic acid immediately dissociates into bicarbonate ions and hydrogen ions, the hydrogen ions in turn combining with hemoglobin. An additional small portion of the carbon dioxide combines directly with hemoglobin to form carbaminohemoglobin. When the blood arrives in the lungs, where the Pco_2 of the alveolar air (40 mmHg) is lower than that of blood (45 mmHg) these chemical reactions are rapidly reversed, and the carbon dioxide diffuses out of the blood into the alveoli.

REGULATION OF RESPIRATION

Respiratory Rhythm. The continual respiratory rhythm is caused by intermittent nerve impulses originating in the *respiratory center,* which is located in the brain stem in the reticular substance of the medulla and the pons. This center has a basic oscillating mechanism that causes it to emit rhythmic impulses to the respiratory muscles. However, the intensity of this rhythmic excitation of respiration can be increased or decreased by changes in the chemical composition of the blood described below and also by sensory signals from the lungs.

A special reflex that is important in helping to regulate the respiratory rhythm is the *Hering-Breuer reflex.* This reflex is initiated by nerve receptors that detect the degree of stretch of the lungs. When the lungs become overly inflated, the receptors send signals into the respiratory center to inhibit inspiration and to excite expiration. Obviously, this reflex prevents overinflation of the lungs.

Control of the Alveolar Ventilation by Carbon Dioxide. The rate of alveolar ventilation is normally about 4.2 liters per minute, but this can be increased for short periods of time to higher than 150 liters per minute, or it can be decreased to zero. By far the most powerful stimulus for increasing both the rate and the depth of respiration, and therefore increasing the rate of alveolar ventilation, is carbon dioxide. When increased quantities of carbon dioxide are formed in the body cells and these collect in the body fluids, the ventilation sometimes increases to as high as ten times normal. This in turn blows off the extra quantity of carbon dioxide from the lungs.

Regulation of Alveolar Ventilation by Blood pH. Earlier in the chapter, in connection with the discussion of acid–base balance, it was pointed out that an increase in hydrogen ion concentration (that is, a decrease in *p*H) stimulates the respiratory center and increases alveolar ventilation. This causes increased quantities of carbon dioxide to be blown off from the blood which in turn decreases the amount of blood carbonic acid. Also, since carbonic acid is in constant equilibrium with hydrogen ions of the blood, the hydrogen ion concentration also decreases back toward normal.

Regulation of Alveolar Ventilation by Oxygen Lack. Lack of oxygen in the blood can also increase the rate of alveolar ventilation. However, unlike the effects of carbon dioxide and hydrogen ion concentration, oxygen lack does not directly stimulate the respiratory center. Instead, it excites special nerve receptors called chemoreceptors located in minute carotid and aortic bodies that lie, respectively, in the carotid bifurcations and along the aorta. Each of these bodies has a special artery that supplies abundant amounts of arterial blood to the chemoreceptors. When the arterial oxygen concentration falls, signals from the chemoreceptors are transmitted to the respiratory center where they cause an increase in alveolar ventilation.

The oxygen lack stimulus for increasing alveolar ventilation is a weak one compared with stimulation by excess carbon dioxide and low *p*H. Maximal increase in carbon dioxide can increase alveolar ventilation about tenfold; maximal increase in hydrogen ion concentration can increase it about fivefold; but maximal oxygen lack (under acute conditions) can increase alveolar ventilation only by about one and two thirds.

One often wonders why the evolutionary processes have made oxygen lack such a poor stimulus of respiration in comparison with carbon dioxide and hydrogen ions. However, oxygen concentration in the tissues is regulated principally by the hemoglobin buffer mechanism discussed above, while carbon dioxide concentration is regulated almost entirely by alveolar ventilation, and hydrogen ion concentration is also regulated to a major extent in this way as was discussed earlier. Therefore, there is less need for oxygen to control respiration than for carbon dioxide and hydrogen ion concentration to control it.

Regulation of Respiration in Exercise. In exercise, alveolar ventilation sometimes increases as much as 30-fold, which is even more than the increase that occurs as a result of maximal carbon dioxide or maximal hydrogen ion stimulation. The precise cause of the greatly increased respiration during exercise has not been determined, but it is believed to result from nerve signals transmitted during exercise from other centers of the brain that are simultaneously providing nervous drive for the exercise itself, and possibly from sensory signals originating in the active muscles.

PHYSIOLOGY OF RESPIRATORY DISORDERS

Hypoxia. The term hypoxia means insufficient availability of oxygen to support normal tissue metabolism. If we very rapidly review the mechanisms of oxygen transport to the tissues, we can readily understand the different possible causes of hypoxia: (1) too little oxygen in the inspired air, (2) obstruction of the respiratory passageways, (3) decreased diffusing capacity of the lungs caused by destruction of large portions of the lung or thickened pulmonary membranes, (4) too little blood flow to the tissues to carry adequate oxygen, (5) absence of or diminished blood flow through large portions of the lungs, (6) too little hemoglobin in the blood to carry oxygen to the tissues, (7) too few capillaries in a particular tissue area to allow adequate tissue oxygenation, and (8) too few oxidative enzymes in the cells for the oxygen to be used (or poisoned enzymes—due to cyanide poisoning, for example).

Oxygen Therapy in Hypoxia. In certain types of hypoxia, administration of high concentrations of oxygen in the respiratory air can relieve the hypoxic condition. This is particularly true of atmospheric hypoxia, obstructive hypoxia, and hypoxia caused by diminished diffusing capacity of the lungs, for, in all of these, an increase in the oxygen concentration increases the P_{O_2} in the alveoli and thereby promotes increased oxygen diffusion into the blood. In other types of hypoxia the problem is mainly diminished transport of oxygen to the tissues or diminished use of oxygen by the tissues. In these types of hypoxia, oxygen therapy may be of slight benefit but not nearly so much as in the types mentioned above.

AVIATION PHYSIOLOGY

Hypoxia at High Altitudes. The main problem in aviation physiology is a progressive decrease in P_{O_2} at higher and higher altitudes. A normal person often becomes lethargic and loses much mental alertness at about 12,000 to 15,000 feet. At 18,000 feet, a person can become so disoriented that judgment is lost; pilots may actually fly still higher rather than returning to a lower level to correct the hypoxic condition. And at about 23,000 feet an unacclimatized aviator will become comatose in 20 to 30 minutes. If pure oxygen is used rather than normal air, a pilot can ascend to an altitude of about 45,000 feet before becoming hypoxic, because the oxygen replaces the nitrogen that normally fills the major amount of space in the alveoli.

Acclimatization to Hypoxia. Though an aviator almost never remains at a high altitude long enough to become adjusted to the altitude, mountain climbers often become acclimatized sufficiently that they can live and work at altitudes many thousand feet higher than normal persons. Acclimatization results from three major physiologic changes:

1. The oxygen lack mechanism for control of pulmonary ventilation normally increases ventilation only about 65%, but after a person remains at high altitudes for several days, this mechanism becomes progressively more effective and increases ventilation about 400% instead of the normal 65%, thus providing much greater amounts of oxygen for the alveoli.

2. When one stays at a high altitude for several weeks, the hypoxia causes greatly increased production of red blood cells by the mechanism explained earlier in the chapter, sometimes increasing the total red cell mass to as much as 80% above normal and the hematocrit to 50% above normal. This obviously increases

the ability of the blood to transport oxygen to the tissues.

3. Associated with the increased blood cell mass is a slight increase in the number of blood vessels in the tissues or in their sizes so that increased quantities of blood can flow through the tissues, thus again increasing the available oxygen in the tissues.

Acceleratory Forces in Aviation. Another major problem in aviation is *centrifugal acceleration,* which means that a person tends to be displaced in one direction or another when the airplane turns to one side or up or down. Centrifugal acceleration is of special importance when one comes out of a dive or when one goes through a tight turn. Sometimes the aviator is pressed downward against the seat of the airplane with a force many times the weight of his or her body. The normal weight of the body is said to be 1 gravity (g), but if the total force against the seat is two times body weight, the acceleration is 2 g. A person can withstand up to about 4 g without harm, but 5 g or more for only 10 seconds usually causes blackout because of "centrifuging" the blood out of the head and into the vessels of the legs and abdomen.

SPACE PHYSIOLOGY

Survival in space is mainly an engineering problem, for the person will have to exist in a pressurized chamber or in a pressurized suit that contains an adequate supply of oxygen. Other problems have to do with linear acceleration or deceleration, weightlessness, radiation hazards, and provision of a complete life cycle.

The problem of *linear acceleration* exists principally when the space ship leaves the earth, for the ship must be accelerated to the velocity required to escape the pull of earth's gravity. Approximately the highest degree of linear acceleration developed is about 9 g—that is, the body is pushed backward against the seat with a force about nine times its own weight. The human body can stand 9 g in a horizontal or reclining position though not in the upright position. Therefore, takeoff has to be accomplished with the body horizontal to the line of takeoff. Linear deceleration occurs during reentry, and the problems are the same.

Weightlessness occurs in space because both the space ship and the human are traveling through space at the same speed, both of them affected by the same forces so that nothing pulls the human toward the bottom, the top, or the sides of the space ship. He or she simply floats in the ship. This has not proved to be a severe physiological problem, mainly an engineering one to provide means for keeping the body properly oriented in the ship. However, it does cause decalcification of the bones and loss of fluid from the tissues of the lower body.

The radiation hazard of space travel is likely to prevent prolonged space travel in a zone 500 to 20,000 miles above the earth. The play of cosmic particles on the stratosphere at this height creates a very strong field of gamma rays.

By far the greatest problem of space survival is that of providing a continuous supply of oxygen, water, and food for the traveler, particularly since interplanetary space travel may well require months to years. This is expected to be accomplished by installing a complete life cycle in the space ship. Algae or some other type of plant life will be used to convert carbon dioxide, with use of the sun's energy, into oxygen and food. In turn, the excreta from the human being will be used as nutrients for the plant life. Thus survival can continue indefinitely.

DEEP-SEA DIVING PHYSIOLOGY

Effects of High Gaseous Pressures on the Body. When a person descends deep under the sea, air must be pumped into the lungs with progressively more and more pressure so that the chest can withstand the pressure of the water on the outside; otherwise, the chest would collapse. At a depth of 10 m, the pressure must be two times normal atmospheric pressure; at 20 m, 3 atmospheres; at 30 m, 4 atmospheres; and so forth.

When air is compressed into the lungs under more than about 8 to 10 atmospheres of pressure, both the oxygen and the nitrogen become toxic. High pressures of oxygen cause mental disorientation, presumably because of excessive usage of oxygen by certain of the neuronal cells. The person first becomes quite irritable, and this is often followed by convulsions and coma. Obviously, if such should occur at great depths, it would be disastrous.

High nitrogen pressures have an anesthetic effect, causing first a lethargic state, then a somnolent state, and finally total anesthesia. The deepest sea depth that a person can survive while breathing pure air for more than an hour is about 300 feet, at which depth the pressure is 10 atmospheres. At this pressure the nitrogen narcosis effect approaches the somnolent level, and the oxygen effect approaches the convulsion level. For safety's sake, a person rarely works below 250 feet even for short periods of time when breathing compressed air. For deeper levels, the nitrogen and part of the oxygen are replaced by helium, which causes little or none of the narcotic or convulsive effects of nitrogen or oxygen.

Bubble Formation on Ascent—Decompression Sickness. Another major problem in deep-sea diving physiology is the tendency for divers to develop bubbles in their body fluids as they ascend from the depths. When the body is exposed to high pressure, the inert gases of the breathing mixture—such as nitrogen or helium—become dissolved in high concentrations in all the body fluids. Then, when the person is again exposed to low pressure, these gases must diffuse out of the tissue spaces into the blood and then through the lungs into the expired air. This "degassing" process sometimes requires as much as 6 or more hours, and, if the pressure around the body is decreased rapidly rather than slowly, these gases will simply form bubbles in the body fluids rather than diffusing out through the lungs. Therefore, it is essential that the diver ascend from depths slowly or that he be decompressed slowly over a long period in a decompression chamber.

The development of bubbles in the body fluids can cause serious damage in the tissues or can cause gas emboli in the circulating blood. Two of the most distressing effects are (1) air emboli in the pulmonary vessels, which causes the "chokes," and (2) disruption of nerve pathways in the nervous system, which causes serious pain or even paralysis. This condition is generally called *decompression sickness,* the bends, caisson disease, or diver's paralysis.

CENTRAL NERVOUS SYSTEM

BASIC ORGANIZATION OF THE CENTRAL NERVOUS SYSTEM

The central nervous system is a rapidly acting control system for the body. Control of the different bodily functions depends basically upon (1) sensory receptors that apprise the nervous system of the conditions in the body, (2) effector organs that perform functions dictated by the nervous system, and (3) integrative mechanisms in the central nervous system to determine the effector responses to receptor signals.

Sensory Receptors. The sensory receptors include any type of nerve ending in the body that can be stimulated by some physical or chemical stimulus originating either outside or within the body. These receptors include (1) the rods and the cones of the eyes for detection of light; (2) the cochlear nerve endings of the ear for detection of sound; (3) the taste endings in the mouth for detection of taste; (4) the olfactory endings in the nose for detection of smell; (5) the sensory nerve endings in the skin for detection of touch, pain, warmth, cold, pressure and tickle; (6) sensory endings deep in the body for detection of deep pressure, position of the limbs, vibratory impulses, and so forth; (7) stretch receptors in the walls of the arteries for detection of arterial pressure; (8) stretch receptors in the veins, the lungs, and other visceral organs; (9) chemical receptors in different portions of the brain, such as in the vasomotor center and the hypothalamus, as well as in outlying organs such as the carotid and aortic bodies; and (10) a variety of other specialized receptors. Thus, we have a long list of different types of receptors that can detect almost any type of normal stimulus to the body.

Effector Organs. These include every organ that can be stimulated by nerve impulses. Perhaps the most important effector system is the skeletal muscular system. In addition, the smooth muscle of the body and the glandular cells are among the important effector organs. However, all cells of the body react to circulating hormones in the body fluids, some of which are secreted in response to nerve impulses. For instance, sympathetic stimulation causes the adrenal medulla to release large amounts of epinephrine and norepinephrine. These are transported throughout the entire body and increase the metabolism of every known type of cell. In this sense, then, every cell of the body is an effector organ, though some cells are far more important in the scheme of nervous control than are others.

Reflex Arc. One basic means by which the nervous system controls functions in the body is the reflex arc, in which a stimulus excites a receptor, appropriate impulses are transmitted into the central nervous system where various nervous reactions take place, and then appropriate effector impulses are transmitted to an effector organ to cause a reflex effect.

Some reflexes are very simple with the effect following the stimulus within a fraction of a second. An example of such a reflex is the withdrawal of the hand from a hot stove. Other reflexes act extremely slowly. For instance, a person may see something he or she might desire in a store window today but not initiate the effector responses to buy the object until many months later. Nevertheless, this, in a sense, is still a reflex that requires many months of storage of information before the final effect occurs.

Integrative Centers of the Nervous System. Those parts of the nervous system that put many different types of sensory signals together before causing a reaction or that first store the information and later cause a reaction are called the integrative centers of the nervous system. For instance, even in the simple reflex that causes a person to withdraw his hand from a hot stove, the areas of the spinal cord that are concerned with this withdrawal reaction are known as the centers for integration of the withdrawal reflex. At a much higher level of complexity are the integrative centers of the cerebral cortex that have to do with memory and thinking. The medulla is the integrative center for most respiratory control, for most control of arterial pressure and for control of swallowing; the motor area of the cerebral cortex, the cerebellum, the basal ganglia and large parts of the reticular substance of the brain stem are major parts of the integrative centers for control of muscular movement.

FUNCTION OF THE SINGLE NEURON

The nervous system contains between 100 and 200 billion neurons, one of which is illustrated in Figure 3-12. The sum of all the actions of the single neurons determines the overall function of the brain. Therefore, it is necessary to understand the functional abilities of single neurons in order to comprehend the manner in which these operate together to give the integrative functions of the nervous system.

The Synapse. The neurons of the nervous system are arranged so that each neuron stimulates other neurons, and these in turn stimulate still others until the functions of the nervous system are performed. The point of contact between successive neurons, illustrated in Figure 3-13, is called a synapse, and the terminal endings of the nerve filaments that synapse with the next neuron are called *presynaptic terminals, synaptic knobs, boutons,* or simply *end feet.* Usually, there are many thousand presynaptic terminals on each neuron, these having originated from preceding neurons. Each terminal secretes a particular hormone called a transmitter substance that may either excite the next neuron or inhibit it. These hormones are called *excitatory* or *inhibitory transmitters.*

Function of a Transmitter Substance at a Synapse. Over thirty different types of transmitter substances have been described, and undoubtedly many more will yet be described. Each presynaptic terminal generally secretes one characteristic trans-

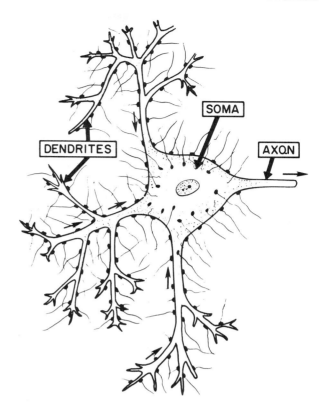

Fig. 3-12. A typical neuron of the central nervous system, showing presynaptic terminals on the neuronal soma and dendrites. Note also the single axon. (Guyton AC: Textbook of Medical Physiology, 7th ed. Philadelphia, WB Saunders, 1986)

mitter substance but often more than one. Each transmitter is synthesized within the terminal and stored in thousands of small vesicles. When an action potential spreads over the end of the nerve fiber, the depolarization of the terminal causes mi-

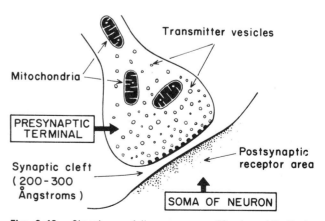

Fig. 3-13. Structure of the synapse. (Guyton AC: Textbook of Medical Physiology, 7th ed. Philadelphia, WB Saunders, 1986)

gration of a few of the vesicles to the membrane surface of the terminal, and these vesicles then extrude their contents of transmitter substance into the synaptic cleft between the terminal and the membrane of the succeeding neuron. The transmitter then combines with a receptor (a protein molecule) that is an integral part of the subsequent neuronal membrane. This opens a channel through the receptor protein in the membrane and allows ions to move through the channel. The receptor may be either an *excitatory receptor* or an *inhibitory receptor*. If it is excitatory, it opens sodium pores and allows sodium ions to move selectively to the inside of the membrane, which partially depolarizes the neuron and therefore stimulates it. In the case of the inhibitory receptor, the pores become permeable to chloride and potassium ions. Movement of these ions through the membrane *hyperpolarizes* the neuron (makes the inside of the membrane more negative), and this inhibits the neuron rather than exciting it.

Thus, whether a transmitter substance will be excitatory or inhibitory depends on the receptor substance as well as the transmitter. Some transmitters can be either excitatory or inhibitory, depending on the receptor substance with which it reacts. On the other hand, other transmitters are almost always either excitatory or inhibitory.

Excitatory Transmitters. An excitatory transmitter that is released by a large number of presynaptic terminals in the central nervous system is acetylcholine. This stimulates the successive neuron in exactly the same way that it stimulates a muscle fiber at the neuromuscular junction, that is, by increasing the permeability of the neuronal membrane to sodium. The sodium leaks rapidly to the interior of the cell, causing a sudden change in electrical potential across the membrane. However, stimulation of a single excitatory synapse almost never causes the neuron to "fire," for the amount of excitatory transmitter secreted at one synapse will not cause sufficient depolarization of the membrane to initiate an action potential. Each type of neuron is different in the number of synapses that must fire on its membrane to cause excitation. Certain neurons might require only five simultaneous firings; others might require as many as 100 to 1000 synapses discharging simultaneously. Thus, certain neurons allow signals to pass very easily, while others allow passage only with great difficulty. In this way, incoming signals can be channeled in the proper direction through the neuronal circuits of the brain.

Other transmitter substances that often function as excitatory transmitters include norepinephrine, epinephrine, glutamic acid, enkephalin, and substance P. However, some of these also function as inhibitory transmitters in the presence of inhibitory receptor substances.

Inhibitory Transmitters. Many presynaptic terminals secrete inhibitory transmitters rather than excitatory transmitter. In fact, there are far more inhibitory synapses in the central nervous system than most people realize, for function of large parts of the brain, including the cerebral cortex, the basal ganglia, the thalamus, and the cerebellum, depend almost as much on inhibition of neurons as upon excitation. It is probable that as many as a third or even more of the synapses are of the inhibitory type rather than of the excitatory type.

Two inhibitory hormones that are secreted at large numbers of synapses are gamma aminobutyric acid (GABA) and glycine. Other transmitters that sometimes but not always serve as inhibitory transmitters (in the presence of inhibitory receptors) include norepinephrine, epinephrine, serotonin, and dopamine.

Excitability of the Neuron. Whether or not a neuron will be excited depends on three major factors: (1) the basic nature of the neuron itself, whether it tends to be an excitable type of neuron or a relatively dormant type; (2) the number of excitatory synapses firing in any given time; and (3) the number of inhibitory synapses firing at any given time. In certain parts of the brain highly excitable neurons perform rapid and easily elicited actions; in others, relatively dormant neurons respond only when tremendously strong signals reach them. Thus, the integrative capabilities of the neurons differ in different parts of the brain.

FUNCTIONS OF "POOLS" OF NEURONS

Each part of the brain usually contains large numbers of similar types of neurons that lie close to each other and are interconnected by means of many fine nerve filaments. Each such group of neurons is called a *neuronal pool*. Different patterns of nerve filament interconnections exist in different pools, and the type of pattern in turn determines the manner in which the pool operates in the overall function of the brain. In general, three basic types of circuits occur in neuronal pools: (1) the diverging circuit, (2) the converging or integrative circuit, and (3) repetitive firing circuits.

Diverging Circuit. This circuit is the simplest of all that occur in the neuronal pools. It is simply a circuit in which the nerve fibers entering the pool divide many times so that a few impulses entering the pool cause a large number of impulses to leave the pool. This type of circuit is typified by the nervous control of muscular activity, for stimulation of a single large neuron in the motor cortex can stimulate many interneurons in the spinal cord, and these in turn might then stimulate as many as 50 to 100 anterior motor neurons, which in turn stimulate thousands of muscle fibers.

Converging or Integrative Circuit. An integrative circuit is one that, after receiving incoming signals from several sources, determines the level of reaction that will occur. That is, impulses "converge" into the pool, some from inhibitory nerves, some from excitatory nerves, some from peripheral nerves and some from parts of the brain. The different factors that enter into the response of the pool are (1) the basic excitability of the neurons in the pool, (2) the number of excitatory impulses entering the pool, (3) the number of inhibitory impulses entering the pool, (4) whether or not there might be some diverging circuits also in the pool, (5) the distribution of excitatory and inhibitory impulses to the different neurons, and so forth. From this list of possible factors that can affect the output from the neuronal pool, one can readily understand that basic differences in the anatomic organization of different neuronal pools can give thousands of different responses to incoming signals. For instance, the pool may be a high threshold pool into which many excitatory impulses must arrive before an effect will occur. It might be a low threshold pool into which only a few impulses must arrive before an effect will occur. The low threshold circuit is typified by the neuronal response that causes withdrawal of a limb when only a few pain receptors are stimulated, while the high threshold circuit is typified by withdrawal of a hand only when tremendous numbers of touch receptors are stimulated.

Repetitive Firing Circuits. Among the most important types of circuits in the nervous system are the repetitive firing circuits. In these, impulses entering a pool of neurons cause the pool to emit a series of impulses lasting long after the incoming signal is over. Three types of circuits can cause this: The first is a pool of neurons consisting of very excitable neurons, each one of which has a natural tendency to fire repetitively. The second is a *long chain of neurons* arranged one after another so that an incoming stimulus activates each one in succession. From each neuron of the chain a nerve fiber extends to some outlying neuron. Thus, this outlying neuron receives repetitive impulses from the successive neurons of the chain, but after all these

have fired the repetitive firing from the output neuron ceases.

Third, probably the most important type of repetitive firing circuit is the *reverberating circuit* in which an incoming impulse is passed along a succession of neurons until finally one of the neurons restimulates an earlier neuron in the succession. This causes the impulse to go around the circuit again and again. Every time around the circuit, collateral impulses are emitted into outgoing nerve fibers that spread to other parts of the nervous system. Theoretically, this type of circuit might continue to oscillate indefinitely, but more usually the oscillation ceases when some of the neurons in the circuit become too fatigued to continue. The continual respiratory rhythm represents a continually reverberating circuit, while the thought processes of the cerebral cortex probably represent circuits that revertebrate for short periods until neurons in the circuit fatigue or are inhibited so that the thought ceases.

To summarize, the nervous system is actually made up of many neuronal pools, each one of which has specific circuit characteristics that allow it to emit a certain pattern of output impulses in response to incoming signals. By combining the functional characteristics of the many different pools in the nervous system one can achieve almost any type of integrative function in one portion of the nervous system or another.

THE PROCESS OF CEREBRATION

Thoughts. The bases of *cerebration* are the individual thoughts, many of which occur directly as a result of incoming sensory impulses. For instance, the impulses from the eyes when a person is looking at a beautiful scene certainly generate a number of different thoughts.

The precise mechanisms of thoughts in the brain are not understood, but one of the suggestions is that a thought represents a pattern of impulses passing through particular neurons in multiple simultaneous areas of the conscious brain.

Memory. Memory simply means storage of information in the brain. The precise mechanism by which information is stored for long periods is not known, though it is believed to result from permanent facilitation of synapses. This means simply that excitation of a synapse repetitively over a time will cause that synapse to become more and more effective in stimulating the neuron. In other words, the fact that an impulse passes through a synapse once makes it easier for successive impulses to pass through the same synapse. Therefore, if a thought pattern is evoked over and over again by incoming sensory stimuli, eventually the pathway for transmission of impulses through that particular thought channel becomes facilitated so that even the slightest stimulus entering this pathway at a later time can elicit the entire thought. For instance, such a facilitated thought pathway might develop in response to seeing the beautiful scene referred to above. Then a year later, some stray impulse from another part of the brain might enter this particular thought pathway and allow the person to see the scene again in his mind. This is believed to be the basis of memory.

The portion of the brain most concerned with memory seems to be the *cerebral cortex,* since all through this structure are located neuronal pools that can be facilitated by sensory impulses so that subsequent signals entering these pools will evoke specific reactions. Furthermore, the storage of information in the brain is mostly lost when the cortex is gone.

"Programming" of the Thoughts. Now that we have discussed the possible basis of thoughts and memory, we still need to develop some understanding of the manner in which these are used in the thinking process. Everyone is familiar with the fact that different thoughts usually occur in rapid succession, and that each succeeding thought usually has some association with the preceding thought. Many sequences of thoughts are initiated by incoming sensory signals, whether these originate from the skin, from the eyes, from the ears, and so forth. For instance, a sudden knife cut on the leg would elicit first a thought of pain, then another thought that localizes the cut on the body, this followed by integrative processes that make the person turn the eyes and head to look at the pained area, followed by visual input impulses that combine with the previous thoughts to determine the nature of the stimulus causing the pain, and, finally, a series of integrations that cause motor movements to remove the painful object from the body. In this sequence of cerebration, the person must call forth memories from past experiences in order to understand why and how the leg is being pained, for, if he or she has never seen a knife before and is not familiar with its cutting capabilities, simply looking at the leg and seeing a knife against the skin will not explain the cause of the pain. In short, for cerebration to occur, the thoughts must be programmed. Some part of the brain must determine where the attention of the mind will be directed, whether it will be directed to the incoming sensory signals from the leg, to the movement of the head and the eyes, or to one of the

memory circuits to call forth information. The nature of this programming system of the brain is still unclear. However, the anatomic locations of the thalamus and the reticular substance of the mesencephalon have made many neurophysiologists point to these two areas as possible programming centers. Also, stimulation of specific points in these two areas cause highly specific patterns of reaction in other parts of the brain and cord.

THE SOMATIC SENSORY SYSTEM

The somatic sensory portion of the nervous system, illustrated in Figure 3-14, transmits sensory signals from all parts of the body into the central nervous

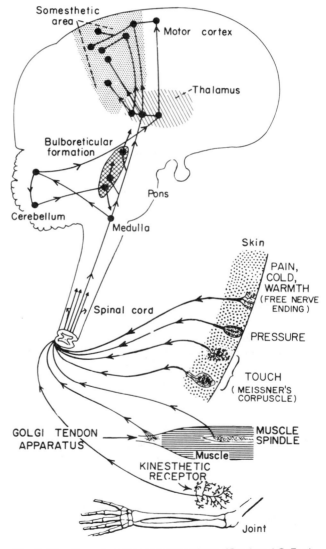

Fig. 3-14. The somatic sensory system. (Guyton AC: Textbook of Medical Physiology, 7th ed. Philadelphia, WB Saunders, 1986)

system. It is often subdivided into three different systems: the *exterioceptive system,* which transmits impulses from the skin; the *proprioceptive system,* which transmits impulses mainly from the muscles and joints relating to the momentary physical condition of the body; and the *visceral sensory system,* which transmits impulses from the viscera.

Modalities of Sensation. It is common knowledge that many different types of sensations can be perceived from the skin, including light touch, tickle, pressure, pain, cold, and warmth. These are called modalities of sensation. Proprioceptive modalities of sensation include sense of position of the limbs, degree of tension in the muscle tendons, degree of stretch of the muscle fibers, and deep pressure on different parts of the body. In addition to these, other modalities that are not transmitted by the somatic sensory system are sight, hearing, equilibrium, smell, and taste.

Sensory Receptors. Each modality of sensation is usually detected by a particular type of nerve ending. The most common nerve ending is the *free nerve ending,* illustrated in Figure 3-14, which is nothing more than a filamentous end of a nerve usually interwoven with other filamentous nerve endings. Different types of free nerve endings can detect pain, crude touch, tickle, heavy pressure, and probably warmth. In addition to the free nerve endings, the skin contains a number of specialized endings that are adapted to respond to some specific type of physical stimulus. For instance, one of these endings, called a *Meissner's corpuscle,* responds specifically to light touch.

Sensory endings deep in the body that subserve the different proprioceptive sensations are the *joint receptors,* which detect degree of angulation of the joints; *pacinian corpuscles,* which detect very rapid changes in pressure; *Golgi tendon apparatuses,* which detect degree of tension in the tendons; and *muscle spindles,* which detect degree of stretch of the muscle fibers.

Pathways or Transmission of Somatic Sensations into the Central Nervous System. The impulses generated in the sensory receptors are transmitted first into the spinal nerves and then through the dorsal roots of the spinal nerves into the spinal cord. In general, the proprioceptive impulses are transmitted by large *type A nerve fibers,* which can transmit at velocities as high as 100 m per second. This rapid velocity is especially important when a person is moving rapidly, for he needs to know during each split second the position of all parts of his body.

On the other hand, many of the aching type pain impulses are transmitted by the very small *type C fibers,* which transmit impulses at velocities less than 1 m per second. Here, rapidity of response is not needed. On the other hand, sharp pain is transmitted by intermediate velocity fibers, which allows rapid response to stimuli that might be damaging to the tissues.

Once the sensory fibers enter the spinal cord, most of them terminate there on *second order neurons* that then transmit impulses either to other areas of the cord or all the way to the brain. However, many sensory signals pass through several neurons in the spinal cord before ascending to the brain, but some sensory fibers pass all the way to the medulla where they end in the cuneate and the gracile nuclei, which in turn send second order nerve fibers to higher centers of the brain. Most of the second order nerve fibers of the somatic system terminate in the ventrobasal complex of the thalamus, and third order neurons pass from this area to the cerebral cortex, especially to the somatic sensory cortex and the somatic sensory association cortex, which lie behind the central sulcus of the brain.

It should be noted particularly that along the entire course of the sensory fibers from the cord to the cerebral cortex many collateral fibers spread in all directions. Especially abundant are (1) collateral fibers that spread in the cord itself, (2) collateral fibers that spread into the cerebellum and into all parts of the reticular substance of the brain stem, and (3) collaterals that spread from the sensory neurons of the thalamus to most other portions of the thalamus, the hypothalamus, and other closely associated nuclei. Thus, the "trunk line" sensory system carries sensory signals into essentially all parts of the brain.

The Labelled-Line Law. If a sensory nerve fiber is stimulated by an electrical stimulus, a person will perceive only one particular modality of sensation. For instance, excitation of a pain fiber will cause pain, excitation of a warmth fiber will cause the sensation of warmth, and so forth. Thus, each type of sensory nerve fiber transmits only one modality of sensation, and this is called the labelled-line law.

However, it is not the type of fiber that determines the modality of sensation transmitted, but, instead, it is the point in the central nervous system to which the fiber connects that determines the modality. For instance, pain fibers end in a slightly different point in the thalamus from the warmth fibers, and in a different point from the cold fibers.

Since some modalities of sensation can still be perceived even when the sensory portions of the cerebral cortex are removed, it is believed that sensory centers in the brain stem and the thalamus can determine at least some of the different sensory modalities, especially pain, cold, warmth, and crude touch. On the other hand, a person cannot localize sensations in different parts of his or her body accurately when the sensory portions of the cerebral cortex have been destroyed. Therefore, discrete localization is principally a function of the somatic sensory cortex, though the thalamus by itself is capable of crude localization to general areas of the body.

PAIN

The Basic Pain Stimulus; Threshold for Pain Perception. Pain fibers are stimulated any time a tissue is being damaged or being overstressed by mechanical force. However, once the damage is complete, the pain sensation gradually disappears in a few minutes or sometimes even in a few seconds. Pain nerve endings can be stimulated by mechanical trauma to the tissues, excess heat, excess cold, chemical damage, certain types of radiation damage, such as the pain associated with sunburn, and even lack of adequate blood flow to a tissue area, which causes ischemic pain.

Threshold for Pain Perception and Reactivity to Pain. Frequently, it is said that some people perceive pain far more easily than others. This is not true, for actual research on various degrees of injury in relation to the perception of pain shows that all persons begin to perceive pain at almost exactly the same degree of injury.

However, once the pain is perceived, the degree of transmission of pain signals in the nervous system, as well as the reactivity of different persons to the pain, varies tremendously. The reactivity to pain is partly an inherited characteristic of certain people, but it is also greatly influenced by previous training.

Control of Pain by Central Nervous System Mechanisms. The brain has the capability to control the sensitivity of pain pathways. It does this by sending centrifugal inhibitory signals from the brain to the brain stem and spinal cord to control pain signal transmission.

One of the controlling centers for pain is an area extending from near the third ventricle in the hypothalamus downward into the *central gray region* around the aqueduct of Sylvius in the mesencephalon. The perception of pain can be inhibited by *enkephalins* and *endorphins,* which are morphine-like substances found in this area of the brain. Therefore, they are believed to be an intrinsic brain opiate system for pain control. When the central gray area is stimulated by enkephalins, signals are transmitted to a thin midline nucleus called the *raphe magnus nucleus,* located in the lower pons and upper medulla. This nucleus in turn transmits nerve signals all the way to the spinal cord, where they terminate on neurons in the *dorsal horn gray matter.* It is through this same dorsal horn area that pain signals are transmitted into the central nervous system. The endings of the nerve fibers from the raphe magnus nucleus secrete serotonin, which in turn excites other dorsal horn neurons to secrete enkephalin; the enkephalin then acts on the pain-conducting neurons to block the pain signals.

VISCERAL SENSATION

Visceral Pain and Referred Pain. Essentially all internal organs of the body are supplied with pain nerve endings, but these are usually far more sparse than in the skin. Therefore, in general, sharp pain is much less likely to occur from the viscera than is the generalized aching or burning type of pain. The different types of stimuli that are particularly prone to cause visceral pain are (1) overdistention of a hollow viscus, (2) spasm of the smooth muscle of a viscus, (3) too little blood flow to the viscus, and (4) chemical damage such as that produced by spillage of acid gastric juice into the peritoneal cavity through a ruptured peptic ulcer. It is especially interesting that most deep tissues of the body, including even the organs of the abdomen, are relatively insensitive to a sharp knife cut, indicating that there are insufficient pain endings in any minute area to cause pain. Therefore, visceral pain usually occurs only on stimulation of pain endings over a wide area. However, this is not true in the periosteum of the bones, in the walls of the arteries, in the parietal pleura, and in the parietal peritoneum; these areas are almost equally as susceptible to pain as the skin.

Pain in a visceral organ is not always felt directly over the organ itself but may be referred to a distant area of the body. For instance, pain originating in the heart is often felt in one or both arms. This is called referred pain. Referred pain usually results from collateral neuronal connections between the visceral pain fibers and the somatic pain pathways in the cord, the visceral impulses exciting the somatic pathways and the person feeling the pain in some nonvisceral part of the body.

Other Visceral Sensations. There are few other types of visceral sensation besides pain that reach the conscious portions of the brain. However, many visceral sensations, such as stretch of arterial walls, stretch of the lungs, stretch of the gut, and so forth are of particular importance in reflex control of the specific organs. These reflexes and their initiating receptors are discussed at different points in this chapter in relation to the different organ systems.

CORD REFLEXES

Many central nervous system functions occur locally in the spinal cord without the aid of the brain. The cord integrates many specific reflexes that help to control muscle movements.

The Stretch Reflex. The simplest cord reflex, called the stretch reflex, is initiated by the muscle spindles. These receptors continually send impulses into the spinal cord to excite the anterior motor neurons; these in turn transmit impulses back to the respective muscle. This continual flow of impulses helps to maintain a certain amount of basal tone in the muscle.

The stretch reflex is elicited by stretching the muscle. In its simplest form, the stretch reflex involves only two neurons, the neuron from the muscle spindle to the anterior motor neuron and the anterior motor neuron back to the muscle. Stretch of the muscle spindles increases the number of impulses transmitted by the spindles, and this increases the number of impulses transmitted by the anterior motor neurons back to the muscle. Therefore, muscle stretch enhances the contractile tension in the muscle. This tension in turn tends to shorten the muscle back to its initial length. Thus, the stretch reflex opposes changes in muscle length.

The stretch reflex has both a dynamic and a static component, called respectively the *dynamic stretch reflex* and the *static stretch reflex.* The dynamic effect occurs only when the muscle is stretched rapidly because the spindles are very strongly stimulated during the actual instant of stretching; the strong signal from the spindle causes extreme feedback contraction of the muscle to oppose the sudden stretch. The static stretch reflex is much weaker than the dynamic reflex, but it maintains muscle contraction for minutes or hours when the muscle remains stretched beyond its normal length.

The muscle spindles themselves are provided with excitory nerve fibers from the spinal cord called *gamma efferent fibers,* and these in turn are controlled by signals from the reticular formation of the brain stem. Impulses transmitted through the gamma fibers can increase the degree of activity of the muscle spindle and therefore can also increase the intensity of either the dynamic stretch reflex on the static reflex. In this way, signals from the brain stem can alter the overall reactivity of the muscles.

The Withdrawal Response. Withdrawal reflexes can function in each part of the body to pull that part away from any painful object. For instance, if the hand is placed on a hot stove, impulses are transmitted from the pain receptors to the cord and immediately back to the flexor muscles of the arm to withdraw the hand. Because the flexor muscles are involved in this instance, this particular withdrawal reflex is called a *flexor reflex.*

Part of the withdrawal response involves impulses transmitted to the opposite side of the body to extend the opposite limb, thereby pushing the whole body away from the vicinity of the painful object. This extensor effect is called the *crossed extensor reflex.*

The withdrawal response is different for each part of the body. For instance, a painful stimulus applied to the lower back will cause forward arching of the back, or if the right deltoid region of the shoulder becomes pained, the whole upper body shifts to the left and the shoulder drops. Even in persons with the spinal cord transected in the neck, most of these withdrawal reflexes can still occur in a crude fashion. However, the human being has additional reflexes that go all the way to the brain and back that aid in the withdrawal response.

The Positive Supportive Reflex. Pressure on the bottoms of the feet causes the extensor muscles of the legs to tighten, which helps the legs to support the weight of the body against gravity. This reflex is integrated entirely in the few segments of the spinal cord that control the activity of each respective limb.

Walking Reflexes. Even walking movements can be performed by the limbs of a lower animal whose spinal cord has been transected. In an opossum with a transection in the thorax, the hind limbs can "walk" but without coordination with the movements of the forelimbs. If the cord is transected in the neck, rhythmic to-and-fro coordinated walking movements among all four limbs can occur. Occasionally, trotting movements also occur and, very rarely, galloping movements. However, with a neck transection, equilibrium cannot be maintained, so that the animal cannot actually make forward progression.

Thus, the basic patterns for walking and other movements of locomotion are integrated in the spinal cord. The nerve fiber tracts that coordinate the functions of the superior and the inferior segments of the cord are the *propriospinal fiber pathways* that lie near the gray matter and account for approximately one half of all the fiber tracts in the cord.

FUNCTIONS OF THE BRAIN STEM

Support of the Body Against Gravity. Even though the spinal cord is capable of providing the positive supportive reflex that helps to support the body against gravity and also of supplying walking reflexes, the human body still cannot stand and certainly cannot walk without the aid of higher central nervous system centers. With progression from lower phylogenetic types to the higher types, more and more of the control systems have gradually shifted from the cord toward the brain. As stated above, a lower animal, such as an opossum, can still walk quite well with its hind limbs even when its spinal cord is transected in the thorax. In the dog, basic walking movements can occur in the hind limbs with the thoracic cord transected, but these cannot be coordinated sufficiently to provide functional walking. In the human being, even these walking reflexes are crude when the cord is cut.

Located in the brain stem are a number of centers that help the limbs support the body against gravity. These transmit impulses especially to the extensor muscles, tightening the muscles of the trunk, the buttocks, the thighs, and the lower legs to allow the body to stand in an upright position. Therefore, it is frequently said that the brain stem supplies the nervous energy required for supporting the body against gravity. It is principally the vestibular nuclei and the reticular nuclei of the mesencephalon and the pons that are responsible for this function.

Maintenance of Equilibrium—Function of the Vestibular Apparatus. Closely associated with the support of the body against gravity is the maintenance of equilibrium. The vestibular and reticular nuclei of the brain stem can vary the degree of tension in the different extensor muscles in proportion to the need for maintenance of equilibrium. To do this these nuclei in turn are controlled by the vestibular apparatuses located on the two sides of the head in close association with the ears.

The vestibular apparatuses contain two types of receptor organs: One of these is the *macula* of the *utricle* and *saccule,* which contain large numbers of small calcified crystals called *otoliths* that lie on "hairs" projecting from sensory receptor cells called *hair cells.* Leaning of the head to one side or forward or backward causes these otoliths to fall toward the direction of leaning, thus bending the hairs. Because the different hair cells are oriented in all the different directions, this bending of the hairs causes signals to be transmitted into the brain informing the brain of the position of the head in relation to the direction of gravitational pull.

The second receptor system of the vestibular apparatus is the *semicircular canals,* which consists of three canals on each side of the head. Each of the canals is oriented in one of the three planes of space. The canals are filled with fluid so that any time the head rotates in any plane, inertia of the fluid causes it to move through one or more of the canals and thereby to stimulate hair cells located in the *ampullae* of the semicircular canals. Thus, rotating movements of the head are also made known to the nervous system.

From the vestibular apparatus signals are transmitted to the vestibular nuclei in the medulla, to the reticular nuclei of the brain stem, and into the flocculonodular lobes of the cerebellum. From the flocculonodular lobes the signals are transmitted back into the vestibular and reticular nuclei of the brain stem. After appropriate integration, the final necessary signals are emitted from the reticular and vestibular nuclei to cause shifts in tension of the different postural muscles, thereby causing the person's body to remain in a constantly upright position in relation to the pull of gravity.

Visceral Functions of the Brain Stem. Earlier in this chapter it was noted that the brain stem contains centers for respiratory control and vasomotor control. Also located in the brain stem are nerve centers for regulation of swallowing, secretion by some of the gastrointestinal glands, motor movements of the gastrointestinal tract, and emptying of the urinary bladder—all functions that are discussed at further length elsewhere in the chapter. Thus, the brain stem controls many subconscious visceral functions in addition to providing subconscious support of the body against gravity and maintenance of equilibrium.

INTEGRATION OF SENSORY AND
MOTOR FUNCTIONS IN THE CEREBRAL CORTEX

Primary Sensory Areas of the Cortex. Signals from each type of sensory receptor are transmitted to a specific area of the cerebral cortex. For instance, the somatic sensations are relayed by the thalamus directly to the somatic sensory cortex. Visual sensations are relayed from the optic tract by the lateral geniculate bodies of the thalamus directly to the visual cortex in the calcarine fissure area of the occipital lobes. Auditory impulses from the auditory nerves are relayed by the medial geniculate bodies of the thalamus to the auditory cortex in the central portion of the superior temporal gyri. Taste impulses are relayed through the nuclei of the tractus solitarius and the thalamus to a small area of the cerebral cortex deep in the fissure of Sylvius, and olfactory sensations are relayed to the amygdala (a subcortical mass of neurons in the anterior temporal lobe) and the pyriform area of the cortex.

In the visual system each minute area of the retina is connected directly to a minute area of the visual cortex. In the somatic sensory system each point on the surface of the body connects with a specific point in the somatic sensory cortex, as illustrated in Figure 3-15, so that stimulation of a finger, for instance, will excite only a minute area of the cortex. In the auditory cortex certain sound frequencies stimulate the anterior portion of the auditory cortex, while others stimulate the posterior auditory cortex.

In general, therefore, the types of information transmitted into the cerebral cortex by the different sensory systems are (1) the locations in the body from which the signals are arriving, (2) the types of receptors detecting the sensations, and (3) the intensities of the sensory stimuli. Once this information has entered the primary sensory areas, signals are relayed to other portions of the brain where the different types of information begin to be assembled into usable thoughts.

Sensory Association Areas. Located immediately adjacent to the primary sensory areas are the sensory association areas, which receive direct communications from the primary sensory areas. In the sensory association areas many memories of past sensory associations are stored, and here the new information arriving from the primary sensory areas is compared with information that has been stored from the past. In this way the significance of the new sensory signals is determined. For instance, when a person hears a word, he or she will not know that it is a word unless memory of that word has been stored in the auditory association areas. Likewise, when a person sees an airplane, the primary visual cortex is unable to determine the nature of the object, but, on transmission of appropriate information into the visual association areas, the person becomes aware that he is seeing an object that he has seen before and perhaps classifies it as an airplane. Similar functions are performed by somatic, taste, and smell association areas.

Gnostic Function of the Brain—Wernicke's Area. Brain surgeons have found that destruction of the posterior part of the superior gyrus of the temporal lobe, an area called **Wernicke's area,** in the left hemisphere of the right-handed person will destroy the ability to put together information from the different sensory association areas and thereby determine the overall meaning. For this reason, this region of the brain has been called the **gnostic center,** which means simply the "knowing center." This area is well located for this purpose because it lies at the juncture of the temporal, the parietal, and the occipital lobes in very close association with most of the sensory association areas of the cortex.

Ideomotor Function of the Brain. Once all the information from the different sensory association areas has been integrated into a distinct conscious meaning, the brain then decides what type of physical reaction should occur—from no reaction at all to very violent reaction. This is called the ideomotor function of the brain. Again, in neurosurgical patients it has been found that damage to Wernicke's area will cause a person to lose ideomotor ability.

After all sensory information is put together, appropriate signals are then sent to the motor portion of the brain, which in turn causes muscular movements.

THE MOTOR PATHWAYS

Primary Motor Cortex. Figure 3-16 illustrates the motor axis of the nervous system. A strip of the cortex averaging about 2 cm in width and lying horizontally all the way across the cortex, located immediately in front of the central sulcus of the brain, is called the primary motor cortex. Stimulation of discrete points in the primary motor cortex will cause contraction of discrete muscles in the body. For instance, stimulation of the primary motor cortex at a point on top of the brain where it dips into the longitudinal fissure will cause contraction of a leg muscle on the opposite side of the body, while

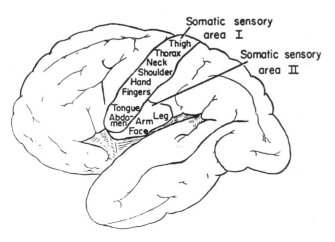

Fig. 3-15. Localization of sensory perception in the cerebral cortex. (Guyton AC: Textbook of Medical Physiology, 7th ed. Philadelphia, WB Saunders, 1986)

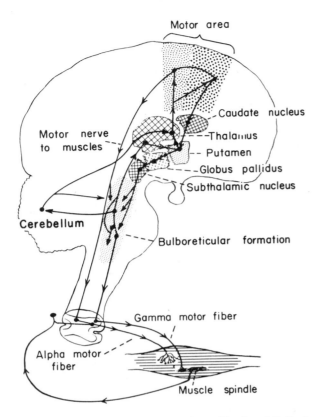

Fig. 3-16. The motor nervous system. (Guyton AC: Textbook of Medical Physiology, 7th ed. Philadelphia, WB Saunders, 1986)

stimulation of the primary motor cortex where it begins to dip into the fissure of Sylvius will contract a muscle somewhere on the opposite side of the face.

Pyramidal System and Pyramidal Tracts. In the primary motor cortex of each hemisphere are some 30,000 large neuronal cells called *pyramidal* or *Betz cells.* Fibers from these cells pass downward through the *pyramidal tracts* all the way into the spinal cord. There they synapse mainly with *interneurons* located in the lateral gray matter of the cord. The interneurons also receive many nerve endings from (1) sensory nerve fibers entering the spinal cord through the spinal nerves, (2) propriospinal fibers originating in other segments of the cord, and (3) other nerve fibers from the brain. The interneurons, after integrating the signals from all these sources, in turn transmit impulses to the *anterior motor neurons* located in the anterior gray matter of the cord. These neurons receive additional impulses directly from (1) proprioceptive nerve fibers from the spinal nerves, (2) a few nuclei in the brain stem, and (3) other segments of the spinal

cord. After integrating these signals, the anterior motor neurons in turn send impulses through the peripheral nerves to all the skeletal muscles of the body.

Premotor Cortex. Located anterior to the motor cortex is still another strip averaging about 2.5 cm in width called the premotor cortex. Stimulation of a discrete point in the premotor cortex usually does not cause contraction of a discrete muscle but, instead, causes a "pattern" of muscle contraction. That is, it might cause the whole arm to rise upward, or it might cause the whole hand to flex forward, or stimulation of still another point might cause the thumb and the forefinger to move toward each other as if cutting with scissors.

There is reason to believe that different patterns of movements can be learned and stored in the premotor cortex and that essentially all movements of the body consist of sequences of such learned movements. It is believed that the ideomotor function of the cortex from Wernicke's area controls the sequence of patterns of movement. Perhaps not more than a few hundred different patterns of movement are stored in the normal premotor cortex. However, considering the thousands to millions of different combinations into which these patterns of movement can be organized, even this few number of movements could allow almost any type of activity.

Extrapyramidal Pathways. To cause many of the actual muscle movements, the premotor cortex transmits signals into the primary motor cortex, which in turn controls the actions of the discrete muscles. However, some gross patterns of movement, such as those involving the trunk of the body, are transmitted through the *extrapyramidal system,* the nerve tracts of which pass first to lower centers of the brain and then from these through additional pathways to the spinal cord. For instance, one major extrapyramidal pathway is from the motor and premotor cortex to the reticular formation of the brain stem and from there through the reticulospinal tracts to the spinal cord. Another extrapyramidal pathway is from the motor and premotor cortex to the basal ganglia, then to the brain stem, and finally to the spinal cord.

FUNCTION OF THE BASAL GANGLIA

The basal ganglia are aggregates of neuronal cells that lie to the sides of the thalamus and beneath the cortex. They have very extensive neuronal connections with the premotor and primary motor portions of the cortex, with the somatic sensory cortex, with the thalamus, and with some nuclei of the brain stem. Unfortunately, little is known about the basic neurophysiology of these structures, though from a clinical point of view they are known to have four particular functions:

1. They operate in association with the premotor and the motor cortex to help control most of the patterns of movements. Damage to certain areas of the basal ganglia will cause abnormal and often continuous movements such as choreiform movements, writhing movements, and so forth.

2. The basal ganglia help to control the basal degree of activity of the entire motor system. Damage to certain areas of the basal ganglia can cause portions of the motor system to become greatly overexcitable, resulting in intense tonic contraction of either localized portions of the body or of the whole body. This results in a state of rigidity.

3. The basal ganglia operate in conjunction with the nuclei of the brain stem to damp the antagonistic movements of the postural muscles. For instance, if an extensor muscle should attempt to extend a limb, this would immediately elicit certain proprioceptive reflexes that would make flexor muscles tend to contract. This in turn would tend to make the extensor muscles contract again, and, as a result, a continuous state of oscillation would develop. However, this effect is normally damped by some of the lower basal ganglia so that antagonistic movements throughout the body are normally very smooth rather than tremorous. But in patients who have **Parkinson's disease,** which results from damage to the **substantia nigra,** one of the brain stem nuclei connected with the basal ganglia, a continuous tremor exists between the antagonistic pairs of muscles either in the entire body or in certain affected areas.

4. Recent studies show that when a person performs voluntary muscle activity the basal ganglia become activated before the primary motor cortex; still other studies have shown that, before the onset of muscle activity, portions of the sensory cortex also become activated even before the basal ganglia. Therefore, a suggested scheme to explain voluntary motor activity is: First, the nature of the motor act is probably conceived in the sensory cortex. Then signals are sent to the middle regions of the brain's motor system such as the basal ganglia, the reticular formation in the brain stem, and even the cerebellum to initiate the more gross aspects of the motor act. Finally, the primary motor cortex is called into play to control the more discrete actions of the peripheral parts of the body, such as the hands, fingers, and feet.

FUNCTION OF THE CEREBELLUM

The cerebellum receives collateral signals from the pyramidal and extrapyramidal fibers whenever they are stimulated by the primary motor cortex, by the premotor cortex, and by the basal ganglia, and it also receives impulses from proprioceptor nerves originating in all peripheral parts of the body. Thus, every time a motor movement is instituted by the brain, the cerebellum receives direct information of the projected movement from the cerebrum and receives information from the peripheral parts of the body telling it whether the movement has been accomplished and how much so. Putting these different types of information together, the cerebellum helps the motor system to stop the movements when the mission has been accomplished. To do this, the cerebellum performs two basic functions: First, it performs a **predictive function.** From the proprioceptor impulses it can tell how rapidly a part of the body is moving and from this can predict when the part will get to a desired position. As it approaches the appropriate point, impulses are transmitted from the cerebellum through the thalamus to the motor cortex and basal ganglia, there initiating the motor signals that stop the movement.

A second function of the cerebellum closely associated with the predictive function is its **damping function.** By starting to stop the movement of a limb before it gets to the desired point, the momentum of the limb will not carry it beyond its intended position. However, if the cerebellum has been destroyed, the momentum will carry the limb beyond the position. Then the other areas of the brain attempt to bring it back again to the desired position, but again the limb overshoots, and this continues several times until the intended movement is finally accomplished. Thus, in cerebellar damage, tremors occur that are very similar to those that result from basal ganglia damage. However, there is one particular difference: the basal ganglia tremor continues almost all the time when the person is awake, while the cerebellar tremor occurs only during movements associated with specific voluntary motor acts such as intentional movement of the hand from one point to another.

Failure of the predictive and the damping functions of the cerebellum causes a person to walk with ataxic movements, causes hand movements to be jerky if they are performed rapidly, and even causes speech to become dysarthric, which means that some sounds are overemphasized or held too long while other sounds are underemphasized to such an extent that the words are frequently unintelligible. It should be emphasized, though, that a person without a cerebellum can still perform most functions, even with precision, if he or she performs them very, very slowly. Therefore, the cerebellum is a system for helping to control rapid motor movements while they are actually occurring, keeping them precise despite rapidity of movement.

AUTONOMIC NERVOUS SYSTEM

Sympathetic System.   The motor impulses from the central nervous system to the visceral portions of the body are transmitted differently from those to the skeletal muscles. These pass through two differ-

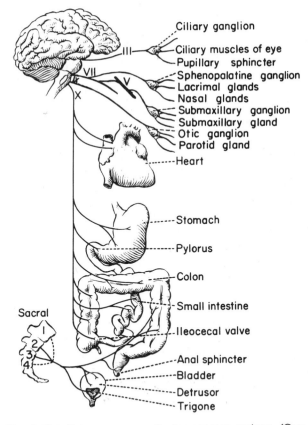

Fig. 3-18. The parasympathetic nervous system. (Guyton AC: Textbook of Medical Physiology, 7th ed. Philadelphia, WB Saunders, 1986)

ent divisions of the autonomic nervous system called the sympathetic and the parasympathetic systems, which are illustrated in Figures 3-17 and 3-18.

The sympathetic nervous system originates in neurons located in the lateral horns of the gray matter in the spinal cord between the first thoracic cord segment and the second lumbar segment. Nerve fibers pass by way of the anterior spinal roots first into the spinal nerves and then immediately into the sympathetic chain. From here, fiber pathways are transmitted to all portions of the body, especially to the different visceral organs and to the blood vessels.

Most sympathetic nerve endings secrete a hormone called norepinephrine that excites most of the visceral structures but inhibits a few. In general, it excites the heart and most of the blood vessels of the body, causing increased force of cardiac contraction and increased total peripheral resistance, with a resultant rise in arterial pressure. It inhibits the activity of the gastrointestinal tract, thereby

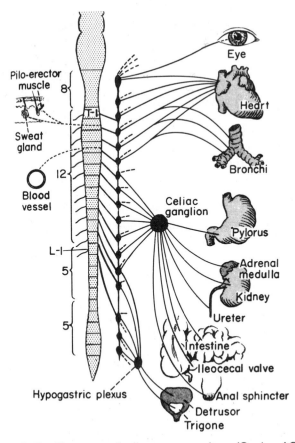

Fig. 3-17. The sympathetic nervous system. (Guyton AC: Textbook of Medical Physiology, 7th ed. Philadelphia, WB Saunders, 1986)

slowing peristalsis, and it inhibits the urinary bladder, dilates the pupil of the eye, excites the liver to cause release of glucose, and increases the rate of metabolism of essentially all cells of the body.

Secretion of Epinephrine and Norepinephrine by the Adrenal Medullae. Sympathetic nerves control the rate of secretion of both epinephrine and norepinephrine by the adrenal medullae, the central portions of the two adrenal glands. These hormones are carried by the blood and cause essentially the same effects in most parts of the body as those caused by direct sympathetic stimulation in each respective part. Furthermore, these hormones reach some cells that have no sympathetic nerve supply. They especially increase the rate of metabolism in all cells of the body.

The adrenal medullae represent a second means by which the central nervous system can cause sympathetic effects throughout the body. When sympathetic nerves to some organs have been destroyed, these hormones can still elicit the usual sympathetic functions when the overall sympathetic nervous system is excited.

Parasympathetic System. The parasympathetic fibers pass mainly through the vagus nerves, though a few fibers pass through several of the other cranial nerves and through the anterior roots of the sacral segments of the spinal cord. Parasympathetic fibers do not spread as extensively through the body as do sympathetic fibers, but they do innervate some of the thoracic and abdominal organs, as well as the pupillary sphincter and ciliary muscles of the eye and the salivary glands.

The parasympathetic nerve endings secrete acetylcholine, which, like norepinephrine, stimulates some organs and inhibits others. In general, it inhibits the heart and those very few blood vessels that have parasympathetic innervation, but it excites the ciliary and the pupillary sphincter muscles of the eye, the glandular and motor functions of the gastrointestinal tract, the urinary bladder, and the gallbladder.

Control of the Autonomic Nerves by the Central Nervous System. The activities of the sympathetic and the parasympathetic nerves are controlled in four different levels in the central nervous system: (1) in the cord, (2) in the brain stem, (3) in the hypothalamus, and (4) in the cortex. The autonomic cord reflexes have to do principally with local reactions in discrete parts of the body. For instance, excess filling of the rectum causes a parasympathetic reflex from the sacral cord that promotes emptying of the rectum. Visceral pain from the small intestine causes reflex sympathetic inhibition of the gastrointestinal tract, and excess heat to a skin area causes reflex sympathetic vasodilatation of the localized blood vessels, which helps to reduce the local skin temperature.

In the brain stem such factors as blood pressure, swallowing, vomiting, salivary secretion, stomach and pancreatic secretion, and, to a certain extent, emptying of the urinary bladder are all controlled. These different functions are discussed in relation to different systems of the body at other points in the chapter.

The autonomic centers of the hypothalamus control such functions as body temperature, degree of overall excitability of the body, and various responses of the viscera to emotions. To perform these functions the hypothalamus transmits signals into the lower brain stem and thence either into the vagus nerves or down into the spinal cord to stimulate the spinal autonomic centers.

Centers in the cerebral cortex can elicit almost any type of autonomic response. These responses are often of an emotional nature, such as fainting caused by widespread vasodilation through the body. Also, some are associated with muscular exercise, such as a rise in blood pressure and vasodilation in the muscles. The responses caused by the cerebral cortex are transmitted mainly through the autonomic centers in the hypothalamus and the lower brain stem.

EYE

OPTICS OF THE EYE

Function of the Eye as a Camera—the Lens System. The eye is constructed very much like a camera, as illustrated in Figure 3-19. The *retina* is analogous to the film in a camera, the *cornea* and the *lens*

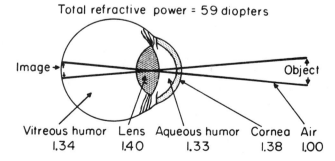

Fig. 3-19. The eye as a camera. The numbers are the refractive indices, which are the reciprocals of the light velocities. (Guyton AC: Textbook of Medical Physiology, 7th ed. Philadelphia, WB Saunders, 1986)

of the eye are analogous to the lens system of a camera, and the *pupil* is analogous to the diaphragm of a camera.

Because light rays travel at different velocities in the eye fluids, the cornea, and the lens, they are refracted—that is, they are bent—at four different corneal and lens surfaces: (1) the anterior surface of the cornea, (2) the posterior surface of the cornea, (3) the anterior surface of the lens, and (4) the posterior surface of the lens. This bending of the light rays allows an image of the scene in front of the eyes to be focused on the retina in exactly the same way that an image is focused by the lens system of a camera on the film. The image is upside down and reversed to the opposite side from the orientation of the object in front of the eyes.

Mechanism of Focusing. For a clear image to be formed on the retina, the surfaces of the cornea and of the lens of the eye must have the appropriate curvatures in relation to the distance of the retina behind the lens system. That is, the image must be focused on the retina. The eye can change the curvature of the lens in the following way: Attached around the periphery of the lens are approximately 70 ligaments that pull continually to the side, keeping the lens normally in a flattened, ovoid shape. The lens itself is a very elastic structure so that when these ligaments are loosened, it assumes a round, globular shape. When an object comes close to the eye, the more rounded shape of the lens is required to focus a clear image on the retina. To achieve this a muscle called the *ciliary muscle* is tightened. This muscle is a circular sphincter extending all the way around the peripheral attachments of the ligaments, and on contraction the circle of the sphincter becomes smaller so that the ligaments are loosened. This automatically allows the lens to change from its normal ovoid shape to a more rounded shape, thereby assuming far greater curvature and allowing adequate focusing of the images of nearby objects.

Yet, the tension on the lens ligaments must be controlled very exactly, or the lens might become too round for adequate focusing. This is controlled by the cerebral cortex. If the image is in poor focus, the visual image in the brain is indistinct, and appropriate impulses are transmitted back through the visceral nucleus of the third nerve and finally through the third cranial nerve to the ciliary muscle to adjust the degree of contraction.

The diameter of the pupil of the eye is controlled by a nervous reflex originating in the retina called the *light reflex.* Signals caused by strong light on the retina are transmitted along the optic nerve and op-

tic tract into the pretectal nuclei of the midbrain, from there to the visceral nucleus of the third nerve, and then back to the pupillary constrictor to decrease the pupillary aperture thus decreasing light intensity on the retina. Conversely, in darkness, lack of light signals from the retina reverses the reflex and causes the diameter of the pupil to increase.

Another importance of the pupil is that it alters the *depth of focus* of the eye. When the image on the retina is not in exact focus, the light rays passing through the peripheral edges of the lens will be much more out of focus than those passing through the very center of the lens. However, as the pupillary diameter becomes smaller, the light rays entering the peripheral edges of the eye are blocked and do not reach the retina. Therefore, by constricting the size of the pupil, which occurs in bright light, a person whose lens is not in exact focus will still have fairly clear vision; that is, he or she has increased "depth of focus."

FUNCTION OF THE RETINA

Rods and Cones. The light sensitive receptors of the retina are millions of minute cells called *rods* and *cones.* The rods distinguish only the white and the black aspects of an image while the cones are capable of distinguishing its colors as well.

In general, from 50 to 400 rods are connected to a single optic nerve fiber while, in the central portion of the retina, a single cone is connected to a single optic nerve fiber. As a result, minute points of light on the retina can be localized to very discrete positions by the cones but can be localized far less acutely by the rods. Thus, very acute and clear vision of objects is mediated by the cones, while only a diffuse type of vision is mediated by the rods. The central portion of the retina, only 0.4 mm in diameter and called the *fovea centralis,* has only cones, which allows this portion to have very sharp vision, while the peripheral areas, which contain progressively more and more rods, have progressively more diffuse vision.

Rhodopsin–Retinal Cycle of the Rods. For a person to see an image, the light energy entering the eye must be changed into nerve impulses. In the rods this is accomplished by means of a chemical system called the rhodopsin–retinal cycle. Large quantities of the light-sensitive substance *rhodopsin,* also known as *visual purple,* are present in the rods. When light impinges on these, a small portion of the rhodopsin is transformed immediately into another substance called *lumi-rhodopsin,* which is a very unstable compound that lasts in the rods for only a fraction of a second. Instead, it degenerates through a series of chemical steps to form two substances called *retinal* and *scotopsin* (a protein). But, during the split second while the rhodopsin is being degraded, the rod becomes excited, sending nerve impulses from the retina into the optic nerve.

The retinal and scotopsin are gradually recombined by the metabolic processes of the rod to reform rhodopsin, thereby continually supplying the rod with new rhodopsin.

Retinal is derived from vitamin A; therefore, when a person has a very serious deficiency of vitamin A in the diet, the retina is likely to become relatively insensitive to light, causing the condition known as *night blindness.*

Dark and Light Adaptation. The retina is capable of adapting its sensitivity so that the eye can see almost equally as well in both very bright light and in dim light. This adaptation is a far more powerful mechanism than the pupillary adaptation discussed above, though it requires several minutes to several hours to develop fully each time the person changes to a new level of light intensity. The mechanism of dark and light adaptation is the following:

When a person remains in very bright light for a long time, extremely large quantities of rhodopsin are split into retinal and scotopsin; this reduces the quantity of rhodopsin in the rods and therefore makes them become insensitive to light, which is called *light adaptation.* Conversely, when a person spends a long time in darkness, only very small amounts of rhodopsin are split while the metabolic systems of the rods are continually building more and more rhodopsin. Consequently, rhodopsin collects in very high concentrations after a while and greatly increases the sensitivity of the retina; this is called *dark adaptation.*

One might wonder why it is important for the sensitivity of the retina to change so much. However, it must be remembered that to see an image clearly there must be dark areas in the image as well as light areas. If the retina should remain highly sensitive all of the time and a person should then go out into the bright sunlight, all portions of the image would be so bright that everything would appear white without any dark areas.

Color Vision. The cones of the eye function in very much the same way as the rods except that the light sensitive chemicals are slightly different from rhodopsin and are called *iodopsin.* These chemicals still utilize retinal as the basis for light sensitivity, but the retinal combines with a different *photopsin* for each of the three primary colors rather than with scotopsin. Each photopsin, like scotopsin, is a protein, but slightly different from other photopsins. The nature of this protein determines the color sensitivity of the light sensitive chemical. There are three major groups of cones that respond especially intensely to certain colors of light. These cones are classified as *blue cones, green cones,* and *red cones.*

The eye determines the color of an object by the relative intensities of stimulation of the different types of cones. For instance, yellow is a color with a wavelength midway between green and red. Therefore, it stimulates the green and the red cones about equally, which gives one the sensation of seeing the color yellow. Orange has a wavelength somewhat closer to that of red light than of green light. Therefore, it stimulates the red cones about twice as much as it does the green cones, giving the sensation of orange. Finally, pure red light stimulates the red cones very strongly while stimulating the green and blue cones only weakly. This gives the sensation of red. The same principles hold true for the different shades of color between green, blue, and yellow.

Transmission of Signals from the Retina to the Cerebral Cortex. Each point of the retina connects with a discrete point in the *visual cortex* of the brain located in the calcarine fissure area of the occipital cortex. Therefore, every time a single point on the retina is stimulated, a corresponding point is stimulated in the visual cortex. From here other signals pass to the visual association areas and also to Wernicke's area for analysis of the visual images, as described earlier in the chapter.

The visual image begins to be analyzed even before it leaves the retina. In the retina are several other types of neuronal cells in addition to the rods and cones. These are the bipolar cells, the horizontal cells, the amacrine cells, and the ganglion cells. Some of these are inhibitory while others are excitatory. By combining excitatory and inhibitory signals from the excited rods and cones, the signals that finally reach the ganglion cells of the retina are initiated almost entirely by three types of visual effects: (1) spots or borders in the retinal image where there is a sudden change from light to dark or dark to light—that is, sudden change in contrast in the image, (2) sudden increases or decreases in light intensity from one instant to another, and (3) changes in color from one area to another. In other words, those portions of the visual image that do not have any contrasts in intensity or color in them do not stimulate the ganglion cells to a great extent. It is only where contrast borders occur that the ganglion cells are strongly stimulated. Also, some ganglion cells are stimulated strongly when there is a sudden change in light intensity. Thus, these contrast borders and the changes in light intensity send most of the signals to the primary visual cortex.

In the primary visual cortex, similar interactions occur between excitatory and inhibitory neurons. This allows the primary visual cortex to be stimulated by short lines of specific orientations, some of the neurons being stimulated by lines oriented in one direction while other neurons are stimulated by lines oriented in still different directions. Then, in the visual association areas, still more complex patterns are required to stimulate the neurons, such as a line of distinct length or a line oriented in a single direction. In other instances an angulated line is necessary to stimulate a particular neuron.

It is the recent research studies on this manner in which the visual brain analyzes images that have given us our greatest understanding of basic mechanisms of brain function.

EAR

Transmission of Sound from the Tympanum to the Cochlea.

Figure 3-20 illustrates the functional parts of the ear. Sound is caused by compression waves that travel through the air at a velocity of about 1/5 mile per second. As each compression wave strikes the *tympanic membrane* (or "ear drum"), the membrane is forced inward, and between compressions it moves outward. The center of the tympanic membrane is connected to the *ossicular system,* which consists of three bony levers (the malleus, incus, and stapes) that transmit the sound vibrations into the cochlea at the oval window. The tympanic membrane and the ossicular system function as a sound "transformer," because

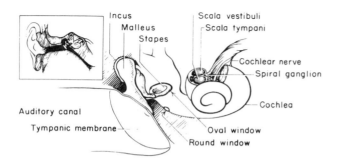

Fig. 3-20. The tympanic membrane, the ossicular system of the middle ear, and the inner ear. (Guyton AC: Textbook of Medical Physiology, 7th ed. Philadelphia, WB Saunders, 1986)

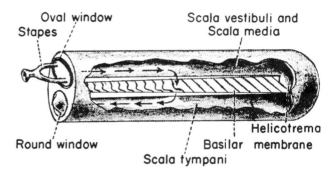

Fig. 3-21. Vibration of the basilar membrane in response to sound. (Guyton AC: Textbook of Medical Physiology, 7th ed. Philadelphia, WB Saunders, 1986)

the tympanic membrane has a surface area some 20 times the surface area of the oval window, giving a total increase in force of the sound vibrations against the oval window of about 20-fold.

Resonance in the Cochlea—Determination of Pitch.

Figure 3-21 illustrates the fluid system in the cochlea. The cochlea is composed of two major fluid-filled tubes, the scala vestibuli and the scala tympani, which lie side by side in a coil and are separated by the basilar membrane. Inward movement of the stapes against the oval window, which is at the end of the scala vestibuli, pushes the fluid into the scala vestibuli, and this in turn causes the basilar membrane to bulge and push the fluid in the scala tympani. Finally, the fluid in the scala tympani pushes outward against the round window, which is at the end of this scala. Thus, every time the stapes moves inward, the round window bulges outward into the middle ear.

Low frequency sound causes the stapes to move back and forth very slowly, which allows the pressure waves to travel far up into the scala vestibuli before maximum bulging of the basilar membrane into the scala tympani occurs. On the other hand, high frequency sound waves cause very rapid vibration of the stapes, and the waves have enough time between waves to travel only a short distance into the scala vestibuli before maximum bulging occurs. In this way a form of resonance occurs in the cochlea, with low frequency waves causing maximum back-and-forth vibration of the basilar membrane near the far tip of the cochlea and high frequency sound causing vibration of the basilar membrane near the base of the cochlea, that is, close to the oval and round windows. The brain determines the pitch of the sound mainly from the portion of the basilar membrane that vibrates—high pitch near the base of the cochlea and low pitch near the apex.

Stimulation of the Hair Cells—Determination of Loudness. Located on the surface of the basilar membrane are many hair cells similar to those in the vestibular apparatus discussed earlier. When the basilar membrane vibrates, these cells are stimulated—the more forceful the vibration the greater the rate of nerve impulses. The loudness of the sound is determined by this rate of impulses transmitted from the hair cells into the brain.

Transmission of Auditory Impulses into the Brain. Approximately 25,000 nerve fibers are attached to the hair cells of the cochlear apparatus. The auditory signals in the auditory nerves go first to the cochlear nuclei located in the brain stem; from here they pass upward to the inferior colliculus, then to the medial geniculate body, and finally to the auditory cortex in the superior temporal gyrus of the temporal lobe. The spatial orientation of the nerve fibers is maintained all the way from the basilar membrane to the auditory cortex so that one sound frequency excites one area of the auditory cortex while another sound frequency excites another area. The meanings of the auditory signals are then interpreted in the auditory association areas immediately adjacent to the primary auditory cortex.

CHEMICAL SENSES

TASTE

Taste Buds and the Primary Sensations of Taste. Located on the surfaces of the tongue, especially on the papillae and most importantly on the circumvallate papillae which lie in a V line on the posterior part of the tongue, and also in small numbers on the lateral walls of the pharynx, are many small taste receptor organs called taste buds. One of these is illustrated in Figure 3-22. Each taste bud has a hollow cavity that communicates through a small *taste pore* with the mouth. Lining the cavity are sensory taste receptor cells, and cilia called taste "hairs" protrude from the ends of these cells into the pore. Certain types of chemicals diffuse into the taste pores and excite the hairs of the taste cells.

Four different types of taste buds are known to exist, each of these responding principally to (1) saltiness, (2) sweetness, (3) sourness, and (4) bitterness. The first three of these taste sensations help the person to select the quality of food that he eats and in some instances even makes him desire certain substances such as salt that may be deficient in

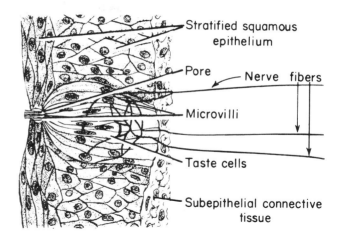

Fig. 3-22. The taste bud. (Guyton AC: Textbook of Medical Physiology, 7th ed. Philadelphia, WB Saunders, 1986)

his body. The last of the taste sensations, bitterness, is principally for protection, because most of the naturally occurring poisons among plant foods elicit a bitter taste that normally will cause an animal to reject the food.

Transmission of Taste Signals into the Brain. Most of the taste signals are transmitted by way of the chorda tympani into the seventh nerve and then into the brain stem; the remainder are transmitted through the ninth and tenth nerves into the brain stem. The signals pass first to the nucleus of the tractus solitarius, then to the thalamus, and finally to the primary taste cortex, which lies laterally in the parietal cortex immediately posterior to the central sulcus of the brain and deep in the fissure of Sylvius (also called the lateral fissure).

SMELL

The Olfactory Epithelium and Its Stimulation. Located in the superiormost part of each nostril is a small area having a surface of about 2.5 cm² called the olfactory epithelium. This contains large numbers of nervous receptors called *olfactory cells* that send long cilia ("olfactory hairs") into the mucus on the surface of the epithelium. Almost any chemical substance that can diffuse through the mucus and then into these cilia will stimulate one or more of the olfactory cells. Since the cilia themselves have lipid membranes, lipid-soluble substances stimulate the cells much more readily than non-lipid-soluble substances. The precise types of chemicals that stimulate different olfactory cells are not known, for it has been very difficult to study by either subjective or objective means the olfactory stimulus from a single olfactory cell. It is believed that there might be seven or more primary sensations of smell and that the many hundreds of different smells to which we are accustomed are actually combinations of these primary sensations.

TRANSMISSION OF OLFACTORY SIGNALS INTO THE BRAIN

From the olfactory cells signals are transmitted first to the olfactory bulb of the first cranial nerve and then through the olfactory tract into several midline nuclei of the brain that lie superior and anterior to the hypothalamus, and also into the pyriform cortex and amygdala. The midline nuclei control the crude functions of smell, such as eliciting salivation or licking the lips. The pyriform cortex and amygdala deal with olfactory conditioned reflexes that determine appetite and the more social responses to food.

GASTROINTESTINAL TRACT

Figure 3-23 illustrates the alimentary tract, which is more commonly referred to as the gastrointestinal tract, though the gastrointestinal tract is only part of the entire tract.

Fig. 3-23.   The alimentary tract. (Guyton AC: Textbook of Medical Physiology, 7th ed. Philadelphia, WB Saunders, 1986)

Physiologically, the important features of the alimentary tract are (1) the movement of food and secretions through the tract, (2) the secretion of the digestive juices and digestion of the foods, and (3) the absorption of the digestive products. Therefore, we shall discuss each of these separately.

MOTOR MOVEMENTS OF THE GASTROINTESTINAL TRACT

Propulsive Movements.   There are two general types of movements in the gastrointestinal tract: the propulsive movements that propel food forward along the tract and the mixing movements that keep mixing the intestinal contents.

The principal propulsive movement is *peristalsis,* which can occur in almost all smooth muscle tubes. That is, stimulus of a single section of the gut causes a constrictive ring to move forward along the gut, pushing any material in the gut ahead of the constriction. A nerve plexus in the wall of the gut called the *myenteric plexus* provides most of the control of the peristalsis, keeping the peristaltic movements oriented principally in the analward direction along the gut rather than in the upward direction, and also strengthening the peristalsis.

Peristalsis occurs in all segments of the gastrointestinal tract, but the intensity and frequency of

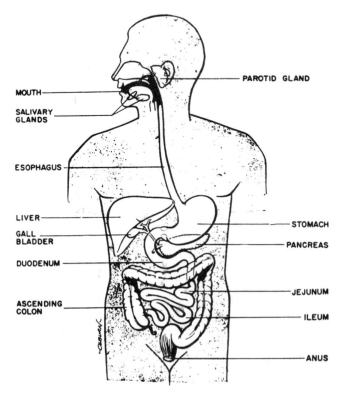

PAROTID GLAND

MOUTH

SALIVARY GLANDS

ESOPHAGUS

LIVER

GALL BLADDER

DUODENUM

ASCENDING COLON

STOMACH

PANCREAS

JEJUNUM

ILEUM

ANUS

peristalsis vary tremendously from one part of the tract to another. The types of stimuli that cause peristalsis are usually either distention of the gut by a bolus of food, irritation of the mucosa, or nervous increase in the excitation of the gut by the myenteric plexus.

In the stomach, the intensity of peristalsis is usually sufficient to cause movement of the food through the stomach within 1 to 3 hours after a meal. In the small intestine the peristaltic waves are usually very weak and spread downward along the intestinal tract only 10 cm to 15 cm at a time. Therefore, 3 to 10 hours is usually required to move the food all the way through the small intestine. In the large intestine, the propulsive movements are a modified type of peristalsis, often very strong but lasting only a fraction of an hour out of each day. As a result, the intestinal contents remain for many hours in the large intestine, allowing reabsorption of all or almost all of the electrolytes and water before expulsion of the feces.

At night, or at other times after the small intestine has been mainly emptied of food, about every hour and a half a series of peristaltic waves, called the *migrating complex,* sweeps slowly downward over the small intestine, carrying along to the large intestine any residual food and accumulations of secretions that may have collected in the meantime.

Swallowing is a special type of propulsive movement. When food is pushed into the back of the mouth by the tongue, nerve receptors in the pharynx elicit an automatic swallowing process. Signals are transmitted from these receptors to the brain stem, integrated there, and a sequence of swallowing signals is then transmitted back through the pharyngeal and vagus nerves to the pharynx and upper esophagus. A peristaltic wave begins in the pharyngeal constrictors, the glottis closes so that food cannot pass into the trachea, the upper esophageal constrictor muscle at the opening of the esophagus relaxes so that the food will enter the esophagus, and then the peristaltic wave proceeds downward along the upper esophagus, all of this controlled directly by nerve impulses from the brain stem. On reaching the lower half of the esophagus, the natural peristaltic process of the myenteric plexus in the gastrointestinal tract takes over and propels the food the rest of the way to the stomach.

The Mixing Movements. Special movements promote mixing of the food with gastrointestinal secretions. In the stomach these are mainly peristaltic waves that are not strong enough to propel the food through the pylorous but are strong enough to keep mixing the food with the secretions. The mixture of food and secretions that results is called *chyme.*

In the small intestine, intermittent constrictive rings occur as often as several times a minute, dividing the intestine into segments. Then the constrictions relax and others occur at other points. In this way the chyme is chopped again and again into small portions. These movements are called *segmenting contractions.* In the large intestine similar but much slower contractions called *haustrations* occur; these slowly roll the fecal matter over and over, allowing almost complete absorption of the water and electrolytes.

SECRETION IN THE GASTROINTESTINAL TRACT

Secretion of Saliva. Saliva is secreted principally by the parotid, the submaxillary, and the sublingual glands. Their secretion is controlled by the salivatory nuclei in the brain stem, and these in turn can be stimulated either by nerve impulses from the mouth when food is eaten or by psychic stimuli from the cerebral cortex.

Secretion in the Stomach. As illustrated in Figure 3-24, stomach secretion occurs in response to either nervous stimuli or hormonal stimuli. About half of the secretion is caused by vagal impulses transmitted from the dorsal motor nuclei of the vagi in the brain stem. These in turn are caused by (1) impulses from the cerebrum initiated by the thought of food or the smell of food, (2) impulses from the mouth during the chewing process, and (3) impulses from the stomach when food is actually in the stomach; this last is the stimulus that causes as much as half of all the stomach secretion.

The hormonal mechanism operates in the following way: Certain types of food, especially those that have a high degree of taste, extract a hormone called *gastrin* from the mucosa of the lower end of the stomach, the **antrum.** This hormone then passes by way of the blood stream to the *gastric glands* located in the upper three-quarters of the stomach, called the *fundus* and *body,* to cause secretion of a very highly acid gastric juice.

Secretion by the Pancreas. The pancreas, like the stomach, is also stimulated by both nervous and hormonal stimuli, but mainly by the hormonal stimuli. The same factors that cause nervous impulses to the stomach also cause impulses to the pancreas and thereby promote secretion of digestive enzymes.

Stimulation of the pancreas by hormonal mechanisms occurs as follows: The chyme, on entering the small intestine, extracts two different hormones

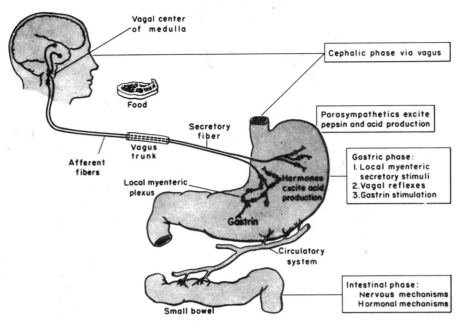

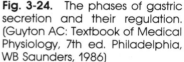

Fig. 3-24. The phases of gastric secretion and their regulation. (Guyton AC: Textbook of Medical Physiology, 7th ed. Philadelphia, WB Saunders, 1986)

from the intestinal mucosa, **secretin** and **cholecystokinin,** and these are carried in the blood to the pancreatic acini. Secretin causes the pancreas to secrete large amounts of highly alkaline, watery solution, and cholecystokinin causes the pancreatic cells to release large quantities of digestive enzymes into this solution. Secretin is released from the intestinal mucosa mainly in response to acid emptied from the stomach into the duodenum; the alkaline pancreatic secretion in turn neutralizes the acid. The cholecystokinin is released mainly in response to the presence of fats and proteins in the chyme, and the secreted enzymes in turn help to digest the proteins and fats.

Secretion in the Small Intestine. Almost all of the secretion in the small intestine is caused by local stimulation of the intestinal glands. This results from either mechanical stimulation of the mucosa by the chyme or distention of the gut, both of which elicit very rapid flow of intestinal juices mainly by way of intramural nervous reflexes in the submucosal and myenteric plexuses.

Secretion of Mucus. Mucus is secreted in all parts of the gastrointestinal tract, from the salivary glands all the way to the mucosal glands of the large intestine. Mucus is an excellent lubricant and is also very resistant to chemical destruction either by the intestinal juices or by different types of foods. Therefore, it provides excellent protection for the mucosa of the gastrointestinal tract.

DIGESTION IN THE SMALL INTESTINAL TRACT

The chemical processes of digestion are all processes of **hydrolysis** of the different foods. This means that the food molecule splits into two smaller molecules, and at the same time a hydrogen atom from a water molecule combines with one of the food products at the point of splitting while the remaining hydroxyl radical from the water combines with the other food product. The carbohydrates are hydrolyzed into monosaccharides, the fats into glycerol and fatty acids, and the proteins into amino acids. Hydrolysis of the different types of foods is catalyzed by different types of enzymes called the digestive enzymes.

Digestion of carbohydrates is begun by salivary amylase secreted in the saliva, and their digestion is carried still further by pancreatic amylase secreted in the pancreatic juice. After the action of these two, the carbohydrates will have been split principally into disaccharides. Then four enzymes in the epithelial cells of the small intestinal mucosa, sucrase, maltase, isomaltase, and lactase, split the disaccharides into monosaccharides, principally glucose, fructose, and galactose.

The fats are split into glycerol and fatty acid molecules by lipases secreted mainly in the pancreatic juice but to a very slight extent in other digestive secretions.

Protein digestion begins in the stomach under the

influence of pepsin and hydrochloric acid. Then it continues in the upper small intestine under the influence of trypsin and chymotrypsin secreted by the pancreas. At this point, the proteins will have been digested into large polypeptides. Then several different peptidases secreted in the pancreatic juice or located in or on the surfaces of the intestinal epithelial cells split the polypeptides into amino acids.

ABSORPTION FROM THE GASTROINTESTINAL TRACT

Role of the Intestinal Villi in Absorption. Located on the mucosal surface of the small intestine are millions of small intestinal villi, each of which projects about 1 mm into the intestinal lumen as shown to the left in Figure 3-25. These villi increase the surface area of the small intestine about 10-fold. The end-products of digestion are absorbed through the epithelial cells lining these villi into sublying villar blood vessels and lymphatics.

In addition to the increased surface area caused by the presence of the villi, each epithelial cell has approximately 600 microvilli, each 1 micron in length. These increase the surface area exposed to the intestinal materials another 20-fold. In all, the total area for absorption is about 250 m² for the entire small intestine.

Active Absorption. Certain substances can be actively absorbed from the gastrointestinal tract. This means that the molecules are transported through the intestinal mucosa by a chemical process that greatly enhances the rate of absorption. This active absorption is very similar to that which occurs in the urinary tubules, which was explained earlier in the chapter. Substances that can be actively absorbed are most monosaccharides (especially glucose, fructose, and galactose), the amino acids, sodium ions, and several other ions.

Passive Absorption. Passive absorption means absorption of substances simply by diffusion through the membrane. When substances in the chyme are actively absorbed, such as glucose, the amount of osmotically active substances increases in the fluids on the outer side of the intestinal membrane while the amount decreases in the chyme. As a result, tremendous quantities of water are osmotically absorbed from the gut. Also, when positively charged ions such as sodium ions are actively absorbed, a positive charge builds up on the other side of the membrane, and this pulls negatively charged substances such as chloride ions through the membrane. The most important substances passively absorbed are water, chloride ions, and some fats.

Portal and Lymphatic Routes of Absorption. Almost all of the water-soluble substances are absorbed directly into the blood capillaries of the villi, and they then pass with the portal blood through the liver into the general circulatory system. This is called the portal route of absorption, and the substances absorbed in this way are (1) most of the water and electrolytes, (2) the carbohydrates, and (3) the amino acids.

Fatty acids are not absorbed into the blood of the villi but, instead, while passing through the epithelium of the villus, recombine with glycerol to form neutral fat. This then passes into the lymphatics and is transmitted upward along the thoracic duct in the form of minute fatty globules called *chylomicrons* to be emptied into the veins of the neck.

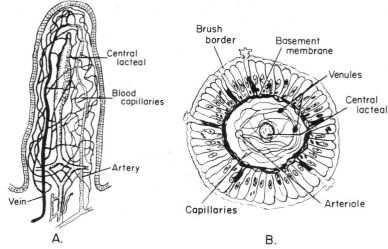

Fig. 3-25. Structure of the intestinal villus. (*A*) Longitudinal section; (*B*) cross-section. (Guyton AC: Textbook of Medical Physiology, 7th ed. Philadelphia, WB Saunders, 1986)

GASTROINTESTINAL DISORDERS

Peptic Ulcer. The digestive enzymes in the stomach juice can digest the mucosa of either the stomach itself or of the duodenum, if the secretions ever penetrate the mucous cell coat of the mucosal lining. Ordinarily, especially large quantities of mucus are secreted by the entire mucosal surface of the stomach and duodenum. Furthermore, the acidity of the stomach secretions is immediately neutralized by alkaline pancreatic juice when the secretions enter the duodenum. However, the protective barrier against the stomach juice sometimes loses some of its effectiveness. For instance, continued sympathetic stimulation reduces the secretion of mucus by the glands of Brunner in the upper duodenum and therefore predisposes this area to the development of a *duodenal ulcer.* Also, some persons have been shown to secrete five or more times as much stomach juice as the normal person during the interdigestive period between meals, the normal person usually secreting only a few milliliters during the whole night. Obviously, the excess acid in the stomach juice is difficult to neutralize in the absence of food in the stomach to combine with much of the acid; therefore, this is perhaps the most common cause of *peptic ulcer.* Worry and anxiety commonly increase this interdigestive secretion.

Diarrhea and Constipation. Almost any irritation of the gastrointestinal mucosa greatly increases the local rate of secretion of intestinal juices and also the intensity of peristalsis. This causes a "washout" phenomenon, the material in the irritated area flowing rapidly toward the anus. Thus, the most common cause of *diarrhea* is mucosal irritation, often due to bacterial infection but sometimes to irritative foods.

Diarrhea can also result from excessive activity of the parasympathetic nervous system, because parasympathetic stimulation increases the secretory and propulsive activities of the entire GI tract but especially so of the latter half of the large intestine. This, too, results in rapid "washout" of the gut.

Exactly the opposite effects can cause *constipation.* Sympathetic stimulation, for instance, decreases the activity of the gastrointestinal tract throughout its entire extent and can result in serious constipation. Also, spasm of the gut at some point in the descending colon or the sigmoid colon is a common cause of constipation; spasm of even a small area in this region can prevent adequate emptying of the large intestine even though colon activity elsewhere may be completely normal. Such spasm is often caused by local irritation.

Achalasia and Megacolon. Two gastrointestinal disorders have been shown to be caused by either lack of or dysfunction of the myenteric plexus in the intestinal wall. One of these is *achalasia,* which results from neuronal dysfunction at the lower half of the esophagus, and the other is *megacolon,* which results from lack of or deranged myenteric plexus in the sigmoid colon. In either instance, the propulsive movements through the affected area are either greatly inhibited or blocked. In achalasia the food piles up in the esophagus, sometimes causing an extreme enlargement of the esophagus called *megaesophagus.* In the case of megacolon, the failure of feces to pass through the sigmoid causes progressive dilatation of the colon, sometimes resulting in bowel movements as infrequently as once every several weeks.

METABOLISM AND ENERGY

METABOLISM OF CARBOHYDRATES AND SYNTHESIS OF ADENOSINE TRIPHOSPHATE

Glucose as the "Common Denominator" in Carbohydrate Metabolism. The digestive products of essentially all carbohydrates are glucose, fructose, and galactose. Much of the fructose is converted to glucose as it is absorbed by the intestinal epithelium, and the galactose, after being absorbed, is transmitted by the portal blood mainly to the liver where it is almost all also converted into glucose. Then this glucose eventually passes back out of the liver cells into the blood to join the glucose that is absorbed directly from the gastrointestinal tract. Therefore, it is in the form of glucose that essentially all carbohydrates are made available to the cells to be metabolized.

Storage of Glycogen in the Liver. Large quantities of glucose, either that converted from fructose and galactose or that directly absorbed from the gastrointestinal tract, can be stored in the liver cells in the form of glycogen granules, glycogen being a polymer of glucose. Special enzymes in the liver cells cause the polymerization of glucose into glycogen. When the glucose level in the blood falls too low, the glycogen is split by still other enzymes back into glucose, which then passes into the blood to be utilized elsewhere in the body. In this way extra glucose is removed from the blood when the blood glucose concentration is too high and then is returned when the blood glucose falls too low. Thus, the liver provides a blood glucose-buffering function.

Entry of Glucose into the Cells—Effect of Insulin. Glucose is transported through the cell membrane by a facilitated diffusion mechanism, as was discussed in the early part of the chapter. The activity of this mechanism for glucose transport is controlled by the amount of insulin secreted by the pancreas. Large amounts of insulin increase the rate of glucose transport to about 15 times the rate when no insulin is available. When the pancreas fails to secrete insulin, very little glucose can enter most cells, but when excess insulin is secreted, glucose enters the cells so rapidly that the blood glucose level falls to very low.

Glycolysis and Synthesis of Adenosine Triphosphate. After entry into the cells, glucose can be polymerized into glycogen and stored temporarily as glycogen granules, or it can be used immediately to provide energy for cellular functions. The initial process for providing energy is principally *glycolysis,* which means splitting each molecule of glucose to form pyruvic acid. This occurs by a series of chemical reactions involving several stages of phosphorylation and several transformations all catalyzed by protein enzymes in the cells.

During the different stages of glycolysis, a net of two molecules of adenosine triphosphate (ATP) are synthesized for every molecule of glucose converted into pyruvic acid. In this way a small portion (about three per cent) of the energy stored in the glucose molecule is transferred to adenosine triphosphate molecules. The ATP in turn is very highly reactive and can provide immediate energy to other functional systems of the cells as needed.

Citric Acid Cycle and the Release of Carbon Dioxide and Hydrogen from Pyruvic Acid. The two molecules of pyruvic acid formed from glucose in the glycolysis process still contain about nine tenths of the energy originally in the glucose molecule. To make this available to the cell, each molecule of pyruvic acid is first split into carbon dioxide and hydrogen. This occurs principally by means of a series of chemical reactions called by various names: the *Krebs cycle,* the *tricarboxylic acid cycle,* or the *citric acid cycle.*

The pyruvic acid is first decarboxylated to form *acetyl coenzyme A,* and this immediately combines with oxaloacetic acid to form citric acid. Then the citric acid is progressively decomposed, liberating carbon dioxide and hydrogen atoms. The carbon dioxide diffuses out of the cells and is blown off by the lungs into the expired air. However, the hydrogen atoms are made available to react with oxygen, a process that provides tremendous amounts of energy to the cell, as will be discussed below. After the carbon dioxide and hydrogen atoms have been removed, the residue of the citric acid molecule is a new molecule of oxaloacetic acid that can be used over and over again in the citric acid cycle.

All the chemical reactions in the citric acid cycle are catalyzed by another series of enzymes called *decarboxylases* (which remove the carbon dioxide) and *dehydrogenases* (which remove the hydrogen atoms).

Oxidation of Hydrogen and Synthesis of More Adenosine Triphosphate. Most of the hydrogen that is released during the breakdown of pyruvic acid combines with nicotinamide adenine dinucleotide (NAD) and from this is then rapidly passed to another substance, a flavoprotein. Then the hydrogen leaves the flavoprotein to become hydrogen ions, each hydrogen losing one electron in the process. The electrons removed from the hydrogen atoms are passed rapidly through a series of electron carriers, including cytochrome B, cytochrome C, cytochrome A, and cytochrome oxidase, and finally combined with water and the dissolved oxygen in the fluids of the cell to convert these into hydroxyl ions. The presence of both hydrogen and hydroxyl ions in the same fluid allows immediate combination of the two to form water. The water in turn diffuses out of the cell and eventually is excreted by the kidneys or evaporates from the body.

The important feature about this oxidation of hydrogen is not the formation of water but, instead, the use of energy from the hydrogen and oxygen atoms for synthesis of (ATP). Thirty-six molecules of adenosine triphosphate are formed for each molecule of glucose oxidized, 18 times as many molecules as are formed by the process of glycolysis alone. Therefore, this final oxidation of pyruvic acid is the main source of energy for the cells.

Role of the Mitochondria in the Citric Acid Cycle and in "Oxidative Phosphorylation." The overall process by which hydrogen ions are oxidized and the released energy is used to generate ATP is called oxidative phosphorylation. This entire process occurs inside the mitochondria. It begins with transport of acetyl coenzyme A, which is formed from pyruvic acid, through the double membrane wall of the mitochondrion into the mitochondrial cavity. It is here that the chemical reactions of the citric acid cycle occur and hydrogen atoms are released. The manner in which the hydrogen atoms are then utilized to cause the formation of adenosine triphosphate is as follows. The first step is ionization of the hydrogen atoms and passage of the electrons removed during the ionization process through the electron carrier system. The electron carriers are large protein molecules that are integral parts of the inner wall of the mitochondrion. As the electrons pass from one carrier to the next, they give up energy, and the energy is used to pump the hydrogen ions from the central cavity of the mitochondrion into the outer chamber between the two mitochondrial walls. This creates a high concentration of hydrogen ions in this outer chamber. Then the large hydrogen ion gradient across the inner wall of the mitochondrion causes the hydrogen ions to leak back through the inner wall toward the central cavity. This flow of hydrogen ions through the inner wall of the mitochondria from the outer mitochondrial chamber to the central cavity occurs through very large protein molecules called **ATP synthetase.** Each of these molecules is an ATPase enzyme capable of using the energy derived from the flow of hydrogen ions through its molecular matrix to convert adenosine diphosphate plus a phosphate radical into ATP—that is, to cause synthesis of ATP. Thus, in this roundabout way, the tremendous energy that had been present in the glucose molecule is finally used to form ATP, which itself stores a large portion of this energy and uses it later to energize almost all intracellular reactions.

This mitochondrial mechanism for synthesis of ATP is called the **chemiosmotic mechanism.**

Functions of Adenosine Triphosphate. Adenosine triphosphate is a highly labile compound, the formula for which is the following:

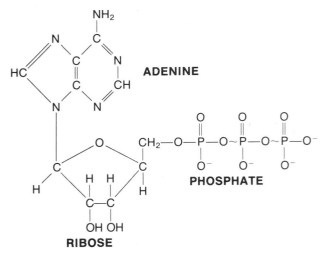

At each point where the last two phosphate radicals attach (indicated by the curving bonds, called

"high energy phosphate bonds") from 7,000 to 12,000 calories of energy are available for each mole of adenosine triphosphate, the exact amount depending on concentrations and other conditions of the reactants. The two phosphate radicals on the end of the molecule can split away with great ease and can transfer this energy to other chemical processes in the cells. Thus, adenosine triphosphate is almost an explosive compound that is ready to act immediately. As it is used up, more adenosine triphosphate is formed by the processes described above.

Some of the specific functions of adenosine triphosphate are (1) to provide the immediate energy needed for contraction of muscle cells, (2) to provide the energy needed to pump sodium out of nerve and muscle cells so that action potentials can be transmitted along the membranes, (3) to provide the energy needed to synthesize new proteins by the ribosomes in the cytoplasm, and (4) to provide the energy needed for synthesis and secretion of almost all substances formed by the glands. These are only a few of the functions of adenosine triphosphate; without adenosine triphosphate almost no chemical reactions can occur in cells.

METABOLISM OF FATS

Transport of Fat in the Plasma—the Lipoproteins. Most fatty substances are not soluble in the body fluids. Therefore, most of the fatty substances in the blood are in the form of minute suspended particles, only a fraction of a micron in size, called lipoproteins. The fatty substances in the lipoproteins are loosely bound with varying amounts of protein. The proteins in turn, being miscible with water, increase the suspension stability of the lipoproteins in the plasma and prevent excessive adherence of them to each other or to the endothelium.

Free Fatty Acid. A very small amount of fatty acids, about 10 mg per 100 ml is present in the plasma in combination with the albumin of the plasma proteins. These are called *free fatty acids.* Despite this very small concentration, this free fatty acid is transferred extremely rapidly back and forth with the tissue fats, as much as one half of it transferring every 2 to 3 minutes. Such rapid mobility makes this the principal means of transport of most of the fat from one area of the body to another.

Chylomicrons. After absorption of fatty acids from the small intestine, these immediately recombine in the intestinal epithelial cells with glycerol to form minute particles of neutral fat (triglycerides) that then aggregate with small amounts of protein to form minute fat globules called chylomicrons. These pass into the intestinal lymphatics and along the thoracic duct to empty into the blood. Within an hour or so after a meal has been completely absorbed most of the chylomicrons will have been removed from the circulating blood, some of them being absorbed by the liver cells and a very large portion being split by an enzyme, lipoprotein lipase, into fatty acids that are either metabolized for energy or are resynthesized into fat by the fat cells and stored.

Fat Depots. All the fat cells of the body are known collectively as fat depots. Fat can remain stored in the fat cells for hours, days, or months. When the amount of circulating fatty acid falls very low in the blood during the interdigestive period between meals, the stored fat is split by tissue lipoprotein lipase into fatty acid and then transported in the blood to other cells of the body where it may be needed.

Use of Fat for Energy—Synthesis of Adenosine Triphosphate. Fat is used by the body to provide energy in almost the same way that carbohydrates are used. The chemical processes for deriving energy from fats include the following stages: (1) The neutral fat is split inside the fat cells into glycerol and fatty acids. The glycerol, having a chemical composition very similar to that of certain glucose breakdown products, can easily be oxidized to energize the formation of adenosine triphosphate molecules. (2) The fatty acid molecules are partially oxidized, mainly in the liver cells, by a process called beta carbon oxidation, which causes the fatty acid to split and form many acetyl coenzyme A molecules. These in turn enter the mitochondria where they are decomposed by the citric acid cycle and then completely oxidized by the oxidative phosphorylation process to synthesize large numbers of ATP molecules in exactly the same way that the acetyl coenzyme A derived from pyruvic acid is used for the same purpose. Thus, fats provide energy in nearly the same manner as carbohydrates except that the initial stage for splitting carbohydrates is mainly the glycolysis mechanism while the initial stage for splitting fats is principally the beta carbon oxidation mechanism.

A large share of all fatty acid degradation begins in the liver, but only a small portion of the acetyl coenzyme A formed in the liver cells is used for energy in the liver itself. Instead, it is transported away from the liver by the blood in the form of *acetoacetic acid,* a condensation product of two molecules of acetyl coenzyme A. This in turn is absorbed by the other cells of the body where it is split again into two molecules of acetyl coenzyme A, then enters the citric acid cycle and is used for energy.

Phospholipids. All cells of the body synthesize phospholipids, which are chemical substances derived mainly from fat and have certain of the physical and chemical characteristics of fats, but most of these are synthesized in the liver or intestinal epithelial cells. The phospholipids are used by the cells to form part of the cellular membrane, different intracellular membranes, and other intracellular structures. One of the most important features of all cellular life is the different compartments into which each cell is divided by lipid membranes. The physical characteristics of the phospholipids and other fatty substances in these membranes make it possible for the membranes to separate the cytoplasm from the extracellular fluid, the nucleoplasm from the cytoplasm, the fluids of the mitochondria from the cytoplasm, and so forth.

Cholesterol. Another substance derived from fats is cholesterol; it, too, has many physical and chemical characteristics similar to those of fat. Like phospholipids, cholesterol is synthesized by all cells of the body and is used along with phospholipids and small amounts of neutral fat in composing the different membranous structures of cells. An especially large amount of cholesterol is formed by the liver, and about 80% of this is then used by the liver to synthesize bile acids that are secreted in the bile into the small intestine. These in turn promote emulsification of fats in the gastrointestinal tract so that they can be digested, and they also promote fat absorption.

Also, cholesterol is used by the sex glands and the adrenal cortex for synthesis of different steroid hormones.

Atherosclerosis. Unfortunately, large quantities of cholesterol are occasionally either synthesized by the walls of the arteries or are deposited there from the blood. As a result, large plaques of cholesterol frequently develop in the arterial walls and protrude through the intima into the flowing arterial blood. This disease is called *atherosclerosis.* Blood clots often develop on the protruding cholesterol plaques, at times becoming large enough to occlude completely the lumen of the vessel. This is the cause of most acute coronary occlusions that bring about heart attacks.

The rate at which cholesterol is deposited in the walls of the arteries is directly proportional to the intake of calories in the diet, especially when this is above the daily requirements for energy. Atherosclerosis also seems to be more severe when most of the intake of calories is in the form of highly saturated fats rather than in the form of unsaturated fats, proteins and carbohydrates. Certain persons are genetically inclined to very severe atherosclerosis.

METABOLISM OF PROTEINS

Transport and Storage of Amino Acids. The amino acids, which are the end products of protein digestion in the gastrointestinal tract, are absorbed into the portal blood and then are disseminated into all parts of the body. Some of the amino acids are transported into the liver cells and are temporarily stored there, though this is of minor importance in comparison with the storage of glucose and fat by the liver. Most of the amino acids are rapidly absorbed directly into all the cells of the body.

Cellular Synthesis of Proteins. Once inside the cells, most amino acids are rapidly synthesized into proteins. This process is controlled by messenger ribonucleic acid molecules that act as templates for the formation of the protein molecules in the ribosomes. This overall mechanism was described at the beginning of this chapter in the discussion of cellular physiology.

Essential Amino Acids. The usual proteins of the body contain 20 different amino acids, and these are available in almost all protein foods that are eaten. However, an occasional protein of the diet has a deficiency of one or more of the usual amino acids. Often one of the available amino acids can be converted into the missing one, but 10 of the 20 amino acids cannot be formed this way and must be present in the diet in order for the cells to synthesize their normal complements of proteins. These 10 amino acids are called essential amino acids.

Synthesis of Other Substances from Amino Acids. Many special chemical substances needed in the cells are synthesized from amino acids. For instance, many of the hormones are either modified amino acids or polypeptides, including thyroxine, norepinephrine, parathyroid hormone, posterior pituitary hormones, and insulin. In addition, such important substances as adenosine triphosphate and creatine phosphate derive parts of their structures from proteins.

Catabolism of Proteins in the Cells. Catabolism of proteins means splitting of the proteins back into amino acids. A small concentration of amino acids, about 30 mg per 100 ml, is always maintained in the plasma and interstitial fluid. When this amount decreases, amino acids are transported out of the cells, and this causes the proteins of the cells

to begin to be catabolized into amino acids. This catabolism is catalyzed by intracellular enzymes called *cathepsins,* which are digestive enzymes released from lysosomes in the cells. In this way a small concentration of amino acids is always maintained in the body fluids. Then, if a particular cell becomes damaged or for some other reason needs an immediate source of amino acids to repair its structural and enzyme systems, the amino acids are available. Thus, amino acids can be mobilized from one part of the body to another by this process—to wherever the need is momentarily greatest. Amino acid mobilization is greatly accelerated by glucocorticoid hormones.

Deamination of Amino Acids and Their Use for Energy. If a person eats more protein than the amount needed to maintain adequate protein stores in the cells, all the excess amino acids are degraded and then used for energy as carbohydrates and fats are used. The first stage in this process is deamination, which means removal of the amino radical from the amino acid. This is accomplished by a specific enzyme system in the liver cells. The amino radical is then synthesized into urea, which is excreted through the kidneys into the urine.

Many of the resultant deaminated amino acids are similar to pyruvic acid and can enter the citric acid cycle either directly or after a few stages of minor alterations. In this way, the amino acids become oxidized in very much the same way as carbohydrates and fats, and large quantities of adenosine triphosphate are formed to be used as an energy source everywhere in the cells.

NUTRITION

The Energy Equivalent of Foods—Calories. In the above sections it has been noted that carbohydrates, fats, and proteins can all supply energy to the cells. Energy is generally expressed in terms of Calories (spelled with a capital C), which are equivalent to kilocalories. However, the different types of food are not equal in their capabilities for supplying energy. One g of carbohydrate or 1 g of protein supplies 4.1 Calories of energy to the body, while 1 g of fat supplies 9.3 Calories of energy. Therefore, it is evident that over twice as much carbohydrate or protein must be eaten to provide the same amount of energy as a specified quantity of fat.

Energy Requirements. A normal adult requires about 1,600 Calories of energy each day simply to exist even without sitting up or walking around. To provide the energy needed for sitting, another 200 to 400 Calories is required; and for walking and working a moderate amount, still another 500 Calories. The total daily energy requirement for the average person adds up to about 2,500 Calories. This is called the *metabolic rate* of the body. For performing very heavy physical labor this can occasionally be as great as 6,000 to 7,000 Calories per day.

Basal Metabolic Rate. The basal metabolic rate is the metabolic rate of an awake person whose body is as inactive as possible. To attain the *basal state* a person must have had essentially no exercise for the past 8 to 10 hours, no food for the past 12 hours, and he must have quiet conditions and normal room temperature. The normal basal metabolic rate of the young male adult is about 40 Calories per m^2 of body surface area per hour or a total of about 70 Calories per hour for the whole body.

Daily Protein Requirement. About 30 g of amino acids are degraded each day and used by the body mainly for synthesizing various necessary intracellular substances. Even when a person is starving, this degradation of amino acids continues. Therefore, simply to maintain normal protein stores of the body, about 30 g of proteins are needed in the diet per day. And, if these proteins do not contain the correct ratios of amino acids, or if they are not utilized completely by the body, still larger amounts of protein are required.

Regulation of Food Intake. Food intake is regulated by two mechanisms, one called short-term regulation of intake and the other long-term regulation.

Short-term regulation of food intake is a function of the gastrointestinal system itself. That is, whenever the gastrointestinal system becomes overly filled, nervous signals passing from the intestinal tract to the brain diminish one's desire for food and therefore diminish the intake of food. Particularly important is the degree of distention of the stomach and upper portions of the small intestine. It is this short-term mechanism that makes a person begin to lose his or her appetite for food toward the end of a meal.

Long-term regulation of food intake is mainly a function of nervous centers in the hypothalamus. Located in the lateral nucleus of the hypothalamus is a *feeding center,* which, when stimulated, increases the food intake. Located in the ventromedial nucleus of the hypothalamus is a center that makes a person feel satisfied and therefore inhibits food intake; therefore, this center is called the *satiety center.* The degree of activity of the feeding center of the hypothalamus is determined by the metabolic status of the body. When a person becomes overweight, the activity of the feeding center diminishes. On the other hand, in starvation, the feeding center becomes greatly activated. Yet, the exact feedback signals to the feeding center that activate or inactivate it are not too well understood. It is known, though, that one of the signals is an increase in circulating glucose and amino acids in the blood, both of which will inhibit feeding, while diminished quantities of these excite feeding. It is possible that the level of fatty acids in the circulating blood also is an important factor in controlling the activity of the feeding center.

Obesity. Obesity means simply the storage of excess amounts of fat in the body. When more energy foods are ingested than are utilized each day, the extra amount is stored in the form of fat. Even excess carbohydrates and proteins are converted into fat and then stored. Thus, obesity actually develops from an excess intake of energy each day over utilization of energy. Unfortunately, certain people have far more insatiable appetites than others, often an inherited genetic trait, which causes them to continue eating far beyond their energy needs. This results from abnormal function of the feeding centers in the hypothalamus.

Starvation. In starvation, the stored energy substances in the body are utilized very rapidly. Sufficient glycogen is stored in the liver and muscle cells to provide significant amounts of energy for about ½ to 1 day. Beyond that, almost all the energy made available to the body at first comes from the stored fat, this sometimes lasting for as long as 3 to 8 weeks. However, during the entire process of starvation, a small amount of body protein is continually degraded and used for energy as well, and when the fat stores begin to run out, tremendous amounts of protein then begin to be used for energy. When this happens, the functional state of the cells quickly deteriorates, and death soon follows. However, it is fortunate that most of the proteins are spared until the last.

Functions of the Vitamins. Vitamins are substances ingested in the food in only minute quantities but that play key roles in the metabolic systems of the body. The functions of some of the important vitamins are the following:

Vitamin A is used to synthesize rhodopsin, which was discussed earlier as a necessary chemical for vision. It also aids in the normal growth of cells, especially epithelial cells.

Thiamine operates as part of a cocarboxylase for removal of carbon dioxide from foods being used by the cells.

Niacin functions in the body in the forms of nicrotinamide adenine dinucleotide (NAD) and nicotinamide adenine dinucleotide phosphate (NADP). These act as hydrogen acceptors when hydrogen is removed from the foods; therefore, they are important in the oxidation of food.

Riboflavin is used to form flavoprotein, which is also a hydrogen carrier in the oxidation of foodstuffs.

Vitamin B_{12} and folic acid were discussed earlier in the chapter as substances needed for the maturation of red blood cells in the bone marrow.

Pantothenic acid is a precursor of *coenzyme A,* which is needed for acetylation of many substances in the body. It is especially needed for the formation of acetyl coenzyme A prior to oxidation of both glucose and fatty acids.

Pyridoxine is used as a coenzyme in many reactions involving amino acid metabolism, one of which acts to transfer amino radicals from one substance to another, and another of which causes deamination.

Ascorbic acid (vitamin C) is a strong reducing compound that probably acts in several metabolic processes in which electrons are exchanged with oxidative chemicals. Though the precise nature of these specific chemical reactions is not known, the major physiologic function of ascorbic acid is to maintain normal intercellular substances, including normal collagen fibers and normal intercellular cement substance between the cells.

Vitamin D is needed for absorption of calcium from the gastrointestinal tract.

Vitamin K, which was discussed in connection with blood coagulation, is needed in the synthetic processes of the liver for formation of prothrombin, Factor VII, and several other factors that are utilized in blood coagulation.

REGULATION OF BODY TEMPERATURE

Body temperature is controlled by the balance between the rate of heat production in the body and the rate of heat loss. If the rate at which heat is produced is greater than the rate at which it is lost, the body temperature will rise. On the other hand, if the rate of loss is greater, then the body temperature will fall.

Heat Production and Its Control. All the metabolic processes of the body produce heat as a by-product, for almost all the energy in the food eventually becomes heat after it has performed its other functions. Thus, in the average person about 2,500 Calories of heat are formed each day. In other words, the rate of heat production is controlled by the metabolic rate of the body.

Under the basal conditions it is mainly the internal organs—the brain, the heart, the kidneys, the gastrointestinal tract, and especially the liver—that produce most of the heat. However, when a person uses muscles for various activities, these produce tremendous amounts of heat. During extreme muscular activity the total heat production of the body can increase temporarily to as much as 15 times normal, over 90% of the heat then coming from the muscles.

Heat Loss. Normally, the most important means by which the skin loses heat to the surroundings is by *radiation;* that is, heat waves, a type of electromagnetic radiation, are transmitted from the surface of the body to surrounding objects. A large portion of the heat is also lost by **conduction** to objects touching the body or to the surrounding air and then **convection** of the heated air away from the body. Finally, when a person sweats, very large amounts of heat are consumed to cause *evaporation* of the water in the sweat.

The skin is supplied with an abundant vasculature, but the amount of blood that flows through these vessels is controlled very exactly by the sympathetic nervous system so that when the body becomes overly heated skin blood flow will be tremendous, and when the body is underheated skin blood flow will be negligible. Rapid flow of blood heats the skin, allowing large amounts of heat to be lost to the surroundings. Also, sympathetic stimuli to the sweat glands increase sweat production and consequently greatly increase the evaporative loss of heat. Slow blood flow prevents heat loss because the internal heat of the body cannot be carried to the skin, and the skin temperature falls rapidly to approach that of the surroundings.

Regulation of Body Temperature by the Hypothalamus. Portions of the hypothalamus are sensitive to changes in body temperature, so that whenever the blood becomes too hot or too cold, appropriate readjustments in the rates of heat production and heat loss return the body temperature to normal.

Located in the preoptic area of the hypothalamus is a small region called the *heat center.* When this becomes too cold, a decrease in the signals transmitted from here to the posterior hypothalamus causes three effects: (1) it reduces the rate of heat loss by constricting the blood vessels to the skin; (2) it transmits additional signals into the brain stem and spinal cord to stimulate the skeletal muscles throughout the body; this in turn increases muscle tone and causes shivering, which increases the muscle metabolic rate, sometimes increasing heat production as much as 300%; and (3) it increases heat production by exciting the sympathetic nervous system and causing release of epinephrine, which effects an increase in the rate of metabolism of all cells in the body, sometimes increasing heat production as much as 20% to 40%. As a result of all these effects, the body temperature rises back toward normal.

When the preoptic area becomes too hot, this same temperature control system functions in exactly the opposite manner. It decreases heat production by reducing the tone of the skeletal muscles throughout the body and reducing the sympathetic release of epinephrine. More important, however, it increases the rate of heat loss in two ways: (1) lack of sympathetic vasoconstriction allows the blood vessels of the skin to become greatly dilated; the skin temperature rises, and increased amounts of heat are lost to the surroundings; and (2) stimulation of a sweat center, also located in the heat center of the hypothalamus, causes sweating over the entire body, with resultant evaporative loss of heat.

In summary, if the preoptic area of the anterior hypothalamus becomes too hot, heat production is decreased while heat loss is increased, and the body temperature falls back toward normal. Conversely, if the preoptic area becomes too cold, heat production is increased, while heat loss is decreased so that the body temperature now rises toward normal.

Effect of Skin Temperature Signals on Body Temperature Regulation. Not only do signals from the preoptic area of the hypothalamus play an important role in body temperature regulation, but temperature signals from the skin do also. When the skin becomes too warm, nerve impulses are transmitted from the skin warm receptors all the way to the preoptic area of the hypothalamus to increase sweating, and this obviously increases body heat loss. Conversely, when the skin becomes too cold, signals from the skin cold receptors are transmitted to the posterior hypothalamus where they activate shivering, which in turn helps to increase the body temperature back toward normal. Therefore, body temperature control is vested in an integrated mechanism in which the hypothalamus is the central integrator, but reacts to signals both from the preoptic area and from the skin.

Local reflexes from the skin to the spinal cord and then back to the skin to control the degree of local sweating and local vasodilatation or constriction also play a minor role in temperature control.

ENDOCRINE GLANDS

The endocrine glands secrete *hormones* that control many of the body's functions. Hormones function in three major ways: (1) by controlling transport of substances through cell membranes, (2) by controlling the activity of specific cellular genes, which in turn determine the formation of specific enzymes and other cellular factors, and (3) by controlling directly some metabolic systems of cells.

Some hormones perform their functions by first activating an *intracellular hormonal mediator* called a *second messenger* that then performs the specific intracellular function. One of the most important of the second messengers is *cyclic adenosine monophosphate* (cyclic AMP), illustrated in Figure 3-26. To activate this intracellular mediator, the general hormone first binds with a receptor on the surface of the membrane of the target cell. This receptor in turn activates the enzyme adenylcyclase in the membrane, and this in turn causes formation of cyclic AMP inside the cell. And, finally, the cyclic AMP performs a specific function within the cell such as causing an increase of enzymes, alteration of cell permeability, or modification of chemical reactions within the cytoplasm.

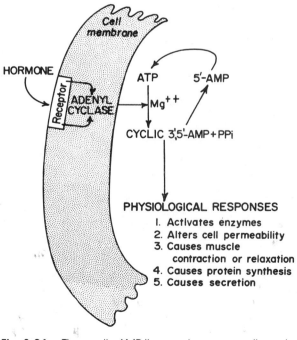

Fig. 3-26. The cyclic AMP "second messenger" mechanism by which hormones often control cell function. (Guyton AC: Textbook of Medical Physiology, 7th ed. Philadelphia, WB Saunders, 1986)

PITUITARY HORMONES

The pituitary gland secretes hormones that regulate a wide variety of functions in the body. This gland is divided into two major divisions: the anterior pituitary gland and the posterior pituitary gland. Six well-known hormones are secreted by the anterior pituitary gland—growth hormone, thyroid stimulating hormone, adrenocorticotropic hormone, prolactin, and two gonadotropic hormones, luteinizing hormone and follicle-stimulating hormone. Two well-known posterior pituitary hormones are secreted—antidiuretic hormone, also called vasopressin, and oxytocic hormone.

Control of Pituitary Hormone Secretion by Hypothalamic Hormones. When the anterior pituitary gland is separated from the hypothalamus, secretion of most of its hormones, with the exception of prolactin, decreases to very small amounts. This occurs because secretion by the anterior pituitary gland is controlled mainly by hormones formed in the hypothalamus and that are then conducted to the pituitary through the *hypothalamic-hypophyseal venous portal system* illustrated in Figure 3-27. This system consists of small veins that carry blood (and hormones) from capillaries to the lower hypothalamus to the venous sinuses of the anterior pituitary gland. Here, the hormones from the hypothalamus act directly on the anterior pituitary cells to control secretion of the pituitary hormones. Most of the hormones from the hypothalamus have a positive effect on the anterior pituitary cells, causing release of the pituitary hormones, but some of them have a negative effect, inhibiting release.

The important hypothalamic hormones that control the function of the anterior pituitary gland are the following:

Growth hormone-releasing hormone, which causes release of growth hormone
Corticotropin-releasing hormone, which causes release of adrenocorticotropic hormone
Thyrotropin-releasing hormone, which causes the release of thyroid-stimulating hormone
Luteinizing hormone-releasing hormone, which causes release of the two gonadotropins, luteinizing hormone and follicle-stimulating hormone
Prolactin inhibitory hormone, which inhibits the release of prolactin (in the absence of this hormone, the rate of prolactin secretion increases to about three times normal)

Growth Hormone. Growth hormone causes growth of the body. It is secreted by the anterior pituitary gland throughout life, not merely while a person is growing, but slightly more during the growing phase. It causes enlargement and proliferation of cells in all parts of the body, resulting in progressive growth of the body stature until adolescence. At this time the epiphyses of the long bones unite with the shafts of the bones so that further increase in height of the body cannot occur. However, certain of the "membranous" bones and soft tissues, such as the bones of the nose and certain bones of the skull, as well as the tissues of some of the internal organs, still continue to grow.

The precise mechanism by which growth hormone exerts its effects on the cells is not clear.

Fig. 3-27. The hypothalamic–hypophyseal portal system. (Guyton AC: Textbook of Medical Physiology, 7th ed. Philadelphia, WB Saunders, 1986)

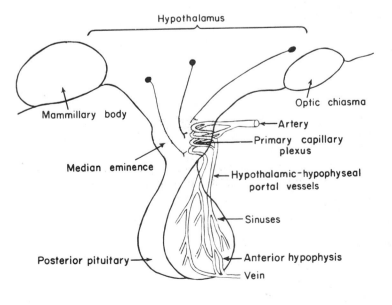

However, it is known to act on the liver to cause formation of several small protein substances called *somatomedins.* It is these substances that in turn cause growth of the bones and perhaps also cause many or most of the other effects of growth hormone.

Growth hormone specifically promotes transport of some amino acids through cell membranes, thereby making more of these available to the cells. In addition, it (1) activates the RNA translation process to cause increased formation of proteins by the ribosomes, (2) increases the rate of DNA transcription to increase the amount of messenger RNA, (3) increases the replication of DNA which causes increased reproduction of the cells themselves, and (4) decreases the rate of breakdown of proteins in the cells. Thus, growth hormone has a potent effect to enhance all aspects of protein synthesis and storage in the cells of the body. It is presumably this effect that is most important in promoting growth.

After adolescence, growth hormone continues to be secreted at about two-thirds the preadolescent rate. Though most growth in the body stops at this time, primarily because the growth potential of the long bones ceases when the epiphyses unite with the shafts, the other metabolic effects of growth hormones continue.

Growth hormone also affects carbohydrate metabolism, though not nearly as much as protein metabolism. It increases the blood sugar and decreases the rate of metabolism of carbohydrates by the cells. Growth hormone affects fat metabolism as well. It increases the rate of breakdown of fats into fatty acids and increases their use for energy by all the cells.

Growth hormone secretion is controlled by growth hormone-releasing hormone that is secreted in the hypothalamus and transported to the anterior pituitary gland through the hypothalamic-hypophyseal portal system. When nutritional debility causes protracted hypoglycemia or decreases the body's protein stores, the secretion of growth hormone-releasing hormone and therefore also the rate of growth hormone secretion are increased. Also, other types of physical stress or mental stress often greatly increase the rate of growth hormone secretion.

Thyroid-Stimulating Hormone. Thyroid-stimulating hormone stimulates the thyroid glandular cells in many ways: (1) it increases the rate of synthesis of thyroglobulin, (2) it increases the rate of uptake of iodide ions from the blood by the glandular cells, and (3) it activates all the chemical processes that cause thyroxine production and release

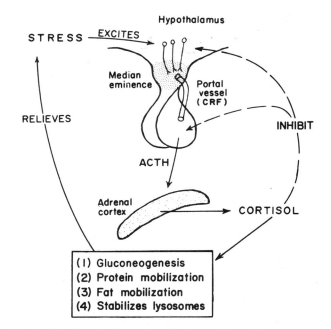

Fig. 3-28. Regulation of cortisol secretion. (Guyton AC: Textbook of Medical Physiology, 7th ed. Philadelphia, WB Saunders, 1986)

by the thyroid gland. Therefore, indirectly, thyroid-stimulating hormone increases the overall rate of metabolism of the body, for, as will be discussed later, this is the principal effect of thyroxine.

The degree of activation of the anterior pituitary gland to secrete thyroid-stimulating hormone is controlled principally by a negative feedback effect of thyroxine on the hypothalamus. When the thyroxine concentration is high, this decreases the rate of secretion of thyrotropin-releasing hormone by the hypothalamus and also decreases the activity of the anterior pituitary glandular cells to produce thyroxine. Therefore, when excess thyroxine is already present in the blood, this feedback effect turns off further production.

Adrenocorticotropic Hormone. As illustrated in Figure 3-28, adrenocorticotropic hormone (ACTH) strongly stimulates *cortisol* production by the adrenal cortex, and it stimulates the production of other adrenocortical hormones to a much less extent. Cortisol in turn has many different metabolic effects in the body, including especially degradation of proteins in the tissues, release of amino acids into the circulating blood, conversion of many of these amino acids into glucose (the process of gluconeogenesis), and decreased utilization of glucose by tissue cells. These effects will be discussed later in relation to the adrenal hormones.

Figure 3-28 also shows that the secretion of adrenocorticotropic hormone by the anterior pituitary is controlled mainly by *corticotropin-releasing hormone* (CRF) from the hypothalamus. The rate of secretion of this hormone, in turn, is strongly stimulated by stressful states such as disease, trauma to the body, and even emotional excitement. Also, when excessive quantities of cortisol are present in the blood, these have a feedback effect on the hypothalamus and anterior pituitary cells to decrease the rate of secretion of adrenocorticotropic hormone, thus providing a negative feedback mechanism for controlling the concentration of cortisol in the blood.

The Gonadotropic Hormones. The anterior pituitary gland secretes two hormones called gonadotropic hormones that regulate many male and female sexual functions. These are follicle-stimulating hormone and luteinizing hormone. The rates of secretion of these hormones are controlled mainly by luteinizing hormone-releasing hormone from the hypothalamus. However, feedback effects from the sex hormones also help to control their rates of secretion. The gonadotropic hormones will be discussed in more detail later in the chapter in relation to the male and female functions.

Prolactin. Prolactin plays an important role in the development of the breasts during pregnancy and also in promoting milk secretion by the breasts after birth of the baby. These functions will be discussed in more detail in relation to milk production.

The secretion of prolactin is controlled mainly by prolactin inhibitory hormone from the hypothalamus. Prolactin secretion increases about 10-fold during pregnancy. Its rate of secretion is also increased by suckling of the nipples by the baby; this in turn causes production of more milk.

Posterior Pituitary Hormones. Two different hormones are secreted by the posterior pituitary gland. The first of these is *antidiuretic hormone* (ADH), which was discussed earlier in relation to water reabsorption from the renal tubules. Briefly, when the body fluids become excessively concentrated, neuronal cells in or near the supraoptic nucleus of the hypothalamus, called osmoreceptors, cause antidiuretic hormone to be released from the posterior pituitary gland. On reaching the kidney, this hormone enhances the rate of water reabsorption from the renal tubules and tends to correct the overconcentration of the body fluids.

Antidiuretic hormone also constricts the arterioles and causes the arterial pressure to rise, for which reason it is also called vasopressin. Finally, this hormone can also cause contraction of many other smooth muscle structures throughout the body.

The second posterior pituitary hormone, *oxytocin,* causes contraction especially of the uterus and, to a lesser extent, some of the other smooth muscle structures of the body. Oxytocin is released by the posterior pituitary gland in increased amounts during parturition, and it may play a significant role in initiating birth of the baby. Oxytocin also plays a role in lactation in the following ways: Sucking on the breast initiates nerve impulses that pass all the way from the nipple to the hypothalamus, which then sends signals to the posterior pituitary gland to cause release of oxytocin. The oxytocin in turn stimulates myoepithelial cells in the breasts that constrict the alveoli of the breasts in a manner that makes the milk flow into the ducts. This is called *milk ejection* or *milk letdown.*

ADRENOCORTICAL HORMONES

The adrenal cortex secretes three different types of steroid hormones that are chemically similar to each other but physiologically widely different. These are: (1) the *mineralocorticoids,* which are represented principally by aldosterone, (2) the *glucocorticoids,* which are represented mainly by cortisol, and (3) the *androgens,* which have masculine sexual effects.

Mineralocorticoids—Aldosterone. The mineralocorticoids have significant effects on electrolyte balance in the body. Several such hormones are secreted by the adrenal cortex, but 95% or more of the total mineralocorticoid activity is due to aldosterone.

Aldosterone was discussed earlier in this chapter in relation to reabsorption of sodium from the renal tubules and tubular secretion of potassium. Briefly, aldosterone enhances sodium transport from the tubules into the peritubular fluids, and at the same time enhances potassium transport from the peritubular fluids into the tubules. Therefore, aldosterone causes conservation of sodium in the body and excretion of potassium in the urine.

Aldosterone also causes increased reabsorption of chloride ions and water from the tubules in the following ways: When sodium is reabsorbed, this transfers a positive charge to the outside of the renal tubules that pulls the negative chloride ions through the membrane. When increased amounts of sodium and chloride are resorbed, the osmotic concentration of the tubular fluid decreases, while the osmotic concentration of the peritubular fluids increases. As a result, large quantities of water are absorbed by osmosis into the extracellular fluid, and the total extracellular fluid volume increases.

The important factors for control of aldosterone secretion are: (1) An increase in potassium ion concentration has an especially powerful effect to cause increased aldosterone secretion. This provides a negative feedback system for controlling the extracellular fluid potassium ion concentration because the aldosterone then promotes excretion of the excess potassium from the extracellular fluid into the urine. (2) Angiotensin also can strongly stimulate the secretion of aldosterone. This controls the total extracellular fluid volume in the following way: When the extracellular fluid volume decreases, the arterial pressure also tends to decrease. This then causes the kidney to form renin and angiotensin, as was explained earlier in the chapter. The angiotensin stimulates aldosterone secretion, which in turn causes absorption of sodium, chloride, and water, thus increasing the extracellular fluid volume back toward normal. (3) Decreased sodium ion concentration in the extracellular fluid also stimulates aldosterone secretion. This may occur because decreased sodium also stimulates angiotensin formation. (4) Adrenocorticotropic hormone from the pituitary gland has a slight effect to increase aldosterone secretion.

Glucocorticoids—Cortisol. Several different glucocorticoids are secreted by the adrenal cortex, but almost all of the glucocorticoid activity is caused by cortisol, also called *hydrocortisone.* Glucocorticoids affect the metabolism of glucose, proteins, and fats.

Cortisol decreases glucose uptake into cells and also decreases the rate of utilization of glucose by the cells. In addition, it increases the rate of *gluconeogenesis* in the liver cells, which converts amino acids into glucose that is then emptied into the blood. Thus, several different effects cause the blood concentration of glucose to increase.

Cortisol also causes degradation of proteins and decreases protein synthesis in most tissues of the body. This causes amino acids to be released from the cells and therefore increases their concentration in the blood. The liver, however, is different from the other tissues because cortisol increases amino acid uptake by liver cells. There they are used to synthesize increased quantities of plasma proteins, to provide metabolic energy for the liver, and to be converted into glucose by the process of gluconeogenesis as noted above.

Cortisol causes increased use of fat for energy. This results mainly from an effect of cortisol to activate *hormone sensitive lipase* in the fat cells, which causes splitting of the fat and release of fatty acids into the circulating blood.

In an animal that does not secrete cortisol, the body's tissues are very susceptible to cellular destructive processes. However, stress of almost any type—such as trauma, surgical operations, disease, mental stresses, and so forth—causes increased secretion of cortisol. This cortisol in turn seems to be essential for repair of damaged tissues. However, the manner in which cortisol stimulates tissue repair still is not understood. Perhaps it is the increase in availability of amino acids and glucose in the blood induced by cortisol that is mainly responsible for this effect.

Cortisol can also suppress inflammation. One of the most important mechanisms of this is that cortisol stabilizes the cellular lysosomes, preventing them from rupturing and releasing their digestive enzymes, histamine, bradykinin, and other factors that promote the inflammation process. Cortisol also decreases the permeability of capillary membranes, which minimizes leakage of fluid into the tissues during inflammation.

Androgens. The androgens are steroid hormones that cause masculinizing effects in the body. Though the most important androgen is testosterone secreted by the testis, the adrenal cortex also secretes several other androgenic hormones. These are normally of minor importance, but, when an adrenal tumor develops or when the adrenal glands become hyperplastic and secrete excess quantities of hormones, the amounts of androgens then secreted occasionally become great enough to cause even a child or an adult female to take on adult masculine characteristics, including growth of a beard, change of the voice to a bass quality, and increased muscular size and strength.

THYROID HORMONES

Formation and Release of Thyroxine and Triiodothyronine. The thyroid gland is composed of follicles lined with thyroid glandular cells, illustrated in Figure 3-29. These cells secrete a very large glycoprotein called thyroglobulin to the inside of the follicle. They also absorb iodide ions from the circulating blood and secrete these in an oxidized form into the follicles along with the thyroglobulin. This oxidized iodine combines with tyrosine amino acid molecules that are integral parts of the key thyroglobulin molecule. In this manner, large quantities of thyroxine (and smaller quantities of triiodothyronine) are formed within the thyroglobulin molecule, and the thyroglobulin then remains

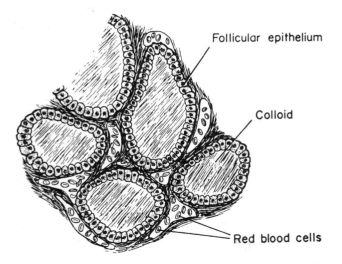

Fig. 3-29. Structure of the thyroid gland. (Guyton AC: Textbook of Medical Physiology, 7th ed. Philadelphia, WB Saunders, 1986)

stored in the thyroid follicles for an average of about 6 weeks. As thyroid hormones are needed in the circulating blood, some of the thyroglobulin is reabsorbed back into the glandular cells by the process of pinocytosis. Then the thyroglobulin is digested by proteases released from lysosomes in the cells, thus releasing thyroxine and triiodothyronine into the blood.

The rate of formation of the thyroid hormones, thyroxine, and triiodothyronine, and especially their rate of release from thyroglobulin, is controlled by thyroid stimulating hormone (TSH) from the anterior pituitary gland, as was discussed earlier.

Once the thyroid hormones have been released into the blood, they combine with several different plasma proteins. Then during the next week they are slowly released from the blood into the tissue cells.

Effect of Thyroxine and Triiodothyronine on the Cells. Thyroxine increases the rate of activity and metabolism of almost all cells in the body. It also increases the breakdown of all cellular foodstuffs and the rate of heat release from the cells. Triiodothyronine has the same effects as thyroxine except that it acts more rapidly.

Unfortunately, the exact manner in which thyroxine and triiodothyronine perform their functions in the cells is still unknown. However, they increase the rate of synthesis of proteins in most cells and especially the rate of synthesis of many different enzymes that in turn are the basis for the increased metabolic activities of the cells. They also

increases the sizes and numbers of mitochondria in the cells, and these in turn increase the rate of production of ATP, which might be another factor that promotes enhanced cellular metabolism.

Hyperthyroidism. An excess of thyroid hormone secretion above that needed for normal function of the body is called hyperthyroidism. Briefly, this causes excessive activity of essentially all the functional systems of the body including (1) greatly increased rate of metabolism throughout the body, (2) increased heart rate and increased cardiac output, (3) increased gastrointestinal secretion and gastrointestinal motility, (4) increased activity of the nervous system, sometimes causing a fine tremor of all the muscles, (5) increased respiratory rate, (6) often abnormal glandular secretion by the other endocrine glands, and (7) severe loss of weight in extreme cases.

Hypothyroidism. The opposite of hyperthyroidism is hypothyroidism; it results from too little secretion of thyroid hormone. It causes greatly inhibited activity of almost all the functional systems, including (1) a decrease in metabolic rate to as low as 40% below normal, (2) sometimes such lethargy that the person sleeps 14 to 16 hours per day and even when awake has difficulty cerebrating, and (3) collection of a mucinous fluid in the tissue spaces between the cells, creating an edematous state called *myxedema.*

PANCREATIC HORMONES—INSULIN AND GLUCAGON

The pancreas has thousands of small clusters of cells called *islets of Langerhans,* one of which is illustrated in Figure 3-30. These islets secrete two different hormones, *insulin* and *glucagon,* the first of which is of extreme importance to normal function of the body. Insulin is a small protein, molecular weight about 6000, formed by the beta cells of the islets of Langerhans. Glucagon likewise is a small protein, molecular weight about 3500, formed by the alpha cells of the islets of Langerhans.

The Metabolic Role of Insulin. Insulin is often called the "storage hormone" because its secretion is greatly increased immediately after a meal, and it causes cellular storage of all of the different foodstuffs including carbohydrate, fat, and protein.

Effect of Insulin on Carbohydrate Metabolism. Insulin has an especially large effect to cause glucose storage following a meal. Approximately 60% of this is stored in the liver, and about 15% is stored in the muscles, while most of the remainder is used for energy. The mechanism by which insulin

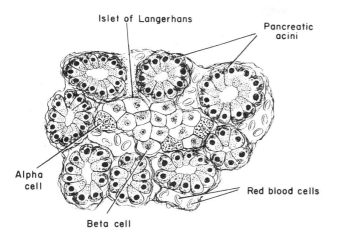

Fig. 3-30. Anatomy of an islet of Langerhans in the pancreas. (Guyton AC: Textbook of Medical Physiology, 7th ed. Philadelphia, WB Saunders, 1986)

promotes glucose storage in the liver is quite different from the mechanism in muscle. In the liver, glucose diffuses through the cell membrane with ease but is trapped in the hepatic cells by being converted first into glucose phosphate and then into glycogen. Insulin promotes this effect by greatly increasing the activities of two liver enzymes, glucokinase and glycogen synthetase. In muscle and most other cells of the body (besides the liver and the brain) insulin increases the permeability of the cell membranes to glucose. In the presence of large amounts of insulin, the membrane of resting muscle is about 15 times as permeable to glucose as it is when there is no insulin. Insulin also moderately increases the activity of the enzymes in these cells both for storing glucose in the form of glycogen and also for increased metabolic usage of the glucose.

Insulin has little or no effect on transport of glucose into the brain cells. Instead, the rate of glucose diffusion into these cells is directly proportional to blood glucose concentration.

The insulin system plays the most important role of all the hormones in maintaining a normal blood glucose concentration. The large amounts of insulin secreted after each meal prevent the glucose concentration from rising too high by causing storage of almost all of the absorbed glucose in the liver. Then, between meals, in the absence of insulin, most of this glucose returns to the blood because of a continual breakdown of glycogen in the liver when insulin is not present. It is especially important that the blood glucose concentration be regulated in this manner because it assures a relatively unvarying rate of delivery of glucose to the brain. Unfortu-

nately, the brain cells are special in that they utilize fats and proteins very poorly for energy. Therefore, the regulation of blood glucose concentration—which is performed principally by the action of insulin—helps to maintain a steady rate of neuronal activity.

Effect of Insulin on Fat Metabolism. Insulin has both direct and indirect effects on fat metabolism. The direct effect is to decrease the rate of fatty acid release from fat tissues into the body fluids. The mechanism of this is mainly intense depression of hormone sensitive lipase by insulin; this prevents the hydrolysis of triglycerides in the fat tissue and therefore prevents fatty acid release. Conversely, when there is little insulin, this enzyme becomes excessively active and causes large quantities of fatty acids to be released into the tissue fluid. In this way, fatty acids become mobilized and are utilized for energy in place of glucose that cannot be utilized in most tissues of the body without insulin.

The indirect effect of insulin on fat metabolism occurs secondarily to insulin-induced changes in carbohydrate metabolism. Insulin has the same effect on fat cells that it has on muscle cells to cause increased glucose transport into the fat cells. This causes some increase in formation of fatty acids in these cells and then storage of these in the form of triglycerides. However, the most important effect is that the glucose inside the fat cells is used to form the glycerol portion of the stored triglycerides. In addition, much larger quantities of fatty acids are synthesized in the liver when there is excess blood glucose and insulin. These fatty acids are then transported to the fat cells where they combine with the glycerol to form still more triglycerides that are then stored.

When, in the absence of insulin, large quantities of fatty acids are released from the fat cells, many of these are transported to the liver where they form excessive quantities of (1) stored fat in the liver, (2) cholesterol, phospholipids, and triglycerides that are then released into the blood, and (3) acetoacetic acid that is also released into the blood. In prolonged periods of no insulin secretion, the acetoacetic acid can become so great that it causes severe acidosis.

Effect of Insulin on Growth and Protein Metabolism. Insulin is absolutely essential for growth. Even growth hormone will not cause a significant amount of growth in an animal in the absence of insulin. Insulin probably has this effect because it increases the formation of protein in cells. It does this by promoting active transport of some of the amino acids through the cell membrane to the interior of the cell, by increasing the number of functional ribosomes for forming proteins, and by increasing the activity of the DNA–RNA system that controls protein formation.

Control of Insulin Secretion.   The rate of secretion of insulin by the pancreas is controlled mainly by the concentration of glucose in the circulating blood but also by the concentration of amino acids. At a high concentration of glucose, large quantities of insulin are secreted, and the insulin in turn promotes storage of glucose in the body cells, especially in the liver. At a low concentration of blood glucose, the rate of insulin secretion decreases, and glucose is then transported out of the liver back into the blood.

Diabetes Mellitus.   Failure of the pancreas to secrete sufficient amounts of insulin results in diabetes mellitus. In this disease, the metabolism of all the basic foodstuffs is altered. The basic effect on glucose is to prevent its uptake by essentially all cells of the body besides those of the brain. As a result, blood glucose concentration rises very high, while cellular utilization of glucose falls lower and lower. Fat utilization rises higher and higher to make up the difference. Four principal sequelae often result from these basic effects:

First, the very high blood glucose concentration causes far more glucose to filter into the renal tubules than can be reabsorbed. Because this unreabsorbed glucose creates osmotic pressure in the tubules, it also prevents reabsorption of much of the tubular water, thereby promoting very rapid diuresis, with loss of large quantities of extracellular fluid into the urine and resulting dehydration.

The second effect, which can be more detrimental than the first, results from the increased utilization of fats for energy. This causes the liver to release acetoacetic acid into the plasma far more rapidly than it can be taken up and oxidized by the tissue cells. As a result, the patient develops severe acidosis, which, in association with the dehydration, causes diabetic coma. This leads rapidly to death unless the condition is treated immediately with large amounts of insulin.

A third effect is to cause, over a prolonged period of time, depletion of the body's proteins. Also, failure to utilize glucose for energy leads to decreased storage of fat as well. Therefore, a person with severe untreated diabetes suffers rapid weight loss and often death within a few weeks without treatment.

Fourth, also over a long period of time, the excess fat utilization in the liver causes very large amounts of cholesterol in the circulating blood and also increased deposition of cholesterol in the arterial walls. This leads to severe arteriosclerosis and other vascular lesions.

Glucagon.   Glucagon has the opposite effect on blood glucose to that of insulin, sometimes causing it to double in as little as 20 minutes. It causes this effect mainly by increasing the rate of breakdown of glycogen in the liver cells. Over a longer period of time, it also causes marked increase in gluconeogenesis, which is the process by which amino acids are converted into glucose. The mechanism by which glucagon causes glucose release from the liver cells is believed to be the following: Glucagon activates adenylcyclase in the liver cell membranes. This in turn causes formation of cyclic AMP in the cells, which then activates phosphorylase, the enzyme that causes glycogen to split into glucose molecules.

When the blood concentration of glucose falls below normal, the pancreas secretes large amounts of glucagon. The blood glucose raising effect of glucagon then obviously helps to correct the hypoglycemia. Therefore, glucagon is important for control of blood glucose concentration, though over long periods of time not nearly so important as insulin.

PARATHYROID HORMONE AND PHYSIOLOGY OF BONE

Formation of Bone.   Before the function of parathyroid hormone can be explained, we must first discuss the basic physiology of bone and its relation to calcium and phosphate in the extracellular fluids. Bone is formed by *osteoblasts,* which line the outer surfaces of all bones and are also present inside most of the bone cavities. The osteoblasts secrete a very strong *protein matrix,* comprised mainly of collagen fibers, which gives the bone its toughness. This matrix has the special property of causing phosphate ions to combine with calcium ions, precipitating a complicated salt of calcium and phosphate called *hydroxyapatite* in the protein matrix to make it extremely hard. The extreme strength of the collagen fibers gives the bone tremendous tensile strength, while the hardness of the bone salt gives it tremendous compressive strength.

When calcium is not available in large quantities in the body fluids, bone is poorly formed. Calcium is difficult to absorb from the gastrointestinal tract, and when it fails to be absorbed, phosphate is also poorly absorbed because the two substances form insoluble compounds in the gut. However, vitamin D greatly increases calcium absorption, which in turn allows increased phosphate absorption. Therefore, lack of vitamin D decreases the amount of available calcium and phosphate for bone formation and can result in such poor mineralization of the bones that they no longer resist compressive forces. This is the disease known as rickets. Before vitamin D can increase calcium absorption by the gastrointestinal tract, it must be converted from its natural form into the substance **1,25-dihydroxycholecalciferol.** The first stage of this conversion occurs in the liver and a second stage in the kidney; the second stage requires the presence of parathyroid hormone. Therefore, severe liver disease, kidney disease, or lack of parathyroid hormone can lead to diminished calcium absorption by the intestinal tract.

Absorption of Bone. Bone is also continually absorbed by large numbers of *osteoclasts* present in the bone cavities. This absorption of bone has two major functions: (1) In all bones the protein matrix gradually becomes aged and loses its toughness, thus allowing the bone to become brittle. The osteoclastic absorptive process removes the aging bone, which is then continually replaced by new bone formed by the osteoblasts. (2) Absorption of bone provides a means by which calcium ions can be made available rapidly to the extracellular fluids.

Function of Parathyroid Hormone. Parathyroid hormone is principally concerned with the regulation of calcium ion concentration in the body fluids. It does this to a great extent by regulating the activity of the osteoclasts—the greater the parathyroid secretion, the greater becomes the number of osteoclasts and the greater their rates of activity, thereby markedly accelerating the osteoclastic absorption of bone. In this way, parathyroid hormone in large quantities can increase the calcium ion concentration in the extracellular fluid as much as 50% in as little as 4 hours. Another means by which parathyroid hormone increases calcium ion concentration in the extracellular fluid is to promote increased absorption of calcium ions from both the gastrointestinal tract and the renal tubules. A large part of the increased absorption from the intestine results from the effect of parathyroid hormone to activate vitamin D as explained earlier.

Large quantities of phosphate are also released into the blood by the absorption of bone. However, parathyroid hormone also accelerates the rate of phosphate excretion by the kidneys so that extracellular phosphate concentration, in contradistinction to the calcium concentration, usually does not rise but may actually fall when parathyroid hormone is administered.

This regulation of calcium ions by parathyroid hormone is extremely important because almost all of the excitable tissues of the body, including nerves, muscle fibers, the heart, and all smooth muscle organs, depend upon a well-regulated calcium ion concentration for normal function. For instance, a low calcium ion concentration causes such extreme increase of irritability in the peripheral nerves that they begin to emit impulses spontaneously, these causing a state of continual muscular contraction called *tetany.* Also, greatly decreased calcium ion concentration reduces the contractility of the cardiac muscle. Parathyroid hormone secretion is the principal method by which normal calcium ion concentration is maintained in the body fluids at all times, and the bones act as a large reservoir of calcium to be used for this purpose.

Regulation of Parathyroid Hormone Secretion. Whenever the calcium ion concentration in the body fluids falls too low, this causes proliferation of and increased secretion by the parathyroid cells. Among the conditions that increase the output of parathyroid hormone are: (1) low calcium ion concentration in rickets, (2) low calcium ion concentration in osteomalacia (adult rickets), (3) lactation, in which large amounts of calcium are secreted in the milk, and (4) low calcium diet.

Calcitonin and Its Role in Regulation of Calcium Ion Concentration. The hormone calcitonin, when injected into an animal, causes rapid deposition of calcium in the bones and therefore rapid decrease in calcium ion concentration in the body fluids. This hormone is secreted by special cells located between the follicles in the thyroid gland in the human. Its rate of secretion increases when the calcium ion concentration rises above normal. Therefore, it functions in exactly the opposite manner to parathyroid hormone, returning the calcium ion concentration back toward normal when this concentration rises too high. Furthermore, it responds much more rapidly than does parathyroid hormone. However, the quantitative role of calcitonin in calcium ion regulation is far less than that of parathyroid hormone. Also, it is doubtful that its effect can continue for more than a few hours to a few days.

REPRODUCTIVE FUNCTIONS OF THE MALE

Spermatogenesis. The basic reproductive function of the male is the formation of sperm by the testes. The *seminiferous tubules* of the testes contain a basal layer of *germinal epithelium,* the cells of which divide through several stages and gradually form the sperm. During formation, essentially all of the cytoplasm is lost from the cell, and the cell membrane elongates in one direction to form a tail. Also, at one stage of division, the 23 pairs of chromosomes split into two sets of unpaired chromosomes, one of these sets going to one sperm and the other to the second sperm. One pair of chromosomes, called the *XY pair,* is known as the sex pair. After separation of the chromosomal pairs in the process of sperm formation, half of the sperm carry an X chromosome and the other half a Y chromosome. The X chromosome causes a female child to be formed, while the Y chromosome causes a male child to be formed. Thus, the sex of the offspring is determined by the type of sperm that fertilizes the ovum. Furthermore, this division of the chromosomes allows half of the genes of the father to be inherited by the child, while the other half come from the mother.

In addition to germinal cells, the seminiferous tubules contain large *Sertoli cells* from which the developing sperm obtain nutrient substances during their development.

Testosterone. Large quantities of testosterone are formed by the *interstitial cells* of the testes located between the seminiferous tubules. This testosterone has a local effect in the testes to promote the production of sperm by the seminiferous tubules, and without it spermatogenesis cannot occur. However, in addition to its effect on spermatogenesis, it also is secreted into the blood and causes development of the sexual and secondary sexual characteristics of the male, including (1) formation of the penis when the fetus is developing, (2) descent of the testes into the scrotum during intrauterine life, (3) development of the enlarged musculature of the male, (4) increase in the thickness of the skin, (5) bass quality of the male voice, (6) growth of a beard on the face and of hair on many other areas of the body, and (7) baldness in those male individuals who are genetically predisposed to this.

Regulation of Testicular Function by the Anterior Pituitary Gland. At least two *gonadotropic hormones* secreted by the pituitary gland help to control spermatogenesis and testosterone secretion by the testes. During childhood, essentially no gonadotropic hormones are secreted by the anterior pituitary gland, but at puberty both follicle stimulating hormone and luteinizing hormone begin to be secreted, the follicle stimulating hormone promoting division of the germinal cells to initiate spermatogenesis, while luteinizing hormone stimulates the interstitial cells to produce testosterone. The testos-

terone in turn is required for proper development of the sperm and for their maturation. The testes continue to produce both sperm and testosterone from puberty until death, though beyond approximately the 40th year of life the rates of production gradually decline.

Regulation of Gonadotropic Hormone Secretion—Role of Luteinizing Hormone Releasing Hormone. The rate of secretion of gonadotropic hormones by the anterior pituitary gland is controlled mainly by luteinizing hormone releasing hormone, a hormone formed in the hypothalamus and transported to the anterior pituitary gland through the hypothalamic-hypophyseal venous portal system. This hormone causes both luteinizing hormone and follicle stimulating hormone to be released from the anterior pituitary gland.

Testosterone secreted by the testes inhibits the formation of luteinizing hormone releasing hormone by the hypothalamus, thus providing a negative feedback mechanism for control of testosterone secretion. In addition, a substance called *inhibin* is secreted by the seminiferous tubules; this has an effect on the anterior pituitary gland to diminish the rate of secretion of follicle stimulating hormone, thus providing a feedback mechanism for controlling the formation of sperm.

During childhood, the rate of secretion of luteinizing hormone releasing hormone is very low because the hypothalamus is extremely sensitive to the inhibitory effects of even minute amounts of circulating testosterone. However, at approximately the age of 12, the hypothalamus loses most of this inhibitory sensitivity, and large amounts of luteinizing hormone releasing hormone then begin to be secreted, and the sex life of the male begins. This is the period of *puberty.*

Storage of Sperm and Ejaculation. After sperm are formed in the seminiferous tubules, they then pass into the *epididymis* where they must remain for approximately a day while they mature within this new environment. From there, they pass into the *vas deferens* and the *ampulla,* where they are stored. During coitus, sexual stimulation transmits impulses to the spinal cord that cause reflex (parasympathetic mediated) erection of the penis. Then, at the height of sexual stimulation, rhythmic peristalsis (sympathetically mediated) begins in the epididymis and spreads up the vas deferens, into the ampulla and seminal vesicles, and finally through the prostate gland. This expels the semen into the posterior urethra, a process called *emission.* Then, rhythmical contractions of the bulbocavernosus muscle cause rhythmic compression of the urethra, and about 3 ml of semen is expelled. This process is called *ejaculation.*

The *ejaculate* is composed of a mixture of: (1) sperm from the testes; (2) a highly mucid and nutritive fluid from the seminal vesicles; and (3) a highly alkaline fluid from the prostate gland. The alkalinity of the prostate fluid causes the sperm to become immediately motile by activating movement of the sperm tail, causing the sperm to travel at a velocity as much as 1 mm to 4 mm per minute, which allows the sperm to pass upward through the uterus and the fallopian tubes to fertilize the ovum.

Failure of the male to ejaculate more than 60 to 80 million sperm in each ejaculate usually results in sterility. This may be caused by the lack of sufficient hyaluronidase and various proteolytic enzymes that are secreted by the sperm. These enzymes dissolve the mucous plug of the cervix and possibly also help to break granulosal cells away from the surface of the ovum, thereby allowing a sperm to penetrate the ovum.

REPRODUCTIVE FUNCTIONS OF THE FEMALE

Ovarian Cycle and Oogenesis. Oogenesis means the formation of ova. The newborn female child has approximately two million *primordial ova* in her two ovaries. Many of these degenerate during childhood so that only about 300,000 remain at puberty. At that time, under the stimulation of gonadotropic hormones from the anterior pituitary gland, a rhythmic monthly sexual cycle begins. At the beginning of each month, cells surrounding a few of the ova, the *granulosal* and the *thecal cells,* begin to proliferate, and these secrete large quantities of *estrogens,* one of the female sex hormones. Fluid is also secreted by the granulosal and thecal cells, forming cavities around these few ova called *follicles.* After approximately 14 days of growth, one of the growing follicles breaks open and expels its ovum into the abdominal cavity. Then, all the other growing follicles begin to degenerate within a few hours, a process called *atresia.* Presumably, this results from some type of inhibiting hormonal action on the ovaries after ovulation occurs. Nevertheless, the result is the release of one single ovum each month at approximately the 14th day of the female sexual cycle.

Immediately after the ovum has been expelled, the granulosal and thecal cells undergo rapid fatty changes and considerable swelling, a process called *luteinization,* and they begin to secrete large amounts of progesterone in addition to estrogens. This modified mass of cells, now called a *corpus luteum,* persists for approximately another 14 days, at the end of which time it degenerates. Then a new set of follicles begins to develop, and at the end of another 14 days another ovum is expelled into the abdominal cavity, the cycle continuing on and on.

At about the same time that the ovum is expelled from the follicle, the nucleus of the ovum divides two times in rapid succession. During one of these divisions, the pairs of chromosomes separate, and half of them are expelled from the ovum, leaving only 23 unpaired chromosomes in the final *mature ovum,* which is then ready for fertilization.

Effects of Estrogens and Progesterone on the Endometrium. The estrogens and the progesterone secreted by the ovaries have very important effects on the uterine endometrium, preparing it for implantation of a fertilized ovum. The estrogens secreted during the first half of the monthly ovarian cycle cause very rapid proliferation of the endometrial stroma and glandular cells. Then during the second half of the monthly cycle progesterone causes both the stromal and the glandular cells to enlarge and the glandular cells to begin secreting a serous fluid while the stromal cells store large quantities of protein and glycogen in preparation for supplying nutrition to the developing ovum.

Menstruation. When the corpus luteum degenerates at the end of the monthly cycle, almost no estrogens or progesterone are then secreted by the ovaries for the next few days. Lack of the normal stimulatory effect of these hormones causes the endometrial cells to lose their stimulus for increased activity. One of the results is that the blood vessels to the endometrium become spastic, which causes very rapid necrosis of the superficial two-thirds of the endometrium, the dead tissue sloughing away and being expelled through the vagina along with about 50 ml of blood plus several times this much additional serous exudate. This process, called menstruation, normally lasts about 4 days. By the end of menstruation, new follicles have begun to develop in the ovary and are beginning to secrete estrogens once again. Under the influence of these estrogens the endometrium begins a new cycle of development.

Effects of Estrogens and Progesterone on Other Tissues. In addition to the effects of estrogens and progesterone on the endometrium, these hormones, particularly the estrogens, have a number of other effects throughout the body. Estrogens cause proliferation and enlargement of the smooth muscle cells in the uterus, increasing the uterine size after puberty to about double the childhood size. Estrogens also cause proliferation of the glandular cells of the breast and cause deposition of fat in the breast tissues, thus giving the characteristic growth of the female breasts. They cause fat deposition on the hips and in other points peculiar to the female. They cause very rapid growth of the bones immediately after puberty but also promote early uniting of the epiphyses with the shafts of the long bones so that the final height of the female, despite her rapid growth immediately after puberty, is less than it otherwise would have been. Finally, they cause enlargement of the external genitalia.

Progesterone has very much the same effect on the breasts that it has on the uterine endometrium, causing the glandular cells to increase in size and to develop secretory granules in their cells. In addition, it causes accumulation of fluid and electrolytes in the breast tissue, making them swell during the latter half of each monthly sexual cycle.

Regulation of the Female Sexual Cycle by the Hypothalamus and Anterior Pituitary Gland.

Until the female is approximately 12 years of age, the anterior pituitary gland secretes no gonadotropic hormones, as is also true in the male. This is believed to result from exquisite sensitivity of the hypothalamus to inhibition by even the minutest amounts of estrogen and progesterone secreted by the ovaries. However, at this age, the age of puberty, the hypothalamus loses this inhibitory sensitivity and begins to secrete luteinizing hormone releasing hormone, in the same manner that occurs in the male. This hormone in turn stimulates the secretion of both luteinizing hormone and follicle stimulating hormone in a monthly cycle by the anterior pituitary gland, as illustrated by the lower curves of Figure 3-31. It is the follicle stimulating hormone that causes initial growth of the ovarian follicles during the first few days of the monthly ovarian cycle. Then this hormone, aided by luteinizing hormone as well, causes the thecal cells, and possibly also the granulosal cells, to secrete estrogens (the "estradiol" curve in the upper portion of the figure) plus large quantities of fluid into the developing follicles.

At about the 13th day of the ovarian cycle, an especially large amount of luteinizing hormone is secreted by the anterior pituitary gland, which is called the *luteinizing hormone surge*. The excess luteinizing hormone, in some way not completely understood, causes ovulation about 24 hours later. The luteinizing hormone also causes the granulosal and thecal cells to change into *lutein cells* which in the aggregate become the corpus luteum. Luteinizing hormone then stimulates the corpus luteum to produce large quantities of both progesterone and

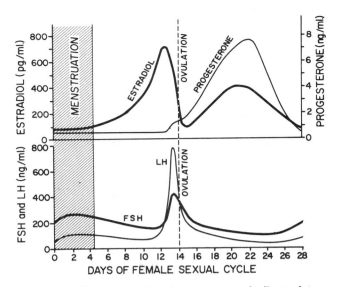

Fig. 3-31. Changes in the plasma concentrations of gonadotropins and ovarian hormones during the normal menstrual cycle. (Guyton AC: Textbook of Medical Physiology, 7th ed. Philadelphia, WB Saunders, 1986)

estrogen during the latter half of the female sexual cycle. Finally, when the corpus luteum degenerates at the end of the cycle, the resulting lack of progesterone and estrogen production leads to menstruation as described above.

It is not clear exactly how the successive changes in secretion of follicle stimulating hormone, luteinizing hormone, estrogen, and progesterone during the monthly female sexual cycle are controlled. However, it is known that estrogen in particular, and progesterone to a less extent, normally causes feedback inhibition of luteinizing hormone releasing hormone secretion by the hypothalamus. Therefore, during the latter part of the ovarian cycle, when large amounts of progesterone and estrogen are secreted by the corpus luteum, secretion of both follicle stimulating hormone and luteinizing hormone by the anterior pituitary gland becomes diminished. This in turn leads to degeneration of the corpus luteum and cessation of production of the large quantities of progesterone and estrogen. Next, lacking the feedback inhibition from these two hormones, the hypothalamus and the pituitary gland become active once again during the next few days, and the rates of secretion of follicle stimulating hormone and luteinizing hormone rise once more, thus beginning a new cycle.

However, it is still difficult to understand what causes the midmonthly luteinizing hormone surge, but it is believed to occur in the following way: Experiments have shown that when large quantities of estrogen circulate in the blood for several days, this has exactly the opposite effect on the hypothalamus and anterior pituitary gland from its normal inhibiting effect. That is, it causes a positive feedback effect instead of negative feedback and actually stimulates the production of more luteinizing hormone releasing hormone; this in turn leads to massive production of luteinizing hormone by the anterior pituitary gland. And this leads to ovulation, followed by development of the corpus luteum and the subsequent events described above.

Menopause. At 40 to 50 years of age essentially all of the ova in the ovaries have been used up, a few expelled into the abdominal cavity by ovulation and vast numbers degenerated in situ in the ovaries. Therefore, no follicles or any corpus luteum can develop in the ovaries to secrete either estrogens or progesterone. The anterior pituitary gland continues to secrete large quantities of gonadotropic hormones, but since no estrogen or progesterone can now be secreted to inhibit the hypothalamus or the pituitary, no monthly sexual cycle occurs thereafter.

Loss of the female sex hormones sometimes causes rather drastic psychic and psychosomatic effects, resulting often in depressive states, hallucinatory states, and "hot flashes" of the skin. This period in the life of the female is called the menopause.

PHYSIOLOGY OF PREGNANCY

Fertilization and Implantation. After coitus, millions of motile sperm make their way upward through the uterus and fallopian tubes. These sperm are capable of living in the genital tract of the female for as long as 72 hours but are very fertile for only about 24 hours. If during this time an ovum is expelled from the ovary, or, if an ovum has been expelled up to 24 hours prior to coitus, then a sperm can cause fertilization. In the process of fertilization, the head of the sperm combines with the nucleus of the ovum. Since each of these contains 23 unpaired chromosomes, the combination restores the normal cellular complement of 23 pairs of chromosomes. This allows the ovum to begin a process of division, the first division occurring approximately 30 hours after fertilization. Subsequent divisions then take place at a rate of about once every 18 to 24 hours.

The ovum usually passes shortly before fertilization into one of the two fallopian tubes, the fimbriated ends of which lie in approximation to the ovaries. The cilia that line the fallopian tube beat toward the uterus and slowly move the dividing ovum downward along the tube to reach the uterus in about 3 days.

The dividing ovum develops an outer layer of *trophoblast cells;* these are capable of phagocytizing nutrient materials from the secretions of the fallopian tube and the uterus, thus making nutrients available to the developing mass of cells. The trophoblast cells also secrete proteolytic enzymes that allow the developing mass of cells to eat its way into the endometrium and thereby implant itself.

Function of Chorionic Gonadotropin in Pregnancy. When the corpus luteum degenerates at the end of the normal monthly menstrual cycle, the endometrium of the uterus sloughs away, and menstruation occurs. However, when the ovum becomes fertilized, it is important that the endometrium remain intact in order for the early developing fetus to implant and grow. Fortunately, the trophoblast cells secrete a hormone called *human chorionic gonadotropin* that has almost the same effects on the corpus luteum as luteinizing hormone from the pituitary gland. Therefore, this hormone keeps the corpus luteum from degenerating and keeps it secreting large quantities of estrogens and progesterone; as a result, menstruation does not occur. Instead, the endometrium actually grows thicker and is gradually phagocytized by the growing fetal tissues, in this way providing the major portion of the nutrition for the fetus during approximately the first 8 to 12 weeks of pregnancy.

After the first 2 to 4 months of pregnancy, the placenta begins to secrete large quantities of estrogens and progesterone. From then on the corpus luteum is not needed.

Function of the Placenta. During the early weeks of pregnancy, the trophoblast cells and other fetal tissues gradually develop the placenta. This organ contains several very large chambers filled with the mother's blood, and into these project millions of small villi containing blood capillaries from the fetus. Trophoblast cells cover the surfaces of the villi, and these actively absorb many nutrients from the mother's blood and transport them into the fetal blood during the earlier weeks of pregnancy. However, after this time by far the greater proportion of the necessary nutrients is absorbed passively from the mother's blood into the fetal blood. That is, the concentrations of the nutrients are greater in the mother's blood than in the fetal blood, and as a result they simply diffuse through the placental membrane into the fetal blood. Conversely, excretory substances such as urea, uric acid, and creatinine accumulate in higher concentrations in the fetal blood and then diffuse backward through the placental membrane into the mother's blood, and then excreted by the mother's kidneys.

Hormones Secreted by the Placenta. In addition to secreting human chorionic gonadotropin, which was discussed above, the placenta also secretes several other important hormones, especially estrogens and progesterone. After approximately the third month, the rate of secretion of human chorionic gonadotropin becomes greatly reduced, and the corpus luteum begins to degenerate. Therefore, from that time onward the estrogens and progesterone from the placenta are essential for the maintenance of pregnancy. Toward the end of pregnancy, the rate of secretion of estrogens is as much as 100 times that during the normal ovarian cycle, and the rate of secretion of progesterone is about ten times as great. The estrogens and the progesterone are also essential for growth and development of the fetus.

The progesterone secreted by the placenta is formed from cholesterol derived from the mother's blood. However, secretion of estrogens by the placenta requires a double stage process. The first stage is the formation of large quantities of androgens by greatly enlarged adrenal cortices in the fetus. These androgens are then carried in the blood to the placenta and there converted into several different types of estrogens, including estradiol, the most potent of all the estrogens.

The placenta also produces large quantities of another hormone called **human chorionic somatomammotropin.** This hormone has several important effects: First, it promotes growth of the fetus. Second, it causes increased use of fatty acids by the mother for energy and decreased use of glucose; this makes the excess glucose of the mother available for use by the fetus, an important effect because the fetus is especially geared for utilization of glucose. Third, human chorionic somatomammotropin also aids in the growth and development of the breasts during pregnancy, thus preparing the breasts for lactation following birth of the baby.

Growth of the Fetus. During the first few weeks of pregnancy the fetus hardly grows at all, though the surrounding fetal membranes, especially the placenta, develop very rapidly. After 4 weeks, however, the length of the fetus increases approximately directly in proportion to the time of gestation, and the weight increases with the cube of the time. Thus, at 6 months, the length is approximately six-ninths the final length, but the weight is still only one-fourth the final weight. It can be seen, then, that by far the greatest growth in weight of the fetus

occurs in the last 3 months, and during this time, pregnancy makes many demands on the mother for nutritive substances needed by the baby, including especially proteins, vitamins, large amounts of calcium for the bones, and iron for the red blood cells.

Parturition. When the fetus is fully formed, approximately 9 months after fertilization, the uterus suddenly becomes far more excitable than usual, labor begins, and the baby is expelled. This is called parturition. The precise factors that initiate parturition have never been determined, but it seems that it results from a combination of several different factors that progressively increase the excitability of the uterine musculature as follows: (1) Near term the placenta begins to secrete a progressively higher ratio of estrogens to progesterone. Since estrogens normally excite uterine activity while progesterone inhibits it, this change in ratio increases the excitability of the uterine musculature. (2) The fetus itself increases in size, which stretches the uterine musculature, thus also increasing its excitability. (3) The head of the fetus presses downward against the cervical opening of the uterus and begins to stretch the cervix; this, too, seems to increase the excitability of the uterus. (4) The posterior pituitary gland begins to secrete increased quantities of oxytocin, and at the same time the sensitivity of the uterine musculature to oxytocin increases greatly, both of which together further increase the excitability of the uterine musculature. As a result of the combination of all of these factors, the rhythmic contractions of the uterus become stronger and stronger. Finally, they become strong enough to begin pushing the baby into the birth canal. This in turn stretches the cervix very rapidly, which causes a still greater increase in the excitability of the uterus itself, making the uterus contract still harder. Also, sensory signals from the cervix to the hypothalamus cause progressively increasing secretion of oxytocin that in turn excites the uterus still more. Thus a cycle is set up as follows: strong uterine contraction, stretching of the cervix, stimulation of still stronger uterine contraction caused by this stretch, still more stretch of the cervix, and so forth until the baby is expelled.

Changes in the Baby Immediately upon Birth. Prior to birth, the baby receives its nutrition and oxygen through the placenta. Normally the first function performed by the newborn baby is rapid expansion of its lungs to aerate its own blood, thereby allowing it to lead an independent existence. A baby can usually go as long as 4 to 6 minutes without breathing before damage occurs. However, beyond this time many neuronal cells of the brain are likely to be destroyed.

In the fetus, blood bypasses the lungs by two routes: (1) Some of it flows from the right atrium through the foramen ovale directly into the left atrium. (2) Most of the remaining blood that does not take this route is pumped by the right ventricle into the pulmonary artery and then through the ductus arteriosus directly into the aorta rather than through the lungs. However, birth of the baby changes these directions of blood flow in the following ways: (1) Loss of blood flow through the placenta after birth greatly increases the total peripheral resistance in the baby's systemic circulatory system. (2) Expansion of the lungs expands the pulmonary blood vessels and in this way greatly reduces the resistance to blood flow through the pulmonary circulation. As a result, the ratio of resistance in the systemic circulation to resistance in the pulmonary circulation increases several fold, allowing much easier flow of blood through the lungs, but considerably more difficult flow through the systemic circulation. Because of this, the pulmonary arterial pressure falls, while the systemic arterial pressure rises so that blood now begins to flow backward from the aorta through the ductus arteriosus rather than forward. This brings arterialized blood, containing a high oxygen concentration, into contact with the ductus, and the oxygen constricts the ductus causing functional closure within a few hours. Then fibrous tissue grows into the ductus walls and causes permanent closure in 1 to 2 months in all babies except one in several thousand.

Also, immediately after birth, the increased resistance in the systemic circulation increases the load on the left heart and therefore increases the left atrial pressure. At the same time the decreased resistance in the lungs decreases the right atrial pressure. This higher pressure in the left atrium than in the right atrium closes a valvelike structure over the foramen ovale, preventing further flow through this route. Thus, these two changes in the circulatory system now provide normal blood flow through the lungs.

LACTATION

All during pregnancy large quantities of estrogens and progesterone are secreted either by the corpus luteum or the placenta. The estrogens cause proliferation of the glandular tissues of the breasts, and the progesterone causes development of the alveoli as well as storage of nutrient materials in the glandular cells. Other hormones that also help to promote breast development during pregnancy include prolactin and growth hormone from the mother's anterior pituitary gland, insulin from her pancreas, glucocorticoids from her adrenal glands, and human chorionic somatomammotropin from the placenta. However, the progesterone and estrogens also inhibit actual milk production despite their effect on breast proliferation. Therefore, before birth of the baby, the mother does not secrete milk. Loss of the placenta from the mother's body when the baby is born removes the source of the progesterone and estrogens so that the breasts are now no longer inhibited; within 24 to 48 hours milk begins to flow.

During pregnancy, the mother's anterior pituitary gland produces increasing quantities of prolactin, increasing to about 10 times the normal rate of secretion. This hormone is especially required to cause final development of the breasts and also to cause them to secrete milk. After birth of the baby, continued removal of milk from the breasts causes the anterior pituitary gland to continue producing large quantities of prolactin, and this in turn stimulates the breasts to continue producing milk. When milk is no longer needed by the child and is no longer removed from the breasts, the anterior pituitary gland stops producing prolactin, and milk production ceases within a few days.

Oxytocin secreted by the posterior pituitary gland is also important for lactation, causing milk ejection from the breast alveoli, which was discussed earlier in relation to the posterior pituitary hormones.

QUESTIONS IN PHYSIOLOGY

General

What is meant by homeostasis?

What are the differences between extracellular and intracellular fluids?

What is meant by the internal environment of the body?

List the functional systems of the body and describe the manner in which each helps to provide homeostasis.

The Cell

Describe the parts of the cell.

What is the function of the chromosomes and the genes in the cells?

Describe the principal mechanism by which energy is released in the cell, and give the function of the mitochondria.

How do the genes regulate protein synthesis by the cell?

What are the functions of codons?

Describe the functions of the special types of cells throughout the body.

How does cellular reproduction come about?

Body Fluids

How are the body fluids distributed between the extracellular and the intracellular compartments, and how does the blood fit into these two compartments of fluid?

What is the difference between the ionic composition of extracellular fluid and intracellular fluid?

Describe the structure of the cell membrane.

Explain the mechanism of diffusion through the cell membrane, and list the common substances that normally pass through the membrane in this manner.

What is meant by active transport through the cell membrane? Give the mechanism of active transport.

What is the significance of the sodium pump?

Explain the mechanism of osmosis through the cell membrane, and explain how osmotic pressure can develop across a semipermeable membrane.

What is meant by isotonicity, hypotonicity, and hypertonicity?

Explain how different types of intravenous fluids are partitioned between the extracellular and the intracellular fluids when administered intravenously.

What are the functional differences between the capillary membrane and the cellular membrane?

What is the difference between colloid osmotic pressure at the capillary membrane and total osmotic pressure at the cellular membrane?

Explain the law of the capillaries. How do capillary pressure, tissue pressure and tissue colloid osmotic pressure enter into the law of the capillaries?

Outline the abnormalities in capillary dynamics that can cause interstitial fluid edema.

How is lymph formed?

List the functions of the lymphatic system.

What part does the lymphatic system play in the control of tissue fluid protein concentration?

Trace the flow of fluid in the cerebrospinal fluid system.

Describe the mechanisms of formation and absorption of fluid in the eye. How is the pressure in the eye regulated?

What is meant by a potential fluid space, and under what conditions can transudates appear in the potential fluid spaces?

Kidneys

Describe the nephron, and give the hemodynamics of blood flow through the kidneys.

Describe the mechanism by which glomerular filtrate is formed in a nephron.

Explain how solutes are reabsorbed from the tubules, and explain the difference between absorption by diffusion and by active absorption.

Explain the clearance concept in relation to the formation of urine.

How is sodium ion concentration in the extracellular fluids regulated?

How are the concentrations of chloride and potassium ions regulated in the extracellular fluids?

Explain the role of aldosterone in the control of body fluid electrolytes.

Explain the mechanism of the osmoreceptor system and its importance in the regulation of total concentration of solutes in the extracellular fluids.

Explain the role of arterial pressure in regulating the extracellular fluid volume.

What are the functions of atrial natriuretic factor (ANF)?

How does the thirst mechanism enter into the regulation of electrolyte concentration in the body fluids?

Explain the chemical mechanism of an acid-base buffer.

How does the respiratory system regulate hydrogen ion concentration?

What are the different mechanisms by which the kidneys help to regulate hydrogen ion concentration?

Blood and Immunity

What are the normal concentrations of red and white cells in the blood, and what is meant by the hematocrit?

How is the concentration of the red cells in the blood regulated?

What are the nutritive factors that are necessary for red blood cell formation?

Give the basic functions of the different types of white blood cells.

Describe the mechanisms by which blood coagulation occurs. What is the importance of tissue thromboplastin, and what is its origin?

What is the significance of prothrombin, fibrinogen, Factor VII, calcium ions, and platelets in blood coagulation?

Explain the cause of bleeding in hemophilia, in thrombocytopenia and in prothrombin deficiency.

Explain the mechanism of the immune process by which a person develops adaptive immunity.

Explain the difference in function of antibodies and T cells in the process of immunity.

What is meant by immunologic tolerance?

What is the basic cause of autoimmune disease?

What is the significance of IgE antibodies in allergy?

How does histamine enter into allergic reactions?

Describe the effects of a transfusion reaction.

What is meant by the A-B-O blood groups, and how can mismatching of these groups cause transfusion reactions?

How do the Rh blood types differ from the A-B-O blood groups in causing transfusion reactions?

Explain the problems of transplantation of tissues from one person to another.

Nerve and Muscle

How does a membrane potential develop across the nerve membrane?

Explain the mechanism of the action potential. How does an action potential spread along a nerve membrane?

What is meant by the all-or-nothing law?

If oxidative metabolism in the nerve suddenly stops, can the nerve continue to transmit nerve impulses?

Describe the mechanism by which an impulse is transmitted through a neuromuscular junction.

Explain the "amplification" function of the neuromuscular junction.

Describe the ultramicroscopic structure of a skeletal muscle fiber and explain the mechanism of contraction.

How is contraction initiated in a skeletal muscle fiber?

Explain the mechanism of muscle tetanization.

Explain the mechanisms by which different strengths of muscle contraction can be achieved.

How does smooth muscle differ from skeletal and cardiac muscle?

How does cardiac muscle differ from smooth and skeletal muscle?

Explain the significance of tone and plasticity of smooth muscle.

Heart

Explain the basic mechanisms for control of rhythmicity in the heart and explain the "pacemaker" function of the S-A node.

Trace the conduction of the cardiac impulse through the heart.

What is the significance of the junctional fibers in the Purkinje system?

What is meant by heart block and how does it come about?

Explain the circus movement in the heart, and describe the mechanisms of flutter and fibrillation.

What is the significance of the P-Q interval in the electrocardiogram?

What types of conditions can cause abnormal QRS waves in the electrocardiogram?

What conditions can cause abnormal T waves in the electrocardiogram?

How does a "current of injury" affect the electrocardiogram?

What is the function of the atria in the pumping action of the heart?

Explain the mechanisms of pumping by the ventricles.

Give the Frank-Starling law of the heart, and explain its significance.

Describe the nervous control of the heart.

What is the difference between sympathetic and parasympathetic control?

Circulation

Explain the "circuit" concept of the circulation.

Outline the distribution of blood in the different segments of the circulation.

Give the formula relating blood flow to blood pressure and resistance.

What are the factors that determine the resistance of a blood vessel?

What are the mean pressures in the different parts of the systemic circulation?

How is blood flow regulated in local tissue areas by the arterioles?

Explain the possible mechanisms of autoregulation of blood flow.

What are the blood reservoirs, and what is their significance?

Under what conditions is nervous regulation of blood flow important in the systemic circulation?

How is blood flow in the skeletal muscles regulated?

How is blood flow through the skin regulated to control body heat?

What is the relationship of carbon dioxide to the regulation of cerebral blood flow?

What is the relationship of the portal circulatory system to ascites?

List the mean pressures in the different parts of the pulmonary circulation.

How does increasing the blood flow through the lungs affect the resistance to blood flow in the pulmonary circulation?

Under what conditions do large quantities of blood shift from the pulmonary circulation to the systemic circulation and vice versa?

Explain why the pulmonary alveoli normally remain empty of fluid.

Under what conditions will pulmonary edema develop?

Describe the renal-body fluid volume mechanism for regulation of mean arterial pressure.

Describe the renin-angiotensin mechanism for control of arterial pressure.

How do the different cardiovascular reflexes enter into the regulation of mean arterial pressure?

Give the mechanism of the baroreceptor reflex control of arterial pressure.

What conditions of the kidneys can cause renal hypertension?

List the different types of hormonal hypertension.

Discuss the possible basic mechanisms of essential hypertension.

What are the factors that are of importance in the regulation of cardiac output?

How can the pumping action of the heart be increased or decreased in different conditions?

What are the factors that regulate venous return?

What is the significance of the mean systemic filling pressure, and how does sympathetic stimulation affect venous return?

How is venous pressure regulated?

Explain the mechanism of the venous pump.

What is meant by low cardiac output failure?

How can the nervous system compensate for mild degrees of cardiac failure?

Under what conditions can fluid retention be of value, and under what conditions can it be of harm in heart failure?

What conditions can cause left heart failure, and what conditions can cause right heart failure? Also, what are the differences that occur in the circulation in these two types of failure?

Describe the dynamics of the circulation in aortic stenosis, aortic regurgitation, mitral stenosis, and mitral regurgitation.

What is meant by a right-to-left shunt, and how does this affect the circulation?

What are the dynamics of cardiac shock?

What are the significant differences between hypovolemic shock and neurogenic shock?

Explain why circulatory shock is progressive in nature.

Under what conditions does circulatory shock become irreversible?

How long can a person tolerate circulatory arrest, and what is the significance of coagulation in the circulation in circulatory arrest?

Respiratory System

Define and give the values for tidal air, minute respiratory volume, vital capacity, maximum rate of pulmonary ventilation, alveolar ventilation per minute, dead space, and functional residual capacity.

What is the importance of the functional residual capacity?

List the concentrations and the partial pressures of the different gases in the alveoli.

Why is it important that gases utilized by the respiratory system be expressed in terms of partial pressure?

Why does carbon dioxide diffuse through the pulmonary membrane far more rapidly than does oxygen?

Define the "diffusing capacity" of the lungs and give its value for oxygen.

Explain the mechanism by which hemoglobin transports oxygen in the blood.

Give the different mechanisms by which carbon dioxide is transported in the blood.

What causes the continual respiratory rhythm?

How do carbon dioxide, blood pH, and oxygen lack increase pulmonary ventilation?

List the different causes of hypoxia.

In what hypoxic conditions is oxygen therapy particularly valuable?

How does pneumonia affect the respiratory system?

How does emphysema affect the respiratory system?

How does atelectasis affect the respiratory system?

How high can an aviator ascend without developing coma from hypoxia?

What are the mechanisms by which a person becomes acclimatized to hypoxia?

What is meant by an acceleratory force of 5 g, and approximately how much centrifugal acceleratory force can an aviator stand?

What are the particular physiologic problems involved in space travel?

What are the toxic effects of high oxygen pressure and high nitrogen pressure on the body?

What is decompression sickness, and what is its cause in deep sea diving?

Central Nervous System

List the different types of sensory receptors.

List the different types of effector organs.

Describe the basic mechanism of the reflex arc.

What is meant by the integrative centers of the nervous system?

Describe the synapse and its functions.

What is meant by an excitatory transmitter, and under what conditions will it excite a neuron?

What is meant by an inhibitory transmitter, and how does it function at the synapse?

What factors determine the excitability of the neuron?

Explain how an amplifying circuit in a neuronal pool works.

Explain the mechanism and the significance of a converging or an integrative circuit in a neuronal pool.

Give the types of repetitive firing circuits in a neuronal pool. What are the specific characteristics of each?

Describe a possible mechanism by which thoughts occur in the central nervous system.

Describe a possible mechanism of memory.

What is meant by programming of thoughts?

What is meant by modality of sensation? List the different modalities.

What determines the modality of sensation that will be felt when a nerve fiber is electrically stimulated?

Trace the pathways for transmission of different types of somatic sensations into the central nervous system.

What is meant by the ''labelled-line'' law?

What is the basic stimulus necessary to cause pain?

Distinguish between the threshold for pain perception and reactivity to pain.

What types of stimuli can cause visceral pain?

Explain the mechanism of referred pain.

How is pain intensity controlled by the central nervous system?

Describe the stretch reflex, and give its functions.

What are the functions of the gamma efferent fibers?

Describe the withdrawal response and explain its relationship to the flexor reflex and the crossed extensor reflex.

Describe the positive supportive reflex and explain its importance.

How are walking reflexes integrated in the spinal cord?

Explain the function of the brain stem in the support of the body against gravity.

What is the difference between the functions of the macula of the utricle and the semicircular canals in equilibrium?

List the different visceral functions of the brain stem.

List the locations of the primary sensory areas of the cerebral cortex.

What is meant by sensory association areas, and what are the functions of the somatic, the auditory, and the visual sensory association areas?

What is meant by the gnostic function of the brain?

What is the ideomotor function of the brain?

Explain the functions of Wernicke's area.

Trace the pyramidal system from the motor cortex to the spinal cord.

What is the function of the premotor cortex in the control of muscular movements?

Trace the extrapyramidal pathways from the cerebral cortex to the spinal cord.

List the functions of the basal ganglia in the control of muscular movements.

How does the cerebellum damp the movements of the body?

Why does cerebellar dysfunction frequently cause ataxic movements?

What are the hormones secreted by the sympathetic and the parasympathetic nerve endings?

How does the central nervous system control the autonomic nerves?

Eye

What are the four refractive surfaces of the eye?

Explain the mechanism by which the eye focuses images on the retina.

What is the relationship of the pupil to the depth of focus of the eye?

Give the mechanism of the pupillary light reflex.

Distinguish between the functions of the rods and the cones.

Explain how the rhodopsin-retinal cycle of the rods operates.

Explain the mechanism of dark and light adaptation.

Explain the method by which the eye distinguishes different colors.

Trace the transmission of nerve impulses from the retina to the cerebral cortex.

Ear

Explain the mechanics of sound transmission from the tympanum to the cochlea.

How does resonance occur in the cochlea?

Explain the mechanism by which the cochlea determines the pitch of a sound.

Explain how the cochlea determines the loudness of a sound.

Trace the transmission of auditory impulses into the brain.

Chemical Senses

What are the four different types of taste buds?

Trace the transmission of taste impulses into the brain.

What types of substances can stimulate the olfactory cells?

Trace the transmission of olfactory impulses into the brain.

Gastrointestinal Tract

What are the major types of movements in the gastrointestinal tract?

Explain the mechanism of peristalsis and its control.

Describe the mechanism of swallowing.

Explain how the intestinal contents are mixed in the stomach, in the small intestine, and in the large intestine.

Describe the mechanisms by which gastric secretions are controlled.

Explain how pancreatic secretion is controlled.

What is the major mechanism by which small-intestinal secretion is controlled?

What is the importance of mucus secretion throughout the gastrointestinal tract?

Explain the mechanisms of digestion of carbohydrates, fats, and proteins in the gastrointestinal tract.

What substances are actively absorbed from the gastrointestinal tract?

What substances are absorbed by diffusion?

What substances are absorbed into the portal blood, and what substances are absorbed into the lymphatic system from the gastrointestinal tract?

What abnormal conditions can cause peptic ulceration?

What abnormal conditions can cause diarrhea and constipation?

What is the basic abnormality of achalasia or megacolon?

Metabolism and Energy

Explain why glucose is called the common denominator in carbohydrate metabolism.

What is the importance of glycogen storage in the liver?

How is glucose transported into cells, and how does insulin affect this transport?

What is meant by glycolysis, and what is meant by the citric acid cycle?

What are the significance and the functions of adenosine triphosphate in the metabolic scheme?

Describe the mechanisms by which adenosine triphosphate can be formed in the cells.

How are fats transported in the plasma?

What are chylomicrons, and how are they removed from the blood?

What are fat depots?

How can fat be utilized to synthesize adenosine triphosphate?

What are the functions of phospholipids and cholesterol in the body?

Discuss what is known about the cause of atherosclerosis.

How are amino acids transported, and how are they stored in the body?

What is meant by an essential amino acid?

Under what conditions does catabolism of proteins occur in the cells?

Why must deamination of amino acids occur before these can be used for energy?

Explain the energy equivalent of foods and give the energy equivalents for carbohydrates, fats, and proteins.

What are the daily energy requirements of the body under different physiologic conditions?

What is meant by the basal metabolic rate?

What is the cause of obesity?

What types of stored foods are utilized by the body in starvation?

Give the functions of vitamin A, thiamine, niacin, riboflavin, vitamin B_{12}, folic acid, pantothenic acid, pyridoxine, ascorbic acid, vitamin D, and vitamin K.

What are the mechanisms by which heat is produced in the body?

What are the mechanisms by which heat is lost from the body?

Explain the hypothalamic mechanism for automatic control of body temperature.

Endocrine Glands

Explain how cyclic AMP acts as an intracellular hormonal "second messenger."

List the six significant anterior pituitary hormones.

Explain the control of anterior pituitary hormone secretion by the hypophyseal hormones.

List the functions of growth hormone.

How does growth hormone promote tissue growth?

How does thyroid-stimulating hormone affect the thyroid gland?

How does adrenocorticotropin affect the adrenal cortices?

How is the secretion of adrenocorticotropin by the anterior pituitary gland controlled?

What are the two posterior pituitary hormones, and what are their functions?

How does aldosterone function in the body?

What is the function of cortisol, and how is its secretion regulated?

What are the adrenal androgens, and under what conditions are they important?

What are the basic effects of thyroxine on the cells?

List the physiologic abnormalities in hyperthyroidism.

What portions of the pancreas secrete insulin and glucagon?

What are the basic functions of insulin?

How does insulin affect the overall aspects of carbohydrate metabolism?

How does insulin affect the overall aspects of fat and protein metabolism?

What physiologic abnormalities result from diabetes mellitus?

What are the significant functions of glucagon?

Outline the principal steps in the formation of bone.

Under what conditions are bones absorbed in the body?

Explain how parathyroid hormone regulates calcium ion concentration in the extracellular fluids.

Describe the function of calcitonin.

What factors can cause increased secretion of parathyroid hormone?

Describe the formation of sperm in the testes.

What are the physiologic functions of testosterone?

Describe the secretion of testosterone and the regulation of testicular function by the anterior pituitary gland.

Explain the process of ejaculation.

Explain maturation of the ovum.

Describe the events in the ovarian cycle during the female sexual month.

How do estrogens and progesterone affect the endometrium?

Explain the cause of menstruation.

What are the effects of estrogens and progesterone on the tissues of the body other than the sex organs?

Explain the regulation of the female monthly sexual cycle by the hypothalamus and the anterior pituitary gland.

How does the ovum become fertilized and later implanted in the uterus?

Why is human chorionic gonadotropin necessary for the continuation of pregnancy?

Describe the nutritive functions of the placenta.

Outline the schedule of growth of the fetus during gestation.

Explain the mechanism of parturition.

Describe specifically the changes that occur in the baby's respiration and in its circulation immediately after birth.

List the factors that cause growth of the mother's breasts and then milk secretion following birth of the baby.

What is the function of oxytocin in lactation?

Multiple Choice Questions

Choose the *best* answer. Answers are at the end of this chapter.

1. What is the probable structure of pores in the cell membrane?
   (a) A cylindrical hole through the membrane
   ✓ (b) A protein molecule in the membrane with a channel through it
   (c) A phospholipid molecule entrapped in the membrane
   (d) A large polysaccharide molecule entrapped in the membrane
   (e) A slit in the membrane
2. The ribosomes are formed in:
   (a) The Golgi apparatus
   ✓ (b) The endoplasmic reticulum
   (c) The lysosomes
   (d) The mitochondria
   (e) The nucleolus in the nucleus
3. Cardiac muscle:
   (a) Has a velocity of conduction of acton potentials of .3 m to .5 m per second
   (b) Never contracts for more than .12 second
   (c) Is not influenced by norepinephrine
   (d) Has a longer duration of contraction during tachycardia
   (e) All of the above
4. During the middle of diastole:
   (a) The second heart sound is heard
   (b) The mitral valve is closed

(c) Aortic pressure is falling

(d) All of the above

5. During the middle of systole:
   (a) The pulmonic valve is open
   (b) The QRS complex is occurring
   (c) Ventricular volume is increasing
   (d) All of the above

6. An irregular, rapid heart rate with normal QRS complexes and no P waves suggests:
   (a) Sinus arrhythmia
   (b) Second degree heart block
   (c) Paroxysmal tachycardia with a ventricular pacemaker
   (d) Atrial fibrillation

7. The delay between the P wave and the Q wave in the normal electrocardiogram is primarily caused by:
   (a) A slow transmission through the A-V node and junctional fibers
   (b) Delay at the internodal pathways
   (c) Circus movement
   (d) The slow rate of conduction in atrial heart muscle

8. A stronger than normal heart might be observed during:
   (a) Sympathetic stimulation
   (b) Myocardial ischemia
   (c) Stokes-Adams syndrome
   (d) Atrial fibrillation

9. The Purkinje fibers:
   (a) Are myelinated axons
   (b) Have a conduction velocity about five times that seen in heart muscle
   (c) Have action potentials about a tenth as long as those in heart muscle
   (d) All of the above

10. The heart is predisposed to ventricular fibrillation:
    (a) When action potentials follow a short, but circular pathway
    (b) During sinus bradycardia
    (c) If conduction velocity through the myocardium is decreased
    (d) All of the above

11. Which of the following statements is *incorrect?*
    (a) Blood flow velocity in the capillaries is greater than in the large veins.
    (b) Total surface area of the capillaries is much greater than of the the large veins.
    (c) Reduced oxygen tension in the tissues tends to relax precapillary sphincters.
    (d) Increased sympathetic nerve stimulation tends to constrict the small arterioles.

12. Which of the following changes tend to cause accumulation of fluid (edema) in the tissues?
    (a) Increased precapillary vascular resistance
    (b) Decreased postcapillary vascular resistance
    (c) Increased plasma colloid osmotic pressure
    (d) Increased venous pressure

13. Which of the following changes would probably occur as a result of a two-fold increase in the net filtration of fluid into the tissues?
    (a) A marked increase in lymph flow rate
    (b) Approximately a two-fold increase in interstitial fluid volume
    (c) A decrease in interstitial fluid colloid osmotic pressure
    (d) Both (a) and (b)
    (e) Both (a) and (c)

14. Vitamin B_{12} is essential for what aspect of blood cell reproduction?
    (a) Formation of hemoglobin
    (b) Extrusion of the nucleus from the normoblasts
    (c) Formation of DNA
    (d) Activation of erythropoietin
    (e) Promotion of iron absorption from the intestinal tract

15. What cells found in lymph nodes phagocytize unwanted particles in the lymph?
    (a) Neutrophils
    (b) Lymphocytes
    (c) Plasma cells
    (d) Microphages
    (e) Macrophages

16. In a person with type O blood, what type or types of agglutinins does he have in his plasma?
    (a) None
    (b) Anti-A
    (c) Anti-B
    (d) Alpha and beta

17. In most instances of erythroblastosis fetalis:
    (a) The mother is Rh positive, the father Rh negative, and the baby Rh negative.
    (b) The mother is Rh negative, the father Rh positive, and the baby Rh negative.
    (c) The mother is Rh negative, the father Rh negative, and the baby Rh negative.
    (d) The mother is Rh positive, the father Rh positive, and the baby Rh positive.
    (e) The mother is Rh negative, the father Rh positive, and the baby Rh positive.

18. Contraction of which of the following muscles is most important for causing forceful expiration?
    (a) Internal intercostals
    (b) Diaphragm
    (c) External intercostals
    (d) Sternocleidomastoids
    (e) Abdominals

19. The major cause of the hyperpnea of muscular exercise is:
    (a) Stimulation of the respiratory center by the cerebral cortex and the joint proprioceptors
    (b) Hypercapnia
    (c) Hypoxemia
    (d) Alkalosis
    (e) Peripheral chemoreceptors

20. Which of the following factors has no direct stimulatory effect on the medullary respiratory center?
    (a) Changes in arterial P_{CO_2}
    (b) Changes in arterial pH
    (c) Changes in arterial PO_2
    (d) Changes in the nervous output from the joint proprioceptors

21. In which of the following diseases would you expect to find an increase in thickness of the respiratory membrane?
    (a) Emphysema
    (b) Asthma
    (c) Pulmonary artery thrombosis
    (d) Skeletal abnormalities of the chest
    (e) Pulmonary edema

22. Which of the following would *not* be expected to cause hypoxia?
    (a) Hypoventilation
    (b) Abnormal ventilation to perfusion ratio
    (c) Hyperpnea
    (d) Diminished diffusing capacity for O_2
    (e) Excessive blood flow through venous to arterial shunts

23. The peripheral vasculature under the least control of the sympathetic nervous system are the:
    (a) Arteries
    (b) Arterioles
    (c) Capillaries
    (d) Venules
    (e) Veins

24. Baroreceptor impulses:
    (a) Inhibit the vagal center
    (b) Increase in number with decreased carotid arterial pressure
    (c) Result in increased heart rate
    (d) Excite the sympathetic vasoconstrictor center
    (e) None of the above

25. Which of the following changes would tend to *decrease* glomerular filtration rate?
    (a) Increased afferent arteriolar resistance
    (b) Increased glomerular capillary filtration coefficient
    (c) Decreased hydrostatic pressure in Bowman's capsule
    (d) Decreased plasma colloid osmotic pressure

26. The bicarbonate buffer system is important in regulating extracellular fluid H^+ concentration because:
    (a) The concentrations of CO_2 and HCO_3^- in the extracellular fluid are very high.
    (b) The pK of the bicarbonate buffer system is close enough to the pH of the extracellular fluid to allow good buffering.
    (c) The two elements of the bicarbonate buffer systems (CO_2 and HCO_3^-) are regulated by renal and respiratory mechanisms.
    (d) Both (a) and (c)
    (e) Both (b) and (c)

27. Which of the following statements is *incorrect?*
    (a) Countercurrent flow in the vasa recta minimizes solute loss from the medulla of the kidney.
    (b) There is net movement of water out of the descending limb of the loop of Henle.
    (c) The thick ascending limb of the loop of Henle is highly permeable to water.
    (d) Blood flow through the vasa recta is very slow, compared to blood flow through peritubular capillaries of cortical nephrons.

28. Vasodilation of the *efferent* arterioles of the kidney *tends to:*
    (a) Increase renal blood flow
    (b) Decrease glomerular filtration rate
    (c) Decrease peritubular capillary colloid osmotic pressure
    (d) Decrease glomerular capillary hydrostatic pressure
    (e) All of the above

29. Which of the following changes would *not* occur under *steady-state conditions* in a normal person as a result of a 50% decrease in sodium intake?
    (a) Increased plasma concentration of angiotensin II

(b) Increased plasma aldosterone concentration

(c) Approximately a 50% decrease in sodium excretion

(d) A large (greater than 10%) decrease in plasma sodium concentration

30. For which of the following substances would you expect the renal clearance to be the *lowest,* under normal conditions?
    (a) Urea
    (b) Creatinine
    (c) Sodium
    (d) Glucose
    (e) Water

31. Which of the following changes would *not* occur as a result of dehydration (loss of water, but not solute)?
    (a) Increased secretion of antidiuretic hormone
    (b) Increased plasma sodium concentration
    (c) Decreased permeability of the collecting ducts to water
    (d) Increased solute concentration in the renal medulla

32. If a person has a tidal volume of 411 ml, a physiological dead space volume of 100 ml, and a respiratory minute ventilation of 3600 ml/min, what is his approximate alveolar ventilation?
    (a) 3600 ml/min
    (b) 3000 ml/min
    (c) 2700 ml/min
    (d) 1500 ml/min
    (e) 900 ml/min

33. The major factor regulating alveolar ventilation during rest is:
    (a) Arterial Po_2
    (b) Arterial Pco_2
    (c) Arterial pH
    (d) Nervous output from the joint proprioceptors
    (e) None of the above

34. Which one of the following effects in the heart would *not* be a result of increased vagal nerve activity?
    (a) Acetylcholine release at the nerve endings
    (b) Decreased S-T interval
    (c) Bradycardia
    (d) Hyperpolarization of the S-A node

35. Increased venous return leads to increased cardiac output by way of the Frank-Starling mechanism. Which one of the following would *not* happen?

(a) Increased enddiastolic sarcomere length

(b) Increased myocardial tension during systole

(c) Increased stroke volume

(d) Decreased enddiastolic volume

36. Just before atrial depolarization and contraction:
    (a) The heart is completely polarized.
    (b) A period of diastasis occurs.
    (c) The pulmonic valve is closed.
    (d) Left ventricular pressure is less than 20 mmHg.
    (e) All of the above occur.

37. A possible cause of sinus bradycardia is:
    (a) Complete heart block
    (b) Decreased sympathetic outflow
    (c) Atropine
    (d) Decreased vagal outflow
    (e) All of the above

38. Secretory granules in secretory cells are mainly formed by which intracellular organ?
    (a) Mitochondria
    (b) Golgi complex
    (c) Endoplasmic reticulum
    (d) Lysosomes
    (e) Microtubules

39. What is the maximum concentration of hemoglobin normally found in red blood cells?
    (a) 5%
    (b) 10%
    (c) 16%
    (d) 20%
    (e) 34%

40. When infection occurs in a tissue, what type of white blood cell is first attracted from the blood into the tissue by the process of chemotaxis?
    (a) Neutrophils
    (b) Monocytes
    (c) Eosinophils
    (d) Basophils
    (e) Plasma cells

41. What is the first important event in hemostasis following severe tissue injury?
    (a) Blood coagulation
    (b) Formation of a platelet plug
    (c) Vascular spasm
    (d) Formation of thromboplastin
    (e) Formation of prothrombin activator

42. If a nerve membrane of a large type A nerve fiber is not able to pump sodium and potassium ions through the membrane but otherwise it is in the normal resting state, approximately how many nerve impulses can be

transmitted by the nerve fiber before it cannot transmit any more impulses?
(a) 1
(b) About 10
(c) About 5,000
(d) Usually 50,000 or more

43. Skeletal muscle contraction is excited when the intracellular concentration of which ion rises above 10^{-5} moles per liter in the sarcoplasm of the muscle cells?
(a) Na
(b) K
(c) Mg
(d) Ca
(e) Cl

44. With normal cardiac function, a 10 mmHg change in which of the following pressures would have the greatest effect on cardiac output?
(a) Pressure in the carotid arteries
(b) Pressure in the renal artery
(c) Aortic pressure
(d) Right atrial pressure
(e) Pulmonary artery pressure

45. Following acute failure of the left ventricle of the heart in humans, pulmonary edema generally begins to appear when left atrial pressure approaches:
(a) 7 mmHg
(b) 15 mmHg
(c) 20 mmHg
(d) 30 mmHg
(e) 50 mmHg

46. The factors that cause arterial pressure to recover from moderate degrees of hemorrhagic shock include:
(a) Formation of angiotensin
(b) Baroreceptor reflexes
(c) Absorption of fluid from interstitial spaces of the body
(d) Release of vasopressin
(e) All of the above

47. When a normal person suddenly changes from recumbent to standing posture:
(a) Blood pressure falls dramatically
(b) Renin secretion is suppressed
(c) Blood pools in the jugular vein
(d) Heart rate increases.

48. The partial pressure of water vapor in the lungs:
(a) Increases with hyperventilation
(b) Is relatively constant with changes in altitude
(c) Is proportional to the CO_2 concentration

(d) Becomes negative when barometric pressure falls below 47 mmHg

49. What type of ions is probably most important in causing release of transmitter vesicles at nerve endings?
(a) Sodium ions
(b) Potassium ions
(c) Magnesium ions
(d) Calcium ions
(e) Chloride ions

50. The type of nerve fiber that has a conduction velocity of approximately 1 meter per second is:
(a) Type A alpha
(b) Type A beta
(c) Type A gamma
(d) Type A delta
(e) Type C

51. Kinesthetic sensations are detected mainly by what type of receptors?
(a) Muscle spindles
(b) Golgi tendon apparati
(c) Skin receptors
(d) Joint receptors

52. The Betz cells of the primary motor cortex are located in which layer of the cortex?
(a) Layer II
(b) Layer III
(c) Layer IV
(d) Layer V
(e) Layer VI

53. Which primary cortical sensory area is located in the middle of the superior temporal gyrus?
(a) Vision
(b) Hearing
(c) Somatic sensation
(d) Taste
(e) Smell

54. Damaging what area of the brain is likely to cause anterograde amnesia?
(a) Prefrontal cortex
(b) Occipital cortex
(c) The amygdala
(d) The hippocampus
(e) The thalamus

55. When a person wishes to speak a certain thought, where does the thought originate?
(a) In Broca's area
(b) In Wernicke's area of the temporal cortex
(c) In the supramarginal gyrus
(d) In the facial region of the motor cortex
(e) In the prefrontal cortex

56. In what layer of the retina is a large store of vitamin A found?
    (a) The choroid
    (b) The pigment layer
    (c) The outer nuclear layer
    (d) The outer plexiform layer
    (e) The inner nuclear layer

57. Which type of cone has a peak absorbancy at a light wavelength of 430 millimicrons?
    (a) Red cones
    (b) Green cones
    (c) Blue cones

58. The red cones and the green cones are stimulated approximately equally. What color will the person see?
    (a) Red
    (b) Yellow
    (c) Green
    (d) Purple
    (e) Blue

59. The type of taste that is most sensitive to minute concentrations of the substance to be tasted is:
    (a) The sour taste
    (b) The salty taste
    (c) The sweet taste
    (d) The bitter taste

60. What hormone causes contraction of the gall bladder?
    (a) Secretin
    (b) Gastrin
    (c) Villikinin
    (d) Cholecystokinin
    (e) Bradykinin

61. Which of the following enzymes requires an acid pH of approximately 2.0 to function optimally?
    (a) Trypsin
    (b) Chymotrypsin
    (c) Pepsin
    (d) Pancreatic lipase
    (e) Parotid amylase

62. What is the usual cause of megacolon (also called Hirschsprung's disease)?
    (a) Infection in the colon
    (b) Excessive parasympathetic stimulation
    (c) Excessive sympathetic stimulation
    (d) Congenital absence of the myenteric plexus in the sigmoid

63. Approximately what proportion of the bile salts is normally reabsorbed and then resecreted by the liver?
    (a) 5 %
    (b) 15%

(c) 40%
(d) 70%
(e) 95%

64. What substance in gallstones causes them to be sometimes x-ray opaque?
    (a) Bile salts
    (b) Bilirubin
    (c) Cholesterol
    (d) Calcium
    (e) Phospholipids

65. At normal room temperature most body heat loss is by:
    (a) Convection
    (b) Direct conduction
    (c) Radiation
    (d) Sweating

66. The hormone responsible for increased body temperature after ovulation is:
    (a) Luteinizing hormone
    (b) Progesterone
    (c) Increased estrogen
    (d) Androgens

67. Secretion of estriol during pregnancy:
    (a) Is dependent on both a viable fetus and a functioning placenta
    (b) Is largely produced by the maternal ovaries
    (c) Is not dependent on a viable fetus
    (d) Is lower than the secretion rate of estriol in the nonpregnant female

68. In the female rat, selective neutralization of follicle-stimulating hormone with anti-FSH antibodies:
    (a) Increases estrogen and progesterone secretion by the corpus luteum
    (b) Causes early uniting of the epiphyses
    (c) Prevents early follicular growth
    (d) Suppresses the secretion of hypothalamic releasing factors

69. Toxemia of pregnancy:
    (a) Is caused by abnormal hormone production
    (b) Is associated with retention of salt and water
    (c) Is associated with hypotension
    (d) Always results in eclampsia

70. In the female rat, selective neutralization of estrogen with antiestrogen antibodies just prior to midcycle:
    (a) Prevents menstruation
    (b) Prolongs the female sexual cycle
    (c) Inhibits ovulation
    (d) Prevents the preovulatory surge of gonadotropins

71. What probably causes stimulation of the thermal receptors?
    (a) Change in the membrane permeability caused by heat or cold
    (b) Change in the number of protein receptors in the nerve ending
    (c) Change in the viscosity of the fluid surrounding the neuron
    (d) Change in the concentration of sodium ions outside the neuron caused by changes in temperature

72. The energy levels in two different sounds differ from each other by 10,000 times; how much difference is this in decibels?
    (a) 10,000
    (b) 4
    (c) 40
    (d) 20
    (e) 80

73. Which theory probably explains long-term memory the best?
    (a) The theory that it causes actual physical or chemical changes at the synapses
    (b) The theory that there is change in RNA inside the soma of the neuron
    (c) The theory that the glial cells around the neuron change
    (d) The theory that the ionic composition of the neurons change
    (e) The theory that the electrical potential of the neuron changes

74. Which of the basal ganglia plays the greatest role in initiating and regulating gross intentional movements of the body?
    (a) The substantia nigra
    (b) The globus pallidus
    (c) The subthalamic nucleus
    (d) The claustrum
    (e) The striate body

75. What part of the lower regions of the brain probably plays the most significant role in directing one's attention to one particular type of brain activity?
    (a) The thalamus
    (b) The hypothalamus
    (c) The mesencephalon
    (d) The pons
    (e) The septal region of the limbic system

76. Motor aphasia results from damage to:
    (a) The general interpretative area
    (b) Broca's area
    (c) The angular gyrus area
    (d) The superior temporal cortex
    (e) The prefrontal area

77. Very light stimulation of the primary somatic sensory cortex is most likely to cause:
    (a) Movement of an area of the body to which the sensory cortex is connected
    (b) Pain in the area of representation
    (c) A feeling that someone has touched the area of representation
    (d) A mild electric, tingling feeling in the area of representation
    (e) A hot feeling in the area of representation

78. Amino acids are transported in the blood mainly in the form of:
    (a) Plasma proteins
    (b) Lipoproteins
    (c) In combination with a carbohydrate carrier
    (d) In combination with a phospholipid carrier
    (e) Amino acids themselves

79. If the baroreceptor reflexes are fully functional when upright posture is assumed:
    (a) The blood vessels of the arms will become vasodilated.
    (b) Arterial pressure in the foot will be maintained at 120/80 mmHg.
    (c) Bradycardia will occur.
    (d) Cerebral blood flow will not change appreciably.

80. Menstruation is caused by the:
    (a) Surge of LH just prior to midcycle
    (b) Failure of the corpus luteum to involute
    (c) Sudden reduction of progesterone and estrogen at the end of the ovarian cycle
    (d) Excessive secretion of estrogen and progesterone at the end of the ovarian cycle

81. The onset of puberty in the male is caused by:
    (a) The sudden "ripening" of the testicles with secretion of large quantities of testosterone
    (b) Spontaneous secretion of FSH and LH by anterior pituitary gland at the age of 12
    (c) An aging process of the hypothalamic sexual control centers
    (d) A sudden sharp decrease in hypothalamic sensitivity to testosterone

82. Oxygen debt:
    (a) Cannot be incurred when breathing pure oxygen
    (b) Can never occur in a healthy individual
    (c) Is often evidenced by an increase in lactic acid concentration in the blood

(d) Is caused by lack of anaerobic metabolism

83. If a person whose normal core body temperature is 98.6°F is placed in a tub of water that is 98°F, and the person is breathing air that is 98°F and 100% humidified:
    (a) The person's core temperature will rise.
    (b) The person's core temperature will fall to 98°F.
    (c) Shivering is likely.
    (d) Sweating will occur and maintain constant body temperature.

84. The most important factor that tends to collapse the lungs (the recoil tendency) is the:
    (a) Elastic fibers in the lungs
    (b) Intrapleural fluid pressure
    (c) Total intrapleural pressure
    (d) Surface tension of the alveolar fluid
    (e) Tension in the intercostal muscles

85. Oxygen therapy has significant value in all the following types of hypoxia *except:*
    (a) Atmospheric hypoxia
    (b) Hypoventilation hypoxia
    (c) Hypoxia due to pulmonary edema
    (d) Hypoxia due to decreased hemoglobin in the blood
    (e) Histotoxic hypoxia due to cyanide poisoning

86. The blood vessels of the systemic circulation responsible for most of the resistance to blood flow in the circulation are the:
    (a) Aorta and large arteries
    (b) Arterioles
    (c) Capillaries
    (d) Venules
    (e) Venae cavae and large veins

87. After drinking a large amount of *hypotonic* fluid and after absorption of the fluid from the gut into the blood, which of the following changes would you expect?
    (a) Increased secretion of antidiuretic hormone
    (b) A decrease in collecting duct permeability to water
    (c) A marked decrease in glomerular filtration rate
    (d) A marked increase in sodium excretion

88. If one loses a large quantity of saliva externally, which of the following ions would be lost in the greatest amount in relation to its concentration in plasma?
    (a) Sodium
    (b) Chloride
    (c) Potassium

89. The hormone generally considered to be the major stimulus for enzyme secretion by the pancreas is:
    (a) Cholecystokinin
    (b) Secretin
    (c) Trypsin
    (d) Gastrin

90. Failure to absorb bile salts in the distal ileum causes:
    (a) Constipation
    (b) No effect
    (c) Diarrhea

91. The absence of lactase in the intestine would cause failure to digest completely:
    (a) Steak
    (b) Beer
    (c) Milk
    (d) Table sugar

92. A large, greasy, smelly stool usually indicates failure of digestion of:
    (a) Carbohydrates
    (b) Fats
    (c) Proteins
    (d) Peptones

93. Sudden exposure of an unacclimatized subject to 25,000 feet would produce after 10 minutes?
    (a) Improved night vision
    (b) Falling pH
    (c) Helium bubbles in the blood
    (d) Coma
    (e) All of the above

94. The maximum number of ribosomes that a messenger RNA molecule can be attached to at any one time is:
    (a) 0
    (b) 1
    (c) 2
    (d) More than 2

95. Which of the following is correct about the energy required to cause diffusion through a cell membrane?
    (a) No energy is required.
    (b) The energy that causes the diffusion comes from chemical reactions in the cell membrane.
    (c) Energy for diffusion is required only when a net rate of diffusion must occur against a concentration gradient.
    (d) The energy that causes the diffusion comes from the kinetic energy of the particles of the solution.

96. The sodium concentration in extracellular fluid is progressively decreased. What hap-

pens to the degree of positivity of the plateau in the monophasic cardiac action potential?
(a) It increases.
(b) It decreases
(c) There is essentially no change.

97. When energy is derived from creatine phosphate to cause muscle contraction, what is the first step in this transfer of energy?
(a) The creatine phosphate transfers its energy to the cross bridges to cause them to become cocked.
(b) The creatine phosphate causes the power stroke of the cross bridges.
(c) The creatine phosphate transfers its energy to the actin filament.
(d) The creatine phosphate transfers its energy to the myosin filament.
(e) The energy of the creatine phosphate is used to convert ADP into ATP.

98. What provides most of the energy used to maintain a normal resting membrane potential of about 70 millivolts inside the neuronal soma?
(a) The chloride pump
(b) The bicarbonate pump
(c) The sodium-potassium pump
(d) The calcium pump
(e) Diffusion of chloride ions

99. When temporal summation occurs at the neuronal soma, which of the following will cause the greatest degree of summation?
(a) Fiber stimulus frequency of 1,000 impulses per second
(b) Fiber stimulus frequency of 100 impulses per second
(c) Fiber stimulus frequency of 10 impulses per second
(d) Fiber stimulus frequency of 1 impulse per second

100. To what part of the brain do most of the signals from the Golgi tendon apparati and muscle spindles go?
(a) The somesthetic cortex
(b) The thalamus
(c) The basal ganglia
(d) The motor cortex
(e) The cerebellum

101. In what part of the central nervous system do the signals probably originate to provide most of the support of the body against gravity?
(a) The pontile and mesencephalic reticular formation
(b) The basal ganglia

(c) The motor cortex
(d) The cerebellum
(e) The spinal cord

102. Where are the centers located for causing such gross stereotype body movements as rotational movements of the head, raising movements of the head and body, flexing movements of the head and body, and turning movements of the body?
(a) Motor cortex
(b) Cerebellum
(c) Amygdala
(d) Mesencephalon

103. Damage to which area of the cerebral cortex is likely to cause the greatest degree of loss of intellectual capabilities in a right-handed person?
(a) The frontal lobes
(b) The left somesthetic sensory and sensory association areas
(c) The right somesthetic sensory and sensory association areas
(d) The left posterior superior temporal gyrus
(e) The right posterior temporal and angular gyrus regions

104. What determines whether norepinephrine circulating in the body fluids will be excitatory or inhibitory in a particular organ?
(a) The nature of the receptor in the cells of the organ
(b) The intensity of nerve stimulation of the organ
(c) The chemical changes that occur in the norepinephrine before it excites the cells
(d) The position on the cells where norepinephrine is secreted by the nerve endings

105. When rhodopsin is decomposed by light energy, what happens to change the membrane potential of the rod?
(a) The activity of the sodium pump is increased.
(b) Membrane permeability in the outer segment is increased.
(c) The membrane permeability for potassium greatly increases.
(d) Membrane permeability for sodium ions in the outer segment is decreased.
(e) The activity of the potassium pump is increased.

106. Integration of temperature information by the nervous system occurs mainly in the:
(a) Spinal cord
(b) Hypothalamus

(c) Amygdala
(d) Peripheral receptors
107. The arterial pulse pressure in the femoral artery is normally:
    (a) Less than the pulse pressure in the upper aorta
    (b) Less than 20 mmHg
    (c) Greater than the pulse pressure in the upper aorta
    (d) Equal to the pulse pressure in the upper aorta
    (e) None of the above
108. Macrophages are the mature form of:
    (a) Neutrophils
    (b) Eosinophils
    (c) Basophils
    (d) Monocytes
    (e) Lymphocytes
109. Hemophilia is most commonly caused by deficiency of which of the following clotting factors?
    (a) Platelet factor 3
    (b) Factor V
    (c) Thromboplastin
    (d) Factor VIII
    (e) Factor XII
110. Troponin is believed to play what role in the muscle contractile process?
    (a) It provides the major amount of elastic tension during the contractile process.
    (b) It is believed that in the resting state it covers or in some other way inactivates the active sites on the actin strands of the actin helix.
    (c) Combination of this complex with myosin excites the activity of the "power stroke."
    (d) Combination of calcium with the troponin is believed to trigger muscle contraction.
111. The endoplasmic reticulum has which of the following functions?
    (a) Formation of glucose by the granular portion of the reticulum
    (b) Formation of proteins by the agranular portion of the reticulum
    (c) Digestion of proteins by all portions of the reticulum
    (d) Transport of protein molecules in some cases from one part of the cell to another part
112. What portion of the cell membrane acts as a barrier to limit the movement of water and water-soluble substances through the membrane?

(a) The lipid portion
(b) The protein portion
(c) The mucopolysaccharide portion
(d) The pores
(e) The membrane enzymes
113. The concentration of sodium on the first side of a membrane is two times as great as on the second side of the membrane. This concentration is now increased to five times as great on the first side as on the second side. How many times does the net rate of sodium diffusion through the membrane increase?
    (a) 5 times
    (b) 4 times
    (c) 2.5 times
    (d) 2 times
    (e) 1.25 times
114. A solution contains 1 gram-mole of magnesium sulfate per liter. Assuming full ionization of this compound, calculate the osmotic pressure of the solution (1 mosmole/liter concentration is equivalent to 19.3 mmHg osmotic pressure).
    (a) 19.3 mmHg
    (b) 38.6 mmHg
    (c) 19,300 mmHg
    (d) 38,600 mmHg
    (e) 57,900 mmHg
115. In a self-excitable tissue such as the sinoatrial node of the heart where the rhythm of the heart is generated, what causes the pause between successive action potentials?
    (a) Prolonged increased permeability of the sodium channels during this period
    (b) Prolonged excess permeability of the potassium channels during this period
    (c) Increased leakage of calcium ions to the interior of the fiber during this period
    (d) Excessive gating potential on the potassium channels during this period of time
    (e) Excessive gating potential on the sodium channels at this time
116. Which of the following cortical layers is stimulated most by the diffuse thalamocortical system?
    (a) Layer 2
    (b) Layer 3
    (c) Layer 4
    (d) Layer 5
    (e) Layer 6
117. If the connections are cut between the cortex and the thalamus, which one of the following types of brain waves can still be recorded in the cortex?

(a) Alpha waves

(b) Beta waves

(c) Theta waves

(d) Delta waves

118. Almost all of the cerebral cortex has direct two-way communication with which one of the following subcortical structures?

(a) Cerebellum

(b) Thalamus

(c) Hypothalamus

(d) Bulboreticular facilitory area

(e) Putamen

119. Under resting conditions the ganglion cells of the retina discharge at approximately what rate?

(a) 1 per second

(b) 5 per second

(c) 25 per second

(d) 125 per second

(e) 1250 per second

120. Stimulation of the hair cells in the cochlea is caused by:

(a) Compression of the hair cells by the sound waves

(b) Vibration of the hair cells by the sound waves

(c) Movement of the hair cells back and forth so that the hairs are bent by fluid or the tectorial membrane

(d) The electrical current generated by potential differences between the endolymph and the perilymph

(e) Nerve stimuli originating from the cochlea nerve

121. What of the following statements is *not* true about brain waves?

(a) The brain wave of petit mal epilepsy is a spike and dome pattern.

(b) Grand mal epilepsy is characterized by high frequency high voltage waves.

(c) Psychomotor epilepsy is characterized by lower than normal frequency waves.

(d) Deep sleep is characterized by alpha waves.

122. Which of the following statements is true?

(a) The transmitter secreted at the endings of the sympathetic preganglionic neurons is norepinephrine.

(b) The transmitter secreted at the endings of the preganglionic neurons of the parasympathetic neurons is epinephrine

(c) The transmitter secreted at the postganglionic neuron endings of the parasympathetic neurons is atropine.

(d) The transmitter secreted at most postganglionic neuron endings of the sympathetic nervous system is norepinephrine.

123. Which of the following is *not* important in dark adaptation?

(a) Conversion of retinal into rhodopsin

(b) Conversion of vitamin A into retinal

(c) The pupillary reflex

(d) Conversion of retinal into lumirhodopsin

124. Two basic types of electrical waves in smooth muscle of the gastrointestinal tract are:

(a) Fast waves and spikes

(b) Short and long waves

(c) Slow waves and spikes

(d) Slow waves and fast waves

125. The most frequent stimulus of peristalsis is:

(a) Distention

(b) Sympathetic stimulation

(c) Acid chyme

(d) Alkaline chyme

126. The principal function of the lower esophageal spincter is:

(a) To allow stomach acid into the esophagus

(b) To maintain food in the esophagus for digestion

(c) To prevent reflux of stomach contents

127. Hydrochloric acid is secreted by the:

(a) Paneth cells

(b) Goblet cells

(c) Chief cells

(d) Parietal cells

128. The three phases of gastric secretion are:

(a) First, second, and third

(b) Cephalic, gastric, and intestinal

(c) Ptylin, gastrin, secretion

(d) Gastric, intestinal, colonic

129. A transmitter substance is applied to the surface of a neuron, and this causes the pores to open up, with greatly increased permeability to chloride ions and potassium ions but no increase in permeability to sodium ions. However, the potential across the cell membrane does not change when the pores open up. What happens to the excitability of the neuron?

(a) The neuron is facilitated.

(b) The neuron is inhibited.

(c) There is no change in degree of facilitation or inhibition.

(d) The neuron is facilitated but there is a long latent period for development of the excitation.

(e) The neuron is inhibited but there is a long

latent period for development of the inhibition.

130. What is the most important deficit that occurs when the somatic sensory association area is removed?
    (a) Loss of tactile sensation
    (b) Loss of thermal sensation
    (c) Loss of pain sensation
    (d) Loss of three dimensional conception of the body
    (e) Loss of ability to localize sensations on the surface of the body

131. The portion of the vestibular system that is most important for preventing a person from suddenly falling if he makes a sudden turn while moving forward is the:
    (a) Saccule
    (b) Utricle
    (c) Cochlea duct
    (d) Otoconia
    (e) Semicircular canals

132. Where is motor activity probably initiated in the brain?
    (a) Motor cortex
    (b) Premotor cortex
    (c) Basal ganglia
    (d) Cerebellum
    (e) The somatic sensory cortex

133. Braxton Hicks contractions:
    (a) Are a positive feedback system
    (b) Are another term for labor contractions
    (c) Occur during most of the months of pregnancy
    (d) Result in hypoxia of the fetus

ANSWERS TO MULTIPLE CHOICE QUESTIONS

1. b	35. d	69. b	103. d
2. e	36. e	70. c	104. a
3. a	37. b	71. a	105. d
4. c	38. b	72. c	106. b
5. a	39. e	73. a	107. c
6. d	40. a	74. e	108. d
7. a	41. c	75. a	109. d
8. a	42. d	76. b	110. d
9. b	43. d	77. d	111. d
10. c	44. d	78. e	112. a
11. a	45. d	79. d	113. b
12. d	46. e	80. c	114. d
13. e	47. d	81. d	115. b
14. c	48. b	82. c	116. a
15. e	49. d	83. a	117. d
16. d	50. e	84. d	118. b
17. e	51. d	85. e	119. b
18. e	52. d	86. b	120. c
19. a	53. b	87. b	121. d
20. c	54. d	88. c	122. d
21. e	55. b	89. a	123. d
22. c	56. b	90. c	124. c
23. c	57. c	91. c	125. a
24. e	58. b	92. b	126. c
25. a	59. d	93. d	127. d
26. e	60. d	94. d	128. b
27. c	61. c	95. d	129. b
28. e	62. d	96. b	130. d
29. d	63. e	97. e	131. e
30. d	64. d	98. c	132. e
31. c	65. c	99. a	133. c
32. c	66. b	100. e	
33. b	67. a	101. a	
34. b	68. c	102. d	

4

Biochemistry

Robert Roskoski, Jr., M.D., Ph.D.
Professor and Head
Department of Biochemistry and Molecular Biology
Louisiana State University Medical Center
New Orleans, Louisiana

INTRODUCTION TO BIOCHEMISTRY AND MOLECULAR BIOLOGY

Biochemistry is the study of life at the molecular level. It includes a study of the molecular composition of living systems and the chemical reactions that they undergo. Biochemistry is also concerned with the production and utilization of fuel molecules, which provide living organisms with the chemical energy required to maintain their highly organized state. In addition to the chemical energy required for biosynthesis, biochemistry considers the mechanisms responsible for the work of transport, intracellular movement, and locomotion. The subject also entails a consideration of replication, differentiation, development, maintenance, healing or repair, and aging.

In addition to addressing physiological processes, biochemistry plays an important role in understanding the pathogenesis of diseases. A complete understanding of pathological processes occurs only after the biochemical mechanisms have been discovered. In perusing current health science literature, the titles of many articles convey the importance of biochemistry as illustrated by the frequent reference to enzymes, biochemical reactions, or the elucidation of the structure of a gene associated with a disease.

The complexity of living systems and attempts to understand the biochemistry of humans and human pathogens is sometimes daunting and bewildering. The large number of components involved adds to the difficulty. The realization, however, that all forms of life are made up of about 50 fundamental building blocks and their derivatives constitutes a major step in simplifying the science of biochemistry. A list of additional unifying principles is listed in Table 4-1; these can be reviewed with the appropriate section in this chapter.

The Cell

Humans, other animals, plants, and microorganisms are composed of fundamental units called cells (see Table 4-1). All cells are surrounded by a semipermeable plasma membrane. The plasma membrane is the boundary between the cell interior and the surrounding environment. It regulates and limits the influx and efflux of fuel molecules such as glucose and ions such as sodium and potassium. Intracellular metabolites such as glucose-6-phosphate and citrate bear electrical charges and pass through the plasma membrane with difficulty, if at all. Those charged molecules that cross the plasma membrane are transported by specific proteins.

Cells arise from other cells by the process of cell division. Organisms are divided into two major classes based on the presence or absence of a discrete cell nucleus. Humans and other organisms whose cells contain a nucleus are called *eukaryotes;* cell division occurs by mitosis. Microorganisms such as *Escherichia coli* or *Streptococcus pneumoniae* lack a well-defined nucleus and are called *prokaryotes;* these cells divide by binary fission.

TABLE 4-1. Fundamental Principles of Biochemistry and Molecular Biology

1. All forms of life are constructed from fundamental units called cells (the cell theory of Schleiden and Schwann).
2. Cells obey the laws of chemistry and physics.
3. Biochemical reactions are catalyzed by enzymes.
4. Enzymes are protein catalysts (Sumner's law).
5. The sun is the ultimate source of energy for life on earth.
6. Biochemical processes proceed with the liberation of free energy.
7. ATP is the common currency of energy exchange in all forms of life (Lipmann's law).
8. The final common pathway in the oxidative metabolism of aerobic organisms is the Krebs citric acid cycle.
9. A proton motive force furnishes the energy for ATP synthesis in (1) oxidative phosphorylation in aerobes and (2) photophosphorylation in photosynthetic organisms (Mitchell's chemiosmotic theory).
10. ATP hydrolysis provides energy for establishing ion gradients. Ion gradients provide energy for metabolite transport.
11. NADH is the hydrogen carrier in most catabolic processes; NADPH is the hydrogen carrier or reductant in most anabolic processes.
12. Activated monomers are the precursors for condensation and polymerization reactions.
13. The generation of inorganic pyrophosphate and its subsequence hydrolysis catalyzed by pyrophosphatase serves to pull biochemical reactions toward completion. This explains why ATP with its two high-energy bonds and not ADP with its single high energy bond is the common currency of energy exchange.
14. The primary structure of a protein governs its secondary and tertiary structure (Anfinsen's law).
15. Biomolecules that interact have complementary structures (Fischer's lock and key hypothesis).
16. Enzymes may be regulated by noncovalent or allosteric agents (theory of Monod, Wyman, and Changeux) and by covalent modification.
17. Metabolic regulation and molecules with regulatory activities (allosteric effectors) follow a pattern which makes physiological sense (the molecular logic of the cell).
18. Various forms of life are continually giving rise to slightly different forms, some of which are adapted to multiply more effectively (Darwin's theories of evolution and natural selection).
19. A single gene codes for one enzyme or polypeptide (The one gene—one enzyme hypothesis of Beadle and Tatum).
20. DNA is the molecule of heredity (law of Avery, MacLeod, and McCarty). In some viruses RNA performs this function (law of Gierer and Schramm).
21. DNA biosynthesis is semiconservative (law of Messelson and Stahl).
22. The flow of information in biological systems is from DNA to DNA and from DNA to RNA to protein (Crick's law of molecular biology). In some cases information flows from RNA to DNA (Temin's law).
23. The genetic code is triplet in nature (a sequence of three nucleotides encodes one amino acid) and mRNA is read in the 5'- to 3'-direction.
24. The genetic code is (almost) universal.
25. Complementary nucleotide base pairing is antiparallel in nature.
26. Nucleic acid elongation reactions proceed in the 5' to 3' direction; amino acid elongation reactions in protein synthesis proceed from the amino to carboxyl terminus.
27. Eukaryotes possess interrupted genes. Intervening sequences in RNA are removed by splicing reactions.

A diagram of a prototypic animal cell is shown in Figure 4-1. The constituent parts and the biochemical reactions associated with each are adumbrated in Table 4-2. This table can be used as a reference for other sections of this chapter. The *nucleus* is the repository of genetic information, which is composed of DNA. *Chromatin* refers to a combination of DNA, histone and nonhistone proteins, and nascent RNA. The nucleus is surrounded by a double membrane that contains nuclear pores (see Fig. 4-1).

The mitochondria contain an *outer membrane* that is freely permeable to small organic molecules and some larger proteins. The *inner mitochondrial membrane,* in contrast, exhibits restricted permeability. Except for a few uncharged substances such as oxygen, carbon dioxide, and urea, the passage of

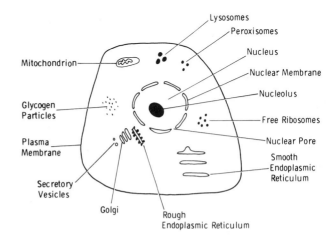

Fig. 4-1. Diagram of a prototypical human cell and its subcellular components.

TABLE 4-2. Properties of Eukaryotic Cell Components

COMPONENT	GENERAL PROPERTIES	ASSOCIATED BIOCHEMICAL PROCESSES	PERCENT VOLUME	NUMBER PER CELL
Cytosol	Nonsedimentable	Glycolysis, glycogenesis, glycogenolysis, pentose phosphate pathway, gluconeogensis, fatty acid synthesis, steroid synthesis, purine and pyrimidine formation, carbamoyl phosphate synthetase II, protein synthesis (free ribosomes)	54	1
Nucleus	Repository and expression of genes	DNA replication, RNA synthesis and processing; contains chromatin, histones, and nonhistones	6	1
Mitochondrion	Powerhouse of the cell; major site of ATP formation.	Citric acid cycle; β-oxidation of fatty acids; oxidative phosphorylation and ATP synthesis; pyruvate dehydrogenase, citrate synthase, carbamoyl phosphate synthetase I (liver); some DNA, RNA, and protein synthesis; metabolic water formed here	22	1700
Lysosome	Waste basket of the cell	Acid phosphatase, cathepsins (degrade several classes of proteins), DNASe, RNASe, hexosaminidase, and many other hydrolytic activities	1	300
Peroxisome	Hydrogen peroxide metabolism	Catalase, peroxidase	1	400
Rough endoplasmic reticulum and Golgi	Synthesis of membrane proteins and proteins for export	Membrane-bound ribosomes, protein processing, and glycosylation	9	1
Smooth endoplasmic reticulum	Complex lipid biosynthesis	Cytochrome P-450 electron transport, steroid hydroxylation, fatty acid desaturation, phospholipid biosynthesis	6	1
Plasma membrane	Boundry between cell exterior and interior	$Na^+ + K^+$ ATPase, adenylate cyclase, many receptors (e.g., insulin, β-adrenergic, HDL receptor), ion channels, glucose, and amino acid transport proteins		1

metabolites through the mitochondrial inner membrane is mediated by specific transport proteins. For example, a specific protein carrier translocates adenosine triphosphate (ATP) in exchange for adenosine diphosphate (ADP). This is an example of *antiport:* one substance moves in one direction and the other moves in the opposite direction. In a *symport* process both substances move in the same direction. The transport of glucose into many cells, for example, is accompanied and driven by the cotransport of sodium. The impermeability of the inner membrane to protons is important in the mechanism of biosynthesis of ATP as noted later. The infoldings of the inner mitochondrial membrane are *cristae.* This represents one way for increasing membrane surface area. The compartment within the inner mitochondrial membrane is called the mitochondrial *matrix.*

Membranes are composed of phospholipid *bilayers* with a hydrophilic exterior and hydrophobic interior. *Integral membrane proteins* are imbedded in or course through the membrane. The lipids and proteins readily move laterally in a two-dimensional plane; this is termed *fluidity.* The existence of proteins within the lipid scaffold is termed a *mosaic.* Both properties are important and have given rise to the *fluid-mosaic model* of membranes.

The interior of *lysosomes* is acidic (pH 5) relative to the cytosol (pH 7). The degradative enzymes found in lysosomes exhibit an acid pH optimum. The hereditary absence of specific enzymes is associated with several lysosomal diseases including Niemann–Pick and Tay–Sachs disease as noted later.

The *endoplasmic* (inside the cell) *reticulum* (network) is a membranous structure that participates in a wide variety of functions (see Table 4-2). When associated with ribosomes *(rough endoplasmic reticulum),* it plays a role in protein synthesis. The ribosomes attached to the endoplasmic reticulum exhibit a studded or roughened appearance as observed by electron microscopy. Many reactions of lipid synthesis occur in the *smooth endoplasmic reticulum* because of the solubility of lipids in membranes.

The dimensions of cells vary considerably. A cuboidal liver cell is about 20 μm $\times$ 20 μm $\times$ 20 μm. The circular mature human erythrocyte is about 7 μm in diameter and 2 μm thick. Erythrocytes serve as an important relative standard when viewing tissues by microscopy with their 7 μm diameter. An *E. coli* cell and a liver mitochondrion are about 1 μm in width and 3 μm in length.

The mammalian erythrocyte lacks a nucleus, mitochondria, an endoplasmic reticulum, and other membranous organelles. It cannot participate in DNA, RNA, or protein synthesis. It contains hemoglobin at a concentration of 5 mM; it also contains 2,3-bisphosphoglycerate at a comparable concentration. Hemoglobin accounts for about 90% of the protein of the erythrocyte. Erythrocytes function in both oxygen and carbon dioxide transport.

The Structural Chemistry of Biomolecules

ELEMENTS

The elementary components of matter that constitute humans can be subsumed as (1) elements of organic matter and water, (2) bulk minerals, and (3) trace minerals. The identity of these elements and their approximate mass in a 70-kg human is given in Table 4-3. Oxygen is the most abundant element in the body (in terms of mass, not number of atoms). The lean body mass is about two thirds water (H_2O), and this accounts for the preponderance of oxygen. Although calcium is predominantly extracellular (as solid hydroxyapatite in bones and teeth and as a 2-mM solution in the extracellular space), it plays an important regulatory role within cells. Changes in intracellular concentration from 10^{-8} M to 10^{-7} M or more trigger muscle contraction and other cellular processes. The other elements will be mentioned as appropriate in the text and will be considered again under nutrition.

CHEMICAL BONDS

There are four types of chemical bonds important in the formation of molecules in biological systems. These consist of (1) covalent bonds, (2) ionic bonds

TABLE 4-3. Elements of the Human Body

ELEMENT	MASS IN 70-Kg HUMAN	COMMENTS
Organic matter and water		
Carbon	12.6 kg	Organic chemicals
Hydrogen	7.0 kg	Organic chemicals and water
Oxygen	45.5 kg	Organic chemicals and water
Nitrogen	2.1 kg	Nucleic acids and amino acids
Phosphorous	0.7 kg	Nucleic acids and many metabolites; constituent of bones and teeth
Sulfur	0.175 kg	Connective tissue and proteins
Bulk minerals		
Sodium	105 g	Principal extracellular cation
Potassium	245 g	Principal intracellular cation; diffusion through cell membrane generates, in part, the negative intracellular electromotive force; obligatory loss of 40 mEq/day in urine
Magnesium	35 g	Cofactor for ATP and other nucleotide reactants; a calcium antagonist; $MgSO_4$ used in treatment of ecclampsia to decrease nerve excitability
Calcium	1050 g	Constituent of teeth and bones; intracellular second messenger; triggers muscle contraction and exocytosis
Chloride	105 g	Major extracellular anion; activates amylase
Fluoride	8 g	Increases hardness of bones and teeth; excess produces dental fluorosis
Trace minerals		
Manganese	20 mg	Activator of arginase and phosphatases
Iron	3000 mg	Found in hemoglobin, myoglobin, cytochromes, iron–sulfur proteins; transported as transferrin and stored as ferritin; deficiency leads to a microcytic anemia
Cobalt	5 mg	Constituent of vitamin B_{12}
Copper	100 mg	Component of cytochrome a,a$_3$ and tyrosinase (in melanin formation); transported in blood by ceruloplasmin; bound to erythrocuprein of the red blood cell; Wilson's disease (hepatolenticular degeneration) is a rare hereditary disorder involving brain and liver with abnormal copper metabolism
Zinc	2300 mg	Cofactor for carbonic anhydrase, carboxypeptidase, and RNA polymerase
Molybdenum	Trace	Xanthine oxidase of purine metabolism and aldehyde oxidase in catecholamine metabolism
Iodine	Trace	Required for production of thyroid hormones T_4 and T_3 (formed from thyroglobulin); deficiency of thyroid hormone produces cretinism in children and myxedema in adults; hyperthyroidism with thyroid hyperplasia is treated with radioiodine
Selenium	Trace	Glutathione peroxidase

(salt bridges), (3) hydrogen bonds, and (4) hydrophobic bonds. ***Covalent bonds*** are composed of a pair of electrons; they are strong (100 kcal/mole) and account for the stability of carbohydrates, fats, proteins, and nucleic acids. In aqueous solution ***salt bridges*** are weak (5 kcal/mole). ***Hydrogen bonds*** refers to a sharing of a hydrogen atom between electronegative oxygen, nitrogen, or a combination of the two. The hydrogen atom is covalently linked to one of the atoms of the pair and interacts electrostatically with the second. The strength of hydrogen bonds is very dependent upon direction. Although individually weak (2–5 kcal/mole), formation of a large number of these bonds promotes stability. ***Hydrophobic*** (water-fearing) ***bonds*** are apolar bonds between hydrocarbon-containing compounds. It is energetically more favorable to sequester hydrocarbons in hydrophobic domains and minimize their contact with polar water molecules in solution. Although individually weak, formation of a large number of such bonds also results in a stable structure.

FUNCTIONAL GROUPS IN BIOCHEMICALS

In considering the reactions of metabolism, it is important to understand the chemistry of the participating functional groups. To examine the precise bonds that are made and broken during a chemical transformation aids in our understanding and analysis of a biochemical process. The main functional groups include hydrocarbons, alcohols, amines, sulfhydryls, carbonyl groups of various types, multifunctional compounds, phosphates and their derivatives, and sulfates and their derivatives (Table 4-4). Most of these are familiar from organic chemistry. Organic chemistry is often described as the chemistry of carbon. Bond making and breaking usually involves a carbon atom. In biochemistry, on the other hand, reactions often involve processes at phosphorus and oxygen as well as carbon.

Most biomolecules, as we shall see, contain more than one functional group. ***Carbohydrates,*** for example, contain an aldehyde or ketone and two or more alcohol groups. ***Amino acids,*** as their name indicates, contain both amino and carboxylic acid groups. Although there is an incredible diversity in all forms of life, there are about 50 fundamental residues that constitute the major mass of living organisms. This unity in nature makes our task easier. In addition to the fundamental building blocks, there are a few hundred other metabolites that constitute the vast majority of compounds with which biochemists are concerned. The diversity of protein molecules in an organism, for example, greatly exceeds that of the low molecular weight compounds or metabolites.

Proteins and Amino Acids

Proteins perform a number of essential functions in all forms of life. The name, in fact, is derived from the Greek ***protos*** meaning first or primary. Proteins

(text continues on p. 300)

TABLE 4-4. Functional Groups in Biochemicals

GROUP		EXAMPLE WITH GROUP
Hydrocarbons		
Alkyl groups	$CH_3(CH_2)_n^-$	Leucine
Alkenes	$\diagdown C = C \diagup$	Fumarate
Aromatic	⬡	Phenylalanine
Alcohol		
R—OH		Ethanol
Amines		
R—NH₂		Glycine
Sulfur Derivatives		
Sulfhydryl group (mercaptan)	R—SH	Cysteine
Disulfide	R—S—S—R¹	Cystine
Thioether	R—S—R¹	Methionine
Sulfate	$HO{-}\overset{\displaystyle O}{\underset{\displaystyle O}{\overset{\|}{\underset{\|}{S}}}}{-}O^-$	

(Continued)

TABLE 4-4. Functional Groups in Biochemicals (*Continued*)

GROUP		EXAMPLE WITH GROUP
Sulfate ester	$R\!-\!O\!-\!\overset{\displaystyle O}{\underset{\displaystyle O}{S}}\!-\!O^-$	Chondroitin sulfate

Carbonyl groups

	$R\!-\!C\!\!\overset{\displaystyle O}{\diagdown}$	
Aldehyde	$R\!-\!C\!\!\overset{\displaystyle O}{\underset{\displaystyle H}{\diagdown}}$	Glyceraldehyde-3-phosphate
Ketone	$R\!-\!C\!\!\overset{\displaystyle O}{\underset{\displaystyle R^1}{\diagdown}}$	Dihydroxyacetonephosphate
Carboxylic acid	$R\!-\!C\!\!\overset{\displaystyle O}{\underset{\displaystyle OH}{\diagdown}}$	Palmitic acid
Ester	$R\!-\!C\!\!\overset{\displaystyle O}{\underset{\displaystyle OR^1}{\diagdown}}$	Triglyceride
Amide	$R\!-\!C\!\!\overset{\displaystyle O}{\underset{\displaystyle NH_2}{\diagdown}}$	Glutamine
Thioester	$R\!-\!C\!\!\overset{\displaystyle O}{\underset{\displaystyle SR^1}{\diagdown}}$	Acetyl-CoA

Combinations

Hemiacetal	$R\!-\!\underset{\displaystyle OR^1}{\overset{\displaystyle OH}{C}}\!-\!H$	Glucopyranose
Acetal	$R\!-\!\underset{\displaystyle OR^1}{\overset{\displaystyle OR^{11}}{C}}\!-\!H$	Glycogen
Hydroxyacid	$R\!-\!\underset{\displaystyle H}{\overset{\displaystyle OH}{C}}\!-\!C\!\!\overset{\displaystyle O}{\underset{\displaystyle OH}{\diagdown}}$	Lactate
Ketoacid	$R\!-\!\overset{\displaystyle O}{\overset{\displaystyle \|}{C}}\!-\!\overset{\displaystyle O}{\overset{\displaystyle \|}{C}}\!\!\underset{\displaystyle OH}{\diagdown}$	Pyruvate

(Continued)

TABLE 4-4. Functional Groups in Biochemicals (*Continued*)

GROUP		EXAMPLE WITH GROUP
Dicarboxylate	$^-OOC-\overset{\overset{\displaystyle H}{\mid}}{\underset{\underset{\displaystyle H}{\mid}}{C}}-\overset{\overset{\displaystyle H}{\mid}}{\underset{\underset{\displaystyle H}{\mid}}{C}}-COO^-$	Succinate
Phosphates		
Phosphoric acid (Pi)	$HO-\overset{\overset{\displaystyle O}{\|}}{\underset{\underset{\displaystyle O^-}{\mid}}{P}}-O^-$	
Pyrophosphate (PPi)	$HO-\overset{\overset{\displaystyle O}{\|}}{\underset{\underset{\displaystyle O^-}{\mid}}{P}}-O-\overset{\overset{\displaystyle O}{\|}}{\underset{\underset{\displaystyle O^-}{\mid}}{P}}-O^-$	
Phosphomonoester	$R-O-\overset{\overset{\displaystyle O}{\|}}{\underset{\underset{\displaystyle O^-}{\mid}}{P}}-O^-$	Glucose-6-phosphate
Phosphodiester	$R-O-\overset{\overset{\displaystyle O}{\|}}{\underset{\underset{\displaystyle O^-}{\mid}}{P}}-O-R^1$	Cyclic AMP, DNA, RNA
Bisphosphate	$\underset{\underset{\displaystyle PO_3^=}{\mid}}{\overset{\overset{\displaystyle PO_3^=}{\mid}}{-}}\overset{\overset{\displaystyle \mid}{}}{\underset{\underset{\displaystyle O}{\mid}}{C}}-\overset{\mid}{C}-$	2,3-Bisphosphoglycerate
Trisphosphate	$^=O_3PO-\overset{\mid}{C}-\underset{\underset{\displaystyle PO_3^=}{\mid}}{\overset{\overset{\displaystyle \mid}{}}{\underset{\underset{\displaystyle O}{\mid}}{C}}}-\overset{\mid}{C}-OPO_3^=$	Inositoltrisphosphate
Diphosphate	$R-O-\overset{\overset{\displaystyle O}{\|}}{\underset{\underset{\displaystyle O^-}{\mid}}{P}}-O-\overset{\overset{\displaystyle O}{\|}}{\underset{\underset{\displaystyle O^-}{\mid}}{P}}-O^-$	Adenosine diphosphate (ADP)
Triphosphate	$R-O-\overset{\overset{\displaystyle O}{\|}}{\underset{\underset{\displaystyle O^-}{\mid}}{P}}-O-\overset{\overset{\displaystyle O}{\|}}{\underset{\underset{\displaystyle O^-}{\mid}}{P}}-O-\overset{\overset{\displaystyle O}{\|}}{\underset{\underset{\displaystyle O^-}{\mid}}{P}}-O^-$	Adenosine triphosphate (ATP)
Phosphoenol group	$CH_2=\underset{\underset{\displaystyle OPO_3^=}{\mid}}{C}-COO^-$	Phosphoenol pyruvate
Phosphoamidate	$R-\underset{\underset{\displaystyle H}{\mid}}{N}-PO_3^=$	Creatine phosphate
Acyl-phosphate	$R-\overset{\overset{\displaystyle O}{\|}}{C}{\diagdown}_{OPO_3^=}$	1,3-Bisphosphoglycerate

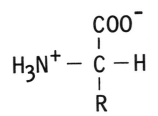

Fig. 4-2. Structure of an α-amino acid.

serve a structural role within the cell (cytoskeleton) and within the connective tissue and skeleton of the whole organism. Proteins also function, *inter alia,* as catalysts, receptors, transporters, antibodies, and hormones. Perhaps 20% of the human body is protein in nature. It is noteworthy that **collagen,** a connective tissue protein, is the most abundant protein in humans. ***Proteins*** are polymers of α-amino acids. There are 20 amino acids that are genetically encoded and serve as precursors for protein biosynthesis on ribosomes. Some of these are modified or derivatized after biosynthesis (posttranslational modification). Specific protein serines, for example, are phosphorylated to produce a phosphoseryl residue; phosphoserine *per se* is not incorporated into the nascent or growing polypeptide chain. Other modifications include hydroxylation, carboxylation, methylation, glycosylation, and acetylation.

AMINO ACIDS

Let us now consider the identity and structures of the 20 genetically encoded amino acids. The amino acids that are found in proteins are α-amino acids (Fig. 4-2). With the exception of glycine, which lacks asymmetric carbon atom (a carbon atom with four different substituents), the amino acids found in proteins possess the **L-*configuration*** (the absolute configuration corresponds to the standard L-glyceraldehyde).

The amino acids with hydrocarbon side chains are shown in Figure 4-3. Glycine is the simplest of the amino acids and is so named because of its sweet taste (Gly, sugar). The side chains of valine, leucine, and isoleucine are hydrophobic. Four amino acids are dicarboxylic acids (aspartate and glutamate) or their derivatives (asparagine and glutamine) and are polar (Fig. 4-4). Asparagine was first isolated from asparagus. Three amino acids contain basic, nitrogen-containing, polar side chains. These consist of lysine, arginine, and histidine (Fig. 4-5). Three amino acids are aromatic (phenylalanine, tyrosine, and tryptophan). These are hydrophobic in nature (Fig. 4-6). Two amino acids contain sulfur: cysteine and methionine (Fig. 4-7). Two amino acids contain a polar alcohol side chain (serine and threonine, Fig. 4-8). The last of

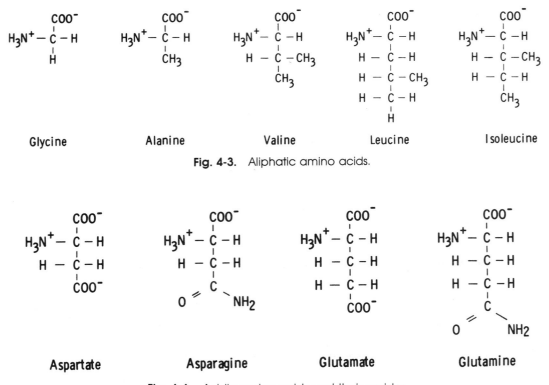

Fig. 4-3. Aliphatic amino acids.

Fig. 4-4. Acidic amino acids and their amides.

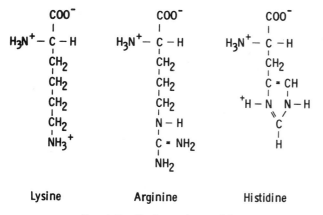

Fig. 4-5. Basic amino acids.

the genetically encoded amino acids is in reality an *imino* acid named proline (Fig. 4-9). The nitrogen atom is linked to two carbon atoms accounting for the term imino. There are a large number of amino acids in nature that are not found in proteins. Examples include ornithine and citrulline, which are important intermediates in urea biosynthesis.

As noted above, glycine lacks an asymmetric carbon atom. Two amino acids, isoleucine and threonine, contain two asymmetric carbon atoms. The β-carbon atom in each case constitutes the second asymmetric center. The amino acids are desig-

nated by a three-letter abbreviation or a single-letter designation (Table 4-5).

The reaction of an α-amino group of one amino acid with the carboxyl group of a second amino acid with the elimination of water results in the formation of a *peptide bond.* The resulting compound is a *dipeptide.* A *tripeptide* contains three amino acid residues, an *oligopeptide* contains a few, and a *polypeptide* contains many amino acids residues. The peptide bond is planar. The carbonyl group and substituted amine occur in a plane, and rotation about the C—N bond is prohibited. This limits the conformation that a polypeptide chain may assume.

Proteins are polypeptides consisting of amino acid residues. The hormone insulin contains 51 amino acids (30 in the A chain and 21 in the B chain). Many biochemists consider this molecule as a protein, and others regard it as a polypeptide. The reader should thus be aware that the distribution between polypeptide and protein is not absolute. All proteins are polypeptides and not vice versa. An average polypeptide chain in a protein contains about 500 amino acid residues; a few contain more than 2,000 amino acid residues. The range of molecular weights of single polypeptide chains ranges from about 5,000 to 300,000. To determine the approximate number of amino acids in a protein, di-

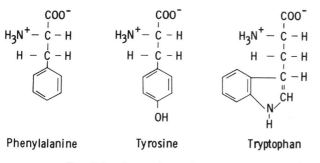

Fig. 4-6. Aromatic amino acids.

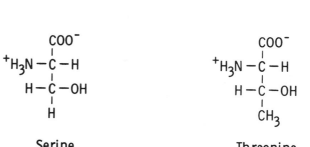

Fig. 4-8. Hydroxyl-containing amino acids.

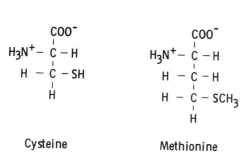

Fig. 4-7. Sulfur-containing amino acids.

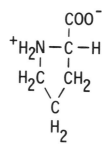

Proline

Fig. 4-9. Proline, an imino acid.

TABLE 4-5. Genetically Encoded Amino Acids

NAME	ABBREVIATION		NUMBER OF CODONS	pKa OF SIDE CHAIN	COMMENTS
Aliphatic					
Glycine	Gly	G	4		Every third residue of collagen
Alanine	Ala	A	4		
Valine	Val	V	4		Hydrophobic
Leucine	Leu	L	6		Hydrophobic
Isoleucine	Ile	I	3		Hydrophobic
Carboxylate Related					
Aspartate	Asp	D	2	4	Anionic
Glutamate	Glu	E	2	4	Anionic
Asparagine	Asn	N	2		
Glutamine	Gln	Q	2		
Basic					
Lysine	Lys	K	2	10.5	Cationic
Arginine	Arg	R	6	12.5	Cationic
Histidine	His	H	2	6	
Aromatic					
Phenylalaine	Phe	F	2		Hydrophobic
Tyrosine	Tyr	Y	2	10.1	Rarely phosphorylated
Tryptophan	Trp	W	1		Hydrophobic; single codon
Sulfur Containing					
Methionine	Met	M	1		Initiator of protein synthesis
Cysteine	Cys	C	2	8.3	Oxidized to cystine
Hydroxyl Containing					
Serine	Ser	S	6		Chief phosphorylated residue of proteins
Threonine	Thr	T	4		Occasionally phosphorylated
Imino					
Proline	Pro	P	4		Occurs at bends in protein chain

vide the molecular weight by 120. This approximates the average molecular weight of an amino acid residue in an average protein.

Proteins consist of one or more polypeptide chains. *Myoglobin,* an intracellular oxygen storage protein containing heme, consists of a single polypeptide chain and is a monomer. Hemoglobin, the oxygen-transport protein found in erythrocytes, consists of two pairs of identical subunits, which form a tetramer. *Hemoglobin* contains two α-chains and two β-chains and the tetramer is denoted as $\alpha_2\beta_2$.

PROTEIN STRUCTURE

The structure of proteins is considered in a hierarchical fashion utilizing four levels (primary, secondary, tertiary, quaternary). The *primary structure* refers to the sequence of amino acids and the nature and position of any covalently attached derivatives. Peptides have a directionality with an amino group (not in peptide linkage) at one end and a carboxyl group (not in peptide linkage) at the other. These groups may be free or derivatized. By convention, structures are written with the amino terminus on the left and carboxyl terminus on the right. The dipeptide Gly-Ala differs from Ala-Gly.

The *secondary structure* of a protein refers to the patterns of hydrogen bonding. There are two major classes associated with secondary structure. The first to be described, the *α-helix,* refers to a helix stabilized by hydrogen bonding between a carbonyl group of one peptide bond and the N—H group on the peptide bond on the chain four residues away (*i.e.,* the residues are close together). The second form of secondary structure to be described was called the *β-pleated sheet.* Here N—H and carbonyl groups form residues very far apart on the polypeptide chain or even residues on a different polypeptide chain form hydrogen bonds. Two varieties of β-pleated sheet are recognized depending on the polarity of the participating polypeptide chains. When the chains are going in the same direction from the amino to carboxyl end of the molecule, the structure is a *parallel* β-pleated sheet. When the participating chains are going in opposite directions with respect to the amino and carboxyl termini, the structure is an *antiparallel* β-pleated sheet.

The *tertiary* structure refers to the three-dimensional arrangement of the atoms of the molecule in space. For a monomeric protein such as myoglobin, this is the highest order of structure. The *quaternary structure* refers to the manner in which subunits of a multimeric protein interact. During the oxygenation of hemoglobin, a tetrameric protein, the subunits move relative to each other. This aspect of structure is the quaternary structure.

The physiologically active conformation of a protein is called the *native* structure. The forces responsible for maintaining the active conformation include covalent bonds, salt bridges, hydrogen bonds, and hydrophobic bonds. The contributions of the latter three in maintaining the active conformation probably varies among proteins. When these forces are disturbed as a result of exposure to extremes of pH (acid or alkali), high temperature (60°C or greater), 6 M urea (an unphysiological concentration), or treatment with charged detergents such as sodium dodecylsulfate, the native conformation is destroyed and a *denatured* structure results. The native state corresponds to one or a few active conformations, but the denatured state may be associated with multiple but inactive conformations.

The sequence of amino acids in a polypeptide chain determines the properties of the protein. Secondary, tertiary, and quaternary structures are determined by the primary structure. This is a statement of Anfinsen's law (see Table 4-1). The substitution of an amino acid by a similar one, for example, replacement of leucine by valine is usually not of great consequence. Substitution by unlike residues, however, can result in a protein with greatly different properties. Substitution of valine for glutamate at position 6 (from the amino terminus) in the β-chain of human hemoglobin, for example, produces *hemoglobin S* (sickle cell hemoglobin). Deoxygenated sickle cell hemoglobin assumes an abnormal conformation and is poorly soluble under physiological conditions. This leads to hemolysis and the circulatory abnormalities in the disease of *sickle cell anemia*.

pH-and the Henderson–Hasselbalch Equation

The properties of water are very important in the maintenance of life's processes. Water constitutes 60% to 70% of the lean body mass of humans, and it is an essential nutrient. Water dissociates into a proton and a hydroxyl group:

$$H_2O \rightleftharpoons H^+ + OH^-$$

In pure water $[H_2O] = 55.6$ M $(1000 \div 18)$.

$$[H^+] = 10^{-7}M$$

$$[OH^-] = 10^{-7}M$$

The concentrations of $[OH^-]$ and $[H^+]$ are in reciprocal relationship to each other. When $[H^+]$ increases, $[OH^-]$ decreases and vice versa. Their product is 10^{-14}.

$$[H^+] \times [OH^-] = 10^{-14}$$

When $[H^+] = 10^{-4}$, for example, then $[OH^-] = 10^{-10}$.

The pH is defined by the following equation:

$$pH = -\log [H^+]$$

At neutrality (when $[H^+] = [OH^-]$):

$$pH = -\log [10^{-7}]$$
$$= -(-7) = +7$$

The pH of blood and physiological fluids is 7.4.

$$7.4 = -\log [H^+]$$

$$3.98 \times 10^{-8} = [H^+]$$

The pH of blood is maintained at 7.4 ± 0.05. *Buffers* are substances that lessen the change in pH when acid or alkali are added to a solution. Buffers are composed of weak acids and their salts or weak bases and their acids. The physiologically important buffers in blood and saliva are (1) $H_2CO_3 - HCO_3^{-1}$, (2) $H_2PO_4^{-1} - HPO_4^{-2}$, and (3) protein–protein^{-1}.

The *Henderson–Hasselbalch equation* provides a convenient way to describe and think about buffers and pH. It is given by the following:

$$pH = pKa + \log \frac{[\text{unprotonated species}]}{[\text{protonated species}]}$$

or equivalently

$$pH = pKa + \log \frac{[\text{salt}]}{[\text{acid}]}$$

For the phosphate system:

$$H_2PO_4^- \rightleftharpoons H^+ + HPO_4^{-2}$$

$$pH = pKa + \log \frac{[HPO_4^{-2}]}{[H_2PO_4^{-1}]}$$

When $[HPO_4^{-2}] = [H_2PO_4^{-1}]$ the concentration of

the protonated form equals that of the unprotonated form and their ratio is 1.

$$pH = pKa + \log 1$$
$$pH = pKa$$

For phosphate at physiological ionic strength the $pKa = 6.8$. The pKa is the pH at which the concentration of salt and acid is identical. Having this value, we can calculate the pH when the concentrations of $[HPO_4^{-2}]$ and $[H_2PO_4^{-1}]$ are known. At a given pH we can calculate the ratios of the two forms. When $[HPO_4^{-2}]/[H_2PO_4^{-1}] = 10$, then

$$pH = 6.8 + \log 10$$
$$= 6.8 + 1$$
$$= 7.8$$

When $[HPO_4^{-2}]/[H_2PO_4^{-1}] = 0.1$, then

$$pH = 6.8 + \log 0.1$$
$$= 6.8 - 1.0$$
$$= 5.8$$

The CO_2 system can be expressed as follows:

$$CO_2 + H_2O \rightleftharpoons H_2CO_3$$
$$H_2CO_3 \rightleftharpoons H^+ + HCO_3^-$$
$$pH = 6.1 + \log \frac{[HCO_3^-]}{[CO_2 + H_2CO_3]}$$

The pKa of the CO_2 system is 6.1. At pH 7.4 the ratio of $[HCO_3^-]/[CO_2 + H_2CO_3]$ is about 20.

When we say that the pKa of an aspartyl group in a protein is 4.1, this means that the residue is half protonated (and half unprotonated) at pH 4.1. When we increase the pH to 7.4, protons are liberated and the aspartyl group bears a net negative charge. When we say that a lysyl residue in a protein has a pKa of 8.3, this means that at pH 8.3, the concen-

trations of R—NH$_2$ and R—NH$_3^+$ of the lysyl group are the same. When we lower the pH to 7.4, more lysyl residues become protonated (since the solution is relatively more acid) and bear positive charges. The imidazole of histidine is the only side chain with a pKa in the physiological range near 7 (see Table 5-4). If one has a pK of 6.9, then at this pH it is half protonated (bearing a positive charge) and half unprotonated (uncharged). At pH 7.4 about a third of the imidazoles are positively charged. The pKa of the side chain of amino acids varies with the protein and the specific residue in the protein. It generally differs from that of the free amino acid. For this reason, the pKa values given in Table 4-5 are only representative or approximate.

Enzymes

GENERAL PROPERTIES

One important function of proteins is that of a catalyst. Almost all reactions of a biochemical nature occur under physiological conditions of temperature and pH because of the existence of protein catalysts (see Table 4-1). An **enzyme** is the term ascribed to a **protein catalyst**. The definition of a protein was considered in the previous section and is a polypeptide made up of α-amino acids. A **catalyst** is a substance that alters the rate of a chemical reaction without itself being permanently changed into another compound. A catalyst increases the rate at which a thermodynamically feasible reaction attains its equilibrium without altering the position of the equilibrium. The rate of a catalyzed reaction ranges from 10^3- to 10^{11}-fold greater than that of an uncatalyzed reaction. A catalyst accelerates a reaction by decreasing the free energy of activation denoted by $\Delta G^{\ddagger}$ (Fig. 4-10). An enzyme provides an

Fig. 4-10. A catalyst lowers the free energy of activation of a reaction.

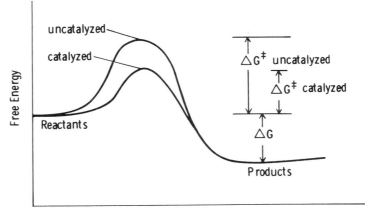

alternative and more speedy reaction route. The development of the science of biochemistry has proceeded concurrently with the development of the science of enzymology.

Enzymes fall into two general classes. Some are *simple proteins* that contain only amino acids. Examples include the digestive enzymes ribonuclease, trypsin, and chymotrypsin. Others are *complex proteins* that contain amino acids and a non-amino-acid cofactor. The complete enzyme is called a *holo-enzyme,* and it is made of a protein portion (apoenzyme) and cofactor.

holo-enzyme = apoenzyme + cofactor

A metal ion may serve as a cofactor. Zinc, for example, is a cofactor for the enzymes carbonic anhydrase and carboxypeptidase. An organic molecule such as pyridoxal phosphate or biotin may serve as a cofactor. Cofactors such as biotin, which are covalently linked to the enzyme, are called *prosthetic groups* (prostithenai, to add to).

In addition to their enormous *catalytic power,* which accelerates reaction rates, enzymes exhibit exquisite *specificity* in the types of reactions that each catalyzes as well as specificity for the substrates upon which they act. Phosphofructokinase catalyzes a reaction between ATP and fructose-6-phosphate. The enzyme does not catalyze a reaction between other nucleoside triphosphates and other sugars to a physiologically meaningful extent. Hexokinase catalyzes a reaction between ATP (and not other nucleoside triphosphates) and glucose, fructose, or mannose (but not galactose). It is noteworthy that *trypsin* catalyzes the hydrolysis of peptides and proteins only on the carboxyl side of polypeptidic lysines or arginines (positively charged, basic residues). *Chymotrypsin* catalyzes the hydrolysis of peptides and proteins on the carboxyl side of polypeptidic phenylalanine, tyrosine, and tryptophan (aromatic residues). Many enzymes exhibit trypsinlike specificity. These include blood-clotting factors and enzymes that are important in processing hormonal peptides.

Enzymes are divided into six classes based upon the type of reaction that they catalyze (Table 4-6). Oxidation–reduction reactions are important in energy metabolism. Kinases are a class of transferase, and they catalyze the transfer of the terminal phosphoryl group of ATP to acceptor substrates. Transfer of acyl groups and amino groups are prevalent in biochemistry. *Hydrolases* catalyze the hydrolysis (lysis or cleavage by water) of proteins, nucleic acids, and a variety of other compounds. *Lyases* (lyein, to loosen or release) catalyze the nonhydro-

TABLE 4-6. Enzyme Classification

CLASS	REACTION
Major Classes	
Oxidoreductases	Transfer hydrogen atom or hydride ion ($H:^-$); act on H_2O_2; act on O_2
Transferases	Transfer carbon, phosphoryl, glycosyl, acyl, and amino groups
Hydrolases	Cleave wide variety of substrates by adding water across bond
Lyases	Cleave carbon bound to carbon, nitrogen, or oxygen
Isomerases	Racemases, epimerases, intramolecular oxidoreductases, intramolecular transferases
Ligases	ATP- or nucleoside triphosphate–dependent condensation reaction
Selected Subclasses	
Kinases	Transfer phosphoryl group from ATP and other nucleotides; transferases
Mutases	Move phosphoryl or other group intramolecularly; isomerases
Phosphorylases	Cleave by adding phosphate across bond; transferases
Decarboxylases	Carboxylate liberated as CO_2; lyases
Hydratases	Add water to double bond and the reverse; lyases
Synthetases	ATP (or equivalent nucleotide)-dependent synthesis; ligases
Synthases	ATP-independent synthesis (e.g., UDPG + glycogen $\rightarrow$ glycogen$_{n+1}$ + UDP); transferases

lytic cleavage of molecules (and the reverse reunification reaction). Aldolase is an example of this class of enzyme. *Isomerases* catalyze the conversion of aldehydes to ketones and of L-compounds to D-compounds. *Ligases* (ligate, to bind, to tie) catalyze the ATP-dependent condensation of one molecule to another. The combination of an amino acid with its corresponding transfer RNA is one example.

KINETICS AND INHIBITORS

There is an increase in reaction velocity with an increase in substrate concentration. In many cases a plot of velocity as a function of substrate concentration yields a *rectangular hyperbola* (Fig. 4-11). At increasingly higher substrate concentrations, the increase in activity is progressively smaller. Such data demonstrate that enzymes exhibit saturation. This was interpreted to mean that the substrates interact with a finite number of catalytic molecules and are converted into products. In an uncatalyzed process the reaction would increase indefinitely as reactant concentration increased. Under defined

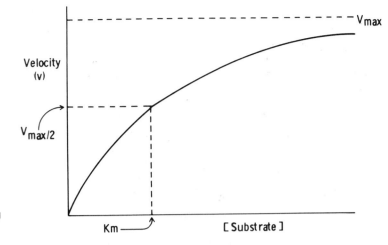

Fig. 4-11. A rectangular hyperbola illustrating saturation kinetics.

conditions and specific amounts of protein, an enzyme exhibits a ***maximum velocity*** (V_{max}), which approaches a limit as the substrate concentration approaches infinity. The K_m ***(Michaelis constant)*** is the substrate concentration at half the maximal velocity ($V_{max}/2$) as illustrated in Figure 4-11. The ***Michaelis–Menten equation*** is an expression for the reaction velocity (v) as a function of substrate concentration ([S]) and the kinetic constants (V_{max} and K_m) as follows:

$$v = \frac{(V_{max} + [S])}{(K_m + [S])}$$

When $v = V_{max}/2$, the reader can verify the result that $K_m = [S]$. It is difficult to estimate the K_m and V_{max} from a rectangular hyperbola. Several methods are available for obtaining accurate values for these parameters including the use of computers. A traditional way for determining the kinetic constants is through the use of a double reciprocal equation. When the reciprocal of the substrate concentration (1/S) is plotted versus the reciprocal of

the velocity (1/v), results similar to those in Figure 4-12 are obtained. The value of $1/V_{max}$ is obtained by extrapolation, and it corresponds to an infinite substrate concentration. The plot also yields $-1/K_m$. Because this is a reciprocal plot, note that a larger V_{max} corresponds to a smaller value of the ordinate (y-axis). Similarly, a larger K_m corresponds to a less negative value of the abscissa (along the x-axis).

Double reciprocal plots are also helpful in studying enzyme inhibition. Enzyme inhibitors are classified as reversible and irreversible. ***Irreversible inhibitors*** usually react covalently with an enzymic amino acid residue and render the enzyme inactive. The rate constants for this reaction can be measured. ***Reversible inhibitors*** generally interact noncovalently and virtually instantaneously with an enzyme; the interactions of this class of inhibitor with enzyme can be studied by steady-state enzyme kinetics. There are two major classes of reversible inhibitor: competitive and noncompetitive. ***Competitive inhibitors*** are structural analogues of the

Fig. 4-12. A double reciprocal or Lineweaver–Burk plot.

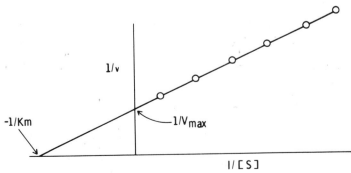

substrate whose concentration is being varied. Consider the following hypothetical enzyme-catalyzed reaction:

$$A + B \rightleftharpoons X + Y$$

Let us assume that B^1 is a substrate analogue of B which interacts with the enzyme but fails to undergo a reaction. If we measure the velocity as a function of the concentration of B at a few fixed concentrations of B^1 and in its absence, we find that at a higher concentration of B (fixed B^1) the magnitude of inhibition is decreased. In fact at infinite concentrations of B (determined by extrapolation), inhibition is abrogated. The location on an enzyme where catalysis occurs is termed the ***active site.*** In this case, a portion of the active site corresponds to A and another portion corresponds to B. B^1 inhibits the enzyme by interacting with the enzyme at the site corresponding to B, and it thereby prevents catalysis. By increasing the concentration of B, its effect overrides that of B^1 and inhibition is overcome. This is illustrated by the unchanged V_{max} for competitive inhibition shown in Figure 4-13.

Let us now consider the effects of varying the concentration of A while keeping B constant. Increasing B^1 increases the degree of inhibition. Increasing concentrations of A, however, cannot completely override the effects of B^1, and the V_{max} at infinite A is lessened (noncompetitive, see Fig. 4-13). This is because A and B^1 do not bind to the same site. No matter how large the concentration of A, B^1 may still bind to and inhibit the enzyme. This type of inhibition cannot be overcome by increased concentrations of substrate not analogous to the reversible inhibitor. Moreover, B^1 does not alter the K_m for A. In the case of competitive inhibition, B^1 increases the apparent K_m of B (see Fig. 4-13).

In examining double reciprocal plots to determine the type of inhibition (see Fig. 13), examine the V_{max}. If the V_{max} is unchanged, the inhibition is competitive. If the V_{max} is decreased and the K_m is unchanged, inhibition is noncompetitive. If similar experiments are carried out with an irreversible inhibitor, a pattern similar to that of noncompetitive inhibition is seen. The irreversible inhibitor inactivates some of the enzyme. The underivatized enzyme is normal (no change in K_m), but there is less active enzyme, and this is reflected by a decrease in V_{max}. As noted above, the chief utility of steady-state enzyme kinetics is in the study of instantaneous, reversible inhibitors and not in the study of irreversible inhibitors.

One of the concepts to emerge from a theoretical consideration of steady-state enzyme kinetics is

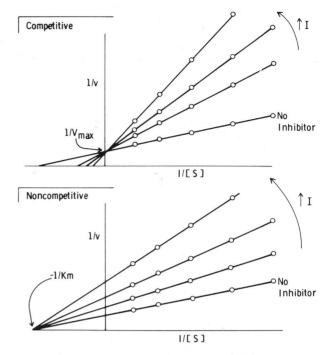

Fig. 4-13. Double reciprocal plots illustrating the effects of competitive and noncompetitive inhibitors.

that the enzyme binds with a substrate to form an enzyme–substrate complex. The enzyme is said to contain an ***active*** or ***catalytic site.*** Following binding of the substrate(s), the enzyme promotes a reaction and the products dissociate. The active site contains residues that participate in the reaction. Amino acids that have been shown to participate in enzymic catalysis include the serine hydroxyl, the cysteine sulfhydryl, the γ-carboxyl of aspartate, the imidazole of histidine, and the ε-amino group of lysine as well as others. Only one, two, or three residues usually participate in reactions in a particular enzyme-active site; additional residues may participate in binding the substrate to the enzyme.

ACTIVITY REGULATION

The activity of enzymes in the cell is subject to a variety of regulatory mechanisms. The amount of enzyme can be altered by increasing or decreasing its synthesis or degradation. Enzyme ***induction*** refers to an enhancement of its synthesis. ***Repression*** refers to a decrease in its biosynthesis. Enzyme activity can also be altered by ***covalent modification*** (see Table 4-1). Phosphorylation of specific serine residues by protein kinases increases or decreases catalytic activity depending upon the enzyme. Proteolytic cleavage of proenzymes (chymotrypsinogen, trypsinogen, proelastase, clotting factors) converts an inactive form to an active form. Enzyme activity can also be regulated by **noncovalent or allosteric mechanisms** (see Table 4-1). Isocitrate dehydrogenase is an enzyme in the Krebs tricarboxylic acid cycle which is activated by ADP. ADP is not a substrate or a substrate analogue. It is postulated to bind to a site distinct from the active site called the **allosteric site.** Allosteric regulation is common, and the changes in activity in response to allosteric effectors make physiological sense (see Table 4-1). When it is realized that one of the primary functions of the Krebs cycle is to provide reducing equivalents for ATP biosynthesis, then we can rationalize its regulation by ADP. When the concentration of ATP is decreased, the concentration of ADP increases and serves as a signal to activate ATP formation. ADP regulates one of the early reactions of the Krebs cycle and promotes greater activity. In addition to activation, some enzymes are subject to **allosteric inhibition.** In *E. coli,* for example, threonine deaminase catalyzes the first step in the reaction pathway for isoleucine biosynthesis. When isoleucine is plentiful, it produces **feedback inhibition** of the first enzymatic reaction and the committed step of the pathway. This decreases the synthesis of an already abundant compound.

Some enzymes fail to conform to simple saturation kinetics and do not exhibit a rectangular hyperbola when velocity is measured as a function of substrate concentration. In the most common case, a sigmoidal curve is observed (Fig. 4-14). A sigmoidal curve is the *sine qua non* for **positive cooperativity.** This is the condition where the binding of one substrate (or ligand) makes it easier for the second to bind. In the case of four binding sites per protein, binding of the second molecule facilitates binding of a third molecule, and this facilitates the binding of the fourth molecule. This is reflected by the increasing slope on the initial portion of the sigmoidal curve. The sigmoidal curve indicates only positive cooperativity. Oxygen binding to hemoglobin is cooperative. Allosteric enzymes often exhibit positive cooperatively but not invariably. A sigmoidal binding curve does not indicate that an enzyme is allosteric in nature. This is a common misconception in the study of biochemistry.

Bioenergetics

FREE ENERGY CHANGES

Bioenergetics is the study of energy changes that accompany biochemical reactions. A **chemical reaction** is the process whereby one or more substances are converted into other substances. For example, dihydroxyacetonephosphate (one biochemical compound) is converted into glyceraldehyde-3-phosphate (another compound) in the cell. The reaction is catalyzed by triosephosphate isomerase. The most important thermodynamic parameter in bioenergetics is the **free energy change** denoted by ΔG (G is named for J. Willard Gibbs, who made fundamental contributions to the study of thermodynamics). This is a change occurring at constant temperature and pressure (the usual case for biochemical reactions). The expression corresponding to this reaction is:

$\Delta G = \Delta G° + RT \ln [\text{G-3-P}]/[\text{DHAP}]$
ΔG = free energy change
$\Delta G°$ = standard free energy change
R = gas constant (1.98 cal K^{-1} M^{-1}) where K is the absolute temperature ($273 + C°$, $C°$ corresponds to degrees Celsius)
T = absolute temperature
$[\text{G-3-P}]$ = concentration of glyceraldehyde-3-phosphate (the product)
$[\text{DHAP}]$ = concentration of dihydroxyacetone phosphate (the reactant)

For a reaction $A + B \rightleftharpoons C + D$:

$$\Delta G = \Delta G° + RT \ln \frac{[C][D]}{[A][B]}$$

The $\Delta G°$ corresponds to the free energy change when a mole of each reactant is converted to a mole of product and all are present at 1 M concentration. Since biochemical reactions occur in dilute aqueous

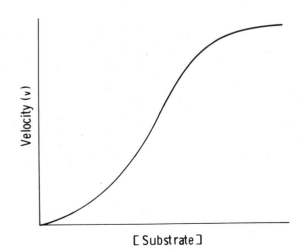

Fig. 4-14. A sigmoidal curve illustrating positive cooperativity.

solution, the effective concentration of water is given a value of 1. When $[H^+]$ is a reactant or product, it is also given a value of 1 because its concentration under physiological conditions (10^{-7} M) is also rather constant. The constant pH is usually designated by including a prime (') with ΔG and $\Delta G°$ as ΔG^1 and $\Delta G°^1$.

Thermodynamically favorable reactions proceed with the liberation of free energy and are exergonic (see Table 4-1). The free energy of the products is less than that of the reactants, that is, ΔG is negative.

ΔG = free energy of products −

free energy of reactants

At equilibrium $\Delta G = 0$ and the reaction is isogonic. When the free energy of the products is greater than that of the reactants, the reaction is thermodynamically unfavorable (endergonic), and ΔG is positive (Table 4-7).

At equilibrium no free energy is derivable, and ΔG is zero. The following important result can then be derived:

$$\Delta G = \Delta G° + RT \ln \frac{[C][D]}{[A][B]}$$

$$0 = \Delta G° + RT \ln \frac{[C][D]}{[A][B]}$$

$$\Delta G° = -RT \ln \frac{[C][D]}{[A][B]}$$

Since the reaction is at equilibrium, the values of A, B, C, and D reflect this and are the concentrations at equilibrium.

$$\Delta G° = -RT \ln K_{eq}$$

From the K_{eq} or equilibrium constant, one can calculate $\Delta G°$ and vice versa. ΔG can be larger or smaller than $\Delta G°$; increasing the concentrations of reactants decreases ΔG (it is more exergonic) and vice versa.

A note of caution is appropriate here. The free energy changes indicate whether or not a reaction under specified conditions is thermodynamically feasible. It fails to provide any information about the rate or kinetics of a reaction. Many thermodynamically feasible reactions are unimportant or irrelevant in biochemistry because of the absence of an enzyme to mediate the reaction in a reasonable time.

A nonbiological example may help to clarify this point. The reaction of oxygen with gasoline to form CO_2 and H_2O is exergonic and proceeds with the liberation of considerable free energy. The gasoline, however, is stable in the presence of oxygen for a very long time. The reaction occurs only under appropriate conditions, such as encountered in an internal combustion engine with an electrical spark initiating the process. The system (gasoline and oxygen) is said to be kinetically stable (unreactive) but thermodynamically unstable (exhibiting the potential for reacting).

ENERGY-RICH COMPOUNDS

The complete oxidation of glucose to carbon dioxide and water is associated with the liberation of 686 kcal of free energy ($\Delta G° = -686$ kcal). These changes in living systems occur in a graded and not explosive fashion. Energy is released in a stepwise fashion and is coupled to the biosynthesis of ATP from ADP and inorganic phosphate (Pi). The ATP-ADP couple receives and distributes chemical energy in all living systems. This is a statement of **Lipmann's law** and is a cornerstone of biochemistry (see Table 4-1). ATP serves as the common currency of energy exchange in living systems.

ATP is an energy-rich compound and serves as a donor of chemical energy for locomotion, muscle contraction, ion transport, and for biosynthetic reactions. The structure of ATP is shown in Figure 4-15. It is composed of a nitrogen-containing base (adenine), a five-carbon sugar (ribose), and three phosphates. The three phosphates are designated α, β, and γ from ribose to the terminus. The β and γ linkages are **acid anhydrides** (water removed from phosphoric acid). These bonds are **energy rich** in nature and are associated with the following reactions: (1) ATP + H_2O → ADP + Pi, and (2) ADP + H_2O → AMP + Pi. The $\Delta G°^1$ for these reactions is about −7 kcal/mole. Compounds with a standard free energy of hydrolysis of −7 kcal/mole or more negative are classified as energy-rich compounds. The reaction ATP + H_2O → AMP + PPi (inorganic pyrophosphate) is also associated with the liberation of considerable free energy (about −7 kcal/mole). The α-phosphate bond (AMP + H_2O → adenosine + Pi) is low energy (−3 kcal/mole) and is

TABLE 4-7. Free Energy Changes and Reaction Directionality

ΔG	DIRECTION OF REACTION FAVORED	CATEGORY
Negative	Toward products	Exergonic
Zero	Equilibrium	Isogonic
Positive	Toward reactants	Endergonic

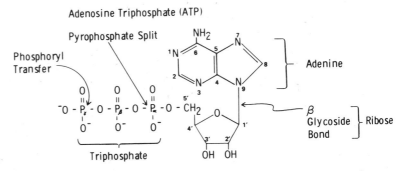

Fig. 4-15. Structure of adenosine triphosphate (ATP).

a phosphate ester (phosphoric acid + alcohol) and not an acid anhydride. The pyrophosphate (1), ADP (1), ATP (2), phosphoenolpyruvate (PEP) (1), acyl-phosphate as found in 1,3-bisphosphoglycerate (1), and phosphoamidate as found in creatine phosphate (1) are high-energy compounds, where the number denotes the quantity of high-energy bonds per molecule. Thioesters, such as acetylcoenzyme A (acetyl-CoA), also contain a high-energy bond.

The following examples illustrate the utility of energy-rich and energy-poor compounds in understanding whether a reaction is favorable (exergonic) or unfavorable (endergonic). Isogonic reactions are equipoised and may proceed in either direction depending upon the circumstances. The following is a prominent reaction in biochemistry:

ATP (2) + glucose (0) →
                ADP (1) + glucose-6-phosphate (0)

The number of high-energy bonds on the left side is two and on the right side is one as indicated. The reaction proceeds with the loss of a high-energy bond; the reaction is exergonic and proceeds to the right. The reaction from right to left is endergonic and does not proceed to a physiologically significant extent. Another example involves the interconversion of two low-energy compounds:

glucose-6-phosphate (0) ⇌
                fructose-6-phosphate (0)

The structures and energy richness of the two compounds is similar and the reaction is isogonic.

A similar analysis obtains for the case where the number of high-energy bonds is the same:

ADP (1) + 1,3-bisphosphoglycerate (1) ⇌
                ATP (2) + 3-phosphoglycerate (0)

This reaction is approximately isogonic, and the reaction proceeds without providing or utilizing much free energy.

The hydrolysis of both energy-rich and energy-poor compounds is exergonic, and the equilibrium

constant is much greater than 1. The reverse reaction is endergonic and is thermodynamically unfavored. Decarboxylations are exergonic; carboxylation reactions usually require the input of energy in the form of ATP. Simple dehydrogenation reactions (not associated with decarboxylation) are generally reversible in nature. Reactions with molecular oxygen are exergonic, and the reverse reaction fails to occur to a meaningful extent.

INTRODUCTION TO METABOLISM

Metabolism refers to all the chemical reactions undergone by an organism. The term metabolism is derived from a Greek word meaning change. Nearly all reactions in living systems are catalyzed by enzymes (see Table 4-1). The chemical reactions or metabolism of living organisms are not random; rather, they are directed along specific sequences called *metabolic pathways*. A metabolic pathway may be composed of from 2 to 20 enzyme-catalyzed steps necessary for the conversion of a molecule into a product. Each of the participant compounds is a *metabolite.*

The process of *catabolism* refers to the conversion of large, complex molecules to simpler small molecules. Some of these reactions release chemical energy; a portion of this chemical energy is captured as ATP is formed from ADP. *Anabolism* refers to the conversion of small molecules to larger ones in the process of biosynthesis. These reactions require chemical energy, which is ultimately derived from ATP.

In general, the pathway for biosynthesis of a compound is not the simple reversal of its pathway for catabolism. The pathways may be completely independent, or they may share common intermediates. The conversion of glucose to pyruvate involves 12 specific enzyme-catalyzed reactions. The conversion of pyruvate to glucose requires 13 reactions. Of these reactions, nine are common to both synthesis and degradation and the others are unique. The different or unique steps occur in such a fashion that the reactions are bioenergetically favorable and exergonic.

A second consequence of this biochemical strategy is that it permits independent regulation of the flux of metabolites through the pathway. For example, the biosynthetic rates can be increased and degradative rates can be decreased because of the occurrence of reactions unique to biosynthesis and degradation. If all the steps were common, alteration of an enzyme activity would increase or decrease both pathways simultaneously. Regulatory enzymes are generally unique to the synthetic or degradative pathway. Moreover, regulation generally occurs at the first or early step in a metabolic sequence. The regulated reaction is often physiologically irreversible and usually constitutes a committed step in metabolism.

We will shortly consider the subject of **intermediary metabolism.** This topic traditionally includes glycolysis and the conversion of pyruvate and fatty acids to acetyl-CoA, the oxidation of acetyl-CoA in the citric acid cycle, and the reactions of electron-transport phosphorylation yielding ATP. In electron-transport or oxidative phosphorylation, reducing equivalents are transported sequentially and stepwise to oxygen. Electron transport is exergonic. Some of the energy is conserved as a proton gradient across a membrane. Protons move down their electrochemical gradient to drive ATP formation from ADP and Pi. The latter is an endergonic process energized by the proton motive force. Amino acids are also degraded to pyruvate, acetyl-CoA, or intermediates of the tricarboxylic acid cycle and then oxidized.

Carbohydrate Chemistry

Carbohydrates are polyhydroxy aldehydes or ketones. Formulas representing D-glucose, the most common sugar in nature, are shown in Figure 4-16.

The middle figure is the open-chain form, and it shows the positions of the hydroxyl group on each of the asymmetric carbon atoms in the Fischer projection. The asymmetric hydroxyl group on carbon atom five forms a hemiacetal adduct with the carbonyl group (carbon one), and a stable six-membered ring results. This generates another asymmetric carbon atom at position one. It occurs with the α- or β-configuration as shown. It is noteworthy that glucose with the β-configuration is one of the most stable sugar structures in nature. First, the six-membered ring is itself stable. Second, the hydroxyl groups occupy equatorial positions and are as far apart from one another as possible.

The ring structures are shown in the Haworth projection format. If one recognizes and can draw the structure of the β-enantiomer of D-glucose, then the other common hexoses can be deduced from it. If one draws the six-membered ring (five carbons and one oxygen) and places the number six carbon with its hydroxyl group above the ring, then the other hydroxyl groups alternate from top to bottom in regular fashion on carbons four (bottom), three (top), two (bottom), and one (top) as shown. If the configuration of the hydroxyl on carbon atom one is altered, then the α-anomer results. Mannose differs from glucose by the hydroxyl configuration about carbon two; galactose differs at carbon four (Fig. 4-17). These three compounds are epimers. **Anomers** refer to differences of configuration at the hemiacetal or hemiketal carbon; **epimers** refer to differences of configuration at the other carbons.

The aldehyde of glucose, mannose, and galactose or the ketone of fructose constitutes a reducing component in alkaline copper solutions. These substances are reducing sugars. The disaccharide lactose contains a hemiacetal group, which also makes it a reducing sugar (Fig. 4-18). In the disaccharide sucrose, the hemiacetal and hemiketal groups are further derivatized to form a glycoside bond. The absence of a simple hemiacetal or hemiketal bond

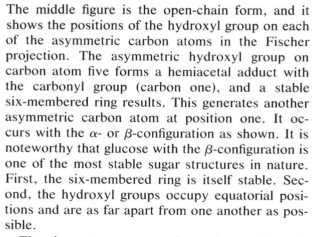

Fig. 4-16. Forms of glucose in aqueous solution.

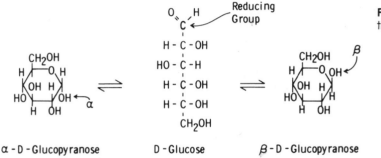

α - D - Glucopyranose   D - Glucose   β - D - Glucopyranose

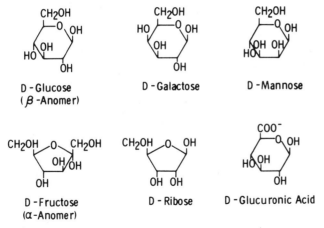

Fig. 4-17. Structure of some physiologically important sugars.

makes sucrose a nonreducing sugar in alkaline copper solution.

Glycolysis

The initial steps in the catabolism of glucose constitute the **Embden–Meyerhof glycolytic pathway.** This pathway and its enzymes are present in all human cells and are located in the cytosol (see Table 4-2). The overall reaction is abbreviated:

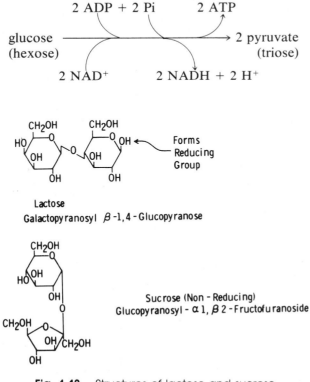

Fig. 4-18. Structures of lactose and sucrose.

During the stepwise conversion of glucose to pyruvate, two molecules of nicotinamide-adenine dinucleotide phosphate (NADH) are formed, and there is a net production of two ATP molecules. In the first stage of glycolysis, two ATPs are consumed in priming reactions to produce fructose-1,6-bisphosphate. This substance is cleaved into two triose phosphates. Two moles of glyceraldehyde-3-phosphate undergo an oxidation to yield two moles of NADH and two of 1,3-bisphosphoglycerate. The latter compounds contain an energy-rich acyl-phosphate linkage, which will be donated to two ADPs to yield two ATPs. Subsequently, two PEP molecules are formed, which will donate their energy-rich phosphoryl group to two ADPs to yield two additional ATPs. Two net ATPs result ($-2 + 4 = 2$). Let us now consider the reactions in this process.

The first step in glycolysis involves the phosphorylation of glucose by ATP (Fig. 4-19). The enzyme that catalyzes this exergonic and irreversible reaction is **hexokinase,** and it is found in all cells. Hexokinase will also catalyze the phosphorylation of mannose and fructose to yield the respective hexose-6-phosphate. Liver contains a second enzyme that catalyzes glucose phosphorylation named **glucokinase.** It will not catalyze the phosphorylation of the other two hexoses. It exhibits a higher K_m for glucose than hexokinase (20 mM vs. 50 μM) and is thus not saturated by the high glucose concentrations delivered to the liver by the portal vein. Glucokinase is also not inhibited by glucose-6-phosphate as is hexokinase.

Phosphohexose isomerase then catalyzes the conversion of glucose-6-phosphate to fructose-6-phosphate. The interconversion of these two energy-poor compounds is nearly isogonic. **Phosphofructokinase** (PFK) catalyzes the second phosphorylation. This reaction is exergonic and physiologically irreversible. PFK catalyzes the rate-limiting or pacemaker reaction of glycolysis. Aldolase then catalyzes the cleavage of fructose-1,6-bisphosphate to glyceraldehyde-3-phosphate and dihydroxyacetone phosphate. **Triose phosphate isomerase** catalyzes the interconversion of these two compounds. **Glyceraldehyde-3-phosphate dehydrogenase** mediates a reaction between the designated compound, nicotinamide-adenine dinucleotide (NAD$^+$), and Pi to yield 1,3-bisphosphoglycerate. Next, **phosphoglycerate kinase** catalyzes the reaction of the latter, an energy-rich compound, with ADP to yield ATP and phosphoglycerate. **Phosphoglycerate mutase** catalyzes the transfer of the phosphoryl group from carbon three to carbon

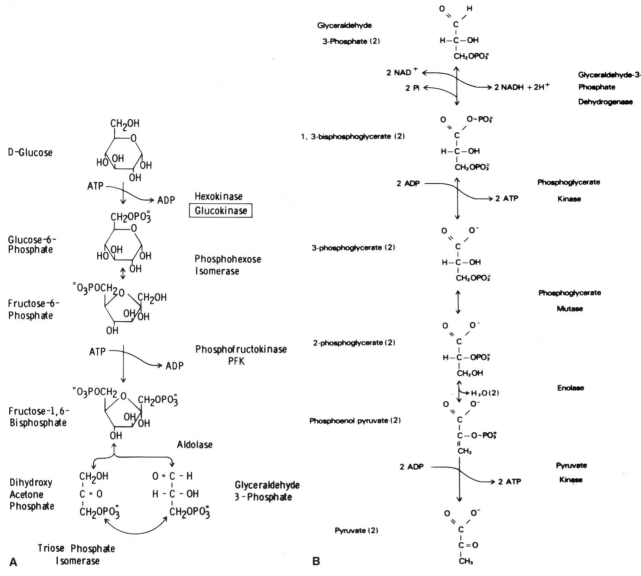

Fig. 4-19A,B. Embden–Meyerhof glycolytic pathway.

two to yield 2-phosphoglycerate. This compound contains an energy-poor phosphoester linkage. *Enolase* catalyzes an isogonic dehydration to yield PEP. This compound contains a very energy-rich phosphate bond. Its standard free energy of hydrolysis is -14.8 kcal/mole. This compound then donates its phosphoryl group to ADP to yield ATP and pyruvate in a reaction catalyzed by *pyruvate kinase*. Although the number of high-energy bonds is the same in the reactants and products (two), the reaction is highly exergonic and is physiologically irreversible.

To recapitulate, the three irreversible steps of glycolysis include the reactions catalyzed by hexokinase, PFK, and pyruvate kinase. PFK is the rate-limiting enzyme of the pathway. It is also the main regulatory enzyme. It is activated by *adenosine monophosphate* (AMP), and *fructose-2,6-bisphosphate* and inhibited by ATP and citrate. Note that ATP is both a substrate and allosteric modulator. One function of glycolysis is to generate chemical energy as ATP. When the cellular concentrations of ATP are high, glycolysis is inhibited. When ATP levels fall, ADP and AMP are formed and the latter activates PFK. During conditions where fatty acids serve as a fuel, citrate levels increase and glycolysis decreases. The regulatory role of fructose-2,6-bisphosphate will be considered under gluconeogenesis. Fluoride, at high and nonphysiological concentrations, inhibits the enolase reaction. The ATP formed in glycolysis results from *substrate level phosphorylation.* An energy-rich metabolite is produced, and it leads to ATP formation. This is in contrast to *oxidative phosphorylation* where ATP is produced by reactions involving electron transport, a proton motive force, and an ATP synthetase.

A note regarding nomenclature is appropriate here. When phosphates are linked together as in ADP and ATP, the appropriate prefix is *di* or *tri,* respectively. When the phosphates are not attached to one another, as in fructose-1,6-bisphosphate or inositol trisphosphate, the prefix *bis* or *tris* is appropriate (see Table 4-4).

HEXOSE METABOLISM

We now consider the metabolism of other hexoses. Two other important sugars are fructose and galactose. In addition to hexokinase, the liver contains a specific *fructokinase,* which catalyzes its phosphorylation by ATP to yield *fructose-1-phosphate* in an exergonic and physiologically irreversible process. The product is cleaved in a reaction catalyzed by aldolase to form glyceraldehyde and dihydroxyacetone phosphate. A specific kinase mediates the phosphorylation of the latter to yield glyceraldehyde-3-phosphate.

The catabolism of galactose is more complex than that of the sugars covered to this point. Galactose (see Fig. 4-17) is derived from the disaccharide lactose (see Fig. 4-18) found in milk (lac). Lactose is hydrolyzed by a digestive enzyme (lactase), absorbed by the gut, and transported to the liver. In the liver it is phosphorylated by ATP in a reaction catalyzed by *galactokinase* to yield ADP and galactose-*1*-phosphate. Galactose is the only common aldohexose that is not a substrate for hexokinase. The reaction is also unusual in that the hydroxyl group of a hemiacetal linkage is derivatized (the hydroxyl of fructose on carbon one is not in hemi-acetal linkage). Galactose-1-phosphate reacts with uridine diphosphoglucose (UDPG) to yield UDP-gal and glucose-1-phosphate. The reaction is catalyzed by a *galactose-1-phosphate uridyltransferase* (Fig. 4-20). Glucose-1-phosphate is converted to glucose-6-phosphate by *phosphoglucomutase* in an isogonic reaction. It is metabolized by the reactions of the Embden–Meyerhof pathway as previously considered.

UDP-gal must be converted to UDPG to regenerate the initial reactant. This reaction is catalyzed by an epimerase that converts the hydroxyl on carbon

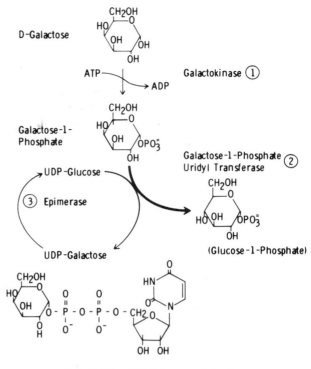

Fig. 4-20. Galactose catabolism.

four to a ketone and then reduces it to give the hydroxyl of the alternative configuration (UDPG) shown in Figure 4-20. The epimerase contains tightly bound NAD^+ as cofactor. The UDPG can now react with a second molecule of galactose-1-phosphate to yield glucose-1-phosphate and UDP-gal. The UDP moiety is thus used repeatedly in a cyclic fashion to mediate the conversion of appreciable galactose-1-phosphate to glucose-1-phosphate. The UDPG is said to function in a catalytic fashion; UDPG is regenerated after every reaction.

The human disease called *galactosemia* is due to a deficiency of *galactose-1-phosphate uridyltransferase.* Excessive galactose-1-phosphate accumulates in cells with consequent deleterious effects. A diet lacking milk and milk products (specifically lactose) constitutes treatment. Galactose forms an essential component of many carbohydrate-containing glycoproteins. Withholding galactose is not harmful because the epimerase can catalyze the formation of UDP-gal from UDPG as necessary. A milder form of galactosemia is due to a hereditary deficiency of galactokinase. It is a less severe disease because there is not an accumulation of charged intracellular metabolites.

For continued glycolysis, it is necessary to regenerate ADP and NAD^+. ATP is utilized in many of the cell's reactions as the common currency of energy exchange resulting in the formation of ADP. We will briefly consider the metabolism of NADH.

In erythrocytes, which lack mitochondria, and in other cells where NADH production exceeds the capacity for electron transport, NAD^+ is regenerated by the *lactate dehydrogenase* reaction. Pyruvate and $NADH + H^+$ react to yield lactate and NAD^+. The regenerated NAD^+ can participate again in glycolysis. The lactate is released from the erythrocyte or exercising skeletal muscle and is carried to the liver by the circulation. Under opportune conditions, lactate reacts with NAD^+ to yield NADH and pyruvate. Pyruvate may be reconverted to glucose by the process of gluconeogenesis. The glucose can be released from the liver and return to other tissues. The conversion of glucose to lactate in extrahepatic tissues, the resynthesis of glucose from lactate in liver and subsequent transport to extrahepatic tissues is called the **Cori cycle**. The reoxidation of NADH to NAD^+ under aerobic conditions by the *malate shuttle* system will be considered in a later section.

Pyruvate Dehydrogenase

The complete oxidation of pyruvate occurs within mitochondria. Pyruvate is transported through the inner mitochondrial membrane by a specific carrier protein or translocase. Pyruvate is oxidized to acetyl-CoA and CO_2 by the *pyruvate dehydrogenase* multienzyme complex found in the mitochondrial matrix (see Table 4-2). A *multienzyme complex* is an aggregate of enzymes that catalyze a series of reactions. The intermediates in the sequence are covalently bound to the complex and are not free to diffuse throughout the surrounding solution. The pyruvate dehydrogenase complex contains three enzyme activities and five cofactors (see Table 4-8).

Pyruvate is converted to CO_2 and a two-carbon hydroxyethyl moiety covalently linked to the thiamine pyrophosphate of E1. The hydroxyethyl group is transferred to lipoate on E2. In the process it becomes the more oxidized acetyl group and it is covalently linked to sulfur (as an energy-rich thioester). E2 transfers the acetyl group to coenzyme A yielding acetyl-CoA. E3 catalyzes the oxidation of reduced lipoate as flavin adenine dinucleotide (FAD) is converted to reduced FAD ($FADH_2$). $FADH_2$ is then oxidized to FAD; $NADH + H^+$ result. Following this reaction the enzyme complex is now in its original form. Pyruvate dehydrogenase catalyzes the net reaction:

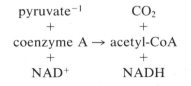

$$
\begin{array}{ccc}
\text{pyruvate}^{-1} & & CO_2 \\
+ & & + \\
\text{coenzyme A} & \rightarrow & \text{acetyl-CoA} \\
+ & & + \\
NAD^+ & & NADH
\end{array}
$$

The reaction is highly exergonic and physiologically irreversible.

The enzyme is activated by NAD^+ and coenzyme A and inhibited by NADH and acetyl-CoA. The mechanism, however, is indirect. A *pyruvate dehydrogenase kinase* is a specific protein kinase associated with the dehydrogenase in mitochondria. Following phosphorylation by ATP, pyruvate dehydrogenase exhibits less activity. Acetyl-CoA and NADH activate this protein kinase; coenzyme A and NAD^+ inhibit it. A phosphoprotein phosphatase catalyzes the hydrolytic removal of phosphate from pyruvate dehydrogenase to generate the initial enzyme form.

The Krebs Citric Acid Cycle

The Krebs citric acid or tricarboxylic acid cycle is often called the final common pathway of metabolism. The catabolism of glucose and fatty acids yields acetyl-CoA; metabolism of amino acids yields acetyl-CoA or actual intermediates of the cycle. The *citric acid cycle* provides a pathway for the oxidation of acetyl-CoA. The reactions occur in the mitochondria of eukaryotes (see Table 4-2). The pathway includes eight discrete steps. Seven of the enzyme activities are found in the mitochondrial matrix; the eighth (succinate dehydrogenase) is associated with the electron-transport chain within the inner mitochondrial membrane.

The net reaction catalyzed during each revolution

TABLE 4-8. The Pyruvate Dehydrogenase MultiEnzyme Complex

ENZYME	COFACTOR	VITAMIN
E1 Pyruvate decarboxylase	Thiamine pyrophosphate	Thiamine
E2 Dihydrolipoyltransacetylase	Lipoate	
	Coenzyme A	Pantothenate
E3 Dihydrolipoyldehydrogenase	Flavine adenine dinucleotide (FAD)	Riboflavin
	Nicotinamide adenine dinucleotide (NAD^+)	Niacin

of the tricarboxylic acid cycle can be depicted as follows:

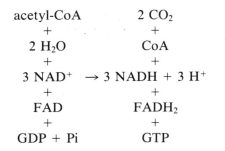

$$
\begin{array}{ccc}
\text{acetyl-CoA} & & 2\ CO_2 \\
+ & & + \\
2\ H_2O & & CoA \\
+ & & + \\
3\ NAD^+ & \rightarrow & 3\ NADH + 3\ H^+ \\
+ & & + \\
FAD & & FADH_2 \\
+ & & + \\
GDP + Pi & & GTP
\end{array}
$$

The CO_2 is an end product of metabolism. Coenzyme A can be reutilized for a variety of reactions. The reduced cofactors will donate their reducing equivalents to the electron-transport chain and oxygen to yield H_2O and the oxidized cofactors. Guanosine triphosphate (GTP) is formed by substrate-level phosphorylation. It is bioenergetically equivalent to ATP and serves a variety of functions. An overview of the cyclic pathway indicates the location of carbon dioxide production and NADH and $FADH_2$ formation (Fig. 4-21). The production of 11 ATP equivalents by oxidative phosphorylation and 1 GTP by substrate-level phosphorylation is also indicated.

The reactions of the cycle are shown in Figure 4-22. *Citrate synthase* catalyzes a reaction between acetyl-CoA, citrate, and water to yield citrate (a tricarboxylic acid) and coenzyme A. This reaction is associated with the hydrolytic removal of CoA, which is a highly exergonic process and renders the reaction physiologically irreversible. The distinc-

tion between *synthases* and *synthetases* is that the latter require ATP or an equivalent nucleoside triphosphate as energy source (see Table 4-6). *Aconitase* catalyzes an isogonic isomerization to yield isocitrate. Although citrate lacks an asymmetric carbon, it is prochiral and the hydroxyl is moved away from the two-carbon end just derived from the acetyl group. Isocitrate undergoes an oxidative decarboxylation reaction involving NAD^+ catalyzed by *isocitrate dehydrogenase;* the products include α-ketoglutarate, CO_2, NADH, and H^+. The reaction is modestly exergonic. The high ratio of $NAD^+ : NADH$ in mitochondria pulls the reaction in the forward direction. Isocitrate dehydrogenase is the rate-limiting enzyme in the pathway. ADP serves as a positive allosteric effector. High ADP levels serve as a signal to enhance the flux of substrates through the cycle.

Alpha-ketoglutarate dehydrogenase catalyzes the reaction between substrate, NAD^+, and CoA to yield succinyl-CoA, CO_2, NADH, and H^+. The enzyme consists of a multienzyme complex that is fully analogous to the pyruvate dehydrogenase complex considered in the previous section. The reaction is highly exergonic and physiologically irreversible. This reaction ensures that the cycle is unidirectional. The next reaction is catalyzed by *succinate thiokinase*. It is an example of substrate-level phosphorylation conserving the energy-rich thioester bond of succinyl-CoA as the terminal phosphoanhydride bond of GTP. Succinyl-CoA, Pi, and guanosine diphosphate (GDP) form succinate and GTP. (Since GDP + Pi $\rightarrow$ GTP + H_2O, this

Fig. 4-21. Overview of the Krebs citric acid cycle.

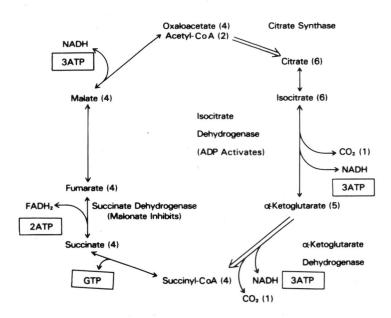

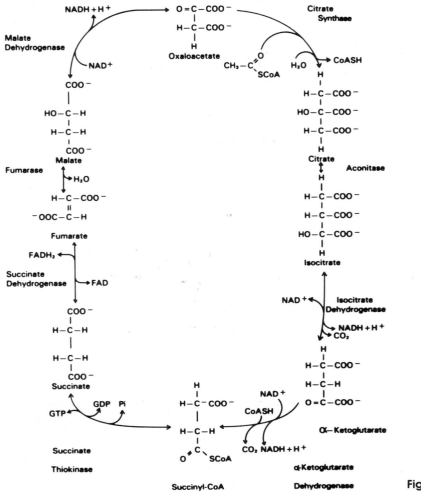

Fig. 4-22. Krebs citric acid cycle.

reaction serves indirectly as a source of water in calculating the stoichiometry of the cycle). *Succinate dehydrogenase* has three properties worth remembering. First, it is the only enzyme of the Krebs cycle found within the inner mitochondrial membrane. It is thus localized contiguous to the electron-transport chain where it passes its reducing equivalents. Second, only two ATPs are produced by electron transport (in contrast to three ATPs from NADH) from the enzyme's flavin adenine nucleotide (FAD) prosthetic group. Third, this enzyme is competitively inhibited by malonate ($^-$OOCCH$_2$COO$^-$). This was an important property that helped H. A. Krebs discover and elucidate the nature of the cycle. Succinate dehydrogenase mediates the conversion of substrate to fumarate (note that fumarate has the transconfiguration at the double bond). *Fumarase* catalyzes the addition of water to fumarate (a hydration) yielding malate. The reac-

tion is isogonic. *Malate dehydrogenase* catalyzes the regeneration of oxaloacetate by reduction of NAD$^+$ to NADH and H$^+$. Although the reaction is readily reversible, it is moderately endergonic.

To recapitulate, the citrate synthase and α-ketoglutarate dehydrogenase reactions are physiologically irreversible. Isocitrate dehydrogenase is the pacemaker and is allosterically activated by ADP. Succinate thiokinase catalyzes a substrate-level phosphorylation. The two molecules of CO$_2$ given off during a single turn of the cycle are not those immediately derived from the acetyl group.

In addition to its role in catabolism, metabolites of the Krebs cycle serve as precursors for the biosynthesis of amino acids. A process playing a role in both catabolism and anabolism is called *amphibolic.* The following reaction, catalyzed by *pyruvate carboxylase,* plays the important role of replenishing intermediates that are utilized for biosynthesis. The reaction involves ATP, HCO_3^-, and pyruvate; oxaloacetate, ADP, and Pi are products. The cofactor for the enzyme is **biotin.** It is covalently linked to the enzyme and is a prosthetic group. The enzyme is allosterically activated by acetyl-CoA. The overall reaction is expressed by the following chemical equation:

$$
\begin{array}{ccc}
\text{pyruvate}^- & & \text{oxaloacetate}^{-2} \\
+ & & + \\
\text{ATP} & \underset{\leftarrow}{\rightarrow} & \text{ADP} + \text{Pi} \\
+ & & \\
HCO_3^- & &
\end{array}
$$

The reaction is isogonic.

Oxidative Phosphorylation

The term **oxidative phosphorylation** refers to reactions associated with oxygen consumption and the phosphorylation of ADP to yield ATP. Oxidative phosphorylation is associated with an **electron-transport chain** or **respiratory chain** which is found in the inner mitochondrial membrane of eukaryotes (see Table 4-2). A similar process occurs within the plasma membrane of prokaryotes such as *E. coli.* The importance of oxidative phosphorylation at this juncture is that it accounts for the reoxidation of reducing equivalents generated in the reactions of the Krebs cycle as well as in glycolysis; this process accounts for the preponderance (90% or more) of ATP production in humans. The electron-transport chain transfers electrons from reductants to oxygen in a series of exergonic reactions. According to **Mitchell's chemiosmotic theory** a portion of the liberated free energy drives protons from inside to outside of the inner mitochondrial membrane (or the plasma membrane of prokaryotes). Such reactions result in energy conservation or storage in the form of a proton gradient. The **proton motive force** exhibits a voltage component (inside negative) and a concentration component (external pH < internal pH). The protons then move down their electrochemical gradient (from outside to inside) in an exergonic process and drive the conversion of ADP +

Pi to ATP + H_2O in a reaction catalyzed by an **ATP synthetase** (see Table 4-1). The enzyme is located on the inner face of the inner mitochondrial membrane; it catalyzes a reversible reaction and can synthesize or hydrolyze substrate (ATPase) depending upon the experimental conditions. Its function in humans *in vivo* is ATP synthesis.

ELECTRON-TRANSPORT PATHWAY

The following are components of the electron-transport chain: iron–sulfur proteins, cytochromes c_1, c, b, aa_3, and coenzyme Q or ubiquinone. The pathway of electrons along the chain is shown in Figure 4-23. Reducing equivalents can enter the chain at two locations. Electrons from NADH are transferred to NADH dehydrogenase. In reactions involving iron–sulfur proteins, electrons are transferred to coenzyme Q; protons are translocated from the interior to exterior of the mitochondrion during this process. Electrons entering from succinate dehydrogenase ($FADH_2$) are donated to coenzyme Q. This is not associated with proton translocation. Electrons are transported from reduced coenzyme Q to cytochrome b and then cytochrome c_1. This process is also associated with active proton translocation. Electrons are then carried by cytochrome c to cytochrome aa_3. Cytochrome aa_3 is also known as **cytochrome oxidase,** and it catalyzes a reaction of electrons and protons with molecular oxygen to produce water. Cytochrome oxidase also actively translocates protons across the inner mitochondrial membrane.

The three sites for active proton translocation are called sites I, II, and III. The precise localization of these sites is not as well established as their designations might signify. Site I occurs between NADH dehydrogenase and coenzyme Q, site II occurs between coenzyme Q and cytochrome c, and site III occurs between cytochrome c and molecular oxygen. The sites were named on the basis of the effects of inhibitors of electron transport and prior to the notion of discrete proton pumping sites. The specific inhibitors are given in Table 4-9. Rotenone

Fig. 4-23. Mitochondrial electron-transport chain.

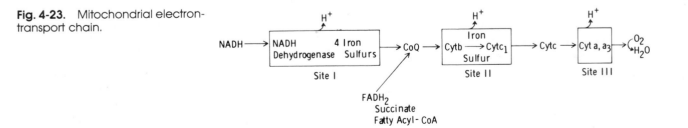

TABLE 4-9. Inhibitors of the Electron-Transport or Respiratory Chain

SITE	INHIBITOR
I	Rotenone
II	Antimycin A
III	Cyanide (CN⁻)
	Azide (N₃⁻)
	Carbon monoxide (CO)

is commonly used as a rat poison. Cyanide is a powerful inhibitor of cytochrome oxidase, and this accounts for its toxic and lethal effects. Carbon monoxide also binds tightly to cytochrome oxidase. Its major toxicity, however, is related to the formation of a complex with hemoglobin, which abolishes its oxygen-binding capacity.

Cytochrome c is a small (molecular weight = 10,000), water-soluble, heme protein. All the other proteins of the electron transport chain are water insoluble and are found embedded in the inner mitochondrial membrane. Coenzyme Q is a lipid soluble organic compound. NAD^+, FAD, and coenzyme Q are two-electron carriers; the cytochromes (with their iron–heme), and iron–sulfur proteins are one-electron carriers. Cytochrome oxidase contains two iron atoms, which are thought to function in one-electron transfers in series. It is not yet known how the reduction of water catalyzed by cytochrome oxidase occurs. This involves a four-electron reaction.

Note that more than 90% of oxygen consumed by humans involves a reaction catalyzed by cytochrome oxidase. When oxygen transport to tissues is blocked as the result of an arterial occlusion, serious pathology or death ensues. The occlusion produced by coronary artery disease resulting in a myocardial infarction (heart attack) or cerebral vascular disease resulting in a stroke cogently illustrates the importance of the cytochrome oxidase reaction. The product of oxygen reduction is water. In humans, this accounts for the production of about 300 ml of metabolic water per day.

The precise mechanism of proton translocation at each of the three sites is unknown. Uncertainty exists over the number of protons transported per electron per site. It seems to be two to three. An important aspect of the chemiosmotic theory is that a membrane is required, and the membrane must be relatively impermeable to protons. Protons are transported by specific transport proteins and do not simply diffuse through the membrane. Next we address the issue of how the proton motive force drives ATP synthesis.

ATP SYNTHESIS

A complex enzyme called **ATP synthetase** is associated with the inner aspect of the inner mitochondrial membrane. As protons move down their electrochemical gradient in an exergonic fashion, they provide the energy for the reaction of ADP and Pi to give ATP and H_2O (see Table 4-1). In one scheme it is postulated that the protons move through the multisubunit protein constituting the ATP synthetase. The synthetase is made up of two domains. The F_o domain (o stands for oligomycin—an inhibitor of the overall synthetase reaction) is embedded in the inner membrane. The F_1 complex forms a knoblike structure in association with F_o. In the intact structure the membrane is proton impermeable. When F_1 is removed from F_o, the membrane transmits protons. This observation provides evidence that protons course directly through the ATP synthetase. The F_1 complex contains binding sites for ATP, ADP, and Pi. Movement of protons down their thermodynamic gradient provides the energy to drive the endergonic portion of the reaction $(ADP + Pi \rightarrow ATP + H_2O)$. The number of protons that must move down their gradient to drive ATP synthesis is uncertain. It seems to be two to three. The elucidation of the biochemistry of ATP synthesis represents an exciting challenge to contemporary investigators.

One of the triumphs of the chemiosmotic theory is the explanation of the necessity of a membrane in oxidative phosphorylation. It also explains the effects of uncouplers of oxidative phosphorylation. **2,4-Dinitrophenol** is the prototype of this class of compound. It does not inhibit electron transport from reductant to oxygen; if anything, it enhances the rates observed in experimental systems. It does, however, abolish phosphorylation or ATP formation. This is the meaning of the term "uncoupler" since oxidation occurs, but phosphorylation does not. 2,4-Dinitrophenol and other uncouplers dissipate the proton gradient. They ferry protons across the membrane and abrogate the proton motive force. In the absence of a proton gradient, proton pumping is not restrained, and electron transport to oxygen is increased. Parenthetically, 2,4-dinitrophenol was used in the treatment of human obesity in the 1930s. Because of its low therapeutic index, several deaths ensued and the practice was abolished.

Experiments in the early 1940s showed that the P:O ratio (number of ATPs formed from ADP + Pi per gram atom of oxygen consumed) was 3 using NADH as substrate. Subsequent experiments indicate that the P : O ratio with succinate as substrate is 2. Each site (I, II, and III) is associated with the generation of a proton gradient sufficient for the formation of one ATP. Succinate circumvents site I and results in the production of only two ATPs (see Fig. 4-23).

To recapitulate this section on oxidative phosphorylation, we note four properties of the process. First, transport of electrons from reductant to oxygen along the respiratory chain is a very exergonic process. Second, part of the chemical energy is conserved as protons are pumped from the inside to the outside of the inner mitochondrial membrane to establish a gradient. Third, the membrane is not freely permeable to protons. Fourth, protons then move down their electrochemical gradient (an exergonic process) and drive ATP formation in a process involving the ATP synthetase of the inner mitochondrial membrane.

TRANSPORT ACROSS THE INNER MITOCHONDRIAL MEMBRANE

The lipid portion of the inner mitochondrial membrane is relatively impermeable to ionic metabolites, phosphate, hydroxide, and even protons. It is important in metabolism to transport compounds generated in one cellular compartment into another. Specific proteins, sometimes called translocases, mediate transport across membranes. The identification of a number of such translocases and their physiological role are considered in this section.

First of all, ATP is generated within the mitochondrion and functions predominantly in the cytosol. In the cytosol, ADP and Pi are formed. Two different translocases are necessary for transporting these substances. ATP is transported out in exchange for ADP (an antiport system). Both ATP and ADP are transported down a concentration gradient. Under physiological conditions, ADP is transported down its gradient into the mitochondrial matrix. These processes are inhibited by a plant-derived toxin called **atractyloside.** Phosphate is transported into the mitochondrion in exchange for hydroxide. The mitochondrial hydroxide concentration exceeds that of the cytosol. Carriers also exist for the exchange of α-ketoglutarate for malate, citrate for malate, phosphate for malate, and aspartate for glutamate. Transport proteins do not exist for the following substances and the biochemical ramifications will be considered in appropriate sections: NAD$^+$, NADH, NADP$^+$, NADPH, coenzyme A, acyl-CoA, and oxaloacetate.

We will now consider the transport of reducing equivalents. One important source of cytosolic reductant includes the NADH (two per mole of glucose metabolized) generated during glycolysis. Only a small proportion of NAD$^+$ is regenerated by the lactate dehydrogenase reaction in nearly all cells (except mature erythrocytes) under aerobic conditions. Since a translocase for NADH is nonexistent, the cell utilizes an indirect method called the **malate–aspartate shuttle.** Two membrane translocases are required: one is specific for malate and α-ketoglutarate, and the second exchanges the amino acids aspartate and glutamate. Two sets of two enzymes also are also required: mitochondrial and cytosolic malate dehydrogenase and aspartate aminotransferase.

Let us consider the various aspects of this shuttle for reducing equivalents beginning with NADH in the cytosol, shown on the lower left of Figure 4-24. Malate dehydrogenase catalyzes a reaction between oxaloacetate and NADH + H$^+$ to yield NAD$^+$ and malate. The NAD$^+$ can now participate in the glyceraldehyde-3-phosphate dehydrogenase reaction of glycolysis. Malate is translocated into the mitochondrial matrix, and α-ketoglutarate is transported outward. Inside the mitochondrion, malate dehydrogenase catalyzes a reaction of substrate with NAD$^+$ to yield oxaloacetate and NADH + H$^+$. The latter serves as reductant for the respiratory chain and leads to the formation of three ATPs. Two NADH equivalents in the cytosol generated from a mole of glucose (two moles of triose phosphate) will yield six ATPs. If a malate–oxaloacetate exchange protein occurred, the shuttle would be much less complex. Such a system, however, does not exist and additional processes are necessary to re-establish the initial conditions. Oxaloacetate (derived from malate) reacts with glutamate to yield aspartate and α-ketoglutarate. Aspartate is transported in exchange for glutamate. To resume the initial conditions, external aspartate reacts with α-ketoglutarate to yield oxaloacetate and glutamate.

ATP YIELD

We have seen that the conversion of 1 mole of glucose to 2 moles of pyruvate during glycolysis results in the net formation of two ATP equivalents. Let us now consider the energy yield following the complete oxidation of glucose by the Krebs cycle and oxidative phosphorylation. We can also determine the yield of ATP from selected intermediates. We noted that intramitochondrial NADH yields three ATPs and FAD containing enzymes such as succinate dehydrogenase, which feed reducing equiva-

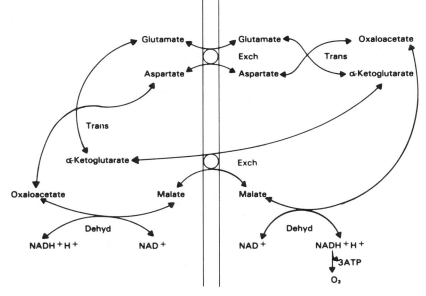

Fig. 4-24. Malate-aspartate shuttle for transporting reducing equivalents into the mitochondrion.

lents into the respiratory chain at the level of coenzyme Q yield two ATPs. Table 4-10 summarizes the various reactions in the catabolism of glucose indicating that this process is associated with the formation of 38 ATPs/mole of glucose. We can also calculate that a mole of pyruvate yields 15 ATPs, and one of acetyl-CoA yields 12 ATP equivalents. The reader should verify the correctness of these values.

Glycogen Metabolism

Before considering the catabolism of lipids and amino acids, we will consider some additional aspects of carbohydrate metabolism. We will first consider the pathways for glycogen formation (glycogenesis) and glycogen degradation (glycogenolysis). In the next sections we will discuss the pentose phosphate pathway and gluconeogenesis. The latter term refers to the pathway for glucose biosynthesis from pyruvate, lactate, and citric acid cycle intermediates.

Glycogen serves as a reservoir or storage form of carbohydrate. It is a polymer of glucose residues and is found in all cells except mature erythrocytes. The major stores of glycogen in human occur in liver and muscle tissues. Liver glycogen serves as a source of glucose in blood. Muscle glycogen is a source of fuel for muscle contraction. Glycogen is a branched, treelike molecule with a large molecular weight (up to 1 million). The straight chain portions are composed of α-1,4-glycosidic bonds, and the branch points occur at α-1,6 bonds. Branches occur about every 10th residue (Fig. 4-25).

Glycogen biosynthesis begins with glucose-6-phosphate. Phosphoglucomutase (PGM) catalyzes the isogonic conversion of glucose-6-phosphate to glucose-1-phosphate. The next reaction is designed to produce an activated high-energy form of glucose for biosynthesis, which is UDPG. A UDPG

TABLE 4-10. ATPs Generated During the Complete Oxidation of Glucose and Other Substances by Glycolysis with the Malate–Asparate Shuttle, Citric Acid Cycle Reactions, and Oxidative Phosphorylation

PROCESS OR REACTION	ATP YIELD	
Glycolysis (glucose → 2 pyruvate)	2	
Two NADH from glyceraldehyde-3-phosphate dehydrogenase and malate shuttle	6	
Pyruvate dehydrogenase (2 NADH)	6	
Isocitrate dehydrogenase (2 NADH)	6	
α-Ketoglutarate dehydrogenase (2 NADH)	6	
Succinate thiokinase (2 substrate level)	2	
Succinate dehydrogenase (2 FADH₂)	4	
Malate dehydrogenase (2 NADH)	6	
	38	ATP yield per hexose
NADH (1)	3	
FADH₂ (1)	2	
Acetyl-CoA (1)	12	
Pyruvate (1)	15	

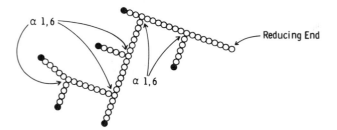

Fig. 4-25. Branched structure of glycogen.

pyrophosphorylase catalyzes a reaction between uridine triphosphate (UTP) and glucose-1-phosphate to produce UDPG and PPi. This reaction is isogonic. We see for the first time a reaction in which PPi is a product. Its only known metabolic fate in humans is hydrolysis to yield two Pi molecules; the reaction is catalyzed by a ubiquitous and separate inorganic pyrophosphatase. This hydrolytic reaction is exergonic and physiologically irreversible. The formation of PPi and its hydrolysis represents one mechanism for pulling a specific reaction forward. This happens to be a rather general and noteworthy principle of metabolism (see Table 4-1). Many reactions are associated with the so-called pyrophosphate split, and invariably the bioenergetics and principles are those enunciated here.

The glycosidic bond between a sugar and pyrophosphate as found in UDPG is energy rich with a standard free energy of hydrolysis of −7 kcal/mole. Two enzyme activities are required for glycogen biosynthesis. The first involves the formation of linear chains, and the second is responsible for the formation of branch points. *Glycogen synthase* cata-

lyzes the reaction between glycogen$_n$ containing n glycosyl residues and UDPG to yield glycogen$_{n+1}$ and UDP; the high energy bond of UDPG is converted into a low-energy glycosidic bond, and the reaction is exergonic and physiologically irreversible (Fig. 4-26). After 12 to 16 glucosyl residues are added distal to a branch point, then a *branching enzyme* transfers a block of six or so residues to yield a new branch. Both ends of the branch can now be elongated in reactions catalyzed by glycogen synthase. Hepatic glycogen synthesis occurs postprandially from the glucose substrate transported by way of the hepatic portal vein.

Two enzymes are necessary for glycogenolysis (the degradation or lysis of glycogen). *Glycogen-phosphorylase* (usually called phosphorylase) catalyzes a reaction between Pi and glycogen to yield glucose-1-phosphate and glycogen$_{n-1}$ (Fig. 4-27). This phosphorolysis (lysis by phosphate) reaction occurs at α-1,4-glycosidic bonds and is modestly exergonic. Note that this is not a hydrolysis reaction. The reaction occurs until a glucose residue about four residues from a branch point is reached. Then a single protein with two enzymatic activities, called *debranching enzyme,* mediates the elimination of the branch. A glucosyltransferase activity moves three glucosyl residues as a block leaving a single glucose in α-1,6 linkage at a branch point; the glycosyl group is added elsewhere to extend a straight chain with the α-1,4 bond (Fig. 4-28). Then the debrancher catalyzes the hydrolytic removal of glucose at the branch point to yield free glucose and the remainder of the glycogen molecule (Fig. 4-29).

Most of the glucosyl residues from glycogen are released as phosphate esters by the phosphorylase

Fig. 4-26. Glycogen synthesis.

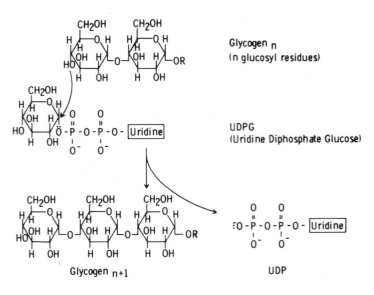

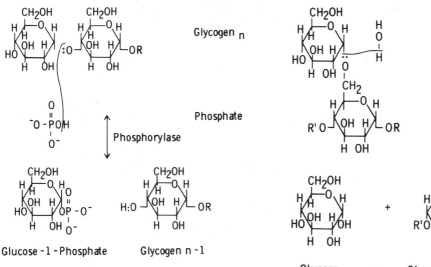

Fig. 4-27. Glycogen phosphorylase catalyzes a phosphorylytic cleavage of glycogen to yield glucose-1-phosphate.

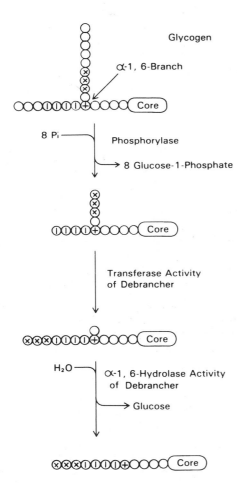

Fig. 4-28. Glycogenolysis requires phosphorylase and debrancher activities.

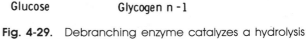

Fig. 4-29. Debranching enzyme catalyzes a hydrolysis reaction yielding free glucose.

reaction. The resulting glucose-1-phosphate is converted to glucose-6-phosphate by PGM. About 10% of the residues are hydrolytically released as free glucose by the debranching reaction. For the metabolism of free glucose, it must be phosphorylated by ATP to form glucose-6-phosphate in a reaction catalyzed by hexokinase or glucokinase. An additional noteworthy property of phosphorylase is that it requires pyridoxal phosphate as cofactor. Several inborn errors of metabolism, called glycogen-storage diseases, have been described. Their names and associated enzyme deficiencies are given in Table 4-11.

GLYCOGENESIS AND GLYCOGENOLYSIS REGULATION

The biosynthesis and degradation of glycogen are the result of distinct enzyme-catalyzed reactions. This allows for enhancement of the activity of one process with concomitant inhibition of the other. It was through the study of the regulation of these processes that the metabolic regulation by the cyclic AMP second messenger system was first enunciated by Earl W. Sutherland, Jr. The initial problem centered on the mechanism of hyperglycemia following epinephrine secretion. We now know that epinephrine activates a specific receptor (the β-adrenergic receptor) found in the liver cell membrane. The activated receptor interacts with a G_s protein (guanine nucleotide–binding protein, stimulatory). G_s is composed of three subunits (α, β, and γ). The

TABLE 4-11. Glycogen-Storage Diseases

TYPE	NAME	DEFICIENCY	COMMENTS
I	von Gierke*	Glucose-6-phosphatase	Liver and kidney have increased glycogen of normal structure
II	Pompe*	α-1 → 4 Glucosidase	Lysosomal disease
III	Cori	Debrancher	Highly branched glycogen
IV	Andersen	Brancher	Sparsely branched glycogen
V	McCardle*	Muscle phosphorylase	Proved role of glycogen synthase in glycogenesis
VI	—	Liver phosphorylase	—

* Noteworthy.

α subunit exchanges GTP for GDP and dissociates from the β and γ subunits and interacts with adenylate cyclase and activates it. Adenylate cyclase catalyzes the formation of cyclic AMP and PPi from ATP. Cyclic AMP then activates a cognate protein kinase (cyclic AMP–dependent protein kinase). The following equation describes this activation:

$$R_2C_2 + 4 \text{ cyclic AMP} \rightleftharpoons 2\ C + R_2 - \text{cyclic AMP}_4$$
(less active)   (more active)

R designates a *r*egulatory subunit, and C designates a *c*atalytic subunit.

Let us first consider how this process activates glycogenolysis, and then we will consider how it inhibits glycogenesis. The catalytic subunit of a cyclic AMP–dependent protein kinase catalyzes the phosphorylation of a second protein kinase called phosphorylase kinase. The activity of phosphorylase kinase is thereby increased. This enzyme now catalyzes the phosphorylation of the enzyme (glycogen) phosphorylase. The phosphorylated enzyme, called **phosphorylase a,** is the more active form. The unphosphorylated enzyme is called **phosphorylase b** and is less active. Phosphorylase a then catalyzes the degradation of glycogen. Consider the role of glycogenolysis *in vivo.* The major metabolite, glucose-1-phosphate, is converted into glucose-6-phosphate, which can in turn be hydrolyzed to glucose and released into the blood stream. The enzyme catalyzing this reaction is glucose-6-phosphatase, which is present in the liver and, to some extent, the kidney. All other tissues lack this enzyme. The liver is the most important organ in releasing stored carbohydrate into the blood stream as glucose. Other organs are unable to do so because they lack this enzyme.

An enhancement of the activity of the degradative enzyme represents one side of the coin. Let us now consider how epinephrine decreases the rate of biosynthesis of liver glycogen. The regulatory scheme parallels that described above in that an activation of cyclic AMP–dependent protein kinase

occurs. The inhibition of the chief biosynthetic enzyme, namely glycogen synthase, is produced in a direct fashion without the intermediacy of another protein kinase. The activated cyclic AMP–dependent enzyme catalyzes the phosphorylation of glycogen synthase. Following phosphorylation, glycogen synthase is less active. The phosphorylated, less active form is *d*ependent upon glucose-6-phosphate for its activity and is called the D-form. The unphosphorylated form is *i*ndependent of glucose-6-phosphate and is the I-form. As in the case of phosphorylase, regulation of glycogen synthase depends upon a combination of covalent and allosteric effectors.

Epinephrine is the hormone of "flight or fright" and produces hyperglycemia in preparation for or to sustain the response. When the stimulus subsides, let us examine the processes that reestablish the initial state of the enzymes. Decreasing epinephrine concentration decreases β-receptor occupation. The α-subunit of G_s catalyzes the hydrolysis of GTP to GDP and Pi. The α-subunit then recombines with the $\beta\gamma$-subunits and adenylate cyclase activity returns to unstimulated or basal levels. A phosphodiesterase catalyzes the hydrolysis and destruction of cyclic AMP by converting it to 5′AMP. A decrease in cyclic AMP concentration favors the reassociation of the catalytic and regulatory subunits of cyclic AMP–dependent protein kinase rendering the enzyme less active. Both phosphorylase kinase and glycogen synthase are regenerated from their phosphorylated forms following hydrolytic reactions catalyzed by phospho-protein phosphatases.

To summarize this section, two enzymes are required for glycogen biosynthesis, and two are required for its degradation. The synthetic enzymes are glycogen synthase and brancher; the catabolic enzymes are phosphorylase and debrancher. Glucose-1-phosphate is the product of phosphorylase, and free glucose results from the action of debrancher. Cyclic AMP and its cognate protein kinase enhance glycogenolysis by protein phosphorylation. Phosphorylase kinase is the target enzyme. It then catalyzes the phosphorylation and activation of phosphorylase. Cyclic AMP–dependent protein kinase catalyzes the direct phosphorylation of glycogen synthase rendering it less active. Protein phosphorylation can change the activity of the target enzyme in positive or negative direction—the result depends upon the enzyme.

Other mechanisms come into play in the regulation of glycogen metabolism. These include the concentrations of circulating glucose and the concentrations of the hormones insulin and glucagon. Glucose *per se* also decreases phosphorylase activity in an allosteric fashion and thereby inhibits glycogenolysis. Higher blood glucose levels stimulate the release of insulin from the β-cells of the pancreas. Insulin promotes glucose transport from the extracellular space into muscle and adipose tissue; it has no direct effect on glucose transport into liver or brain cells. Insulin may increase glycogen synthase activity in liver cells by enzyme induction. Glucagon release is enhanced at low blood glucose concentrations. It interacts with its specific receptor in the liver cell membrane, and this in turn activates adenylate cyclase. The mechanism for stimulating glycogenolysis and inhibiting glycogenesis is the same as that described for epinephrine. Note that the epinephrine receptor and glucagon receptor, although different molecules, activate adenylate cyclase by a similar mechanism by interaction with a G_s protein.

Gluconeogenesis

The supply of hepatic glycogen is limited, and other fuels must be utilized to maintain normal blood glucose levels following even an overnight fast. *Gluconeogenesis* is the process responsible for converting lactate (produced by red blood cells, muscle, and other tissues), glycerol (produced from lipolysis or triglyceride catabolism), pyruvate, and intermediates of the tricarboxylic acid cycle (derived from amino acid catabolism) into glucose. Lactate is also produced by muscle during anaerobic conditions and functions as part of the Cori cycle mentioned earlier. Gluconeogenesis occurs in the liver and to a lesser extent in the kidney. The pathway is absent in muscle, heart, and brain tissue, and in other organs. Although muscle and heart tissue can utilize other metabolic fuels such as free fatty acids and ketone bodies *(vide infra)*, the brain is completely dependent upon circulating glucose, and it is for this reason that adequate blood glucose levels must be maintained.

We will first consider the conversion of pyruvate to glucose. As noted earlier, nine enzyme-catalyzed reactions are shared by glycolysis and gluconeogenesis. Three reactions of glycolysis are highly exergonic and biochemically irreversible. These are the reactions catalyzed by hexokinase, PFK, and pyruvate kinase. The process of gluconeogenesis can be more easily understood if we consider how these reactions are bypassed.

First, we will consider the conversion of pyruvate to PEP. The very large negative free energy of hydrolysis of PEP (-14.8 kcal/mole) is an indication that it is very energy rich in nature. The direct phosphorylation of pyruvate by ATP does not occur to a physiologically important extent. To overcome the thermodynamic barrier, nature has utilized a two-step pathway. *Pyruvate carboxylase* catalyzes a reaction between ATP, pyruvate, and bicarbonate to yield oxaloacetate, ADP, and Pi as considered earlier. The reaction is isogonic. This reaction occurs within the mitochondrion. The subsequent reactions of gluconeogenesis take place in the cytosol. As noted previously, oxaloacetate *per se* is not transported across the inner mitochondrial membrane. It is converted to malate, transported outside the mitochondrion, and oxidized to yield oxaloacetate. *Phosphoenolpyruvate carboxykinase* (PEP carboxykinase) catalyzes a reaction between oxaloacetate and GTP to yield PEP, GDP, and Pi. This reaction is nearly isogonic. Two high-energy bonds ($\Delta G^{\circ l}$ of hydrolysis of -7.3 kcal/mole) are expended to form the energy-rich linkage of PEP ($\Delta G^{\circ l} = -14.8$ kcal/mole). The enzymes of glycolysis catalyze the formation of fructose-1,6-bisphosphate. To circumvent the PFK reaction, *fructose-1,6-bisphosphatase* catalyzes the hydrolysis of this compound to yield fructose-6-phosphate and Pi; this is an exergonic reaction and is physiologically irreversible. Following a reaction catalyzed by phosphohexose isomerase, *glucose-6-phosphatase* catalyzes the hydrolysis of its substrate to yield glucose and Pi; the reaction is physiologically irreversible.

The stoichiometry for the gluconeogenesis pathway is as follows:

$$
\begin{array}{ccc}
2\ \text{pyruvate} & & \text{glucose} \\
+ & & + \\
2\ \text{NADH} + 2\text{H}^+ & & 2\ \text{NAD}^+ \\
+ & & + \\
2\ \text{GTP} & \rightarrow & 2\ \text{GDP} \\
+ & & + \\
2\ \text{ATP} & & 2\ \text{ADP} \\
+ & & + \\
4\ \text{H}_2\text{O} & & 4\ \text{Pi}
\end{array}
$$

Note that four high-energy bonds are expended and that 2 moles of reduced NADH are required.

Let us next consider the regulation of this pathway. When glucose and insulin levels are low, there is an increase in catabolism of fatty acids in the liver. This is accompanied by an increase in the concentrations of citrate and acetyl-CoA. *Acetyl-CoA* activates pyruvate carboxylase (the first step in gluconeogenesis). Acetyl-CoA also inhibits pyruvate dehydrogenase activity by activating a pyruvate dehydrogenase kinase. Furthermore, citrate inhibits PFK and decreases catabolism by glycolysis. *Fructose-2,6-bisphosphate* is another allosteric regulator of glycolysis and gluconeogenesis; it interacts with PFK and fructose-1,6-bisphosphatase. Fructose-2,6-bisphosphate activates PFK and inhibits fructose-1,6-bisphosphatase. Its presence favors glycolysis. Under conditions favoring gluconeogenesis, the concentration of fructose-2,6-bisphosphate declines. This removes a stimulus for PFK and an inhibitor of fructose-1,6-bisphosphatase.

Fructose-2,6-bisphosphate is formed in a reaction involving fructose-6-phosphate and ATP; ADP is the other product. Fructose-2,6-bisphosphate is degraded by hydrolysis to form fructose-6-phosphate. A single protein contains the kinase and phosphatase activities that catalyze these reactions. The phosphorylation of this protein by cyclic AMP–dependent protein kinase increases the phosphatase activity and decreases the fructose-6-phosphate 2-kinase activity. This occurs under conditions of low plasma glucose and insulin, or high glucagon levels. Agents that elevate cyclic AMP levels in the liver promote gluconeogenesis, and this observation can be used to rationalize the reciprocal effects and levels of fructose-2,6-bisphosphate.

The simultaneous operation of two opposing pathways such as glycolysis and gluconeogenesis is called a *futile cycle.* The net transformation of metabolites fails to occur; it is associated with the loss of ATP as illustrated by the following:

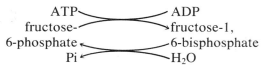

Regulatory mechanisms apparently operate to minimize futile cycles *in vivo.*

Let us now consider the pathway for other substances that serve as substrates for gluconeogenesis. Lactate is converted to pyruvate by the lactate dehydrogenase reaction in one step as considered previously. Alanine is converted into pyruvate by alanine aminotransferase in one step as will be considered in a later section. Alanine is one of the most important substrates for human gluconeogenesis. It is mobilized from muscle. Amino acids which can be converted into tricarboxylic acid cycle intermediates also serve as substrates for gluconeogenesis. They can be converted to oxaloacetate in the Krebs cycle, and the subsequent reactions of gluconeogenesis follow.

The β-oxidation of fatty acids containing an even number of carbon atoms (the most common case) yields acetyl-CoA. In humans, acetyl-CoA cannot lead to a net increase in glucose and other carbohydrates. This is because of the unidirectional nature of the tricarboxylic acid cycle. Following the reaction with oxaloacetate to yield citrate, two carbon atoms are eliminated during the conversion to oxaloacetate (see Fig. 4-21). Due to the lack of a net increase in the number of carbon atoms in the resulting metabolite, acetyl-CoA cannot serve as a source for the net production of carbohydrate. This is the explanation for the often cited and noteworthy aphorism that fat (fatty acids) cannot be converted to carbohydrate in humans.

Pentose Phosphate Pathway

In addition to the Embden–Meyerhof glycolytic pathway, the pentose phosphate pathway represents a second scheme for the metabolism of glucose-6-phosphate. The function of the pathway is twofold. First, it is responsible for the production of biosynthetic reducing equivalents as NADPH. One of the noteworthy principles of human biochemistry is that NADPH is used in biosynthetic reactions, and NADH is produced in catabolic reactions (see Table 4-1). NADPH is important in fatty acid and steroid biosynthesis. The tissues and organs that exhibit high activities of the enzymes of the pentose phosphate pathway include adipose tissue, the liver (an important organ for fatty acid and cholesterol biosynthesis), adrenal cortex (steroid hormone biosynthesis), and lactating mammary gland (lipid biosynthesis). The second major function of this pathway is the generation of pentose sugars. These occur in nucleotides such as ATP, NAD^+, $NADP^+$, RNA, and DNA. We will see that NADPH is produced concomitantly with pentose phosphates. The requirement for NADPH, however, is generally much greater than that of the pentose phosphates. Enzymes exist which convert the pentose phosphates to triose phosphate and glucose-6-phosphate to affect conversion of the five-carbon sugar derivatives. The pentose phosphate pathway is a very flexible one and allows for the interconversion of many carbohydrate intermediates.

The pentose phosphate pathway can be divided into two portions. The first is the **oxidative branch** and is associated with NADPH production. The second is the **nonoxidative branch** and is associated with the interconversion of several pairs of sugar phosphates. These range from trioses to heptoses. A simplified stoichiometry of the pathway is given by the following:

$$
\begin{array}{ccc}
\text{3 glucose-6-phosphate} & & \text{2 glucose-6-phosphate} \\
+ & & + \\
\text{6 NADP}^+ & \rightarrow & \text{3 CO}_2 \\
& & + \\
& & \text{1 glyceraldehyde-} \\
& & \text{3-phosphate} \\
& & + \\
& & \text{6 NADPH + 6 H}^+
\end{array}
$$

Let us first consider the oxidative branch. **Glucose-6-phosphate dehydrogenase** catalyzes a reaction between substrate and NADP$^+$ to form 6-phosphogluconolactone and NADPH + H$^+$ in a reversible fashion. Next, a specific **lactonase** catalyzes the hydrolysis of the lactone to yield 6-phosphogluconate in an irreversible hydrolytic reaction. **6-Phosphogluconate dehydrogenase** catalyzes an oxidative decarboxylation yielding **ribulose-5-phosphate,** CO$_2$, NADPH, and H$^+$. Two moles of NADPH are generated per hexose phosphate. This concludes the oxidative branch.

Let us now consider the nonoxidative branch of the pathway. It involves four enzymes: two catalyze specific reactions, and two catalyze general reactions. The specific enzymes include a **3-epimerase,** which mediates the reversible interconversion of ribulose-5-phosphate and xylulose-5-phosphate. The second is a **ketoisomerase,** which catalyzes the reversible interconversion of ribulose-5-phosphate (a ketopentose) and ribose-5-phosphate (an aldopentose). The two general enzymes are **transaldolase** and **transketolase.** The former contains an essential lysine residue that mediates the transfer of a three-carbon fragment from a donor to an acceptor. Transketolase contains **thiamine pyrophosphate** as an essential cofactor and mediates the transfer of a two-carbon ketonyl fragment to an appropriate acceptor. From the reactants and products of a reaction, one can deduce whether the enzyme is a transketolase (two-carbon transfer) or transaldolase (three-carbon transfer).

Next let us consider the pathway for the transformation of 3 moles of ribulose-5-phosphate (15 carbons) to 2 moles of glucose-6-phosphate (12 carbons) and 1 mole of glyceraldehyde-3-phosphate (3 carbons). Two moles of ribulose-5-phosphate are transformed into xylulose-5-phosphate by the 3-epimerase, and one is transformed into ribose-5-phosphate by ketoisomerase. Then transketolase transfers a two-carbon fragment from xylulose-5-phosphate to ribose-5-phosphate to form sedoheptulose-7-phosphate and glyceraldehyde-3-phosphate. Transaldolase then operates on these two substrates and transfers a three-carbon fragment from sedoheptulose-7-phosphate to glyceraldehyde-3-phosphate yielding fructose-6-phosphate and erythrose-4-phosphate. Fructose-6-phosphate can be metabolized by glycolysis or converted to glucose-6-phosphate and metabolized by the pentose phosphate pathway. Transketolase then catalyzes the transfer of a two-carbon fragment from xylulose-5-phosphate and erythrose-4-phosphate to yield fructose-6-phosphate and glyceraldehyde-3-phosphate. Both compounds are intermediates for glycolysis or gluconeogenesis and will be further metabolized depending upon metabolic need. Despite extensive investigation, little is known about the mechanism of regulation of the pentose phosphate pathway.

The pentose phosphate pathway plays an important role in maintaining the mature erythrocyte. It provides NADPH for the reduction of oxidized glutathione. **Glutathione** is a tripeptide (γ-glutamyl-cysteinylglycine). It exists as the reduced (G-SH) and oxidized forms (G-S-S-G). **Glutathione reductase** converts the oxidized to the reduced form:

$$
\begin{array}{ccc}
\text{GSSG} & & \text{2 GSH} \\
+ & \rightarrow & + \\
\text{NADPH + H}^+ & & \text{NADP}^+
\end{array}
$$

Reduced glutathione is a substrate for **glutathione peroxidase** (selenium is a cofactor):

$$
\text{2 GSH} + \text{H}_2\text{O}_2 \rightarrow \text{GSSG} + \text{2 H}_2\text{O}
$$

This reaction plays an important role in destroying H$_2$O$_2$ in the erythrocyte. Recall that the mature erythrocyte lacks membranous cellular organelles, such as peroxisomes, which are found in nucleated cells. Catalase in peroxisomes mediates the conversion of hydrogen peroxide to water and molecular oxygen (H$_2$O$_2 \rightarrow$ H$_2$O + 1/2 O$_2$). Glutathione peroxidase functions in the red blood cell to destroy hydrogen peroxide as catalase functions in other cells. A deficiency of glucose-6-phosphate dehydrogenase is associated with drug-induced hemolytic anemias produced by primaquine (an antimalarial agent) and other substances. Hemolysis may be related to deficient NADPH production for the glutathione peroxidase reaction.

Fatty Acid Oxidation and Biosynthesis

The important classes of lipids in humans include triacylglycerols (triglycerides), phospholipids, and steroids. Triacylglycerol serves as the main storage form of metabolic fuel in humans. It is the most concentrated form of metabolic energy (9 kcal/g); moreover, it is stored in an anhydrous state and represents 10% to 15% or more of the total body mass. It can subserve humans for weeks or months of starvation. In contrast, stored carbohydrate is depleted in a day or so and must be replenished by gluconeogenesis. Glycogen is extensively hydrated, and this increases its bulk. A gram of tissue glycogen contains an equivalent amount of bound water. Glycogen does not represent as efficient an energy storage form as triglyceride. Amino acids and proteins are not stored to any appreciable extent.

Fatty acids stored in adipose tissue are released from triglycerides by hydrolysis reactions catalyzed by triglyceride lipase. This is also called *hormone-sensitive lipase* because it responds to circulating epinephrine by undergoing phosphorylation by cyclic AMP–dependent protein kinase and concomitant activation. The liberated fatty acids are transported in the circulation as a complex with albumin and are taken up by most organs or tissues (except the brain). After entering the cells, the fatty acids must be derivatized as thioesters with coenzyme A prior to metabolism. A family of *fatty acyl coenzyme A synthetases* and *pyrophosphatase* catalyze these reactions in the cytosol.

(a)   fatty acid + ATP + coenzyme A $\rightleftharpoons$
           fatty acyl-CoA + AMP + PPi
(b)   PPi + H$_2$O $\rightarrow$ 2 Pi

The first reaction *(a)* involves the formation of an intermediate fatty acyl-adenylate and PPi. Coenzyme A displaces the adenylate to yield fatty acyl-CoA and AMP. The family of enzymes differs in the chain length specificity. Long chain (16 carbons or more), intermediate chain (6–14 carbons), and short chain (2–4 carbons) specific enzymes have been described. Thioesters are energy-rich bonds. To pull the reaction forward as mentioned in Table 4-1, pyrophosphatase (a separate enzyme) catalyzes the hydrolysis of PPi to yield two Pi molecules in an exergonic and biochemically irreversible reaction *(b)*.

As noted previously, coenzyme A and its derivatives do not pass through the inner mitochondrial

membrane. To effectuate the transfer of fatty acids into the mitochondrial matrix (the site of fatty acid oxidation; see Table 2-4), the formation of fatty acyl-carnitine is required. This isogonic process is catalyzed by carnitine acyl transferase I:

fatty acyl-CoA   fatty acyl-carnitine
        + $\rightleftharpoons$ +
    carnitine   coenzyme A

The fatty acyl-carnitine is transported into mitochondria in exchange for carnitine. Once inside the mitochondrion, carnitine acyltransferase II catalyzes the reverse reaction yielding fatty acyl-CoA and free carnitine. Carnitine ($(CH_3)_3N^+CH_2CH-(OH)CH_2COO^-$) forms an ester linkage through its —OH group with the carboxyl group of the fatty acid.

BETA-OXIDATION

The conversion of fatty acyl-CoA to acetyl-CoA requires the action of four enzymes. The stoichiometry for the conversion of steroyl-CoA (18-carbon atoms) to 9 moles of acetyl-CoA is as follows:

steroyl-CoA   9 acetyl-CoA
     +   +
  8 FAD   8 FADH$_2$
     + $\rightarrow$ +
  8 NAD$^+$ 8 NADH + 8 H$^+$
     +
8 coenzyme A

The cyclic pathway for β-oxidation is illustrated in Figure 4-30. An *acyl-CoA dehydrogenase* catalyzes an isogonic oxidation to yield the trans-enoyl-CoA and FADH$_2$. The reducing equivalents are donated to the electron-transport chain at the level of coenzyme Q and will provide energy for the formation of two ATPs. Next, an *enoyl-CoA hydratase* catalyzes an isogonic hydration yielding an L-β-hydroxyacyl-CoA. The resulting compound is oxidized by NAD$^+$ in a reaction catalyzed by *hydroxyacyl-CoA dehydrogenase* to yield β-ketoacyl-CoA, NADH, and H$^+$. Oxidation of NADH by the respiratory chain yields three ATPs. Next, *β-ketothiolase* (thiolase) catalyzes an exergonic cleavage or thiolysis by coenzyme A to yield acetyl-CoA and an acyl-CoA lacking the two carbon atoms. For steroyl-CoA, the β-oxidation cycle (see Fig. 4-30) occurs eight times with the stoichiometry shown in the previous paragraph.

This series of reactions can be more easily remembered and understood when it is realized that they are analogous to three reactions in the Krebs

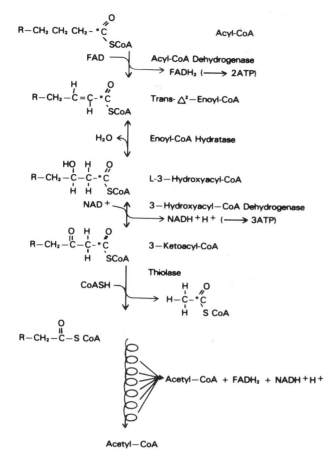

Fig. 4-30. β-oxidation of fatty acyl-CoA.

TABLE 4-12. ATP Yield From the Complete Oxidation of Stearic Acid (18C)

PROCESS		ATP RESULTING
8 FADH$_2$	8 × 2	16
8 NADH + 8 H$^+$	8 × 3	24
9 Acetyl-CoA	9 × 12	108
		148
ATP required for steroyl-CoA formation*		−2
Net ATP production		146

*ATP → AMP + 2 Pi.

citric acid cycle. The pattern of the first oxidation in β-oxidation by FAD is analogous to the succinate dehydrogenase reaction (with two ATPs resulting by oxidative phosphorylation). The hydration reaction in β-oxidation parallels that catalyzed by fumarase. Finally the oxidation of an alcohol by NAD$^+$ to form a ketone parallels that of the malate dehydrogenase reaction. Three ATP molecules result from the NADH formed by this process.

Let us now consider the number of ATPs formed from ADP and Pi as a result of the β-oxidation of the 18-carbon stearic acid and reactions of the Krebs cycle and oxidative phosphorylation. This is shown in Table 4-12. The net production takes into account the fact that the fatty acid must be converted to a coenzyme A derivative with the expenditure of two high-energy bonds (ATP → AMP + 2 Pi).

A small percentage of fatty acids in the human diet contain an odd number of carbon atoms. They undergo β-oxidation and yield propionyl-CoA and acetyl-CoA following the final thiolytic cleavage.

Propionyl-CoA is also produced during the catabolism of several amino acids; the pathway for its metabolism is quantitatively more important for amino acid metabolism than in the metabolism of the uncommon odd-chain fatty acids. This pathway requires the participation of vitamin B$_{12}$.

Propionyl-CoA carboxylase catalyzes a reaction between substrate, bicarbonate, and ATP to yield D-methylmalonyl-CoA, ADP, and Pi (Fig. 4-31). This ATP-dependent carboxylation reaction, like several others, involves a biotin prosthetic group. An ***epimerase*** catalyzes an isogonic conversion of D-methylmalonyl-CoA to the L-isomer. ***Methylmalonyl-CoA mutase*** (a vitamin B$_{12}$–dependent enzyme) catalyzes the conversion of L-methylmalonyl-CoA to succinyl-CoA. The carbonyl-SCoA is transferred to the carbon marked with the asterisk to yield the final product (see Fig. 4-31). Succinyl-

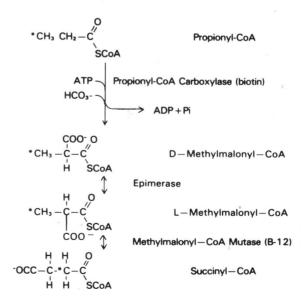

Fig. 4-31. Conversion of propionyl-CoA to succinyl-CoA.

CoA is an intermediate in the tricarboxylic acid cycle and is metabolized by familiar reactions. The association of **vitamin B₁₂** with **methylmalonyl-CoA mutase** is noteworthy.

Two other enzyme activities are important in fatty acid catabolism. One is a Δ3-cis, Δ2-trans-enoylisomerase. Most naturally occurring fatty acids contain cis double bonds. When a Δ3-cis bond forms as a result of the thiolytic cleavage of unsaturated fatty acids, this isomerization is necessary for subsequent reactions. When a Δ2-cis enoyl-CoA forms during the metabolism of unsaturated fatty acids (note that a Δ2-trans enoyl-CoA forms during β-oxidation), the enoyl hydratase will catalyze the hydration reaction resulting in the formation of a D-β-hydroxylacyl-CoA. This compound, however, is not a substrate for the dehydrogenase. A hydroxy-acyl-CoA epimerase catalyzes the formation of L-hydroxyacyl-CoA, which is a substrate for the dehydrogenase.

BIOSYNTHESIS

The reactions of fatty acid biosynthesis take place on a **fatty acid synthase multienzyme complex.** A priming reaction utilizing acetyl-CoA initiates the process. Then malonyl-CoA adds successive two-carbon fragments to the primer. Following each addition, four reactions convert a β-ketoacyl compound to the reduced acyl derivative. NADPH serves as reductant. The fatty acid synthase contains **acylcarrier protein** (ACP). This is a small protein containing covalently bound **4'-phospho-panthetheine.** The latter constitutes part of the molecular structure of coenzyme A. The ACP carries covalently linked intermediates from the various active sites necessary for biosynthesis. The —SH group of ACP is called the **central thiol.** An enzymic cysteine constitutes a **peripheral thiol.** After the 16-carbon palmitoyl group is formed, free palmitate is released by hydrolysis.

Let us now consider the pathway for palmitate biosynthesis. Acetyl-CoA initiates the process by reacting with the multienzyme complex to yield an acetyl-enzyme thioester intermediate involving the peripheral thiol group. This acetyl group will contribute carbon atoms 15 and 16 of the 16-carbon palmitate. They are at the omega end of the fatty acid, that is, furthest removed from the carboxyl group. The other 14-carbon atoms are contributed by malonyl-CoA. Let us consider its formation as catalyzed by **acetyl-CoA carboxylase:**

$$\text{ATP} + \text{HCO}_3^- + \text{acetyl-CoA} \rightleftharpoons \text{malonyl-CoA} + \text{ADP} + \text{Pi}$$

This is the rate-limiting step in fatty acid biosynthesis and is activated by citrate. Malonyl-CoA reacts with the acetyl–fatty acid synthase complex to yield coenzyme A and the malonyl group bound to the central thiol of ACP (Fig. 4-32).

The sequential series of reactions begins as the α-carbon of malonyl-ACP attacks the carbonyl group of acetyl-CoA in a condensation reaction catalyzed by **3-ketoacyl synthase** (see Fig. 4-32). A β-ketoacyl group is attached to the central thiol as the peripheral thiol is freed. CO_2 also is displaced. This decarboxylation renders the process exergonic in nature. This accounts for the formation and utilization of the malonyl group; the carboxyl activates the tail of the acetyl group for this condensation reaction. A **3-ketoacyl reductase** catalyzes a reaction with NADPH + H⁺ to form the D-β-hydroxyacyl-ACP and NADP⁺. A **dehydratase** catalyzes the elimination of water yielding a 2,3-unsaturated acyl-ACP. An **enoyl reductase** catalyzes a reaction with NADPH + H⁺ to yield the acyl-ACP. The acyl group, now elongated by two carbons, is transferred to the peripheral thiol. Next, malonyl-CoA reacts with the acyl-enzyme, and the malonyl group is linked to the central thiol. This is followed by another condensation reaction resulting in the formation of a β-ketoacyl group elongated by two carbon atoms. CO_2 is the other product. The sequence of reactions is repeated as a reduction, dehydration, and second reduction occurs. The acyl group is transferred to the peripheral thiol. A total of seven condensation reactions is required to produce the palmitoyl enzyme. A thioesterase catalyzes the hydrolytic cleavage and release of palmitate, and the free enzyme is regenerated. That fatty acids longer than palmitate cannot be synthesized by the complex is probably related to a limitation in the size of one of the active sites of the complex.

A comparison of fatty acid oxidation and synthesis is given in Table 4-13. The separate pathways and intracellular localization permit independent regulation of the processes. Although CO_2 as bicarbonate is required for malonyl-CoA formation, the added carbonyl group is released during the condensation reactions, and bicarbonate is not a direct source of the carbon atoms in fatty acids. All of the carbon atoms are derived from acetyl-CoA; the two on the omega end are derived directly from acetyl-CoA, and the others are derived from malonyl-CoA.

Let us now consider the source of NADPH and acetyl-CoA used as substrates for biosynthesis. Most of the NADPH is derived from the pentose phosphate pathway. Additional NADPH results

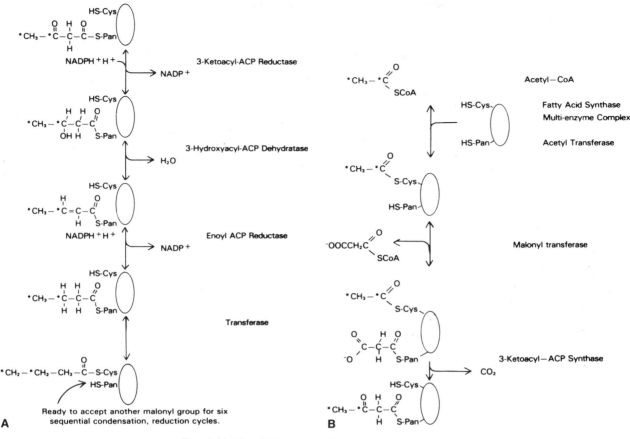

Fig. 4-32A,B. Pathway for fatty acid biosynthesis.

from the reaction catalyzed by **malic enzyme** (NADP malate dehydrogenase) shown here:

$$
\begin{array}{ccc}
\text{malate} & & \text{pyruvate} \\
+ & \rightarrow & + \\
\text{NADP}^+ & & \text{CO}_2 \\
& & + \\
& & \text{NADPH} + \text{H}^+
\end{array}
$$

The producers and consumers of NADPH occur within the cytosol, so that no barrier to effective utilization occurs.

The provision of cytosolic acetyl-CoA, however, requires transport across the mitochondrial membrane. Glucose serves as the source of carbon atoms for much of fatty acid biosynthesis. Glucose is converted to pyruvate by glycolysis. Pyruvate is transported into the mitochondria by its specific translocase and is converted to acetyl-CoA. Coenzyme A and its derivatives are not directly transportable through the inner membrane. The transport of acetyl groups occurs by citrate. Citrate is formed by the usual Krebs cycle reaction. It is transported through the inner mitochondrial membrane in exchange for malate. Once in the cytosol, **citrate lyase** (citrate cleavage enzyme) catalyzes a reaction with substrate, coenzyme A, and ATP to yield acetyl-CoA, oxaloacetate, ADP, and Pi. Acetyl-CoA then functions as a precursor for fatty acid formation. Oxaloacetate is reduced to malate and

TABLE 4-13. Comparison of Fatty Acid Oxidation and Synthesis

	OXIDATION	SYNTHESIS *de novo*
Acetyl-CoA required	+	+
Malonyl-CoA required	−	+
NAD⁺	+	−
NADPH	−	+
Coenzyme A	+	+
ACP (acyl carrier protein)	−	+
Mitochondria	+	−
Cytosol	−	+
Multienzyme complex	−	+
L-Hydroxyacyl intermediate	+	−
D-Hydroxyacyl intermediate	−	+

can be transported into the mitochondrian in exchange for citrate.

The provision of cytosolic acetyl-CoA by mitochondrial citrate provides a possible explanation for the regulation of the tricarboxylic acid cycle at the isocitrate dehydrogenase reaction. This allows for the biosynthesis of citrate and still permits the regulation of the tricarboxylic acid cycle by ADP at a distal step, that is, at the isocitrate dehydrogenase reaction. Recall that cytosolic citrate activates the acetyl-CoA carboxylase reaction (the rate-limiting reaction in fatty acid biosynthesis).

Lipid Biosynthesis and Degradation

TRIACYLGLYCEROL BIOSYNTHESIS

The substrates for triglyceride synthesis include 3 moles of fatty acyl-CoA and glycerol phosphate. The palmitic acid produced by synthesis *de novo* is thioesterified as palmitoyl-CoA in a reaction catalyzed by fatty acyl-CoA synthetase. Fatty acid,

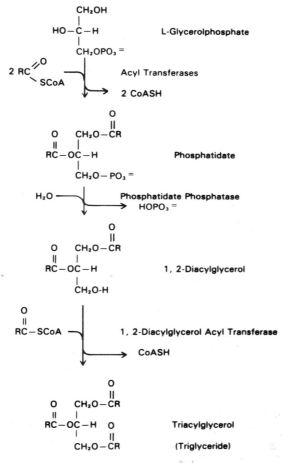

Fig. 4-33. Biosynthesis of triacylglycerol.

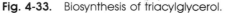

ATP, and coenzyme A are reactants and fatty acyl-CoA, AMP, and PPi are products. Palmitoyl-CoA acid may also be elongated, desaturated, or both prior to incorporation into triglyceride. Dietary fatty acids, derived from triacylglycerol, are also a major precursor of stored triglyceride. Glycerol phosphate can be obtained by the reduction of dihydroxyacetone phosphate catalyzed by **glycerol phosphate dehydrogenase** or by the ATP-dependent phosphorylation of glycerol as catalyzed by **glycerol kinase.** The fatty acyl-CoA groups are energy-rich and activated forms of fatty acids, which are logical donors in biosynthetic reactions. Four reactions yield the final product. Glycerolphosphate acyltransferase catalyzes the first reaction between fatty acyl-CoA, which is activated like a warhead, and glycerol-3-phosphate to yield 1-acylglycerol-3-phosphate. An acyltransferase catalyzes the addition of the next acyl group from fatty acyl-CoA (usually unsaturated) to yield 1,2,diacylglycerol-3-phosphate (also called phosphatidate) as shown in Figure 4-33. Next, a phosphatidate phosphatase catalyzes a hydrolysis to yield 1,2-diacylglycerol and Pi. Finally, 1,2-diacylglycerol acyltransferase catalyzes a reaction of diacylglycerol with fatty acyl-CoA to yield triacylglycerol and coenzyme A. Each of the four reactions is highly exergonic. The fatty acid thioesterified to coenzyme A constitutes a high-energy and activated form of the fatty acid. Activated monomers serve as energetically favorable precursors in condensation reactions (see Table 4-1).

PHOSPHOLIPID BIOSYNTHESIS

The important phospholipids include phosphatidylcholine (lecithin), phosphatidylserine, and phosphatidylethanolamine. The latter two compounds can be converted into phosphatidylcholine. Let us consider the pathway for phosphatidylcholine formation beginning with free choline and 1,2-diacylglycerol. This is called the salvage pathway since preformed choline is salvaged or reutilized. This will be in contrast to the *de novo* pathway (from the beginning) where choline will be formed from phosphatidylethanolamine.

Choline is first phosphorylated by ATP to yield phosphocholine and ADP in a reaction catalyzed by choline kinase (Fig. 4-34). Phosphocholine must now be converted to an activated or energy-rich form prior to its combination with an acceptor molecule (see Table 4-1). The activated form is cytidine diphosphate-choline (CDP-choline). The diphosphate linkage is that of an acid anhydride and is

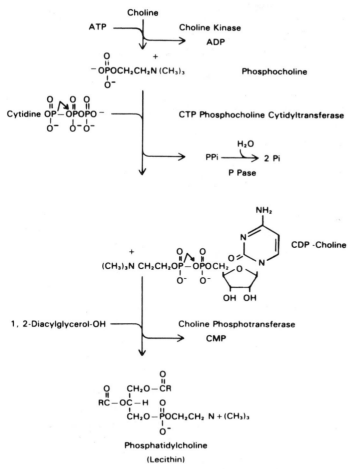

Fig. 4-34. Phosphatidylcholine biosynthesis by the salvage pathway.

energy-rich in nature with a $\Delta G^{\circ\prime}$ of hydrolysis of -7 kcal/mole. The activation process involves a reaction of cytidine triphosphate (CTP) and phosphocholine to yield CDP-choline and PPi and is catalyzed by CDP phosphocholine cytidyltransferase. This is an isogonic reaction. The process is coupled to the hydrolysis of PPi catalyzed by pyrophosphatase, which serves to pull the reaction forward (see Table 4-1). CDP-choline reacts with 1,2-diacylglycerol to yield phosphatidylcholine and cytidine monophosphate (CMP) in a reaction catalyzed by a choline phosphotransferase.

The pathway for phosphatidylethanolamine biosynthesis is analogous to that for choline biosynthesis. Ethanolamine is phosphorylated by ATP to form ethanolamine phosphate (Fig. 4-35). The latter reacts with CTP to form CDP-ethanolamine. It reacts with 1,2-diacylglycerol to form phosphatidylethanolamine. This substance occurs in the lipid bilayer of cell membranes as does phosphatidylcholine. Phosphatidylethanolamine can be converted into phosphatidylcholine in three successive trans-

methylation reactions involving S-adenosylmethionine (see Fig. 4-35).

Another cytidine derivative important in lipid metabolism is CDP-diacylglycerol. It results from a reaction involving phosphatidate and CTP and yields CDP-diacylglycerol and PPi. This reacts with inositol (a hexitol) to form phosphatidylinositol and CMP. Phosphatidylinositol is phosphorylated by ATP to form ADP and phosphatidylinositol-4-phosphate. The latter is phosphorylated by ATP to form ADP and phosphatidylinositol-4,5-bisphosphate. The latter is an important precursor for two intracellular second messengers: 1,4,5-inositoltrisphosphate and 1,2-diacylglycerol. The physiological roles of these agents are considered later.

SPHINGOLIPID BIOSYNTHESIS

This group of phospholipids contains a complex amino alcohol named sphingosine; these substances lack glycerol. **Sphingosine** is formed in a three-step process from palmitoyl-CoA and serine. In a reac-

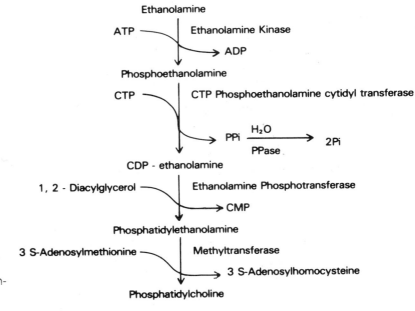

Fig. 4-35. Phosphatidylcholine biosynthesis *de novo.*

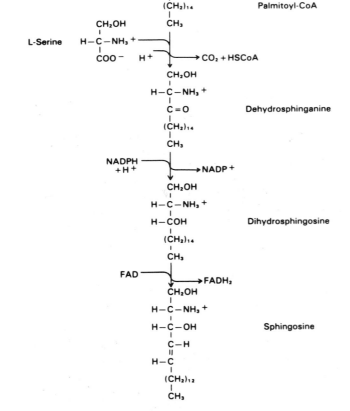

Fig. 4-36. Conversion of palmitoyl-CoA and serine to sphingosine.

tion catalyzed by a pyridoxal phosphate-dependent enzyme, the 16-carbon palmitoyl-CoA reacts with the 3-carbon serine to yield the 18-carbon dehydrosphinganine, CO_2 (from serine), and coenzyme A (Fig. 4-36). This intermediate is reduced by $NADPH + H^+$ to dihydrosphingosine, which is then oxidized to yield an unsaturated $\Delta 4$ alkene linkage in sphingosine.

Following a reaction with acyl-CoA catalyzed by an *N*-acyltransferase, sphingosine is converted to ***ceramide*** (Fig. 4-37). Ceramide (*N*-acylsphingosine) is a key intermediate in sphingolipid biosynthesis. It is converted to ***sphingomyelin*** (*O*-phosphocholine ceramide) following a reaction with CDP-choline. Ceramide is also converted to ***cerebrosides*** and ***gangliosides***. The alcohol group of ceramide reacts with an activated, UDP-sugar to yield cerebroside and UDP (see Fig. 4-37). The addition of several (up to five) sugars to ceramide yields a family of gangliosides. These are glycolipids (sugars attached to lipid).

PHOSPHOLIPID HYDROLYSIS

The specificity of several phospholipases is indicated in Figure 4-38. Two phospholipases have been implicated in several regulatory processes. Phospholipase A_2, for example, catalyzes the hydrolysis of the fatty acid at position 2. Arachidonate and other polyunsaturated fatty acids often occur in this position. Arachidonate is converted into biologically active eicosanoids (prostaglandins [PGs], pros-

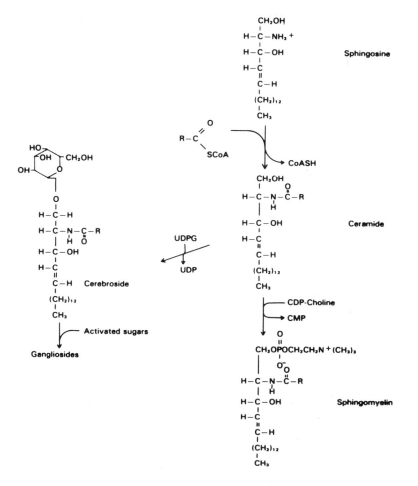

Fig. 4-37. Sphingomyelin and glanglioside biosynthesis.

tacyclins [PGIs], thromboxanes [TXs], and leuko- trienes [LTs]). Phospholipase C catalyzes the removal of a sugar alcohol at position 3. Important products derived from phosphatidylinositol-4,5-bis- phosphate include inositol trisphosphate and dia- cylglycerol; their actions will be considered later.

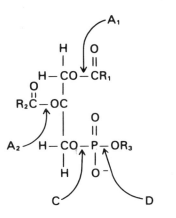

Fig. 4-38. Bonds hydrolyzed by phospholipases A_1, A_2, C, and D.

SPHINGOLIPID HYDROLYSIS

A number of diseases, called sphingolipidoses, are caused by a deficiency of enzymes that catalyze the hydrolysis of sphingolipids. These are listed in Ta- ble 4-14. The enzymes normally occur within the lysosomes. In the absence of activity, the sphingoli- pid that cannot be degraded accumulates and pro- duces the characteristic pathology. The diseases have been known much longer than the existence and functions of lysosomes. Basic research has pro- vided an intellectual and scientific framework for understanding these disorders. The design of cura- tive or effective palliative treatment remains for the future.

Ketone Body Metabolism

A group of three related biochemicals are generi- cally called **ketone bodies**. These three substances are **acetoacetate, β-hydroxybutyrate,** and **acetone.** The condition of ketosis occurs during carbohy- drate deprivation and starvation. A more severe

TABLE 4-14. Enzyme Deficiencies in Selected Sphingolipidoses

DISEASE	ENZYME	SITE OF DEFICIENT REACTION (DENOTED BY /)
Gaucher*	β-Glucosidase	Cer/Glc
Krabbe	β-Galactosidase	Cer/Gal
Niemann–Pick*	Sphingomyelinase	Cer/P-Choline
Metachromatic leukodystrophy	Arylsulfatase A	Cer-Gal/OSO$_3^-$
Tay–Sachs*	Hexosaminidase A	Cer-Glc-Gal(NeuAc)/GalNac

* Noteworthy.
    Cer = ceramide.
    Glc = glucose.
    Gal = galactose.
  NeuAc = N-acetylneuraminic acid.
 GalNAc = N-acetylgalactosamine.

form is that of diabetic ketoacidosis. Ketosis occurs in humans during the extensive mobilization of fatty acids. Ketone bodies are synthesized, but not utilized, by the liver. They are transported to extrahepatic tissues where they are consumed. Although a paradoxical contradiction in terms, ketone bodies can be considered as water-soluble lipids.

Let us first consider the biosynthesis of these substances. Like fatty acids, ketone bodies are derived from acetyl-CoA. Two moles of acetyl-CoA condense to yield acetoacetyl-CoA and coenzyme A. This constitutes the reversal of the thiolase reaction and is endergonic. Acetoacetyl-CoA is also produced by β-oxidation. One might envisage the synthesis of acetoacetate by hydrolysis of its coenzyme A thioester. This pathway, however, is not prominent or is nonexistent. The absence of such a hydrolytic enzyme prevents the loss of acetoacetyl-CoA formed during the course of the β-oxidation of fatty acids. Acetyl-CoA condenses with acetoacetyl-CoA followed by hydrolysis of one thioester bond to yield coenzyme A and 3-hydroxy-3-methylglutaryl-CoA (HMG-CoA) in a highly exergonic reaction catalyzed by **HMG-CoA synthase.** HMG-CoA is a substrate for **HMG-CoA lyase,** which catalyzes the dismutation (not hydrolysis) of substrate to form acetoacetate and acetyl-CoA. HMG-CoA synthase and lyase are found in liver mitochondria. This accounts for the exclusive production of ketone bodies by the liver. These reactions occur under conditions favoring fatty acid oxidation.

A portion of acetoacetate is reduced to form β-hydroxybutyrate by a specific dehydrogenase. This enzyme is found in liver and extrahepatic tissues. The reaction is reversible and functions in vivo in both directions depending upon metabolic need. Acetoacetate undergoes a nonenzymatic decarboxylation reaction to yield CO_2 and acetone. Acetone constitutes a metabolic dead end and is excreted in the urine or exhaled by the lungs. It does not form to a significant extent during human fasting. It does form, however, during diabetic ketoacidosis. A suggestive diagnosis of ketoacidosis can be made by smelling acetone in the breath of a comatose patient. It is reminiscent of the odor associated with fruity chewing gums. Cigarette smoke in the environment can mask the odor.

Beta-hydroxybutyrate and acetoacetate are transported from the liver to extrahepatic organs where they are taken up by cells. The β-hydroxybutyrate is oxidized to acetoacetate. It is derivatized in mitochondria in a reaction catalyzed by succinyl-CoA:acetoacetyl-CoA transferase; the coenzyme A is transferred from succinyl-CoA yielding succinate and acetoacetyl-CoA. The latter is a substrate for thiolase and yields 2 moles of acetyl-CoA. The HMG-CoA synthase and lyase in the liver explain its synthesis there. Liver tissue lacks the coenzyme A transferase; it is present in extrahepatic tissues, and this explains why it is not metabolized in the liver but is metabolized in other tissues.

Cholesterol Metabolism

Cholesterol and cholesterol esters are an important constituent of the membranes of human cells. **Cholesterol** and its ester make up about 40% by weight of the golgi and plasma membranes. It is present to a lesser extent in the endoplasmic reticulum and nuclear membranes. Cholesterol is converted into **bile acids,** which are important in lipid digestion and absorption. Cholesterol is also converted into important steroid hormones including estrogens, progesterone, testosterone, and adrenocortical hormones. The structure and numbering system for the 27-carbon compound is shown in Figure 4-39. There

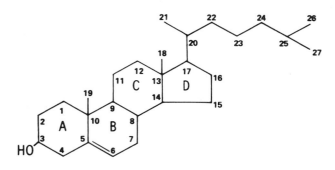

Fig. 4-39. Structure of cholesterol.

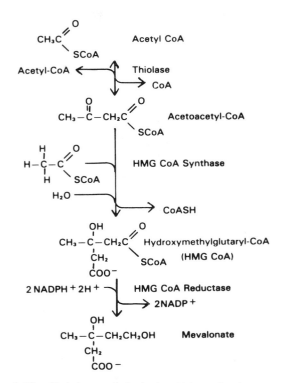

Fig. 4-40. First stage of cholesterol biosynthesis: conversion of acetyl-CoA to mevalonate.

are two sources of cholesterol in humans; it is synthesized *de novo* in all nucleated animal cells and is obtained from animal products in the diet. About 1 g per day is synthesized *de novo,* and 0.3 g per day is absorbed from the gut.

Animals lack the ability to degrade the steroid nucleus or ring system (see Fig. 4-39) to CO_2 and H_2O. Conversion of cholesterol into bile acids and excretion into the feces represents the quantitatively important route of its elimination. Conversion to steroid hormones, although important biologically, constitutes a quantitatively minor route of metabolism.

BIOSYNTHESIS

Cholesterol is derived entirely from acetyl-CoA. Acetyl-CoA is converted into the six-carbon HMG-CoA (Fig. 4-40) as previously described for ketone body formation, except that the reactions occur in the cytosol (see Table 4-2) and not in mitochondria as in the case of ketone bodies. We will consider only a few of the steps in cholesterol biosynthesis in detail. First, let us consider the committed step in the pathway, which is catalyzed by **HMG-CoA reductase.** It involves a reaction between substrate and two molecules of NADPH to form 2 $NADP^+$ and *mevalonate* (see Fig. 4-40). Mevalonate undergoes three successive phosphorylation reactions by ATP yielding mevalonate phosphate, mevalonate pyrophosphate, and mevalonate-3-phospho-5-pyrophosphate (Fig. 4-41). The latter compound undergoes a decarboxylation and elimination of Pi to yield *isopentenylpyrophosphate* (isopentenyl-PPi).

Isopentenyl-PPi undergoes an isomerization reaction to form *demethylallyl pyrophosphate.* The conversion of these isoprenoid compounds to cholesterol is outlined in Figure 4-41. Two 5-carbon

fragments (isopentenyl-PPi and dimethylallyl-PPi) condense to form the 10-carbon *geranyl-PPi*. The latter reacts with the 5-carbon isopentenyl-PPi to yield the 15-carbon *farnesyl-PPi*. Two of these react to form the 30-carbon *squalene* (first isolated from shark tissue). In a reaction involving molecular oxygen, squalene is converted into the four-membered ring system of steroids in the form of the 30-carbon *lanosterol*. Formate is released in an oxygen-dependent reaction, and this is followed by two decarboxylations resulting in the 27-carbon *zymosterol*. This is converted in two steps to the 27-carbon cholesterol.

Eicosanoids

Arachidonate (5,8,11,14 eicosatetraenoate) and other unsaturated fatty acids give rise to eicosanoids (20-carbon acids) including PGs, PGIs, TXs, and LTs. Humans cannot synthesize arachidonate *de novo*. It can be derived from linoleate or linolenate. These two fatty acids *(linoleate, linolenate)* are termed **essential fatty acids** to reflect the fact that they cannot be synthesized in humans. The eicosanoids have multiple and diverse effects. TXs, for example, are synthesized in platelets and pro-

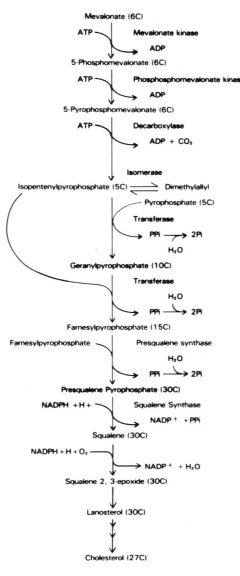

Fig. 4-41. Second stage of cholesterol biosynthesis.

duce vasoconstriction and platelet aggregation. PGIs are produced by blood vessel walls and inhibit platelet aggregation. PGs increase cycle AMP in platelets, the anterior pituitary and lung, but lower cyclic AMP levels in renal tubules and adipose cells. LTs are produced in leukocytes, platelets, and macrophages. They attract and activate leukocytes and are thought to play a role in inflammation and hypersensitivity reactions including asthma. The eicosanoids are synthesized on demand (not stored) and are released and act locally in an autocrine or paracrine fashion. These compounds also have an evanescent existence. Only the general pathway for biosynthesis is considered here.

Arachidonate is derived from phospholipids in the plasma membrane following its hydrolytic removal catalyzed by phospholipase A_2 (see Fig. 4-38). This is the rate-limiting enzyme in the pathway. Phospholipase A_2 activity is stimulated by angiotensin II, bradykinin, epinephrine, and thrombin under specific conditions. It is inhibited by anti-inflammatory corticosteroids. Arachidonate exists at a branch point in metabolism. Under the action of cyclo-oxygenase, it reacts with 2 moles of oxygen to form a prostanoid termed PGG_2. This compound is converted to one of the PGs, PGIs, or TXs by specific enzymes (Fig. 4-42). Cyclo-oxygenase is inhibited by aspirin and indomethacin.

Arachidonate, under the action of lipoxygenase, is converted to 5-hydroperoxyeicosatetraenoate (5-HPETE; see Fig. 4-42). This is converted to 5-hydroxyeicosatetraenoate (5-HETE) or to the LTs. LTs are potent constrictors of bronchial smooth muscle. Leukotriene A_4 forms a covalent adduct by a thioether linkage with glutathione to yield leukotriene C_4. Glutamate is hydrolytically removed yielding leukotriene D_4, and glycine is hydrolytically removed to yield leukotriene E_4. Sophisticated chemical techniques including gas chromatography/mass spectrometry were required to elucidate the reactions outlined in Figure 4-42, which is given for reference purposes.

Lipid Transport and Lipoproteins

Glucose and other monosaccharides, amino acids, and ketone bodies are very soluble in aqueous solution. In contrast, fatty acids, triglycerides, and cholesterol esters are sparingly soluble in water. A specialized and complex transport system has evolved to mediate the transport of lipids in the extracellular compartments between the intestine, liver, adipose tissue, and other peripheral organs. There are two general processes for affecting transport of lipids. Free fatty acids are transported as a complex with albumin. This system has a low capacity for fatty acids and an even lower capacity for cholesterol. A second system with larger capacity for triacylglycerol and cholesterol is composed of four classes of lipoproteins. The lipoproteins are made up of a hydrophilic phospholipid monolayer exterior, specific proteins (apolipoproteins) associated with the phospholipid surface, and an apolar lipid core. The principle of lipoprotein solubility and transport is dependent upon the hydrophilic nature of the particle exterior. In addition to solubility, the proteins that constitute the various classes of lipoprotein particles are endowed with properties important in se-

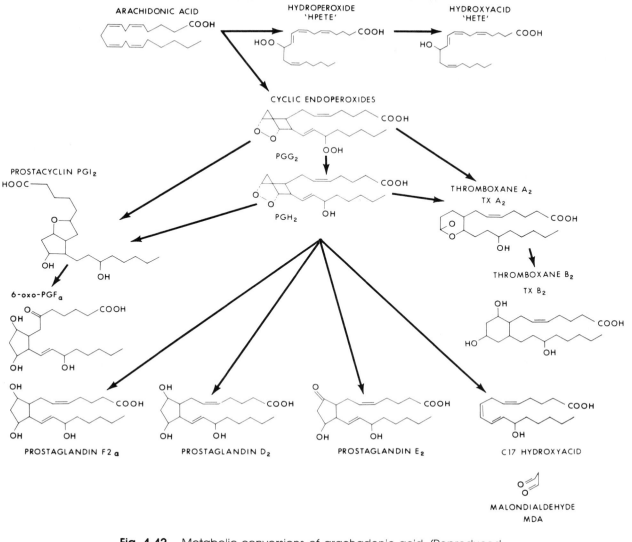

Fig. 4-42. Metabolic conversions of arachadonic acid. (Reproduced with permission from Moncada S, Vane JR: Mode of action of aspirinlike drugs. In Stollerman GH et al (eds): Advances in Internal Medicine, Vol 24. Copyright © 1979 by Year Book Medical Publishers, Chicago)

cretion, cell recognition, and activation of participating enzymes. Let us first consider the transport of free fatty acids.

FREE FATTY ACID TRANSPORT

Adipose tissue is made up of triacylglycerol and serves as a storage depot for this substance. A **hormone-sensitive lipase** catalyzes the hydrolysis of two of the three fatty acids of triacylglycerol. A second enzyme catalyzes the removal of the third fatty acid. The fatty acids are released into the circulation where they are transported as a complex with albumin. Nearly all organs except the brain will take up fatty acid. This furnishes between one quarter and one half of the required metabolic energy under fasting conditions. The plasma content of underivatized fatty acid (bound to albumin) is about 0.5 mM postabsorptively and 0.8 mM after an overnight fast.

TRIACYLGLYCEROL AND CHOLESTEROL TRANSPORT

There are four major classes of lipoproteins. These include (in order of increasing density and decreasing percent of lipid) **chylomicrons,** very low density lipoprotein **(VLDL)** low density lipoprotein **(LDL),** and high density lipoprotein **(HDL).** The major

TABLE 4-15. Composition and Function of the Major Classes of Lipoproteins

PARTICLE	FUNCTION	ORIGIN	FATE	APOLIPOPROTEINS
Chylomicron	Transports dietary triglyceride and cholesterol from gut to other tissues	Gut and HDL	Liver and HDL	Apo B-48 Apo A Apo CI, CII, and CIII Apo E
VLDL	Transports triglyceride from liver to other tissues	Liver	Converted into LDL	Apo B-100 Apo CI, CII, CIII Apo E
LDL	Transports cholesterol from liver to other tissues (bad cholesterol)	Formed from VLDL by liver	Taken up by target cells	Apo B-100
HDL	Transports cholesterol to liver from other tissues (good cholesterol)	From chylomicrons and liver	Liver	Apo A Apo B

function of chylomicrons is to transport triacylglycerol and cholesterol, derived from the diet, from the intestine to other tissues (Table 4-15). They are synthesized by the intestine but derive some apolipoproteins from HDL. Lipases in the capillary endothelium throughout the body catalyze the hydrolysis of triglyceride to fatty acids, which are then taken up by cells of the tissues or organs. The enzyme is called *heparin-sensitive lipase.* The stimulation by heparin is pharmacological in nature and probably plays no significant role in regulation *in vivo.* Chylomicron remnants return apoproteins to HDL and are taken up and destroyed by the liver.

The function of VLDL is to transport triglyceride from the liver to extrahepatic tissues. Heparin-sensitive lipase catalyzes the hydrolysis and release of fatty acids from the core triacylglycerol. VLDL is synthesized by the liver and also receives apoproteins from HDL. After transporting a portion of its triglyceride, and after returning specific apoproteins to HDL, VLDL is converted into LDL by the liver.

The main function of LDL is to transport cholesterol from the liver to extrahepatic tissues. This process has been implicated as a potential factor in atherogenesis, and sometimes LDL is called "bad cholesterol." The LDL complex is recognized by specific plasma membrane receptors in most cells. The LDL is taken up by the cell by receptor-mediated endocytosis and is delivered to the lysosomes. The latter degrade the apoproteins and hydrolyze cholesterol ester to cholesterol. Cholesterol acts to decrease the synthesis of HMG-CoA reductase and thereby decreases intracellular cholesterol formation. The LDL receptor is nonfunctional in a hereditary disease named *familial hypercholesterolemia.* These individuals develop atherosclerosis as children and generally succumb to the disease.

HDL transports cholesterol from extrahepatic tissues to the liver. It is sometimes called "good

cholesterol" because it removes cholesterol from peripheral tissues. It is synthesized in the liver and donates and receives components from chylomicrons and VLDL. It is apparently degraded by the liver. These properties are summarized in Table 4-15.

Amino Acid Metabolism and Urea Biosynthesis

Oxidation of the carbon skeletons of amino acids accounts for about 15% of the metabolic energy of humans. The amino groups are converted to ammonia and urea. The metabolism of some of the amino acids involves complex pathways and will be covered in abbreviated form. The amino acids are derived from the breakdown of body proteins and of dietary protein. About 85% of the amino acids resulting from the breakdown of endogenous body proteins are reutilized for protein biosynthesis. The breakdown of proteins into amino acids and their reutilization for protein synthesis is called *turnover.*

The metabolism of amino acids was initially studied in whole animals. Amino acids are designated as *glycogenic* if they lead to carbohydrate formation, *ketogenic* if they lead to ketone body formation, and *both* glycogenic and ketogenic if they lead to increases in both types of compound. This classification was derived from experiments performed by administering each amino acid and determining whether there was an increase in glucose (glycogenic amino acid), circulating ketone bodies (ketogenic amino acid), or both. Ketogenic amino acids are catabolized to acetyl-CoA, acetoacetyl-CoA, or both. The general classification of amino acids in this fashion is given in Table 4-16. Note that *leucine* is the sole amino acid that is ketogenic only. The aromatic amino acids, lysine, and isoleucine are both glycogenic and ketogenic and the remainder

TABLE 4-16. Classification of Glycogenic and Ketogenic Amino Acids

GLYCOGENIC ONLY		BOTH GLYCOGENIC AND KETOGENIC	KETOGENIC ONLY
Gly	Arg	Ile	*Leu
Ala	His	Lys	
Val	Ser	Phe	
Asp	Thr	Tyr	
Asn	Cys	Trp	
Glu	Met		
Gln	Pro		

* Noteworthy.

are glycogenic only. Before examining the fate of the carbon skeletons of the amino acids, we will consider (1) transamination reactions, (2) ammonium ion production, and (3) urea biosynthesis.

TRANSAMINATION REACTIONS

These reactions, which are isogonic, are pivotal for both the degradation and biosynthesis of the majority of the genetically encoded amino acids. The following is representative of all the reactions.

$$H_3N^+{-}\underset{R1}{\overset{COO^-}{C}}{-}H + O{=}\underset{R2}{\overset{COO^-}{C}} \rightleftharpoons O{=}\underset{R1}{\overset{COO^-}{C}} + H_3N^+{-}\underset{R2}{\overset{COO^-}{C}}{-}H$$

There are several enzymes that catalyze this reaction, and *pyridoxal phosphate* is the cofactor. They generally demonstrate a preference for one of the pairs of the amino group donor and acceptor and exhibit a varying latitude for the reciprocal cognate pair. The involvement of glutamate and α-ketoglutarate as the substrates for one transaminase is prevalent and pivotal. Enzymes preferring alanine and pyruvate, and aspartate and oxaloacetate, also are important. The ability of most amino acids to donate their amino groups to α-ketoglutarate to form glutamate is responsible in part for the central role of glutamate in nitrogen metabolism. Glutamate is also a common amino group donor in the formation of many other amino acids. The transaminase enzymes occur in the cytosol and mitochondria of all human cells. They also occur in low activities in human blood plasma. An increase in serum transaminases occurs during hepatitis, other forms of liver disease, and following the tissue necrosis of a myocardial infarction. Clinical chemistry laboratories commonly measure SGOT (*s*erum *g*lutamate *o*xaloacetate *t*ransaminase) and SGPT (*s*erum *g*lutamate *p*yruvate *t*ransminase).

Glutamate is also a source of free ammonium ion. ***Glutamate dehydrogenase*** catalyzes a reversible reaction involving the following components:

$$\begin{array}{ccc} \text{glutamate} & & \alpha\text{-ketoglutarate} \\ + & & + \\ NAD(P)^+ & \rightleftharpoons & NAD(P)H \\ + & & + \\ H_2O & & NH_4^+ \end{array}$$

Both NAD^+ and $NADP^+$ are substrates for this reaction. It is amphibolic and can function in biosynthesis or degradation depending upon metabolic need.

UREA BIOSYNTHESIS

The most important excretory product of nitrogen metabolism in humans is urea. A human consuming about 100 g of protein daily excretes about 16.5 g of nitrogen per day. About 80% to 90% of this is in the form of urinary urea. A small proportion is excreted as uric acid and free ammonium ion. An additional 5% is excreted in complex organic molecules in the feces. Urea is synthesized in the liver (and to a lesser extent in the kidney) but not in other tissues or organs. The precursors of urea are shown in Figure 4-43. One nitrogen of urea is derived from ***ammonium ion,*** and the second is derived from ***aspartate.*** The carbonyl group is derived from CO_2 (as bicarbonate). Amino groups are funneled into glutamate (see Fig. 4-43). Glutamate is oxidized and one precursor (ammonia) is formed; glutamate donates its amino group to oxaloacetate to yield the second precursor (aspartate).

The pathway for urea biosynthesis was elucidated by H. A. Krebs and a medical student (Kurt Henseleit) in 1932. The process involves a cyclic metabolic pathway called the Krebs urea cycle or urea cycle. This constitutes the first cyclic pathway and represents the intellectual cornerstone resulting in the conception of the citric acid cycle. The latter often is called simply the Krebs cycle.

The pathway involves a complex interplay of mitochondrial and cytosolic reactions. The stoichiometry of the overall process is given as follows:

$$\begin{array}{ccc} NH_3 & & 2\ ADP + 2\ Pi \\ + & & + \\ HCO_3^- & & AMP + PPi \\ + & & + \\ \text{aspartate} & \rightarrow & \text{fumarate} \\ + & & + \\ 3\ ATP & & \text{urea} \\ + & & \\ H_2O & & \end{array}$$

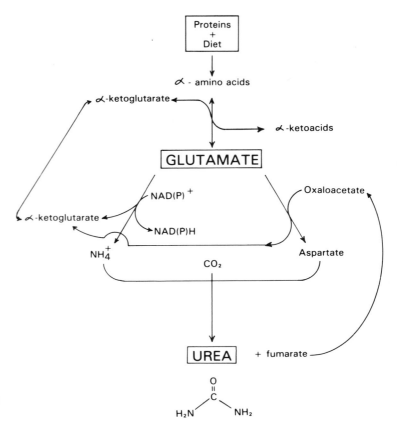

Fig. 4-43. Glutamate plays a central role in amino acid metabolism.

The first steps in the cycle involve the formation of active carbamate as ***carbamoyl phosphate.*** Its formation requires the expenditure of two high-energy bonds from two ATPs and is catalyzed by carbamoyl phosphate synthetase I in mitochondria.

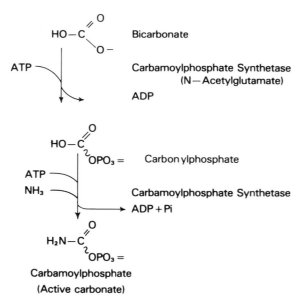

Fig. 4-44. Synthesis of carbamoyl phosphate.

This enzyme requires **N-acetylglutamate** as an allosteric activator. It is distinct from the cytosolic enzyme that is involved in pyrimidine formation (carbamoyl phosphate synthetase II). The reaction is shown in Figure 4-44. Active carbamate reacts with ornithine in a reaction catalyzed by ***ornithine transcarbamoylase*** to yield citrulline. ***Citrulline*** is transported into the cytosol (in exchange for ornithine) prior to the subsequent reactions of urea formation (Fig. 4-45). Aspartate, ATP, and citrulline react to form AMP, PPi, and argininosuccinate in a reaction catalyzed by ***argininosuccinate synthetase.*** PPi is hydrolyzed by pyrophosphatase to pull the reaction forward. Next, ***argininosuccinase*** catalyzes a lyase (not hydrolase) reaction to yield arginine and fumarate. ***Arginase*** catalyzes the hydrolysis of arginine to form urea and ornithine. Ornithine is transported into the mitochondria in exchange for citrulline.

From the stoichiometry of the cycle, we see that three ATP molecules and four energy-rich bonds are expended (2 ATP → 2 ADP + 2 Pi (2) and ATP → AMP + 2 Pi (2)). The overall process is exergonic. Renal disease is often associated with an elevation of the ***blood urea nitrogen*** (BUN). In severe liver disease, there is an elevation of blood ammo-

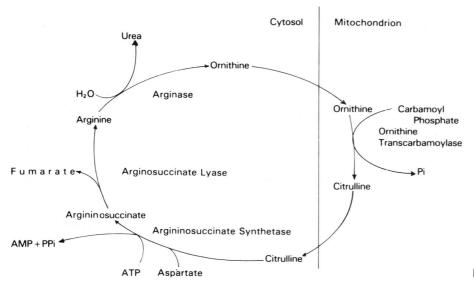

Fig. 4-45. The urea cycle.

nia. The mechanism of toxicity of ammonia is thought to be due to the depletion of mitochondrial citric acid cycle intermediates by converting α-ketoglutarate to glutamate in the reaction catalyzed by glutamate dehydrogenase. Krebs citric acid cycle function is especially important in the brain, and ammonium toxicity leads to hepatic encephalopathy with confusion, stupor, or even coma and death. A few inborn errors of metabolism associated with the urea cycle are given in Table 4-17.

CATABOLISM OF THE CARBON SKELETONS OF THE AMINO ACIDS

Amino acids that give rise to pyruvate and intermediates of the citric acid cycle (α-ketoglutarate, succinyl-CoA, fumarate, and oxaloacetate) are glyco-genic. These compounds are able to furnish substrates for gluconeogenesis. In contrast, those amino acids that directly yield acetyl-CoA or aceto-acetyl-CoA can not support gluconeogenesis. These compounds yield ketone bodies. We will consider the metabolism of amino acids. Several amino acids also exhibit multiple pathways of metabolism, which are not considered here.

Five amino acids (alanine, threonine, glycine, serine, and cysteine) are converted to pyruvate. *Alanine* undergoes a transamination reaction and yields pyruvate directly. *Threonine* undergoes an NAD^+-dependent dehydrogenation and decarboxylation to form aminoacetone, CO_2, NADH, and H^+. This reaction is catalyzed by threonine dehydrogenase. Monoamine oxidase catalyzes the oxidative conversion of aminoacetone to pyruvalde-

TABLE 4-17. Inborn Errors of Urea Cycle and Amino Acid Metabolism

NAME	ENZYME DEFICIENCY	METABOLISM AFFECTED
Argininosuccinaturia	Argininosuccinase	Urea cycle
Citrullinemia	Argininosuccinate synthetase	Urea cycle
Hyperammonemia I	Ornithine transcarbamoylase	Urea cycle
Hyperammonemia II	Carbamoyl phosphate synthetase	Urea cycle
Alkaptonuria*	Homogentisate oxidase	Phe, Tyr
Argininemia	Arginase	Arg
Cystathionuria	Cystathionase	Cys, Met, Ser
Histidinemia	Histidase	His
Homocystinuria	Cystathionine synthase	Cys, Met, Ser
Maple syrup urine* disease	Branched chain ketoacid dehydrogenase	Val, Leu, Ile
Phenylketonuria*	Phenylalanine hydroxylase	Phe

* Noteworthy.

hyde. Oxygen is the other reactant, and ammonia and hydrogen peroxide are the other products. Aldehyde dehydrogenase catalyzes the $NAD(P)^+$-dependent conversion of pyruvaldehyde to pyruvate and $NAD(P)H$ and H^+. *Glycine* reacts with N^5,N^{10}-methylenetetrahydrofolate and water to yield *serine* and tetrahydrofolate. Serine dehydratase catalyzes a pyridoxal phosphate-dependent elimination of ammonia with a rearrangement to yield pyruvate. Note that the initial steps in the catabolism of threonine, glycine, and serine do not involve transaminations. The main pathway for *cysteine* metabolism in humans involves oxidation of the thiol group to sulfinate ($R-SO_2^-$), transamination, and then hydrolysis (releasing $HO-SO_2^-$) yielding pyruvate.

Five amino acids (proline, arginine, histidine, glutamine, and glutamate) are metabolized to α-ketoglutarate. *Proline* is dehydrogenated (NAD^+) forming a double bond in the ring between the α-carbon and nitrogen (Δ1-pyrroline-5-carboxylate) and is hydrolyzed between these atoms yielding L-glutamate semialdehyde. A specific dehydrogenase (NAD^+) oxidizes the aldehyde on carbon five to yield glutamate. *Glutamate* is converted into α-ketoglutarate by transamination or by dehydrogenation (glutamate dehydrogenase). *Arginine* is hydrolyzed to urea and ornithine. Ornithine undergoes a transamination reaction to form L-glutamate semialdehyde, whose metabolism we have just considered. *Histidine* metabolism is too complex to consider fully. Histidase catalyzes the elimination of ammonia to form urocanate (first isolated in canine urine). This undergoes two successive hydrolysis reactions to yield N-formimino-L-glutamate (FIGLU). This reacts with tetrahydrofolate to form L-glutamate and N^5-formiminotetrahydrofolate. In folic acid deficiency, FIGLU is excreted in the urine and forms the basis of a diagnostic test following a large dose of histidine. Glutaminase catalyzes the hydrolysis of the amide group of *glutamine* to yield glutamate and ammonia. It is noteworthy that the glutaminase reaction in the kidney is responsible for the generation of the majority of ammonium ion excreted in the urine. Glutamate is converted into α-ketoglutarate in one step by transamination or dehydrogenation.

Valine, isoleucine, and methionine are metabolized to succinyl-CoA. The pathway from *valine* to succinyl-CoA consists of eight steps and will not be covered in its entirety. The first step is a transamination to form α-ketoisovalerate. This undergoes an oxidative decarboxylation involving NAD^+ and coenzyme A. The reaction is catalyzed by a *branched chain keto-acid dehydrogenase,* discussed

later. The reaction is analogous to the pyruvate dehydrogenase and α-ketoglutarate dehydrogenase reactions. Subsequent steps eventually yield methylmalonyl-CoA, which is metabolized in a vitamin B_{12}-dependent pathway that was considered in the metabolism of fatty acids with an odd number of carbon atoms (see Fig. 4-31). Methylmalonyl-CoA is converted to succinyl-CoA in this process.

Isoleucine is first transaminated to α-keto-β-methylvalerate, and it undergoes an oxidative decarboxylation by the same branched chain keto-acid dehydrogenase mentioned above. After several more steps, a thiolytic cleavage produces propionyl-CoA and acetyl-CoA. Propionyl-CoA is converted to succinyl-CoA by the B_{12}-dependent pathway (see Fig. 4-31). Propionyl-CoA is glycogenic and acetyl-CoA is ketogenic, accounting for its classification in Table 4-16.

The complete metabolism of *methionine* is rather complex; we shall consider the reactions of its derivative, *S*-adenosylmethionine, in some detail later. *S-Adenosylmethionine* is an important methyl donor in several reactions. The conversion of phosphatidylethanolamine to phosphatidylcholine, for example, was considered previously (see Fig. 4-35). *Homocysteine,* which forms after transmethylation and hydrolysis, is a four-carbon homologue of cysteine with the thiol group on the γ-carbon. Homocysteine reacts with serine to yield *cystathionine* ($HOOCCH(NH_2)CH_2CH_2SCH_2CH(NH_2)COOH$) and water. Cystathionine is cleaved in a lyase reaction catalyzed by cystathionase to form cysteine, ammonia, and α-ketobutyrate; the latter is derived from the four carbons of methionine following hydrolysis of the amino group. *Alpha-ketobutyrate* undergoes an oxidative decarboxylation (not by the branched chain keto-acid dehydrogenase) involving NAD^+ and coenzyme A and yields propionyl-CoA. The latter is converted to succinyl-CoA by the vitamin B_{12}-dependent pathway (see Fig. 4-31). Valine, isoleucine, and methionine constitute the succinyl-CoA family.

Phenylalanine and tyrosine are converted to fumarate (glycogenic) and acetoacetyl-CoA (ketogenic). *Phenylalanine* (essential) is converted into tyrosine (nonessential) in a reaction catalyzed by *phenylalanine hydroxylase,* which occurs only in the liver. *Tetrahydrobiopterin* is the reductant, and molecular oxygen is required. The products include tyrosine, dihydrobiopterin, and water. The hereditary deficiency of phenylalanine hydroxylase is associated with the disease called *phenylketonuria* (PKU). This is one of the more common inborn errors of metabolism. Tyrosine undergoes a transamination reaction with α-ketoglutarate to yield 4-hydroxyphenylpyruvate and glutamate; the enzyme catalyzing this reaction is *tyrosine aminotransferase*. In a reaction involving molecular oxygen, 4-hydroxyphenylpyruvate is decarboxylated, hydroxylated, and re-arranges to produce *homogentisate.* This undergoes a reaction with oxygen catalyzed by *homogentisate oxidase,* which opens the aromatic ring yielding *maleylacetoacetate*. This undergoes an isomerization to *fumarylacetoacetate*. A lyase then catalyzes the formation of *fumarate* and *acetoacetate.* Acetoacetate is transported from the liver for metabolism in extrahepatic tissues as a ketone body.

Asparagine and asparatate are metabolized to oxaloacetate. Fortunately the metabolism is simple. Asparaginase catalyzes the hydrolysis of the amide group of *asparagine* to yield ammonia and aspartate. *Asparate* undergoes transamination and yields oxaloacetate.

Leucine, lysine, and tryptophan are converted to acetoacetyl-CoA. *Leucine* is converted to *α-ketoisocaproate* by transamination. This substance undergoes an oxidative decarboxylation by the branched chain keto-acid dehydrogenase and yields isovaleryl-CoA. (We see that this enzyme operates on valine, isoleucine, and leucine metabolites). In three enzyme-catalyzed reactions, 3-hydroxy-3-methylglutaryl-CoA is formed from isovaleryl-CoA. HMG-CoA lyase catalyzes its dismutation to acetyl-CoA and acetoacetate. It is noteworthy that leucine is the only genetically encoded amino acid that is entirely ketogenic (see Table 4-16).

Lysine metabolism is complex and incompletely understood. Alpha-ketoadipate (a six-carbon dicarboxylic acid) is an intermediate metabolite. This is converted in several steps to acetyl-CoA. How lysine contributes to glycogenesis is unclear.

Tryptophan metabolism is also complex. The first reaction in its catabolism involves a reaction with both atoms of an oxygen molecule, which opens the five-membered ring of imidazole and yields N-formyl kynurenine. Following the hydrolytic cleavage of formate, L-*kynurenine* results. This undergoes a hydroxylation (O_2 and NADPH are reactants) and is followed by the elimination of alanine (glycogenic) and the formation of *3-hydroxyanthranylate*. This has two possible fates. The intermediate can be converted into α-ketoadipate as occurs in lysine metabolism. It is noteworthy, however, that 3-hydroxyanthranylate is also converted into quinolinate. This can be converted into *nicotinic acid ribose phosphate.* Nicotinic acid is a vitamin in humans because this pathway fails to provide physiologically adequate amounts of nicotinic acid. This pathway decreases the requirement for nicotinic acid, and such a process is called *sparing.*

There are a large number of inborn errors in the metabolism of amino acids. The most common is phenylketonuria, and its incidence is 1 : 10,000 live births. Classical *phenylketonuria* is due to a relative deficiency of phenylalanine hydroxylase (see Table 4-17). Since phenylalanine cannot be degraded, alternative metabolites accumulate. These include phenylpyruvate (the phenylketone excreted in urine), phenyllactate, and phenylacetate. Although several commercial methods are available as screening tests for this disorder, a definitive diagnosis requires a determination of plasma phenylalanine levels. The treatment includes a diet deficient in phenylalanine. Variants of phenylketonuria exist. One is due to a deficiency of dihydropteridine reductase activity. This enzyme is responsible for converting the product of the reaction, dihydrobiopterin, to the reactant, tetrahydrobiopterin. *Alkaptonuria* is another disorder of phenylalanine and tyrosine metabolism. It is attributable to a deficiency in *homogentisate oxidase;* homogentisate is excreted in the urine. Several diseases associated with defects in cysteine metabolism with consequent *homocystinuria* are known. *Maple syrup urine* disease is a very rare genetic disorder. It is associated with a deficiency in the branched chain α-keto-acid dehydrogenase involved in the metabolism of valine, leucine, and isoleucine (see Table 17). There are elevated levels of each of these three amino acids and their corresponding α-keto-acids in plasma. The disease received its name by the odor of urine in affected individuals, which is reminiscent of maple syrup.

Amino Acid Biosynthesis

There are 20 genetically encoded amino acids. If one of these amino acids is present in inadequate amounts, then protein synthesis is correspondingly diminished. *Nonessential amino acids* can be produced in sufficient quantity from endogenous metabolites. *Essential amino acids* cannot be derived from endogenous metabolites in required amounts and must be obtained from the diet. A relative deficiency of an essential amino acid impairs protein synthesis and leads to a *negative nitrogen balance* (nitrogen excretion exceeds nitrogen intake). In healthy adults *nitrogen balance* exists (intake equals excretion). In growing children where nitrogen intake exceeds excretion, *positive nitrogen balance* occurs. Negative nitrogen balance also occurs in a variety of nonphysiological conditions including infections, burns, and postsurgical stress. This is related in part to increased glucocorticoid secretion from the adrenal cortex.

Experiments with normal adult volunteers indicated that 8 of the 20 amino acids are essential and must be provided in the diet. These same amino acids are required in rats. Growing rats also need two additional amino acids for optimal growth (histidine and arginine); it is thought that human infants also require these two amino acids. A mnemonic for the essential amino acids is the acronym PVT TIM *HA*LL (private Tim Hall). This corresponds to phenylalanine, valine, threonine, tryptophan, isoleucine, methionine, histidine, arginine, leucine, and lysine. If one remembers that tyrosine is nonessential, since it is derived from phenylalanine (essential), then the mnemonic is less ambiguous. HA is italicized to signify that these are the two additional amino acids needed for growing humans. The case for the essentialness of arginine in humans is not universally accepted, but it is included for completeness.

In this section we will adumbrate the pathways for the synthesis of the nonessential amino acids. The pathways for the biosynthesis of essential amino acids that occur in plants and microorganisms are generally very complex; these will not be considered. Glycine is formed by multiple pathways including that from serine by way of the hydroxymethyltransferase reaction involving tetrahydrofolate. Alanine is formed by transamination of pyruvate. Glutamate and aspartate are formed by transamination of α-ketoglutarate and oxaloacetate, respectively. Glutamate is also formed through the action of glutamate dehydrogenase as noted earlier. This important reaction converts free ammonia to an organic amino function. Glutamate then serves as amino donor in a variety of reactions.

The biosynthesis of glutamine and asparagine requires ATP. In the former case, ADP and Pi result. In the latter, AMP and PPi are formed. *Glutamine synthetase* catalyzes a reaction between ATP, glutamate, and ammonia to yield glutamine, ADP, and Pi (Fig. 4-46). A intermediate γ-phosphoglutamate is an activated acyl-phosphate intermediate that undergoes a reaction with ammonia.

In the *asparagine synthetase* reaction, aspartate, the amido group of glutamine, and ATP react to form asparagine, glutamate, AMP, and PPi. The amido group of glutamine serves the important function as a nitrogen donor. The K_m of the human enzyme for ammonia is very high, and ammonia is not a physiologically important donor in this reaction.

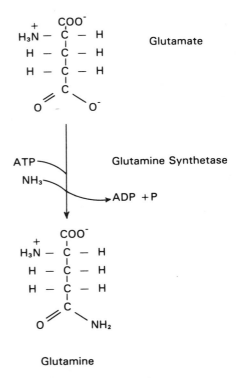

Fig. 4-46. Glutamine biosynthesis.

There are two pathways for the conversion of 3-phosphoglycerate (an intermediate in glycolysis) to serine. The main pathway involves an NAD^+-dependent dehydrogenation of 3-phosphoglycerate to phosphohydroxypyruvate. It undergoes a transamination reaction to form O-phosphoserine. This undergoes a hydrolysis to form serine and Pi. Although phosphoserine is found in proteins, the amino acid is added to the nascent polypeptide chain as a seryl group. A post-translational phosphorylation catalyzed by protein kinases mediate the phosphorylation of the protein–serine to yield the phosphoseryl residue.

Proline is derived from glutamate. The pathway requires two reductions and a dehydration, but the precise enzymology in mammals has not been determined; $\Delta1$-pyrroline-5-carboxylate is an intermediate. Cysteine is derived from methionine (essential) and serine (nonessential). Methionine is converted to homocysteine, forms an adduct with serine called cystathionine, and it is cleaved to form cysteine and homoserine. Tyrosine is formed from phenylalanine (essential) in the phenylalanine hydroxylase reaction.

Porphyrins, Heme, and Bile Pigments

Porphyrins are tetrapyrroles linked by methenyl

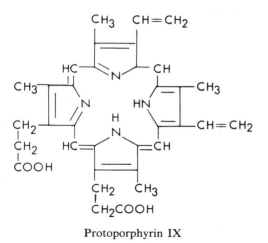

CH₃   CH=CH₂

Protoporphyrin IX

Fig. 4-47. Structure of protoporphyrin IX.

(=CH—) bridges. **Heme** is the iron derivative of **protoporphyrin IX** (Fig. 4-47). Heme occurs in hemoglobin, myoglobin, cytochromes, and catalase. The precursors for heme biosynthesis include succinyl-CoA, glycine, and iron. The rate-limiting reaction in porphyrin biosynthesis is catalyzed by **δ-aminolevulinate synthase** (ALA synthase). The reactants are glycine and succinyl-CoA; δ-aminolevulinate, coenzyme A, and CO_2 are products. Two molecules of δ-aminolevulinate condense to form **porphobilinogen.** Four of these condense to produce the tetrapyrrole. After additional decarboxylations and oxidation, protoporphyrin IX is produced. The insertion of iron to produce heme is catalyzed by **ferrochelatase.** Heme combines with its apoprotein to form the heme–protein derivative.

The activity of the pathway is regulated by increasing or decreasing the biosynthesis of ALA synthase by enzyme induction or repression.

Following degradation of heme proteins, heme is catabolized to **bile pigments.** Heme oxygenase catalyzes the opening of the tetrapyrrole ring to form **biliverdin.** Biliverdin is reduced to form **bilirubin.** These degradative reactions occur in the reticuloendothelial system. Following transport to the liver as a complex with albumin, bilirubin reacts with 2 moles of UDP-glucuronate to form **bilirubin diglucuronide** (conjugated bilirubin). The latter is more water soluble than free bilirubin. Conjugated bilirubin is excreted in the bile. Intestinal flora catalyze the transformation of bilirubin to numerous **bile pigments,** most of which are excreted in the feces. The remainder are absorbed and are subsequently excreted in the urine.

One-Carbon Metabolism

The reactions of *S*-adenosylmethionine, biotin, and folate derivatives are important in the transfer of one-carbon groups in metabolism. *S*-Adenosylmethionine is important in many methyl-transfer reactions. The methyl group represents the most reduced form of carbon (Table 4-18). Biotin, covalently linked to proteins, also serves as an intermediary of one-carbon carboxyl-transfer reactions. This represents the most oxidized form of carbon. Derivatives of tetrahydrofolate (THF) play a role in a variety of one-carbon transfers of varying oxidation states. One-carbon groups transferred by tetrahydrofolate include methyl, methylene, hydroxymethyl, methenyl, formyl, and formimino groups

TABLE 4-18. Oxidation States of One-Carbon Groups

MOST REDUCED ──────────────────────────→ MOST OXIDIZED

CH_4 Methane	CH_3^- Methyl	$^-CH_2^-$ Methylene	$^-C^=$ Methenyl	CO_2 Carbon dioxide
		H—C—H (=O) Formaldehyde	H—C—OH (=O) Formic acid	HO—C—OH (=O) Carbonic acid
		HO—C— (H, H) Hydroxymethyl	H—C— (=O) Formyl	HO—C— (=O) Carboxy
			H—C— (=NH) Formimino	
			C=O Carbon monoxide	

(see Table 4-18).

Let us first consider the biochemistry of S-adenosylmethionine (CH$_3$S$^+$(5'-adenosyl) CH$_2$CH$_2$CH-(NH$_2$)COOH). It is formed in a very unusual reaction between ATP, methionine, and water. In this reaction, triphosphate is displaced and is hydrolyzed to Pi and PPi prior to its release from the enzymic-active site. PPi is then hydrolyzed to two Pi molecules by a separate pyrophosphatase activity. Two high-energy bonds and a low-energy bond are consumed during the overall process.

The standard free energy of hydrolysis of the methyl group of S-adenosylmethionine is -7 kcal/mole and is of the high-energy variety. S-Adenosylmethionine represents one form of an activated methyl group. It transfers its methyl group to a variety of acceptors to yield S-adenosylhomocysteine and a methylated compound. Methylated products include choline, creatine, epinephrine, spermine, spermidine, and 5-methylcytosine in DNA.

Let us next consider the role of biotin in ATP-dependent carboxylation reactions. Biotin forms a covalently linked prosthetic group in *propionyl-CoA carboxylase, pyruvate carboxylase,* and *acetyl-CoA carboxylase.* The substrate bicarbonate presumably forms an activated carboxyl-phosphate (acid anhydride) intermediate and ADP in the first part of the reaction. It reacts with the biotin prosthetic group to form an activated carboxyl-biotinyl group. The activated carboxyl group is transferred to an acceptor such as propionyl-CoA, pyruvate, or acetyl-CoA, depending upon the reaction, to produce the carboxylated compound and regenerated enzyme.

THFs are made up of tetrahydropterin, para-aminobenzoate, and glutamate. In humans the glutamyl group is covalently linked to additional glutamate residues. The one-carbon groups are linked to N^5, N^{10}, or both nitrogen atoms. Serine is the major donor of one-carbon groups in humans in a reaction catalyzed by serine hydroxylmethyltransferase. The reaction involves serine and THF and yields N^5,N^{10}-methylene-THF, glycine, and water.

Methylene-THF can be reduced by NADPH to yield N^5-methyl-THF. This can transfer its methyl group to homocysteine in a vitamin B$_{12}$–dependent reaction catalyzed by methyl-THF : homocysteine transmethylase to form methionine. This is the precursor of S-adenosylmethionine, an important methyl donor as noted previously. Methylene-THF also serves as methyl donor and reductant for *thymidylate* synthesis as noted later. Thymidylate is

incorporated into DNA. N^5,N^{10}-Methylene-THF can be oxidized by NADP$^+$ to yield N^5,N^{10}-methenyl-THF. This serves as a one-carbon donor in purine biosynthesis. This can also be formed from formimino-THF.

Purine and Pyrimidine Nucleotide Structures

Purine and pyrimidine nucleotides are small, nitrogen-containing, aromatic compounds with many important biological functions. Nucleotides serve as carriers of metabolic energy (ATP) and as coenzymes in oxidation–reduction reactions (NAD$^+$, NADP$^+$). They also are constituents of DNA, RNA, and serve as metabolic second messengers (cyclic AMP).

The structures of the common purine and pyrimidine bases are shown in Figure 4-48. These compounds are called bases since they contain nitrogen, and the latter accept protons. Under physiological conditions, however, these nitrogen atoms rarely bear a frank positive charge as does the ammonium ion. The bases are aromatic and planar. *Adenine* and *guanine* occur in both DNA and RNA. *Cytosine* and *thymine* occur in DNA; *cytosine* and *uracil* occur in RNA. *Nucleosides* are made up of a base and sugar. The sugar is *ribose* in RNA and in the common coenzymes. The sugar is *2-deoxyribose* in DNA. *Nucleotides* are *phosphorylated nucleosides.* AMP is a nucleo*side* monophosphate. This is mistakenly called nucleotide monophosphate; the term nucleotide already signifies the presence of phosphate. The terminology of bases and derivatives is based on historical precedents and is an understandable source of confusion. Table 4-19 gives a

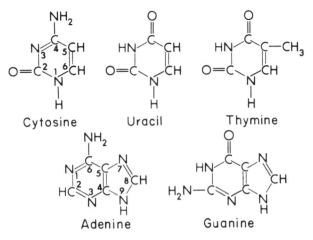

Fig. 4-48. The pyrimidine and purine bases.

TABLE 4-19. Nomenclature of the Common Purines and Pyrimidines

BASE (ABBREVIATION)	NUCLEOSIDE; BASE-SUGAR	NUCLEOTIDE; NUCLEOSIDE MONOPHOSPHATE (ABBREVIATION)	NUCLEOSIDE TRIPHOSPHATE (ABBREVIATION)
Purine			
Adenine (A)	Adenosine	Adenosine monophosphate (AMP)	Adenosine triphosphate (ATP)
Guanine (G)	Guanosine	Guanosine monophosphate (GMP)	Guanosine triphosphate (GTP)
Hypoxanthine (H)	Inosine	Inosine monophosphate (IMP)	Inosine triphosphate (ITP)
Xanthine (X)	Xanthosine	Xanthosine monophosphate (XMP)	Xanthosine triphosphate (XTP)
Pyrimidine			
Cytosine (C)	Cytidine	Cytidine monophosphate (CMP)	Cytidine triphosphate (CTP)
Uracil (U)	Uridine	Uridine monophosphate (UMP)	Uridine triphosphate (UTP)
Thymine (T)	Thymidine*	Thymidine* monophosphate (TMP)	Thymidine* triphosphate (TTP)

*Refers to the deoxyribo derivative; the unusual ribose derivative is called ribothymidine; dTMP = TMP; dTTP = TTP.

list of the bases and the corresponding nucleosides and nucleotides.

Pyrimidine and Purine Biosynthesis

Like amino acid biosynthesis and degradation, nucleotide biosynthesis can be divided into two categories: simple and complex. Pyrimidine biosynthesis is simple when compared with purine biosynthesis. We shall first consider pyrimidine formation and then sketch the pathway for purine biosynthesis. The bases of the pyrimidines are derived from two precursors, namely, aspartate and carbamoyl phosphate. This is illustrated in Figure 4-49. We will divide the pathway for pyrimidine biosynthesis into four portions: (1) the formation of carbamoyl phosphate, (2) the pyrimidine ring, (3) the addition of the sugar phosphate, and (4) the formation of the various pyrimidine derivatives.

PYRIMIDINE BIOSYNTHESIS

The formation of active carbamate is catalyzed by *carbamoyl phosphate synthetase II*. This differs in three ways from the enzyme that participates in urea biosynthesis. The pyrimidine enzyme (1) is found in the cytosol (see Table 4-2) of all nucleated cells (and not just in liver and kidney mitochondria), (2) utilizes glutamine as amido donor, and (3) is not regulated by *N*-acetylglutamate. The reaction is given by the following chemical equation:

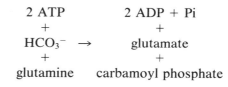

$$
\begin{array}{ccc}
2\text{ ATP} & & 2\text{ ADP} + \text{Pi} \\
+ & & + \\
\text{HCO}_3^- & \rightarrow & \text{glutamate} \\
+ & & + \\
\text{glutamine} & & \text{carbamoyl phosphate}
\end{array}
$$

Aspartate transcarbamoylase catalyzes the reaction between aspartate and carbamoyl phosphate to yield *N*-carbamoyl aspartate (see Fig. 4-49). Dihydro-orotase then catalyzes a condensation reaction with the removal of the elements of water to produce dihydro-orotate. This is oxidized by NAD^+ in a dihydro-orotate dehydrogenase (orotate reductase) catalyzed reaction to form orotate. This enzyme is a flavoprotein found in the outer face of the inner mitochondrial membrane.

Next, we must consider the reaction responsible for adding the ribose-phosphate to the pyrimidine ring. The donor is phosphoribosylpyrophosphate (PRPP), and we consider the pathway for its formation. The reactants include ribose-5-phosphate (from the pentose phosphate pathway) and ATP, and the enzyme is *PRPP synthetase*. The pyrophosphoryl group is transferred to the hemiacetal oxygen on carbon one; PRPP and AMP are the products.

PRPP represents active phosphoribose; the standard free energy of hydrolysis of PRPP to ribose-5-phosphate and PPi is about −7 kcal/mole. PRPP reacts with orotate to yield orotidine monophosphate (OMP) and PPi. The latter is hydrolyzed to

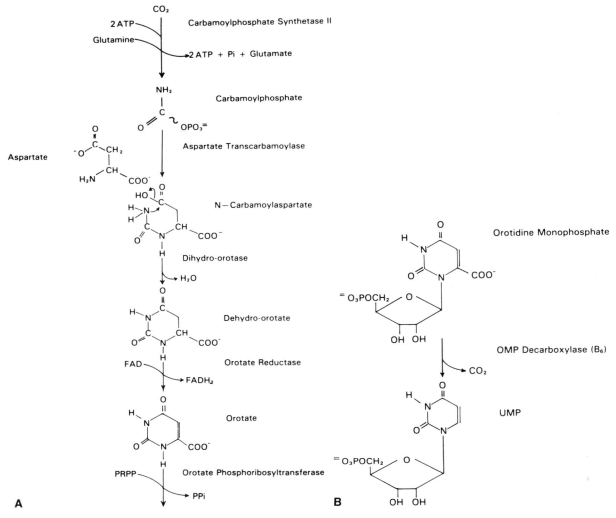

Fig. 4-49A,B. Pyrimidine biosynthesis.

two Pi molecules by a separate pyrophosphatase that helps to pull the reaction forward (see Table 4-1). OMP is decarboxylated in a vitamin B_6–(pyridoxal phosphate)–dependent fashion to form uridine monophosphate (UMP) and CO_2. Myokinase catalyzes an isogonic reaction of UMP and ATP to yield UDP and ADP.

UDP is a key intermediate in pyrimidine metabolism. Nucleoside diphosphokinase catalyzes an isogonic reaction between UDP and ATP to form UTP and ADP. UTP is a precursor for RNA biosynthesis and numerous uridine diphosphate sugar compounds utilized in carbohydrate metabolism. UTP is also converted to CTP. **CTP synthetase** catalyzes a reaction between UTP, ATP (an energy source), and glutamine (an amido donor) to yield CTP, ADP, and glutamate. CTP is a precursor of RNA and nu-

merous CDP derivatives important in lipid biosynthesis.

UDP is also a precursor of thymidylate. Ribonucleotide reductase catalyzes the reduction of UDP to deoxyuridine diphosphate (dUDP). **Ribonucleotide reductase** catalyzes a reaction between nucleoside **diphosphates** and reduced thioredoxin to form the corresponding deoxynucleoside diphosphate and oxidized thioredoxin (Fig. 4-50). The latter is reduced by NADPH and H^+ in a reaction catalyzed by **thioredoxin reductase.** Ribonucleotide reductase is extremely important because of its obligatory participation in the synthesis of DNA precursors. Uridine nucleotides, however, are not genuine constituents of DNA. Deoxyuridine diphosphate is converted to dUTP by phosphorylation and then hydrolyzed to dUMP and PPi. De-

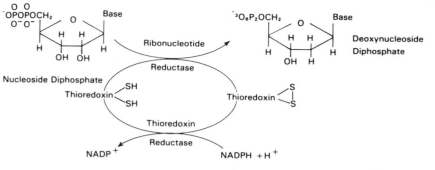

Fig. 4-50. The ribonucleotide reductase reaction.

oxyuridine diphosphate is a substrate for the important **thymidylate synthase** reaction (Fig. 4-51). It reacts with N^5,N^{10}-methylene-THF to yield TMP and *di*hydrofolate. In this reaction methylene-THF serves as a one-carbon donor and a reductant. This sequence of reactions is important in understanding the mechanism of action of antifolates such as methotrexate. Methotrexate is a drug used in the treatment of children with acute lymphocytic leukemia and is used in a number of other neoplastic disorders. It is a structural analogue of dihydrofolate and binds avidly to **dihydrofolate reductase.** It inhibits the conversion of dihydrofolate to THF and thereby diminishes the levels of the fully reduced and active form of folate. The therapeutic effectiveness of this and other drugs is dependent upon the differential sensitivity of normal and tumorigenic cells. Although neoplastic tissues may initially be sensitive to the action of methotrexate, resistance may develop. One form of resistance is related to overproduction of the enzyme dihydrofolate reductase.

PURINE BIOSYNTHESIS

In contrast to the simple pathway for pyrimidines, that for purines is rather complex. We shall consider only the initial steps in any detail. We shall see that the purine ring is built upon the ribose phosphate backbone. This contrasts with pyrimidine formation where the sugar phosphate is added after formation of the ring. The source of atoms found in the purine ring, illustrated for inosine monophosphate, is indicated in Figure 4-52.

The first and committed step in the pathway is catalyzed by PRPP glutaminyl aminotransferase. The reactants are PRPP, an activated form of the 5-phosphoribosyl group, and glutamine. The products include glutamate, PPi, and 5-phosphoribosylamine. Note that inversion at carbon one of ribose has occurred (see Fig. 4-52). It has gone from the α-configuration in PRPP to the β-configuration in the product. Next, the carboxylate group of glycine condenses with the amino function in an ATP-dependent reaction. Glycine contributes atoms four,

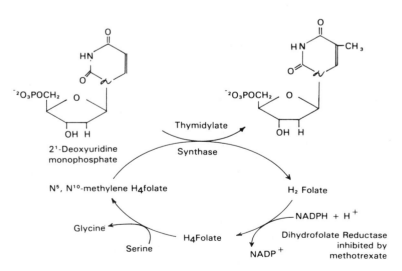

Fig. 4-51. Thymidylate biosynthesis.

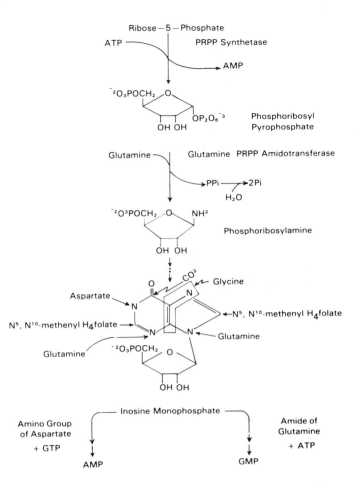

Fig. 4-52. Overview of purine biosynthesis.

five, and seven of the final structure. Methenyl-THF (-H_4folate) then donates carbon eight. Glutamine then contributes nitrogen three in an ATP-dependent reaction (ATP → ADP + Pi). The five-membered ring is formed in an ATP-dependent reaction yielding ADP and Pi. This constitutes a mechanism for removing the elements of water from the precursor to yield the five-membered imidazole ring. Carbon six is derived from CO_2 in an ATP-independent reaction. Nitrogen one is derived from aspartate in a reaction analogous to that seen in urea biosynthesis. The amino group of asparate condenses with a carboxylate to yield an N-succinylamide in an ATP-dependent process. Unlike the reaction in urea biosynthesis, in purine formation ATP is converted to ADP and Pi. As in urea formation, a lyase catalyzes the elimination of fumarate. In summary, to add nitrogen, aspartate reacts with a compound in an ATP-dependent reaction and then fumarate is eliminated. Next, N^5,N^{10}-methenyl-H_4folate donates carbon two. In older textbooks (prior to 1982), formyl-THF is des-

ignated as the precursor; subsequent work indicated that methenyl-THF serves as donor. Closure of the six-membered ring occurs with the elimination of water; no ATP is required for this reaction. The product of the reaction is inosine-5'-monophosphate (IMP) as shown in Figure 4-52.

IMP serves as a precursor of AMP and GMP and occupies a branch point for these processes (see Figure 4-52). A two-step reaction is required to convert IMP to **AMP.** This involves the replacement of an oxygen (or hydroxyl group of the tautomer) by an amino group. The amino donor is again aspartate utilizing a familiar motif. IMP condenses with aspartate (as **GTP** is converted to GDP + Pi) to form N-succinyladenylate. A specific lyase catalyzes the elimination of fumarate to form AMP. Two steps are also required to convert IMP to GMP. First, IMP is oxidized in a reaction involving IMP, H_2O, and NAD^+. The products are NADH + H^+ and xanthosine monophosphate (XMP). Glutamine serves as the amido donor to yield the amino group found on carbon two of the purine ring. The reactants are XMP, glutamine, and ATP; the products are GMP, glutamate, AMP, and PPi. Note that ATP is required for GMP formation, and GTP is required for AMP formation. Kinases catalyze the phosphorylation of the purine nucleoside monophosphates to the corresponding diphosphates with ATP as donor. The nucleoside diphosphates are substrates for ribonucleotide reductase to yield the corresponding deoxyribonucleotides as necessary (see Fig. 4-50). GTP, dGTP, and dATP are formed from the corresponding diphosphates and ATP. Several mechanisms exist for the formation of ATP from ADP by substrate-level and electron-transport phosphorylation.

In addition to the synthesis of purines from low molecular weight precursors (*de novo* synthesis), salvage pathways exist. The preformed bases (adenine, hypoxanthine, guanine) resulting from degradative reactions are reutilized for anabolic pathways. Two enzymes catalyze the salvage reactions. *Adenine phosphoribosyl transferase* (APT) catalyzes a reaction of substrate with PRPP to form AMP and PPi. *Hypoxanthine-guanine phosphoribosyl transferase* (HGPRT) catalyzes a reaction of either base with PRPP to form IMP (from hypoxanthine) or GMP. The physiological importance of salvage pathways was not fully appreciated until it was discovered that Lesch–Nyhan syndrome is due to a hereditary deficiency of HGPRT. This human genetic disorder is associated with extreme aggression and self-mutilation. It is X-linked, recessive, occurs in males, and is fortunately rare.

The metabolism of PRPP is central in both purine and pyrimidine metabolism and is important in metabolic regulation. *PRPP synthetase* is subject to complex allosteric regulation by purine nucleotides. AMP and GMP are inhibitory. The committed step in purine formation is catalyzed by *PRPP glutaminyl amidotransferase*. It is also allosterically inhibited by AMP and GMP. Pyrimidine biosynthesis

in humans is regulated at *carbamoyl phosphate synthetase*. This enzyme is inhibited by pyrimidine nucleotides and activated by purine nucleotides. In contrast to humans, the regulatory step of pyrimidine biosynthesis in *E. coli* is at the level of the aspartate transcarbamoylase reaction. The conversion of IMP to AMP and GMP is differentially regulated. AMP inhibits its synthesis, and GMP inhibits its own synthesis in the first step of the pathway from IMP.

Purine and Pyrimidine Catabolism

The end product of purine metabolism in humans is **uric acid** or its salt **urate.** There are multiple pathways for converting AMP and GMP into xanthine and thence urate. Some of these enzyme activities are listed in Table 4-20. Through the action of various deaminases and a general 5'-nucleotidase and purine nucleoside phosphorylase, purine bases result. These include adenine, hypoxanthine (from adenosine by inosine [a nucleoside]), and guanine. About 90% of these are reutilized by the salvage pathway in reactions with PRPP. The remaining 10% of these purines are converted to uric acid. Hypoxanthine is oxidized to xanthine in a reaction catalyzed by *xanthine oxidase.* Guanosine is deaminated (by hydrolysis) to yield xanthine. Xanthine oxidase also catalyzes the oxidation of xanthine to uric acid.

A common derangement of purine metabolism in humans is that of gout. Its incidence is about 3 per 1000 persons. It is associated with hyperuricemia. Gouti tophi in joints and urate calculi in the kidney occasionally result. Individuals are frequently treated with allopurinol, which is an inhibitor of xanthine oxidase. The biochemical lesion in most cases of gout has not been identified.

Pyrimidines are first converted to *dihydrouracil* prior to their complete metabolism. Deaminases

TABLE 4-20. Selected Enzymes Of Purine Catabolism

ENZYME	REACTION	COMMENTS
5'-Nucleotidase	5'-nucleotide + H_2O → nucleoside + Pi	Will operate on all 5'-nucleotides and 5'-deoxynucleotides including IMP and XMP
AMP deaminase	AMP + H_2O → NH_3 + IMP	
Adenosine deaminase	Adenosine + H_2O → NH_3 + Inosine	Hereditary deficiency associated with fatal immunodeficiency syndrome
Purine nucleoside phosphorylase	Purine nucleoside + Pi → purine + ribose-1-phosphate or deoxyribose-1-phosphate	Generates free base
Guanine deaminase	Guanine + H_2O → xanthine + NH_3	
Xanthine oxidase	Hypoxanthine + O_2 + H_2O → xanthine + H_2O_2 Xanthine + O_2 + H_2O → urate + H_2O_2	

and nucleoside phosphorylase result in the conversion of the ribo- and deoxyribopyrimidines to uracil. Uracil is converted to dihydrouracil by NADPH and H^+ in a reaction catalyzed by dihydrouracil dehydrogenase. It is hydrolyzed to β-ureido propionate. This is hydrolyzed to CO_2, ammonia, and β-alanine. Thymine catabolism yields β-aminoisobutyrate instead of β-alanine.

INTRODUCTION TO MOLECULAR BIOLOGY

Biology is the science of life. Its subjects include the nature of living organisms and how they reproduce, develop, function, adapt, and evolve. It is the goal of molecular biology to understand these biological phenomena at the molecular level. It has been known for millennia that progeny resemble their parents. During the past century the science of genetics has made prodigious advances; progress continues at an accelerating pace. The science of *molecular biology* concerns the structure, function, and expression of the gene. The *gene* is the unit of inheritance. Fifty years ago, the gene was a biological concept. As progress in science has occurred, we now know that genes are made up of DNA. Genes are specific sequences of bases (A, T, G, and C), along a sugar phosphate backbone, which code for specific RNAs and proteins or which play a regulatory role in genetic expression.

In the next section we shall consider the structure of DNA and how it is replicated. We will see that the information present in parental DNA is used to direct the synthesis of two daughter molecules identical to the parent in the process called *replication.* The pathway for the direction of information flow in biological systems was given in Table 4-1 and is shown in Figure 4-53. The information in the parental sequence of DNA serves as the source of information for progeny DNA in replication. It also dictates the sequence of nucleotides of RNA during gene *transcription* in RNA biosynthesis. RNA in turn directs the synthesis of proteins during *translation.* The 4-letter alphabet of nucleic acids (corresponding to four bases) is translated into the 20-

letter alphabet of proteins (corresponding to the 20 genetically encoded amino acids).

Messenger RNA (mRNA) dictates the sequence of amino acids found in proteins. *Transfer RNA* (tRNA) has two important functions. It combines with its corresponding amino acid to produce a bioenergetically activated species of amino acid. Second, it serves as an adapter in translating serial nucleic acid hydrogen-bonding patterns into an amino acid sequence of a protein. A third type of RNA, *ribosomal RNA* (rRNA), forms a scaffold for the ribosome and perhaps plays a functional role in ribosome action during protein synthesis. Following ribosomal protein synthesis (translation), proteins are subject to translocation to another part of the cell, exocytosis from the cell, and covalent modifications. The latter are called post-translational or processing reactions and include, *inter alia,* proteolytic cleavage, glycosylation, phosphorylation, hydroxylation, methylation, carboxylation, and acetylation.

In addition to these physiological events, important advances in manipulating DNA and RNA in the laboratory have developed during the past 15 years. It has been possible to obtain considerable amounts of purified DNA for analysis and study. The techniques involve the production of *recombinant DNA* molecules. New DNA molecules (recombinant DNA) are often constructed from any DNA of interest *(target DNA)* and a *vehicle DNA,* which can be combined with the target DNA. The vehicle serves as a molecular handle and provides a means of amplifying DNA by cloning procedures to produce adequate amounts for study. Vehicles are often bacterial *plasmids* (extrachromosomal DNAs that replicate autonomously) and bacterial *viruses.* Sometimes animal virus sequences are added to recombinant DNA, so that one can propagate the DNA in either bacterial or animals cell in culture. Recombinant DNA can also be used to produce *chimeric genes,* which encode products that are derived from two different organisms. The design of DNA molecules with specific properties is called *genetic engineering.*

DNA, moreover, can be sequenced by techniques developed since 1975. This permits the deduction of amino acid sequences of proteins (both normal and mutant) through the use of the *genetic code.* The class of enzymes that revolutionized the study of DNA and permitted the production, manipulation, and analysis of recombinant DNA molecules are *restriction endonucleases.* These molecules cleave DNA only at specific nucleotide sequences. It is also possible to prepare radioactive segments of

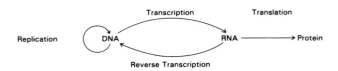

Fig. 4-53. Information transfer; the central dogma of molecular biology.

DNA. These interact with related sequences of DNA obtained from the genome by complementary base pairing or annealing. This has permitted the development of genetic fingerprinting techniques and is playing a role in the diagnosis of a variety of diseases through the use of *restriction fragment length polymorphisms* (RFLPs).

It has been possible to introduce human DNA into *E. coli* and other microorganisms; this process is called *transformation.* By appropriate genetic engineering, cells can be induced to produce large amounts of protein corresponding to the human DNA. Human insulin produced by recombinant DNA technology is currently available for treatment of diabetes mellitus. Human growth hormone, tissue plasminogen activator, interferons (α, β, and γ), blood-clotting factors, and erythropoeitin are among future possible therapeutic agents produced by this technology. In addition to having the protein with the human sequence (as opposed to that of another species), the shortcoming that only minuscule amounts can be obtained from human sources is obviated.

DNA and RNA Structures

DNA is the molecule of heredity (see Table 4-1). DNA is a long thin macromolecule made up of a large number of deoxynucleotides. It can be made up of millions of deoxynucleotides depending upon the species or particular chromosome of a species. The specificity and uniqueness of a DNA molecule is determined by the sequence of bases constituting each deoxynucleotide (base-sugar-phosphate) unit. The information of a DNA molecule corresponds to the sequence of bases in the same way that the information in this sentence depends upon the sequence of letters of the alphabet constituting the sequence. The structure of a tetranucleotide is shown in Figure 4-54. It illustrates the sugar phosphate backbone with bases (A, T, G, and C) attached to the 1'-carbon of deoxyribose by a glycosidic bond. The bonds between the sugars are phosphodiesters linking a 3'-group to the 5'-group in an adjacent nucleotide unit. Linear molecules have a directionality or polarity from the 5'-end to the 3'-end. The 5'-end lacks a phosphodiester involving the 5'-sugar, and the 3'-end is that with a 3'-hydroxyl not in phosphodiester linkage. Some DNAs (prokaryotic and mitochondrial) form covalently closed circles. If an arrow is drawn from the 5'- to 3'-carbon on the same sugar, the direction of the arrow shows the 5'- to 3'-polarity (see Fig. 4-54).

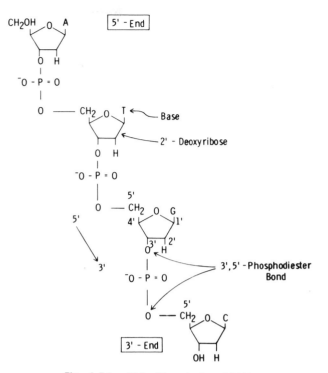

Fig. 4-54. 5' to 3' polarity of DNA.

Human DNA and almost all other DNA is double stranded in nature (that of a few viruses exists as a single strand but forms a double strand during replication). The nature of the double-stranded or duplex DNA was described by James D. Watson and Francis H. C. Crick in 1953. The double-stranded DNA forms a *right-handed double helix;* the strands of the helix ascend as a right hand is turned clockwise (Fig. 4-55). The two strands of the double helix are composed of *complementary polydeoxynucleotides.* The sugar phosphate backbone of each strand is on the exterior and is represented by the ribbons; the bases face the interior and are represented by the lines. The hydrogen bonds between bases are represented by the vertical lines (see Fig. 4-55). The key aspect of the Watson–Crick structure is the formation of *complementary base pairs.* The complementary bases pairs are *A* and *T* (adenine and thymine) and *G* and *C* (guanine and cytosine) (Fig. 4-56). The complementary nature is associated with specific base pairing involving hydrogen bonds (two with A = T and three with G = C). Each complementary pair is composed of a purine and pyrimidine (and not two purines or two pyrimidines). Analysis of DNA molecules from a variety of species has shown that the mole fraction of adenine equals that of thymine; the mole fraction of

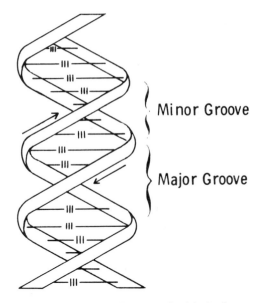

Fig. 4-55. DNA forms a double helix.

guanine also equals that of cytosine. This is called **Chargaff's rule.** The G + C content, however, varies from about 30% to 70% in all species (it is constant in a given species).

The two strands of the double helix exhibit opposite polarity. One courses in the 5'- to 3'-direction, and the complementary strand extends in the opposite direction. This is indicated by the arrows in Figure 4-55. This property is called **antiparallel.** In addition to complementary hydrogen bonding be-

tween double strands in DNA, complementary base pairing occurs between DNA and RNA (during transcription) and between RNA and RNA (intramolecularly in the tRNA cloverleaf and intermolecularly between the anticodon of tRNA and the codon of mRNA). In all known instances, complementary base pairing is antiparallel in nature (see Table 4-1).

The existence of a double-stranded DNA structure with complementary base pairing has a number of theoretical and practical consequences. First, if we know the sequence of bases along one strand, then we can immediately determine the sequence of bases along the other as A base pairs with T and G with C. The sequence has the opposite polarity when compared with its complementary strand. Second, the duplex structure suggests a replication mechanism. If each strand serves as a template for the biosynthesis of a complementary strand, then two daughter DNA duplexes will result, and each will be identical with the parent duplex. Third, methods have been developed for studying the complementary interaction of natural or artificial segments of DNA or RNA with any DNA or RNA of interest. When nucleic acids form a complementary duplex, the polynucleotides are said to **anneal** or **hybridize.** The natural, functional DNA duplex exists in its native conformation. It can be converted into two single-stranded polynucleotides by denaturation. The denatured form is produced by treatment with heat, alkali, or selected organic solvents such as formamide. Under appropriate conditions,

Fig. 4-56. Watson–Crick complementary base pairing.

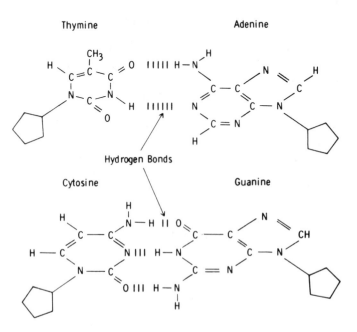

the denatured DNA can reanneal to form a native duplex.

The familiar DNA double helix exists in the B-form. This corresponds to a specific structure determined from its x-ray diffraction pattern. One complete turn of the double helix occurs every 3.4 nm. There are *10* base pairs for each complete turn, and each pair occupies 0.34 nm. This form of DNA also exhibits a major and minor groove when viewed from the side (see Fig. 4-55). Recent x-ray diffraction studies have revealed the existence of another form of DNA called **Z-DNA** (for zig zag). The major difference between the B-form and Z form is that the latter forms a left-handed helix; it still retains the Watson–Crick complementary base pairing property. The sugar phosphates reside on the exterior, and the bases occur on the interior. The Z form is elongated and slimmer when compared with B-DNA. In Z-DNA, there are 12 base pairs per turn of the helix; one full turn is 4.6 nm in length. The physiological role of Z-DNA is still under investigation.

Diploid nuclear DNA of human somatic cells contains about 7×10^9 base pairs. It is distributed among 23 pairs of linear chromosomes. The haploid genome consists of 3.5×10^9 base pairs in the 23 individual chromosomes. It is thought that the DNA in each chromosome consists of a single, linear DNA duplex. Each human mitochondrion contains a small, circular DNA molecule. The mitochondrial DNA carries the information for only a few mitochondrial protein subunits. The **genome** of a cell or organism refers to its total DNA. A gene is a portion of DNA that codes for a functional unit; it may code for a polypeptide chain, a tRNA or rRNA, or it may play a regulatory role.

Let us now consider the manner in which the DNA of a cell is packaged, namely, its structural organization. The length of the DNA in a single human cell exceeds 2 m. The length of a typical human cell, however, is only 20×10^{-6} m or 20 μm. DNA must be condensed into a compact structure. Since the DNA is found in the nucleus, and since the nucleus represents only a portion of the cell (see Table 4-2), the condensation required is even more formidable. **Chromatin** is the term applied to the condensed DNA–protein complex. Proteins in chromatin are divided into two classes: histones and nonhistones. The mass of DNA and protein in chromatin is nearly equal. In humans, **histones** are the most abundant proteins associated with DNA. Histones are a class of proteins that are rich in the positively charged lysine and arginine residues. This presumably allows the interaction of the nega-

tively charged phosphates along the DNA backbone with the positively charged regions of histone proteins. The lowest order of condensation and that which is best understood relates to the formation of nucleosomes. **Nucleosomes,** which resemble beads on a string when observed by electron microscopy, contain two loops of DNA containing about 150 base pairs wrapped around a protein core. The protein core consists of two molecules each of histone H2A, H2B, H3, and H4. These molecules form an octomer. Adjacent nucleosomes are connected by a 60 base pair region, associated with two molecules of histone H1, called the **linking region.** Higher order fibrils and chromatin fibers have been described. These structures account for only a small proportion of packaging necessary to delimit 2 m of DNA in an 8 μm-diameter nucleus.

Nearly the entire chromosome (4×10^6 base pairs) of *E. coli* contains information corresponding to proteins or functional RNA molecules. It was surprising to find that only a small proportion of human DNA consists of sequences corresponding to functional protein or RNA. The quantity of DNA in the human haploid genome is sufficient to encode for 3×10^6 proteins. The actual number of proteins that humans produce in their lifetime, however, corresponds to 3×10^4 to 10×10^4. The function of the apparently excessive DNA, if any, is unknown.

Human DNA consists of various classes based on their copy number in a haploid genome. About 20% to 30% of human DNA is unique and occurs only once. There are two classes of repetitive DNA: highly repetitive and moderately repetitive. **Highly repetitive DNA** occurs in unit lengths of 5 to 500 base pairs and constitutes from 1 to 10 million copies per haploid genome. These are clustered in the centromere (center) and telemeres (ends) of chromosomes. The **moderately repetitive sequences** (less than 10^6 per haploid genome) constitute two subclasses. **Long interspersed repeats** occur in unit lengths of 5000 to 7000 base pairs. **Short interspersed repeats** consist of a few to only several hundred base pairs. The Alu family is one example. (Alu is a restriction enzyme used in characterizing this family; *vide infra*). There are 5×10^5 copies of the Alu family in humans, and it constitutes 5% to 6% of the haploid genome. Similar families exist in other eukaryotes.

Let us now consider the chemical structure and function of **RNA.** It is a polyribonucleotide consisting of a sugar phosphate 3',5'-phosphodiester backbone to which either of two purine or pyrimidine bases are attached. It shares many properties with

TABLE 4-21. General Classes of Eukaryotic and Prokaryotic RNA

CLASS	SIZE		COMMENTS
Eukaryotic ribosomal RNA	18S	1900 Bases	18S, 28S, and 5.8S rRNA derived from common precursor; RNA polymerase I transcript
	28S	4700 Bases	18S found in small ribosomal subunit; other three occur in large subunit
	5.8S	160 Bases	
	5S	120 Bases	RNA polymerase III transcript
Prokaryotic ribosomal RNA	16S	1541 Bases	Small subunit
	23S	2904 Bases	Large subunit
	5S	120 Bases	Large subunit
Prokaryotic and eukaryotic transfer RNA	75–90 Bases		About 40 different tRNAs in cytosol of human cells; many bases modified posttranscriptionally; products include: ribothymidine, dihydrouracil, pseudouridine, 4-thiouridine, inosine, and isopentenyladenosine among others
Prokaryotic messenger RNA	600 Bases and greater		5% of total cellular RNA; short half-life (minutes); may be polycistronic (translated into more than one protein)
Eukaryotic mRNA	600 Bases and greater		5% of total; half-life from minutes to days; contains 5'-7 methyl G cap and poly A 3'-tail; derived from hnRNA; monocistronic.
Eukaryotic heterogeneous nuclear RNA	May contain 100 kb of nucleotide or more		95% degraded in nucleus; precursor of mRNA; undergoes splicing reactions; RNA polymerase II transcript
Eukaryotic small nuclear RNA (snRNA)	100–300 Bases		At least 10 classes exist; each present at 10^5–10^6 copies/cell; RNA polymerase III transcript

DNA, but it also possesses some unique attributes. First, the pentose sugar in RNA is ribose. The presence of ribose confers alkaline lability to the molecule (0.1 N NaOH). This property is utilized to advantage experimentally. Second, while both RNA and DNA contain adenine, guanine, and cytosine, RNA contains uracil in place of thymine. Third, RNA is single stranded and does not exist as a duplex. As a corollary, the content of guanine does not necessarily equal cytosine, nor does adenine equal uracil. The *primary structure* of DNA and RNA refers to the sequence of bases along the molecule. By convention, sequences of each are given in the 5'- to 3'-direction from left to right unless specified otherwise. The *secondary structure* of RNA refers to hydrogen-bonding properties. The single-stranded RNA molecule forms intramolecular loops when segments are self-complementary. These are prominent in tRNA.

There are three major classes of RNA in all living organisms. Eukaryotes, including humans, possess two additional classes. The three universal classes are tRNA, rRNA, and mRNA. Some of their properties are adumbrated in Table 4-21. Eukaryotes also contain heterogeneous nuclear RNA (hnRNA). This is the precursor of mRNA. Eukaryotes, moreover, contain small nuclear RNAs (snRNA), some of which may play a role in splicing reactions (removal of intervening sequences of RNA).

Replication: DNA Biosynthesis

REQUIRED COMPONENTS

We will first consider the properties of the various enzymes and proteins necessary for DNA replication. We will concentrate on the replication process in *E. coli*. The biochemistry and genetics of this system has been extensively characterized. We will also consider the properties of mammalian replication enzymes. After the known components have been described, we will correlate biochemistry and cell biology and describe a working model of replication. We will also consider mechanisms for repairing DNA that has undergone an alteration resulting from the inherent instability of the bases or as a result of an environmental insult.

The classes of enzyme activities that are required for replication in *E. coli* include the DNA polymerases and DNA ligase. Another enzyme, called primase, is required for the formation of a polynucleotide primer. The 3'-exonuclease activity of *E. coli* DNA polymerases catalyzes the stepwise hydrolysis of deoxynucleotides from the 3'-end and plays a role in proofreading or editing. Their 5'-exonuclease activity degrades DNA stepwise (or in blocks of up to 10 residues in length) and is important in excising the primer and in repair of DNA. A *helicase* is an ATP-dependent enzyme that separates the bases of the double strand ahead of the site

TABLE 4-22. Replication Proteins in *E. coli*

PROTEIN	ROLE
DNA polymerase III	Synthesizes DNA
DNA polymerase I	Degrades primer and fills gaps; repair synthesis
DNA ligase	Eliminates nicks in phosphodiester backbone; NAD$^+$ serves as a source of phosphate bond energy
Primase	Initiates polymerization with hybrid ribodeoxyribonucleotides
Helicase	ATP-dependent separation of base pairs in the replication fork
DNA gyrase	A topoisomerase that introduces superhelical twists
Single-strand binding protein (SSB)	Stabilizes single-stranded regions in replication fork

of polydeoxyribonucleotide biosynthesis. A **DNA gyrase** is an enzyme that alters the supercoiling of DNA, which facilitates the polymerization reactions (Table 4-22). Otherwise identical molecules of DNA with different degrees of supercoiling are called **topological isomers**. **Topoisomerases** catalyze the interconversion of these various forms. DNA gyrase is one type of topoisomerase.

Let us consider the elongation reactions in DNA biosynthesis. The generic name for enzymes that catalyze these reactions is **DNA polymerase**. In *E. coli*, three polymerases have been described and are designated I, II, and III in the order of their discovery. It appears that DNA polymerase III is responsible for the preponderance of DNA synthesis *in vivo*. DNA polymerase I is required for replacing the primer (a mixed ribo-deoxyribonucleotide segment) and for repair synthesis. The function of DNA polymerase II is unknown. Three mammalian DNA polymerases have been described: DNA polymerases α, β, and γ. Polymerase α is thought to mediate the preponderance of nuclear DNA synthesis and polymerase β functions in nuclear repair synthesis. DNA polymerase γ carries out replication within the mitochondrion (Table 4-23).

TABLE 4-23. Replication Proteins in Humans

PROTEIN	FUNCTION
DNA polymerase α	Synthesizes DNA
DNA polymerase β	Repair synthesis
DNA polymerase γ	Mitochondrial DNA synthesis
DNA ligase	Eliminates nicks in phosphodiester backbone; ATP serves as a source of phosphate bond energy
Topoisomerase II	ATP-dependent topoisomerase that introduces superhelical twists

All known DNA polymerases (both eukaryotic and prokaryotic) exhibit the following properties. They catalyze the elongation of an existing polynucleotide (designated as the **primer**) in the **5'- to 3'- direction** (see Table 4-1). The enzyme requires all four deoxynucleoside triphosphates as substrates (as the Mg^{2+} complex). The sequence of deoxyribonucleotides in the growing chain is determined by a **template** strand of DNA by the principle of Watson–Crick base pairing. If a C is present in the template strand, then G is added to the growing chain (Fig. 4-57) and vice versa. If T is present in the template strand, then A is added to the growing chain (and vice versa). The template strand is antiparallel to the growing polynucleotide chain (see Fig. 4-57). The chemistry of the elongation reaction is shown in Figure 4-58. (This diagram contains a deceptively large amount of information and should be mastered by the reader.) It shows that the 3'-hydroxyl group of the growing chain attacks the α-phosphorous of the incoming deoxynucleoside triphosphate. A new phosphodiester bond forms, and PPi is displaced. From this diagram, we can readily see that chain growth is in the 5'- to 3'-direction. The polarity of the growing polynucleotide is such that the last residue added contains a free 3'-hydroxyl group.

DNA polymerases from bacteria exhibit a 3'-exonuclease activity. This apparently paradoxical activity catalyzes the hydrolytic removal of the last polynucleotide added to the growing nucleotide chain. The product is a polynucleotide with one fewer residue and a free 3'-hydroxyl group. The best substrate for this 3'-exonuclease activity is a molecule that contains a mismatched 3'-deoxynucleotide (Fig. 4-59). For example, if G were added

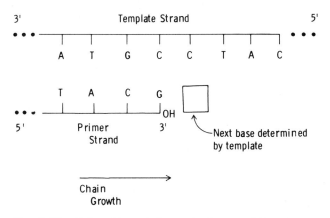

Fig. 4-57. Role of template and primer in DNA biosynthesis.

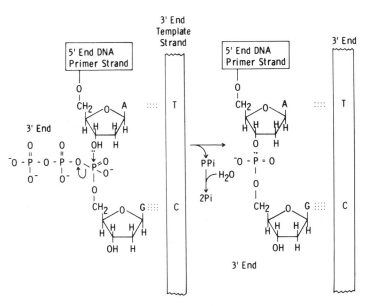

Fig. 4-58. Chemistry of the chain elongation reaction of DNA biosynthesis.

in a position complementary to T, then deoxyguanosine monophosphate constitutes a very good substrate for prompt hydrolytic removal. This is called the *editing* or *proofreading* function of DNA polymerase. Following this correction, A is then incorporated. This feature increases the fidelity of enzymatic DNA replication. The polymerase selects the appropriate deoxynucleoside triphosphate by the base-pairing principle. The selection is monitored a second time by the proofreading function, and the occasional mistake is eliminated. The error frequency is reduced to $1 : 10^8$ by this mechanism. It is puzzling that mammalian DNA polymerases lack this 3'-exonuclease activity. The fidelity of replication, however, is at least as great as that for *E. coli*.

DNA polymerases from bacteria also exhibit 5'-exonuclease activity. The enzyme can remove monomers and somewhat higher segments (perhaps up to 10) by a single hydrolytic cleavage. The en-

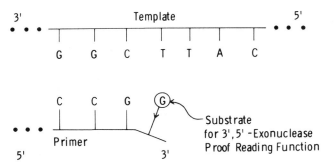

Fig. 4-59. Substrate for the 3',5'-exonuclease proofreading activity of DNA polymerase.

zyme is capable of degrading polynucleotide segments by 5'-exonuclease activity and filling in the resulting gaps by polymerase activity. This property is thought to be important in removing the mixed ribo-deoxyribonucleotidyl primer whose formation is mediated by primase. The occurrence of this activity in eukaryotes has not been established with certainty.

Let us now consider the action of **DNA ligase.** This activity is responsible for linking a free 3'-hydroxyl with an adjacent 5'-phosphate occurring in a DNA duplex (Fig. 4-60). It eliminates a nick from DNA. This is important for both replication and repair. For humans DNA ligase catalyzes the adenylylation of the 5'-phosphate (Fig. 4-61). This results in the activation of the 5'-phosphate: the molecule contains an acid anhydride, high-energy bond. The enzyme catalyzes the reaction between the nucleophilic 3'-hydroxyl with the activated phosphate to produce a phosphodiester bond (the nick is eliminated). AMP is released. PPi is the other product, and it is degraded by hydrolysis. The reaction in *E. coli* is analogous except that NAD+ (nicotinamide-ribose-phosphate-phosphate-adenosine) is the adenylyl (phosphoryl-adenosine) donor.

We noted above that DNA polymerase requires a prefabricated polynucleotide (primer) in order to catalyze the formation of any phosphodiester bonds. **Primase** is an enzyme that is able to initiate polynucleotide formation. It utilizes both nucleoside and deoxynucleoside triphosphates as substrates, and it also requires a template. Chain growth is in the 5'- to 3'-direction, and the reaction

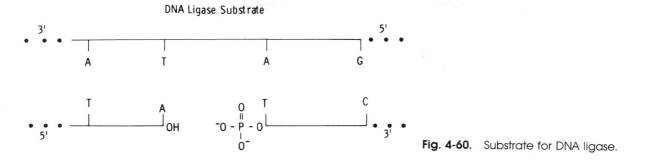

Fig. 4-60. Substrate for DNA ligase.

catalyzed is analogous to that shown in Figure 4-58. After a primer of 10 to 50 residues is produced, polymerase III (in *E. coli*) utilizes the resulting primer and catalyzes the template-directed synthesis of polydeoxyribonucleotide (Fig. 4-62). The primer is recognized by cellular proteins as being distinct from the product of the elongation or polymerization reaction since the primer contains ribonucleotides. The primer is removed by DNA polymerase I 5'-exonuclease activity; this enzyme also fills the resulting gap (polymerase activity). DNA ligase completes the process by combining a free 3'-hydroxyl with a 5'-phosphate.

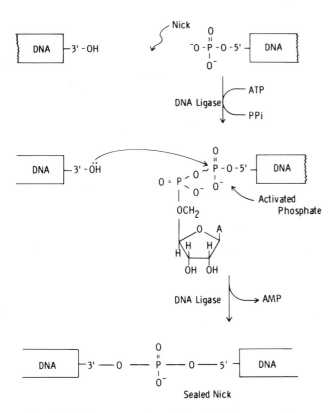

Fig. 4-61. Bioenergetics of the DNA ligase reaction.

REPLICATION

Next, we consider the process of DNA replication from a higher structural order. Replication in *E. coli* (and in mammals) involves the synthesis of DNA complementary to both strands of the DNA duplex, and replication forks move in both directions from a replication origin. In *E. coli* there is a unique sequence of DNA that serves as a replication origin. In eukaryotic cells there are thousands of replication origins on each chromosome. Multiple origins of replication are illustrated in Figure 4-63. The following components play a role in the replication process in *E. coli*. A helicase separates the strands at the cost of one ATP per base pair. DNA gyrase (a topoisomerase) introduces supercoils to relieve the torsion. Single-strand binding (SSB) proteins stabilize the single-stranded regions. Primase initiates synthesis off one strand toward the right. Polymerase III continues synthesis. Elongation toward the right is 5' to 3', and synthesis proceeds continuously for the leading strand (Fig. 4-64).

A major dilemma results when considering the synthesis of the opposite strand as the replication fork moves to the right. All DNA polymerases catalyze polymerization in the 5'- to 3'-direction. The solution to this quandary emerged when it was dis-

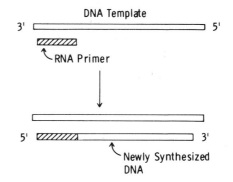

Fig. 4-62. An RNA primer is required to initiate DNA biosynthesis.

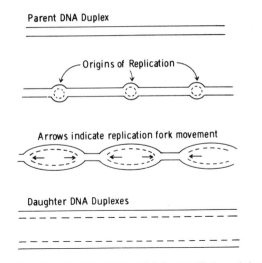

Fig. 4-63. Eukaryotic DNA exhibits multiple origins of replication.

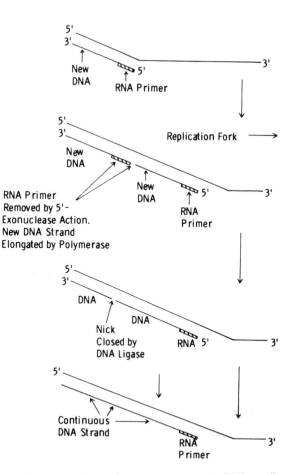

Fig. 4-65. Lagging strand biosynthesis in DNA replication.

covered that one strand of DNA is synthesized in short fragments (*Okazaki fragments*) in a discontinuous fashion (see Fig. 4-64; Fig. 4-65). For this to occur, primase starts on the right and polymerase III synthesizes the complementary strand toward the left. Primase then initiates synthesis of another segment farther to the right, and synthesis continues toward the left (see Fig. 4-65). In this fashion both strands are elongated as the replication fork proceeds rightward. The trick employed by nature is to synthesize the lagging strand in short (1000-nucleotide) stretches to the left. This procedure emphasizes the importance of polymerase I in physiological synthesis. At the many primer sites on the lagging strand, its 5'-exonuclease activity degrades the primer portion, and its polymerase activity fills the gap. DNA ligase then seals the nick, and a continuous strand thereby results (see Fig. 4-64).

An analogous situation exists on the replication fork progressing leftward. Primase can initiate chain growth toward the left, and polymerase can

continue it in a continuous fashion on one of the two strands. Synthesis using the opposite strand as template begins on the left and continues to the right. A second strand begins farther to the left and continues to the first strand. Then 5'-exonuclease activity of polymerase I removes the ribonucleotide–deoxyribonucleotide portion and fills the gap. DNA ligase seals the nick. As chain growth continues, the parental strands separate. The daughter DNA contains one parental strand and one newly synthesized strand. This property is referred to as *semiconservative replication* (conservative replication refers to the nonexistent situation where both parent strands and both daughter strands are found together). DNA gyrase aids in the unraveling process by converting the supercoiled DNA into more favorable topological isomers. It removes twists that are produced by the unwinding process.

The previous description reflects current knowledge of the process of replication in *E. coli* and other bacterial chromosomes. This process proba-

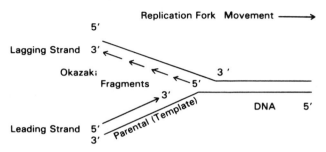

Fig. 4-64. Leading and lagging strands in DNA replication.

bly applies to eukaryotic DNA replication. Our knowledge of the proteins involved, however, is less complete. It seems probable that activities in addition to these given in Table 4-23 are required. Unlike *E. coli*, with a single origin of replication, thousands of replication origins exist in mammals. Proteins or factors may exist that cause initiation at specific and presently uncharacterized sites. Eukaryotic chromosomes also possess nucleosomes with their associated histones; bacterial chromosomes lack histone and the nucleosome structure. The negative charges of DNA phosphate in bacteria are neutralized by metals (Mg^{2+}, K^+) and organic cations such as spermine and spermidine. The histones associated with the parent eukaryotic DNA duplex become associated with the leading strand and its template strand where reformation of nucleosomes occurs. Newly synthesized histones become associated with the lagging strand and its template strand. Eukaryotic DNA polymerases progress along their templates about 10 times more slowly than those in *E. coli*. The discontinuous strands, called Okazaki fragments, in eukaryotes are 10% to 20% the length of those in *E. coli*. These differences may be related to the presence of nucleosomes and the greater degree of compactness of eukaryotic DNA when compared with that of *E. coli*.

DNA Repair

DNA is inherently unstable. It is thus subject to change by physical and chemical agents in the environment. Altered DNA is repaired by mechanisms considered in this section. These repair mechanisms rely on the fact that information is originally contained in two strands. If only one strand is modified, information residing on the other can be used to affect the repair process. If both strands of the duplex are altered, then a recombinational process involving an allele on the other chromosome of the pair may provide the information to achieve repair. If neither of these occur, then the damage is retained as a mutation (an inheritable change in DNA, which is passed on to progeny cells). Such insults accumulate in humans and have been postulated to be important factors in aging, tumorigenesis, and perhaps cell death.

Let us consider the types of structural modifications that DNA undergoes and then the process of repair. The amino groups of cytosine and adenine in DNA undergo spontaneous (nonenzymatic) hydrolysis and form uracil and hypoxanthine, respectively. These structures are recognized by cellular proteins or enzymes as abnormal. An AP-glycosi-

dase catalyzes the hydrolytic removal of the abnormal base leaving an intact sugar phosphate backbone. The result is an AP site where AP is an abbreviation for apurinic (lacking A or G) or apyrimidinic (lacking C or T). One of a family of endonuclease activities catalyzes the hydrolysis of a phosphodiester bond on the 5'-side and near the AP site. 5'-Exonuclease activity then removes a segment of the polynucleotide containing the AP site. A repair polymerase, utilizing a newly created 3'-hydroxyl group, fills the gap. Then DNA ligase seals the nick, and the original base sequence is restored. A similar sequence of reactions involving *excision repair* results when a purine is spontaneously hydrolyzed from one of the strands. Alterations produced by ionizing radiation, the chemical modification of bases by alkylating agents, and the formation of thymine dimers by ultraviolet light can also be corrected by this excision–repair process.

Transcription: RNA Biosynthesis

RNA is transcribed from DNA. The enzymes that catalyze RNA biosynthesis are **DNA-dependent RNA polymerases.** We shall consider the reaction catalyzed by prokaryotic and eukaryotic RNA polymerases. Then we will consider the structural differences in enzymes isolated from *E. coli* and from mammals. Following biosynthesis the primary RNA transcript may be chemically modified in processing reactions. We will consider later the signals in DNA that are important in dictating the start site for transcription and the sequences that play a regulatory role in determining the frequency of initiation.

RNA polymerase, unlike DNA polymerase, is readily able to initiate polynucleotide synthesis, that is, a primer is not required. The elongation reactions are highly analogous to those catalyzed by DNA polymerase. Chain growth proceeds in the 5'-to 3'-direction (see Table 4-1). The sequence of nucleotides in the resulting RNA is determined by Watson–Crick base-pairing principles with the substitution of uracil (RNA) for thymine (DNA). The base-pairing rules are as follows: template A yields U, T yields A, G yields C, and C yields G. The RNA strand is antiparallel to its template. During replication both strands of DNA serve as a template to produce two duplex molecules. In RNA synthesis only one of the two strands of a particular genetic DNA duplex functions as a template. One strand of the DNA duplex serves as template in some genes, while the opposite strand is the template strand in other genes. The template strand, however, is anti-

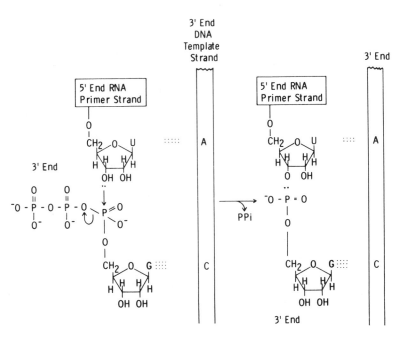

Fig. 4-66. Chemistry of the RNA polymerase reaction.

parallel to the RNA in all cases. RNA polymerases also lack the 3' to 5' proofreading exonuclease function. The physiological consequence of an error in RNA synthesis is not as great as that for DNA synthesis.

In addition to the DNA template, the four nucleoside triphosphates (as their magnesium complex) are required as substrates. The chemistry of the elongation reaction is illustrated in Figure 4-66. From this diagram we can see that chain growth occurs in the 5'- to 3'-direction. This scheme contains a deceptively large amount of information and should be understood by the reader.

Let us consider the properties of the **RNA polymerase** isolated from E. coli. The holoenzyme consists of four different protein subunits. These are present with the stoichiometry $\alpha_2\beta\beta'\sigma$ (Table 4-24). The $\alpha_2\beta\beta'$ component constitutes the **core enzyme.** It possesses RNA polymerase activity. The **sigma subunit** (σ) confers the property of specific initiation to the core enzyme. Following initiation the sigma

subunit dissociates from the complex and can combine with another core enzyme to initiate synthesis of another chain. When the core enzyme approaches a transcriptional stop signal, a factor named **rho** interacts with the core polymerase and results in appropriate chain termination.

In contrast to E. coli with its single RNA polymerase, eukaryotes have three RNA polymerases that catalyze the biosynthesis of different classes of RNA in the cell nucleus. Each of the three polymerases has more subunits (>10) than the bacterial enzyme. The functions of the subunits, however, have not yet been determined. In addition to the polymerases, several auxillary proteins called **transcription factors** are required for initiation of RNA synthesis at the correct sites on DNA. The three classes of eukaryotic RNA polymerase are designated by Roman numerals I, II, and III. **RNA polymerase I** is responsible for rRNA synthesis in the nucleolus. RNA polymerase II mediates the formation of hnRNA; polymerase III catalyzes the formation of 5S RNA and other small RNAs (see Table 4-21). The three polymerases also differ with respect to their sensitivity to a fungal toxin named α-amanitin. Polymerase II is most sensitive, and polymerase III is somewhat sensitive to this substance. Polymerase I, on the other hand, is insensitive to α-amanitin.

The primary transcripts of all three classes of RNA in eukaryotes undergo additional modifications; these are called processing reactions. The conversion of hnRNA to mRNA by processing is

TABLE 4-24. RNA Polymerase Subunits and Transcription Factors in E. coli

SUBUNIT	NUMBER IN ENZYME	FUNCTION
β (Beta)	1	Catalytic site
β' (Beta prime)	1	DNA binding
α (Alpha)	2	Unknown
σ (Sigma)	1	Promotor recognition, initiation
ρ (Rho)	1	Termination

the most complex. Prior to chain completion, the nascent chain reacts with GTP to form a 5' to 5' guanosine triphosphate terminus (Fig. 4-67). This is methylated by *S*-adenosylmethionine and is called the 5'-*cap*. After chain termination, the 3'-end reacts with several (>100) ATPs to form a poly A tail structure (a series of covalently linked adenylate residues) and PPi. The cap is probably necessary for mRNA to interact with the ribosome; the poly A tail may stabilize the message. Occasional mRNAs, such as those encoding histones, lack the poly A tail. Heterogeneous nuclear RNA also undergoes splicing reactions. During this process, intervening sequences are removed by excision. It is imperative that splicing be performed accurately; otherwise an aberrant protein would result. Small nuclear RNAs apparently play a role in aligning the hnRNA to ensure accurate splicing (see Fig. 4-67). These processing reactions occur in the cell nucleus prior to transport to cytoplasmic ribosomes.

The signals for splicing out intervening sequences consist of canonical sequences of about nine bases consisting of 5'-donor and 3'-acceptor sites within the hnRNA. The first two bases of the excised RNA are GT and the last two are AG. Canonical sequences in the 3'-region of hnRNA (AAUAAA) specify the site for adding the 3' poly A tail 10 to 30 nucleotides downstream.

Rifamycin is a drug that inhibits the initiation of RNA biosynthesis in prokaryotes, but not elonga-

tion. It binds specifically to the β subunit. This suggests that the interaction of the β and σ subunits are important during the initiation process. Rifamycin is currently one of the three drugs employed for the treatment of persons with tuberculosis. It does not inhibit initiation in eukaryotes. ***Actinomycin D*** is a drug that binds to DNA and inhibits RNA elongation reactions in both eukaryotes and prokaryotes. This substance is used in the treatment of several types of malignant tumors. It fails to inhibit DNA elongation reactions.

Translation: Protein Biosynthesis

Crick's law of molecular biology (often called the central dogma of molecular biology) states that information flows from DNA to RNA to protein (see Table 4-1). The alphabet of nucleic acids consists of four letters: A, T, G, and C in DNA and A, U, G, and C in RNA. The alphabet of proteins consists of 20 letters corresponding to the 20 amino acids that participate in ribosomal protein synthesis (see Table 4-5). The conversion of the 4-letter nucleic acid alphabet to the 20-letter protein alphabet is called ***translation.*** It requires very elaborate biochemical machinery consisting of more than 150 molecular components.

Three classes of RNA are involved in translation: rRNA, tRNA, and mRNA. The rRNA constitutes about half the mass of ribosomes, and protein constitutes the remainder. Ribosomes are made up of two subunits: a small subunit and a large subunit. Ribosomes are the subcellular machines where peptide bond formation and protein synthesis occurs. Transfer RNAs have two functions. They serve as adaptors that recognize the nucleic acid code, and they carry activated amino acids bound through a high-energy bond. Messenger RNA carries information as a specific sequence of bases (codons), which specify the sequence of amino acids found in the corresponding protein. Enzymes (amino acid–tRNA synthetases) catalyze the attachment of the amino acids to their corresponding tRNAs. Several nonribosomal proteins participate in protein biosynthesis. These include initiation factors, elongation factors, and termination or release factors. Before considering the steps involved in protein synthesis, let us first consider the properties of the genetic code.

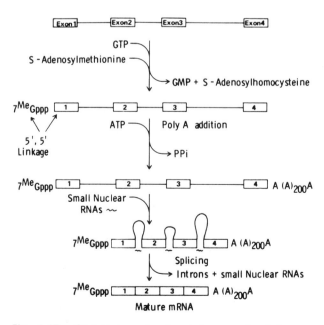

Fig. 4-67. Capping, polyadenylation, and splicing reactions are involved in mRNA formation.

GENETIC CODE

A two-letter code constructed from any 4 letters (A, T, G, or C in DNA or A, U, G, or C in RNA) yields

4^2 or 16 different code words or *codons*. This is insufficient to uniquely specify the 20 different amino acids. A 3-letter or triplet code yields 4^3 or 64 different codons. This is more than adequate to specify the 20 different amino acids. Extensive experimentation has shown that the genetic code is triplet in nature; the codons and their corresponding amino acids are tabulated in Table 4-25. Based on the methodology used to decipher the code, the codons are expressed as a sequence of RNA beginning from the 5'-end of each triplet. During protein synthesis mRNA is translated triplet by triplet in the 5'- to 3'-direction.

Of the 64 possible codons, all but 3 (*i.e.*, 61) correspond to an amino acid. The three exceptions (UAG, UAA, UGA) are stop codons and code for chain termination. Methionine (AUG) and tryptophan (UGG) have a single codon. **AUG** is the initiating codon for protein biosynthesis, and **methionine** is the initiating amino acid in eukaryotes and prokaryotes. AUG also codes for the methionine residues that occur on the interior of proteins. The 18 other amino acids are represented by more than one codon, and this property is called **degeneracy**. Nine of the amino acids are represented by two codons. In this group of nine, the first two bases are the same, and the third position is either a pyrimidine (Py) or a purine (Pu). The codons are XYPy or XYPu. Five amino acids are represented by four codons. In each case the first two bases are the same, and the third base can be any of the four (A, U, G, or C). Three amino acids are represented by six codons. These constitute a combination of four

codons and two codons with the above-mentioned properties (see Table 4-25). Isoleucine is the only amino acid represented by three codons (see Table 4-5). Again, the first two bases are the same (see Table 4-25).

Because of the variation in the third position of the codon and because it participates in some non-standard Watson–Crick base pairing with the tRNA anticodon, the third codon position is called the **wobble** position. Because of this property, some tRNAs are able to interact with (adapt to) two or even three different codons. On the order of 40 tRNAs will interact with the 61 codons. We will not consider the precise nature of wobble base-pairing here. The interaction of tRNA with mRNA occurs in an antiparallel orientation. The wobble position is on the 3'-end of the mRNA codon; this corresponds to the 5'-end of the anticodon triplet.

As mentioned previously, AUG codes for the first and initiating amino acid, which is methionine. The genetic code is read triplet by triplet in the 5'- to 3'-direction until a termination or stop codon is reached. No punctuation signal is required to indicate the end of one codon and the beginning of the next (the code is **commaless**). Each base of the triplet is used only once per polypeptide synthesized (the code is **nonoverlapping**). The genetic code is (almost) **universal**. It is the same for both prokaryotes and eukaryotes. That for mitochondrial protein synthesis is exceptional and is somewhat different from that given in Table 4-25.

THE RIBOSOME

The ribosome is the biochemical machine on which protein biosynthesis occurs. It is here where mRNA and aminoacyl-tRNAs interact; it is also here where peptide bond formation occurs. The size of ribosomes and their subunits are expressed by their sedimentation coefficients (Svedberg or S values). The *E. coli* ribosome is a 70S ribosome. It is composed of a large subunit (50S) and a small subunit (30S). The composition is shown in Table 4-26. Eukaryotic ribosomes are 80S in nature and also consist of a large (60S) and small (40S) subunit (Table 4-27). The primary structures of the rRNAs and most of the ribosomal proteins have been determined.

Ribosomes contain two functional sites termed the **A site** and the **P site**. Aminoacyl-tRNA binds at the A site; peptidyl-tRNA and the initiating methionine tRNA bind at the P site. The small and large subunits make contributions to both sites. The **peptidyltransferase** activity, which catalyzes peptide bond formation, resides on the large subunit.

TABLE 4-25. Genetic Code

FIRST POSITION (5'-END)	SECOND POSITION				THIRD POSITION (3'-END)
	U	C	A	G	
U	Phe	Ser	Tyr	Cys	U
	Phe	Ser	Tyr	Cys	C
	Leu	Ser	Stop	Stop	A
	Leu	Ser	Stop	Trp	G
C	Leu	Pro	His	Arg	U
	Leu	Pro	His	Arg	C
	Leu	Pro	Gln	Arg	A
	Leu	Pro	Gln	Arg	G
A	Ile	Thr	Asn	Ser	U
	Ile	Thr	Asn	Ser	C
	Ile	Thr	Lys	Arg	A
	Met	Thr	Lys	Arg	G
G	Val	Ala	Asp	Gly	U
	Val	Ala	Asp	Gly	C
	Val	Ala	Glu	Gly	A
	Val	Ala	Glu	Gly	G

TABLE 4-26. Composition of the Ribosomes of *E. coli*

PROPERTY	RIBOSOME	SMALL SUBUNIT	LARGE SUBUNIT
Sedimentation coefficient	70S	30S	50S
RNA		16S	23S
			5S
Protein		21 Polypeptides	31 Polypeptides

AMINO ACID ACTIVATION

The enzymes that catalyze the formation of amino-acyl-tRNA are termed ***aminoacyl-tRNA synthetases*** (or ligases). There is 1 enzyme in *E. coli* and 1 cytoplasmic enzyme in eukaryotes corresponding to each of the 20 genetically encoded amino acids. These enzymes attach the specific amino acid to each of the tRNAs that correspond to that amino acid. The degeneracy of the genetic code necessitates the utilization of more than one tRNA for several amino acids. The tRNAs that correspond to a given amino acid are called isoacceptors. The mechanism of amino acid activation is analogous to that for fatty acid activation. It involves a pyrophosphate split from ATP to yield an aminoacyl-AMP intermediate. This reacts with its corresponding tRNA to form aminoacyl-tRNA and AMP. The reaction can be outlined as follows (where aa denotes amino acid).

$$aa + ATP \rightleftharpoons aa\text{-}AMP + PPi$$

$$aa\text{-}AMP + tRNA \rightleftharpoons aa\text{-}tRNA + AMP$$

Both steps are catalyzed by a single enzyme. There is no loss of energy-rich bonds in this process. The hydrolysis of PPi catalyzed by a separate pyrophosphatase serves to pull the reaction in the forward direction (see Table 4-1). The 3'-sequence of eukaryotic and prokaryotic tRNAs ends with . . . CCA in all known cases. The amino acid is covalently linked to the 2'- or 3'-hydroxyl of ribose on the 3'-terminal adenine nucleotide of tRNA through an energy-rich bond.

TABLE 4-27. Composition of Mammalian Ribosomes

PROPERTY	RIBOSOME	SMALL SUBUNIT	LARGE SUBUNIT
Sedimentation coefficient	80S	40S	60S
RNA		18S	28S
			5.8S
			5S
Protein		33 Polypeptides	49 Polypeptides

TABLE 4-28. Factors Involved in Protein Synthesis in *E. coli*

FACTOR	MOLECULAR WEIGHT	FUNCTION
Initiation Factors		
IF1	9,000	Unknown
IF2	100,000	Binds GTP and formyl-met-tRNA[i]
IF3	23,000	mRNA binding
Elongation Factors		
EF-T is made of		Transfer
EF-Tu	43,000	unstable; binds amino-acyltRNA/GTP
EF-Ts	74,000	stable; displaces GDP
EF-G	77,000	GTPase; translocates mRNA along ribosome
Release Factors		
RF1		Recognizes UAA, UAG
RF2		Recognizes UAA, UGA

PROTEIN SYNTHESIS FACTORS

The reactions of protein synthesis are conveniently divided into initiation, elongation, and termination. There are protein factors that transiently associate with the ribosome to perform specific functions. In prokaryotes the *initiation factors* are designated IF, the *elongation factors* are EF, and the *termination* or *release factors* are called RFs. The factors in eukaryotic systems are similarly designated with an e prefix for eukaryotic (*e.g.,* eIF). The various factors are given in Tables 4-28 and 4-29.

TABLE 4-29. Factors Involved in Protein Synthesis in Mammals

FACTOR	FUNCTION
Initiation Factors	
eIF1	Assists mRNA binding
eIF2	Binds initiator met-tRNA[i] and GTP
eIF3	Binds mRNA
eIF4A	Assists mRNA binding
eIF4B	Assists mRNA binding
eIF4C	Unknown
eIF5	Releases eIF2 and eIF3
eIF6	Prevents association of large and small subunit
Elongation Factors	
EF1	Binds aminoacyl-tRNA and GTP
EF2	Translocates mRNA along ribosome; hydrolyzes GTP
Release Factor	
eRF	GTP–binding activity and hydrolysis (GDP + Pi) accompanies hydrolysis of peptidyl-tRNA

Three initiation factors are required in prokaryotes, and several more occur in eukaryotes. The functions of the first three in each class are similar. IF2 binds GTP and formyl-met-tRNA^I (where I refers to a special, Initiator molecule) in prokaryotes; eIF2 binds GTP and met-tRNA^I in eukaryotes. These factors place the initiator methionine-tRNA^I into the P site of the ribosome during the initiation process. N-Formyl-methionine-tRNA^I (f-met-tRNA^I) is the initiating residue in prokaryotes, and met-tRNA^I (unformylated) is the initiator in eukaryotes. The formyl group in prokaryotes is added after methionine has been linked to its cognate tRNA; THF is the formyl donor. Methionine-tRNA^{met} is not formylated in either case. The initiation factors do not form a complex with methionine-tRNA^{met}; the latter is the source of the methionine placed into internal positions of nascent polypeptide chains. EF-Tu in prokaryotes and eEF-1 in eukaryotes form a complex with GTP and methionine-tRNA^{met} and all other aminoacyl-tRNAs (one at a time) required for protein biosynthesis. These factors place the aminoacyl-tRNA into the A site during protein synthesis. Let us now consider the various steps of protein synthesis.

PROTEIN SYNTHESIS REACTIONS

To initiate the biosynthetic process, mRNA must form a complex with the ribosome and f-met-tRNA^I (prokaryotes) or met-tRNA^I (eukaryotes). The initiating AUG codon is not at the 5'-end of mRNA but is 50 to 100 nucleotides or more from the 5'-end. The following is a description of protein synthesis in prokaryotes. To initiate synthesis, the small ribosomal subunit binds near the initiation codon in a process negotiated by IF3. Next, IF2/GTP/f-met-tRNA^I binds to the mRNA–small subunit complex. The large subunit then binds to these components. GTP is hydrolyzed to GDP and Pi; IF2 dissociates from the complex. At the end of this process, f-met-tRNA^I is bound to the P site of the ribosome with its anticodon bound in an antiparallel fashion with the initiating AUG of mRNA.

Following the formation of the initiation complex, a series of repetitive elongation relations occur. For a protein containing 300 amino acids, there is a unique initiation event followed by many elongation events and a unique termination event. A series of ternary complexes of EFTu/GTP/aminoacyl-tRNAs interact with the A (aminoacyl-tRNA) site of the ribosome (eEF1/GTP/aminoacyl-tRNAs in eukaryotes). When a match between the triplet codon immediately after the AUG (on the 3'-side) and the corresponding aminoacyl-tRNA anticodon occurs, then GTP is hydrolyzed and EFTu dissociates from the ribosome. The appropriate aminoacyl-tRNA is implanted in the A site. Next, the endogenous peptidyltransferase activity of the large ribosomal subunit catalyzes a reaction between the amino group in the A site with the activated carboxyl group in the P site to form the first peptide bond. Following this reaction the dipeptidyl-tRNA is bound to the A site, and free tRNA is found in the P site. Prior to the next elongation reaction, EFG/GTP interacts with the complex and mediates the translocation of mRNA and peptidyl-tRNA from the A site to the P site. In the process GTP is hydrolyzed to GDP and Pi, and the free tRNA is ejected from the P site. This completes the first elongation cycle. The dipeptidyl-tRNA now occupies the P site. The second and subsequent cycles of elongation occur as described for the first. Aminoacyl-tRNA is brought to the A site as a complex with EF-Tu and GTP. Following interaction of the matching codon with anticodon, GTP hydrolysis occurs. Peptide bond formation and translocation follow. The process in eukaryotes is analogous and is shown in Figure 4-68.

The reaction catalyzed by peptidyltransferase is the same in prokaryotes and eukaryotes and is shown in Figure 4-69. This diagram contains a deceptively large amount of information and should be mastered by the reader. From the diagram, one can determine that chain growth occurs from the amino to carboxyl terminus. One can also see that peptidyl-tRNA occupies the A site following the peptidyltransferase reaction. This necessitates a translocation reaction as illustrated in Figure 4-68.

The elongation cycles continue until a termination or stop codon occupies the A site. A release factor interacts with the complex and discharges the polypeptide from tRNA by hydrolysis; the ribosomal subunits dissociate, and the tRNA is liberated. The process in prokaryotes and eukaryotes is analogous. Several antibiotics inhibit specific steps of translation; the actions of several of these are given in Table 4-30. Diphtheria toxin, moreover, catalyzes a reaction between eEF-2 and NAD$^+$ to give ADP ribosyl-eEF2 and nicotinamide. The covalently bound ADP ribosyl group inactivates the eukaryotic elongation factor. The potent toxin, made in $Corynebacterium diphtheriae,$ has no effect on bacterial protein synthesis.

Let us now consider the bioenergetic cost of peptide bond formation. Two high-energy bonds of ATP are expended to form aminoacyl-tRNA (ATP → AMP + 2 Pi). One GTP is hydrolyzed (to

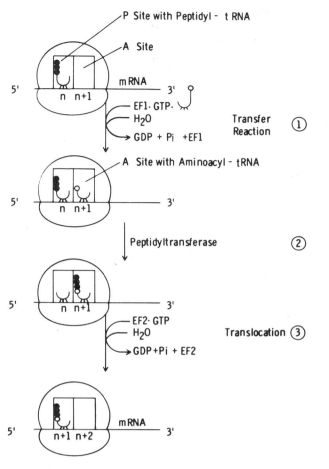

Fig. 4-68. Topography of elongation and translocation reactions in protein biosynthesis: the A and P sites.

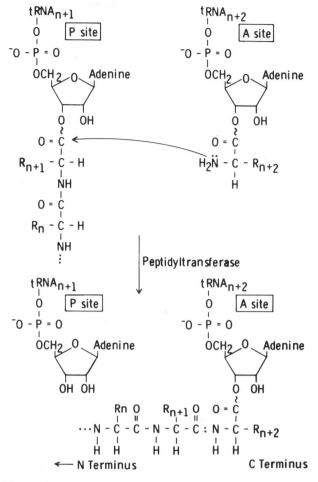

Fig. 4-69. Chemistry of the elongation reaction of protein synthesis.

GDP and Pi) in the transfer reaction where aminoacyl-tRNA is placed in the A site. Peptide bond formation *per se* does not require any additional energy expenditure. The high-energy bond of aminoacyl-tRNA is converted to the low-energy peptide bond in an exergonic reaction. A fourth high-energy bond is expended as GTP is hydrolyzed (to GDP and Pi) in the translocation reaction. A total of four high-energy bonds are thus expended per peptide bond formed. The cost of peptide bond formation is considerable. The chemical energy and the complex ribosomal machinery are required to convert the language of the 4-letter nucleic acid alphabet to the 20-letter alphabet of proteins.

Reverse Transcription: RNA-Dependent DNA Synthesis

The direction of biological information was initially thought to flow from DNA to DNA (replication), DNA to RNA (transcription), and RNA to protein

(translation) as noted in Table 4-1. Later work with the avian Rous sarcoma virus (one of a large number of tumor viruses) showed that the viral genetic RNA possesses a DNA intermediate. Furthermore, the intermediate integrates into the host cell

TABLE 4-30. Antibiotics That Inhibit Protein Synthesis

ANTIBIOTIC	SENSITIVE ORGANISMS	PROCESS INHIBITED
Streptomycin	Prokaryotes	Initiation; produces mistakes in translation
Tetracycline	Prokaryotes	Aminoacyl-tRNA attachment to the ribosome
Chloramphenicol	Prokaryotes	Ribosomal peptidyltransferase
Puromycin	Prokaryotes and eukaryotes	Causes premature chain termination
Cycloheximide	Eukaryotes	Ribosomal peptidyltransferase

genome. The synthesis of DNA from RNA templates is termed reverse transcription, and this family of viruses is called retroviruses. The enzyme that catalyzes the reaction is **reverse transcriptase.** It requires the four deoxynucleoside triphosphates and an RNA template. Like DNA polymerases it can not initiate DNA synthesis *de novo;* a primer is required. The enzyme reverse transcriptase, the RNA template (the genome), and the primer (a tRNA) are carried by the infectious virus. The elongation reactions proceed in the 5'- to 3'-direction.

A large number of retroviruses produce cancer in a variety of species. Only a few human cancers are known to be associated with retroviruses. The human disorder named acquired immunodeficiency syndrome (AIDS) is a result of infection by a retrovirus now called HIV-1 (human immunodeficiency virus, type 1). The study of retroviruses has been helpful in the study of tumorgenesis and AIDS. Reverse transcriptase, moreover, is an extremely important tool in molecular biology and biotechnology as noted below.

Post-Translational Protein Modification

Two common post-translational modifications occurring either during or shortly after synthesis of polypeptides include proteolytic cleavage and glycosylation. Although methionine is the universal initiating amino acid, it is found on the amino terminus of only a small proportion of proteins. It is hydrolytically removed by the action of an aminopeptidase. Acetylation of the resulting amino terminus by acetyl-CoA to give an *N*-acetylpolypeptide is a common post-translational modification in humans and other mammals. Additional post-translational modification is common in proteins destined for secretion from the cell, insertion into the plasma membrane, or translocation into the lysosome. Proteins with these properties are synthesized on ribosomes found in the rough endoplasmic reticulum. We shall consider the properties of proteins that lead to their synthesis at this location under the rubric of the signal peptide hypothesis.

SIGNAL PEPTIDE HYPOTHESIS

Proteins destined for secretion or insertion into membranes exhibit a leader sequence of 20 to 30 hydrophobic amino acids at their amino terminus. Translation begins on free ribosomes and stops shortly after the leader or signal sequence has been synthesized. A **signal recognition particle** (SRP) is responsible for arresting biosynthesis as it recog-

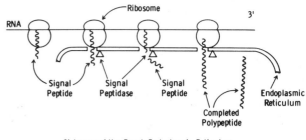

Cisternae of the Rough Endoplasmic Reticulum

Fig. 4-70. The signal peptide directs nascent proteins to the rough endoplasmic reticulum.

nizes the hydrophobic leader sequence and binds to the nascent polypeptide/ribosome complex. The SRP consists of 6 discrete polypeptides and a 300-nucleotide RNA. The arrested complex binds to an SRP receptor in the rough endoplasmic reticulum. This allows biosynthesis to resume as the nascent polypeptide chain with its signal sequence is directed into the lumen of the endoplasmic reticulum (the precise mechanism for this is unknown). Before translation is complete, the signal sequence is hydrolyzed from the precursor or the preprotein to produce the protein within the lumen of the rough endoplasmic reticulum. A **signal peptidase** catalyzes the hydrolytic removal of the leader sequence. These steps are illustrated in Figure 4-70.

Let us briefly consider the mechanism of insulin biosynthesis in the β-cells of the pancreas. It is synthesized as a precursor called **preproinsulin.** The order of synthesis of preproinsulin is leader sequence, B chain, connecting peptide, and finally A chain. All of these are initially on a single polypeptide; the discrete chains form as a result of proteolytic processing. After synthesis is initiated, preproinsulin is channeled into the lumen of the rough endoplasmic reticulum in a process involving a signal peptide sequence (the presequence of preproinsulin), the SRP, and its receptor on the rough endoplasmic reticulum membrane as just described. A signal peptidase catalyzes the hydrolytic removal of the signal sequence, and synthesis continues to yield **proinsulin.** The three disulfide bonds found in native insulin (two between the A and B chain, and one within the A chain) form within the single polypeptide chain constituting proinsulin. The polypeptide is cleaved at paired basic residues at two sites by an enzyme or enzymes with trypsinlike specificity to yield a C or connecting peptide and insulin made of its two chains (A and B). An enzyme with carboxypeptidase activity removes extra carboxy terminal basic residues on the B chain to yield insulin. Insulin is packaged into secretory vesicles, stored, and released upon demand. It undergoes no further post-translational modifications.

PROTEIN GLYCOSYLATION

Many proteins found in the plasma membrane and many circulating proteins such as antibodies and hormones (thyroid-stimulating hormone, luteinizing hormone, follicle-stimulating hormone) are glycoproteins. Glycosylation of proteins occurs within the Golgi complex and prior to their migration into secretory vesicles (see Fig. 4-1). Albumin, the most abundant plasma protein, is synthesized in and secreted by the liver. It is not glycosylated. This indicates that glycosylation is not a requirement for secretion.

There are two major classes of glycoprotein. A single protein, however, can be a member of both groups. The two classes of glycoprotein are O-linked (involving protein–serine or threonine) and N-linked (involving protein–asparagine residues). The O-linked class, which is the simpler of the two, is considered first. There are 80 types of sugar linkages in glycoproteins. Each type of linkage is determined by enzyme specificity. The donor substrates are listed in Table 4-31. Formation of these oligomeric sugar derivatives is unlike that of nucleic acids because the sequence is not determined by a template mechanism.

The ABO blood group pentasaccharide is an example of a carbohydrate attached to protein by an O-linkage. A specific transferase catalyzes the addition of each residue to its acceptor substrate. Biosynthesis is specified and determined by enzymes acting sequentially. For the ABO oligosaccharide, N-acetylgalactosamine is attached to an acceptor protein–serine or threonine. Then galactose, sialic acid (N-acetylneuraminic acid), fucose, and a second galactosamine are added sequentially to yield the final product.

The oligosaccharides attached at N-linkages are larger than those attached at O-linkages, and the mechanism of biosynthesis is more formidable. There are two subclasses of N-linked oligosaccharides: **high mannose** and **complex.** The latter is derived from the former by additional reactions. The pathway for biosynthesis of high mannose chains involves the following three processes: (1) formation of a 14-member oligosaccharide linked to dolichol by a pyrophosphate linkage, (2) transfer of the oligosaccharide to the acceptor protein, and (3) hydrolytic cleavage of specific sugars. The subsequent addition of several sugars from nucleotides to the high mannose class results in the formation of the complex class of oligosaccharide. These processes begin in the endoplasmic reticulum and are completed in the Golgi (see Fig. 4-1).

Let us consider the first phase. **Dolichol** is a polyisoprenoid compound (17–20 five-carbon units) with an alcohol at one terminus. It is found within the membranes of the endoplasmic reticulum. The alcohol group is phosphorylated by ATP to form ADP and dicholphosphate. This reacts with UDP-N-acetylglucosamine to form dolichol diphospho-N-acetylglucosamine and UMP. Six additional sugars are transferred from nucleotide donors, and then seven sugars are transferred from dicholphosphate derivatives. The 14-member core is transferred en block to the acceptor protein asparagine. This occurs at sites in the acceptor protein in the sequence . . AsnXSer (Thr) . . . where X is nearly any amino acid. Terminal glucosyl residues (four) are removed by hydrolysis reactions catalyzed by specific glycosidases. A single mannose is removed. When the process stops here the product is a **high mannose oligosaccharide.** To form the **complex chain oligosaccharide,** N-acetylgluco-

TABLE 4-31. Carbohydrate Donors Required for O-Linked and N-Linked Glycoprotein Synthesis

DONOR	BOTH O- AND N-LINKED OR N-LINKED	COMMENTS
UDP-galactose	Both	
CMP-sialic acid	Both	A nine-carbon sugar acid; same as N-acetylneuraminic acid
GDP-fucose	Both	
UDP-N-acetylgalactosamine	Both	
UDP-glucose	N	Glucose present as an intermediate but eliminated in final product
GDP-mannose	N	
UDP-N-acetylglucosamine	N	

samine, fucose, galactose, and sialic acid are added from the derivatives indicated in Table 4-31. These activated monomers serve as precursors or donors for condensation or polymerization reactions (see Table 4-1).

Regulation of Gene Expression

Gene regulation lies at the heart of the processes of differentiation, development, maintenance, and perhaps even aging. Tremendous advances in our understanding of gene regulation have been made with the advent of gene isolation, sequence analysis, and recombinant DNA methodologies as described in the next section. Before considering the process of gene regulation, we must introduce a few terms. As previously stated, DNA-dependent RNA synthesis is called transcription. The *promoter* represents the RNA polymerase binding site on genetic DNA. The *terminator* is the region of genetic DNA downstream from the promoter where RNA synthesis stops. The *transcription unit* extends from the promoter to the terminator. The RNA product resulting from transcription is called the *primary transcript*. A *cistron* is a unit of gene expression. In prokaryotes the product of several contiguous genes may be transcribed to produce a *polycistronic message*. A single mRNA, for example, in *E. coli* codes for three proteins called β-galactosidase, permease, and acetylase. Initiation and termination of protein synthesis from a polycistronic message occurs independently for each of the components. In contrast to prokaryotes, messages for eukaryotes are generally *monocistronic.*

EUKARYOTIC TRANSCRIPTION SIGNALS

Through DNA sequence analysis and functional studies, *consensus* or *canonical sequences* for func-

tional elements of DNA have been established. These constitute the predominant base at each position of the functional unit. About 25 nucleotides upstream from the start sites of eukaryotic hnRNA is an AT-rich region called the TATA box (Fig. 4-71). It corresponds to the following canonical sequence: TATAAAAG. The AT-rich region is thought to participate in local strand separation to allow for template-directed RNA biosynthesis. The energy of duplex formation is proportional to GC content and inversely related to AT content. About 75 nucleotides upstream from the transcription start site is the CAAT (pronounced cat) box with its specific consensus sequence (see Fig. 4-71). Both CAAT and TATA sequences provide information on *where* hnRNA synthesis should originate.

Another class of sequences called *enhancers* or *silencers* play a role in determining the *frequency* of transcription initiation. These sequences, which may be 50 to 100 nucleotides long, can be effective hundreds or thousands of nucleotides from the promoter (either upstream or downstream). Moreover, they are effective in both orientations: left to right or *vice versa* with respect to the promoter. *Regulatory elements* represent DNA sequences that affect transcriptional regulation of hormones or second messengers such as cyclic AMP. Other genetic elements play a role in tissue-specific expression so that a given gene is transcribed only in liver, or pancreas, or the hematopoietic system, and not in other cells. Research is currently underway to determine the canonical sequences that limit synthesis to specific cell types. The mechanisms utilized by various classes of genetic regulatory sequences is unknown. Proteins that bind to specific DNA sequences have been implicated in the overall process.

Fig. 4-71. Organization of a eukaryotic gene encoding an mRNA.

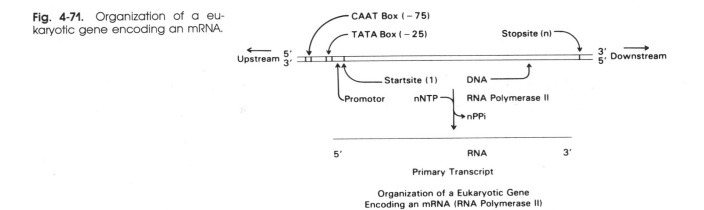

Organization of a Eukaryotic Gene
Encoding an mRNA (RNA Polymerase II)

PROKARYOTIC TRANSCRIPTION SIGNALS

Bacteria such as *E. coli* have a Pribnow or TATA box about eight nucleotides upstream from an mRNA transcription start site. They also have a TTGACA consensus sequence 35 nucleotides upstream from start sites.

THE LAC OPERON OF E. COLI

E. coli grown on glucose as a carbon source possess low levels of three proteins required to metabolize lactose. When the growth medium is changed to lactose as a carbon source, the levels of these three lactose-related proteins increase by several orders of magnitude. This system proved convenient for the study of the regulation of gene expression, and the concepts are adumbrated here.

The *lac operon* constitutes the regulatory and structural genes that play a role in lactose metabolism. The following genes are involved. A continuous DNA segment includes an operator gene and the z, y, and a genes, which encode for β-galactosidase, galactoside permease, and acetylase, respectively. An i gene, which is separated from these four genes, is also involved. The operator gene is a regulatory gene and does not code for a protein. The other genes are structural genes and code for proteins. A group of contiguous genes controlled by a single operator is called an *operon.*

The i gene codes for a *repressor.* The repressor is a protein that binds to the operator (a specific 17-nucleotide sequence) and inhibits transcription of the z, y, and a genes. In the presence of lactose, it or a metabolite (allolactose) binds to repressor. The sugar/repressor is inactive and can no longer bind to the operator. Transcription and translation of the proteins of the z, y, and a genes then transpires. The corresponding proteins are synthesized, and their levels increase by several orders of magnitude. The three proteins participate in the utilization of lactose as a fuel to support cellular metabolism. The operator lies between the promoter and start site of the z gene. The binding of the repressor inhibits gene expression and is a *negative regulator.* Examples of positive regulators are known in bacterial and animal systems.

Recombinant DNA Technology and Restriction Fragment Length Polymorphisms

In the previous sections we have reviewed the general principles of genetic chemistry. A field of recombinant DNA technology and genetic engineering was initiated in the mid-1970s. In addition to advances in our understanding of physiological and pathological processes, the use of these methodologies has led to advances in diagnosis and understanding of a variety of genetic disorders. It is the purpose of this section to give a general overview of progress in this rapidly emerging field.

RESTRICTION ENZYMES

Scientists have isolated more than 100 enzymes called restriction endonucleases from several bacterial species. *Restriction endonucleases* catalyze the hydrolysis of a phosphodiester bond in each of both strands of DNA which contain a specific sequence of nucleotide bases. The great utility of these enzymes is that cleavage is sequence specific and not random. The sequence recognized by restriction endonucleases constitutes a palindrome. A *palindrome* is a word, sentence, or number that reads the same forward or backward. Examples include: Otto, Able was I ere I saw elba, and 1881. In the case of nucleic acids, a palindrome occurs when the sequence on one strand of nucleic acid (from 5' to 3') is identical to its complement (from 5' to 3'). This is illustrated by the following examples:

$$5' \text{ GGCC } 3'$$
$$3' \text{ CCGG } 5'$$

$$5' \text{ GAATTC } 3'$$
$$3' \text{ CTTAAG } 5'$$

In each case the sequence of the bottom strand is identical to that of the top strand. One convenient way to recognize palindromes is to identify bases where identities occur in adjacent positions on opposite strands. Then determine whether sequence identities occur when reading in opposite directions from the center of symmetry on the complementary strands. Consider the second example. G differs from T, A differs from T, but A is identical to A. This represents a center of symmetry. To determine its extent, read in opposite directions from the point of symmetry on opposite strands. Going leftward on the top strand, we see that AAG (3' to 5') is the same as going rightward on the lower strand (AAG, 3' to 5'). Similarly TTC (5' to 3') on the top strand is the same as TTC (5' to 3') on the bottom. This is easier than comparing six bases on one strand with six on the other strand one segment at a time. It is much easier to confirm the identification of these palindromes because only the relevant sequence is given; it is more difficult to identify palindromes in long sequences of DNA by inspection. Computers are used in practice to analyze sequences of many kilobases (kb) in length for palindromes and other structural characteristics.

The sequences and positions of cleavage of a few restriction endonucleases are given in Table 4-32. Some enzymes nick or hydrolyze the DNA at staggered positions, for example, Bam Hl; other enzymes produce blunt ends, for example, Bal l. The ends produced by Bam Hl are self-complementary and are called *cohesive* or "sticky" ends. The product of the Bam Hl cleavage has an extended 3'-end termed a 3'-overhang. That from the Pst 1 has a 5'-overhang. If we mixed two different DNA's (*e.g.*, human and bacterial) treated with the same restriction endonuclease that produces cohesive ends, some strands of human DNA will combine at their cohesive end with the complementary ends of *E. coli* DNA. This is one of the important strategies used in producing *recombinant DNA molecules.* The restriction endonucleases yield a strand with a 5'-phosphate, and the other contains a free 3'-hydroxyl group. Annealed cohesive ends are *bona fide* substrates for DNA ligase, so that the recombinant strands can be covalently attached to one another.

The probability of having a tetranucleotide sequence of GGCC in a DNA molecule is $1 : 4 \times 4 \times 4 \times 4$ or $1 : 256$. This sequence would occur on a random basis once every 256 nucleotides. In contrast, the probability for restriction endonuclease sites for CTGCAG is $1 : 4 \times 4 \times 4 \times 4 \times 4 \times 4$ or $1 : 4096$. The number and size of the DNA fragments produced by restriction endonucleases depend upon the actual DNA sequence. SV40 DNA (from an animal virus) is 5226 nucleotides long and contains a single EcoRI restriction enzyme cleavage site. Bacteriophage T7 DNA is 40,000 nucleotides long but it lacks a single EcoRI site.

TABLE 4-32. Restriction Endonuclease Cleavage Sites

SOURCE	ENZYME DESIGNATION	SEQUENCE 5' → 3' / 3' ← 5'
Bacillus amyloliquefaciens H	Bam Hl	G'GATCC / CCTAGG
Brevibacterium albidum	Bal l	TGG'CCA / ACCGGT
Escherichia coli RY13	EcoRi	G'AATTC / CTTAAG
Haemophilus aegyptius	Hae lll	GG'CC / CCGG
Providencia stuartii 164	Pst 1	CTGCA'G / GACGTC

NUCLEIC ACID RESOLUTION BY ELECTROPHORESIS

Negatively charged DNA and RNA migrate in an electric field toward the anode. The distance of migration is inversely related to the molecular weight or number of monomeric residues in the polymer. Small molecules migrate more rapidly than large molecules. The matrix or medium in which the macromolecule is electrophoresed is a carbohydrate polymer called agarose or a synthetic polyacrylamide. The concentration and composition of the matrix is varied depending upon the size of the nucleic acid of interest. In some cases, nucleic acids of 2 kb to 10 kb or larger are under study, and in others the size ranges from 30 to 300 nucleotides.

DNA samples can be characterized by *Southern blotting.* A sample of DNA, for example human DNA, might be treated with a restriction endonuclease and then subjected to agarose gel electrophoresis. The resulting fragments are resolved on the basis of size. The DNA on the gel is transferred to a thin support system such as nitrocellulose paper by capillary action. Buffer moves through the slab gel and nitrocellulose; in the process DNA (or RNA) is transferred from the gel and is retained by nitrocellulose. The DNA (or RNA) is bonded to the nitrocellulose by heat or ultraviolet light treatment. The mechanics are such that the relative positions of DNA or RNA on the gel are maintained on the nitrocellulose paper.

The resolution of DNA by electrophoresis and transfer to nitrocellulose is called a *Southern blot* (named after the originator). A similar analysis of RNA was dubbed a *Northern blot.* Electrophoresis and transfer of proteins is called a *Western blot.* The principles involve electrophoretic resolution of macromolecules based on size and a transfer to a bonding agent by a method that ensures maintenance of resolution. In the next section we will consider methods for identifying specific DNA or RNA segments by annealing or hybridization.

PREPARATION OF RADIOACTIVE DNA PROBES AND HYBRIDIZATION

Southern blotting of an EcoRI restriction endonuclease enzyme digest of a sample of human DNA might yield 850,000 different fragments. To identify the fragment of interest requires the use of a probe. This is generally accomplished by preparing a radioactive (^{32}P) DNA sample. There are two strategies for achieving this. If we could obtain the primary structure of the DNA from the literature, we would chemically synthesize a complementary DNA of 15 to 25 nucleotides in length. This can be labeled at the free 5′-hydroxyl group in a reaction between radioactive ATP and the synthetic oligonucleotide catalyzed by *polynucleotide kinase.*

oligonucleotide + [γ^{32}P]ATP →
$$[^{32}P]oligonucleotide + ADP$$

If we know the primary structure of a segment of protein of interest, we could synthesize corresponding oligonucleotides based on the genetic code. Because of codon degeneracy, we would have to make a family of oligomer's corresponding to each possible codon.

If we possessed a larger, double-stranded or duplex DNA of a cloned gene, we could label the probe by *nick translation.* A nick is a discontinuity. These can be produced by using low concentrations of purified DNAse. The other components in a nick translation system include DNA polymerase I from *E. coli* and four deoxynucleoside triphosphates (one or more of which is labeled with ^{32}P in the α-position). DNA polymerase adds successive nucleotides beginning at the original nicks so that the resulting strand contains radioactivity. The process is called nick translation since the position of the nick is moved from its origin. Following the polynucleotide kinase reaction or nick translation, the resulting labeled probe is resolved from the radioactive precursors.

Next, the Southern or Northern blots are incubated with the radioactive probe under specific temperatures and salt concentrations. During this procedure the probe hybridizes or anneals to any immobilized complementary DNA (Southern) or RNA fragments (Northern) present on the filter. After hybridization the blot is washed with buffer to remove unbound probe. The samples are then subjected to autoradiography to locate the position of the complementary nucleic acids. Standard nucleic acids are run in parallel so that the length or size of the DNA or RNA bands can be ascertained.

When a restriction enzyme digest of DNA from several humans is performed, the resulting Southern blots might show different patterns in response to a specific DNA probe. This might reflect RFLPs or different forms of a gene (alleles). Some individuals may show a 10-kb band, and others may show a 6-kb fragment. It might be that one form is closely associated with a specific disease. RFLPs associated with Huntington's disease, cystic fibrosis, and Duchenne's muscular dystrophy have been described. It is not necessary that the restriction enzyme cleave the defective gene; oftentimes the altered site is near the defective gene and serves as a

marker. Similar tests are feasible in diagnosing hereditary diseases in cells isolated from amniotic fluid following amniocentesis. Extensive experimentation is required to establish and validate such diagnostic tests.

PLASMIDS AND DNA CLONING

Plasmids are small, autonomously replicating circular DNA molecules; we will consider only bacterial plasmids. Many copies (up to 50) of small plasmids (4 kb or kilobases) can be present per bacterium and replicate independently of the main chromosome. Many naturally occurring plasmids carry genes that confer antibiotic resistance; this property has been used in the production of genetically engineered plasmids for recombinant DNA research. Plasmids are used as vectors for cloning foreign DNA as will be described shortly. When we speak of cloning the DNA of a gene, this refers to the process of preparing a large number of identical DNA molecules. A *clone* is an exact copy of the original form. Plasmids can be used to clone DNA up to 4 kb or 5 kb in length. Other vehicles are used to produce DNAs of longer length. Bacteriophage lamda, for example, can be used to clone DNAs of 10 kb, and cosmid vectors can be used to prepare DNAs up to 50 kb in length.

Because eukaryotic genes are interrupted and contain sequences that are removed by splicing from the primary transcript, the DNA corresponding to mRNA is contained in a much longer stretch of nucleotides. For example, the 2-kb mRNA of phenylalanine hydroxylase is derived from a DNA sequence of nearly 100 kb. The 1.8-kb mRNA of tyrosine hydroxylase is derived from a DNA sequence of 10 kb. One reason that scientists are interested in cloning large DNAs is to obtain segments that contain the entire gene, which may extend many kilobases.

A diagram of pBR322, a commonly used plasmid, is shown in Figure 4-72. This contains 4362 base pairs and genes that code for resistance to ampicillin and tetracycline. These genes contain unique restriction enzyme sites. If we mix a sample of target DNA previously treated with Pst I endonuclease with pBR322, also treated with this enzyme, then a certain proportion of the pBR322 will anneal with the target DNA. A covalently closed circle results following treatment with (bacteriophage) T4 DNA ligase and ATP. Some pBR322 will reanneal (not bind to target DNA). Some target DNA will reanneal (not bind to pBR322 DNA), and some recombinant DNAs will result (target DNA and pBR322

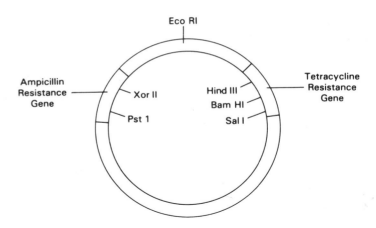

Fig. 4-72. Diagram of the genome of a bacterial plasmid (pBR322).

DNA). Bacteria *(E. coli)* lacking antibiotic resistance genes are exposed to the plasmids (in the presence of $CaCl_2$), and some of them take up the DNA (they are transformed). The cells are grown in the presence of tetracycline. Untransformed cells do not grow under such conditions because they lack the antibiotic resistance gene. Individual cells with a plasmid form colonies of cells containing identical copies (clones) of the original plasmid. Cells containing a target DNA inserted into the ampicillin resistance gene can be identified by their sensitivity to ampicillin.

A *gene library* refers to a collection of plasmids, phage, or cosmids containing the DNA corresponding to the entire genome of an organism. A bacteriophage lamda library of 250,000 is sufficient to contain the entire human genome. This can be contained in a single drop of media. To identify the DNA sequence or gene of interest requires ingenuity, and there are a number of successful strategies. One common procedure is to screen thousands of plasmid-containing bacterial colonies corresponding to a library to ascertain the few that hybridize to a radioactive DNA probe of interest. The positive colonies are taken for further study.

COMPLEMENTARY DNA PREPARATION

Complementary DNA (cDNA) generally denotes DNA that is complementary to RNA. It is easier to clone, sequence, and manipulate DNA in the laboratory than it is to perform these functions with RNA. A cDNA library corresponds to many clones of DNA complementary to a mixture of starting RNA. In some instances it is possible to enrich or purify RNA so that the cDNA produced is limited. In the case when a cDNA corresponding to mRNA is wanted, mRNA can be resolved from rRNA and tRNA through the use of oligo-dT cellulose chromatography. Most mRNA binds to oligo-dT by way of its 3' poly A tail. Ribosomal RNA and tRNA, however, fail to bind. A few mRNAs including those for histones lack the 3' poly A tail and fail to bind.

The first step in preparing cDNA is to incubate RNA with the four deoxynucleoside triphosphates, reverse transcriptase (RNA-dependent DNA polymerase derived from animal retroviruses), and a primer such as oligo-dT. After synthesis of the first strand (an RNA–DNA hybrid results), the sample is treated with NaOH. RNA is hydrolyzed by alkali, but DNA is stable. After neutralization to physiological *p*H, DNA polymerase I and the deoxynucleoside triphosphates are then added to effectuate synthesis of the second strand of DNA. As previously noted, DNA polymerase requires a primer and will not synthesize DNA *de novo*. Apparently the first strand folds back on itself (making a hairpin loop) and serves as a primer. Following the synthesis of the second strand, the product is treated with S1 exonuclease. This is specific for single-stranded nucleic acids; it hydrolyzes the phosphodiesters constituting the non-double-stranded portions of the hairpin loop and produces linear duplex DNAs.

There are a number of procedures for combining the cDNA with plasmid or bacteriophage DNA for molecular cloning. Synthetic oligonucleotide linkers can be attached to the duplex DNA by bacteriophage T4 ligase. The sequence of the linkers can be designed to produce cohesive ends complementary to the cloning vector following treatment with the appropriate restriction enzyme. A second procedure is also available. The cDNA can be incubated with dCTP or dGTP and polydeoxynucleotide terminal transferase. This adds a poly-dC or poly-dG tail on the 3′-hydroxyl group of cDNA by extension. Synthesis is independent of template. The alternative, complementary tail can be added to the plasmid or cloning vector. The poly-dC tail on one anneals with the poly-dG tail on the other, and recombinant DNA molecules (cDNA and plasmid) are formed. These can be introduced into *E. coli* host cells to produce clones. In contrast to the case with restriction enzyme fragments, self-annealing is absent.

DNA SEQUENCE ANALYSIS

One of the greatest technical advances in biochemistry during the past 15 years was the development of methods for rapidly determining the sequence of large molecules of DNA. It has become possible to determine the sequence of hundreds of residues in a day. From such sequences, one can determine the sequence of corresponding proteins by using the genetic code. What might require several years' work in protein sequencing might be accomplished in a few months by DNA sequence analysis. Because of the ability to clone and amplify DNA, it is not unusual to determine the sequence of proteins, which cannot be obtained in purified form in sufficient quantity to sequence by chemical methods. Computers are helpful and necessary in analyzing the sequence of DNA and the corresponding protein.

The **dideoxynucleotide** or **chain termination** method is described in abbreviated form. DNA of interest is subcloned into a single-stranded bacteriophage (M13) in segments of 200 to 300 bases adjacent to a specific sequence of nucleotides. A synthetic oligonucleotide is annealed to this specific sequence of the phage DNA and serves as primer. This complex is divided into four identical reaction mixtures. To each are added the four deoxynucleoside triphosphates (one or more of which contains ^{32}P in the α-position) and DNA polymerase I. A different chain terminator is included in each of the four mixtures. These include: ddATP, ddTTP, ddGTP, and ddCTP where dd indicates dideoxy. These lack hydroxyl groups at both the 2′- and 3′-carbons of ribose. When these dideoxynucleotides are incorporated into the nascent chain at positions complementary to the cloned insert, elongation is impossible (there is no free 3′-hydroxyl group) and termination results. In the case where ddATP is included, chain termination occurs randomly at every position complementary to a thymine residue, and a family of polydeoxynucleotides results. The incorporation of the other dideoxynucleotides indicates the positions corresponding to their complementary

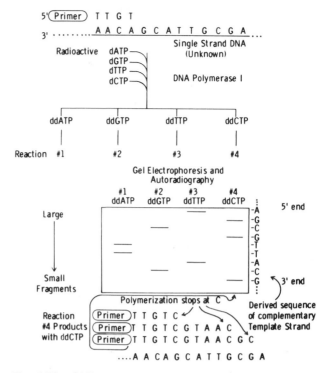

Fig. 4-73. DNA sequence analysis by the dideoxy chain termination technique.

base. The four mixtures are subjected to gel electrophoresis and autoradiography. The gels resolve every polydeoxynucleotide by size. It is possible, for example, to resolve a polynucleotide of 197 from one of 198 bases. One can read from the shortest to longest and identify the residues terminating in A, T, G, or C by the order of their appearance on the autoradiograph. The information can be entered into a computer data bank for full analysis. The steps are shown in Figure 4-73. The figure illustrates many fundamental aspects of DNA biosynthesis and is therefore worth all the time it takes to understand the principles outlined. These principles are more important to the reader than the DNA sequencing procedure itself.

NEUROCHEMISTRY

The brain and spinal cord constitute the **central nervous system.** The **peripheral nervous system** lies outside of the skull and vertebral column. It is made up of the voluntary nervous system (nerves to skeletal muscle), the autonomic nervous system, and sensory nerves. The neurotransmitter of the voluntary or motor nervous system is acetylcholine. Acetylcholine is also the neurotransmitter of the preganglionic sympathetic and pre- and postganglionic parasympathetic nervous system. Norepinephrine is the neurotransmitter of the postganglionic sympathetic nervous system. The identity of the neurotransmitters of the sensory nervous system has not yet been definitively established.

Considerable work has been performed to ascertain the identity of the neurotransmitters of the central nervous system. These include acetylcholine, the catecholamines (dopamine, norepinephrine, and epinephrine), serotonin, glutamate and aspartate, GABA (γ-aminobutyric acid), and several neuropeptides. Each of these substances is present in the brain, but their role in neurotransmission or neuromodulation has been established to only a varying degree. We shall consider the biochemistry and metabolism of most of these agents.

Acetylcholine Metabolism

Acetylcholine synthesis is limited, for practical purposes, to nerves that are *cholinergic* in nature. Mature noradrenergic nerves, for example, do not synthesize acetylcholine. The enzyme that catalyzes acetylcholine formation is *choline acetyltransferase.* It catalyzes the reaction between acetyl-CoA and choline as indicated:

$$\text{acetyl-CoA} + \text{choline} \rightleftharpoons \text{acetylcholine} + \text{CoA}$$

Acetyl-CoA is an energy-rich donor of the acetyl group. Acetylcholine is packaged into synaptic vesicles. When a nerve action potential invades a cholinergic nerve terminal, acetylcholine is released in discrete quanta or packets in a calcium-dependent fashion by exocytosis. Acetylcholine diffuses across a synapse or a junctional region, interacts with an effector cell, and brings about the biological response.

To effect this response, acetylcholine and other neurotransmitters interact with their cognate receptor (Table 4-33). There are two major classes of *acetylcholine receptor:* nicotinic and muscarinic. They differ in their molecular structure, anatomic location, and action; they also exist in subclasses. The *nicotinic receptor* occurs at the neuromuscular junction, on postganglionic autonomic cell bodies, and in the central nervous system. The receptor at the neuromuscular junction has been extensively studied. It is made up of four different polypeptide chains with the following composition: $\alpha_2\beta\gamma\delta$. The nicotinic receptor acts as an ion channel or gate. After binding acetylcholine, Na^+ flows into a cell through the receptor. The human disease, *myasthenia gravis,* is due to the adventitious production of

TABLE 4-33. Neurotransmitter Receptors and Their Subtypes

GENERIC RECEPTORS AND SUBTYPES	COMMENTS
*Cholinergic**	
Muscarinic	Postganglionic parasympathetic effector; major cholinergic receptor in brain
Nicotinic	Neuromuscular junction; preganglionic sympathetic and parasympathetic effector
*Dopaminergic**	
D_1	Stimulates adenylate cyclase
D_2	Inhibits adenylate cyclase
*Adrenergic**	
α_1	Alters intracellular calcium
α_2	Inhibits adenylate cyclase
β_1	Stimulates adenylate cyclase; cardiac stimulation
β_2	Stimulates adenylate cyclase; bronchodilation
Serotinergic	
5-HT$_1$	Regulated by guanine nucleotides
5-HT$_2$	Prominent in prefrontal cortex
GABAergic	
GABA A	Chloride conductance
GABA B	
Excitatory amino acids	
A1	N-Methyl-D-aspartate (NMDA) is a pharmacological agonist; prominent in cerebral cortex and hippocampus
A2	Quisqualate agonist
A3	Kainate agonist
Opiate	
Mu*	Morphine selective
Delta*	Enkephalin selective
Kappa*	Dynorphin selective
Sigma	N-Allylnormetazocine selective

* Noteworthy.

antibodies against the nicotinic receptor at the neuromuscular junction. A second type of acetylcholine receptor is the *muscarinic receptor.* It is responsible for the actions of acetylcholine liberated from the postganglionic parasympathetic system; acetylcholine is the postganglionic parasympathetic effector. The muscarinic receptor is specifically blocked or antagonized by atropine.

Neurotransmitters such as acetylcholine can be *excitatory* or *inhibitory;* the action depends upon the receptor and the physiological situation. Activation of the nicotinic receptor at the neuromuscular junction, for example, is excitatory. Activation of the muscarinic receptor in the pancreas is also excitatory. Activation of the muscarinic receptor in the heart, on the other hand, is inhibitory.

Inactivation of acetylcholine is mediated by metabolic degradation. *Acetylcholinesterase,* localized on the exterior of the cell surface of many neural and nonneuronal cells, catalyzes the hydrolysis of acetylcholine:

$$\text{acetylcholine} + H_2O \rightarrow \text{acetate} + \text{choline}$$

Following its liberation in the acetylcholinesterase reaction, choline is transported into nerve cells by a sodium-dependent high-affinity uptake system and can be reutilized. A circulating form of acetylcholine esterase called pseudocholinesterase also exists in humans. Its physiological function is unclear. The hereditary deficiency of pseudocholinesterase results in increased sensitivity to succinylcholine used as a muscle relaxant during surgery. Diisopropylphosphofluoridate is an irreversible inhibitor of acetylcholinesterase. It forms a covalent adduct with an active site serine hydroxyl group. Diisopropylphosphofluoridate has been used in chemical warfare as a nerve gas.

Catecholamine Metabolism

Catecholamines are derived from tyrosine. The first, rate-limiting, and regulatory step is catalyzed by *tyrosine hydroxylase.* Tetrahydrobiopterin and oxygen are the other reactants. Dihydroxyphenylalanine (DOPA), water, and dihydrobiopterin are the products. The enzyme is activated by several protein kinases and is inhibited by the catecholamine end products. *Aromatic amino acid decarboxylase* (a pyridoxal phosphate–dependent enzyme) catalyzes the conversion of DOPA to dopamine and CO_2 (Fig. 4-74). This is the end product in dopaminergic cells of the brain including those of the nigrostriatal pathway. In other cells dopamine reacts with oxygen and ascorbate to yield norepinephrine, water, and dehydroascorbate in a reaction catalyzed by *dopamine β-hydroxylase.* This is the end product in noradrenergic neurons. In other brain cells and in the adrenal medulla, norepinephrine is methylated by *S*-adenosylmethionine to yield epinephrine and *S*-adenosylhomocysteine (see Fig. 4-74). The corresponding enzyme is *phenylethanolamine* **N-methyltransferase** (PMNT). Epinephrine and norepinephrine are the hormones of the adrenal medulla.

Catecholamines are released from cells and interact with their specific receptor (see Table 4-33) and bring about their response. The β-adrenergic receptor activates adenylate cyclase at many locations.

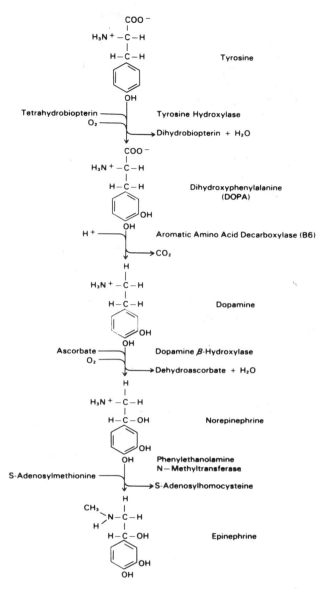

Fig. 4-74. Pathway of catecholamine biosynthesis.

The action of catecholamines, in contrast to acetylcholine, is not terminated by metabolic degradation within the synaptic cleft or junctional region. Catecholamines are inactivated by sodium-dependent uptake or transport systems. The most active systems reside in the plasma membrane of the nerve cells that release the catecholamines by exocytosis.

We now know that transport from the exterior to the interior of cells is the major mechanism for neurotransmitter inactivation. The two exceptions include acetylcholine and the neuropeptides. The inactivation of these two classes of compound is mediated by hydrolytic cleavage catalyzed by specific degradative enzymes. The metabolism (not inactivation) of intracellular catecholamines is mediated by catechol-*O*-methyltransferase, monoamine oxidase, aldehyde reductase, and aldehyde dehydrogenase. The structures of the many intermediates are not considered here. The chief metabolite of norepinephrine is *vanylylmandelic acid* (VMA). This is often measured in the urine of patients with suspected pheochromocytoma (a tumor of the adrenal medulla or abdominal paraganglia [Organs of Zuckerkandl]) to aid in diagnosis.

The nigrostriatal pathway utilizes dopamine as neurotransmitter. *Parkinson's disease* is associated with a degeneration of these neurons and a decrease in dopamine content in these brain regions. The mechanism of degeneration is unknown. The oral administration of L-DOPA constitutes one treatment. It is transported through the blood–brain barrier and is taken up by the surviving cells and is converted into dopamine. Dopamine does not pass through the blood–brain barrier and is ineffective in the treatment of Parkinson's disease.

Serotonin Metabolism

Serotonin is found in the gut and in the brain. In fact most neurotransmitters and neuropeptides are found in both locations. Serotonin is derived from tryptophan in a two-step pathway. First, tryptophan hydroxylase catalyzes a reaction with substrate, oxygen, and tetrahydrobiopterin to yield 5-hydroxytryptophan, water, and dihydrobiopterin. This reaction is analogous to that catalyzed by tyrosine hydroxylase and phenylalanine hydroxylase. The three enzymes exhibit homologous primary structures and constitute a family of aromatic amino acid hydroxylases. Next, 5-hydroxytryptophan is converted to serotonin and CO_2 by aromatic amino acid decarboxylase; this is the same vitamin B_6-dependent enzyme that converts DOPA to dopamine. Serotonin is packaged into synaptic vesicles and released by exocytosis; after diffusion to its receptor to bring about its effect, it is inactivated by uptake. It is metabolized intracellularly to 5-hydroxyindole acetic acid (5-HIAA) by the action of monoamine oxidase and aldehyde dehydrogenase. Quantitation of 5-HIAA in urine is undertaken in patients suspected of having the carcinoid syndrome associated with the production of excessive serotonin.

Excitatory Amino Acids

Considerable physiological and pharmacological evidence suggests that glutamate and aspartate may function as excitatory neurotransmitters in the human brain. They are thought to be packaged into synaptic vesicles, released into the synaptic region to interact with their receptor to bring about their effect, and undergo inactivation by uptake. In contrast to the restricted cellular distribution of acetylcholine, the catecholamines and serotonin, the common amino acids glutamate and aspartate are present in all cells. It is possible that both glutamate and aspartate are released from the same cell; each may also be released from specific neurons.

Gamma-Aminobutyric Acid Metabolism

GABA is thought to be the chief inhibitory neurotransmitter of the human brain. It is formed from glutamate in a one-step reaction catalyzed by glutamate decarboxylase; GABA and CO_2 are the products. Like most decarboxylase reactions, pyridoxal phosphate serves as a cofactor. In the 1950s infants inadvertently fed formulas deficient in vitamin B_6 developed seizures. This was apparently produced by a paucity of inhibitory GABA. GABA is released by exocytosis, acts on its receptor to bring about a response, and is inactivated by its specific high-affinity sodium-dependent uptake system. Its degradation is mediated by a pathway called the *GABA shunt*. GABA undergoes transamination with α-ketoglutarate to form succinate semialdehyde and glutamate as catalyzed by GABA transaminase. Succinate semialdehyde dehydrogenase catalyzes a reaction of substrate with NAD^+ to form succinate, NADH, and H^+. The latter donates electrons to the electron-transport chain, which results in ATP formation.

The content of the biogenic amines (acetylcholine, serotonin, and the catecholamines) in brain is in the micromoles/kilogram range. On the other hand, the content of aspartate, glutamate, and GABA is in the range of millimoles/kilogram.

Neuroactive Peptides

More than 30 peptides are known to exist in the brain as demonstrated by immunochemical techniques. A selected list is shown in Table 4-34. Most of these are small (5 to 50 amino acids). They are synthesized as protein precursors in an mRNA-dependent fashion and converted to the active agent by specific proteolysis. They are packaged, released by exocytosis, interact with their receptor to bring about their physiological effect, and are inactivated by proteolytic degradation. It is unclear whether they function as neurotransmitters or neuromodulators. In any case their function is

TABLE 4-34. Selected Neuroactive Peptides

Angiotensin II	Neurotensin
Cholecystokinin	Oxytocin
Dynorphin*	Secretin
Endorphin*	Somatostatin
Leucine enkephalin*	Substance P
Methionine enkephalin*	Vasoactive intestinal peptide (VIP)
Neuropeptide Y	Vasopressin

* Opoid peptide.

thought to be physiologically important. In addition to their exclusive release from their own specific neurons, they may be coreleased with other low molecular weight neurotransmitters. The list of possible coexistence of neuropeptides and low molecular weight transmitters is long. Some cortical neurons, to cite one example, are thought to contain and corelease GABA and somatostatin.

General Aspects of Nervous System Metabolism

Under physiological conditions the brain utilizes glucose as a metabolic fuel. It is unable to utilize fatty acids, ketone bodies, or other potential sources of chemical energy. The brain may be able to utilize ketone bodies following prolonged starvation. The brain is very dependent upon a continual supply of blood for both glucose and oxygen. A decrease of blood glucose to less than 40 mg/deciliter produces coma. Occlusion of the cerebral blood supply produces a stroke.

The brain contains a small amount of glycogen; it may play an important function under conditions of hypoglycemia. It is clearly inadequate to subserve metabolism under conditions of severe hypoglycemia. As noted earlier, glycogen is stored in a very hydrated state. Substantive changes of the glycogen content of the brain is probably prohibited because increases in volume are limited in the enclosed cranium. Regardless of the underlying mechanisms, the brain is dependent upon the liver to maintain adequate blood glucose levels.

Nearly all cells maintain a high intracellular potassium and a low intracellular sodium concentration. The diffusion of potassium through the plasma membrane accounts, in part, for the negative intracellular electrochemical potential ranging from -50 mV to -70 mV. Sodium is impermeant under resting conditions. During the propagation of a nerve action potential, sodium courses down its electrochemical gradient (from outside to inside), and the polarity is reversed.

The sodium plus potassium ATPase is responsi-ble for generating these ion gradients in nerve, heart, muscle, and other cells. A considerable proportion of ATP generated in nerve cells is required to maintain these ion gradients (see Table 4-1). The ATPase is an integral membrane glycoprotein with the following subunit composition: $\alpha_2\beta_2$. It reacts with ATP to form a phospho-enzyme intermediate and transports three sodium ions to the cell exterior. It then transports two potassium ions into the cell and undergoes a dephosphorylation reaction. The $Na^+ + K^+$ ATPase is a receptor for cardiac glycosides such as digitalis. It is not known how interaction with this enzyme enhances the action of the failing heart.

HORMONES

Hormones are substances produced by **endocrine** cells, released into and transported by the circulatory system to their target organs where they exert their effects. **Paracrine** function, in contrast to endocrine action, involves the release and action of substances on neighboring cells. **Autocrine** function involves the release of a substance that then acts upon the cell that released it. The latter two functions, paracrine and autocrine, do not involve transport by the circulatory system.

Hormones are conveniently classified as lipid soluble and water soluble. The lipid-soluble hormones listed in Table 4-35 include steroid hormones, the thyroid hormones (T_3, triiodothyronine; and T_4, tetraiodothyronine), and 1,25 dihydroxycholecalciferol (synthesized from vitamin D). Although these hormones enter most cells by diffusion, their sites of action are restricted to those cells that possess specific intracellular protein receptors. Following interaction with the hormone, the receptor undergoes a conformational change (called transformation). Except for the thyroid hormone or T_3 receptor, which is located in the cell nucleus, the initial binding and transformation occur in the cytosol. The hormone receptor complex is translocated into the nucleus, interacts with the genome, and enhances the transcription of hormone-responsive genes. Current studies suggest that the hormone receptor complex recognizes a specific sequence of nucleotides upstream from the target genes called a **hormone-responsive element.**

The classes of steroid hormones are adumbrated in Table 4-35; their structures are shown in Figure 4-75. These hormones are synthesized from cholesterol in the appropriate endocrine cell. In contrast to the water-soluble hormones, these substances are not stored to a significant extent. They are syn-

TABLE 4-35. Lipid-Soluble Hormones

HORMONE	STRUCTURAL PROPERTIES	TRANSPORT PROTEIN
Steroid hormones		
Pregnane Group (C21)		
Progesterone	Acetyl group attached to C17	Transcortin
Aldosterone	C18 is an aldehyde group (Ald)	None
Cortisol	11, 17-Dihydroxyl groups	Transcortin
Corticosterone	11 Hydroxyl group	Transcortin
Androstane Group (C19)		
Testosterone	17-Hydroxyl group; no aromatic ring	Sex hormone–binding globulin
Estrane Group (C18)		
Estradiol	Aromatic A ring; 3,17-dihydroxyl groups	Sex hormone–binding globulin
Thyroid hormones		
Triiodothyronine	Three iodines	Thyroxine-binding globulin
Tetraiodothyronine	Four iodines	Thyroxine-binding globulin
Cholecalciferol		
1,25-Dihydroxycholecalciferol	Vitamin D ring system	α_1-Globulin transport protein

thesized and released upon demand. They are effective at nanomolar (10^{-9} M) concentrations.

The water-soluble hormones include catecholamines, small peptides, polypeptides, proteins, and glycoproteins. The biosynthesis of norepinephrine and epinephrine (catecholamines) from tyrosine was considered in the section on neurochemistry (see Fig. 4-74). The others are synthesized by ribosomes in an mRNA-dependent fashion. Removal of signal peptides and processing by peptidases are required to produce the active hormone. Glycosylation may also occur. These modifications occur in the Golgi. Water-soluble hormones are stored in secretory granules and released from the endocrine cell by exocytosis.

Following release into the circulation, these hormones interact with their corresponding target cells through the action of an integral membrane protein receptor located in the plasma membrane. This is in contrast to the receptor for lipid-soluble hormones, which is found intracellularly. The next step in the sequence of events that bring about the physiological response varies. In many cases the hormone, considered the *first messenger,* alters the levels of an intracellular *second messenger.* Second messengers include cyclic AMP, cyclic GMP, calcium, inositol trisphosphate, and diacylglycerol.

The Cyclic AMP Second Messenger System

Following the interaction of norepinephrine and epinephrine with the β-adrenergic receptor present on target cells, the intracellular concentration of cyclic AMP increases. The activated receptor does not directly stimulate the activity of adenylate cyclase (the enzyme that catalyzes the formation of cyclic

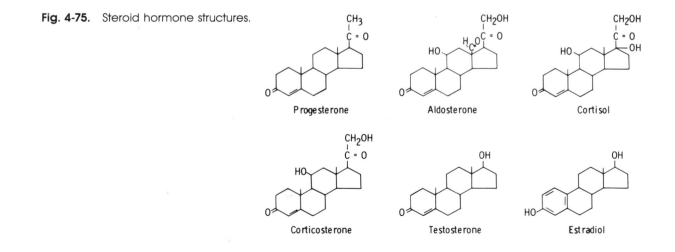

Fig. 4-75.   Steroid hormone structures.

Progesterone   Aldosterone   Cortisol

Corticosterone   Testosterone   Estradiol

AMP from ATP). The activity of adenylate cyclase is regulated by intermediary guanine nucleotide–binding proteins. The β-adrenergic receptor interacts with Gs (stimulatory guanine nucleotide–binding protein); the muscarinic acetylcholine receptor in many, but not all, instances interacts with Gi (inhibitory guanine nucleotide–binding protein).

Gs and Gi consist of three different polypeptides: α, β, and γ. The α-subunits differ; the β- and γ-subunits are similar if not identical. The epinephrine/β-receptor complex activates Gs; activation involves the binding of GTP to α_s and its dissociation from the $\beta\gamma$-dimer. The α_s/GTP complex activates adenylate cyclase. Following hydrolysis of GTP to GDP and Pi, α_s binds to $\beta\gamma$ to form inactive $\alpha\beta\gamma$. It can be reactivated by epinephrine/β-receptor or by other activated stimulatory receptors present in the cell membrane. The interaction of an inhibitory hormone receptor complex with Gi results in the formation of α_i/GTP and a dissociated $\beta\gamma$-dimer; α_i/GTP inhibits adenylate cyclase activity. Hydrolysis of GTP to GDP + Pi is followed by formation of the inactive $\alpha\beta\gamma$-trimer of Gi.

As noted previously in the section on glycogen metabolism, adenylate cyclase mediates the formation of cyclic AMP, which in turn activates its protein kinase (cyclic AMP–dependent protein kinase). The activated protein kinase catalyzes the phosphorylation of acceptor proteins, which then have altered activity (either increased or decreased, depending upon the acceptor protein). To reverse the activation process, *cyclic AMP phosphodiesterase* catalyzes the hydrolysis of cyclic AMP to inactive 5′-AMP. The cyclic AMP–dependent protein kinase returns to the inactive form. *Phosphoprotein phosphatases* catalyze the hydrolytic dephosphorylation of the phosphorylated substrate proteins; the activity of the unphosphorylated form is again expressed.

The predominate residue phosphorylated by cyclic AMP–dependent protein kinase is protein-serine; in a few cases protein–threonine is phosphorylated. A partial list of hormones that increase or decrease cyclic AMP levels in target cells is given in Table 4-36.

The Cyclic GMP Second Messenger System

Most eukaryotic cells also contain cyclic GMP. The components of the cyclic GMP system parallel those for cyclic AMP. These include guanylate cyclase, phosphodiesterase, cyclic GMP–dependent protein kinase, acceptor substrates, and phosphoprotein phosphatases. Adenylate cyclase is local-

TABLE 4-36. Hormones That Affect Cyclic AMP Levels in Appropriate Target Cells by Altering Adenylate Cyclase Activity

Stimulatory
Adrenocorticotrophic hormone (ACTH)
β-Adrenergic catecholamines
Follicle-stimulating hormone (FSH)
Glucagon
Luteinizing hormone (LH)
Thyroid-stimulating hormone (TSH)
Vasopressin (antidiuretic hormone or ADH)

Inhibitory
Acetylcholine (muscarinic)
α_2-Adrenergic catecholamines
Angiotensin II
Somatostatin

ized exclusively in the plasma membrane. In contrast, guanylate cyclase occurs in both a plasma membrane particulate form and a cytosolic form. The function of the two forms is unclear. The identity of the physiological regulators of guanylate cyclase is not as well known as are the regulators of adenylate cyclase. The particulate guanylate cyclase may be regulated by a recently discovered cardiac hormone named cardionatrin I. Cyclic GMP levels are regulated in some cases by the muscarinic cholinergic receptor. Intracellular calcium may play a role in regulating cyclic GMP; the mechanism, however, is unknown.

Cells also possess a cyclic GMP–dependent protein kinase. It is a dimer of identical subunits. It is activated in an allosteric manner by cyclic GMP. In contrast to the cyclic AMP–dependent protein kinase, cyclic GMP–dependent protein kinase does not dissociate into separate catalytic and regulatory subunits. Activation can be expressed in the following fashion:

$$E_2 + 4 \text{ cGMP} \rightleftharpoons E_2 - \text{cyclic GMP}_4$$
$$\text{(less active)} \qquad \text{(more active)}$$

The physiological substrates of cyclic GMP–dependent protein kinase are unknown. In some cases it phosphorylates the same substrates as the cyclic AMP–dependent protein kinases. Other cyclic AMP–dependent protein kinase substrates, however, are phosphorylated poorly if at all by cyclic GMP–dependent protein kinase. It was hypothesized at one time that cyclic AMP and cyclic GMP have antagonistic functions. This notion, however, has fallen out of favor.

The Calcium Second Messenger System

Calcium serves as a very important intracellular regulator. Calcium is required for exocytosis and muscle contraction. Calcium also plays an important role as a second messenger. A number of bioactive substances that exert their action, at least in part, by affecting intracellular calcium levels are shown in Table 4-37.

There are at least two mechanisms by which a first messenger acting through its receptor can increase intracellular calcium. The hormone receptor complex may enhance calcium influx through the plasma membrane in exchange for intracellular sodium. Another recently discovered mechanism involves the phosphoinositide system. The initial substrate for this process is *phosphatidylinositol-4,5-bisphosphate,* and it is present on the inner aspect of the plasma membrane. The hormone receptor complex activates *phospholipase C* (see Fig. 4-38), which in turn catalyzes the hydrolysis of phosphatidylinositol bisphosphate to form 1,2-diacylglycerol and 1,4,5-inositoltrisphosphate. Inositol trisphosphate, liberated into the cytosol, interacts with the endoplasmic reticulum and promotes the release of stored calcium.

To effectuate a response, calcium interacts in many cases with a specific calcium-binding protein called *calmodulin.* This is a low molecular weight protein (17,000 daltons) that binds up to four calcium ions with high affinity (binding constants in the micromolar range). Following this, the protein undergoes a conformational change and alters the activity of specific effectors. Calcium/calmodulin, for example, activates one form of cyclic nucleotide phosphodiesterase. This provides reciprocal interaction of the calcium and cyclic nucleotide second messenger systems. The activity of adenylate cyclase is also subject to regulation by calcium/calmodulin.

The activity of several protein kinases is also enhanced by calcium and calmodulin. Three enzymes have been distinguished by their substrate specific-

TABLE 4-37. Hormones That Affect Calcium Levels in Appropriate Target Cells

ACTH	Histamine (H1)†
Acetylcholine (muscarinic)*	Luteinizing hormone
α_1-Adrenergic catecholamines	Thyrotropin-releasing hormone
Angiotensin II	
Cholecytokinin	Vasopressin
Gastrin	

* Neurotransmitter.
† Autocrine agent.

TABLE 4-38. Some Physiological Substrates of Cyclic AMP–Dependent Protein Kinase

PROTEIN SUBSTRATE	EFFECT
Glycogen synthase	Inhibits
Hormone-sensitive lipase	Activates
Phosphatase inhibitor I	Activates
Phospholamban (muscle)	Activates
Phosphorylase kinase	Activates
Pyruvate kinase (liver)	Inhibits
Tyrosine hydroxylase (nerve)	Activates

ity and are called *calcium/calmodulin–dependent protein kinases I, II, and III* based on their order of discovery. Phosphorylase kinase is made of four different types of subunits: α, β, γ, and δ. The δ-subunits, tightly attached to the others, are actually calmodulin. Phosphorylase kinase is activated as calcium binds to the δ-subunit. Phosphorylase kinase also is activated by the phosphorylation catalyzed by cyclic AMP–dependent protein kinase (Table 4-38).

The Diacylglycerol Second Messenger System

The hydrolysis of phosphatidylinositol bisphosphate generates two second messengers: inositoltrisphosphate (just considered) and diacylglycerol. Diacylglycerol activates its cognate protein kinase, which is called protein kinase C. This enzyme requires phospholipid and calcium for full expression of its activity. The diacylglycerol increases the affinity of protein kinase C for calcium so that it could act at basal intracellular calcium concentrations (0.1 μM). One intriguing finding concerning protein kinase C is that it is specifically activated by tumor promotors including phorbol esters. Tumor promoters alone do not produce cancers. They must be added after an initiating agent such as benzopyrene for tumorigenesis to occur.

Protein–Serine Kinases

All the protein kinases in the previous sections (cyclic AMP–, cyclic GMP–, calcium/calmodulin–, and diacylglycerol–dependent protein kinases) catalyze the phosphorylation of protein–serine residues. In many cases the substrate proteins and even the residue(s) phosphorylated have been determined. Cyclic AMP–dependent protein kinase catalyzes the phosphorylation of phosphorylase kinase (and activates it) and glycogen synthase (and inactivates it). A partial list of its other protein substrates is given in Table 4-38. We know less about the identity of the physiological substrates of cyclic GMP–dependent protein kinase, calcium/calmodulin–dependent protein kinase (I, II, or III) and protein kinase C. The vast majority of phosphate in proteins (>99%) is attached to serine (see Table 4-5). Protein–serine kinases constitute one of the most important means of regulation by covalent modification in humans. A large number of protein–serine kinases are not regulated by these second messengers. One example already considered is pyruvate dehydrogenase kinase. It is regulated by acetyl-CoA and NADH in an allosteric fashion.

Protein–Tyrosine Kinases

Although not as important in a quantitative sense, phosphorylation of protein–tyrosine residues appears to play an important role in the action of several hormones, growth factors, and perhaps in the mechanism of tumorigenesis. The insulin receptor, for example, possesses protein–tyrosine kinase activity. The insulin receptor consists of a tetramer of two α- and two β-chains. The α-chains recognize and interact with insulin on the cell exterior. The β-chains interact with the α-chains, which extend into the cell interior where protein–tyrosine kinase activity occurs. Whether this activity is sufficient to explain all the actions of insulin is unclear. The second messenger, if any, associated with growth hormone, prolactin, or human chorionic gonadotropin is unknown. In addition to insulin, epidermal growth factor and platelet-derived growth factor receptors also possess protein–tyrosine kinase activity. In each case, we lack knowledge of physiological protein substrates.

CARCINOGENESIS

Great advances in understanding the pathogenesis of cancer have been made in the recent decades, and progress is continuing at an accelerating rate. Epidemiological studies have indicated that chemicals such as asbestos (lung), vinyl chloride (liver), benzopyrene (skin and lung), and β-napthylamine (bladder) are carcinogenic. More recent work suggests that many agents undergo oxidation reactions catalyzed by the hepatic cytochrome P-450 system to yield the active carcinogen.

Most carcinogens are also mutagens. The **Ames** test is one method for testing the mutagenicity (possible carcinogenicity) of compounds. The test substance is first incubated with a liver extract containing the cytochrome P-450 system followed by incubation with a histidine-requiring *Salmonella* strain. Mutagens produce revertants not requiring histidine; the mutagens can be further characterized with animal systems. This simple test is about 90% accurate in identifying carcinogens.

Certain DNA and RNA viruses produce tumors in animals. A study of the mechanisms of tumorigenesis by viruses has been enlightening in understanding human cancer. Rous sarcoma virus, for example, contains an oncogene that is responsible for tumorigenesis. The properties of this and other oncogenes have been subjects for investigation. Each viral oncogene (designated v-onc) was originally derived from the host. The host gene is called a proto-oncogene or cellular oncogene (c-onc). The proto-oncogenes are thought to be required for normal growth control or development.

Proto-oncogenes are evolutionarily highly conserved and closely related genes occur in *Drosophila* (fruit flies) and humans. Oncogenes and their gene products fall into a few families. One large family, for example, possesses protein–tyrosine kinase activity (Table 4-39). This is reminiscent of plasma membrane receptors for platelet-derived growth factor, epidermal growth factor, and insulin. The src gene of the Rous sarcoma virus is an example of a protein–tyrosine kinase. The ras gene product is a plasma membrane protein that binds GTP and may be related to the guanine nucleotide protein that activates adenylate cyclase. Myc and fos are nuclear proteins of unknown function. The production of the tumorigenic state might result from abnormal expression of proto-oncogenes or from a mutation producing an abnormal product. Evidence for both processes is found in experimental systems. Moreover, some human bladder carcinomas have been associated with the ras proto-oncogene that has undergone a single base change.

MUSCLE METABOLISM

Muscle accounts for about half the mass of humans. There are three classes of muscle: skeletal, cardiac, and smooth. The former two are striated in microscopic appearance. In this section we will consider the nature of the proteins that constitute muscle as well as the utilization of ATP as a source of chemical energy for muscle contraction.

TABLE 4-39. Oncogenes

DESIGNATION	VIRUS	GENE PRODUCT ACTIVITY OR LOCATION
abl	Abelson murine leukemia	Protein–tyrosine kinase
fes	Feline sarcoma	Protein–tyrosine kinase
fps	Fujinami sarcoma	Protein–tyrosine kinase
src*	Rous sarcoma*	Protein–tyrosine kinase*
erb B*	Avian erythroblastosis	Truncated epidermal growth factor receptor and tyrosine kinase*
sis*	Simian sarcoma	Platelet-derived growth factor B chain*
H-ras*	Harvey murine sarcoma	Binds GTP*
K-ras*	Kirstin murine sarcoma	Binds GTP*
myc*	MC29 myelocytomatosis	Nucleus*
fos	FBJ murine osteosarcoma	Nucleus
erb A	Avian erythroblastosis	Cytoplasm
ets	Avian E26 myeloblastosis	Cytoplasm

* Noteworthy.

Muscle Proteins

The two most abundant proteins in muscle include actin and myosin. Myosin is the chief protein of the thick filament, and actin is found in the thin filament. Some of their properties are adumbrated in Table 4-40. Myosin contains a globular head which contains ATPase activity and a rodlike tail. The two essential and two regulatory light chains of myosin interact with the two heavy chains of myosin in the globular region.

Role of ATP in Muscle Contraction

ATP (Mg^{2+}) interacts with an actin–myosin complex to displace actin and form a complex with myosin. This is hydrolyzed to yield ADP and Pi and an energized state of myosin shown diagrammatically in Figure 4-76. Note that ATP hydrolysis occurs prior to force generation. In response to a nerve impulse, calcium is released from the sarcoplasmic reticulum, and this will trigger muscle contraction according to the following scheme. Calcium binds with troponin C. This produces a change such that tropomyosin rotates out of the path between actin and myosin (Fig. 4-77). Actin then interacts with myosin, and the energized molecule moves relative to actin by a ratchetlike mechanism to generate force and is converted to a de-energized state. The ATPase cycle repeats as many as eight times per second to shorten the sarcomer and generate force. Following the cessation of nerve impulses, calcium is sequestered into the sarcoplasmic reticulum by an ATP-dependent process. The calcium concentration decreases, and troponin reverts to its original conformation. Tropomyosin again blocks the interaction of actin and myosin.

Both skeletal and cardiac muscle, as well as brain, contain creatine phosphate. Creatine phosphate serves as a storage form of energy-rich phos-

TABLE 4-40. Contractile Proteins

COMPONENT	MOLECULAR WEIGHT	STRUCTURE	COMMENTS
Thick filament			
Myosin	520,000	Two heavy chains, four light chains (two essential and two regulatory)	ATPase heads
Thin filament			
Actin	42,000	Globular monomers form fibrous aggregate	Interacts with myosin to generate force
Tropomyosin	70,000	Two coiled subunits that extend the length of seven actin monomers	Blocks binding of actin to myosin
Troponin	76,000		
Troponin I	21,000		Inhibitory
Troponin T	37,000		Binds tropomyosin
Troponin C	18,000		Binds Ca^{2+}

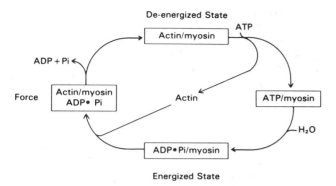

Fig. 4-76. The actin/myosin energy transduction cycle.

phate $(HOOCCH_2N(CH_3)C(=NH)N(H)—PO_3^=)$. Creatine is *N*-methylguanidinoacetic acid. The P—N phosphoamidate bond is of the high-energy or energy-rich variety. Creatine phosphokinase (CPK) catalyzes a reversible reaction between creatine and ATP to from creatine phosphate and ADP. Following contraction and the formation of ADP, CPK catalyzes the phosphorylation of ADP to form ATP. The latter can serve as a substrate for additional muscle contraction. In exercising muscle, the level of creatine phosphate falls prior to the decrease in ATP content. The level of creatine phosphate returns to its initial value during rest. ATP, formed from substrate level and oxidative phosphorylation, serves as the source of chemical energy for this process. CPK is measured in serum samples in the clinical chemistry laboratory. It is commonly elevated following a myocardial infarction and also in muscular dystrophy.

CONNECTIVE TISSUE

In multicellular organisms such as humans, the intercellular space contains an organic matrix rich in proteoglycans. *Proteoglycans* consist of acidic polysaccharides (95% by mass) and proteins (5%). Proteoglycans form the ground substance in which collagen and cells are embedded to form tissues.

Proteoglycans

Proteoglycans are composed of a polysaccharide axis of hyaluronic acid. Many core proteins emanate laterally from the long, thin hyaluronic acid axis. A *link protein* stabilizes the *hyaluronic acid–core protein* complex. Many chondroitin sulfate and keratan sulfate chains are covalently attached to the core proteins and constitute the major mass of the molecule.

There are three types of bonds by which the polysaccharide is covalently linked to the core protein. These consist of (1) an *O*-glycoside bond between xylose and serine, (2) an *O*-glycoside bond between *N*-acetylgalactosamine and serine or threonine, and (3) an *N*-glycosidic bond between *N*-acetylglucosamine and the amide nitrogen of asparagine.

The components of the polysaccharide repeating units are adumbrated in Table 4-41. The following generalizations can be made to simplify the subject. One component of the repeating disaccharide unit consists of either D-glucosamine, D-galactosamine, or one of their derivatives. Except for keratan sulfate (with galactose), the second component consists of a uronic acid; it is either D-glucuronic acid

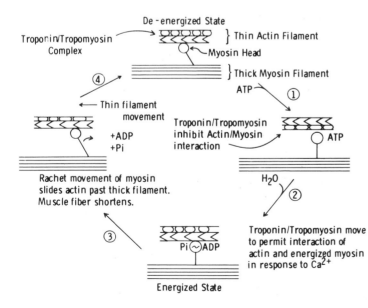

Fig. 4-77. Troponin and calcium mediate the interaction of actin and myosin during muscle contraction.

TABLE 4-41. Properties of the Polysaccharide Components of Proteoglycans

CLASS	COMPOSITION OF REPEATING UNIT	COMMENTS
Hyaluronic acid	Glucuronic acid and N-acetylglucosamine	Widely distributed in animal tissues, synovial fluid, and vitreous of the eye
Chondroitin sulfate	Glucuronic acid and N-acetylgalactosamine as the O-4 or O-6 sulfate	Polysaccharide chains of 20,000 daltons
Keratan sulfate	Galactose and N-acetylglucosamine as the O-6 sulfate	Two forms (I and II) differ in bonding to protein
Heparan sulfate	L-Iduronate O-2 sulfate and glucosamine O-6 and N-2 sulfate or acetate	
Dermatan sulfate	L-Iduronate O-2 sulfate and N-acetylgalactosamine 4-sulfate; glucuronic acid and N-acetylgalactose	Two types of repeating subunit
Heparin	Glucosamine and L-iduronic acid (90%) or glucuronic acid (10%)	Protein core almost all serine and glycine

or its 5-epimer L-iduronic acid. Except for hyaluronic acid, the polysaccharides of proteoglycans contain O-sulfate or N-sulfate esters. The donor of sulfate is phosphoadenosylphosphosulfate (PAPS). The linkages connecting the disaccharides, which are not given here, are specific and determined by the biosynthetic enzyme (specific glycosyl transferases catalyze each addition from a nucleotide sugar). The sulfates and glucuronides account for the acidic nature of this group of complex carbohydrates.

There are several inherited proteoglycan or mucopolysaccharide storage diseases that are the result of deficient activities of lysosomal catabolic enzymes. Some of these are listed in Table 4-42.

Collagen

Collagen is the major macromolecule of connective tissue and the most abundant protein in humans and the animal kingdom. It accounts for perhaps one third of human protein by mass. Collagen is secreted by connective tissue cells called fibroblasts. It forms insoluble fibers of high tensile strength. The most distinguishing property of collagen is that it forms a *triple, left-handed helix* made up of three polypeptide chains. There are three amino acid residues per turn. Three left-handed helices combine to form a right-handed super helix, which is long (300 nm) and narrow (1.5 nm).

Another distinguishing feature of collagen is that every third residue is glycine. This is the only amino acid small enough to exist at the central core of a triple helix. The sequence of the main body of collagen is thus Gly-X-Y where X and Y are residues other than glycine. Of the 1050 residues per chain, about 100 of the X residues are proline, and 100 Y residues are 4-hydroxyproline. Collagen also contains 5-hydroxylysine residues. The collagen helix is stabilized by multiple interchain cross links. The collagens of humans consist of five different molecules composed of seven genetically distinct α-chains given for reference purposes in Table 4-43.

The synthesis of collagen requires a number of post-translational reactions similar to those given previously. Collagen synthesis begins intracellularly, and it is completed extracellularly by proteolytic processing. It is synthesized as a *preprocollagen* in the rough endoplasmic reticulum. The signal peptide is promptly cleaved yielding *procollagen*. Prolyl and lysyl hydroxylation is followed by the subsequent glycosylation of several amino acid residues. The formation of the triple helical structure occurs in the Golgi. The procollagen triple he-

TABLE 4-42. Proteoglycan Storage Diseases (*Mucopolysaccharidoses*)

NAME	ENZYME DEFECT	ALTERNATE DESIGNATION
Hurler	α-L-Iduronidase	MPS I
Hunter	Iduronate sulfatase	MPS II
Sanfilippo A	N-Sulfatase	MPS III A
Sanfilippo B	α-N-Acetylglucosamidase	MPS III B
Sanfilippo C	Acetyltransferase	MPS III C
Morquio	N-Acetylgalactosamine 6-sulfatase	MPS IV

TABLE 4-43. Major Types of Collagen

TYPE	MOLECULAR FORMULA	LOCATION
I	$[\alpha 1(I)]_2 \alpha_2$	Skin, tendon, bone
II	$[\alpha(II)]_3$	Cartilage
III	$[\alpha 1(III)]_3$	Skin, blood vessels, uterus
IV	$[\alpha 1(IV)]_3$ and $[\alpha 2(IV)]_3$	Basement membranes
V	$\alpha A(\alpha B)_2$ or $(\alpha A)_3$ and $(\alpha B)_3$	Widespread in small amounts

lix is secreted from the fibroblast. Procollagen aminopeptidase and procollagen carboxypeptidase are extracellular enzymes that catalyze the hydrolytic removal of amino and carboxy terminal fragments yielding ***tropocollagen.*** The amino terminal and carboxyl terminal fragments, the proprotein sequences, contain disulfide bonds. Tropocollagen and collagen, however, lack cysteine residues. The tropocollagen molecules form regular, parallel arrays and are stabilized by cross-linking reactions involving ε-aldehyde groups formed from lysine and ε-amino groups of lysine to yield collagen.

BLOOD CLOTTING

There is a fine balance between initiating and retarding the formation of blood clots. The physiological purpose of blood clotting is to prevent the extravasation of blood from the circulatory system, which may result from injury or trauma. The blood-clotting scheme involves several protein components. Before considering their specific functions, we will consider the general scheme of blood clotting.

Blood clotting involves a series of reactions where the product of one process initiates a subsequent process the product of which initiates still another. This scheme is termed a ***cascade.*** This process involves at least six distinct proteases with a serine residue at the active site (Factors II, VII, IX, X, XI, and XII). These serine proteases exhibit trypsinlike specificity (hydrolyzing a peptide bond on the carboxyl side of a basic amino acid residue) but of a more restricted nature. In these processes an inactive proenzyme (*e.g.*, factor II) is converted to an active enzyme designated by an a after the factor number (*e.g.*, IIa). The protein substrate for clot formation is fibrinogen (factor I); it is converted into a fibrin clot by proteolysis catalyzed by factor IIa. One of the clotting factors (XIIIa) catalyzes the cross linking of fibrin to form a more stable clot.

Four factors (III, IV, V, and VIII) function as auxiliary components in mediating specific conversions. Factor IV is calcium and factors III, V, and VIII are proteins. Ca^{2+} is necessary for at least five steps in the clotting cascade (formation of IIa, VIIa, IXa, Xa, and XIIIa). The first four of these protein factors contain γ-carboxyglutamyl residues that bind calcium. This residue is a product of posttranslational modification and involves a vitamin K–dependent reaction. Factor VIII is the famous ***antihemophilic factor*** associated with hemophilia A. This is an X-linked bleeding disorder associated historically with European royalty. Factor IX is

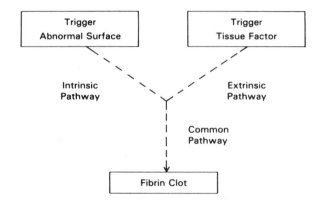

Fig. 4-78. Scheme for the intrinsic and extrinsic clotting pathways.

called ***Christmas factor*** whose name is based on that of a patient who had a disease resembling that of classical hemophilia, but whose biochemical lesion was shown to be different.

There are two clotting pathways: intrinsic and extrinsic. The ***intrinsic pathway,*** which may be initiated by an abnormal surface provided by endothelium *in vivo* or glass *in vitro,* is named because all components are present in blood; no exogenous component is required to initiate or propagate the reaction. In contrast, the ***extrinsic pathway*** requires the addition of an extravascular component (thromboplastin), which results when blood contacts any tissue as a result of injury (Fig. 4-78).

Blood-Clotting Scheme

The reactions involved in the intrinsic and extrinsic pathways are shown in Figure 4-79. The intrinsic pathway is more complex. In response to a condition such as an abnormal surface, factor XII is con-

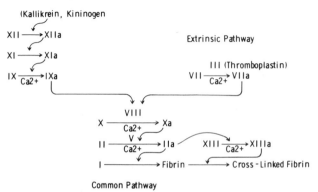

Fig. 4-79. The blood-clotting cascade of reactions.

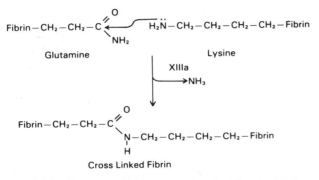

Fig. 4-80. The cross-linking reaction in blood clot formation.

verted to XIIa by proteolysis. Kallikrein and kininogen may participate in this reaction. Factor XI and IX become activated in succession. The coordinate action of IXa, VIII, and Ca^{2+} promote the conversion of X to Xa. Xa, V, and Ca^{2+} then lead to the conversion of prothrombin (II) to thrombin (IIa). Thrombin catalyzes the proteolytic conversion of fibrinogen to fibrin.

Fibrinogen consists of three different polypeptides found with the following stoichiometry: $\alpha_2\beta_2\gamma_2$ and molecular weight of 340,000 daltons. Thrombin hydrolyzes four Arg-Gly bonds in the α- and β-subunits to form four small fibrinopeptides (two A and two B peptides) and fibrin. Fibrin spontaneously associates to form a loose fibrin clot. Thrombin also activates factor XIII by proteolysis to yield XIIIa. XIIIa catalyzes cross-link formation between glutaminyl and lysyl residues (Fig. 4-80). Although the amide bond is not high energy in nature, it provides a modicum of activation to facilitate the cross-linking reaction.

The extrinsic pathway is initiated by the addition of tissue-derived **thromboplastin** (factor III) to blood. Although not a protease, it participates in the proteolytic conversion of VII to VIIa in a calcium-requiring reaction; VIIa, VIII, and Ca^{2+} promote

TABLE 4-44. Blood-Clotting Factors

NAME (DISORDER)	NUMERICAL FACTOR DESIGNATION	SITE OF SYNTHESIS	SERINE PROTEASE	γ-CARBOXY GLUTAMATE	Ca^{2+} REQUIRED	GENERAL PROPERTIES
Fibrinogen (afibrinogenemia)	I	Liver	−	−	−	Converted to fibrin clot by thrombin-catalyzed proteolysis; stabilized by transglutaminyl transferase (factor XIIIa)
Prothrombin (hypoprothrombinemia)	II	Liver	+	+	+	Acts on fibrinogen and factors V, VII, VIII, XIII by proteolysis
Thromboplastin	III	Most tissues	−	−	−	Auxiliary component in factor VII activation
Calcium	IV		−	−		Required for vitamin K−dependent factors (II, VII, IX, X) and activation of XIII
Proaccelerin	V	Liver	−	−	−	Auxiliary to action of Xa
Proconvertin	VII	Liver	+	+	+	Activates IX and X
Antihemophilic factor (hemophilia)	VIII	Liver	−	−	−	Auxiliary to action of IXa
Christmas factor (Christmas disease)	IX	Liver	+	+	+	Activates X
Stuart factor	X	Liver	+	+	+	Activates prothrombin
Plasma thromboplastin antecedent	XI	Liver	+	−	−	Activates IX
Hageman factor	XII	?	+	−	−	Initiates intrinsic pathway
Fibrin-stabilizing factor	XIII	?	−	−	+	Transglutaminase cross links fibrin
Protein C	XIV	Liver	+	−	−	Inactivates V and VII by proteolysis; anticoagulant
Protein S		?	−	−	−	Auxiliary to action of Protein C
Prekallikrein		Liver	+	−	−	Kallikrein activates XII by proteolysis
High molecular weight kininogen		Liver	−	−	−	Accessory to kallikrein
von Willebrand factor (von Willebrand's disease)	VIII Antigen		−	−	−	Carrier of VIII

the proteolytic conversion of X to Xa. The step involving X occurs at the intersection of the intrinsic and extrinsic pathways. Properties of the blood-clotting factors are adumbrated in Table 4-44.

Anticoagulants

The blood contains several natural inhibitors of blood clotting (anticoagulants) including the following: (1) antithrombin III, (2) α_2-plasmin inhibitor, (3) protein C, and (4) α_1-antitrypsin. Antithrombin III, activated by heparin, binds to and inhibits a wide variety of serine proteases including IIa (thrombin), IXa, XIa, and XIIa as well as plasmin, trypsin, and chymotrypsin. Protein C (see Table 4-44) inactivates factors V and VII by proteolysis.

Heparin (by injection) is a pharmacological anticoagulant. It has a rapid onset of action, is short-acting, and its action can be promptly reversed by protamine injection if necessary. Protamine is a cationic protein that binds with anionic heparin. Coumarins are vitamin K analogues that inhibit the vitamin K–dependent carboxylation of several blood-clotting factors; the coumarins require 12 to 24 hours to elicit an anticoagulant effect. Both classes of these agents are used clinically.

Fibrinolysis

After tissue repair has abrogated the need for a clot, it is removed by a process of fibrinolysis. *Plasmin,* a serine protease formed from plasminogen, is a proteolytic enzyme responsible for this process. Plasmin digests or hydrolyzes fibrin. It also degrades factor V and factor VIII. *Tissue plasminogen activator* (TPA) is a serine protease that catalyzes the conversion of plasminogen to plasmin. There is considerable therapeutic interest in producing TPA by recombinant DNA methods for use in restoring coronary artery patency following coronary thrombosis.

NUTRITION

The essential requirements for human growth, development, maintenance, and activity are oxygen, energy-yielding metabolic fuels (mainly carbohydrate and fat), protein, vitamins, minerals, and water.

Water

About 70% of the lean body mass is water. The distribution of water in the various compartments is

TABLE 4-45. Fluid Compartments in Humans

	PERCENT OF LEAN BODY MASS	VOLUME (LITERS)/70-kg BODY MASS
Total body water	70	49.0
Intracellular compartment	50	35.0
Extracellular compartment	20	14.0
Interstitial fluid	15	10.5
Plasma	5	3.5

given in Table 4-45. The interstitial fluid is the intercellular fluid exclusive of that in the arteries, veins, and heart (*i.e.,* it is extracardiovascular). The plasma volume, which amounts to about 5% of the lean body mass, is the extracellular fluid within the cardiovascular system. The latter value is important in calculating some intravenous fluid requirements.

Water balance is the condition when intake is equivalent to output. Representative values are given in Table 4-46. Wide variations in fluid intake in the normal range are possible. Compensating changes in the urinary output maintain balance under physiological conditions. *Metabolic water* is produced by oxidative phosphorylation. Protons, electrons, and oxygen react in the terminal step of respiratory chain phosphorylation in a reaction catalyzed by cytochrome oxidase to produce water. Humans are able to live without oxygen for only a matter of minutes. Water is the next most essential requirement for life. Death from dehydration ensues within several days in the absence of fluid intake.

Caloric and Energy Expenditure

Body weight is determined by the balance between energy expended and energy consumed. If more energy is consumed than expended, then body weight increases. Energy expenditure varies considerably among individuals. It is generally greater in children

TABLE 4-46. Fluid Intake and Output in Humans

Output	
Expired air	800
Feces	200
Perspiration	400
Urine	1200
	2600 ml
Intake	
Food and beverage	2300
Metabolic	300
	2600 ml

TABLE 4-47. Daily Energy Requirements for Adults

Daily energy = BMR + activity
Expenditure
  BMR = weight (kg) × 24 kcal
  Activity: Modest = 0.3 × BMR
         Moderate = 0.4 × BMR
         Heavy = 0.5 × BMR

1 kcal = 1 Calorie of the nutritionist.

than adults, males than females, and young adults than elderly. It is also increased by activity. A general formula for calculating approximate energy requirements in adults is shown in Table 4-47. The *basal metabolic rate* is the energy necessary for maintaining basic physiological activities (heartbeat, brain activity, kidney function, body temperature, and respiratory function). It is approximately 1 kcal/kg/hour or 24 kcal/kg/day. The additional energy required for activity can be much greater than indicated in Table 4-47 for athletes, lumberjacks, and those in other active occupations. The kcal of the biochemist (kilocalorie) is equivalent to the Calorie (capital C) of the nutritionist. The approximate energy requirement for a 70-kg individual with moderate activity is estimated as follows:

$$70 \times 24 = 1680$$
$$0.4 \times 1680 = \underline{672}$$

Total requirement = 2352 kcal or Calories

Since this is an approximation, the figure can be rounded off to 2400 kcal.

Energy Sources

The main sources of energy include carbohydrates, lipids, and proteins. The metabolic energy derivable from 1 g of each is given in Table 4-48. The metabolic energy derivable from carbohydrates, lipids, and alcohol is equivalent to that obtained by oxidation in a bomb calorimeter. The metabolic energy derivable from proteins (4 kcal/g) is about 80% of that obtained by complete oxidation in a bomb calo-

TABLE 4-48. Metabolic Calories Derivable from Foodstuffs

Class	kcal/gram
Carbohydrate	4
Protein	4
Fat	9
Ethanol	7

rimeter. The explanation for this discrepancy is related to the conversion of amino nitrogen to urea *in vivo* and not to nitrogen oxides as in the calorimeter. Note that the caloric value of ethanol is rather substantial. This provides variable amounts of energy for many adults and is not inconsequential.

When energy expenditure exceeds intake, weight loss ensues. The caloric equivalent of a pound of adipose tissue is about 3500 kcal. This is based on a value of 85% fat, 15% water, and negligible carbohydrate and protein per pound of adipose tissue.

$$1 \text{ lb} \times 454 \text{ g lb}^{-1} \times 0.85 \times 9 \text{ Cal g}^{-1} = 3500 \text{ Cal}$$

Triacylglycerol is the major storage form of metabolic fuel in humans.

The caloric energy derived from the average U.S. diet is as follows: carbohydrates, 46%; fats, 42%; proteins, 12%. Various health authorities suggest that decreasing fats to 30% and increasing carbohydrates to 58% would promote health. Others suggest that decreasing fat consumption even further to provide only 20% of the total energy would be more beneficial.

Essential Human Nutrients

Essential nutrients are those that cannot be synthesized in adequate amounts (if at all) and are required in the diet. These are listed in Table 4-49. The essential amino acids can be represented by the acronym PVT TIM *H*ALL (read private Tim Hall). The italicized histidine and arginine indicate that histidine is essential in infants, and the essentialness of arginine has not been rigorously established. Foods vary in protein quality. This reflects the proportion of essential amino acids in them. In general, animal proteins are of higher quality than plant proteins. The recommended dietary allowance for proteins in adults is 56 g/day. The estimated average consumption of proteins in the United States is 101 g/day. The recommended daily allowance for children per unit weight is about twice that for adults.

The most important worldwide nutritional problem is protein–energy malnutrition in children. *Kwashiorkor* develops in children with adequate energy but insufficient protein intake. *Marasmus* develops in children with both inadequate energy and protein intake.

Linoleic and *linolenic* acid are essential in humans. They cannot be synthesized and are therefore required in the diet. They serve as precursors of PGs, LTs, TXs and PGIs as noted earlier.

Carbohydrates can be synthesized from glycogenic amino acids. They can also be formed from

TABLE 4-49. Essential Human Nutrients

AMINO ACIDS	FATTY ACIDS	VITAMINS	MINERALS	OTHER
		Water soluble	**Bulk**	
Phenylalanine	Linoleic	Thiamine (B_1)	Sodium	Water
Valine	Linolenic	Riboflavin (B_2)	Potassium	Energy
Threonine		Niacin	Phosphate	
Tryptophan		Pyridoxine (B_6)	Magnesium	
Isoleucine		Pantothenate	Calcium	
Methionine		Folate	Chloride	
Histidine*		Cobalamine (B_{12})		
Arginine†		Ascorbate (C)	**Trace**	
Leucine		Biotin†	Chromium	
Lysine		Myo-inositol†	Cobalt‡	
			Copper	
			Iodine	
		Fat soluble	Iron	
		A	Molybdenum	
		D	Selenium	
		E	Zinc	
		K	Floride§	

* Essential in infants.
† Human requirement not rigorously established.
‡ As vitamin B_{12}.
§ Promotes stronger teeth and bones; essentialness not established.

glycerol derived from triglyceride. Carbohydrates are a common and abundant source of energy. Individuals on a carbohydrate-free or deficient diet develop ketosis associated with production of the ketone bodies as previously described.

The general properties and functions of the vitamins are adumbrated in Table 4-50. Vitamins are generally divided into two classes: water soluble and insoluble. The latter group includes vitamin A, D, E, and K. Except for vitamin C deficiency and scurvy, deficiencies of a single vitamin are unusual in nature. Deficiencies of two or more vitamins are more characteristic. Pantothenate deficiency, moreover, is unusual in humans. The pan of pantothenate refers to the wide distribution of this compound in nature. A deficiency state occurs only during starvation when symptoms of other avitaminoses are manifest.

Pernicious anemia is more commonly related to a failure to absorb **vitamin B_{12}** than due to inadequate dietary intake. Pernicious anemia develops in individuals who fail to produce a gastric glycoprotein (called intrinsic factor) required for B_{12} (extrinsic factor) absorption. The vitamin B_{12} content of plants is nil. A deficiency state may therefore occur in individuals on a strict vegetarian diet.

The interrelationship of B_{12} and folate metabolism is complex and incompletely understood. Individuals with pernicious anemia develop both anemia and central nervous system lesions. Folate will cor-

rect the anemia but not the neuropathology. The anemia is reversible but not the nervous pathology. Folate is absent from proprietary vitamins to avoid masking the symptomatology of pernicious anemia, which elicits the acquisition of medical attention. The advisability of limiting folate in proprietary vitamins is debatable because many people have marginal folate intake. In humans vitamin B_{12} is necessary for the transfer of the methyl group from methyl-THF to homocysteine. It is unclear whether this is the only interrelationship between folate and vitamin B_{12}.

Provitamin D (7-dehydrocholesterol and ergosterol) require two metabolic transformations (hydroxylations) for conversion to the active form. The first step occurs in the liver and produces 25-hydroxyvitamin D_3. The second occurs in the kidney and produces 1,25-dihydroxyvitamin D_3 (1,25-dihydroxycholecalciferol). This compound is transported in the circulation to act on a variety of tissues and organs such as the kidney, bone, and intestine. It constitutes both a vitamin and hormone.

The biochemical role of vitamin K in clotting has been elucidated in the past 15 years. It is necessary for the carboxylation of glutamyl residues in four blood-clotting factors (see Table 4-44). The production of γ-carboxyglutamyl groups results in residues that bind calcium. The discovery of this post-translational modification was delayed because hydroly-

TABLE 4-50. Major Characteristics of Vitamins

VITAMIN	COFACTOR	DEFICIENCY STATE	BIOCHEMICAL FUNCTIONS	COMMENTS
Water-soluble group				
Thiamine (B_1)	Thiamine pyrophosphate	Beriberi	Oxidative decarboxylation. pyruvate dehydrogenase (pyruvate → acetyl-CoA) α-Ketoglutarate dehydrogenase (α-Ketoglutarate → succinyl-CoA) Ketoacid dehydrogenase Leucine, isoleucine, valine catabolism Transketolase	
Riboflavin (B_2)	FAD FMN		Oxidative decarboxylation reactions listed under thiamine. electron transport	
Niacin Nicotinic acid Nicotinamine	NAD^+	Pellegra	Many hydrogen-transfer redox reactions	Some derived from tryptophan metabolism
Pantothenate	Coenzyme A 4'-phosphopantetheine		Acyl transfer Cofactor of acyl carrier protein in fatty acid biosynthesis	Widely distributed (pan . . .) and isolated deficiency unknown
Biotin	Biotinyllysyl		Acetyl-CoA carboxylase Propionyl-CoA carboxylase Pyruvate carboxylase	
Cobalamine (B_{12})	Methylcobalamine	Perncious anemia	Methylmalonyl-CoA mutase 5-Methyl H_4-folate homocysteine transmethylase	B_{12} = extrinsic factor Not found in plants
Folate	Derivatives of H_4-folate		One-carbon transfer Thymidylate synthase Purine biosynthesis	
Ascorbate (C)	Ascorbate	Scurvy	Prolyl and lysyl hydroxylases (collagen) Dopamine β-hydroxylase	Effectiveness in viral disease controversial
Fat-soluble group				
A, retinol		Night blindness	Forms 11-cis retinal with rhodopsin	Retinal and retinoic acid may play a role in differentiation; possibly beneficial in prevention of some types of cancer
D,7-Dehydrocholesterol, (skin), ergosterol (plants, yeast)	1,25-dihydroxyvitamin D_3	Rickets in children Osteomalacia in adults	Calcium and phosphate metabolism	25 Hydroxylation in liver, 1 Hydroxylation in kidney
E, tocopherol		Unknown	Unknown	
K		Bleeding diathesis	Activated blood-clotting factors II, VII, IX, and X	Mediates formation of γ-carboxyglutamyl protein residues

sis of proteins in HCl, commonly used in biochemical analysis, results in the conversion of the γ-carboxyglutamate to glutamate. It had previously been known that vitamin K is necessary for blood clotting, but the biochemical mechanism was unknown.

The role of minerals in human metabolism is adumbrated in Table 4-3.

QUESTIONS IN BIOCHEMISTRY

Indicate the functions associated with each of the following: cell nucleus, mitochondrion, lysosome, Golgi, peroxisome, endoplasmic reticulum, and cytosol.

Specify the subcellular location of the following: thyroid hormone receptor, insulin receptor, β-adrenergic receptor, malate/α-ketoglutarate exchange protein, succinate dehydrogenase, pyruvate dehydrogenase, $Na^+ + K^+$ ATPase, carbamoyl phosphate synthetase II of pyrimidine biosynthesis, HMG-CoA reductase, HMG-CoA lyase, malate dehydrogenase, phosphofructokinase, phosphorylase, fatty acid synthase, RNA polymerase II, DNA polymerase α, DNA polymerase γ, catalase, adenylate cyclase, β-ketothiolase, fatty acyl-CoA dehydrogenase.

Discuss the primary, secondary, tertiary, and quaternary hierarchical structure of proteins.

Describe the nature of the bonds important in maintaining the primary, secondary, and tertiary structures of proteins.

What is the difference between the native and denatured structures of proteins? DNA? How can the denatured forms be produced?

Name the amino acids whose side chains are charged at physiological pH.

Name the two genetically encoded amino acids that contain a hydroxyl group.

Name the initiating amino acid of protein synthesis.

Name the aromatic amino acids.

Define: enzyme, holo-enzyme, apo-enzyme.

Define pH, pKa, acid, salt, buffer.

Calculate the ratio of $[HPO_4^{-2}]/[H_2PO_4^-]$ at pH 7.4 ($pKa = 6.8$).

Calculate the ratio of $[HCO_3^-]/[CO_2 + H_2CO_3]$ at pH 7.4 ($pKa = 6.1$).

Draw the double reciprocal (1/S vs. 1/v) plot associated with a competitive inhibitor. Noncompetitive inhibitor. Which plot best describes the inhibition of succinate dehydrogenase by malonate?

An enzyme has a V_{max} of 100 μmols/minute and a K_m of 10 μM. Calculate the velocity at the following substrate concentrations: 1 μM, 10 μM, 100 μM, and 1000 μM.

Glucocorticoids induce the formation of hepatic tyrosine aminotransferase. Describe a plausible mechanism for the action of this steroid hormone.

Define positive cooperativity. Hemoglobin binds oxygen in a cooperative fashion. Plot the binding of oxygen to hemoglobin as a function of $[O_2]$. 2,3-Bisphosphoglycerate shifts the binding curve to the right but does not alter its shape. What type of agent is 2,3-bisphosphoglycerate?

Draw the structure of ATP. Indicate the location of its high-energy bonds.

The standard free energy of hydrolysis of ATP to ADP and Pi is −7.3 kcal/mole at 30° and pH 7.0. Calculate the equilibrium constant for this reaction: ATP + H_2O ⇌ ADP + Pi.

Phosphoglucomutase catalyzes the following reaction: glucose-6-phosphate ⇌ glucose-1-phosphate. At equilibrium at 30°C and pH 7, the concentration of glucose-6-phosphate in a sample is 19 mM and that for glucose-1-phosphate is 1 mM. Calculate the standard free energy change ($\Delta G°$). Calculate the free energy change when 1 mole of glucose-6-phosphate is converted to glucose-1-phosphate when the concentrations of each are 1 mM; when the concentration of glucose-6-phosphate is 100 mM and that of glucose-1-phosphate is 1 mM.

Which of the following contain a high-energy phosphate bond: glucose-6-phosphate, phosphoenolpyruvate, dATP, 1,3-bisphosphoglycerate, glyceraldehyde-3-phosphate?

Draw the Haworth projection formulas for D-glucose, D-mannose, D-galactose, D-fructose, lactose (galactosyl-β1, 4-glucose) and sucrose (glucosyl-α1, β2-fructose).

Name the three irreversible enzyme-catalyzed reactions in the Embden–Meyerhof glycolytic pathway. Which enzyme is the chief regulatory enzyme of the pathway? How is its activity affected by ATP, AMP, citrate, fructose-2,6-bisphosphate?

How is the NADH generated in the Embden–Meyerhof glycolytic pathway oxidized under (1) anaerobic and (2) aerobic conditions?

How does the conversion of glucose to lactate differ from the conversion of lactate to glucose?

How can muscle glycogen contribute to the maintenance of blood glucose? What is the Cori cycle?

Describe the pathway for converting galactose to glucose-6-phosphate. What is the enzyme deficiency in galactosemia?

Name the five cofactors required for the conversion of pyruvate to acetyl-CoA.

Name the irreversible steps in the Krebs citric acid cycle. What is the chief regulatory enzyme and its allosteric effector? Name the two enzymes of the cycle that catalyze decarboxylation reactions. Which step is associated with substrate-level phosphorylation? Which step is inhibited by malonate?

Describe the pathway of electron transport from NADH to oxygen. Describe the effect of (1) rotenone and (2) cyanide in this process.

Describe the mechanism for ATP formation in mitochondria. What is the mechanism of action of 2,4-dinitrophenol on this process *in vivo?*

How many ATPs result from the oxidation of pyruvate and acetyl-CoA by the citric acid cycle and oxidative phosphorylation. Account for each molecule formed.

Name the two enzymes necessary for (1) glycogen formation and (2) glycogenolysis. Describe the action of epinephrine on glycogenolysis.

Name the enzyme that catalyzes the following reaction. Identify its cofactor.

xylulose-5-phosphate + ribose-5-phosphate $\rightleftharpoons$
sedoheptulose-7-phosphate +
glyceraldehyde-3-phosphate

Describe the pathway for the conversion of glucose to ribose-5-phosphate.

Compare and contrast fatty acid oxidation and fatty acid biosynthesis.

Calculate the yield of ATP associated with the complete oxidation of (1) palmitate (16-carbon, saturated) and (2) palmitoleate (16-carbon, 1 double bond).

Describe the various processes by which fatty acids originating as triacylglycerol in adipose tissue are subsequently oxidized in the heart.

Describe the biosynthesis of (1) triacylglycerol, (2) phosphatidylcholine, (3) sphingosine, (4) ceramide, (5) sphingomyelin, and (6) cerebroside.

Define (1) transport, (2) symport, and (3) antiport. Give examples of each.

What is the locus of action of phospholipase A_2? Phospholipase C?

Account for the biosynthesis of ketone bodies in the liver and their utilization in extrahepatic tissues.

Lovastatin is a drug that inhibits the rate-limiting reaction in cholesterol biosynthesis. What is this reaction? Name the 10-, 15-, and 30-carbon intermediates in cholesterol formation.

Describe the route for (1) triacylglycerol and (2) cholesterol transport from liver to other tissues. Describe the function of (1) HDL and (2) LDL.

Which amino acid is entirely ketogenic? Distinguish between glycogenic and ketogenic amino acids. How do these concepts relate to the aphorism that fatty acids can not be converted to net quantities of carbohydrate in humans?

Name the sources of atoms present in urea. Outline the pathway for urea biosynthesis.

Name the amino acids converted into oxaloacetate.

Name the vitamin and cofactor required for transamination reactions.

How are intermediates of the citric acid cycle maintained at adequate levels? Define (1) catabolic, (2) anabolic, and (3) amphibolic reactions.

Specify the configuration of (1) amino acids that occur in proteins and (2) glucose that occurs in glycogen relative to D- and L-glyceraldehyde.

What is the amino acid that is the chief source of one-carbon atoms used for purine biosynthesis?

Describe the two roles of vitamin B_{12} in amino acid metabolism in humans.

Describe the processes involved in the conversion of muscle alanine into hepatic glucose.

Describe the conversion of phenylalanine into tyrosine. In which organ does this occur?

Name the precursors of porphyrin.

Outline the pathway for heme degradation.

Name three substances formed by transmethylation from *S*-adenosylmethionine.

Draw the common pyrimidines. Identify the sources of each atom in the ring.

Draw the common purines. Identify the sources of each atom of the ring system.

Distinguish between nucleoside and nucleotide. Name five nucleotides. Name two polynucleotides.

Contrast the general pathways of purine and pyrimidine nucleotide formation.

What is meant by the salvage pathway for purine formation? How is it known that the salvage pathway is operational in human metabolism?

Describe the mechanism of the amination reaction during the conversion of IMP to AMP. Name two other reactions where a similar biochemical strategy is employed.

Describe the biosynthesis of phosphoribosyl pyrophosphate. Describe the reaction for converting ribonucleotides to deoxyribonucleotides.

Describe thymidylate biosynthesis. What is the mechanism of action of methotrexate?

Describe two reactions catalyzed by xanthine oxidase.

Describe the Watson–Crick structure of DNA. Describe or define (1) complementary base pairs, (2) antiparallel structure, (3) phosphodiester bond, (4) hydrogen bond, and (5) Chargaff's rule.

If a sample of duplex DNA contains 20% A, what are the molar ratios of T, G, and C?

The diploid human genome contains 7×10^9 base pairs. Calculate the length of the corresponding DNA if it were all in the B-form.

What is meant by unique DNA?

Describe the polarity of interaction of primer and template DNA and the polarity of the DNA polymerization or elongation reactions.

Describe the chemical structure of RNA. What are the main differences between DNA and RNA?

Define or describe (1) DNA polymerase, (2) 5'-exonuclease activity, (3) 3'-exonuclease activity, (4) DNA ligase, (5) helicase, (6) topoisomerase, (7) single-stranded binding protein, (8) leading strand, (9) lagging strand, (10) template, (11) primer, (12) primase, (13) proofreading or editing function, (14) replication fork, and (15) semiconservative replication.

Describe excision repair of DNA.

Describe the functions of the three eukaryotic DNA polymerases.

What are the chemical energy requirements for the DNA ligase reaction in humans?

Describe the reactions involved in mRNA biosynthesis in *E. coli*.

Describe the reactions involved in mRNA biosynthesis in humans. Describe capping, polyadenylation, and the splicing reactions.

Define mRNA, rRNA, 5S RNA, tRNA, snRNA, and hnRNA. Which eukaryotic RNA polymerases are involved in the biosynthesis of each?

Describe the properties of the genetic code with respect to degeneracy and the wobble. Name the initiation and termination codons.

Describe the ribosome. What are the A site and P site? Where is peptidyltransferase activity located?

Describe the mechanism of amino acid activation.

Recount the role of the soluble (nonribosomal) factors of protein synthesis. Describe how these factors exclude met-tRNA^{met} from the initiation reaction and f-met-tRNA^I (in prokaryotes) or met-tRNA^I (in eukaryotes) from participating in the elongation reactions.

The mRNA for the normal α-chain of hemoglobin ends with the following sequence: ACU UCU* AAA UAC CGU UAA GCU CGA GCC UCG GUA GCA. Specify the sequence of amino acids that corresponds to the indicated triplets. In hemoglobin Wayne, the U denoted with the asterisk is deleted. What is the consequence of this mutation? In hemoglobin Constant Spring, the underlined U is changed to a C. What is the consequence of this?

Describe the reactants that participate in peptide bond formation. In which direction does chain growth occur? Why is a translocation reaction required?

How many high-energy bonds are expended in each polymerization reaction, on the average, in (1) DNA biosynthesis, (2) RNA biosynthesis, and (3) protein biosynthesis?

List several types of post-translational modification. Describe insulin biosynthesis.

Compare and contrast the *O*-glycosylation and *N*-glycosylation reactions. Contrast high mannose and complex glycoprotein formation.

Describe the biosynthesis and secretion of a protein such as albumin.

Define (1) promoter, (2) terminator, (3) primary transcript, (4) monocistronic message, (5) polycistronic message, (6) TATA box, (7) consensus sequence, (8) enhancer, and (9) regulatory element.

How does lactose regulate the expression of the *E. coli* lac operon?

Describe the structure of a eukaryotic gene and its general mode of regulation.

Define (1) restriction enzyme, (2) pallindrome, (3) plasmid, (4) recombinant DNA, (5) Southern blot, (6) Northern blot, (7) hybridization, (8) gene library, and (9) cDNA library.

Write the structures of the family of mRNA oligonucleotides corresponding to the peptide: cys met pro. Write the structure of each DNA complementary to each of these RNAs. How many oligonucleotide structures correspond to the peptide cys leu pro?

There are two general methods for producing recombinant DNA molecules; one involves the use of restriction endonucleases, and the other requires terminal transferase. Self-annealing is possible in one but not other. Explain.

Describe the general procedure for DNA sequence analysis using the dideoxynucleotide chain termination technique. What principles in DNA synthesis are illustrated by this methodology?

What is the mechanism for terminating the action of the following neurotransmitter agents: (1) acetylcholine, (2) dopamine, (3) GABA, (4) glutamate, (5) serotonin, (6) leucine enkephalin, and (7) norepinephrine?

Describe acetylcholine biosynthesis and degradation.

Name the two major types of acetylcholine receptor.

Describe the pathway for norepinephrine biosynthesis.

Name the two major subclasses of adrenergic receptor. Which is associated with activation of adenylate cyclase? Which is associated with calcium mobilization?

What is the neurochemical basis of (1) myasthenia gravis and (2) Parkinson's disease?

Compare the ATP yield in converting α-ketoglutarate to succinate in the Krebs cycle and the conversion of glutamate to succinate by means of GABA in the GABA shunt.

What is the main metabolic fuel for brain metabolism? Which organ plays a role in maintaining adequate blood levels of this fuel? Explain.

What is meant by the Sutherland second messenger hypothesis? Name three first messengers. Name three second messengers.

Define (1) endocrine, (2) paracrine, and (3) autocrine action.

Describe the metabolism and action of cyclic AMP. Describe the mechanism whereby cyclic AMP regulates the activity of cyclic AMP–dependent protein kinase.

Define protein kinases. What amino acid residues accept phosphate? What is the predominant phosphorylated residue in human cells?

Name the main muscle proteins. Which has ATPase activity? How does ATP drive muscle contraction?

Describe the structure of collagen. Describe its pathway of biosynthesis.

Compare and contrast the intrinsic and extrinsic pathway of blood clotting. What is meant by cascade?

Name the blood-clotting factors that are serine proteases. Which factors require Ca^{2+} for action? Which factors contain γ-carboxyglutamate? Which factor has transglutaminase activity?

What is the function of tissue plasminogen activator?

Give the nutritional caloric value of protein, carbohydrate, fat, and ethanol. Why does the nutritional caloric value of protein differ from that obtained by oxidation in a bomb calorimeter?

Estimate the caloric requirements of a 55-kg adult human with modest activity.

What is the composition of the average U.S. diet in terms of carbohydrate, protein, and fat? What types of changes in diet composition are thought by many health authorities to be more optimal?

What is metabolic water? What amount is produced daily in human adults?

Name the lipids essential in humans. Define the term essential.

What are nitrogen balance, negative nitrogen balance, and positive nitrogen balance? Describe circumstances related to each.

What is the importance of the following in humans: (1) cobalt, (2) iodine, (3) fluoride, (4) copper, and (5) iron?

What is marasmus? Kwashiorkor?

Name the vitamin deficiency associated with (1) rickets, (2) beriberi, (3) scurvy, (4) pernicious anemia, and (5) pellegra.

Name the cofactor derived from (1) thiamine, (2) riboflavin, (3) panthothenate, and (4) niacin. Identify the biochemical functions of each cofactor.

Account for the inability of extrahepatic tissues to release free glucose into the circulation.

What is the function of catalase? Where is it located within the cell?

What type of reactions are catalyzed by (1) kinases, (2) hydrolases, (3) phosphorylases, (4) mutases, (5) ligases, (5) lyases, (6) synthetases, and (7) synthases?

Define (1) exergonic and (2) endergonic.

Describe the action of (1) cyanide, (2) tetracycline, (3) rotenone, (4) carbon monoxide, (5) antimycin A, (6) streptomycin, (7) actinomycin D, (8) methotrexate, (9) chloramphenicol, and (10) rifamycin.

Describe the defect associated with the following disorders: (1) von Gierke's disease, (2) Christmas disease, (3) Pompe's disease, (4) Tay-Sachs disease, (5) Gaucher's disease, (6) familial hypercholesterolemia, (7) maple syrup urine disease, (8) phenylketonuria, (9) Hurler's syndrome, (10) hemophilia, (11) Lesch–Nyan syndrome, (12) beriberi, (13) Hunter's disease, and (14) drug-induced hemolytic anemia.

Describe the role of ATP in (1) DNA synthesis, (2) RNA synthesis, (3) protein synthesis, (4) cholesterol synthesis, (5) fatty acid biosynthesis, (6) gluconeogenesis, (7) pyrimidine biosynthesis, and (8) purine biosynthesis.

Describe the role of GTP in (1) RNA synthesis, (2) protein synthesis, (3) purine biosynthesis, (4) gluconeogenesis, and (5) Krebs cycle function.

Describe the role of CTP in (1) RNA biosynthesis and (2) lipid biosynthesis.

Describe the role of UTP in (1) RNA biosynthesis and (2) carbohydrate biosynthesis.

Name a divalent cation indispensable for blood coagulation.

Name a substrate with a $P:O$ ratio of 2.

What is the source of hydrogen for the reductive steps of fatty acid and cholesterol biosynthesis.

Describe Mitchell's chemiosmotic theory.

Describe Blobel's signal peptide hypothesis.

Write the structural formula for cholesterol and indicate the numbering system for its carbon atoms.

How are nucleotides linked in (1) DNA and (2) RNA?

What vitamin is concerned with the synthesis of prothrombin in the liver?

Outline the steps in blood clotting.

Discuss the role of niacin and trytophan in the treatment and prevention of pellegra.

Multiple Choice Questions

ONE-ANSWER TYPE

1. Succinate dehydrogenase is found in the:
   (a) Outer mitochondrial membrane
   (b) Intermembranous space
   (c) Inner mitochondrial membrane
   (d) Mitochondrial matrix
   (e) Cytosol
2. Which of the following amino acids occurs at every third position in collagen?
   (a) Leucine
   (b) Lysine
   (c) Proline
   (d) Alanine
   (e) Glycine
3. Which of the following *lacks* an aromatic component?
   (a) Tyrosine
   (b) Tryptophan
   (c) Adenine
   (d) Hydroxymethylglutarate
   (e) Estradiol
4. Each of the following is transported directly across the inner mitochondrial membrane by a transport system *except:*
   (a) Palmitoyl-CoA
   (b) Citrate
   (c) Malate
   (d) Aspartate
   (e) ATP
5. The energy content of 1 g of fat is _____ kcal.
   (a) 2
   (b) 4
   (c) 7
   (d) 9
   (e) 11
6. The metabolism of 1 mole of acetyl-CoA in mitochondria results in the generation of _____ moles of ATP equivalents.
   (a) 2
   (b) 3
   (c) 12
   (d) 15
   (e) 38
7. Eukaryotic elongation factor 1 (eEF-1) forms a complex with aminoacyl-tRNA and:
   (a) ATP
   (b) CTP
   (c) UDPG
   (d) GTP
   (e) NAD^+
8. The *E. coli* enzyme responsible for removing the primer and repair polymerization reactions of DNA is:
   (a) DNA polymerase I
   (b) DNA polymerase II
   (c) DNA polymerase III
   (d) Primase
   (e) DNA ligase
9. The subcellular location of the Emden–Meyerhof glycolytic pathway is the:
   (a) Nucleus
   (b) Lysosome
   (c) Mitochondrion
   (d) Peroxisome
   (e) Cytosol
10. The RNA polymerase binding site on DNA is called the:
    (a) Repressor
    (b) Operator
    (c) Promoter
    (d) Regulatory element
    (e) Enhancer

POSSIBLY MORE THAN ONE ANSWER

For each of the following questions answer:

   (a) If only 1, 2, and 3 are correct
   (b) If only 1 and 3 are correct
   (c) If only 2 and 4 are correct
   (d) If only 4 is correct
   (e) If all are correct

11. Trypsin cleaves polypeptides on the carboxyl terminal side of which of the following?
    1. Arginine
    2. Leucine
    3. Lysine
    4. Glycine
12. Which of the following activate phosphofructokinase?
    1. AMP
    2. Citrate
    3. Fructose-2,6-bisphosphate
    4. ATP
13. The insulin receptor directly catalyzes the phosphorylation of the following residue in proteins:

1. Serine
2. Methionine
3. Threonine
4. Tyrosine

14. The following blood-clotting factors possess γ-carboxyglutamyl residues:
    1. Prothrombin (Factor II)
    2. Proconvertin (Factor VII)
    3. Christmas Factor (Factor IX)
    4. Stuart Factor (Factor X)

15. The following proteins are found in the thin filament of muscle:
    1. Actin
    2. Troponin
    3. Tropomyosin
    4. Myosin light chain

16. Essential fatty acids include:
    1. Oleate
    2. Linoleate
    3. Palmitoleate
    4. Linolenate

17. The following participates in oxidation–reduction reactions:
    1. Niacin
    2. Ascorbate
    3. Riboflavin
    4. Coenzyme Q

18. The following neurotransmitters are inactivated by a sodium-dependent uptake system:
    1. Norepinephrine
    2. Serotonin
    3. GABA
    4. Acetylcholine

19. Pyridoxal phosphate (vitamin B_6) is a cofactor in the following enzymes:
    1. Glutamate decarboxylase
    2. Aspartate aminotransferase
    3. Aromatic amino acid decarboxylase
    4. Pyruvate dehydrogenase

20. Cyclic AMP–dependent protein kinase catalyzes the phosphorylation and activation of the following:
    1. Phosphorylase kinase
    2. Glycogen synthase
    3. Tyrosine hydroxylase
    4. Phosphorylase

21. The metabolism of the following is altered in individuals with maple syrup urine disease:
    1. Leucine
    2. Isoleucine
    3. Valine
    4. Lysine

22. Electrophoresis of nucleic acids is performed in the following procedures:
    1. Southern blots
    2. DNA sequence analysis
    3. Northern blots
    4. Western blots

23. The following are directly incorporated into the pyrimdine ring system:
    1. Glycine
    2. Aspartate
    3. Serine
    4. Carbamoylphosphate

24. The following contain thiamine pyrophosphate as a cofactor:
    1. Pyruvate dehydrogenase
    2. Transketolase
    3. α-Ketoglutarate dehydrogenase
    4. Transaldolase

25. The following is glycogenic only:
    1. Serine
    2. Methionine
    3. Proline
    4. Glycine

26. Direct precursor of urea:
    1. Ammonium ion
    2. Bicarbonate
    3. Aspartate
    4. N-Acetylglutamate

27. Derived from cholesterol:
    1. Testosterone
    2. Squalene
    3. Bile acids
    4. Bile pigments

28. UDP-glucose is required for the formation of:
    1. Glycogen
    2. Glucose-1-phosphate from galactose-1-phosphate
    3. Gangliosides
    4. Ceramide

29. Irreversible steps of the Krebs citric acid cycle include those catalyzed by:
    1. Malate dehydrogenase
    2. Citrate synthase
    3. Aconitase
    4. α-Ketoglutarate dehydrogenase

30. The following utilize $NADP^+$ as substrate:
    1. Glyceraldehyde-3-phosphate dehydrogenase
    2. Lactate dehydrogenase
    3. Fatty acyl-CoA dehydrogenase
    4. 6-Phosphogluconate dehydrogenase

Each set of the lettered headings below is followed by a list of numbered statements. For each of the numbered statements answer:

(A) If the item is associated with (a) alone

(B) If the item is associated with (b) alone
(C) If the item is associated with both (a) and (b)
(D) If the item is associated with neither (a) nor (b)

(a) Initiation factor 2 in E. coli (IF-2)
(b) Elongation factor T in E. coli (EF-T)
31. Binds GTP.
32. Binds f-met-tRNA^I.
33. Binds ala-tRNA^{ala}.
34. Recognizes an AUG codon.
35. Recognizes an UAA codon.

(a) DNA
(b) RNA
36. Contains thymine.
37. Alkali labile
38. Elongation occurs in the 5′- to 3′-direction.

39. Requires a template for biosynthesis.
40. Found in the nucleus

ANSWERS TO MULTIPLE CHOICE QUESTIONS

1. c	11. b	21. a	31. C
2. e	12. b	22. a	32. A
3. d	13. d	23. c	33. B
4. a	14. e	24. a	34. C
5. d	15. a	25. e	35. D
6. c	16. c	26. a	36. A
7. d	17. e	27. b	37. B
8. a	18. a	28. a	38. C
9. e	19. a	29. c	39. C
10. c	20. b	30. d	40. C

General Microbiology and Immunology

Ronald B. Luftig, Ph.D.
Head, Department of Microbiology,
Immunology and Parasitology,
Louisiana State University Medical Center,
New Orleans, Louisiana

THE MICROORGANISM

Microorganisms of medical importance include various species of bacteria, protozoa, fungi, and viruses.

Bacteria are generally spoken of as *prokaryotes.* The cells of all other organisms, including protozoans, fungi, and higher order species, are said to be *eukaryotic,* that is, their nucleus is enclosed in a membrane, and the cytoplasm contains numerous organelles, including ribosomes (protein synthesis), mitochondria (energy transfer), endoplasmic reticulum (energy transfer and other enzymic functions), lysosomes, Golgi bodies, and a cytoskeleton. All bacterial and eukaryotic cells contain both DNA and RNA. In contrast, viruses may contain either, but never both.

Historical Notes

Antonj van Leeuwenhoek, in 1672, built single-lens microscopes with effective magnification of more than 100× and was the first to see bacteria and protozoa, which he called animalcules, or "little animals." He is often called the "father of bacteriology and protozoology."

Edward Jenner, in 1798, demonstrated that inoculation with active cowpox vesical material conferred immunity to smallpox. As of 1979, smallpox was eradicated as a result of sustained worldwide immunization.

Louis Pasteur (1822–1895), a French chemist interested in the cause of spoilage ("diseases") of beer and wines, entered the controversy concerning spontaneous generation and finally refuted the doctrine by heating infusions in flasks with long, downtwisted necks that excluded dust but were open to the air without any substance between the outer air and the infusion. Such flasks remained sterile until dust was put into them. Pasteur later became interested in the analogy between diseases of beer and wine and human disease and formulated anew the old idea that disease was caused by invasive microorganisms. He also introduced autoclaving to destroy spores and was the first to use synthetic media as well as the first to discover bacteria that can live without air *(anaerobes).* In 1885, Pasteur also successfully developed a vaccine against rabies.

Joseph Lister (1827–1912), an English physician and scientist, contemporary with Pasteur and well acquainted with his ideas on dust in the air as a source of contaminating organisms, conceived the idea of using phenol solutions on surgical wounds to prevent sepsis and, later, of operating in an atmosphere filled with phenol mist. This opened the door to antiseptic surgery and later to aseptic surgery. Lister is the "father of modern aseptic surgery."

Robert Koch (1843–1910), in 1877, provided the first demonstration that a specific bacterium could cause anthrax, an animal disease. Working with the anthrax bacillus, he developed methods for isolating pure cultures on solid media and for staining microorganisms to render them visible under the microscope. Six years later he discovered tubercle bacillus to be the cause of tuberculosis. Koch also set forth postulates that are still used today to determine whether a specific agent is the cause of a particular infectious disease.

Elie Metchnikoff, a Russian pupil of Koch, discovered phagocytosis in 1883.

H. C. J. Gram, in 1884, devised his method for differential staining of bacteria.

Emil A. Von Behring, Shibasaburo Kitasato, and **Albert Fränkel,** in 1890, discovered the phenomena of active and passive immunization against diphtheria and tetanus, which are due to the properties of serum, which we now recognize as a specific antibody.

Iwanowski, in Russia, demonstrated in 1892 the first noncultivable, invisible, and filterable agent of disease—tobacco mosaic virus.

Jules Bordet, in 1895, discovered the heat-labile antibacterial properties of immune serum, which we now ascribe to complement.

F. A. J. Löffler and **Paul Frosch,** in 1898, discovered the agent of hoof-and-mouth disease, the first-described agent of a viral disease of lower animals.

Walter Reed and the U.S. Army Yellow Fever Commission at Havana, in 1899 confirmed the mosquito *(Aedes aegypti)* as vector and discovered the agent of yellow fever, the first virus to be described as the cause of human disease.

K. Landsteiner, in 1900–1901, reported the isohemagglutination reactions that formed the basis for the major (ABO) human blood groups; in 1908, he was the first to transmit poliomyelitis in monkeys by intracerebral inoculation of bacteria-free brain tissue.

Howard Taylor Ricketts, in 1909, discovered the cause of Rocky Mountain spotted fever *(Rickettsia sp.).*

Peyton Rous, in 1911, was the first to demonstrate the transmission of a malignant tumor (chicken sarcoma) by means of cell-free filtrate (Rous sarcoma virus).

Frederick W. Twort, in 1915, and **Felix H. d'Herelle,** in 1917, discovered the bacterial viruses—bacteriophages.

Alexander Fleming, the discoverer of lysozyme, in 1929 isolated *Penicillium notatum* and demonstrated antibacterial activity *in vitro* in culture filtrates. It was not until 1940, however, that **H. W. Florey, E. B. Chain,** and their collaborators at Oxford University showed experimentally that penicillin was nontoxic and highly effective systemically in treating pyogenic infection, thus inaugurating the antibiotic era.

M. Heidelberger and **F. E. Kendall,** in 1929, developed the quantitative precipitin reaction, which underlies the interpretation of most antigen–antibody reactions.

In 1931, **Max Theiler** adapted the virus of yellow fever to embryonated eggs, leading to the development of the 17D attenuated strain of yellow fever virus used in the vaccine.

A. Tiselius and **E. A. Kabat,** in 1939, demonstrated that antibodies were contained in the γ-globulin fraction of serum.

A. H. Coons and his collaborators, in 1942, developed the fluorescent antibody technique.

O. T. Avery, C. MacLeod, and **M. McCarty,** in 1944, demonstrated that the genetic information responsible for transformation of pneumococci was embodied in DNA. This discovery ushered in the era of molecular biology and molecular genetics.

In 1949, **John F. Enders, T. H. Weller,** and **F. C. Robbins** cultivated the virus of poliomyelitis in nonneural tissue explants, making possible the development of poliomyelitis and other attenuated viral vaccines.

The third quarter of this century (about 1950 to 1975) saw a veritable explosion in biomedical knowledge, represented by many signal contributions. To mention only a few, **F. Lipman** and **H. Krebs** contributed fundamental knowledge in the fields of energy metabolism and synthetic pathways in living cells (pentose phosphate pathway and Krebs cycle). In immunobiology, **G. M. Edelman** and colleagues provided the first definitive indication that immunoglobulin G comprised "light" and "heavy" peptide chains; **F. M. Burnet** formulated important theories of antibody formation and the immune response (clonal selection), and **P. B. Medawar** was the first to describe induced tolerance to foreign antigens. **K. Ishizaka** and **T. Ishizaka** identified immunoglobulin E as the agent of reaginic ("immediate")-type hypersensitivity. In microbial and molecular genetics, the contributions of **J. Lederberg, G. Beadle, S. E. Luria, E. Tatum, F. Jacob, A. Lwoff, J. Monod, M. Delbruck,** and **A. D.**

Hershey were seminal. **T. Akiba** and **K. Ochiai** described the phenomenon of simultaneous transfer (from *E. coli* to *Shigella dysenteriae*) of resistance to multiple antibiotics, which **T. Watanabe** subsequently showed to be due to an infectious drug resistance transfer factor (R factor), the first of many types of plasmids to be described. **F. H. C. Crick, J. D. Watson,** and **M. H. F. Wilkins** elucidated the structure of DNA, and **M. W. Nirenberg, H. G. Khorana** and **R. W. Holley** described the genetic code, setting the stage for all of the startling recent advances in "genetic engineering." **H. M. Temin** and **D. Baltimore** identified reverse transcriptase in tumor viruses. In 1975, **G. Kohler** and **C. Milstein** developed the mouse hybridoma procedure for the preparation of monoclonal antibodies, the application of which has had a profound effect in many areas of biomedical science.

Most recently, in 1983 and 1984, two groups, one at the Pasteur Institute headed by **L. Montagnier** and one at the National Institutes of Health (NIH) headed by **R. Gallo** isolated a retrovirus, now designated as human immunodeficiency virus (HIV), as the causative agent of acquired immune deficiency syndrome AIDS.

Classification of Bacteria (Prokaryotes)

Bacteria are single-celled organisms that reproduce by binary fission, have smaller ribosome(s) than eukaryotic cells, and do not contain their DNA within a nuclear membrane. They are classified primarily on the basis of morphology, and on various physiological properties such as pigment, spore formation, staining reactions, motility, enzyme content (*e.g.,* aerobic or anaerobic, proteolytic, fermentative), and DNA analysis. Immunologic properties (antigenic structure) and susceptibility to highly specific bacterial viruses (bacteriophages) are also used in their differentiation and identification.

All medically significant species of bacteria are chemosynthetic and heterotrophic (chemo-organotrophs; see section on bacterial metabolism), having diameters typically <5 μm (usually 1 to 2 μm and less in *Rickettsia* and *Chlamydia*). Unlike viruses, all except rickettsiae and chlamydiae and two or three other species of pathogenic bacteria (*e.g.,* syphilis spirochetes and leprosy bacilli), are cultivable in *inanimate* media. Viruses, rickettsiae, and chlamydiae can multiply only in living cells (cell and tissue cultures, etc.). All bacteria have cell walls of peptidoglycan or murein that contain muramic acid,

a substance unique to the prokaryotes. Medically significant bacteria occur in six orders as follows:

1. *Order Pseudomonadales:* These gram-negative rods grow in simple peptone media at 10°C to 40°C; generally motile with polar flagella, strictly aerobic. Some produce blue pyocyanin, a yellow fluorescent pigment, or both. They characteristically secrete a number of exoenzymes, such as collagenase, lipase, protease, and hemolysin, which allow them to survive in unusual environments such as hot tubs, distilled water, and disinfectants. They also excrete exotoxins, which account in large part for the serious nature of their infections. Representatives: *Pseudomonas aeruginosa, P. pseudomallei.*

2. *Order Eubacteriales:* ("True Bacteria"): Gram-positive or Gram-negative rods or cocci, no helical forms; possess a rigid cell wall; motile species have peritrichous flagella; aerobic, facultative, or strict anaerobes; only two genera (*Clostridium* and *Bacillus*) product heat-resistant endospores; must grow at 37°C in peptone or meat infusion media; some also require blood, yeast extract, or serum. This order contains most of the pathogenic bacteria. Representatives: *Salmonella typhi* and related *Enterobacteriaceae, Streptococcus pyogenes, Staphylococcus aureus, Clostridium tetani, Bacillus anthracis, Neisseria gonorrhoeae.*

3. *Order Actinomycetales:* Exhibit a branching, rod-like or filamentous cells; no motile pathogens; generally Gram-positive; some species are acid-fast; others are the source of many important antibiotics. Representatives: *Mycobacterium tuberulosis, M. leprae, Actinomyces israelii, Nocardia* sp.

4. *Order Spirochaetales:* Helical; flexible; motile without flagella; generally Gram-negative, but preferentially observed with darkfield microscope; contain a central, fibrillar, elastic structure (axial filament) around which the tubular cell is wound. Representatives: *Treponema pallidum, Leptospira icterohaemorrhagiae, Borrelia recurrentis.*

5. *Order Mycoplasmatales:* No cell wall, therefore osmotically fragile and extremely pleomorphic; very small cells (0.2 μm) that pass through filters that retain bacteria; the smallest known living units capable of independent multiplication in inanimate media; nonmotile, though some have flagella; no heat-resistant endospores; colonies on special "enriched me-

dia'' extremely minute, typically with inverted fried egg appearance (except Eaton agent); aerobic or facultative; parasitic species are rich in lipids, mostly steroids, which stabilize and strengthen the cell membrane. Representatives: *Mycoplasma pneumoniae (Eaton agent), M. hominis, Ureaplasma urealyticum.*

6. *Order Rickettsiales:* Bacteria that lack important enzyme systems characteristic of other bacteria, hence their **obligate intracellular parasitism** and extremely minute (0.3 μm) size; only cultivable in cell and tissue cultures, and most in viable chick embryos; prokaryotic, bacterialike cell structure.

Family Rickettsiaceae: Lack several synthetic enzyme systems but can synthesize ATP; multiply by binary fission like other bacteria; have distinct cell walls with muramic acid; morphologically are distinct rods, cocci or filaments. Representatives: *Rickettsia prowazekii, Coxiella burnetii.*

Family Chlamydiaceae: Lack many synthetic enzymes; unlike all other bacteria, *cannot synthesize ATP;* complex intracellular mode of multiplication; cell walls are layered and, like bacteria, contain muramic acid; spheroidal morphology. Representatives: *Chlamydia trachomatis, C. psittaci.*

Classification of Medically Important Protozoa, Fungi, Helminths (Eukaryotes), and Viruses

In addition to bacteria, other groups containing pathogenic microorganisms are listed as follows:

A. Protozoa: Unicellular animals; rarely cultivable on artificial media; five groups differentiated by type of motility:
1. Superclass Sarcodina (move with pseudopodia): *Entamoeba histolytica;* enteric and tissue parasites
2. Subphylum Ciliophora (move with cilia): *Balantidium coli;* enteric
3. Superclass Mastigophora (move with flagella): Arthropod-borne: *Leishmania, Trypanosoma;* blood and tissues; *Trichomonas,* chiefly genitalia
4. Subphylum Sporozoa (ameboid movement in some trophozoites): Alternating sexual and asexual multiplication in different hosts, *e.g.,* humans and mosquito in *Plasmodium* (malaria parasites); blood and tissues
5. Class Toxoplasmea (gliding and flexing motility): Asexual multiplication by binary fission, endogony or sporogony, or both; trophozoites in cysts or pseudocysts. *Toxoplasma gondii, Pneumocystis carinii, Sarcocystis lindemanni*

B. Fungi: Eukaryotic cellular structure; may grow as branching and filamentous forms (mycelia) or single cells (yeasts), or both; nonphotosynthetic (no chlorophyll); chemo-organotrophic; cultivable on inanimate media, *e.g.,* Sabouraud's agar; pathogens are mainly in the division called Fungi Imperfecti or Deuteromycetes, which are not known to reproduce sexually
1. Superficial infections (tinea, athlete's foot, etc.) due to dermatophytes: *Trichophyton* spp; *Microsporum* spp; *Epidermophyton* spp.
2. Deep or systemic infections (histoplasmosis, paracoccidioidomycosis, coccidioidomycosis, blastomycosis) due to yeastlike or dimorphic fungi

C. Helminths (parasitic worms): Eukaryotic cell structure; contain DNA and RNA. Adult helminths are not microscopic, but many of their developmental, infective, and diagnostically important forms are.
1. Platyhelminthes (flatworms)
   a. Trematodes—flukes: Nonsegmented; digenetic (alternate sexual and asexual generations in different hosts); sexual stage in humans; bilaterally symmetrical; dorsoventrally compressed; hermaphroditic except dioecious ($\female$ and $\male$) schistosomes (blood flukes); *e.g.,* liver flukes, lung flukes
   b. Cestodes—tapeworms: Hermaphroditic; consist of enlarged scolex ("head") with suckers (and hooks, depending on species) for attachment to intestinal mucosa; narrow "neck" produces, by budding, successive flat segments; these form the ribbonlike strobilia or chain of from three to several thousand hermaphroditic proglottids, *e.g.,* beef tapeworms
2. Nematodes—roundworms: Nonsegmented; long, slender, cylindrical; dioecious
   a. Intestinal parasites: Typically no intermediate hosts; eggs, larvae or both mature in intestine, on skin, in or on soil; *e.g.,* pinworms, hookworms, Ascaris
   b. Blood and tissue parasites (intermediate hosts necessary)
      (1) *Trichinella spiralis* (pork worm)
      (2) Filaria worms (various species and insect vectors)

D. Viruses: Visible only with the electron microscope; obligate intracellular parasites that grow in cell or organ culture, embryonated eggs, experimental animals; lack intrinsic metabolic mechanisms; contain core of genetic information as DNA or RNA, never both; nucleic acid genome associated with protein (capsid); virus structure has icosahedral, helical, or complex (bilateral) symmetry; some viruses possess an outer envelope containing lipid derived from the host-cell and virus-coded glycoproteins onto which glycosyl residues are incorporated by host-cell transferases; some virus particles contain intravirion nucleic acid transcriptases.

MICROSCOPIC METHODS

The optical microscope commonly used in medical work consists of three principal parts: condenser (with iris diaphragm), objective and ocular or eyepiece; and a source of visible light. Light enters at the lowest part of the optical system and passes upward toward the eye through the object on the stage and the magnifying lenses. Immersion oil is placed between the object and the objective lens to prevent loss of light due to refraction and reflection at the several glass surfaces. An objective lens designed to operate in oil is called an *oil-immersion* objective.

The objective produces a real image magnified about 90 times. The ocular or eyepiece further enlarges it about 10 times, giving a final image about 900 times the size of the object (*i.e.,* 10×90 or $900\times$).

The Electron Microscope

The *resolving power* of the common (optical) microscope is limited by the nature of visible light; images typically obtained in a good-quality research microscope by using a high-power oil-immersion lens are at a magnification of about $1000\times$. To increase the magnification and resolution further, electrons that have a much shorter wavelength than ordinary light (about 0.5 nm or 5 Å) are used. An electron microscope has a much greater resolving power and is capable of giving distinct images at magnifications of 100,000 or more.

The electron microscope uses electromagnetic "lenses" that are functionally analogous to glass lenses in the optical microscope. The electron beam is focused by varying the strength and direction of the electromagnets. Moreover, since electrons travel only in a high vacuum (the mean free path of

electrons in air is about 1 cm, while under an appropriate vacuum it can be more than 10 m), the entire instrument, including the specimen chamber, is designed to be evacuated. This means that specimens, in order to retain their shape, must be chemically fixed (*e.g.,* with aldehydes and/or osmium tetroxide), stained with heavy metal salts (*e.g.,* uranyl acetate) to enhance contrast, and embedded in plastic of high density, such as epoxy resin, which can be cut into ultrathin sections, usually a fraction of a nanometer thick. Additional techniques, such as surface replication, freeze–fracturing, freeze–etching, and negative staining, are also utilized for transmission electron microscopy (TEM). Images generated by transmission of electrons are viewed on a fluorescent screen set below the specimen onto which the electron beam is focused. For micrography, the fluorescent screen is replaced by a photographic plate.

Other Optical Methods

Other optical methods are (1) *phase microscopy,* in which light rays passing *through* the object, and those diffracted *around* it (and therefore out of wavephase with the rays passing through the object) are integrated into a single image, (2) x-ray, and (3) fluorescence microscopy.

For *fluorescence microscopy,* specimens are stained with a fluorescent dye (*e.g.,* fluorescein [FITC] or rhodamine [TMR]), which, in the presence of detergent, penetrates the cell wall of microorganisms such as *Mycobacteria.* FITC preparations are viewed with an ultraviolet light source, which excites the dye to emit yellow–green light.

Darkfield Microscopy

By means of a darkfield condenser or a "stop," central rays of light (usually admitted) are prevented from passing upward through the object to the eye. Peripheral rays (usually eliminated) are refracted by the darkfield condenser to emerge so obliquely from the surface of the slide that they do not reach the eye when the field is devoid of any object. The field therefore appears dark (hence darkfield). When the oblique rays impinge on an object on the slide, *e.g.,* a spirochete or bacterium, they are reflected upward from the surface of the object of the eye through the lenses. The object is then seen brightly outlined by the rays reflected from its surface.

STAINING METHODS

In order to determine the shape of bacteria and also to provide a means of classification, several differential staining techniques have been developed to be used with the light microscope.

Gram's Stain

1. Smear the material to be stained on a slide. Allow to dry in air. Fix by gently heating, which kills the bacteria and allows it to attach to the slide.
2. Apply an appropriate solution of crystal violet. Allow to stain about 1 minute. Wash gently.
3. Apply iodine solution (a mordant, which strengthens the bond between dye and substrate) for 1 minute. Wash gently.
4. Apply 95% ethyl alcohol until all but the thickest parts of the smear are decolorized, or for not more than 10 to 15 seconds. Wash.
5. Counterstain with safranine for 1 minute. Wash. Blot dry.
6. Examine naked smear using the oil immersion lens of the light microscope.
7. Gram-positive organisms are blue–purple and gram-negative bacteria are pink–red.

With the use of Gram's stain, bacteria are differentiated by their ability to either retain or lose the crystal violet–iodine combination in the presence of a decolorizing agent. Those that retain the violet dye are called gram-positive. Those that lose the violet dye (i.e., are decolorized) will take the red safranin counterstain and are called gram-negative. The result of the Gram's stain reaction depends on the type of bacterial cell wall: gram-positive bacteria have a thicker cell wall that is highly cross-linked and can trap the crystal violet–iodine aggregate. In contrast, gram-negative cell walls are thinner and, after alcohol treatment, more easily release the initial dye complex.

Gram-Positive Bacteria

All streptococci
All staphylococci
Pneumococci (Streptococcus pneumoniae)
Diphtheria bacillus (Corynebacterium diphtheriae)
All acid-fast bacilli, such as Mycobacterium tuberculosis
All spore-forming anaerobes (genus Clostridium)
Bacillus anthracis, B. cereus
Listeria, Erysipelothrix, Actinomyces, Nocardia, Streptomyces, Coxiella

Gram-Negative Bacteria

Genus Neisseria
The Enterobacteriaceae, including Salmonella, Shigella, the coliform group
The Hemophilus groups (H. influenzae, H. ducreyi)
Organisms of pertussis (Bordetella pertussis), plague (Yersinia pestis), cholera (Vibrio cholerae)
All species of Pseudomonas, e.g., Pseudomonas aeruginosa
Spirillum minus, Brucella spp., Francisella tularensis, Bacteroides, Fusobacterium, Veillonella, Citrobacter, Proteus, Campylobacter, Legionella

Differences in reaction to the Gram's stain also reflect medically important differences in properties of the organisms, chiefly susceptibility to antibiotics affecting cell wall synthesis (see Table 5-1).

Acid-Fast Stain (Ziehl-Neelsen) and Kinyoun (Cold) Methods

Organisms of tuberculosis and leprosy, and several related saprophytic species of Mycobacterium have the distinctive character called acid-fastness (AF), due to the presence of lipids (waxlike mycolic acid) in the cell wall. They quickly absorb red carbolfuchsin dye when in the presence of a detergent, such as Tween-80, or when warmed, and retain dye after washing with an acidified alcohol solution. All non-acid-fast bacteria, mucus, pus cells, etc., lose the carbolfuchsin when treated with acid alcohol and take a contrasting counterstain, e.g., methylene blue, yellow picric acid, or brilliant green. The acid-fast stain is performed as follows:

1. Fix the smear as for Gram's stain.
2. Flood slide with carbolfuchsin, steam gently for 5 minutes over low flame, do not allow to dry, add more stain if necessary. Cool. Alternatively, carbolfuchsin-containing phenol and alcohol (cool) may be used without heat.
3. Apply 90% alcohol containing 3 to 5% HCl until all but thickest parts of smear cease to give off color (about 1 to 3 minutes). Wash.
4. Counterstain 1 minute with methylene blue. Wash.

Tubercle bacilli are more strongly acid-fast than other members of the acid-fast group, and give a characteristic beaded appearance. Both Gram's stain and acid-fast stain depend on the integrity of the cell wall. Broken or disintegrated bacilli or their parts are neither Gram-positive nor acid-fast.

TABLE 5-1. Antimicrobial Agents That Inhibit Cell Wall Synthesis

DRUG	CHEMICAL GROUP	PRIMARY SITE OF BINDING	ACTIVITY BLOCKED	ACTIVE ON	ADVERSE REACTIONS	SENSITIVITY TO β-LACTAMASES
Penicillin G	β-lactam ring	Periplasmic space (cross-linking enzyme)	Blocks peptidoglycan cross-linking (cidal)	Gram-positive, fastidious gram-negative	Hypersensitivity develops to all penicillins	Gram-positive and gram-negative
Penicillin V	β-lactam ring	Periplasmic space	Blocks peptidoglycan cross-linking	Gram-positive, fastidious gram-negative	Hypersensitivity develops to all penicillins	Gram-positive and gram-negative
Methicillin, Nafcillin, Oxacillin	β-lactam ring	Periplasmic space	Blocks peptidoglycan cross-linking	Staph and other gram-positive	Hypersensitivity develops to all penicillins	Resistant to penicillinase
Ampicillin	β-lactam ring	Periplasmic space	Blocks peptidoglycan cross-linking	Broad spectrum	Hypersensitivity develops to all penicillins	Sensitive to most
Carbenicillin	β-lactam ring	Periplasmic space	Blocks peptidoglycan cross-linking	Broad spectrum (*Pseudomonas*)	Hypersensitivity develops to all penicillins	Resistant to some gram-negative enzymes
Cephalothin	β-lactam ring	Periplasmic space	Blocks peptidoglycan cross-linking	Broad spectrum	Hypersensitivity to all cephalo-sporins	Sensitive to many gram-negative enzymes
Cefamandole, Cefoxitin	β-lactam ring	Periplasmic space	Blocks peptidoglycan cross-linking	Broad spectrum	Hypersensitivity to all cephalo-sporins	Resistant to most
Cycloserine	D-alanine analogue	Cytoplasmic enzyme	Inhibits conversion of D-alanine to L-alanine for sub-unit synthesis	Gram-positive		
Bacitracin	Polypeptide	Cytoplasmic lipid	Inhibits subunit synthesis	Gram-positive	Limited to topical use	
Vancomycin		Cell membrane	Blocks secretion of cell wall subunit	Gram-positive		

Fluorescence Labeling for Detection of Antigen–Antibody Reactions *in Situ*

Antibodies, or protein antigens, can be chemically conjugated with fluorescein without significant loss of specific reactivity. For detection of surface antigens on animal cells, unfixed cells in suspension are treated with fluorescent antibody (FAb) (direct method) or with unlabeled antibody followed by fluorescent antiglobulin (indirect method) of the same species and viewed in the fresh state with ultraviolet illumination. Cells tagged in suspension with FAb can be enumerated by using a light microscope equipped with an epifluorescence accessory or by passage through a fluorescence-activated cell sorter (FACS). To detect both surface and intracellular antigen–antibody reactions, the cells (or tissues) must be fixed in a way that allows penetration of macromolecular reagents through the membrane but causes minimal disruption of ultrastructure. Frozen sections and smears (including those for

bacteriological diagnosis) or cell monolayers fixed in acetone or glutaraldehyde generally meet these requirements. Appropriately fixed preparations are stained by either direct or indirect methods; the latter method has the advantage of requiring only one labeled antiglobulin, provided that all the primary antisera to be used are from the same animal species.

Labeling for Electron Microscopy

Antigen–antibody reactions can be recognized on thin-sections by transmission electron microscopy (TEM) of preparations which have previously been stained with appropriate immunological reagents. However, accurate interpretation of images requires adequate specificity controls for the putative immune reactions. Specific reactions can frequently be identified by the density and distribution of molecular aggregates, particularly on the surface of cells, or by the specific aggregation of antigen particles by antibody, as in immune electron microscopy used in virological diagnosis. Labeling antibody with ferritin greatly increases the ease with which immune reactions are detected, due to the presence of complexed electron-dense iron molecules at the reaction sites. Antibody can be labeled with an enzyme (peroxidase or phosphatase), which, at the sites of combination with antigen yields an electron-dense chromogen by reaction with substrate. The same preparations stained with enzyme-labeled antibody and developed with chromogenic substrate can be fixed and permanently mounted for light microscopy.

THE ANATOMY AND PHYSIOLOGY OF BACTERIA

The Bacterial Genome

The genome of bacterial cells contains double-stranded deoxyribonucleic acid (DNA) predominantly in a B-type supercoiled, double helical conformation. Z-type DNA (the backbone "zigzags" down the molecule) has recently been described in certain, local regions of the DNA. A left-handed DNA helical conformation may have an important role in regulating the interaction of certain regions of genes, i.e., promoters, based on their differential interaction with large proteins that bind to it and that vary in their abundance in different kinds of cells.

Upon separation, each of the two DNA strands is seen to be a long-chain polymer of deoxyribonucleotides, each nucleotide bearing either a purine base: guanine (G) or adenine (A), or a pyrimidine base: thymine (T) or cytosine (C). The nucleotides of each strand are held together lengthwise by strong, covalent, phosphodiester linkages between the sugars while the two strands themselves are held together by relatively weak hydrogen bonds between the bases:

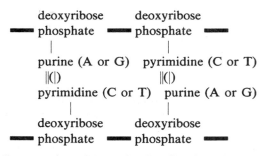

A always pairs with T; C with G. The whole structure can be seen as a helical ladder: the sides are the

firm phosphosugar polymers, the rungs are the separable purine–pyrimidine base pairs. The numbers, sequence, and kinds of nucleotides and their pairing are fixed for each species and constitute its genetic code. The ends of the helix are connected, forming a twisted closed circle, an arrangement important in its replication. The twists in the circle are highly strained, as in a twisted rope. The resulting "supercoils" are released in a controlled manner, which presumably facilitates revolution of the molecule about the helical axis during replication and recombination.

The contrast between prokaryotic and eukaryotic chromosomes is not limited to physical arrangement of molecules, but extends to the organization of the genetic message. The DNA of prokaryotes has few repeated sequences, most of the DNA is transcribed, and there are no intervening sequences within structural genes. Eukaryotic DNA contains many repeated sequences; some repeat millions of times. Much of the DNA is not transcribed; portions of structural genes (exons) are separated from each other by intervening sequences (introns).

Bacterial Cytoplasm

This consists of a fluid matrix containing particulate matter, as well as various ions, enzymes, amino acids, vitamins, nucleotides, tRNA, etc., in solution. Because of the selective permeability of the cell membrane and the action of "one-way" permease enzymes in the cell envelope, many of these substances increase in concentration inside the cell so as to raise the intracellular osmotic pressure to several atmospheres. When the cell (especially a Gram-positive cell) is deprived of its strong wall of peptidoglycan or murein (as by lysozyme or growth in penicillin, cephalothin, etc.), in a hypotonic solution the fragile cell membrane ruptures (see Table 5-2).

Particulate matter includes inert granules of stored food such as polymetaphosphates (volutin); lipids, principally as poly-betahydroxybutyric acid; starchlike granules, etc. The largest portion of cytoplasmic particulate matter of the bacterial cell consists of ribosomes, minute granules of rRNA with some protein. Each 70s ribosome monomer consists of two subunits, 50s and 30s. Ribosomes function in the synthesis of proteins. With the assistance of tRNA anticodons to transfer amino acids, and mRNA codons to carry the genetic code of the nuclear DNA, the sequence of the amino acids in the polypeptides made by the ribosomes are the points

TABLE 5-2. Antimicrobial Agents That Affect Membrane or Nucleic Acid Synthesis

NAME	CHEMICAL FEATURE	SITE OF BINDING	ACTIVITY BLOCKED	RANGE OF ACTIVITY
Polymyxins	Polypeptide ring	Cell membrane	Osmotic properties, detergent-like action	Gram-negative
Nystatin, Amphotericin	Polyene	Cell membrane	Interact with sterols to alter permeability, detergent-like action	Fungi
Sulfanilamide	PAGA-analogue	Cytoplasmic enzyme (dihydrofolic acid synthetase)	Purine and thymidine shortages block RNA and DNA synthesis	Broad
Trimethoprim—Sulfamethoxazole (co-trimoxazole)	—	Cytoplasmic enzymes (dihydrofolic acid reductase)	Purine and thymidine shortages block RNA and DNA synthesis	Broad
Griseofulvin	Guanosine analogue	Unknown	DNA replication	Fungi
Rifampicins	Semisynthetic macrolide	Cytoplasmic enzyme (RNA polymerase)	Transcription of mRNA	Broad
Nalidixic acid, Floxacins	—	Cytoplasmic enzyme (gyrase)	Inhibits DNA unwinding needed for DNA synthesis	Gram-negative
Nitrofurantoin	—	Reduced by microorganisms and reacts with DNA	Integrity of DNA replication	Broad
Metronidazole	—	Reduced by microorganisms and reacts with DNA	Integrity of DNA replication	Anaerobes
Ketoconazole	Synthetic imidazole derivative	Cell membrane	Alters cell membrane permeability by interfering with sterol synthesis	Broad antifungal (hepatotoxic)

of attachment of numerous antibiotics that interfere with protein synthesis (see Table 5-3).

Mesosomes (possibly primitive endoplasmic reticulum) are saccular invaginations of the cytoplasmic membrane and, in contrast with the nuclear material, are associated with cell fission. Mesosomes are absent from mycoplasmas. Bacteria contain no mitochondria, lysosomes, Golgi bodies, or other complex organelles that characterize eukaryotic cells.

BACTERIAL SURFACE COMPONENTS

Fimbriae

Fimbriae, or common pili, are straight, rapid, hairlike microfibrillar structures extending out from the surface and visible only by electron microscopy; they are predominantly found on gram-negative bacteria, particularly those encountered in the oropharynx and the infected urinary tract. They are

TABLE 5-3. Antimicrobial Agents That Block Protein Synthesis

DRUG	CHEMICAL	PRIMARY SITE OF BINDING	STEP BLOCKED	RANGE OF ACTIVITY
Streptomycin, Neomycin, Kanamycin, Gentamicin, Tobramycin, Amikacin	Aminoglycoside	30s ribosomal subunit	Binding of tRNA to ribosome	Broad spectrum
Spectinomycin	Aminocyclitol	30s ribosomal subunit	Binding of tRNA to ribosome	Broad spectrum
Tetracycline	—	30s ribosomal subunit	Binding of tRNA to ribosome	Broad spectrum
Chloramphenicol	—	50s ribosomal subunit	Formation of peptide bond	Broad spectrum
Lincomycin	Macrolide	50s ribosomal subunit	Formation of peptide bond	Gram-positive
Clindamycin	Macrolide	50s ribosomal subunit	Formation of peptide bond	Broad (anaerobes) spectrum
Erythromycin	Macrolide	50s ribosomal subunit	Translocation of ribosome on mRNA	Broad spectrum
Fusidic acid	—	Cytoplasmic soluble protein (elongation factor)	Translocation of ribosome on mRNA	Gram-positive

present in multiple copies (100 to 200) over the entire cell; they are shorter than flagella. Fimbriae allow bacteria to adhere to one another, as seen in the formation of pellicles on the surface of broth cultures. Fimbriae also by virtue of their ability to bind to sugar residues can bind to eukaryotic cell surfaces, *e.g.*, glycoproteins, and thus constitute an important pathogenic mechanism whereby microorganisms initiate infection by adhering to cell and mucosal surfaces (*e.g.*, gonococci in the genitourinary tract) through specific receptors.

F-type pili, or sex pili, are larger, longer and less rigid than common pili and occur in gram-negative "male" donor, or F+, bacteria, in which they serve as conjugation tubes during sexual reproduction (see section on conjugation). When present, F pili are randomly distributed and in fewer numbers than common pili. F pili also serve as receptors for specific bacteriophages, such as the RNA phage f1 or the DNA phage M13.

Slimes and Capsules

Some species of bacteria produce extracellular gels which adhere by noncovalent chemical interactions to the cell as *capsules* or as less dense macromolecular coatings, *slimes*. Capsules most often are polysaccharides (*e.g.*, capsules of pneumococci, meningococci), sometimes polypeptides (*e.g.*, *Bacillus anthracis)*, sometimes glycoprotein (*e.g.*, hyaluronic acid in *Streptococcus pyogenes* of groups A and C). Capsules protect the bacterium from dehydration and phagocytosis, thereby acting as virulence factors. Pathogenic organisms that are encapsulated when first isolated, on further cultivation lose their capsules and become avirulent (*e.g.*, "smooth" to "rough" [S–R] variation in appearance of pneumococcal colonies on agar). Vi, or virulence capsular antigens, seen in *E. coli* and *Salmonella typhi,* are similarly antiphagocytic and are readily removed by heat, or on subcultivation, which concomitantly diminishes virulence.

Bacterial Flagella

Flagella of prokaryotic cells are protein structures that extend out from the bacterial surface. They are attached to the cell membrane by a hook that in turn is bound to a basal body. The flagella impart motility by their characteristic wavelike motion that is governed by chemotactic responses to nutrients or toxic substances through chemoreceptors on the cell surface. The distribution of flagella (whether at one or both poles, over the entire surface of the cell, or in the form of axial filaments as in *Spirillum)* varies with the species of bacteria (there are no motile cocci). Among the *Enterobacteriaceae,* flagellar proteins confer species or type specificity on the cell. Flagellar antigens for these gram-negative bacteria are referred to as H antigens, in contrast to O antigens that reside in the cell wall. Specifically, O antigen specificity is conferred by the lipopolysaccharide (LPS)–protein–phosphatide complexes and this provides for the endotoxic activity characteristic of gram-negative bacteria. In practice, O and H antigens for serodiagnosis (*e.g.*, of salmonellosis) are bacterial suspensions prepared in a manner that on the one hand destroys flagella without affecting somatic (group) antigens (*e.g.*, ethanol at 37°) and on the other hand stabilizes (*e.g.*, dilute formalin) flagella to permit them to react preferentially with type-specific antibody.

Closely related species of bacteria, such as the many serotypes of *Salmonella,* may contain identical O antigens. (Not to be confused with O[H] blood-group antigens. See section on Immunohematology.) Thus, if a person is stimulated antigenically, either by injections of vaccine or by infection with any of the genus *Salmonella,* say *S. typhi,* the blood may contain O agglutinins for several other species of *Salmonella.* This is helpful in diagnosing salmonellosis retrospectively by serum agglutination titrations with any of several group-related species of *Salmonella* (Widal test). With *S. typhi,* it is customary to use both O and H (type) antigens.

Flagella of spirochetes are polar but, unlike the separate flagella of other bacteria, occur in bipolar bundles bent sharply back on the tubular cell, their ends meeting near the midlength. These bundles together form an end-to-end axial filament around which the helical cell is twined. Like other flagella they are attached in the cell wall by hooks and rings.

The Cytoplasmic Membrane

This is commonly of the three-layer, unit-membrane type: a double, inner, lipid leaflet between two outer layers of protein. It acts as a highly selective, semipermeable, osmotic barrier for the cell. In bacteria (except pathogenic mycoplasmas, which have no cell wall) sterols are not present, whereas they are present in pathogenic fungi in which they constitute points of attack by such fungicidal antibiotics as nystatin and amphotericin B (see Table 5-2).

Attached to the cell membrane are many ribosomes, and integrated with it are many enzymes of energy-mediating systems, including cytochromes and the associated oxidative phosphorylation (ATP-producing) systems.

Endospores

Some bacteria can exist either in a vegetative state or as an endospore. These are intracellular, minute, dehydrated, round or oval bodies, only one per cell, with thick, multilayered walls. They contain the essential cell contents in compact form. Endospores cannot take up any form of the Gram's stain and are highly resistant to heat, sunlight, radiation, drying, as well as chemical disinfectants. Under suitable conditions of moisture, nutrition, and warmth, they germinate, much as seeds germinate, and grow into the vulnerable, vegetative form of the organism.

The only known pathogenic organisms forming such highly heat- and disinfectant-resisting spores are species of the aerobic genus *Bacillus (B. anthracis)* and of the anaerobic genus *Clostridium,* including *C. tetani, C. perfringens, C. botulinum* and several species associated with *C. perfringens* in gas gangrene of contaminated wounds. *Coxiella burnetii,* the causative agent of Q fever, also produces an endospore.

The Cell Wall and Periplasmic Space

Prokaryotic cell walls differ from those of eukaryotic green plants and from those of eukaryotic fungi, which contain glycans (*e.g.,* chitin, a homopolymer of *N*-acetylglucosamine). Animal cells have no true cell wall. The cell walls of gram-positive bacteria consist wholly of relatively thick layers of *peptidoglycan* or *murein,* a complex of polymers of *N*-acetylglucosamine (GlcNAc) alternating with N-acetyl muramic acid (MurNAc) and cross-linked by a tetrapeptide through the carboxyl group of MurNAc. The composition of both the glycan and the cross-linking polypeptide may vary among different bacterial species, including additional antigenic polymers (*e.g.,* teichoic acids) linked to peptidoglycan. Certain species contain proteins externally associated with the cell wall that have an important relation to pathogenetic and immune mechanisms (*e.g.,* M proteins of group A streptococci, staphylococcal protein A linked to peptidoglycan).

Gram-negative cells have a rather loosely attached outer membrane (OM) or layer with unit-membrane-type structure that contains the O (LPS, endotoxin) antigen and a relatively thin inner layer of lysozyme-sensitive peptidoglycan in contact with the plasma membrane. The OM acts as a selective permeability barrier, which excludes hydrophobic substances as well as hydrophilic substances above a critical size.

When the rigid cell wall peptidoglycan is lost (*e.g.,* by growth in hypertonic medium with penicillin, which inhibits peptidoglycan synthesis, by treatment with lysozyme, or by mutation), gram-positive bacteria become osmotically fragile *protoplasts.* The analogous form derived from gram-negative species are called *spheroplasts,* which, while retaining cell wall LPS, are less osmotically fragile than protoplasts. Formation and persistent viability of protoplasts *in vivo* (*e.g.,* in the course of penicillin therapy) are thought to have an important role in endogenous recurrence of active bacterial infection (*e.g.,* infective endocarditis, urinary tract infection).

GENETIC TRANSFER IN BACTERIA

Three mechanisms for transfer of bacterial DNA from cell to cell are known: conjugation, transformation, and transduction.

Conjugation

Conjugation, the nearest approach to true sexuality in bacteria, depends on the presence of fertility genes that are often associated with extrachromosomal elements called *plasmids,* some of which confer ability to produce sexual organelles. Such plasmids, through the action of transfer genes, produce sex pili and mediate the intercellular transfer of DNA by the replicative process. An autonomously replicating molecule (replicon) bearing genes for sexual organelles constitutes a self-transferable fertility factor. Furthermore, plasmids bearing transfer genes can transiently insert into other replicons, including the chromosome, and thus promote the transfer by conjugation of the entire genetic complex.

Recent rapid bacterial evolution has been mediated by plasmids and is attributable to their ability to transfer genetic information from cell to cell during conjugation. The importance of plasmids to medicine lies in the fact that they may contain genes for drug resistance and toxin production as well as the means for transferring these traits across interspecies barriers. Moreover, plasmid genes possess *"transposon"* activity, in that genetic information can be freely exchanged from plasmid to plasmid, or from plasmid to chromosome, within the same cell. This property of transposability has served as the basis for constructing new "genetically engineered" strains of bacteria.

In this regard, the emergence of plasmid-born penicillinase genes among clinical isolates of *Haemophilus* and *Neisseria* has caused much concern for the future effectiveness of antibiotic therapy. The DNA responsible has been shown to be derived from Enterobacteriaceae. Based on chronological order of acquired resistance, the information was carried by plasmids from the Enterobacteriaceae into species of *Haemophilus*.

Transformation

In bacteria, this is the transfer of DNA from one cell to another by exposing the recipient cells, *in vitro* or *in vivo*, to contact with DNA derived from a different (but related through adequate base-pair homology of their DNAs) donor cell. This is exemplified by the transformation of *Pneumococcus* serologic (capsular) types and can occur between other related species. Only fragments of DNA from the donor cell enter the recipient cell through the cell wall and membrane. The recipient cell must be in a competent state (*i.e.*, rough, R, or no interfering capsule, etc.) to receive the transforming DNA. Competence also depends on the presence of a particular surface protein.

Note: Do not confuse bacterial transformation with malignant transformation of animal cells due to the integration of oncogenic DNA from animal viruses, such as mouse polyoma viruses or monkey SV40, with the cell chromosome. Oncogenic transformation results in heritable alterations of morphology, the appearance of new tumor specific membrane antigens, due to the release of tumor specific growth factors, and inhibition of movement. The cells pile up, become aneuploid, and when injected into susceptible hosts, such as newborn hamsters, cause the formation of tumors.

Transduction

In early studies with the temperate or lysogenic bacteriophages, such as λ (lambda), a class of defective viruses was discovered (lambda dg) that could not replicate without helper functions supplied by normal phage. Upon subsequent study it was shown that the reason lambda dg particles were defective was because they contained host bacterial DNA in place of an essential lambda gene. Furthermore, this bacterial DNA that had been mispackaged into phage particles could be transmitted to other cells

by viral infection *(transduction)*. Since the error occurred during excision of prophage DNA from a specific bacterial location, this was known as *specialized transduction*. Mispackaging of bacterial DNA can also occur throughout the host genome for viruses such as P1. This is known as *generalized transduction*.

VARIATION AND MUTATION

Phenotypic Changes

The distinguishing characteristics of any cell and its progeny are its phenotype. Because the DNA molecule is remarkably stable, phenotypic characters remain quite constant under ordinary conditions of growth. However, they may be greatly altered by environmental circumstances such as pH, temperature, as well as the presence or absence of certain ions or nutritional or toxic substances. Characters commonly altered by such influences are pigment, slime formation, sporulation, and filamentous growth. Changes of this nature are nonheritable; each cell reverts to its original or unaltered state immediately on removal of the altering influence; the genotype (entire sequences of nucleotides in the chromosome) has remained intact.

INDUCED ENZYMES

A particular type of phenotypic variation is seen in inducible enzyme function. The genotype may code for production of certain enzymes such as β-galactosidase, penicillinase, or certain permeases, but these are suppressed by an intracellular repressor. In the presence of the specific substrate of the enzyme, or of a chemically related substance (*e.g.*, β-galactose or lactose), the repressor is removed or inactivated, and the genetic potentiality is phenotypically expressed. Thus we see formation of lactose by β-galactosidase or destruction of penicillin by penicillinase or admission to the cell of the substrate of the particular permease involved. An important aspect of this is the development of bacteria, notably staphylococci, that, originally susceptible to penicillin, on contact with penicillin produce the enzyme penicillinase, thus becoming wholly resistant to penicillin (see section on drug resistance.) The induced change appears to be permanent though it is not a genetic change. *Inducibility* of an enzyme represents an inherited potentiality under repression; its *induction* is the result of removal of the repressor by an external stimulus.

Lysogenic Conversion

This is a variation in a bacterial property that results when a temperate phage codes for a gene product that alters the host cell, *e.g.*, introduction of the property of toxigenicity into a cell of nontoxigenic *Corynebacterium diphtheriae*. The nontoxigenic cell becomes toxigenic (virulent), but only as long as the converting prophage remains in the cell genome. "Curing" the converted cell of its prophage DNA causes the cell to revert to nontoxigenicity (avirulence). Similar examples of phage-born toxicity are found in other bacterial species, *e.g.*, *Streptococcus pyogenes*.

Colony Variation

Bacteria of virtually any species, when grown on solid agar, may form variant colonies that have differing morphology and biological properties due to variation in their genotype, *i.e.*, alternating mutations and back-mutations.

Smooth, or S-type, colonies are of pasty or butyraceous consistency, smooth, moist-looking, glistening, domed and circular, with even, regular margins. Cells in S colonies tend to be encapsulated and may form long chains (*e.g.*, streptococci in blood broth) or even longer filaments. Growth in broth culture is said to be smooth when the growing organisms impart a more or less even turbidity to the medium.

Rough, or R-type, colonies have a dull, dry looking granular surface, are brittle in consistency, and are rather flat, with crenated, indented, or irregular margins. Bacteria in R colonies are not encapsulated and tend not to form chains or filaments. S to R changes, which are not usually stable, often occur as a result of suboptimal conditions of cultivation. Conversely, R strains passed through an experimental animal (*e.g.*, R pneumococci inoculated into a mouse and subsequently reisolated) may regain capsules, and hence virulence. Pathogenic bacteria (*e.g.*, pneumococci, meningococci) on primary isolation from loci of disease (*e.g.*, purulent sputum, spinal fluid) are always encapsulated.

The capsular substance of S-type cells, usually but not always carbohydrate, is antigenically active and highly specific and, in species such as *Streptococcus pneumoniae*, *Hemophilus influenzae*, and *Neisseria meningitidis* is antiphagocytic and hence associated with virulence. Accordingly, in considering strains to incorporate into a vaccine, it is advantageous to select S variants, which are most likely to produce the largest amounts of protective antigen(s), *e.g.*, capsules in the pneumococcus or meningococcus. In general, R variants, since they are deficient in capsular antigen(s), are of lower virulence than S variants of the same species and retain a broader antigenicity that is more group- than type-specific. These considerations are especially pertinent to the formulation of pertussis or pneumococcal vaccines.

Recombination

It is important to differentiate *recombination,* which involves formation of a new DNA molecule by breakage and joining of two DNA molecules or of two regions within a single DNA molecule and results in a rearrangement of sequences within one or more molecules of DNA, from simple *reassortment* of DNA molecules between cells, such as occurs with plasmid transfer.

The bacterial chromosome is not a fixed structure; all homologous sequences present within the genome will be foci of virtually constant recombinational activity. A strikingly evident example of the consequences of recombination within homologous sequences is the phenomenon of phase variation. The antigenic specificity of the flagella of *Salmonella* alternates periodically between two states. It is now known that this antigenic alteration is due to recombination between homologous DNA sequences (insertion sequences, IS) that bracket the flagellar structural genes. With each recombinational event, the chromosomal sequence of the flagella genes is reversed: When the genes are inserted into the genome in one orientation, the H_1 antigenic phase is expressed; when they are inserted in the other orientation, the H_2 phase is expressed. Many recombinational events go undetected; it is nevertheless becoming apparent that the normal condition of the *E. coli* genome is one of dynamic flux.

Genotypic Changes

These are true genetic mutations; the actual chemical composition of the DNA molecule or genome is altered and if the change is not lethal, as often happens, the change is passed on to the progeny of the cell. Because of the stability of the DNA molecule, most types of spontaneous mutation are rare, ordinarily occurring at frequencies of about 1 in 10^6 or less, unless the frequency is increased by certain mutagenic agents.

The smallest genetic unit, the presence, absence, or alteration of which can result in a mutation, is a single nucleotide, a *muton*. The presence, or structure, of a single nucleotide or base pair may determine a heritable character and be a gene or recombinational unit or *recon,* but genes generally consist of many nucleotides. A gene is defined as any genetically functional segment of the chromosome.

Mutagenic agents may be chemical or physical. Among the most potent physical mutagens are ultraviolet and ionizing radiations. Ultraviolet irradiation, among other effects, tends especially to cause aberrant chemical linkages (dimers) to occur between pyrimidines: T to T, T to C, or C to C. Ionizing radiations can cause destructive effects due to release of free radicals, or mutations due to deletion of nucleotides.

Several chemicals are active mutagens. Alkylating agents such as N and S mustards affect guanine, causing changes that result in erroneous pairing of bases. Nitrosamines are an important possible source of some base analogues, *e.g.,* 5-bromouracil (enol form), which can cause false pairing with G instead of A; AT is thus replaced by GC. Some dyes such as acridine orange cause distortion of the secondary structure of the DNA helix, resulting in faulty replication or recombination.

Potentially lethal lesions occur repeatedly in the DNA of living organisms. Only the presence of error-free DNA repair systems prevents the loss of genetic fidelity. Bacteria continue to provide valuable insights into DNA repair mechanisms and mutagenesis. Bacteria also serve as a principal short-term screen for detection and analysis of environmental mutagens that are responsible for increasing the endogenous load of premutational lesions in mammalian DNA.

The most widely used test (Ames test) has been shown to have highly accurate predictive value for carcinogenic activity in experimental animals. Indeed, of 176 chemical carcinogens tested, 158% or 90% were mutagenic. Conversely, of 108 "noncarcinogens," only 13 were mutagenic. These 13 negatives may reflect the relative lack of sensitivity of tests in animals.

Many mutagens and carcinogens are metabolized to active forms by enzymes present in mammalian cells. Cellular extracts containing these enzymes are often included in the Ames test plates so that compounds requiring activation will not be missed.

As a point of reference, the condensate of the smoke from a single cigarette causes approximately 20,000 mutations when tested in the presence of cellular enzymes.

Auxotrophs

Auxotrophs are deficient mutants that have lost one or more synthetic properties characteristic of the original type ("wild type" or prototype) from which the mutant was derived. Mutations affect antigenic, metabolic, and morphologic properties that form the basis of many diagnostic tests and also determine virulence (*e.g.,* toxigenicity, capsule formation). Resistance to chemotherapeutic agents and, conversely, a metabolic requirement for antibiotics are particularly undesirable mutations. Some of these are transmissible by certain episomes (R or RTF) through conjugation among gram-negative bacteria (see section on antibiotics).

BACTERIAL METABOLISM; BIOENERGETICS

Metabolic Types

All living cells depend on extraneous sources of energy for growth, reproduction, and self-synthesis. Those obtaining energy from the sun, (*e.g.,* green plants, blue-green algae and a few species of nonpathogenic bacteria) are said to be *photosynthetic.* All microorganisms of medical significance (except viruses) obtain energy from exothermic (exergonic) chemical reactions, that is, oxidations; they are said to be *chemosynthetic.* Viruses obtain their energy from the cells they infect.

Some chemosynthetic bacteria of the soil, called *chemolithotrophs,* oxidize only inorganic substrates (*e.g.,* $2NH_3 + 4O_2 \rightarrow 2HNO_3 + H_2O$) as sources of energy. They can use CO_2 as a sole source of carbon. Organisms capable of using CO_2 as a sole source of carbon are often called *autotrophs.* All microorganisms of medical interest, including bacteria, protozoans, and fungi, are chemosynthetic but, unlike autotrophs or chemolithotrophs, can utilize only *organic* substrates as sources of energy *and* carbon, *i.e.,* they are *chemo-organotrophic.* Organisms requiring organic sources of CO_2 are often called *heterotrophs.* Many of these also require CO_2. The various metabolic types may be listed as follows:

Photosynthetic
    Green plants
    Blue–green algae
    Some bacteria of no medical interest
Chemosynthetic
    Chemolithotrophs: oxidize inorganic substrates; use only inorganic N, S, and C (are autotrophic

with respect to C source) (of no medical interest)

Chemo-organotrophs: oxidize only organic substrates; use mainly organic sources of S, N, and C (are heterotrophic with respect to C source); may also require CO_2

Although all pathogenic microorganisms are chemoorganotrophs, some, such as certain enteric species, require only a single organic compound such as glucose if furnished with a complete mineral supplement. Others, like the strict anaerobes, streptococci, and gonococci, require numerous preformed complex substances: peptones, carbohydrates, amino acids, vitamins, and others. Bacteria cannot ingest solid particles of food: their nutrition is entirely by osmosis and diffusion of nutrients in solution. They are said to be *osmotrophic.*

Energy Metabolism of Bacteria

In all chemo-organotrophs, bacterial as well as human, the most generally used source of carbon and energy is glucose. The most common first stage in energy metabolism of glucose is glycolysis by the Embden-Meyerhof scheme. Among bacteria, other systems may also be used, depending on species: the pentose–phosphate pathway, which is thermodynamically less efficient than glycolysis, and the Entner-Doudoroff pathway, found especially in species of *Pseudomonas.* Some species of bacteria can also use numerous other sugars and organic compounds (*e.g.,* phenol and petroleum) as sources of energy and carbon, depending on the enzymic ability of the organism to convert the sugar into a form such that at some point in the metabolic process it can enter the glycolytic or other pathway. These differences are often exploited for diagnostic purposes.

Among bacteria, and depending on species, glucose may be used in one or two of three general types of exergonic reactions: (a) aerobic respiration, (b) anaerobic respiration, and (c) fermentation. In all three the prime source of energy is enzymic (dehydrogenase) removal, from a substrate, of pairs of hydrogen atoms with liberation of their electrons ($H \rightleftharpoons H^+ + e^-$). Removal of electrons is oxidation and yields energy; acceptance of electrons is reduction. In cell metabolism, when hydrogen (e^-) is removed from a substrate by a dehydrogenase, it is transferred to an agent at a higher oxidative potential, commonly nicotinamide-adenine dinucleotide (NAD), which then becomes $NADH_2$. The functioning part of the dehydrogenase is "niacin," which can accept the hydrogen and yield it up. In order to continue to function, the $NADH_2$ must be reoxidized (*i.e.,* 2H removed).

In *aerobic respiration* the $NADH_2$ becomes reoxidized by enzymically transferring the hydrogen to a second O—R system, usually the riboflavin (or flavoprotein) system. Here the electrons are diverted and transferred to a series of four or five enzymes called *cytochromes,* each of greater e^--accepting (oxidizing) potency than the one before it. The coenzymes of the cytochromes are much like heme in having an atom of iron chelated in a porphyrin ring, the iron being able to accept and transfer e^-. In aerobic respiration the final cytochrome of the series, in the presence of the enzyme oxidase and $2H^+$, transfers the $2e^-$ to $\frac{1}{2}O_2$, forming H_2O. The entire series of enzymes and reactions from flavin to, and including, oxidase is called a *respiratory chain.* Many bacteria are restricted to the use of O_2 as a final hydrogen (electron) acceptor; they are called strict or *obligate aerobes.*

Many common organisms (called *facultative*) are capable of respiration under anaerobic conditions as well as under aerobic conditions as above. In the absence of O_2 they can use, as an alternative, several readily reducible inorganic compounds like $NaNO_3$ (substances depending on species) as final hydrogen acceptor in place of O_2: $NaNO_3 + 2H \rightleftharpoons NaNO_2 + H_2O$. Nitrate reduction is a familiar "test" in laboratory microbiology. Nitrite (NO_2) is a toxic product. It is also mutagenic and possibly carcinogenic. Furthermore, it can react with endogenous cellular amines (particularly the ubiquitous compounds spermine and spermidine) to produce nitroso compounds of great mutagenic potency. Some species reduce the nitrite, which is toxic, to N or NH_3 in stepwise reactions.

In *fermentation* two (or more) parts of the same organic substrate molecule (or two similar organic molecules, *e.g.,* the Stickland reaction between two amino acids: alanine + glycine → acetic acid + NH_3 + CO_2) serve as hydrogen (electron) donor and hydrogen (electron) acceptor, respectively, a thermodynamically inefficient mechanism since much less energy is released than in either form of respiration described above.

In aerobic and anaerobic respiration the pyruvate resulting from glycolysis (or alternate pathway) is first combined with acetyl coenzyme A, with liberation of 2H, via NAD, to the respiratory chain. The pyruvate then undergoes the series of changes constituting the Krebs or citric acid or tricarboxylic acid cycle. The overall reaction in bacterial respiration (aerobic or anaerobic) is $C_6H_{12}O_6 \rightarrow 6CO_2 + 6O_2 + 6H_2O$ (plus 34 ATP) and 688 kcal not all of which is available for cell synthesis and reproduction. Some is given off as heat or otherwise lost to entropy.

In fermentation the pyruvate undergoes various alterations different from those seen in aerobic respiration depending on species. There is no respiratory chain of cytochromes; much of the energy is not used. Reoxidation of the $NADH_2$ produced by glycolysis is accomplished by the reduction of cellular metabolites (e.g., pyruvate) followed by excretion of the reduced product (e.g., lactate) from the cell. In this way, the $NADH_2$ is oxidized, but its reducing power is lost to that cell. Some lactic acid bacteria, for example, reduce all of the pyruvate to lactic acid; some produce mainly propionic acid; and others produce a variety of substances, some of which are distinctive: acetylmethyl carbinol (basis of the Voges-Proskauer reaction), ethyl alcohol, acetone, butyric acid, CO_2, and others. All of these products of fermentation contain much of the original energy of the glucose and can serve as energy sources for other species of bacteria and fungi.

ENERGY AND PHOSPHORYLATION

The most important result of any form of energy metabolism for the cell is the phosphorylation of certain organic compounds that, because of the strained state of the phosphate ester bond, become high-energy compounds. Among these are adenosine triphosphate (ATP), guanosine triphosphate (GTP), acetyl phosphate, 1,3-diphosphoglyceric acid, and others. The high-energy ester bond on hydrolysis yields energy to the compound temporarily associated with the high-energy compound. ATP, ADP, and AMP constitute a series of energy transfer compounds, each of the latter two absorbing energy on phosphorylation that is transferred to ATP and H_3PO_4. Together they constitute an almost universally used energy transfer system in the cell.

In the **bacterial respiratory chain,** energy from electrons passing along the chain of cytochromes is transferred to the cell at two or three specific points, forming, with inorganic phosphate, ATP from ADP (oxidative level phosphorylation). Two molecules of ATP are also formed (from ADP + H_3PO_4) during glycolysis, from hydrolysis of 1,3-phosphoglyceric acid to 3-phosphoglyceric acid (substrate level oxidative phosphorylation) and hydrolysis of phosphoenol pyruvic acid to pyruvic

acid. This is almost the entire yield of energy in fermentation.

All forms of exothermic reaction in living cells are sometimes referred to collectively as **bio-oxidations.**

Three other types of bacteria, differing in respect to oxygen requirements, deserve mention: (a) the microaerophils; (b) the indifferent organisms; and (c) the obligate aerobes.

Microaerophils require somewhat lowered oxygen pressures, neither complete anaerobiosis nor full aerobiosis. Probably certain of their enzymes are sensitive to atmospheric oxygen tension. Some pathogens are microaerophils, (e.g., Leptospira, Brucella) when first isolated.

Indifferent species can grow in the presence of air but do not contain cytochrome or the citric acid cycle enzymes. Such species grow better in the absence of free oxygen than aerobically. They have no metabolic pathway to oxygen from glucose. They neither need nor utilize free oxygen, though they can use it for metabolizing glycerol to H_2O_2, which kills them because they do not produce catalase. Neither are they "poisoned" by free oxygen, as are strict anaerobes. They are indifferent to it. Examples are Streptococcus pyogenes and Lactobacillus species.

Strict or obligate anaerobes not only cannot grow but cannot survive in the presence of free oxygen. They are obliged to live in the absence of air (anaerobically). Their metabolism is entirely fermentative. Their sensitivity to free oxygen may depend on certain enzymes or coenzymes that are poisoned by oxygen or must remain in a reduced condition. Typically they do not produce catalase, which decomposes the highly toxic H_2O_2 that is produced by them in contact with O_2. Examples of strict anaerobes are Clostridium tetani, certain hemolytic streptococci, and Bacteroides species. Anaerobic enzyme systems function only at low O—R potentials (e.g., −0.3 volt).

Cultivation of Anaerobes

Cultural conditions suitable for strictly anaerobic bacteria are found in the bottom of tubes filled to a depth of at least 10 cm with chopped animal tissue and covered with broth containing 1% glucose and heated to drive off air (oxygen) shortly before use, or in any organic or tissue medium from which free oxygen is excluded. A plating medium for isolating pure cultures of strict anaerobes consists of meat–infusion glucose agar containing a strong reducing substance, such as cysteine or sodium thioglycollate. In a hermetically sealed "anerobic jar" device, using chemicals in a plastic pack (Gaspak), a combination of oxygen with hydrogen is catalyzed at room temperature without use of electricity or exterior source of hydrogen.

Saprophytes

Not all chemo-organotrophs are pathogens. Some are of great value in the dairy and fermentation industries and in the commercial production of antibiotics. Many are effective scavengers and are called *saprophytes* (Gr. decay-plants). They inhabit the environment in the soil, on plants, and in the oceans and swamps, and in normal animals and humans they constitute the normal flora of the intestinal and genitourinary tracts, the oropharynx, and the external body surfaces. Saprophytes do not commonly invade living tissues or the blood stream unless introduced under circumstances favorable to their survival, such as in immunosuppression, or in contaminated wounds containing devitalized tissue (lowered redox potential) where they grow and secrete toxins (e.g., *Clostridium tetani* and tetanus toxin, or *C. perfringens,* involved in anaerobic cellulitis). Certain soil saprophytes can grow in foodstuffs in which they elaborate toxins (e.g., *C. botulinum*). Thus we may have noninvasive but highly pathogenic saprophytes.

A DESCRIPTIVE CHECKLIST OF IMPORTANT BACTERIA IN MEDICAL MICROBIOLOGY

I. Rod-shaped bacteria
  A. Non-spore-forming
    1. Gram-negative
      a. Enteric bacteria:
        The enteric bacteria include many genera, some of them normal flora and others (*Salmonella* and *Shigella*) exogenous and regularly pathogenic. Enteric organisms are aerobic, ferment a variety of carbohydrates, and possess complex antigenic structures. Because on Gram's stain they all look more or less alike, their identification rests on biochemical reactions, antigenic analysis, susceptibility to colicins (*e.g., Pseudomonas),* and DNA homology analyses. All have endotoxin (LPS); some secrete potent enterotoxins (protein exotoxins). As a group, these organisms are responsible for a large number of nosocomial infections, and many of them are resistant to multiple antibiotics because of their acquisition of drug-resistance plasmids. Most of the enteric organisms are opportunistic pathogens, particularly of the genitourinary tract and central nervous system, in burn patients, and in the compromised host. For all these reasons, careful antibiotic sensitivity testing is central to effective antibacterial chemotherapy.

        The main taxonomic groups (*tribes* and *genera*) of enteric bacteria are:
        Family: Enterobacteriaceae
        Escherichieae—*Escherichia, Shigella*
        Klebsielleae—*Klebsiella* (includes *K. pneumoniae* and other species; nonmotile *Aerobacter aerogenes;* Friedländer's bacillus in older terminology); *Enterobacter* (includes *E. aerogenes* [older name *Aerobacter aerogenes*]); *Serratia* group
        Salmonelleae—*Salmonella, Arizona, Citrobacter*
        Proteae—*Proteus (P. vulgaris. P. mirabilis); Providencia (P. rettgeri, P. stuartii, P. alcalifaciens); Morganella (M. morganii)*
        Family: Vibrionaceae
        Vibrio (V. cholerae, V. parahemolyticus, etc.); Campylobacer (C. fetus)
      b. Respiratory pathogens (see Table 5-4):
        Hemophilus influenzae. Very small, nonmotile, pleomorphic coccobacillus; nonhemolytic; aerobic; requires hemin (X factor) and NADP (V factor) as supplied in "chocolate" agar. Infant tracheobronchitis, epiglottitis, septic meningitis, conjunctivitis (*H. aegyptius).* Virulent strains (type b most frequent) encapsulated. *H. parainfluenzae*—normal oral flora, endocartidis

        Bordetella pertussis. Primary isolation on Bordet-Gengou (BG) agar containing methicillin; hemolytic, pearl-like colonies; identification by immunofluorescence; contain histamine-sensitizing and lymphocytosis-promoting factors, heat-labile toxin and endotoxin (LPS); phase variation. Localized infection or pertussis syndrome; attachment to and immobiliza-

TABLE 5-4. Differential Properties of *Hemophilus* and *Bordetella*

ORGANISM	COLONIES	REQUIREMENT FOR FACTORS X*	REQUIREMENT FOR FACTORS V†	PRODUCTION OF Indole	PRODUCTION OF Catalase	PRODUCTION OF Porphyrins	FERMENTATION OF GLUCOSE	REDUCTION OF NITRATE	MOTILITY
H. influenzae	Small, "dew drop" nonhemolytic‡	+	+	+	+	–	+	+	–
H. parainfluenzae	Small, ± hemolytic	–	+	–	+/–	+			
H. hemolyticus	Small, betahemolytic	+	+	+	+	–	+		
H. ducreyi	Small, weakly hemolytic		–	–	–	–	+/–	–	
H. aegyptius (Koch-Weeks bacillus)	Nonhemolytic	+	+	–	+	–			
B. pertussis	Tiny, hemolytic	niacin		–	–	*Urease*	–	–	–
B. parapertussis	Tiny, hemolytic	cysteine		–	+		–	–	–
B. bronchiseptica		methionine			+		–	+	+

* Hemin.

† Coenzyme 1 or nicotinamide-adenine-dinucleotide (NAD), responsible for "satellite phenomenon" when growing near colonies of *Staphylococcus aureus*.

‡ Typable distinguishable from untypable strains by opalescence (due to capsules) on Levinthal transparent agar. Primary isolation best on chocolate agar (contains free hemin and NAD).

tion of cilia; never invasive. Killed phase I cells in DPT. Related species *B. parapertussis*
c. Genitourinary tract pathogen (other than enterics):
Hemophilus ducreyi. Fastidious; morphologically like *H. influenzae.* Soft chancre (chancroid); in tropics, endemic and commonest cause of genital ulcerative disease
d. Blood and tissue pathogens:
Brucella suis, B. abortus, B. melitensis. Small coccobacilli or rods; nonmotile; biotyped according to metabolism, sensitivity to dyes, antigenic analysis. Primary zoonosis; erythritol (large amounts in fetal tissues of ungulates, not of humans) promotes intracellular localization, infectious abortion in animals; spectrum of acute septicemic to chronic granulomatous human multisystem disease; serodiagnosis based on IgM/IgG agglutinins; cross-reaction with *Francisella tularensis* and *Vibrio cholerae.* Cell-mediated immunity important in recovery and resistance. Tetracycline, streptomycin, rifampin (see Table 5-5)
Francisella tularensis. Small pleomorphic bacillus; fastidious; facultative intracellular parasite. Primary zoonosis; human disease (tularemia), acquired by direct contact or via arthropod vector from diseased animals, has protean manifestations, from localized infection to septicemic pneumonia. Cell-mediated immunity primary factor in recovery and resistance; serodiagnosis by agglutination test. Streptomycin, chloramphenicol, tetracycline

Yersinia pestis (the genus *Yersinia* is in the tribe Yersinieae, included in the family Enterobacteriaceae). Short, ovoid, nonmotile bacillus with bipolar staining. Primary zoonosis in domestic and wild rodents; human disease acquired by direct contact or bites of infected arthropods; septicemic bubonic and pneumonic (100% fatal) plague. Cell-mediated immunity important in recovery and resistance. Streptomycin, tetracyclines and/or chloramphenicol
Bacteroides fragilis group, *B. melaninogenicus* group (black pigment on blood agar). Strict anaerobes; pleomorphic; gas-liquid chromatography useful in speciation. Most produce beta-lactamase. Normal intestinal and oral flora, opportunistic polymicrobic (e.g., *Fusobacterium, Propionibacterium, Peptococcus, Peptostreptococcus*) obstetric–gynecologic infections, infections of central nervous system and thoracic and abdominal cavities, necrotizing cellulitis and metastatic abscesses, septicemia. Chloramphenicol, clindamycin, cefoxitin, moxalactam, metronidazole; also newer penicillins, mezlocillin and piperacillin. Surgical drainage of primary importance (see Table 5-6)
Pseudomonas. Straight or curved rods, chemo-organotrophic; strict aerobes. Normal flora of skin and intestine, environment.
P. aeruginosa produces green pigment (pyocyanin) and is responsible for almost 20% of nosocomial infections. It can adhere to inert solid

TABLE 5-5. Properties of Brucella

ORGANISM	REQUIREMENT FOR CO$_2$ ON PRIMARY ISOLATION*	HYDROGEN SULFIDE PRODUCTION	UREASE ACTIVITY	GROWTH ON AGAR CONTAINING	
				Basic Fuchsin	Thionin
Brucella abortus	+	+	+	+	−
Brucella suis	−	+ +	+ +	−	+
Brucella melitensis	−	−	+	+	+
Brucella canis	−	+	+	−	+

* On Castañeda's double medium.

TABLE 5-6. Nonsporulating Anaerobic Bacilli*

	PREDOMINANT HABITAT(S)	MORPHOLOGY
Gram-positive		
Actinomyces (A. israelii, A. naeslundii)	Mouth, upper respiratory tract	Long, filamentous, irregular branching
Arachnia	Mouth	Pleomorphic, pointed ends
Propionibacterium	Skin	Pleomorphic, chains
Lactobacillus	Mouth, vagina	Short, bifurcated or clubbed ends
Bifidobacterium	Colon, vagina	Pleomorphic, V-shaped arrangements
Eubacterium	Mouth, colon	
Gram-negative		
Bacteroides		
B. fragilis group	Vagina, colon (dominant species)	Long, pleomorphic, vacuoles
B. melaninogenicus group	Mouth	Short, coccobacilli; brown-black pigment formed on blood agar
Fusobacterium	Mouth	Long, tapered ends *(F. nucleatum)* Most species variable

* Account for over 90% of normal intestinal flora. Speciated by gas–liquid chromatography of metabolic products in liquid cultures (pure) and/or immunofluorescence. Direct Gram stain of exudates useful in preliminary diagnosis.

surfaces and thus causes opportunistic urinary (catheter-associated) as well as respiratory tract (respiratory-associated) infections, particularly in debilitated, immunosuppressed, or burn patients. Treatment according to antibiogram. *P. pseudomallai*—motile; characteristic nonpigmented growth; multiple antibiotic resistance. Melioidosis (acute and recrudescent). Tetracycline, chloramphenicol, trimethoprim-sulfamethoxazole

Legionella pneumophila. Major human pathogen of family Legionellaceae; faintly gram-negative; stains with silver impregnation in tissues; facultative intracellular parasite; isolation on charcoal yeast extract agar; identification with immunofluorescence. Infection acquired from environment, acute pneumonia, milder upper respiratory infection, septicemia. Erythromycin

Cat scratch disease bacillus. Found in lymph nodes of affected patients; pleomorphic, gram-negative bacillus found in almost 90% of biopsied lymph nodes examined; stainable with silver impregnation; specific reactivity with convalescent sera; no antigenic relation to *Legionella* or *Rickettsia;* uncultivable; supportive, symptomatic treatment without use of antibiotics is recommended.

2. Gram-positive
   a. Respiratory pathogens:
      Corynebacterium diphtheriae. Methylene blue stain: clublike, beaded, and barred forms; soluble exotoxin, alum-precipitated toxoid (DTP); antitoxin (despeciated horse serum) (see Table 5-21)
      Mycobacterium tuberculosis. Acid-fast, niacin +; nonmotile; obligate aerobe; slow growth on Lowenstein-Jensen egg yolk–glycerine–malachite green medium; virulent strains form "cord factor"; usually isoniazid-sensitive, some strains resistant; distinguish from "atypical" or Runyon-group species; delayed (tuberculin) hypersensitivity; BCG (Table 5-7).
   b. *Mycobacterium leprae.* Obligate intracellular parasite; "lepra" cells; not cultivable on lifeless media. Leprosy (lepromatous, tuberculoid), erythema nodosum, deficient Tc function. Dapsone, rifampin, clofazimine
   c. Blood and tissue pathogens:
      Listeria monocytogenes. A motile "diphtheroid," hemolytic on blood agar. Zoonosis; clinically protean, including amnionitis, perinatal infections, meningitis
      Actinomyces israelii. Branching, filamentous bacterium; strictly anaerobic; found only in humans (bovine species is *A. bovis*); gram-positive but not acid-fast; "sulfur granules" in masses

TABLE 5-7. Differential Properties of *Mycobacterium* Species of Recognized Pathogenicity for Humans

SPECIES (GROUPINGS)	GROWTH TEMPERATURE	PRODUCTION OF NIACIN	NITRATE REDUCTION	TOLERANCE TO 5% NaCl	TWEEN 80 HYDROLYSIS	CATALASE ACTIVITY	RESISTANCE TO ISONIAZID
M. tuberculosis	37	+	+	−	−	−	−
M. bovis (includes BCG strain)	37	+/−	−	−	−	−	−
M. ulcerans	30–33	−	−	−	+	+	(+)
"Atypical" mycobacteria: Group I (photochromogens)*							
M. kansasii	30–37	+/−	+	−	+	+/−	+
M. marinum	30–32	−	−	−	+	+	+
Group II (scotochromogens)†							
M. scrofulaceum	30–37	−	−	−	−	+	+
Group III (nonchromogens)							
M. intracellularis (Battey)	37–44	−	−	−	−	+	+
M. avium							
Group IV (rapid growers; 3–7 days, some scotochromogens)							
M. fortuitum	25–37	−	+	+	Variable	+	+
M. chelonei							

* Produce lemon-yellow pigments on exposure to light.
† Produce yellow-orange to dark-red pigments in the dark.

of "ray fungus" in pus. Actinomycosis, penicillin-sensitive

Nocardia asteroides. Branching forms that readily fragment to bacillus-like or coccoid segments; gram-positive; *N. asteroides* and some others acid-fast in exudates; strictly aerobic; some species form "sulfur-granules" in pus. Madura foot or systemic and pulmonary nocardiosis. Sulfadiazine

B. Spore-forming (special spore stains required; unstained areas in gram-positive bacilli)

Endospores resist 15 minutes or longer boiling at 100°C and 1 hour or more of dry heat at 150°C.

1. Gram-negative: none of medical importance

2. Gram-positive:

a. Aerobic or facultative. Sporulate only in contact with free oxygen

Bacillus anthracis*. Grows well on blood-free media; spores contaminate pastures, hides, wool. Pulmo-

nary anthrax or woolsorters' disease, malignant pustule, septicemia, toxemia, toxoid

b. Anaerobic or microaerophilic. Spores form and germinate only under anaerobic conditions (Table 5-8).

Clostridium species. All inhabit soil, many occur in animal feces; cultivable in the thioglycollate media, etc.; all pathogens motile except *C. perfringens*

C. tetani fecally contaminated wounds; soluble exotoxin affects motor nerve endings; alum-precipitated toxoid prophyl. vs tetanus DTP (see Table 5-21)

C. perfringens "gas bacillus"; associated with *C. novyi, C. histolyticum, C. septicum,* and *C. tetani* in fecally contaminated, deep wounds; exotoxins are various proteolytic and saccharolytic enzymes, collagenases, gas gangrene

C. botulinum. "Snow-shoe" sporulation; grows in soil-contaminated, improperly heat-processed canned foods, forming exotoxin that causes flaccid paralysis; toxin destroyed by 80°C in 15 minutes. Botulism (infant, endogenous)

* Distinguish between the general use of the term "bacillus" in reference to any rod-shaped organism and the generic use of the term *Bacillus* in reference to the genus of aerobic spore-formers, such as *Bacillus anthracis*.

TABLE 5-8. Differential Properties of *Clostridium* Species

ORGANISM	MORPHOLOGY (ALL GRAM-POSITIVE)	MOTILITY	METABOLIC ACTIVITY Lecithinase Activity	Fermentation of Glu-cose	Su-crose	Lac-tose	DISEASES
Histotoxic*							
C. perfringens	Short, thick rods; rare oval subterminal spores; double hemolysis on blood agar	−	+	+	+	+	Myonecrosis, suppuration, cellulitis, septicemia.
C. septicum	Oval, subterminal spores, long thin rods	+	−	+	−	+	(C. perfringens: enterocolitis, food poisoning, intravascular hemolysis)
C. novyi	Oval, subterminal spores	+	+	+	−	−	
C. histolyticum	Oval, subterminal spores, pleomorphic rods	+	−	±	−	−	
Cytotoxic†							
C. botulinum	Large rods, oval subterminal spores	+	−	+	−	−	Botulism (type A, B, E, F toxins) food poisoning; wound botulism; infant botulism
C. tetani	Slender rods, terminal spores, "drumstick"	+	−	−	−	−	Tetanus (neurotoxin)
C. difficile	Oval, terminal spores. Cytotoxins A, B demonstrable in feces. Primary isolation on selective medium (egg-yolk fructose agar, with cycloserine and cefoxitin)	−	(Gas-liquid chromatography)				Antibiotic-associated pseudomembranous colitis (clindamycin, penicillin, cephalosporins) Vancomycin for treatment

* Damage to organized tissues due to local secretion of proteolytic and saccharolytic enzymes.

† Disease due to specific exotoxins disseminated via the blood stream and reactive with target cells (e.g., tetanus toxin and synaptic junctions of anterior horn cells).

II. Coccoid bacteria
   A. Diplococci
      1. Gram-negative:
         Neisseria species. Diplococci; aerobic; colonies indophenol-oxidase positive
         N. gonorrhoeae. Gonococcus (GC) requires chocolate agar on Thayer-Martin selective chocolate agar containing vancomycin, colistin, nystatin under CO_2; 35° to 37°C; isolation essential for diagnosis in females and chronic cases; in smears of exudate GC typically found in polymorphonuclear neutrophils (PMN); oxidase-positive colonies do not utilize maltose. Gonorrhea and septic complications (acute endocarditis, arthritis, proctitis, pharyngitis, meningitis), ophthalmia neonatorum; penicillinase-producing strains (PPNG), chromosome–mediated resistance (CMRNG) to penicillin
         N. meningitidis. Culturally and morphologically like *N. gonorrhoeae* but ferments maltose; found in leukocytes in spinal fluid; serotyping by capsular swelling, agglutination. *Epidemic* meningitis, chronic meningococcemia and septic complications. Polysaccharide vaccine for types A and C
      2. Gram-positive:
         Streptococcus pneumoniae. Green zone (alpha) hemolytic colonies on blood agar; lancet-shaped cocci paired in type-specific polysaccharide capsules; swelling reaction with type-specific serum; optochin-sensitive; inulin-positive. Lobar pneumonia, meningitis, otitis
         S. pyogenes. β-hemolytic: clear zones in blood agar pour plates; cell wall polysaccharides determine Lancefield groups A–U; type specificity determined by M- or T-cell wall proteins. Scarlet fever (erythrogenic toxin, lysogenic streptococci), puerperal sepsis, septicemia, septic sore throat, pyoderma. Nonsuppurative sequelae to group A only: rheumatic fever, glo-

merulonephritis. Group B—neonatal sepsis, meningitis

Group D. Enterococci *(S. faecalis)* and nonenterococci (Table 5-9) urinary tract infections, endocarditis

Viridans group. Heterogeneous; no group-specific carbohydrate. Normal oropharyngeal flora; some secrete dextrans or levans; cause dental plaque *(S. mutans, S. salivarius);* infective endocarditis

Staphylococcus species. Irregular clusters, pairs and single cocci; facultative; catalase-positive; anaerobic use of glucose and pyruvate; grow well on blood-free media at 20°C to 40°C; bacteriophage typing

S. aureus. Golden pigment; most of the pathogenic strains produce coagulase, leukocidin, hemolysin, and other tissue-damaging factors; also ferment mannitol, produce DNase, and liquefy gelatin; penicillin-resistance due to production of penicillinase. Nosocomial, pyogenic infections, endocarditis; thermostable enterotoxin causes food poisoning, toxic shock, and "scalded skin" syndromes. (Differentiate: exotoxin, endotoxin, enterotoxin)

S. epidermis (S. albus). No pigment; coagulase not produced; culturally similar to *S. aureus.* Commensal skin organism, opportunistic endocarditis *(e.g., prosthetic heart valves, long-term central vascular lines)*

III. Helical, flexible bacteria

Treponema species. Four to 14 close, regular spirals; tubular cell wound around an axial filament composed of bundles of modified polar flagella; best seen in darkfield; rotatory and flexing motion; pathogenic species morphologically indistinguishable; antigenically closely related; not cultivable in artificial media; the anaerobically cultivable Reiter treponeme is antigenically similar to *T. pallidum* but not virulent; *T. genitalis, T. microdentium,* and other saprophytes can be confused morphologically with *T. pallidum* in darkfield. *T. pallidum,* syphilis and bejel; *T. pertenue,* yaws; *T. carateum,* pinta. Numerous saprophytic strains are cultivable in vitro.

Borrelia species. Longer, coarser, more open, and irregular spirals than *Treponema;* vigorous lashing motion; stain readily; gram-negative; cultivable microaerophilically in special media. *Ixodes dammini* ticks transmit Lyme disease, caused by *B. burgdorferu.*

Leptospira species. Thinnest (<0.1 μm) and most tightly coiled (12 to 24 turns) of the spirochetes; hooked ends; unifibrillar axial filament; rapid rotatory and progressive motion; cultivable in media with serum; microaerophilic; blood and tissue parasites. Zoonoses source of human infection, "aseptic" meningitis

IV. Bacteria without cell walls

This group includes mycoplasma and pleuropneumonia-like organisms (PPLO). These organisms lack the enzymes that synthesize cell walls, the entire cell (except rare flagella) being enclosed within the thin, pliable, typically bacterial, cell membrane. In general, lack of the strong cell wall leaves them osmotically fragile (*i.e.,* subject to osmotic rupture) unless suspended in special PPLO medium of increased osmotic pressure (*e.g.,* 20% serum, 3% sucrose). Colonies on agar begin growth just below the surface and spread on the surface forming a foamy-looking colony with a fried-egg appearance. As a result of their pliable cell membrane, mycoplasmas are highly pleomorphic, forming cocci, branched filaments, ringforms. Some of the forms are so minute as to be filterable. Lack of cell wall makes mycoplasmas totally resistant to antibiotics that inhibit cell wall formation: penicillin, cephalosporins. They are very sensitive to surfactant substances such as soaps and bile and to tetracyclines. Except for *Mycoplasma pneumoniae,* they are nonhemolytic.

Over 30 species of genus *Mycoplasma* are recognized. These require sterols for growth. Some are associated with a variety of pathologic processes of humans and lower vertebrates: *M. hominis, M. gallisepticum, M. arthritidis, M. agalactiae, M. pneumoniae. Ureaplasma urealyticum* causes "nongonococcal" urethritis (NGU). Of a second genus, *Acholeplasma,* most are saprophytes or of doubtful pathogenicity. They do not require sterols for growth and are osmotically very fragile (*e.g.,* A. laidlawi).

V. Minute Bacteria: Obligate intracellular para-

TABLE 5-9. Properties of Streptococci Most Frequently Isolated from Clinical Specimens (Aerobic)

LANCEFIELD SEROGROUP (SPECIES)	GROUP-SPECIFIC CELL WALL POLYSACCHARIDE	USUAL TYPE OF HEMOLYSIS (SHEEP BLOOD)	GROWTH AT 37°	10°C	45°	FERMENTATION OF Trehalose	Sorbitol	Inulin	HIPPURATE HYDROLYSIS	SENSITIVITY TO Bacitracin†	Optochin	BE‡	TOLERANCE TO 6.5 PER CENT NaCl	DISEASES
A (S. pyogenes)	Rhamnose-GNac	β	+	–	–	+	–	–	–	+				Pharyngitis, tonsillitis, otitis, pyoderma, systemic infections, nonsuppurative sequelae: ARF, AGN
B (S. agalactiae)	Rhamnose-GNH₂	β(α γ)§	+	–	–	+	–	–	+	–(+)		–		Ascending amnionitis, neonatal sepsis, pneumonia, meningitis, nosocomial infections
C (S. equi, equisimilis, dysgalactiae)	Rhamnose-Gal-Nac	β	+	–	–	–	–	–	–	–				Mild URI, puerperal sepsis, endocarditis
D (S. faecalis, bovis, equinus)	Glycerol-teichoic acid-D-ala-glu	Enterococcus (S. faecalis, faecium, durans): α β γ Nonenterococcus (S. bovis, equinus): α γ							v	–	–	+	+	UTI, endocarditis (Enterococci: penicillin resistant)
F (S. milleri, anginosus, minutus, MG)								–	–	–	–	+	–	Respiratory infections, pneumonia
G (S. canis)								+		+				Puerperal, skin, wound infections
VIRIDANS		α									–	–(+)	–	Dental caries, endocarditis
S. salivarius (K)			+	–	+									
S. mitis			+	–	+									
S. mutans			+	–	+									
S. sanguis (H)		(β)	+	–	–									
S. pneumoniae (84 serotypes)	C substance (teichoic acid gal-6P-choline)	α									+	–	–	Pneumonia, septicemia, meningitis, endocarditis, otitis

* Representative species named.
† 5 to 10% of group B and C–G are bacitracin sensitive.
‡ Growth and hydrolysis of esculin on bile–esculin (BE) agar.
§ CAMP test positive.

AGN = acute glomerulonephritis.
ARF = acute rheumatic fever.
URI = upper respiratory infection.
UTI = urinary tract infection.
v = variable.

TABLE 5-10. Diseases Due to Rickettsiae

| DISEASES | GENERA | USUAL VECTOR | WEIL-FELIX REACTION | | | MOLE PERCENT G + C |
			OX19	OX2	OXK	
Typhus group:						
Epidemic typhus	*Rickettsia prowazekii**	Body louse *(Pediculus humanus corporis)*	+ + + +	+	–	29–30
Brill-Zinsser disease	*Rickettsia prowazekii*	Endogenous recrudescent typhus	(variable)			
Murine (endemic) typhus	*Rickettsia typhi** *(mooseri)*	Rat flea *(Xenopsylla cheopis)*	+ + +	+	–	29–30
Spotted fever group:						
Rocky Mountain spotted fever. Other tickborne diseases (e.g., Asian tick typhus, fievre boutonneuse)	*Rickettsia rickettsii**	Dog tick *(Dermacentor variabilis;* rabbit tick *(D. andersoni)*	+ + + +	+	–	32–33
Rickettsialpox	*Rickettsia akari**	Mouse mite *(Allodermanyssus sanguineus)*	–	–	–	32–33
Scrub typhus group:						
Tsutsugamushi (Japanese oriental river or swamp fever; scrub typhus)	*Rickettsia tsutsugamushi**	Harvest (field) mite *(Leptotrombidium deliense, L. akamushi)*	–	–	+ + + +	
Q fever	*Coxiella burnetii†*	Aerosolized fomites; ticks	–	–	–	43
Trench fever	*Rochalimaea quintana‡*	Body louse *(P. humanus corporis)*	(Not applicable)			39

* Grows in chick embryo; cultured mammalian cells.
† Grows in chick yolk sac; eukaryotic phagolysosomes. Develops endospore.
‡ Grows in complex cell-free media and on surface of eukaryotic cells.

sites. All are real bacteria, nonmotile, nonsporing rods or cocci, 0.3 to 0.6 μm. by 0.8 to 2.0 μm. Two orders are now recognized: Rickettsiales and Chlamydiales.

A. Order I. ***Rickettsiales.*** Of three families containing some seventeen genera, only two (genus *Rickettsia* and genus *Coxiella*) contain human pathogens of general importance, though several are of veterinary importance.

Genus *Rickettsia.* Not filterable; normally only arthropod-borne; can synthesize their own ATP. Typhus, Rocky Mountain spotted fever (Table 5-10).

Genus *Coxiella.* Much like *Rickettsia* but filterable: raw milk, dust of barns and cattle yards, infected lochia; probably also several species of ticks. Q fever *(C. burnetii).*

B. Order II. ***Chlamydiales.*** *Chlamydia trachomatis:* trachoma, inclusion conjunctivitis, infant pneumonia (perinatal), lymphogranuloma venereum (L). Nongonococcal urethritis, salpingitis (D–K), well-defined glycogen-rich inclusions, sensitive to sulfonamide, tetracyclines.

C. psittaci. Ornithosis (many species of mammals and birds), no glycogen in inclusions, insensitive to sulfonamide, sensitive to tetracyclines.

Bartonella bacilliformis. Oroya fever, verruga peruana.

STERILIZATION AND DISINFECTION

Sterilization

In relation to microbiology, ***sterilization*** means the destruction of all life. It is often incorrectly used interchangeably with ***disinfection,*** which means the destruction of pathogenic organisms. Thus, milk that is pasteurized (heated at 63°C for 30 minutes and quickly cooled) is disinfected but is not sterile, since many common harmless organisms and spores resist this heating process.

Disinfection

A disinfectant is a substance that kills pathogenic microorganisms but is generally understood not to be sporicidal. A *sporicidal* disinfectant would also be a sterilizing agent, *e.g.*, ethylene oxide, betapropiolactone.

Chemical disinfectants are indiscriminately poisonous. They may combine in cells with a variety of chemical groups, such as carboxyl, sulfhydryl, and hydroxyl. They may act by (1) injuring cell membranes (especially lipid components), causing leakages, rupture or both (*e.g.*, lipid solvents like ethyl or propyl alcohol or emulsifying agents like cationic detergents, *e.g.*, Zephiran), and other surfactants like phenolic compounds (*e.g.*, hexachlorophene, Lysol, Creolin); (2) chemically or physically altering enzymes and other proteins and DNA by breaking hydrogen and sulfide bonds and causing denaturation, coagulation, precipitation (*e.g.*, phenolics, heavy metals like organic mercurials and $AgNO_3$); (3) oxidizing cell components, such as $KMnO_4$; chlorine free or loosely combined as chloramines ($CL_2 + H_2O = HOCl + H^+ + Cl^-$; $HOCl$ a potent oxidizer); (4) toxic combinations, as with I in surfactant iodophers (*e.g.*, Wescodyne) or alkylations as in the presence of ethylene oxide. In many instances the action of any agent is not clearly of one type or another but a combination of effects on different cell components. Factors that affect the action of any disinfectant are kind, numbers and age of bacterial cells present, pH, temperature, time of exposure, concentration. In general, within limits, increase of any of the physical factors increases disinfectant action.

Sepsis; Antiseptics

Sepsis means the presence of pathogenic organisms growing in the tissues or blood. An *antiseptic,* strictly speaking, is a substance that combats sepsis but is generally thought of as a microbicidal or microbistatic substance applicable to exposed living tissues without undue damage to the tissues, *e.g.*, dilute alcohol, surfactant compounds of iodine (iodophors), mild tincture of iodine, and some organic mercurials. Antiseptics are not used internally. The terms antiseptic and disinfectant are often loosely used interchangeably.

Asepsis, strictly speaking, means absence of sepsis, but generally it is used to mean the absence of any living organisms. *Aseptic technique* is any procedure designed to eliminate live organisms and to keep them away. Modern surgical and microbiologic procedures are based on aseptic technique.

Methods

Sterilization may be accomplished by heat, mechanical means such as filtration, and use of sporicidal chemicals, notably ethylene oxide and betapropiolactone. Less widely used are penetrating, ionizing radiations in dosages of 2.5 mrad, chiefly for sterilization of heat-labile drugs, surgical equipment. Ultraviolet (about 260 nm) light has little power of penetration and is best used to control contamination by dust in air in enclosed spaces such as laboratories.

DRY HEAT

1. *Incineration*. Useful for bandages, paper dishes, sputum cups, etc.
2. *Oven Baking*. Useful for articles not containing water or that may be injured by steam. Applied usually to laboratory glassware and to materials not readily permeable by steam, such as petrolatum, mineral oil, sand, wooden articles, and glass syringes. A temperature of 165° C for at least 2 hours is necessary to kill all spores.

MOIST HEAT

1. *Boiling* (100° C at sea level). Some bacterial spores can survive 90 minutes or more of boiling. Hepatitis viruses can survive at least 10 minutes of boiling and probably longer. Therefore, boiling is not satisfactory as a means of sterilization under ordinary circumstances. Boiling for 10 minutes is suitable for disinfection in situations from which (1) spores of pathogenic bacteria and (2) hepatitis viruses are known to be absent.
2. *Autoclaving*. Steam, when compressed, is much hotter than free steam, and at 15 pounds pressure has a temperature of 121°C. An autoclave is a vessel that may be closed hermetically so as to exclude all air but retain steam under pressure. An ordinary household pressure cooker is a miniature autoclave capable of perfect sterilization.

   In autoclaving, steam pressure of 15 to 20 pounds is usually applied from 10 to 30 minutes. All air must escape and all space be filled with steam. Air does not reach the desired temperature. Also, since steam is depended on to bring about *hydrolysis* of bacteria and their spores, mixture with dry air reduces the effectiveness of the process. Autoclaving is generally used for culture media, saline solutions, for surgical supplies, for solutions intended for intravenous injections, and for bandages, dressings. Glassware is often autoclaved. Autoclaving is not used for oils or petrolatum, which cannot absorb steam and therefore remain dry.

SPORICIDAL VAPORS

1. *Formaldehyde* vapor is sometimes used to disinfect (sterilize?) interiors of rooms, ships, but has the disadvantage of polymerizing (paraformaldehyde) on surfaces and being difficult to remove. In high concentration it is sporicidal. It is commonly used dissolved 37% (weight) in water as formalin or formol for tissue fixation and embalming.
2. *Ethylene oxide,* an alkylating agent, is used, diluted about 1 : 10 with CO_2 or other vapor, to reduce toxicity and inflammability, inside autoclaves under conditions of controlled concentration (around 500 mg/liter, of air), pressure (around 10 lb), temperature (around 130°F or 55°C), and relative humidity (around 40%). It is effective but expensive and is useful mainly for objects that are damaged by ordinary methods of heat sterilization.
3. *Betapropiolactone,* liquid at room temperatures, forms a sporicidal vapor in concentrations around 1.5 mg/liter of air at relative humidities around 80% and temperatures around 25°C. Potentially useful (combined with ultraviolet irradiation to remove hepatitis viruses from blood products), but a potent carcinogen.

FILTRATION

Fine-pored filters, long used for mechanical sterilization (*e.g.,* cellulose mixed with asbestos [Seitz disks]; sintered [fused] granular glass), have been supplanted by paper-thin membrane filters that depend chiefly on pore size (about 12 to 0.22 μm) for mechanical sieve action, especially if the perforations in the filters have been made by regulated nuclear bombardment. Such filters also serve to collect microorganisms from fluids for microscopic examination or cultivation directly on the filter when placed on pads saturated with culture medium, often selective media.

MICROBISTASIS (BACTERIOSTASIS)

By this term is meant nonlethal inhibition of growth of microorganisms for hours, days, or years, gener-

ally by interfering with certain enzyme functions. Microbistatic agents may be physical (*e.g.,* refrigeration, freeze-drying, pickling brines, or dehydration), or chemical (*e.g.,* various aniline dyes in media, antibodies, antibiotics, sulfonamide drugs). In selective bacteriostasis in the diagnostic laboratory, such agents are used to inhibit growth of undesired contaminants in specimens such as feces or sputum and permit the desired species to grow. Microbistasis is an inexact term, since, if microorganisms are held "static" long enough, they eventually die, though they may survive for many years under some microbistatic conditions, such as freeze-drying.

Microbistasis is characteristically reversible, for example, by chemical neutralization of the bacteriostatic agent (Hg + H_2S); mechanical removal (washing or dilution); cessation (warming of frozen cells); or rehydrating of dried cells.

Surface Disinfection

Agents that damage bacterial cell membranes may be used to disinfect inert surfaces or the skin. These include cationic (*e.g.,* Zephyran) and anionic (soaps and fatty acids) detergents; phenolic compounds (*e.,g.,* tricresol) emulsified with green soap (*e.g.,* Lysol); diphenyl compounds (*e.g.,* hexachlorophene); alcohols (*e.g.,* 50% to 70% ethanol).

Protein-Denaturing Agents

Denaturing of bacterial cellular proteins, and hence germicidal action, can be achieved with acids (*e.g.,* benzoic acid as food preservative); soluble salts of heavy metals (*e.g.,* merthiolate, silver nitrate, silver sulfadiazine); oxidizing agents (*e.g.,* iodine, hydrogen peroxide); alkylating agents (*e.g.,* formaldehyde; glutaraldehyde as for cold sterilization of instruments; ethylene oxide).

ANTIBIOTICS

Antimicrobial agents used in the treatment of infectious diseases must have deleterious effects on the microorganism with little toxicity for host tissue. This difference in selective toxicity is expressed quantitatively as the therapeutic index. The concept of selective toxicity requires the binding of a drug to a microbial structure or protein that is either absent or significantly different from its counterpart in mammalian cells. The prokaryotic ribosome, which is smaller than its eukaryotic counterpart (70s versus 80s), the peptidoglycan layer of bacterial cell walls, which is unique to these microorganisms and certain special enzymatic stages in bacterial nucleic acid replication or transcription are prime targets.

Mode of Action of Cell Wall Inhibitors

The drugs that inhibit cell wall synthesis are listed in Table 5-1. The inhibition of peptidoglycan synthesis is usually a lethal event for a bacterium because the process of adding new material to the wall is coupled with autolytic digestion of the wall at the anticipated growth sites. In the absence of synthesis, the continued enzymatic digestion weakens the wall until osmotic pressure causes bursting of the cytoplasmic membrane. Cells can survive inhibition of cell wall synthesis if the autolytic enzymes are not functioning, as in nongrowing cells. They can survive also in spite of wall digestion if the osmotic pressure is not sufficient to force lysis, a condition occurring in hypertonic solutions (*e.g.*, pus). These factors support the need for wound drainage concurrent with the institution of antimicrobial therapy.

The process of cell wall synthesis must be understood to appreciate the activity of various antimicrobials. The process includes a cytoplasmic component leading to the synthesis of a peptidoglycan subunit, secretion of this subunit through the cytoplasmic membrane into the periplasmic space, and finally enzymatic addition of subunits to the growing portion of the peptidoglycan and cross-linking by pentaglycine bridges. Each of these three major sets of reactions is subject to selective interference by various antimicrobials. Synthesis of the subunit is blocked by cycloserine and bacitracin. Secretion through the membrane is blocked by vancomycin. Cross-linking of the subunit is blocked by penicillins, semisynthetic penicillins, and cephalosporins.

Problems of Insensitivity and Resistance Related to Antimicrobials That Affect Cell Wall Synthesis

No single antimicrobial agent has effects on all types of microorganisms. There are entire genera in which no species of organism is ever found to be inhibited by a particular drug, that is, these organisms are considered to be inherently *in*sensitive to that drug because of physiological or structural traits common to all members of the group. Accordingly, the degree to which an antibiotic might inhibit such microbes is entirely predictable. On the other hand, most isolates of a given genus or species may be susceptible to a drug, only occasional strains being found to be less sensitive than the majority. These exceptions are generally designated as being *resistant,* that is, insusceptible to concentrations of drug that inhibit other strains of the same organism. Such resistant strains occur at rates that cannot always be predicted, and in such cases, careful *in vitro* susceptibility testing of each isolate is required as a guide to choice of chemotherapeutic agents.

Most gram-negative organisms are insensitive to clinically attainable levels of penicillin G and V. This insensitivity is determined by the impermeability of the lipopolysaccharide layer of the cell wall. Most gram-positive organisms and some of the fastidious gram-negative bacteria allow the penicillins to reach the periplasmic space and exert their lethal action. Some strains of these normally sensitive species resist penicillin because they lack certain proteins in the periplasmic space or because they produce penicillinase. Penicillinase cleaves the β-lactam ring of the penicillin molecule to form penicilloic acid, thereby completely eliminating the activity of the drug. The penicillinases of gram-positive organisms tend to be inducible exoenzymes, whereas the penicillinases of gram-negative organisms remain in the periplasmic space and can be constitutive. Each penicillinase has a range of substrates, most semisynthetic penicillins and cephalosporins being subject to digestion by penicillinases. Chemical substitutions that lead to the protection of the β-lactam ring are partial solutions to the chemotherapeutic problems posed by penicillinase. Nafcillin, methicillin, and oxacillin are resistant to penicillinases common in *Staphylococcus aureus.* Carbenicillin resists some penicillinases of gram-negative rods. Some of the new cephalosporins, for example, cefoxitin and cefamandole, resist a wide variety of penicillinases.

The similarity between penicillins and cephalosporins includes their mechanisms of action but fortunately excludes to a large degree their haptenic properties. Penicillin, like almost all antimicrobial agents, following combination with host proteins, can induce hypersensitivity to the penicillin molecule. A person allergic to penicillin G produces an allergic reaction when exposed to semisynthetic penicillins (*i.e.*, nafcillin, oxacillin, ampicillin). Fortunately, such hypersensitive individuals fail in most cases to react with cephalosporins. Atopic individuals, however, can become hypersensitive to cephalosporins as well as to any of the other drugs.

Vancomycin inhibits cell wall synthesis by blocking the secretion of peptidoglycan subunits into the periplasmic space. Vancomycin should be held in reserve as a valuable drug for use against gram-positive organisms resistant to penicillins and other antimicrobial agents.

Bacitracin and cycloserine, in the bacterial cytoplasm, inhibit cell wall synthesis by different mechanisms. Bacitracin limits the availability of a lipid carrier, the functions of which include binding of newly formed subunits to the internal surface of the cytoplasmic membrane. Cycloserine inhibits synthesis of subunits by blocking the enzymatic conversion of L-alanine to D-alanine.

Mode of Action of Drugs Affecting Nucleic Acid Synthesis

During synthesis, DNA may be cleaved at specific points by endonucleases, which thus allow modifications to be introduced, provided that normal repair mechanisms can act to reconstitute the integrity of the molecule. If normal DNA repair mechanisms are blocked, the nicks caused by endonucleases are lethal to the microorganism.

The inhibitors of nucleic acids act either at the macromolecular level or on the synthesis of nucleic acid bases (Table 5-2).

Several drugs that function at the macromolecular level are *nalidixic acid,* the new quinolones *(floxacins),* and *rifampicin.* Nalidixic acid exerts a bactericidal effect on gram-negative organisms by blocking one enzyme required for normal DNA synthesis. Nalidixic acid binds to the enzyme gyrase, the functions of which include the unwinding of tightly coiled regions of DNA during DNA synthesis. Gyrase-mediated unwinding of DNA is induced by cutting the DNA and allowing relaxation of supercoils and then repair of the nicks. Nalidixic acid binding to this bifunctional enzyme allows the DNA nicking to continue but inhibits repair of the nicks. It is used for gram-negative, non-*Pseudomonas* urinary tract infections. New quinolones, such as norfloxacin and ciprofloxacin, also block gyrase action. They are effective on gram-negative organisms, including *Pseudomonas* and gram-positive organisms, except streptococci. The frequency of mutation is very low ($\leq 10^{11}$).

The action of rifampicin requires its binding to DNA-dependent RNA polymerase of bacteria. This enzyme is composed of a core of four protein subunits plus a separate soluble regulatory protein, sigma (σ). Synthesis of messenger RNA (mRNA) by this enzyme begins when the core binds to the promoter region of a bacterial operon. However, construction of the mRNA requires the binding of protein to the core portion of the enzyme. Rifampicin binds to the core portion of the enzyme, inhibiting the core–sigma interaction required for initiation of mRNA synthesis.

Ansamycin is a new derivative of rifampicin with improved properties for clinical use.

The synthesis of nucleic acid bases in bacteria requires the addition of single carbon units, a reaction mediated by folic acid. Folic acid is synthesized *de novo* in bacterial cells but not in eukaryotic cells, in which it is only consumed or enzymatically modified. Two important enzymatic reactions involved in the synthesis of bacterial folic acid are sensitive to chemotherapeutic agents. The conversion of para-aminobenzoic acid to dihydrofolic acid, a reaction mediated by dihydrofolic acid synthetase, is sensitive to competitive inhibition by "sulfa" drugs, such as sulfanilamide. These drugs do not affect the mammalian cell, which, because it lacks mechanisms for primary synthesis, has a nutritional requirement for dihydrofolic acid.

The second enzymatic reaction in folic acid synthesis that is sensitive to antimicrobial agents is the conversion of dihydrofolic acid to tetrahydrofolic acid. Dihydrofolic acid reductase mediates this reaction in both eucaryotic and bacterial cells. The drug trimethoprim binds about 50,000 times more avidly to the bacterial than to the mammalian enzyme because of differences in structure between the two species of protein. Bacteriostatic concentrations of the drug are therefore well tolerated by the eukaryotic cell. Both sulfonamides and trimethoprim effect a folic acid deficiency, but because they act at different stages in the pathway, a mixture of the two drugs generates a synergistic antibacterial effect and is used for treatment of urinary tract infections, acute otitis media, as well as acute inflammatory diarrhea.

Griseofulvin is an analogue of the purine base guanosine and inhibits DNA synthesis by a mechanism that is not clear. It is an antifungal, used for chitin-containing fungi, especially those in nail infections.

Mode of Action of Drugs Directly Affecting Cell Membranes

Microbial cell membranes resemble those of eukaryotic cells in general organization and chemistry. This fact makes it likely that drugs designed to act directly on cell membrane structure would be unacceptably toxic. However, there are subtle differences that permit selective binding of certain antimicrobial agents (*e.g.,* lack of sterols in bacterial membranes) (Table 5-2). Polymyxins and gramicidin bind to bacterial membranes and cause reorganization of phospholipids around the drug, thereby introducing sites of ionic leakage. Unlike many other bactericidal agents, the polymyxins exert an almost immediately lethal effect, in this respect resembling the action of detergents.

Nystatin (Mycostatin) and amphotericin interact in a detergentlike manner with the membrane of susceptible fungi. The toxicity of nystatin for host tissue, and its relative insolubility limit its application to treatment of surface infections.

Mode of Action of Drugs Affecting Protein Synthesis

Protein synthesis in bacteria begins when the 30s portion of ribosomes, through the action of soluble initiation proteins, binds to mRNA (Table 5-3). The amino acids to be linked into a protein are each bound to species of transfer RNA (tRNA) that in turn recognize specific sequences in mRNA. The binding of tRNA, charged with amino acids, to the 30s portion of the ribosome–mRNA complex is the first stage of protein synthesis susceptible to antibiotic action. Drugs that bind to the 30s subunit and block tRNA recognition include aminoglycosides, spectinomycin, and tetracycline (Table 5-3).

The formation of peptide bonds requires both 30s and 50s portions of the ribosome. The actual formation of peptide bonds may be blocked by certain drugs, such as chloramphenicol, lincomycin, and clindamycin, which bind to the 50s subunit.

In the normal process of protein synthesis, the ribosome moves relative to the mRNA (*i.e.*, translocates), a reaction that requires soluble proteins and GTP for energy. Erythromycin blocks translocation by binding to proteins that form the 50s subunit. Fusidic acid blocks translocation by binding to one of the soluble proteins (elongation factor G) involved in energizing the movement.

The consequences, to the bacterium, of inhibition of protein synthesis, vary depending upon the manner in which the process is inhibited. Inhibition by chloramphenicol is completely reversible and is therefore only bacteriostatic. This implies that continuous protein synthesis *per se* is not absolutely required for bacterial survival. An antibiotic such as streptomycin binds irreversibly to the ribosome, thereby causing nearly complete inhibition of protein synthesis, and hence causing death of the bacterium. The killing effect is related to the production of "mis-sense" proteins, which are synthesized in the presence of the drug and that misfunction because of incorrect amino acid sequences caused by drug-induced alterations of the ribosome. Mis-sense proteins in the cell lead to changes in internal structures or enzymes, thus accounting for the death of the cell.

Major Mechanisms of Antibiotic Resistance

Changes in the structural or physiologic components of an organism that occur by mutation can result in resistance to antibiotics. Significant levels of resistance may occur after a single mutation or after a series of mutations. Antimicrobial drugs do not themselves induce mutation(s), but select out those organisms that have undergone mutation. This sequence is the most common mechanism of resistance to vancomycin, rifampicin, nalidixic acid, and polymyxins. Although resistance to other drugs can emerge as a result of bacterial mutation, acquisition of specific plasmids more often accounts for observed changes in sensitivity to drugs (Table 5-11).

Resistance plasmids (R) govern their own replication and confer resistance on the bacterial host cell. Plasmids that in addition contain a set of transfer genes are called resistance transfer factors (RTF) because they mediate conjugation. The R and RTF plasmids thus differ in size and in ability to initiate conjugation. One bacterium can accommodate a variety of plasmids, and it is not uncommon to encounter mixtures of R and RTF plasmids in a single organism. The R plasmids, although unable to initiate conjugation, can be transferred by conjugation mediated by an RTF in the same organism. In the absence of an RTF, the R plasmid can be transferred only when the organism is infected with a bacteriophage capable of generalized transduction. Because RTF plasmids are not encountered in *Staphylococcus*, the transfer of R plasmids in this organism is dependent on phage. In enteric bacteria, *Hemophilus,* and a variety of other organisms, transfer of R plasmids occurs by either RTF-mediated conjugation or by transduction.

The resistance to antibiotics that is mediated by R and RTF plasmids is determined by a protein product of the plasmid. In the case of penicillins and cephalosporins, this protein has β-lactamase activity and destroys the antibiotic in the periplasmic space or outside of the cell wall. Chloramphenicol, aminoglycosides, and spectinomycin are inactivated because the plasmid protein in the periplasmic space mediates the enzymatic attachment of acetyl, phosphate or adenyl groups. Lincomycin, clindamycin, and erythromycin are inactivated because the plasmid protein mediates the enzymatic

TABLE 5-11. Major Mechanisms of Specific Antibiotic Resistance

DRUG	MECHANISM OF RESISTANCE	GENETIC BASIS OF RESISTANCE
Penicillin	β-lactamase	Plasmid*
Ampicillin	β-lactamase	Plasmid*
Cephalothin	β-lactamase	Plasmid*
Methicillin	Impermeability	Plasmid
Vancomycin	Membrane alteration	Chromosome (mutation)
Sulfanilamide	Novel dihydrofolic acid synthetase	Plasmid*
Trimethoprim	Novel dihydrofolic acid synthetase	Plasmid
Rifampicin	Altered RNA polymerase	Chromosome (mutation)
Nalidixic acid	Altered gyrase enzyme	Chromosome (mutation)
Polymyxins	Altered membrane components	Chromosome (mutation)
Aminoglycosides	Antibiotic-modifying enzyme	Plasmid*
Spectinomycin	Antibiotic-modifying enzyme	Plasmid
Tetracycline	Permeability barrier	Plasmid*
Chloramphenicol	Antibiotic-modifying enzyme	Plasmid*
Lincomycin	Ribosome-modifying enzyme	Plasmid
Clindamycin	Ribosome-modifying enzyme	Plasmid
Erythromycin	Ribosome-modifying enzyme	Plasmid

* Resistance may be part of a transposon.

methylation of an RNA molecule in the ribosome, methylation inhibiting the binding of drug to the ribosome. The plasmid product in some way reduces the uptake of tetracycline drug into the bacterium. In the case of folic acid inhibitors, the plasmid product is a pathway enzyme that is not competitively inhibited by the drug as is the chromosomally produced enzyme.

The single product of a plasmid in some cases reacts with a variety of compounds, that is, a given β-lactamase may destroy ampicillin, penicillin G, and cephalothin, or a given aminoglycoside-modifying enzyme may react with kanamycin, gentamicin, and tobramycin. Thus the expression of resistance to several related drugs is often mediated by one gene product of the plasmid. A single plasmid may contain multiple genes each mediating resistance(s). Because a bacterium can harbor numerous plasmids, the emergence of genetically complex and highly resistant strains is encountered in environments subject to the powerful selective pressure of multiple antibiotics (e.g., a hospital).

One further complication introduced by R and RTF plasmids is that the plasmid gene responsible for resistance may form a transposon. A transposon is capable of "hopping" from the plasmid on which it entered a bacterium to another plasmid, to the chromosome, or even to the DNA of a phage that infects the same cell. Hopping of transposons accounts for the spread of resistance to organisms that are otherwise unable to support the replication of the plasmid originally harboring the resistance gene. This process accounts for the spread of β-

lactamase genes from plasmids of enteric bacteria to species of *Hemophilus* and *Neisseria*.

Methods for Testing Bacterial Sensitivity to Antibiotics

Because of occasional adverse side effects and increasing emergence of antibiotic-resistant organisms, chemotherapeutic agents must be used in critical fashion to safeguard their clinical efficacy. The purpose of testing an organism for sensitivity to several antibiotics is to allow the physician some latitude in the ultimate choice of therapy. This consideration may be important in avoiding undesirable complications attending the use of a particular drug in a given patient (e.g., allergy) and to offer a choice of potentially effective substitutes. The selection of drugs to be tested is based primarily on knowledge of the infection, that is, whether it is in the urinary tract, blood, localized pus, or spinal fluid. In this connection, a carefully done Gram's stain, particularly of pus, spinal fluid, and unspun urine correctly collected, yields vital information about the initial choice of antibiotics that will then be confirmed or modified on the basis of results of sensitivity testing of the organism(s) in question.

The widely used Kirby–Bauer method is based on the inhibition of surface bacterial growth under standard conditions. Several colonies of the organism to be tested are inoculated into Todd–Hewitt broth and grown to a standard optical density. Inoculum from this culture is then spread across the surface of a nutrient agar plate in a manner that gives heavy confluent growth. Disks containing antibiotics are then placed on the agar. After incubation, the diameter of the zone of growth inhibition around each antibiotic disk is measured. Each organism is then scored as sensitive, intermediate or resistant, according to the size of the zone of inhibition, which is a direct function of the sensitivity of the organism to the antibiotic. However, other factors also affect the zone size (*e.g.*, diffusion, stability and concentration of the drug, characteristically of the particular organism, size of inoculum) that collectively impose upper and lower limits within which variations in sensitivity among individual strains of a bacterial species can be judged. Infections due to organisms designated as sensitive to a given antibiotic are more likely to yield clinically to that antibiotic than are infections with strains designated as intermediate or resistant.

It is sometimes important to determine accurately the concentration of an antibiotic that must be achieved to inhibit a particular microorganism. For such determinations, the tube dilution method is used in addition to the Kirby–Bauer method. In this procedure, an antibiotic is serially diluted in growth medium and inoculated with relatively small numbers (10^5/ml) of a particular organism. The lowest concentration of antibiotic that prevents bacterial growth (turbidity) is the minimal inhibitory concentration (MIC).

For antibiotics that are bactericidal, the bactericidal endpoint can be determined by subculturing the tubes in which there is no turbidity and in which viable organisms from the inoculum may have survived. The bactericidal concentration is higher than the bacteriostatic. The MIC refers to the bacteriostatic endpoint. The minimal lethal concentration (MLC) refers to the bactericidal endpoint.

BACTERIAL INFECTIONS

Gram-Negative Enteric Bacteria

For classification, refer to A Descriptive Checklist of Important Bacteria in Medical Microbiology, earlier in this chapter. All but the exogenous pathogens, *Salmonella, Shigella, Yersinia,* and *Vibrio,* are usual members of the normal intestinal flora (along the *Pseudomonas,* anaerobes, *etc.*) but are important causes of opportunistic infections.

SALMONELLOSIS

This term covers infection by any of the several hundred serotypes or bioserotypes of *Salmonella* and covers a wide range of clinical manifestations, including acute gastroenterocolitis (inaccurately referred to as food poisoning), various localized infections (arthritis, myocarditis, abscesses), and typhoid (enteric) fever. The latter is usually regarded as a distinct entity because, unlike common enterocolitis, *S. typhi* is first isolated from the blood and only later from the lower intestinal tract; the disease carries a relatively high morbidity, and despite chemotherapy occasional fatalities occur.

Salmonellae are classified according to their H and O antigens by agglutination reactions with appropriately specific antisera. On this basis (Kauffman–White schema) the genus is divisible into three major species: *S. choleraesuis,* the prototype, *S. typhi* and *S. enteritidis;* the latter makes up the largest number of subspecies. In usual hospital laboratory practice, clinical isolates of *Salmonella* are reported as belonging to groups A, B, C, or D (*S. typhi* only); for final species identification isolates are sent to a central laboratory (*e.g.,* state health department or Centers for Disease Control).

While *Salmonella* grows readily on the usual bacteriologic media, procedures for primary isolation differ according to whether the specimen is a sample of feces, pus, or urine, in which relatively few *Salmonella* might be mixed in with predominant normal flora (cultured on enrichment and selective media), or whether it is from a normally sterile body fluid, such as blood or spinal fluid (cultured directly on blood agar and differential media). Once isolated in pure culture, preliminary identification is achieved on the basis of biochemical reactions (*e.g.,* nonutilization of lactose, selective fermentation of other sugars, motility, hydrogen sulfide formation, lack of urease activity, *etc.*) and serogrouping with polyvalent antisera (to O antigens).

Excepting typhoid fever, salmonellosis is commonly (but not invariably) localized in the intestinal tract, is mild or acute and self-limited. Occasional cases resemble typhoid fever, dysentery, or even cholera, especially in debilitated patients. Neither species nor clinical picture is constant. *S. typhi, S. paratyphi A, S. paratyphi B,* and *S. paratyphi C* are especially invasive.

Meningitis, pneumonia, osteomyelitis, septicemia (especially *S. choleraesuis*) may occur. *Salmonella* infection not infrequently is found in association with debilitating conditions, such as sickle cell anemia, bartonellosis (verruga peruana), or immunosuppression and/or malnutrition.

In typhoid fever, intestinal perforation may occur at necrotic lymphatic areas (Peyer's patches) that are the site of initial localization of *S. typhi.* In typhoid fever, stubborn residual infection of the gallbladder sometimes develops, resulting in cholelithiasis and its complications, one of which is a persistent carrier state, usually curable by cholecystectomy, and especially dangerous in public food handlers ("typhoid Mary").

S. typhimurium, S. choleraesuis, S. oranienburg, and *S. enteritidis* are among species commonly involved in *Salmonella* infection through ingestion of contaminated food. They and others (not *S. typhi,* which is restricted to humans) commonly infect a wide range of wild and domestic animals and poultry, which thus become reservoirs of infection of man via foods: raw meats of infected birds and animals, raw dairy products, raw eggs. All *Salmonella* species are transmitted in human feces (*S. typhi* sometimes also in urine following pyelonephritis and cystitis), hence in sewage and in sewage- or feces-polluted water, food and dairy products; by coprophagic arthropods (flies, ants, roaches, etc.); and by fomites.

In typical *Salmonella* food infection, symptoms commonly begin more than 10 hours following ingestion, that is, long enough for bacterial multiplication to occur, in contrast with food poisoning, especially the common staphylococcal food poisoning, in which symptoms of intense gastroenteritis commonly begin within about 10 hours following ingestion, since the toxin is preformed and growth of staphylococci in the alimentary tract does not ordinarily occur.

Diagnosis. In food infection by *Salmonella* (except *S. typhi*) the organisms occur in the stool early during the enteritis and may be isolated and identified on appropriate media. They usually do not invade the blood stream.

In typhoid fever, on the contrary, the incubation period may be 2 to 3 weeks, symptoms delayed, and the bacilli appear in the blood (2% bile infusion broth and plain infusion broth) during the first 10 days and in the stool or the urine only after the first week. They often persist in the stools up to 12 weeks, and in about 3% of cases they persist more or less intermittently for years. In overt typhoid fever, splenomegaly and rose spots on the trunk are distinctive. Lifelong immunity to *S. typhi* follows documented typhoid fever.

In *serologic diagnosis* of salmonellosis, patients' sera are examined for antibodies against *Salmonella* using standard strains of *S. typhi* as antigen in titered agglutination tests. A significant (greater than 1 : 160) level or a rise (fourfold or greater) in titer with O antigen (*S. typhi* treated so that primarily the somatic antigens are exposed) denotes active infec-

tion. A significant rise in antibody to H antigen (*S. typhi* treated to preserve the flagellar antigens that will then be the primary reactants with antibody) was usually found to follow immunization with typhoid vaccine, which is little used nowadays. Antibodies to a surface (capsular) antigen (Vi) characteristic of some strains of *S. typhi* are thought to be associated with the presence of *S. typhi* as asymptomatic carriers.

Phage Types. Strains of *S. typhi* possessing Vi antigen and antigenically indistinguishable from one another can be further subdivided on the basis of differential sensitivity to bacteriophages. At least 50 phage types are known. This differentiation by phage typing is useful in epidemiologic studies; for example, in tracing possible different sources of infection during a supposedly single-source epidemic. Similar systems of phage typing have been developed for several other groups of bacteria: *Salmonella paratyphi A* and *S. paratyphi B; Shigella; Escherichia coli; Vibrio cholerae; Staphylococcus aureus.*

Treatment. Ampicillin and chloramphenicol are the drugs of choice in the treatment of typhoid fever and systemic infection with other strains of *Salmonella.* Strains resistant to either or both of these antibiotics occur. An alternative choice is trimethoprim-sulfamethoxazole. Uncomplicated *Salmonella* gastroenteritis is usually self-limited; antibiotics are therefore unnecessary and only promote the emergence of drug-resistant strains. Resistance plasmids are extensively shared between human and animal strains of bacteria. Close to half the antibiotics sold in the United States are fed to domestic herd animals and are therefore unwittingly ingested by humans. It is not surprising, therefore, that strains of *Salmonella* isolated from these two sources should show similar antibiograms. Antibiotics fed to livestock thus have a direct role in the rising incidence of multiple drug resistance among members of the Enterobacteriaceae. These multiple resistant strains now represent 20% to 25% of identified cases, in which the fatality rate is much higher than in cases due to sensitive strains.

Prevention of salmonellosis as well as of other communicable diseases of the intestinal tract centers primarily on adequate sanitation and thorough cooking of foods containing animal products or eggs and foods susceptible to contamination by sewage or excreta by avian or mammalian carriers, including humans. Human carriers should not serve as food handlers or nurses. Typhoid carriers are generally registered with, and supervised by, health departments.

Active immunization against typhoid is justified for persons in intimate continued household exposure to a documented typhoid carrier or for travelers to areas in which there is a recognized risk of exposure to typhoid because of poor sanitation practices. The appropriate dosage for adults and children over 10 years of age is 0.5 ml subcutaneously on two occasions 4 weeks apart, and for children younger than 10 years of age, 0.25 ml subcutaneously on two occasions 4 weeks apart. Under conditions of continued or repeated exposure or for indications if more than 3 years after primary immunization, booster (single doses administered subcutaneously as recommended above for each age group) should be given. Only monovalent *Salmonella typhi* vaccine should be used; previous formulations of "TAB" vaccines (combining typhoid and "paratyphoid A and B" antigens) should not be used.

SHIGELLOSIS (BACILLARY DYSENTERY)

Clinical dysentery may be caused by a variety of agents: certain protozoa, viruses, unripe apples, *Salmonella*. Shiga, a Japanese scientist, in 1896 first isolated the bacterium now called *Shigella dysenteriae* during outbreaks of severe dysentery in Japan. Flexner later (ca. 1900) isolated a different species from cases of dysentery in the Philippines. Many varieties were afterward described elsewhere. The various strains were named according to names of discoverers or places where found.

The genus *Shigella* is now classified into four major groups, each with several numbered serotypes based on O antigens:

Group A. *S. dysenteriae*
Group B. *S. flexneri*
Group C. *S. boydii*
Group D. *S. sonnei*

Biochemical reactions serve to differentiate *Shigella* from *Salmonella*. Shigellae do not ferment lactose (except *S. sonnei*, a slow lactose fermenter); are nonmotile; and do not produce H_2S, or gas (except *S. flexneri*) during carbohydrate fermentation. Further species identification depends on numerous additional biochemical reactions and on reactions with group-specific antisera.

Multiplication of dysentery bacilli occurs in the mucosa and the lymph nodes of the lower ileum and colon, with ulceration and sometimes pseudomembrane formation. Acute gastroenteritis is common. Bacteremia is rare. Stools typically contain mucus, pus, and blood. All of the gram-negative enteric bacilli possess lipopolysaccharide (endotoxin) in their cell walls. *Shigella dysenteriae* and *S. flexneri* produce antigenically similar toxins, the former in larger amounts than the latter. The enterotoxin is probably responsible for the watery, small-bowel diarrhea, often severe, that is characteristic of the first few days of shigellosis. *S. dysenteriae* infections cause higher fatality rates (20%) than infections by other *Shigella* species and occur chiefly in epidemic form. They are rare in the United States. In this country *S. flexneri* and *S. sonnei* are the most commonly encountered as the cause of both sporadic and epidemic disease. The fatality rate for shigellosis is relatively low in adults; it is higher in infants, particularly in developing countries, in which it is a leading cause of acute diarrhea in young children. Endemic shigellosis is associated with malnutrition and other concomitants of poor economic and sanitary conditions. Malnutrition-associated complications include hemolytic-uremic syndrome and Reiter's syndrome; in poorly nourished children the organisms may persist for long periods, with clinical relapses. Under ordinary circumstances, the infection is self-limited, and chronic carriers are rare. Control of shigellosis depends primarily on improving sanitary conditions to minimize fecal contamination of food and water sources. A safe or effective vaccine is not yet available.

In laboratory diagnosis, fecal samples and tissue swabs of the rectal mucosa should be cultured and examined microscopically for erythrocytes and leukocytes. Serum agglutinins for *Shigella* when present are of no diagnostic value. Chemotherapy is unnecessary in the usual self-limited form of shigellosis. In severe enteric disease in the presence of malnutrition and dehydration, ampicillin is the drug of choice; when ampicillin-resistant strains are involved, trimethoprim–sulfamethoxazole is used; tetracycline should be reserved for severe disease due to strains resistant to the other two drugs. Transferable multiple drug resistance in *Shigella*, mediated by plasmids, is widespread; complete antibiograms should therefore be done to guide the choice of antibiotic.

INFECTIONS DUE TO ENTEROBACTERIA (*E. COLI* AND OTHER INTESTINAL GRAM-NEGATIVE BACTERIA)

The enteric bacteria are readily cultivable on ordinary media (blood agar; eosin methylene blue agar, which inhibits gram-positive bacteria; and selective media such as McConkey's agar) and are differentiated on the basis of their biochemical reactions in pure culture; all (except for *Proteus* species and *Pseudomonas aeruginosa*) ferment lactose. All may cause opportunistic infection. *E. coli* is responsible for about 85% of cases of cystitis and is the commonest cause of pyelonephritis. The remaining 10% to 15% are accounted for by other *Enterobacteriaceae* (*e.g., Proteus* species, *Klebsiella* species, and *Enterobacter* species) and *Pseudomonas aeruginosa*. Colonization of the urinary tract by certain (pyelonephritogenic) strains of *E. coli* is mediated by attachment of bacterial fimbriae to specific tissue cell receptors. Bacteria defective in cell wall material (so-called L-forms) appear to be important in chronic relapsing pyelonephritis; L-forms do not grow on ordinary culture media and so may escape detection unless specifically searched for. Most of the strains of *E. coli* causing neonatal meningitis carry the K_1 capsular antigen, which is related to the polysaccharide antigen of Group B *Neisseria meningitidis* and is similarly antiphagocytic (*i.e.,* a virulence factor). Infections due to strains resistant to multiple antibiotics carry a relatively high mortality rate. Any of the Enterobacteriaceae (as well as *Neisseria meningitidis, Hemophilus influenzae*) may cause life-threatening septicemia (gram-negative sepsis) in which endotoxic shock is ascribed to lipid A (attached to LPS core polysaccharide common to most gram-negative bacteria). Successful treatment of potentially fatal endotoxic shock with human antiserum to LPS core antigen has been reported. Besides being a frequent cause of nosocomial infection, *Klebsiella pneumoniae* is one of the few gram-negative bacilli that can cause primary lobar pneumonia, particularly in compromised patients in whom the upper lobes are usually involved and undergo cavitation due to the necrotizing infection. Therapy is sometimes successful with a combination of an aminoglycoside and a cephalosporin. Prevalence of multiply resistant strains in a hospital environment is directly related to unregulated and injudicious use of antibiotics.

Certain (enteropathogenic) strains of *E. coli* cause acute diarrheal disease (particularly severe in infants) due to the elaboration of either a heat-labile toxin (LT) or a heat-stable (ST) toxin, both of which are coded for by plasmids. The mechanism of action of LT resembles that of choleratoxin in stimulating the production of adenosine $3',5'$-cyclic monophosphate (cAMP) in small bowel epithelial cells. Certain enteroinvasive strains have been recognized that cause true dysentery (diarrhea with blood and pus) with invasion of the mucosa, in contrast to the cholera-like clinical picture caused by enterotoxin.

The invasive character of these strains is probably also plasmid coded. Serogrouping of *E. coli* outbreaks is of value only as an epidemiologic tool and not in the routine analysis of nonepidemic isolates. Travelers' diarrhea, frequently due to toxigenic *E. coli,* may be prevented (but not treated) by administration of doxycycline (100 mg/day), a long-acting tetracycline analogue.

INFECTIONS DUE TO VIBRIONACEAE

The family Vibrionaceae comprises four genera: *Vibrio, Aeromonas, Plesiomonas,* and *Campylobacter* (Gr. campylo, curved)

The principal agents of cholera are *V. cholerae* and *V. eltor*. *V. cholerae* resembles *Salmonella typhi* in many respects but is common-shaped (*V. comma* in older literature). Whereas all motile Enterobacteriaceae have peritrichous flagella, those of *V. cholerae* are polar. In contrast to *S. typhi, V. cholerae* is proteolytic and grows well in alkaline (*p*H 9) medium (*e.g.* TCBS agar).

V. cholerae resembles *S. typhi* in being an intestinal pathogen restricted to humans, and in modes of transmission, surviving for long periods in polluted water. Also like *S. typhi,* it contains heat-stable O antigens, lipopolysaccharide endotoxin and a heat-labile flagellar antigen.

Antigenic groupings (I to VI) are based on at least three type-specific O antigens: A, B, and C. The Inaba group is designated AC; Ogawa group, AB; Hikojima group, ABC. The Inaba and Ogawa antigenic types are included in vaccines. For diagnosis, an O-group serum with Inaba and Ogawa immunoglobulins is sufficient since all *V. cholerae* and El Tor vibrios are agglutinated by these.

V. eltor causes endemic and epidemic choleralike disease (El Tor cholera), generally with lower death rates than in *V. cholerae* outbreaks. It is of importance in Malaysia and adjacent areas. Both *V. cholerae* and *V. eltor* agglutinate with cholera serum of O group I (A). All may be variants of a common stock. Cholera vibrios also share O antigens with *Brucella,* so that persons who have received cholera vaccine may show significant levels of serum agglutinins for *Br. abortus,* the standard test antigen (see below). The El Tor vibrio produces hemolysin (Greig positive) and its cultures agglutinate chick erythrocytes. Unlike *V. cholerae,* it kills chick embryos, resists polymyxin and group IV choleraphage.

There are saprophytic species of vibrios and some that are pathogenic for lower animals: *V.*

metschnikovi (pigeons); *V. proteus; V. fetus* (sheep, cattle, goats, sometimes humans).

In *V. cholerae,* multiplication of the vibrios is entirely in the gut, with the endotoxin producing intense gastritis and nausea and irritation of the bowel, chiefly the ileum. The exotoxin produced by *Vibrio* is the prototypic enterotoxin, which causes fluid secretion through the activation of tissue adenylcyclase to increase intestinal cAMP concentration. Similar LTs are produced by *E. coli* and all are coded for by transmissible plasmids. Ingestion of contaminated water leads to the penetration of the mucous layer and colonization of the lining epithelium of the small intestine by the vibrios. The epithelium remains intact, but it passes immense quantities of water fluid, turbid with mucus ("rice water" stools), with resulting dehydration, hemoconcentration, electrolyte imbalance, toxemia, and shock. Administration of fluids and electrolytes is of critical importance and is dramatically effective in therapy. Without treatment, mortality in *V. cholerae* outbreaks may range from 5% to 75%.

Epidemic cholera is largely water borne, but sporadic cases may be transmitted by any raw foods contaminated with feces or vomitus of patients or of temporary carriers. Chronic carriers of *V. cholerae* seem to be rare, but convalescent carriers and mild, ambulatory cases seem to be common. The disease is at present absent from the Western Hemisphere but is endemic and epidemic in India and mainland Southeast Asia. Isolated outbreaks in Louisiana have been associated with ingestion of raw oysters taken from contaminated coastal waters.

Control measures are basically as in other enteric bacterial disease. Rigid inspection and control of travelers from endemic and epidemic areas are important in preventing the international spread of cholera.

Vaccines are required for United States travelers to the epidemic or endemic areas. Modern cholera vaccine consists of killed *V. cholerae* suspensions, 10^8 cells per ml, half Inaba, half Ogawa. Studies and experience in the Orient indicate the desirability of including El Tor vibrios. Protection begins about 10 days after vaccination and lasts only about 6 months. It is not very solid and should be reinforced by booster doses each 6 months. The vaccine also evokes antibodies that agglutinate *Brucella* organisms. Toxoid derived from the "permeability factor" or exotoxin is currently under field trial.

Laboratory Diagnosis. Liquid (rice water) stools of patients may be examined microscopically for typical vibrios, blood, mucus, and pus. Cultivation of stools or suspect water in selective (*p*H 9.0) alkaline peptone water often yields prolific growth of the vibrios in a surface pellicle after 6 to 8 hours at 37°C. This pellicle may be examined microscopically and used to inoculate plates of a special thiosulfate–citrate–bile-salts (T-C-B-S) medium containing 1 : 200,000 KTe for selectivity, for isolation of colonies, also for a rapid, preliminary, slide agglutination test. Colonies resemble those of *Shigella.* Final identification depends on morphology, cultural properties, and serologic tests.

Neither serum nor chemotherapy is of recognized value in cholera.

Vibrio parahemolyticus is an inhabitant of saline, estuarine, coastal waters and is very similar to *V. cholerae.* It causes a severe form of gastroenteritis associated especially with consumption of insufficiently cooked or raw shellfish. It differs from *V. cholerae* in requiring 3% to 7% NaCl in the culture medium, growth at 43°C, ability to metabolize chitin, and positive Greig reaction. It is transmitted by the fecal–oral route and by sewage-contaminated foods and water.

Campylobacter infections are important in veterinary medicine; and animal disease (cattle, dogs, fowl) may be an important source of human infection, which may also spread from person to person (*e.g.,* small children with diarrhea in day-care centers). *Campylobacter jejuni* causes enteric disease in any age group. *C. fetus* is a cause of opportunistic infection in debilitated patients and pregnant women; fatal septicemic infections of newborns may be endogenous from the mother.

Also, *C. pyloridis* isolated in 1982 is currently being touted as a cause of 77% of duodenal and gastric ulcers. Thus, antimicrobial treatment together with acid antagonist therapy may prove to be the treatment of choice in the future for these ailments.

Pathogenic, Gram-Positive, Pyogenic Cocci

STREPTOCOCCI

For convenience, three subdivisions of streptococci may be made on the basis of types of hemolytic zones produced around colonies on sheep or rabbit blood agar plates incubated aerobically at 37°C, as follows:

Hemolytic

1. Beta type ("Strep hemolyticus," "beta hemolytic strep," etc.). With one or two exceptions, these comprise the pyogenic group of streptococci. They form a clear, colorless zone of he-

molysis, devoid of intact erythrocytes around small colonies.

2. Alpha type ("Strep viridans," "green strep"). These form a greenish zone of intact erythrocytes around small colonies, with varying degrees of hemolysis at the periphery. The group includes *S. mitis, S. mutans, S. salivarius, S. bovis, S. thermophilus, S. faecium, S. pneumoniae,* and others.

Nonhemolytic

3. Gamma type ("indifferent strep," "nonhemolytic strep"). These produce no visible change in the blood around their colonies. The group includes *S. lactis,* some of the Enterococcus group: *S. faecalis, S. liquefaciens,* etc. (Table 5-9).

Serologic Subdivisions of Streptococci. Lancefield subdivided the **beta-type** hemolytic streptococci into immunologic groups on the basis of cell wall polysaccharide antigens. Grouping is done with highly specific antisera as a precipitin reaction or with counterimmunoelectrophoresis (CIE), using streptococcal extracts, as a coagglutination reaction with antibody-coated staphylococcal cells (protein A) or latex particles, or by ultraviolet light microscopy of bacterial cells stained with fluorescein-labeled antibody (Table 5-5). The Lancefield groups are lettered A to U and, with a few exceptions, are beta hemolytic.

Over 90% of strains isolated from human disease are members of group A, including the classic *Streptococcus pyogenes* from human sources. *S. pyogenes* is the principal human pathogen, causing scarlet fever, septic sore throat, erysipelas, puerperal sepsis, empyema, meningitis. Group A strains are sensitive to bacitracin; most other beta-hemolytic streptococci are resistant. All group A strains are sensitive to penicillin, the drug of choice for therapy and/or prophylaxis of acute rheumatic fever.

Group B strains are a frequent cause of neonatal infections (especially type 3) and are distinguished from all others in producing double-zone ("hot-cold") beta hemolysis, hydrolyzing sodium hippurate, and positive CAMP test. These are mainly *S. agalactiae* strains.

Group D streptococci include enterococci *(S. faecalis)* and are found in miscellaneous human infections such as arthritis, sinusitis, endocarditis, and cystitis, probably as opportunistic invaders. Group D streptococci, although usually indifferently hemolytic (γ), may be viridans or, less frequently, beta-hemolytic. All group D streptococci grow on bile–esculin (B–E) agar with a positive reaction; only enterococci grow in broth containing 6.5% NaCl, which allows one to distinguish them from nonenterococci.

Other groups, through K, Q, and T, occur in lower animals or in dairy products. A few alpha-type and gamma-type *(e.g., S. lactis)* streptococci contain Lancefield group N antigens.

The determination of the Lancefield group of a beta-hemolytic streptococcus is of diagnostic and prognostic value as well as an index to epidemiology and therapy.

A further subdivision of group A streptococci is made into more than 60 numbered serologic types on the basis of precipitin tests with type-specific soluble protein antigens (M proteins) in these streptococci. M proteins are antiphagocytic and therefore are essential to virulence. M protein is the only streptococcal antigen that is protective to the host, in that it protects against reinfection with the same serological type. The M types of group A streptococci are related to certain clinical conditions; for example, types 1, 3, 4, 6, 12 and 25 have been found to predominate in certain epidemics in which acute hemorrhagic nephritis was a prominent complication of acute pharyngitis. Type 2 and a few higher serotypes (49, 55, 57, 59, 60, 61) have been reported as the cause of pyoderma-associated acute glomerulonephritis (AGN). This fact accounts for the sporadic occurrence and geographic localization of AGN in contrast to the relatively constant seasonal incidence of ARF without evident geographic localization in temperate climates. There is little or no cross-immunity between M types. Therefore, repeated group A streptococcal infections may occur in the same individual, each caused by a different M type of streptococcus.

Other cell wall fractions of group A streptococci include acid- and heat-labile but trypsin-resistant T proteins. These can be used as antigens to prepare specific antisera that differentiate some 45 T-agglutinin types. T-agglutination typing is useful in epidemiologic studies on group-A *Streptococcus* infection, especially when M antigens are ill-defined.

Fibrinolysin or *streptokinase* is a protein elaborated by streptococci of groups A, C, and G that activates a serum enzyme, plasmin, able to digest supposedly protective, retaining, fibrin clots that may be formed around infected lesions. *Antifibrinolysin* or *antistreptokinase* appears in the blood of patients recovering from infections with streptococci of these groups and, if increasing in titer, is of diagnostic value.

Beta-type streptococci of group A also produce at least two kinds of soluble hemolysin: S and O. *Streptolysin O* is readily oxidized and appears, in blood agar plates, only around subsurface colonies unless anaerobically incubated. *Streptolysin S* is sensitive to heat, acid, or both, but *not* to oxygen. A significant increase in titer of antistreptolysin O (ASO) or of other antienzymes (streptozyme test) during beta-hemolytic streptococcal infection, especially respiratory infections, is of diagnostic significance in relation to the subsequent emergence of acute rheumatic fever (ARF). *Streptolysin S* is not antigenic.

Capsules and Hyaluronidase. Group A streptococci, especially M types 4 and 22, form protective capsules of hyaluronic acid, a slimy polysaccharide. These capsules may be hydrolyzed by **hyaluronidase,** produced in varying amounts by the streptococci themselves. Although this may offset the antiphagocytic effect of the capsules, it can also digest the ground substance of the connective tissues and has therefore been regarded by some as a spreading factor, permitting invasion of the tissues by the streptococci.

Streptodornase is an enzyme found in cultures of beta-type streptococci that digests deoxyribonucleic acid (hence strepto-*dorn*ase). Much of the slimy, fibrinous exudate in empyema and other conditions consists of fibrin and DNA from lysed leukocytes. Streptokinase and streptodornase have clinical use in chemical debridement of such highly viscous exudates. Antibodies to hyaluronidase and/or to deoxyribonuclease B have the same significance as ASO. In the absence of a significant elevation in one or more of these antienzymes (titer greater than 1/100), a diagnosis of ARF is most unlikely. In streptococcal pyoderma, little or no ASO response may occur, but anti-DNase titers rise.

Infections by Streptococci

Scarlet Fever and Septic Sore Throat. The surface of group A beta-hemolytic streptococci contains lipoteichoic acid residues by which the bacterial cells adhere to specific receptors on mucosal cells in the oropharynx; additional virulence factors (*e.g.,* M protein, numerous extracellular enzymes) interfere with phagocytosis and activation of the alternate C pathway and allow the bacteria to invade the host more deeply. Many strains of *C. pyogenes* (group A) produce an exotoxin (erythrogenic or scarlet-fever toxin) that, when absorbed by the susceptible host, produces the nausea, chills, fever and rash of scarlet fever.

Like the toxin of *Corynebacterium diphtheriae,* erythrogenic toxin is produced only by lysogenic streptococci *(lysogenic conversion).*

Scarlet fever and septic sore throat are two manifestations of the same infection. In both, a septic sore throat is present. Persons susceptible to the erythrogenic toxin also develop a rash and are said to have scarlet fever. Persons insusceptible to the toxin, that is, with antitoxic immunity, have no rash, and such cases are diagnosed as septic sore throat. Reinfections and septic sore throat without rash, due to different M types of toxigenic streptococci, are possible.

Transmission of streptococcal infections is as for respiratory infections in general: oronasopharyngeal secretions and contact.

For diagnostic cultures, swabbings from nose or throat are streaked on blood agar, and undercut or, better, emulsified in broth that is then used to inoculate blood agar pour plates to obtain subsurface colonies. Beta-type hemolytic colonies found after 24 hours at 35°C are fished to blood broth and incubated. Pure cultures may be subjected to appropriate differential tests shown in Table 5-5.

In severe cases septicemia may develop, and blood cultures (10 ml of blood in 150 ml of tryptose broth) are of utmost importance as a guide to treatment.

Acute rheumatic fever is a nonsuppurative sequel to group A streptococcal infection only (acute pharyngitis and tonsillitis and inapparent infection). There is a relatively constant level of incidence up to 3% following all untreated cases regardless of the serotype. Clear delineation of the pathogenesis of ARF has thus far eluded investigators and is made even more difficult by the lack of a suitable experimental animal model. Several factors are thought to have a role in producing tissue damage (*e.g.,* Aschoff bodies characteristically seen in the myocardium, preceded by ''rheumatic inflammation'' of connective tissue). The most important factors are immunological, primarily the incontrovertible role of antecedent upper respiratory tract infection with group A streptococci and the production of antibodies and cell-mediated immune responses to streptococcal antigen(s) (*e.g.,* M protein, protoplast membrane?) cross-reactive with host tissue; some form of autoimmunity has been proposed but remains unproven. Patients with a history of ARF are about 10 times more at risk of recurrence of ARF with each successive acute group A streptococcal infection than are persons without known previous history of streptococcal infection. ARF can be effectively prevented by prompt and adequate penicillin treatment of acute streptococcal pharyngitis.

The pathogenesis of AGN revolves primarily around the subepithelial deposition of immune complexes, containing immunoglobulin and streptococcal antigens, in the glomerular basement membrane, where the C cascade is triggered locally to cause an acute inflammatory reaction and transient impairment of renal function. AGN is usually completely reversible; chronic nephritis rarely if ever results. Circulating immune complexes are also encountered in patients with poststreptococcal AGN. Prompt penicillin treatment of acute pharyngitis caused by nephritogenic strains reduces the incidence of AGN.

Other Streptococcal Infections. Beta hemolytic streptococci of any Lancefield group, but especially groups A, C, and G, may cause various nonepidemic infections, such as otitis media, empyema, sore throat, erysipelas, and meningitis. Puerperal sepsis may be transmitted to parturient women by carriers of beta hemolytic streptococci, which are common, and by unsterile hands, instruments, gloves, dressings, dust.

Group B streptococci (*S. agalactiae,* four serotypes) are found in 25% of normal vaginas and from this source may cause severe and often fatal neonatal infection. "Early onset" disease, due to any of the four serotypes and fatal in up to 60% of cases, occurs during the first postnatal week in association with prematurity and/or obstetric complications; it is characterized chiefly by "respiratory distress syndrome" (pneumonia) and septicemia. "Delayed onset" disease, with lower mortality, is caused usually by type III (either maternally acquired or nosocomial) and is characterized by meningitis, septicemia, and/or more localized infections.

Maternal antibody to group B streptococci protects infants at risk from ascending infection by B streptococci. About 5% of the group B strains are nonhemolytic and may therefore be missed. Up to 30% of the strains may be bacitracin sensitive and thus may be mistaken for group A streptococci. Definitive identification is made by fluorescent antibody techniques and by the CAMP test. Penicillin and related antibiotics are effective in the treatment of these infections in which early diagnosis is life-saving.

Group G beta-hemolytic streptococci may normally inhabit the vagina, oropharynx, gastrointestinal tract, or skin, and from any of these sites (most often the skin) can be introduced into the blood stream and cause serious infection, particularly in patients with neoplastic disease. Maternally derived group G streptococci also may cause neonatal sepsis and respiratory distress syndrome. All strains of group G streptococci are sensitive to penicillin.

Alpha-hemolytic (viridans) streptococci fall into several serogroups and some are untypable. *S. mutans,* by virtue of its capacity to produce high-molecular-weight dextran, is a prime cause of dental plaque formation that, if unchecked, leads directly to dental caries. *S. mitis* and *S. sanguis* are the viridans streptococci most commonly causing endocarditis. All viridans streptococci are universally found in the normal oropharynx and from this site may gain transient entrance into the blood following minor trauma to the supporting periodontal tissues. In patients with damaged endocardial surfaces (healed rheumatic fever, congenital deformities, prostheses), these otherwise noninvasive bacteria of low intrinsic virulence are the primary cause of endocarditis initiated at the site of endocardial discontinuity or denudation. In the same way, group D streptococci account for up to 10% of endocardial infections. If endocarditis is suspected, a persistent effort should be made prior to therapy to recover organisms from the blood. To this end, bidaily cultures should be made until at least three separate blood samples yield the same organisms, for which the minimal inhibitory concentrations of penicillin and streptomycin should be determined. Upon primary isolation, most group D and many viridans streptococci are relatively resistant to penicillin *in vitro* but still yield clinically to adequate dosage of combined antibiotics, usually penicillin and streptomycin with the adjunctive administration of probenecid.

Streptococcus pneumoniae, distinguished from viridans streptococci by sensitivity to optochin, is the most common cause of lobar pneumonia and a frequent cause of meningitis. There are 84 serotypes determined by the capsular swelling reaction with type-specific rabbit antisera. Types 1, 2, 3, 4, 7, 8, 12, and 14 are most virulent. The capsular polysaccharide is antiphagocytic (*i.e.,* the chief virulence factor) and is also the protective antigen.

C polysaccharide is a cell wall group-specific antigen (as opposed to type-specific capsular polysaccharides) which has the unique property of reacting, in the presence of calcium, with a beta-globulin (C-reactive protein, CRP) present in small amounts in normal serum. Serum CRP levels increase in response to any kind of tissue inflammatory reaction (*e.g.,* ARF). CRP in serum is detected and measured by reactivity (precipitin tests, CIE, ELISA) with specially prepared rabbit antisera to CRP (which is readily isolated and purified from human serum). CRP levels are accorded the same significance as other nonspecific "acute phase reactants" (e.g., erythrocyte sedimentation rate). The binding of CRP to C substance in the bacterial cell wall activates complement and promotes phagocytosis; CRP can thus be considered a nonspecific host-protective factor. Certain extracellular pneumococcal enzymes (e.g., neuraminidase) may contribute to virulence.

A vaccine is now available composed of purified capsular polysaccharides of 23 pneumococcal types that account for over 90% of infections. The vaccine is effective in preventing pneumococcal pneumonia in selected high-risk populations in which the case fatality rate of treated bacteremia exceeds 25% (e.g., patients compromised by kyphoscoliosis, diabetes, cellular immune deficiencies, sickle cell disease, splenectomy). Vaccine should not be given to children under 2 years of age or to pregnant women. Most strains of S. pneumoniae are sensitive to penicillin at levels easily achieved in the blood stream. Since 1967, however, strains resistant to penicillin have been encountered with increasing frequency. Resistance to multiple antibiotics has been reported (strain 19A), suggesting that antibiograms should be done on significant clinical isolates.

Respiratory infection with S. pneumoniae is not highly contagious. In contrast to lobar pneumonia, which almost always yields to appropriate antibiotic treatment, pneumococcal meningitis carries a high mortality despite what appears to be adequate treatment. Counterimmunoelectrophoresis is an important aid in diagnosis of meningeal infection when viable organisms cannot be recovered in cultures of the spinal fluid.

PEPTOSTREPTOCOCCI

Strictly anaerobic streptococci are grouped together in the genus *Peptostreptococcus*, in which there are at least six species, identifiable by gas–liquid chromatography of metabolic products. Peptostreptococci are commensal inhabitants of the oral cavity, the lower intestinal tract, and the female genitourinary tract, from any of which sites they can be hematogenously disseminated (by trauma, surgery, etc.) to cause foul-smelling purulent infection in various organs (e.g., lung, paranasal sinuses, brain, liver, pelvic organs) and septicemia. Localized infections are usually polymicrobial, including, besides anaerobic streptococci, other commensal anaerobes such as *Bacteroides*, *Propionibacterium*, *Fusobacterium*, and *Peptococcus*. *Peptococcus* species are similar to peptostrepto-

cocci in that both are anaerobic, gram-positive cocci. They differ in that peptococci tend to grow in clumps, while peptostreptococci grow in chains of cocci. Both are uniformly sensitive to penicillin.

STAPHYLOCOCCI

Staphylococcal Infections. Staphylococci cause numerous types of suppurative inflammatory conditions in any part of the body. They commonly form abscesses and furuncles of the skin and produce a number of metabolites of varying degrees of toxicity. *Staphylococcus aureus* is now a leading cause of frequently fatal endocarditis, particularly in intravenous drug users. In the course of staphylococcal endocarditis, cryoglobulins and circulating immune complexes (CIC) are found, the latter being the triggering mechanism for glomerulonephritis. CIC levels decline when the infection is arrested by chemotherapy. Most pathogenic strains produce β-type hemolysis (but not α type) on blood-agar plates. Staphylococci are much hardier than streptococci (resist drying, can survive a wide temperature range of 4°C to 60°C), grow vigorously on media like those used for streptococci, but are somewhat less fastidious as to temperature (15°C to 40°C) and requirements for blood or serum, though they also require organic N and glucose. Like streptococci, they are facultative anaerobes. Blood agar with mannitol, 7% NaCl, and tellurite is a useful selective medium.

Staphylococci differ from streptococci in producing catalase, having cytochrome systems, and in producing, at 25°C, large opaque, white, cream-colored, or butter-yellow colonies. *S. aureus* tends to produce more yellow pigment than *S. epidermidis*, especially in pus. Resistance of staphylococci to penicillin is transmissible by plasmids that code for penicillinase. Most strains of *S. aureus* pathogenic for humans are characterized by the production of the enzyme coagulase (*bound* or *free*), which induces clotting of citrated or oxalated human or rabbit plasma. Other characters often associated with (but not necessarily the cause of) pathogenicity of *S. aureus* are: fermentation of mannitol; elaboration of acid phosphatase, β-lactamase (penicillinase), protease, hyaluronidase, lysozyme, catalase, deoxyribonuclease; protein A (in cell wall), which binds to Fc portion of immunoglobulins, is antiphagocytic and anticomplementary; several hemolysins or toxins, including exfoliatin (which causes the "scalded skin syndrome") and enterotoxins (causing acute gastroenteritis). In *Staphylococcus au-*

reus, species-specific polysaccharide A is composed of *N*-acetylglucosamine residues attached alpha or beta to a polyribitol phosphate backbone and is associated with cell-wall peptidoglycan. Antibodies to teichoic acids become markedly elevated in staphylococcal septicemia and endocarditis. Measurement of anti-teichoic acid antibody (by CIE) is valuable in gauging antibiotic therapy. Exaggerated hypersensitivity to staphylococcal components develops in certain individuals with persistent staphylococcal infections, particularly chronic furunculosis; in these cases cell-mediated immune responses may contribute to the accentuated inflammatory reactions usually observed. *Staphylococcus epidermidis* species-specific polysaccharide B is composed of polyglycerol P-teichoic acid with beta-linked glycosyl residues.

S. epidermidis and nonpathogenic micrococci are ubiquitous on the human skin. Infections by *S. epidermidis* are typically superficial and rarely severe, except for occasional opportunistic infections (*e.g.,* urinary tract infections resulting from catheterization) and postoperative endocarditis associated with cardiac valve prostheses.

Phage Types and Antibiotic Resistance. Differential sensitivity to 20 or more staphylococcal bacteriophages (divided for convenience into lytic groups I to IV) provides a means of identifying the source and distribution of pathogenic strains, for example, nosocomial infections. Most strains of *S. aureus* in the community, and all hospital strains (*i.e.,* carried asymptomatically by personnel) are resistant to penicillin. Beta-lactamase–resistant drugs (*e.g.,* methicillin, oxacillin, nafcillin, cephalosporins) are used in therapy. Some staphylococcal strains exhibit a type of genome-encoded resistance unrelated to penicillinase, that is, intrinsic resistance (*e.g.,* to methicillin). Patients allergic to penicillin can be treated with vancomycin or trimethoprim-sulfamethoxazole.

Food Poisoning. Some strains of coagulase-positive staphylococci produce a thermostable exotoxin (enterotoxin) that, when ingested, causes acute staphylococcal food poisoning or gastroenteritis. There are at least five antigenic types of staphylococcal enterotoxin (A to E).

Heat-stable enterotoxin is preformed in contaminated food that has been allowed to stand at 20°C to 38°C (room or incubating temperature) for some hours. A wide variety of foods is suitable for growth of staphylococci.

Contamination of foods, resulting in staphylococcal food poisoning, often is traced to food handlers who have abscesses or boils on hands or arms or in the nose. Foods exposed openly in shops and cafeterias may be infected by coughing and sneezing workers or customers.

Intoxication is characterized primarily by the sudden onset of nausea and vomiting after a short incubation period (2 to 6 hours) and is unaccompanied by fever. Dehydration may be severe and even life-threatening, particularly in infants and elderly or debilitated patients. True enterocolitis (bloody diarrhea, necrotizing lesions of small and/or large bowel) as contrasted with acute upper gastroenterointoxication may be caused by antibiotic-resistant strains that colonize the colon, overgrowing the normal flora and producing enterotoxin in situ. Another soluble exotoxin (exofoliatin) produced particularly by strains of phage group II causes the scalded skin syndrome, bullous impetigo, and scarlatiniform rash.

Toxic Shock Syndrome. Toxic shock syndrome (TSS) is an acute and occasionally fatal illness resulting from infection with *Staphylococcus aureus* (usually of phage group I); it is characterized by signs of acute intoxication (fever, hypotension, scarlatiniform rash) and is usually, but not invariably, associated with the use of specific types of vaginal tampons. The product most regularly elaborated by TSS-associated strains of *Staphylococcus* is an exoprotein (TSSE), which has recently been shown to be identical to pyrogenic exotoxin C (PE-C) and enterotoxin F, also elaborated by these lysogenic strains. Toxic shock toxin (TST) has an immunosuppressive effect evidenced by depressed reticuloendothelial system (RES) clearance and IgM synthesis, increased sensitivity to endotoxin (from indigenous gram-negative flora), and enhanced delayed type acquired hypersensitivity possibly accounting for the exfoliation seen in TSS.

Gram-Negative Cocci

INFECTIONS DUE TO NEISSERIA

This genus, found only in humans, is named for Neisser, first to recognize (in 1879) the causative agent of gonorrhea.

Gonorrhea. Although no demonstrable *exo*toxins are produced, the organisms contain endotoxin (LPS) and are highly pyogenic. Gaining entrance to suitable tissues such as glandular or mucosal surfaces of the genitalia, especially those covered by columnar epithelium, they produce an intense inflammatory exudate. Usually within less than 10 (1 to 31) days of infection there is a rapid formation of thick, mucopurulent exudate from the posterior urethra of males or from the cervix. Invasion of neighboring tissues (*e.g.,* prostate and fallopian tubes) often occurs and uncommonly there is bacteremia with arthritis and endocarditis. The gonococci in an infected mother may gain entrance to the conjunctival sac of the infant during birth, causing severe ophthalmia **(ophthalmia neonatorum).** Thus, in males urethritis is most common with a heavy urethral discharge and dysuria, while in females cervicitis with a light to heavy discharge and abdominal pain is commonly seen.

Gonococcal ophthalmia of adults may occur as a result of autoinfection. Gonococci may be found in the urethra, prostate, Bartholin's glands, cervix, vagina, rectum.

N. gonorrhoeae can cause meningitis with septicemia. Disseminated gonococcemia may result in arthritis and/or acute endocarditis. The organism may also be found in the posterior nasopharynx and can cause tracheitis and pneumonitis. *N. meningitidis* can likewise be found in the genital tract and cause essentially all of the same syndromes as *N. gonorrhoeae.* Gonorrhea continues to increase in prevalence, especially among teenagers, in company with syphilis and chlamydial infection. The latter currently exceeds gonorrhea in epidemiological importance.

In the diagnosis of gonorrheal urethritis, gram-stained smears are made of fresh exudate; detection of "gram-negative intracellular diplococci" resembling *N. gonorrhoeae* is good presumptive evidence, which should be confirmed by culture on Thayer-Martin agar (containing vancomycin, colistin, nystatin) incubated in a candle jar or CO_2 incubator. In females, smears are not reliable (many vaginal commensal organisms resemble *N. gonorrhoeae* morphologically); endocervical culture is mandatory. Oxidase-positive colonies detected on primary culture are inoculated into semisolid agar with differential sugars (glucose, maltose, sucrose). *N. gonorrhoeae* ferments only dextrose, *N. meningitidis,* dextrose and maltose; commensal organisms, all three. Definitive identification can be made with fluorescent antibody on appropriately fixed smears of exudate or of cultures. *N. gonorrhoeae* of the small colony types (T1, T2) usually isolated from fresh gonorrheal exudates possess pili that mediate initial attachment to cells and have inherent antiphagocytic (virulence) properties. Pili are the protective antigen of gonococci: antibodies to pili have been shown to protect against experimental infection in primates.

Penicillin is the drug of choice in treatment of gonorrhea; blood levels achieved with high dose (4.8 million units of procaine penicillin G) regimens may be enhanced by the administration of benemid. However, because of the high incidence of concurrent chlamydial infection (in heterosexual as well as homosexual patients), trimethoprim plus sulfamethoxazole and tetracycline are currently recommended to reduce the risk of persistent post-gonococcal chlamydial disease (nongonococcal urethritis, NGU, pelvic inflammatory disease, PID). Penicillin-producing *N. gonorrhoeae* (PPNG) (these are mostly strains imported from the Far East, and not indigenous strains that have acquired penicillinase plasmids) as well as indigenous strains showing chromosomally mediated resistance (CMRNG) to penicillin are being encountered with increasing frequency. Infection due to PPNG or CMRNG is best treated with spectinomycin, resistance to which, although reported, is still infrequent; tetracycline may be added to treat coexistent chlamydial infection. Spectinomycin-resistant gonorrhea should be treated with cefoxitin plus probenecid; for pharyngitis due to PPNG, trimethoprim plus sulfamethoxazole should be used. Norfloxacin (a relative of nalidixic acid) has been used successfully in uncomplicated urethritis due to these resistant strains. Causes of NGU include *Chlamydia trachomatis* and *Ureaplasma urealyticum.* Rapid diagnosis of chlamydial infection is achieved on freshly smeared exudate by staining with specific anti-chlamydial fluorescent antibody (or indirectly with specific monoclonal antibody and fluorescent antiglobulin) and detecting the presence of specifically stained elementary bodies of *C. trachomatis.* Neisserial ophthalmia neonatorum may be prevented by the instillation (mandatory in most states) of 1% silver nitrate solution; neonates born to mothers with known gonococcal infection should receive systemic penicillin therapy. Neonatal infection due to PPNG should be treated with cefotaxime or gentamicin.

Meningococcal Disease. *Neisseria meningitidis* colonizes the posterior nasopharynx in about 5% to 30% of normal individuals; in epidemics carrier rates can approach 95%. From this site; meningococci may spread to cause pneumonia or may invade the blood stream to cause meningitis, purpura, and endotoxic shock. Chronic meningococcemia should suggest itself as a possible cause of unexplained recurrent generalized petechial hemorrhages. Overwhelming meningococcemia with widespread intravascular coagulation and adrenal cortical hemorrhage (Waterhouse–Friderichsen syndrome) may result. Serum antibody to the meningococcus tends to increase with age beyond 6 months to 1 year, as a result of colonization with different species of cross-reactive nonpathogenic *Neisseria*. Maximum incidence of meningitis is from 6 months (no maternal antibody) to about 2 years. (The same general incidence pattern obtains with *Hemophilus influenzae* type b and *Streptococcus pneumoniae*.) Asymptomatic carriers of *N. meningitidis* are the source of infection of contacts via droplets of respiratory secretion. As the carrier rate in a given population increases, the potential for epidemic meningitis intensifies proportionally. The carrier state itself is an immunizing process; carriers rarely if ever contract overt disease. The risk of secondary cases among household contacts of a case of meningitis (meningococcal or *Hemophilus*) is more than 600 times greater than in the general population.

N. meningitidis is divisible into nine serogroups (A, B, C, D, X, Y, Z, W135, 29E) on the basis of capsular polysaccharides. Group B polysaccharide is identical to the K_1 antigen of *E. coli*. Organisms of groups A, B, and C account for most meningococcal disease. Group B meningococci, currently the prevalent type in the United States, are sensitive to sulfadiazine; groups A and C are resistant. Primary isolation is made on chocolate agar; oxidase-positive colonies are transferred to semisolid differential sugar media (*N. meningitidis* ferments glucose and maltose, but not sucrose or lactose). Serotyping is done by agglutination or immunofluorescence. Examination of the cerebrospinal fluid reveals depressed sugar levels (compared with simultaneously drawn and measured blood sugar), and a polymorphonuclear leukocyte count that may be very high. In the absence of cultivable bacteria, spinal fluid should be examined by counterimmunoelectrophoresis (CIE) for polysaccharides of *Meningococcus*, *H. influenzae* type b, *Pneumococcus*, and *Cryptococcus*.

Treatment and Control. Penicillin G is still the drug of choice; chloramphenicol is an effective alternative in penicillin-sensitive patients. Currently an increasing number of sulfadiazine-sensitive strains are being encountered; sulfadiazine may therefore again become useful in treating meningococcal infection. Intimate household (or other) contacts of proven cases of meningococcal meningitis should be carefully watched for early signs; chemoprophylaxis may be undertaken with rifampicin or sulfadiazine (especially group B). Polysaccharide vaccines against groups A, C, Y, and W-135 are available, and their use should be considered in

community outbreaks according to individually assessed risk. Vaccines, however, are not effective in infants under 18 months of age.

INFECTIONS DUE TO BRUCELLA

Brucellosis (Undulant Fever). Undulant fever (Malta fever, Mediterranean fever, Bang's disease in cattle) may be caused by any of three species of the genus *Brucella*: *B. abortus*, *B. melitensis* (Melita, Malta), and *B. suis* (Table 5-5). The species names refer to geographic origin or affinities for respective animal hosts in which infectious abortion is prominant (*B. abortus*, cattle; *B. suis*, swine; *B. melitensis*, goats) and which are the sources of human infection. Brucellosis is contracted by ingestion of raw milk from infected cattle or goats, or by direct contact with effluvia or decidua of infected animals. Brucellosis is therefore an occupational hazard for farm, dairy, and abattoir workers; person-to-person transmission does not occur. Fetal tissues from infected animals contain high concentrations of erythritol (not present in significant amounts in human decidua), which serves as a growth factor for *Brucella*, thus accounting for the predilection of the organisms for animal fetal tissues. *Brucella* have potent endotoxic activity but do not form any exotoxin. These organisms invade the blood stream and localize in lymph nodes, liver, spleen, and glandular tissues; all are facultative intracellular parasites. *B. abortus* tends to form poorly organized granulomata; infections with *B. melitensis* or *B. suis* tend to cause the severest and most protracted clinical illness, which is protean in its manifestations and may include suppurative granulomata with central caseation. Relapses are not uncommon; and serious neurological sequelae have been reported.

A prolonged and variable antibody response characterizes most of these infections and is readily detectable as serum agglutinins for *B. abortus* (broadly cross-reactive with *B. melitensis* and *B. suis*). Agglutinins may be present in the absence of positive blood cultures and, above a certain level (usually about 1:160), are diagnostic. *Brucella* organisms cross-react with *Francisella tularensis* and *Vibrio cholerae*, a fact that must be born in mind in the interpretation of agglutination tests for brucellosis. Primary diagnosis is best made by repeated attempts at recovery of *Brucella* from the blood, from exudates, or from liver biopsy tissue. Blood cultures are taken under CO_2 (required for primary isolation of *B. abortus*) and incubated and periodically subcultured for up to a month. Isolates are speciated by biochemical reactions (Table 5-6) and immunofluorescence. Delayed hypersensitivity is a prominent feature of brucellosis and is concordant with the prolonged intracellular survival of the organisms and with the cell-mediated immune mechanisms involved in pathogenesis and containment of the infection. Diagnostic skin tests with brucellergen, a crude extract of the organism, are no longer recommended because of the risk of severe local and constitutional reactions.

Treatment and Control. Antibiotics of choice in treating proven brucellosis are tetracyclines, with streptomycin. For patients intolerant of tetracyclines, trimethoprim-sulfamethoxazole is used. Therapy should be prolonged well beyond recovery from acute clinical illness. In control of brucellosis, products and tissues of infected animals should be avoided; only pasteurized dairy products should be consumed. Farm animals, particularly cattle, should be tested for brucellosis (Bang's disease) periodically. In the face of threatened infection of a herd, immunization should be undertaken with live attenuated vaccine (attenuated *B. abortus,* strain 19), which itself, however, is the occasional cause of accidental infection in veterinarians and farm personnel. No vaccine is available for human use.

INFECTIONS DUE TO BORDETELLA

Pertussis and Related Diseases. *Bordetella pertussis* is the etiologic agent of pertussis (whooping cough). Syndromes much like classic pertussis, but milder, may be produced by *B. parapertussis* and, rarely, *B. bronchiseptica* (Table 5-4). All these organisms are related antigenically, and all are easily killed by heat, standard disinfectants, and sunlight.

In the initiation of infection in a susceptible individual, organisms enter the upper respiratory tract in droplets of saliva and mucus from patients with active pertussis. The organisms attach by fimbriae to epithelium, immobilizing the cilia. (The bacterial fimbriae also embody the hemagglutinin characteristic of organisms in young cultures and are part of the protective antigen of *B. pertussis*.). Once the respiratory tract has been colonized, there is damage to superficial epithelial layers by both endotoxin (pyrogenic LPS) and a heat-labile exotoxin, as well as by other biologically active substances elaborated by the organism (lymphocytosis-stimulating and histamine-sensitizing factors). As a result of these changes, the mucous membrane of the respiratory tract becomes hyperesthetic, thereby ac-

counting for the persistent and often strangling cough and stridor characteristic of full-blow pertussis. Obstructive edema and some degree of anoxia occur. With intractable coughing, anoxia may become severe and in infants and young children may trigger convulsions. Large numbers of organisms are found in the viscid, mucoid material coughed up during the first 2 to 3 weeks of the disease, but disappear after the fourth week. Carriers are unknown or very rare; bacteremia does not occur. Infection confers lasting immunity, in which both antibody and cellular factors are important.

Control. Infected children should be isolated from susceptibles for 5 weeks after onset. Susceptible children should be isolated for 3 weeks after last exposure unless examined daily by a physician or school nurse. Young children should never come in contact with infectious cases, since postpertussis pneumonia is a frequent cause of mortality in children under 5.

Three rough variants or phases 2, 3, 4 of low virulence and antigenicity occur in cultures undergoing S to R variation and are not associated with human disease. The vaccine in current use is made of phenol-killed encapsulated smooth (S) phase 1 *B. pertussis,* alum precipitated, and usually combined with alum-precipitated diphtheria and tetanus toxoids (DTP). Presently recommended schedules (CDC Advisory Committee on Immunization Practices) call for routine immunization of infants and children by subcutaneous inoculation with DTP at 2, 4, 6, and 18 months of age, with boosters at 4 to 6 years. Adult type D and P toxoids (Td) should be used after the seventh year. Infants and young children who have previously had convulsions (febrile or nonfebrile) are more likely to have seizures following initial pertussis immunization than those without this history. There is no evidence to suggest that seizures temporally associated with vaccine administration predispose to central nervous system damage. However, deferral of pertussis immunization in patients with any seizure history is recommended; severe reactions (*e.g.,* collapse, shock, persistent screaming episode, fever, or any neurological sign) are strong contraindications to the further administration of pertussis vaccine; this does not apply to diphtheria and tetanus toxoids, which can be independently administered.

Laboratory Diagnosis and Treatment. Plates of Bordet–Gengou blood agar, which may be made more selective by inclusion of methicillin and cycloheximide (to inhibit gram-positive organisms and fungi), are inoculated with fresh respiratory secretions obtained by pernasal swab. Plates are incubated at 35°C for at least 6 days and examined frequently for minute, pearly, hemolytic colonies. Colonies are fished to B-G and blood agar, gram-stained, and identified with immunofluorescence. The same material from the swab, smeared and examined directly by immunofluorescence, may yield an early presumptive diagnosis. Lymphocytosis is a frequent and diagnostic sign in the acute "whooping" stage. Antimicrobials have no effect on the clinical course once it has entered the paroxysmal stage. Erythromycin significantly reduces the number of *B. pertussis* in the respiratory tract; corticosteroids may favorably influence severe pertussis.

INFECTIONS DUE TO HEMOPHILUS

The hemophilic group includes *H. influenzae* (meningitis), *H. parainfluenzae* (endocarditis), *H. aegyptius* (conjunctivitis), and *H. ducreyi* (chancroid) (Table 5-4).

Hemophilus influenzae is a common resident of the normal upper respiratory tract; it does *not* cause the disease influenza, although formerly thought to do so; hence, the species misnomer. *H. influenzae* causes several diseases, including "pink-eye" conjunctivitis *(H. aegyptius),* purulent pansinusitis, and severe obstructive epiglottitis and tracheolaryngitis with septicemia. *H. influenzae* type b is the most frequent cause of bacterial meningitis in children 2 months to 5 years of age. This form of meningitis still carries an appreciable mortality, about 35%, and recovery is associated with a substantial incidence of neurological sequelae with 3% to 50% of survivors demonstrating some form of learning disability.

The several serotypes of *H. influenzae* (a to f) are recognized on the basis of capsular polysaccharides (polyribitol phosphate in type b) demonstrable by swelling reactions with type-specific antisera, as with pneumococci; the capsular polysaccharides have antiphagocytic properties and hence are a prime virulence factor. *H. influenzae* produces IgA protease, also possibly an additional factor in virulence. Blood cultures and sputum cultures on chocolate agar are usually positive in acute epiglottitis and laryngotracheobronchitis; blood and spinal fluid cultures are positive in meningitis. On Levinthal transparent agar, typable colonies of *H. influenzae* are immediately recognizable by their characteristic opalescence caused by the massed capsular material. Free capsular polysaccharide can also be detected in cerebrospinal fluid and urine by CIF, an important diagnostic adjunct in the absence of cultivable bacteria. Untypable *H. influenzae* is associated with otitis media in children and with bronchitis and bronchopneumonia in adults suffering from chronic pulmonary disease.

Up to 10% of strains of *H. influenzae* isolated from patients with severe disease are resistant to ampicillin; this resistance is coded for by a plasmid originally derived from *E. coli.* Treatment of meningitis, always life-threatening, should be promptly instituted with chloramphenicol alone or along with ampicillin pending results of the antibiogram. Immunization (after the age of 18 months) with purified capsular polysaccharide of *Hemophilus influenzae* type b has been found to reduce the incidence of meningitis in children between the age of 18 months and 10 years.

Chancroid. Chancroid (soft chancre) is an acute, inflammatory, localized and self-limited necrotizing disease, due to *Hemophilus ducreyi,* occurring on or near the genitalia. It begins as a small pustule, which soon ruptures, leaving an irregular, painful ulcer with undermined edges and a necrotic, erosive, soft base (soft chancre) that spreads rapidly. Like syphilis it usually produces buboes, but, unlike syphilis, these buboes are soft, painful, and often suppurate. Chancroid also differs from syphilitic chancre in the absence of induration and in its violent inflammatory nature. Chancroid-like lesions are sometimes due to (or involve) Herpes simplex virus type 2 and must be differentiated from syphilitic lesions.

Hemophilus ducreyi is typically seen with leukocytes, sometimes in small clusters ("school of fish" pattern) in direct smears, and morphologically resembles *H. influenzae. H. ducreyi* resembles *H. influenzae* also in being very fragile and susceptible to environmental conditions (Table 5-7).

Diagnosis is based largely on clinical findings and history of exposure. Smears of exudate in chancroid, or of pus aspirated from closed buboes, may reveal the organisms. Rabbit blood (25%) infusion agar (3%) under 10% CO_2 is essential for initial isolation of *H. ducreyi.*

Transmission is typically by sexual intercourse, rarely by fomites. The infection is autoinoculable; pus and exudates are infectious. Although broad-spectrum antibiotics (erythromycin) are effective in treatment, the use of antibiotics in any venereal disease entails the danger of masking syphilis, the diagnosis of which should always be excluded by darkfield examination of lesion scrapings and by serology. For this reason, trimethoprim-sulfamethoxazole is considered the treatment of choice.

INFECTIONS DUE TO YERSINIA AND FRANCISELLA

Plague-Like Diseases. This term includes plague, due to *Yersinia pestis;* tularemia, due to *Francisella tularensis;* and hemorrhagic septicemia, due to *Pasteurella multocida.*

All of the above are primarily *zoonoses* (animal diseases transmissible to humans) and are fundamentally alike in pathogenesis. All are, in varying degrees, generalized, hemorrhagic, and septicemic, with localization in various organs and tissues and in lymph nodes that become suppurative, painful buboes. In each disease the organisms occur in pathologic exudates (respiratory, ulcers, draining buboes, etc.).

P. multocida infection is neither common nor serious in man but is highly fatal in animals.

Bubonic Plague and Tularemia. In the advanced, septicemic stage in animals these diseases are transmissible to humans by the bites of arthropods: *Yersinia pestis* by rat fleas (*Xenopsylla cheopis* and others) and by arthropod parasites of ground squirrels and other rodents of forest and prairie (**sylvatic** and **campestral** plague, respectively). Plague-infected household pets, particularly cats, can be the source of infection via cat fleas. *Francisella tularensis* is transmitted by deer flies (*Chrysops discalis*) and various ticks (*Dermacentor variabilis, D. andersoni, etc.*). Human-to-humans transmission may also occur via fleas, *Pulex irritans.* In either disease an infectious pustule develops at the site of the bite. Local buboes develop (hence, "bubonic" plague); in many cases septicemia follows. Tularemia is also transmitted to humans by handling of carcasses of infected animals, notably wild rabbits, resulting in rabbit fever in hunters, market workers, cooks, and others. Lakes and streams contaminated from decaying infected animal carcasses may also be a source of infection by ingestion or inhalation.

The fatality rate in bubonic plague may range from 50% to 80% in untreated cases, but it is much less with early treatment. The less common septicemic plague, which if untreated may go on to pneumonia, is almost invariably fatal. Pneumonic plague may also be contracted by inhalation of respiratory droplets laden with *Y. pestis* from infected patients and is marked by deep cyanosis (the Black Death); when unrecognized and untreated the mortality is 100%.

Tularemia is often very severe, prolonged, and debilitating though rarely fatal if treated early with streptomycin and other broad-spectrum antibiotics. Fatality may range to 5% if untreated. Pulmonary tularemia is especially serious.

Rat flea–borne bubonic plague is prevented by measures that diminish contact between humans and rats (live or dead) and rat fleas. Elimination of open garbage dumps and rat-proofing of buildings are important measures. Dusting rat runways with insecticides to control the fleas, and antirat-poisoning campaigns are often effective. Pneumonic plague is controlled only by prompt diagnosis, immediate and rigid segregation of patients, and expert communicable-disease nursing. Streptomycin, chloramphenicol, and tetracycline are the drugs of choice for the tularemia. Uncomplicated bubonic plague responds to streptomycin, tetracycline, chloramphenicol, or sulfadiazine if treatment is begun early. Streptomycin or tetracyclines are preferred for septicemic plague. A living attenuated vaccine is recommended under special circumstances involving high risk of exposure (*e.g.*, laboratory workers). Chemoprophylaxis of plague contacts (*i.e.*, close household contacts) with either tetracycline or sulfadiazine is recommended.

Recovery from both tularemia and bubonic plague confers high-grade, durable immunity, evidenced by sustained levels of agglutinins, which are cross-reactive with *Fr. tularensis* and *V. cholerae.* Cell-mediated immune responses are important in containment of these infections.

In diagnosis, pathologic material stained with Wayson's stain (methylene blue and carbon fuchsin) reveals the organisms as ovoid rods. *Yersinia pestis* is distinguished by having well-marked bipolar staining, most of the cells resembling a closed safety pin. The other species show this character to a lesser degree. The polar granules tend to disappear in cultures.

Yersinia pestis grows well on any media, is motile, and produces an exotoxin and soluble protein antigen (fraction 1) that is antiphagocytic. The lipopolysaccharides of both *Francisella* and *Yersinia* contribute to clinical manifestations of disease. *Yersinia* exhibit capsules and bipolar staining and can be readily identified with fluorescent antibody. *Francisella tularensis* is difficult to recover on primary isolation, for which blood glucose cysteine agar or other media containing sufficient SH compounds are required; the organism is identified by specific agglutination or by fluorescent antibody. Phagocytized by polymorphonuclear leukocytes, *Y. pestis* is killed; in monocytes it survives, multiplies, forms capsules, and gains virulence. *Y. enterocolytica* is an increasingly recognized cause of diarrheal disease, mesenteric adenitis, and self-limited reactive arthritis (associated with HLA-B27).

Legionellaceae. A group of related bacterial pathogens are now subsumed in a newly established family, *Legionellaceae,* the most important member of which is *Legionella pneumophila,* the cause of legionnaires' disease. This was originally described as a fulminant pneumonia with high morbidity and mortality. It has generally been seen in either apparently healthy older patients (mean age of 55 years) or in high-risk renal dialysis and transplant patients as a nosocomial infection.

"Pontiac fever," a milder form of the disease, is characterized by pleuritis without pneumonia. The etiologic agent of both these entities was identified as a fastidious unencapsulated, aerobic, pleomorphic, motile, nonsporulating rod, capable of surviving intracellularly as well as in the environment, such as aquatic ecosystems. It is the source of human infection by inhalation of infectious droplets or dust. The organism has a worldwide distribution. Person-to-person transmission has not been documented. The organism *(Legionella pneumophila)* is cultivable on buffered charcoal yeast extract (BCYE) agar and identified by direct immunofluorescence. *Legionella* organisms, albeit gram-negative, stain weakly with Gram's stain; the bacterial cells can be demonstrated in tissues and smears of body fluids with silver impregnation stains and by direct immunofluorescence. By the latter technique, six serogroups of *L. pneumophila* are currently recognized. There are at least 23 other species within the genus, some of which cause milder forms of disease. "Pittsburgh fever," caused by *L. micdadei* is a pneumonic form that to date has been described only in immunosuppressed patients. Specific antibody response can be demonstrated by indirect immunofluorescence with paired sera; the duration of immunity to reinfection is unknown. *L. pneumophila* multiplies in human blood monocytes. Cell-mediated immunity is of prime importance and humoral immunity of relatively little importance in the containment of this infection. Antibiotics (erythromycin, rifampicin) that penetrate macrophages inhibit but do not kill *L. pneumophila,* a fact that probably helps explain the relapses that may follow antibiotic therapy. Erythromycin is the drug of choice in the treatment of any form of legionellosis, combined with rifampicin in the severest cases.

Actinomycetes and Related Organisms

INFECTIONS DUE TO *CORYNEBACTERIUM*

Diphtheria. *Corynebacterium* shares cell wall and other characteristics (cord factor, glycolipid, enzymes) with *Nocardia* and *Mycobacteria*. *C. diphtheriae,* the cause of diphtheria, occurs on the oropharyngeal mucosa and in active diseases may spread to larynx, trachea, bronchi, nares, and lips. Strictly aerobic, it is not invasive. However, at the sites of primary infection in the mucosa of the respiratory tract, or on the skin, pathogenic strains produce toxin that has both local and systemic effects on the host. In the respiratory tract, the toxin causes local irritation, an acute inflammatory reaction, and necrosis contributing to pseudomembrane formation. Acute airway obstruction may have to be relieved by intubation or tracheotomy. Toxin absorbed from the local lesion into the lymphatics and blood stream causes myocardial degeneration and peripheral neuritis.

Transmission from person to person occurs via infected respiratory secretions. Patients with active diphtheria should be isolated until two or three successive daily negative posterior nasal cultures have been obtained. If antibacterial chemotherapy has been employed, negative cultures are of no significance until 1 week after the last dose of drug. The age of incidence of diphtheria has shifted in recent years to involve those 30 to 50 years of age. Skin diphtheria is seen not infrequently, especially in the tropics where fungal infections of the skin may become secondarily infected with toxigenic *C. diphtheriae.*

The **Schick test** (undertaken to determine immunity or susceptibility to diphtherial toxin) consists of an intracutaneous injection of active toxin (0.02 guinea pig MLD). A positive reaction, appearing in 24 to 36 hours, consists of slight infiltration surrounded by a red areola 1 to 5 cm in diameter and is caused by the direct dermonecrotic action of the toxin; it is *not* in itself a hypersensitivity reaction. A typical positive reaction does not reach maximal intensity for at least 5 days and may be accompanied by necrosis and sloughing; it indicates that there is less than about 0.01 unit of circulating antitoxin per milliliter, that is, not enough to neutralize either the test toxin or any toxin that might emanate from naturally acquired diphtherial infection. A negative reaction (no erythema) indicates antitoxic immunity. A pseudoreaction, denoting delayed type hypersensitivity to diphtherial protein (engendered by colonization with commensal *Corynebacteria*), recedes after 36 to 48 hours, well before a positive reaction peaks. Persons giving pseudoreactions are immune to the toxin, but allergic to diphtherial protein. Such persons are at risk of having severe adverse reactions to the administration of toxoid. Adults who have a negative Schick test and who are therefore candidates for immunization should be tested first for type IV allergy to diphtherial protein (Moloney test: 0.1 ml. of 1 : 100 fluid toxoid intracutaneously). Positive Moloney reactors may already have antitoxic immunity or will develop it in response to the Moloney test itself. Only those with negative reactions to the Moloney test should be given adult (Td) toxoid.

Laboratory Diagnosis. On slants of Löffler's coagulated-serum medium or Pai's coagulated-egg medium the organisms grows readily at 35°C when inoculated with swabbings from local lesions. Stained with alkaline methylene blue, *C. diphtheriae* has a very distinctive beaded, barred, club-, spindle-, and dumbbell-shaped morphology readily recognized by the experienced bacteriologist. *C. diphtheriae* is readily isolated by streaking throat swabs on blood agar containing about 0.04% of potassium tellurite as a selective agent. Suspicious block colonies are fished to slants for pure culture study, including determinations of type and toxigenicity on freshly prepared Tinsdale (tellurite) agar. *C. diphtheriae* grows in black colonies surrounded by a brown "halo." Staphylococci and commensal *Corynebacteria* (diphtheroids) produce similar black colonies, but without halos. *Listeria monocytogenes* may be misdiagnosed as a "hemolytic diphtheroid."

Suspected diphtheriae-like organisms should be tested for toxigenicity by immunodiffusion (*in vitro* toxigenicity test). A simple form of the latter consists of embedding, in special serum-agar medium in a Petri dish, a strip of filter paper saturated with diphtheria antitoxin. After the agar hardens, the suspected culture is heavily streaked linearly across the agar surface at right angles to the paper. A precipitin reaction, visible as a white line in the agar, develops where toxin diffusing from virulent cultures meets antitoxin diffusing from the paper strip.

All pathogenic (toxigenic) strains of *C. diphtheriae* elaborate antigenically identical toxin. All toxigenic strains of *C. diphtheriae* carry a specific bacteriophage (corynephage beta) that codes for the toxin; strains that are not lysogenic are not toxigenic. The toxin is synthesized as a single polypeptide chain, which can be cleaved by trypsin (and probably tissue enzymes) to yield two portions: fragment A (which, once it is internalized, exerts toxic activity by blocking elongation factors in protein synthesis) and fragment B (which, about twice the size of fragment A, binds whole toxin to cell surfaces and facilitates internalization of toxin molecules). There is striking similarity between diphtherial toxin and other bacterial toxins (e.g., *Shigella* and cholera toxins, *E. coli* enterotoxin, pseudomonas exotoxin A, pertussis, anthrax, tetanus, botulinus toxins) in three general respects: An A–B enzyme-binding structure, receptor-mediated endocytotic penetration into target cells, and ADP-ribosylating activity.

Diphtheria antitoxin is produced commercially by immunization of horses with toxin or toxoid. The globulin fraction is concentrated by standard methods of serum fractionation and is "despeciated" by digestion with pepsin, which reduces its antigenicity by removing most of the Fc portion of the immunoglobulins. The final antitoxin product contains 20,000 units per milliliter and is still allergenic. To be effective (*i.e.*, prevent the effects of toxin on myocardial and neural tissues), antitoxin must be given by intramuscular injection as soon as the diagnosis is established, in order to neutralize free toxin in the circulation; toxin already fixed to tissues can no longer be neutralized. Administration of antitoxin should be preceded by a skin test for hypersensitivity to horse serum (0.1 ml of a 1 : 1000 dilution of antitoxin), and epinephrine should be at hand. Whenever antitoxin is administered, in the absence of demonstrable horse serum sensitivity, the development of serum sickness within a week or 10 days should be anticipated. Antibiotics (erythromycin and/or penicillin) are given to treat the upper respiratory tract infection and eliminate the organism, and hence prevent the carrier state. Tonsillectomy and adenoidectomy may be necessary to eliminate the carrier state which persists despite adequate antibiotic therapy.

Recommended immunization schedules (CDC Advisory Committee on Immunization Practices) for normal infants and children call for DTP at 2 to 3 months of age, followed by two boosters, respectively, at 2-month intervals, and a third at 18 months. DTP may be used through the seventh year, after which only adult toxoids (Td) should be administered in order to avoid severe reactions (see Table 5-21).

INFECTIONS DUE TO ACTINOMYCETALES

Tuberculosis. *Mycobacterium tuberculosis,* var. *hominis,* is the principal pathogen of the genus and the etiologic agent of human tuberculosis, which as recently as 1980 was the leading cause of death among 38 notifiable diseases. More than 10 million persons in the United States are infected, and this number is bound to increase with new immigrants from other areas of the world in which the infection rate is high. Many of the unusual characteristics of the organism are attributable to the extraordinarily high lipid content of the cell and cell wall, for example, resistance to staining, acid-fastness, slow growth rate, resistance to the action of antibodies plus complement, virulence, and resistance to the action of physical and chemical agents.

A primary infection that follows the inhalation of airborne tubercle bacilli induces in the patients a cell-mediated immune response, detectable by the tuberculin skin test. Delayed or tuberculin-type allergy is directly referable to intracellular persistence of tubercle bacilli and greatly affects the course of the disease in either reinfection or reactivation type seen in adults. Resistance to reinfection, which is usually endogenous, depends on the capacity of the host to contain the organism by the same cell-mediated mechanisms that produce the inflammatory response in delayed dermal hypersensitivity, that is, T lymphocytes and lymphokines such as MIF and MAF.

Consequences of infection depend upon the immune status of the host, size of the inoculating dose, and virulence of the bacilli. Progressive tuberculosis is a chronic granulomatous process that may eventually involve multiple organ systems. The concept of tuberculous infection is to be distinguished from that of tuberculous disease. Both generate cell-mediated immune responses.

Specimens collected for smear and culture include 24-hour sputa, gastric washings (especially desirable for infants, for some adults who swallow their sputum, and for sputum-negative individuals with minimal activity), 24-hour urines, cerebrospinal fluid, and other appropriate materials. Microscopic examination of direct smears stained with either the Kinyoun acid-fast or the fluorescent dye techniques may not reveal any acid-fast bacilli. Sediments of specimens concentrated by centrifugation following digestion using one of several standard techniques provide better material from which to isolate tubercle bacilli. Cultures are an absolute necessity for speciation of mycobacteria because identification cannot be accomplished using only microscopic morphology. Growth on solid media such as coagulated egg proteins (e.g., Lowenstein-Jensen medium) or oleic acid–albumin (e.g., Dubos–Middlebrook medium) permits observations regarding colonial morphology, thermal tolerance, and growth rate and also provides organisms for various biochemical tests, for example, niacin production, nitrate reduction, Tween-80 hydrolysis, catalase activity; for virulence tests, for example, serpentine cord formation or presence of cord factor, neutral red binding, guinea pig inoculation; and drug-susceptibility assays (Table 5-7).

M. tuberculosis grows best at 37°C and requires 2 to 4 weeks to produce typical, dry, crumbly, cornmeal-like colonies. The organism is niacin positive, reduces nitrate to nitrite, does not hydrolyse Tween-80, is negative for catalase activity after heating at 68°C for 20 minutes, produces cord factor (serpentine cords), binds neutral red dye, and is virulent for guinea pigs.

Antigens used in the tuberculin skin test are standardized based on milligrams of tuberculoprotein and expressed as tuberculin units (TU), old tuberculin (OT), or purified protein derivative (PPD). One milligram standard PPD contains 50,000 TU. Intermediate strength PPD equals 5 TU (OT 1/2000). The greatest value of the tuberculin skin test is in the detection of those individuals whose reactions have converted from negative to positive. Equivocal reactions may be seen in patients infected with a mycobacterial species other than M. tuberculosis, in which instances, species-specific antigens may be used to aid in the differentiation process. Antituberculous drugs are prescribed for converters with clinical symptoms and may be prescribed for prophylaxis for asymptomatic converters. The latter should be distinguished by their age and the chronology of their responses to PPD-testing from persons who show a "booster" response and who may therefore be presumed to have longstanding infection and should not be treated.

A vaccine (BCG, bacille Calmette-Guérin), prepared from an attenuated strain of M. bovis, is available for prophylactic immunization. The vaccine should be administered only to those who are nonreactive to tuberculin. Although the vaccine is widely used in Europe and other countries, its use in the United States is restricted to certain high-risk groups, such as young children in a household in which there is an open case of tuberculosis. Immunization vitiates the usefulness of the tuberculin test. BCG should not be given to anyone with a positive tuberculin (PPD) skin test.

Many BCG vaccines are available, all derived from the original strain, but varying widely in immunogenicity, efficacy, and reactogenicity. Lasting protection cannot be assured by vaccination. Therefore tuberculosis must be included in the differential diagnosis even in vaccinees.

Treatment usually consists of a combination of drugs (at least two) to increase therapeutic effectiveness and to minimize the emergence of drug-resistant mutants. When the patient's bacterial population is thought to be particularly large, three drugs are frequently used during the early phase of therapy, for instance when there are extensive infiltrates or cavitary lesions and thus bacilli can be found on direct smears of unconcentrated sputum.

Isoniazid (INH), rifampicin, ethambutol, and

streptomycin are generally considered first-line drugs. The most frequently used regimen in the United States is a combination of the first two. Prevention of infection secondary to open cases is effectively achieved by isoniazid, especially if the tuberculin test is negative, indicating maximal susceptibility, or in cases in which tuberculin tests have converted recently from negative to positive. In the latter instance, whether or not roentgenographic evidence of tuberculosis is present, INH is indicated to prevent progression of active disease. With short-course chemotherapy (twice weekly isoniazid and rifampin for 9 months), a 95% success rate has been reported. When drug-resistance is identified, streptomycin and pyrazinamide are added. When there is reason to suspect isoniazid resistance, residence in a developing country or past exposure to antituberculous drugs, therapy should be started with four drugs initially (streptomycin, INH, rifampin, pyrazinamide).

Other mycobacterial species, although less pathogenic for man than *M. tuberculosis,* are capable of causing human tuberculous disease and therefore present diagnostic and therapeutic problems. *M. bovis* causes bovine tuberculosis and at one time was a leading cause of human tuberculosis. *M. avium,* the cause of avian tuberculosis, has been isolated from human pulmonary lesions. *M. ulcerans* is the etiologic agent of chronic cutaneous tuberculosis. Species classified in the Runyon groups I–IV, sometimes called the "atypical mycobacteria," cause both pulmonary disease and chronic cutaneous lesions. Identification of these less virulent mycobacterial species is necessary because many of them exhibit responses to chemotherapeutic drugs which are different from those of *M. tuberculosis.* The close antigenic relationships that exist among the mycobacteria make immunologic differentiation difficult or impossible. Identification therefore depends upon accurate observations regarding colonial morphology, nutritional and environmental influences on growth and growth rate, and precise performance of the variety of biochemical tests described in other literature (Table 5-8).

Leprosy. *Mycobacterium leprae,* the etiologic agent of human leprosy, has never been cultured either on lifeless media or in tissue explants. A generation time of 20 to 30 days has been obtained from serial passages in mouse foot pads. Lesion distribution suggests a diminished ability to multiply in body areas where temperatures exceed 30°C. In tissues, the acid-fast organism closely resembles *M. tuberculosis.* Athymic ("nude") mice offer a good host cell medium for propagation of *Mycobacterium leprae.* The nine-banded armadillo has been shown to develop a chronic infection in which *M. leprae* multiplies to high numbers and with little harm to the animal.

M. leprae is probably as communicable as *M. tuberculosis.* However, the portal of entry, method of spread, genesis of lesions, and manner of dissemination are still unclear. Children are infected more readily than adults. Disease usually occurs in individuals who live in endemic areas, such as Africa, Asia, Pacific islands (in a recent survey, more than 1100 cases in Micronesia, twice the 1977 total), and certain areas of the United States and who have a history of long and close contacts with leprosy patients. An increasing number of new cases is reported annually in the United States, all thought to have been imported from Southeast Asia and Latin America. The usually prolonged incubation period varies from several months to 30 years. Regardless of the portal of entry and incubation period, the bacilli eventually find their way to the mucous membranes, skin, and peripheral nerves, giving rise to cutaneous lesions and peripheral anesthesias.

The tuberculoid or mild form and the lepromatous or progressive form are the two recognized types of leprosy. Tuberculoid leprosy lesions are usually localized and confined to the skin, mucous membranes, and area nerves. Histologically, they resemble tubercles and are comprised of epithelioid cells, lymphocytes, and plasma cells; there is usually no caseation, and organisms are rare. In contrast, lepromatous leprosy lesions appear as cutaneous nodules called lepromas that occur principally on the face and extremities, but may involve the liver, spleen, bone marrow, viscera, and other areas. Histologically, the lepromas are composed of lymphocytes, plasma cells, and lipid-laden macrophages and giant cells (called lepra cells) containing numerous bacilli arranged in bundles or globular masses (globi).

The status of the patient's cellular immune system and the ability to mount a competent cell-mediated immune response determines to a large degree the type of leprosy that will develop. Tuberculoid leprosy is seen in the more resistant patients whereas lepromatous leprosy is seen in patients with T-lymphocyte defects.

Patients with tuberculoid leprosy react positively to intradermal injections of lepromin, an antigen derived from homogenized leprous tissue, and to tuberculin. Lepromatous leprosy patients give a negative response to lepromin, indicating a defect in the cell-mediated immune responses. Normal individuals, persons immunized with BCG, and tuberculosis patients also give a positive reaction to lepromin, indicating cross-reactivity with tuberculoproteins and tissue antigens. The only real value of the lepromin test rests in its ability to identify anergic leprosy patients.

Excepting injuries stemming from peripheral anesthesias, complications of leprosy appear to have an immunologic origin, such as erythema nodosum, erythema necroticans, and others.

Sulfone drugs are most effective in treatment, especially dapsone (DDS, 4'-4'-diamino-diphenyl-sulfone). Rifampin kills *M. leprae* and shows promise as a useful drug. Clofazimine has been shown to suppress the erythema nodosum reaction. Thalidomide has shown promise in clinical trials.

INFECTIONS DUE TO ACTINOMYCES AND NOCARDIA

Actinomyces and *Nocardia* species are gram-positive bacilli that grow slowly producing, delicate, branching filaments that tend to fragment into bacillary elements. These organisms and the infections they cause are usually grouped and studied with the fungi for the reasons stated previously and because they cause chronic infections characterized by suppuration and abscess and granuloma formation. The two genera are classified into separate families, Actinomycetaceae and Nocardiaceae, respectively, based on oxygen requirements, catabolic activities, and cell wall composition. *Actinomyces* species, part of the normal oral flora, are anaerobic, ferment carbohydrates, are non-acid-fast, and their cell walls do not contain diaminopimelic acid (DAP). *Nocardia* species are soil inhabitants, are aerobic, produce acid from carbohydrates oxidatively, are partially acid-fast, and contain meso-DAP and nocardiomycolic acid in their cell walls.

Among the *Actinomyces* species, *Actinomyces israelii*, and *Actinomyces bovis* are the principal etiologic agents of actinomycosis, the former in humans, the latter in cattle. Differentiation of the two species is dependent upon biochemical tests such as nitrate reduction, starch hydrolysis, carbohydrate fermentations; upon serologic tests such as immunofluorescent tests (FA) and immunodiffusion tests (ID); upon the appearance of micro- and macrocolonies; and upon microscopic morphology.

The disease is seen more frequently in cattle than in humans. The organisms are indigenous in humans and probably in cattle, initiating infection following oral tissue trauma. Bovine infections, called "lumpy jaw," usually involve the mandible with the formation of tumefactions, abscesses, fistulas and sinus tracts, producing soft-tissue and bone destruction and marked cicatrization. The disease is chronic, spreading to contiguous tissues rather than involving blood and lymph vessels. The animal's general health is not affected unless mastication or breathing is impaired.

Human actinomycosis occurs as cervicofacial, abdominal, and thoracic infections. Similar to the bovine counterpart in its initiation and clinical picture, the cervicofacial type is the most common and has the best prognosis. Abdominal actinomycosis is thought to arise from swallowing. *A. israelii* bacilli or from abdominal trauma and may occur concurrently with or in the absence of a preexisting cervicofacial infection. Abdominal disease often involves the appendix with spread to nearby tissues. Symptoms are referable to the organ systems involved. Thoracic actinomycosis is thought to arise as an extension through the neck from a cervicofacial infection or as an extension through the diaphragm from hepatic infection or as a primary infection initiated by aspirating organisms present in the mouth. Symptoms are those of a subacute pulmonary infection, often resembling tuberculosis. Disseminated infections may occur, and death may supervene as a result of secondary bacterial infections. Rarely are pure cultures of *Actinomyces israelii* (or *Actinomyces bovis*) obtained from lesions or exudates.

In purulent discharges from the sinus tracts, minute yellow-white granules are found ("sulfur granules"). The granules, crushed under a coverslip and examined microscopically, are composed of tangled, branching filaments with peripheral ends radially arranged and clubbed. After being washed to remove contaminants, the granules should be cultured in a broth medium containing a reducing agent or on blood agar and incubated anaerobically at 37°C. Examination of cultures for microcolonies at 48 hours and macrocolonies at 14 days facilitates identification.

Penicillin, the drug of choice, is administered intravenously in doses that vary from 3 to 20 million units per day, depending upon the severity of the disease. Energetic surgical intervention to incise and drain lesions and to excise lesions and devitalized tissues is highly recommended. Other drugs used for therapy are tetracycline, chloramphenicol, streptomycin, and sulfadiazine. Antibiotic therapy should be continued for 12 to 18 months following surgical procedures.

Nocardiosis is an acute or chronic disease usually caused by *Nocardia asteroides*. It most often begins as a primary pulmonary infection characterized by suppuration, less frequently by granuloma formation. Bacilli are hematogenously disseminated to subcutaneous tissues and other organs, particularly the central nervous system where they produce multiple abscesses in the brain and meninges. Delicate, branching filaments that are gram-positive and acid-fast are seen in sputum, infected tissues, and exudates from abscesses. Granules are not produced.

Nocardiosis is a term usually reserved for primary pulmonary infections or systemic infections resulting from dissemination from a pulmonary locus. Other infections caused by the *Nocardia* are mycetoma, a localized, chronic process characterized by the development of tumefactions, abscesses, fistulas, and sinus tracts, and the lymphocutaneous syndrome characterized by the progression of abscesses along a lymphatic channel, producing a clinical picture similar to that seen in lymphocutaneous sporotrichosis. Granules, composed of fine, radially arranged, branching, acid-fast filaments with or without terminal clubbing, are produced and found in exudates from mycetoma lesions. Granule morphology facilitates a presumptive diagnosis by permitting differentiation between bacterial and fungal etiology. Mycetoma is usually caused by *Nocardia brasiliensis* or *Nocardia caviae*. *N. brasiliensis* is the usual etiologic agent of the lymphocutaneous syndrome. All are soil saprobes, initiating infections following inhalation or traumatic cutaneous implantation of the bacilli.

Sputum from nocardiosis patients and deep-tissue biopsies (preferred because fewer contaminants are present) or granules (processed as are actinomycosis granules) from mycetoma patients are cultured on Sabouraud's dextrose or blood agar without added antibiotics and incubated aerobically and anaerobically at 22°C and 37°C. All three species produce similar colonies that appear as dry, brittle, orange or yellow, cauliflower-like, or cerebriform growths that are often covered with a short-napped mycelium. Speciation of nocardia is based on biochemical reactions, principally casein, tyrosine, and xanthine hydrolysis and oxidative acid production from carbohydrates.

Sulfadiazine, the drug of choice for nocardiosis, is administered in doses of 3 to 10 g/day to achieve a blood level of 9 to 20 mg/100 ml (depending upon the severity of the infection) for 3 to 6 months. Sulfamethoxazole is also effective. Therapy for mycetoma depends upon the etiologic agent; bacterial or actinomycotic mycetoma responds to antibiotic or antibacterial drugs, whereas eumycotic mycetoma

is extremely refractory to antibiotics or antimycotic drugs. Early actinomycotic mycetoma lesions (before bone involvement) respond to sulfadiazine. More advanced cases respond to high doses of penicillin. Surgical intervention to drain abscesses and remove devitalized tissues augments healing.

Pathogenic Anaerobic Bacilli

Improved techniques with prereduced media and specialized apparatus have greatly enhanced our capability to isolate strictly anaerobic bacteria from blood, exudates and affected tissues; the application of gas–liquid chromatography (GLC) has been central to elucidating the distinctive biochemical patterns of these organisms. Their often rigid requirements for anaerobiosis depend on lack of cytochrome respiratory chains, despite the presence of flavoprotein enzymes that transfer hydrogen to free oxygen to form H_2O_2, a very toxic product; and failure of strict anaerobes to form peroxidase or catalase to destroy H_2O_2, or of superoxide dismutase to destroy superoxide radicals. Prominent among the anaerobes are endospore-forming rods, *Clostridium* species (Table 5-8), various species of gram-negative, nonsporulating pleomorphic rods (Table 5-6), and *Peptostreptococcus* and *Peptococcus* (see earlier sections). On initial isolation, these organisms (especially the gram-negative rods) require strictly anaerobic conditions and rich organic media, such as cooked chopped meat, or special anaerobic media. Diseases caused by clostridia are primarily intoxications; those caused by anaerobic gram-negative organisms are always endogenous metastatic pyogenic infections.

DISEASES CAUSED BY CLOSTRIDIA

Tetanus. *Clostridium tetani,* the cause of tetanus or lockjaw, has the general properties of the genus (Table 5-9). It is not invasive but grows well in dead tissue; there it can produce its soluble exotoxin. It normally inhabits superficial layers of the soil, especially of cultivated and manured fields, because of its regular presence in the feces of domestic and wild animals and sometimes of man. The spores of *C. tetani* resist dry heat at 150°C for 1 hour, autoclaving at 121°C for 5 to 10 minutes and 5% phenol for 12 to 15 hours. Protected from sunlight (ultraviolet light), the dried spores remain viable for many years. Toxin interferes with neuromuscular transmission by inhibiting release of acetylcholine from nerve terminals in muscle. Muscle spasms are due to interference, by the toxin, with spinal cord synaptic reflexes, leading to inhibition of antagonists (strychnine-like action). Secondary disturbances of autonomic functions occur.

Tetanus Toxin. Tetanus neurotoxin, the structural gene for which is on a plasmid, has marked affinity for nervous tissue and reaches the central nervous system (spinal cord) via the blood and lymphatics, especially those associated with nerve trunks.

Tetanus bacilli or spores are doubtless frequently introduced into wounds. The nature of the wound determines whether the bacilli can proliferate. Deep (anaerobic), soil-contaminated wounds in which there has been considerable tissue destruction are especially likely to supply these conditions.

Tetanus neonatorum occurs especially when filthy conditions surround parturition with infection of the umbilical stump by feces and soil containing *C. tetani* spores.

In the acute form of tetanus the incubation time ranges from 3 to 14 days; in the chronic form the incubation period may exceed a month.

Recognition of conditions favoring development of tetanus should prompt measures to prevent it, that is, adequate surgical debridement of contaminated wounds supplemented by administration of systemic antibiotics (penicillin or alternative). In individuals without known prior immunization, tetanus immune globulin (TIg, human) should be infiltrated around the wound and given systemically, up to a total of 10,000 units; one dose is usually sufficient. In individuals with known prior immunization, 0.5 ml of tetanus toxoid should be given if the time of injury is more than 3 to 5 years after the last booster. Previously immunized individuals begin to produce adequate levels of antitoxin within 2 to 4 hours after a booster dose of toxoid. Basic primary immunity is achieved by routine immunization of infants with DPT at 2, 4, and 6 months of age (see Table 5-21). Boosters are given at 18 months and at 4 to 6 years of age. After the 6th year, 0.5 ml alum-precipitated toxoid boosters need be given only at 10-year intervals or whenever tetanus-prone injury is sustained more than 3 to 5 years after a booster.

The diagnosis of tetanus is made entirely on clinical grounds and once established (mortality up to 40%) requires intensive supportive care: muscle relaxants, neuromuscular blocking agents (in collaboration with the anesthesiologist), respiratory assistance, attention to fluid balance.

Gas Gangrene (Clostridial Myositis). Gas gangrene may occur when deep (anaerobic), contused wounds are contaminated with soil that contains spores of one or more of several species of clostridia. Devitalized tissue provides an environment with lowered redox potential that favors the germination and multiplication of anaerobic bacteria. *Clostridium perfringens*, the principal agent in gas gangrene, inhabits the mammalian intestine and female genital tract and soil and is nearly always accompanied in infected wounds by one or more other soil clostridia that act synergistically with *C. perfringens: C. putrificum, C. histolyticum, C. novyi, C. fallax, C. septicum,* and others; the bacteriology is rather variable and heterogeneous. *C. tetani* is also commonly present. As in tetanus, whether or not gas gangrene develops depends on the nature of the wound and the virulence of the bacteria present. Approximately 30 species of *Clostridium* have been isolated from human infections. Taxonomic differentiation, usually impractical for the routine diagnostic laboratory, is based on morphologic and cultural characteristics and on gas–liquid chromatography to identify fermentation products.

Clinical manifestations of clostridial infections are highly varied. Clostridial food poisoning ranks second or third on the list of common forms, usually involves ingestion of meat contaminated with *C. perfringens;* and has an attack rate of 50% to 70%. Diarrheal disease is caused by heat-labile protein enterotoxin associated with the spore coat that is released as the ingested vegetative cells are lysed in the intestine. Maximum activity occurs in the ileum. The toxin inhibits glucose transport and causes protein loss into the intestinal lumen. Diagnosis is made by isolation of toxigenic *Clostridium perfringens* from food and/or feces of afflicted patients. Enteritis necrotans is caused by ingestion of meat contaminated with *Clostridium perfringens* type C, the β-toxin of which is the cause of an acute ulcerative process, restricted to the small intestine in which the mucosa is denuded and sloughed. It is accompanied by acute abdominal pain, bloody diarrhea, vomiting, shock, and a high incidence of peritonitis by direct extension; it is frequently fatal. A somewhat similar process has been recognized as occurring in association with prolonged broad-spectrum antibiotic therapy, most often clindamycin, in the presence of which *Clostridium difficile*, a member of the normal flora, overgrows to produce a potent necrotizing toxin, which is heat labile and acid sensitive. Vancomycin is effective in suppressing *C. difficile. Clostridium perfringens* and *Clostridium ramosum* together represent almost half of the total isolates from clostridial infections of soft tissue, which can occur in almost any region of the body and in which devitalization of tissue and polymicrobial contamination promote anaerobic conditions. These include intraabdominal and abdominal sepsis, carcinoma, empyema and pelvic, brain, pulmonary, prostatic, and perianal abscesses. Localized infection of the skin and subcutaneous tissue occurs, particularly in compromised patients such as diabetics and heroin addicts (suppurative myositis), and may develop into diffuse spreading cellulitis and fasciitis, with widespread gas formation, toxemia, shock, renal failure, and intravascular hemolysis, ending in death. *C. perfringens, ramosum,* and *septicum* may be recovered in blood cultures. In contrast to the foregoing, clostridial myonecrosis (gas gangrene) is a process in which muscle destruction is prominent, in association with crepitance and systemic toxemia, and usually follows trauma or a surgical procedure (*e.g.,* elective colon resection, biliary tract surgery). Gram-stained water discharges show myriad gram-positive rods and relatively few inflammatory cells. Blood cultures frequently yield *Clostridia. C. perfringens* accounts for 80% of cases, the remaining being attributable to *C. novyi, septicum,* and *bifermentans.*

Diagnosis rests on the characteristic appearance of affected muscle, which initially is pale, edematous, and devitalized, progressing inward to frank gangrene. The same condition may occur in the absence of evident trauma (nontraumatic myonecrosis) and is occasionally associated with silent colonic carcinoma. Septic abortion and, less frequently, normal delivery may be complicated by uterine myonecrosis, usually signaled by jaundice, massive intravenous hemolysis (due to the α-toxin lecithinase) and renal failure with hemoglobinuria, and hypotension. Uncomplicated clostridial bacteremia may occur in the absence of clear-cut localizing signs of infection.

Central to treatment is adequate debridement, along with judiciously selected antimicrobial therapy, particularly of suppurative infections in which broad-spectrum antibiotics can serve to suppress aerobic as well as anaerobic bacteria in this invariably polymicrobial infection (aerobes: aminoglycosides such as gentamicin, tobramycin, amikacin; anaerobes: clindamycin, chloramphenicol, metronidazole, cefoxitin). Penicillin G is maximally effective against *C. perfringens.* The use of pentavalent clostridial antitoxin is controversial and should be limited to those patients clearly exhibiting toxemia (hemoglobinemia, disseminated intravascular coagulation, shock, renal failure). The decision to use it must be weighed against the hazards of serum sickness or anaphylactic shock. Skin tests should precede the administration of antitoxin (horse serum).

Exchange erythrocyte transfusion to remove damaged erythrocytes has adjunctive therapeutic value. Hyperbaric oxygen, also a controversial topic, has its proponents. Substantial risks are involved and the number of centers with hyperbaric chambers is limited. It cannot replace other modalities of therapy focused on containing and obliterating the source of infection according to good surgical principles.

Botulism (Food Poisoning). Botulism was first described in cases of poisoning by meat sausage (botulus is Latin for sausage). *C. botulinum* may grow in sausages, hams, and canned foods of any sort not too dry and not too acid (limiting pH 4.5) for growth, that are contaminated with soil or marine sediment (E spores); anaerobically packed; and heat processed at a temperature inadequate to kill spores of *C. botulinum,* which are highly resistant to heat and drying. In storage at room temperatures the spores germinate and the growing bacilli form the potent exotoxin. Under commercial canning conditions in the United States, botulism is uncommon.

The ability of organisms to produce botulinus toxin (the most neurotoxic substance known) is mediated by specific bacteriophage. In contrast to most exotoxins, botulinus toxin is not actively secreted into the tissues or growth medium; rather it is produced inside the bacterial cell and released only on the death and lysis of vegetative *C. botulinum.* Types A, B, and, less commonly, E and F affect humans; types C and D affect ungulates, and type E affects avian species. The toxins are antigenically distinct polypeptides with a molecular weight of about 140,000 daltons. The toxins spread hematogenously to the motor nerves, where the large subunit of the toxin molecule binds to specific acceptors on nerve terminal membranes. Toxin is then internalized by the acceptors in an energy-dependent step and, by antagonizing the effects of Ca^{2+}, irreversibly inhibits release of acetylcholine from peripheral nerves. Botulinus toxin is inactivated by boiling for 10 minutes or by heating to 80°C for 30 minutes and by ultraviolet light.

Botulism presents as an afebrile neurological disorder, characterized by symmetrical descending weakness or paralysis (diplopia, photophobia, fixed pupils, dysphonia, dysarthria, dysphagia, respiratory muscle weakness), diminished salivation, oropharyngeal desiccation, ileus, and urinary retention. Any or all of these signs and symptoms may occur beginning 6 hours to 8 days after ingestion of toxin-containing food. Specific diagnosis rests on a demonstration of toxin in the blood or in the stool and/or food, in which *Clostridium botulinum* may also be found (mouse bioassay for toxin). Death is from respiratory failure. Polyvalent antitoxin (horse serum) preceded by a skin test is recommended, 1 vial intravenously, 1 intramuscularly. Expectant supportive care is essential, particularly respiratory care, and may be lifesaving, because intoxication is self-limited. Contamination wounds have been reported as a primary source of botulin. Infantile botulism (the hypotonic or "floppy" infant) and sudden infant death syndrome (SIDS) can both be caused by botulin (types A and B) emanating from organisms that colonize the gastrointestinal tract from some unknown source.

INFECTIONS DUE TO NONSPORULATING ANAEROBIC BACILLI

The indigenous microbiota of humans is heavily weighted in favor of the anaerobes: by factors of 10 : 1 on the skin and in the vagina, 100 : 1 in the oral cavity, and as much as 1000 : 1 in the large intestine (Table 5-6). Life-threatening infections (*e.g.*, lung or brain abscess, peritonitis, septicemia, septic abortion, etc.) caused by endogenous pyogenic anaerobes are now more frequently recognized than disease due to the clostridia. *Kawasaki disease* (mucocutaneous lymph node syndrome), a multisystem disease of young children, is thought to be caused by *Propionibacterium acnes,* a common intestinal and skin inhabitant in older age groups. The disease is not favorably influenced by antibiotics. Recovery of fastidious pyogenic anaerobes from clinical specimens requires correct use of prereduced transport medium for sample collection and, in the laboratory, appropriate anaerobic environmental systems and special media for primary isolation. Speciation of isolates is accomplished by GLC of metabolic products, which gives elution patterns characteristic of each strain of bacteria. The most accessible natural source of these organisms is the oral cavity, where they constitute a major portion of the normal flora, but where they may also be directly related to pathology of periodontal disease, root canal infections, and other localized lesions destructive of teeth and supporting tissues. Each of these pathologic conditions, while of immediate concern for the dental surgeon, may be the source of metastatic systemic infection at distant sites. It may seem paradoxical that strict anaerobes, highly sensitive to oxygen, should normally inhabit the oral cavity, which is constantly exposed to hot air. However, anaerobic conditions (anaerobiosis, lowered redox potential) are maintained by the presence of ne-

crotic tissue in periodontal and crevicular spaces as well as through the utilization of oxygen by commensal aerobic bacteria inhabiting the same microenvironment.

A presumptive diagnosis of anaerobic infection is suggested by foul-smelling putrid exudate or discharge from sites in which anaerobes normally occur, by evident tissue necrosis and gas formation (crepitus), by failure to recover potential pathogens on routine aerobic culture (culture under CO_2 is *not* anaerobic), and, most importantly, by Gram's stain of exudate or pus from the lesion. The latter may be the only clue on which to base therapy pending results of anaerobic culture and GLC analysis.

Pathogenic Aerobic Bacilli

DISEASES DUE TO AEROBIC BACILLI

Anthrax. Anthrax, due to *Bacillus anthracis,* a strict aerobe, is primarily a disease of domestic herbivora grazing on spore-infested pastures. It is contracted by humans usually via skin abrasions, mainly from tissues or body fluids of infected animals and handling spore-contaminated hides or wool from infected animals or fertilizer made from infected bone meal. Spores sometimes occur in dust on sheep's wool or other animal hair, and inhalation of the infectious dust produces a dangerous pneumonic form of anthrax (called wool-sorters' disease). Gastrointestinal anthrax, highly fatal, may also occur. Infection of the face through improperly sterilized shaving brushes and analogous accidents have occurred. A skin lesion (malignant pustule) is most typical.

Most species of *Bacillus* are harmless, motile, ubiquitous saprophytes of the soil and environment. *B. anthracis* is distinctive, being highly pathogenic, nonmotile, and nonhemolytic. *B. cereus* is a hemolytic, harmless species closely similar to *B. anthracis*. Most species of *Bacillus* are more or less strict aerobes or facultative and readily cultivable on simple peptone media or blood agar at 25°C to 40°C. Oval spores occur near the middle of anthrax bacilli without swelling the rod. Anthrax pores are long lived and unusually resistant to heat and chemicals. In infected tissues *B. anthracis* forms a large polypeptide capsule that is antiphagocytic and therefore associated with virulence.

In *cutaneous anthrax,* the most common form, the characteristic ulcer appears within about 24 hours after infection, teeming with bacilli. Its center soon changes into a black, central necrotic area with markedly edematous areola, spreading eschar ("malignant pustule") and painful local lymphadenopathy. With severe local reactions, especially around the head and neck, toxemia may occur ("malignant edema"). Anthrax in any form, but especially pulmonary and gastrointestinal forms with toxemia, is accompanied by bacteremia and may be the source of hematogenous meningitis. Penicillin is the drug of choice in therapy. Cortisone is indicated in cases of malignant edema. Penicillin-allergic patients can be successfully treated with erythromycin, tetracycline, or chloramphenicol.

A potent and complex protein exotoxin consisting of three distinct factors was first discovered in tissues and exudates of infected animals and was later demonstrated in cultures rich in serum and bicarbonate ions, which also increase capsule production. Virulence of *B. anthracis* depends on production of both capsules and toxin. Infection evokes antibodies against both. Nontoxigenic, encapsulated variants occur.

Control. Careful incineration or deep burial of dead animals, their exudates, and contaminated straw is necessary. Animal autopsies should not be performed on farms, as all body fluids and tissues are highly infectious, and exposure to air induces anthrax organisms to sporulate. Legislation requires disinfection of hides, wool, bone meal fertilizer, and brush bristles in commercial use.

During an outbreak, unaffected animals should be immunized with a spore vaccine available for veterinary use and/or a "protective antigen" (PA) vaccine (alum-precipitated toxoid). The latter can be used to immunize persons who may be at particular risk.

Diagnosis. Gram-stained smears of pus or exudate, body fluids, tissues, or blood (from animals moribund or dead of anthrax) show characteristic encapsulated rods. Cultures on ordinary blood agar of these materials readily yield large nonhemolytic colonies, and the diagnosis can be confirmed by immunofluorescence or mouse inoculation.

Pathogenic Spirochetes

The order Spirochaetales (spirochetes) includes spiral, flexible bacteria (contrast with rigid *Spirillum*). Although procaryons, the spirochetes are structurally the most complex of bacteria, consisting of three principal parts: an outer envelope or periplast probably containing murein, on which marked susceptibility of some species to penicillin presumably depends; the cell proper, an elongated cylindrical tube with cytoplasmic membrane; a fibrillar, axial filament arising, like flagella (and, seemingly like them, contractile), from basal granules at one end of the tubular cell and gathered into a bundle constituting an axial filament around which the cell is wound helically. In general, spirochetes are not readily stained and are commonly examined in the living state in moist material by means of the darkfield microscope. (See also Fluorescent Antibody-Staining Technique.)

The order contains numerous saprophytes, and only a few genera are of medical importance.

All pathogenic spirochetes are quite fragile and readily killed by drying, heat, and disinfectants. However, they can survive for years at −76°C.

TREPONEMAL DISEASES

Syphilis. *Treponema pallidum,* the cause of syphilis, is from 4 μm to 20 μm in length and 0.2 μm in diameter. The cytoplasm is surrounded by a trilaminar cytoplasmic membrane, a delicate inner mucopeptide layer (periplast), and an outer lipoprotein membrane containing lipopolysaccharides. Three fibrils are inserted into the tapered ends of the cell. The organism has 4 to 14 coils and differs from *Borrelia* (see below) in the tightness and regularity of its coils. Its distinctive movements consist of occasional rotation about the long axis, slow to-and-fro gliding and occasional sedate bending.

For diagnostic darkfield examination fluid should be taken from a cleanly scraped chancre or, better, punctured bubo and should contain as little blood and solid material as possible. Dried smears, negatively stained with India ink, nigrosin, or other stains in lieu of darkfield for diagnosis can lead to error because distinctive motility permits some degree of differentiation from saprophytic treponemes of the genitalia.

Spirochetes are demonstrated in tissues by the silver impregnation method of Levaditi or Fontana. *Treponema pallidum* has never been cultivated in a virulent state on artificial media, though several readily cultured nonpathogenic strains (notably the Reiter strain) morphologically identical with, and antigenically very closely similar to, *T. pallidum* are well known.

Demonstrable immunity appears in 2 to 4 weeks after appearance of the primary lesion (chancre) when standard serologic tests (SST or STS) become positive. Specific antitreponemal tests also become positive.

Primary (2 to 6 weeks) and secondary stages (4 weeks to 4 months) subside with developing specific resistance. Years later, tertiary gummatous lesions of arteries, central nervous system, bones, viscera, and other organs, with intense cytologic response and necrosis, probably related to allergy, develop. Transplacental transmission leads to congenital syphilis, which continues at a constant level as a cause of neonatal morbidity. A healthy neonate of a syphilitic mother may have syphilitic IgG globulins in its blood since IgG molecules pass the placenta. Syphilitic IgM cannot pass the placenta and appears in the neonate only as a result of active fetal syphilitic infection.

If effective antispirochetal therapy (*e.g.,* penicillin) is instituted early in the disease (before immunity has developed) reinfection can occur. High-grade immunity develops in 2 to 6 weeks. Relapse may occur if the early therapy is not totally effective.

Transmission is by sexual contact (vaginal or oral) or, rarely (0.01%), by contact with *fresh* exudates from any open lesions at any stage; direct blood transfusion or insufficiently aged (less than 4 days) blood-bank blood can transmit during any septicemic stage. Freshly infected needles, syringes, etc., can also transmit the disease to nonimmune persons.

Diagnosis

1. *Darkfield examination* of material from open lesions at any stage, including secondary lesions on mucosal surfaces of oropharynx and vagina.
2. *Nontreponemal standard serologic tests (SSTs)* or serologic tests for syphilis (STS) depend on the presence in the serum of immunoglobulins (IgM or IgG) reactive with a lipoidal antigen prepared from bovine heart muscle (cardiolipin). This antibody (referred to as **reagin** or **reaginic** or **Wassermann** antibody) results from the interaction of the host with *Treponema pallidum* and has nothing to do with IgE, which is also referred to as reagin or reaginic antibody, but is associated with atopic allergy. Wassermann antibody, although also mainly IgG in syphilitic infection, is distinct from antibody to *T. pallidum* and is measured by flocculation with cardiolipin-cholesterol-lecithin antigen in the Venereal Disease Research laboratory (VDRL) test, the rapid plasma reagin (RPR), or the automated reagin test (ART). A positive nontreponemal serologic test may occur in many conditions other than syphilis, from which they must be distinguished by a negative specific test for treponemal antibody (FTA-ABS). "Biological false-positive" STSs occur frequently in infectious

mononucleosis, malaria, granulomatous disease of many etiologies, some viral and chlamydial infections, dysgammaglobulinemias, autoimmune diseases such as rheumatoid arthritis and systemic lupus erythematosus, and malignancies.

3. *Tests for specific antitreponemal antibody.* These antibodies are evoked by and are *specific* for *T. pallidum* and persist throughout the duration of syphilitic infection, including latent syphilis, even when SSTs are negative. Treponemal antibody is detected with the fluorescent treponemal antibody absorption (FTA-ABS) test, in which the indirect or "sandwich" FAb staining procedure is used. Patients' sera and known positive and negative control sera are inactivated at 56°C for 30 minutes and absorbed with material (sorbent) from Reiter spirochetes to remove antibody to commensal spirochetes that cross-react with *T. pallidum*. *T. pallidum* (Nichols strain) grown in rabbit testis, lyophilized and fixed to slides are used as antigen substrate. The microhemagglutination–*Treponema pallidum* (MHA–TP) test, more recently developed, is just as specific and sensitive as the FTA–ABS and is cheaper and simpler to perform. In the MHA–TP test, tanned erythrocytes coated with treponemal antigens are agglutinated in microtiter plates by specific antibody in the test sera. False-positive treponemal antibody tests (FTA–ABS, MHA–TP), due mainly to IgM, are unusual, but may occur in connective tissue disorders (systemic lupus erythematosus, rheumatoid arthritis), leprosy, and infectious mononucleosis; these discrepancies may be resolved by application of the *Treponema pallidum* immobilization (TPI) test, the first specific treponemal test introduced, but also the most difficult because it requires the use of living treponemes. The TPI test now serves chiefly as a standard of reference available at the Centers for Disease Control. It should be remembered that nonsyphilitic treponemal diseases (yaws, bejel, pinta) give *bona fide* positive treponemal antibody tests and must therefore be distinguished from syphilis on clinical and epidemiological grounds.

In the diagnosis of neurosyphilis, the treponemal tests are unreliable, and serodiagnosis is made on the basis of the VDRL test carried out on spinal fluid. VDRL-CSF, however, may be negative in late neurosyphilis. False-positive VDRL reactions on spinal fluid are rare.

Yaws, Pinta, Bejel. These nonvenereal, tropical treponematoses are caused by *Treponema pertenue, T. carateum,* and *T. pallidum,* respectively. Bejel is endemic (nonvenereal) syphilis. The infections are usually acquired in childhood by direct body contact. As with venereal syphilis, all of these diseases are characterized by self-limited primary and secondary lesions, a latent period apparently disease-free and late lesions that frequently are destructive, particularly of bone and skin. In all three diseases, there are at some stage positive VDRL or RPR and/or treponemal antibody (FTA–ABS) tests indistinguishable from those accompanying sexually transmitted syphilis. In yaws, the distinctive "framboise" (French for raspberry) lesion is diagnostic. Yaws confers solid immunity to syphilis. All three of the nonvenereal treponematoses can be diagnosed by darkfield examination, the organisms being morphologically indistinguishable from one another. Unlike syphilis, the diseases are commonly transmitted by fomites and nonvenereal contact, as between mother and child; in addition, yaws is transmitted (probably mechanically) by small flies.

A single injection of long-acting penicillin G (benzathine penicillin G) is effective in the treatment of each of these treponematoses.

ZOONOSES

Zoonoses are diseases that are communicable from animals to humans and may be caused by any of a variety of protozoa, bacteria, intermediate forms and viruses (Table 5-12). In general, the risk to humans is directly proportional to the degree of contact, direct or through vectors, with diseased animals or their discharges (*e.g.,* veterinarians, hunters, farmers). In this section we will confine ourselves to those zoonoses caused by spirochetes of the *Lepstospira* or *Borrelia* genera.

Leptospirosis. Leptospirosis is a zoonotic infection caused by any of approximately 150 serotypes of a single species *(Leptospira interrogans)*. About 40 cases were reported in the U.S. in 1986. Morphologically and culturally, the pathogenic types are distinguishable from one another. The general properties of leptospires are listed elsewhere. There are numerous free-living saprophytic species, often collectively referred to as the *L. biflexa* group. These are commonly found in wet, decomposing materials or domestic drain pipes. They differ markedly from pathogenic species in their resistance to azaguanine, their survival in contaminated cultures and sewage, and their capacity to grow at temperatures from 5° to 15°C.

TABLE 5-12. Zoonoses As Sources of Human Infection

PROTOZOA	BACTERIA	RICKETTSIAE/CHLAMYDIAE	VIRUSES
Babesiosis (2)	Antrhax (2,P)		
Cryptosporidiosis (2,4)	Brucellosis (2m,3,Te+Sm)	Rockey Mountain spotted fever (1,Ch,Te)	Contagious ecthyma (Orf) (2,4)
Echinococcosis	Erysipeloid (2,P)	Q fever (5,Te)	Dengue fever (1)
Larva migrans (2) (cutaneous; visceral [Th])	Listeriosis (?2,P,Am,Er)	Typhus (1,Te,Ch)	Encephalitides (1) (Western esquire, St. Louis, Venezuelan, California, Powassan)
Schistosomiasis (2)	Leptospirosis (3,Te)		
Taeniasis (3)	Plague (2,4,Sm,Te,Ch,Tr/S)		Hemorrhagic fevers (2)
Taenia solium (Pr) (cysticercosis)	Salmonellosis (2,3,Am,Ch)	Psittacosis (5,Te) (ornithosis)	Rabies (2)(5,Te)
Taenia saginata (Ni,Pr)			
Toxoplasmosis (2,3,Py,Tr/S)	Tularemia (1,2,3,5,Sm,[Te,Ch])		Yellow fever (1)
Trichinosis (3,Th)	Relapsing fever *(Borrelia duttoni)* (1,Te)		

Mode of transmission:
1 = Arthropod vector.
2 = Direct contact with infected animal, tissue, discharges.
3 = Ingestion of, or contact with, contaminated material.
4 = Human-to-human transmission possible.
5 = inhalation.

Chemotherapeutic agent(s) used:
Am = ampicillin.
Ch = chloramphenicol.
Cl = clindamycin.
Er = erythromycin.
Ni = niclosamide.
P = penicillin.

Pr = praziquantel.
Py = pyrimethamine.
Sm = Streptomycin
Te = tetracycline.
Th = thiabendazole.
Tr/s = trimethoprim—sulfa methoxazole

Pathogens (generally referred to as the *L. interrogans* complex) grow well only between 30° and 37°C and are readily overgrown by contaminants in culture. Like *Treponema pallidum,* these organisms are extremely sensitive to detergents and acid conditions, although they will survive in urine-contaminated water if not too acid. They will traverse ordinary bacteriostatic filters. The various pathogenic types can be differentiated from each other antigenically.

Leptospirosis is primarily a disease of wild and domestic animals and is readily transmissible to humans (Weil's disease, Fort Bragg fever, rice field fever) by water contaminated with urine from infected rats, dogs, cats, cattle, and humans or through direct contact with infected animal carcasses in abattoirs or infected fowl in poultry-dressing plants. Person-to-person transmission occurs rarely. Leptospires enter the blood mainly via abrasions in the skin or via the oral mucosa during ingestion of contaminated foods or water. Neither endotoxins nor exotoxins have been demonstrated. Following an incubation period of 1 to 2 weeks, a spectrum of systemic symptoms (high fever, chills, headache, generalized myalgias) may supervene, during which the organisms are found in the blood, spinal fluid, and most organs, particularly kidneys and liver. With the development of antibodies, the organisms are cleared and symptoms subside. Subsequently, the organisms may appear in the urine, and meningitis or hepatitis (with or without icterus) may develop. In most cases, the disease is entirely self-limited; immunity is type specific.

Diagnosis can be made presumptively early in the disease by darkfield examination of urine and blood and confirmed by culture of blood in special semisolid media and by darkfield microscopic agglutination tests for antibody in acute and convalescent sera. Due to the presence of lymphocytes in the spinal fluid, this disease may be mistaken for aseptic (viral) meningitis, making darkfield microscopy essential. Penicillin and/or tetracycline is recommended for clinically severe leptospirosis.

Relapsing Fever (Borreliosis). There are up to 19 recognized species within the genus *Borrelia,* all of which are arthropod-borne, and 10 of which cause relapsing fevers (do not confuse with undulant fever, brucellosis) and one that causes Lyme disease (see below). *Borrelia* are distinguished morphologically from treponemes by their course irregular coils and are cultivable, though with difficulty, on Kelly's semisolid medium. *Borrelia* are best observed with darkfield microscopy in blood of febrile

patients, or in blood of rats that have been injected for diagnostic purposes and in which infection may develop rapidly with marked borrelemia. Blood films stained with Giemsa also reveal the organisms.

Transmission is by body lice *(Pediculus humanus)* in south central Europe, India, Asia, and North Africa, and other areas where pediculosis occurs. In these geographical areas, epidemic relapsing fever is due principally to *B. recurrentis,* for which humans are the only hosts. In South Africa, the Balkans, eastern Mediterranean regions, South and Central America, and the western United States, other species, notably *B. duttoni,* are transmitted in the bites, joint (coxal) fluids and feces (depending on the species) of various *Ornithodoros* soft ticks. The tick-borne disease is a true zoonosis (endemic relapsing fever), the animal reservoirs being principally wild rodents, monkeys, armadillos, and opossums, the sources of tangential human infection. If contracted during pregnancy, *Borrelia* may cause intrauterine infection that is fatal to the fetus.

After inoculation into the human host, the organisms multiply in the blood stream, as well as in the tissues. After an initial acute, febrile episode with headache, chills, hepatosplenomegaly, and macular rash, the fever ends by crisis in 1 to 2 weeks, due to the appearance of serum antibody. Examination of blood at this point may reveal agglutinated *Borrelia* in "rosette" formation. The organisms persist in lymphoid tissues, become resistant to antibody, presumably due to the appearance of antigenic mutants, and again invade the blood stream for 1 to 3 weeks, repeating the clinical cycle, though usually with diminished severity. Relapses may occur from 2 to 10 times (depending on the type of *Borrelia*).

Prevention depends on active louse control in areas of epidemic disease prevalence and avoidance of tick-infected rodents and other carriers of endemic borreliosis. Antibiotic treatment (tetracycline and/or chloramphenicol) is effective; if it is given during a febrile attack, Jarisch-Herxheimer–like reactions may occur.

Lyme Disease. Lyme disease is a syndrome that was first recognized in 1975 through a clustering of affected children in Lyme, Connecticut; it is now known to occur in at least 14 states, in Europe, and in Australia. The disease is characterized by a unique red skin lesion (erythema chronicum migrans, ECM) and by arthritis, which appears about a month after onset of acute symptoms, affects one or more joints, and may be recurrent. Erosive and proliferative synovitis may develop that resembles rheumatoid arthritis. Persons with HLA-DR2 histocompatibility antigens are also prone to develop meningoencephalitis and peripheral neuropathies in association with other manifestations of Lyme disease. Disease activity is correlated with serum IgM levels; there is also lymphopenia and lowered response of mononuclear cells to mitogens (e.g., phytohemagglutinin). Immune complexes are found in the blood simultaneously with the skin lesions. The infectious origin of ECM was deduced by the transmission of ECM between human volunteers by injection of tissue of active lesions. Lyme disease is now considered to be caused by Borrelia burgdorferi, which is carried by at least two species of tick, Ixodes dammini and I. pacificus. In 1986 there were 1500 cases, predominantly seen in the Northeast. The organism is cultivable in special medium, in which it grows slowly; it is highly sensitive to high-dose penicillin, which is curative of the infection. Due to increased T-suppressor-cell activity, late manifestations of the disease may mimic any of a number of disorders of immune origin (e.g., rheumatoid arthritis, Reiter's syndrome, multiple sclerosis) due either to autoimmune phenomena or exaggerated immune responses to the spirochete.

MYCOPLASMAS AND L FORMS

Infections Due to Mycoplasmas. *Mycoplasma mycoides*, the first of this group to be discovered (1898), was found to be the cause of contagious bovine pleuropneumonia. Subsequently, similar forms, called pleuropneumonia-like organisms (PPLO), were found in cases of mastitis in sheep and goats and in rodents, often associated with arthritis and lesions of eyes and ears. Mycoplasmas are the smallest known free-living forms of life, with no cell wall and a variable morphology; most inhabit the normal upper respiratory and genitourinary tracts. Only three are of clinical importance: *M. pneumoniae*, *M. hominis*, and *Ureaplasma urealyticum*.

Mycoplasma pneumoniae. M. pneumoniae (Eaton agent), the first of the mycoplasmas proven to be a cause of human disease, is the etiologic agent of "primary atypical pneumonia" (PAP), so called because of its clinical dissimilarity to lobar (typically pneumococcal) pneumonia and its failure to respond to sulfonamides and penicillin. Because of this, PAP was at first thought to have a viral etiology, in accord with the ability of the infectious principal to pass through bacteriostatic filters. However, unequivocal clinical response to broad-spectrum antibiotics in the earliest cases reported, and ultimately the cultivation of the causative organism on lifeless media, clearly substantiated the bacterial nature of the Eaton agent.

M. pneumoniae is a significant cause of lower respiratory tract infection (tracheobronchitis to interstitial pneumonia) characterized by nonproductive cough, persistent fever, absence of leukocytosis, and "walking pneumonia." The infection occurs primarily in temperate climates and may become epidemic, most frequently affecting school-age children and young adults; it is spread by respiratory droplet and close contact. The clinical disease must be distinguished from Q fever, legionnaires' disease, ornithosis (chlamydial), and interstitial pneumonia of viral etiology. Being a surface infection, M. pneumoniae colonizes the respiratory epithelium, interrupting normal ciliary motion; the organism is not invasive and is never recovered from the blood. Recovery and immunity to reinfection are due to local accumulation of secretory IgA and serum IgG antibody. Treatment with tetracyclines or erythromycin is effective; penicillin is ineffective because M. pneumoniae lacks a cell wall. Rarely, central nervous system and other systemic complications may follow proven M. pneumoniae infection.

To establish the diagnosis, M. pneumoniae can be recovered from sputum on special selective agar enriched with animal serum and yeast extract, on which colonies of M. pneumoniae are recognized by their ability to adsorb erythrocytes (hemadsorption) and by direct immunofluorescence. The organisms are too small and fragile to stain with Gram's or Giemsa stain. The clinical diagnosis is confirmed retrospectively by a rise in serum antibody demonstrated by complement fixation or tetrazolium-reduction-inhibition (TRI, metabolic inhibition) tests. In addition to specific antibody, up to 40% of patients with mycoplasmal pneumonia develop serum "cold" agglutinins, that is, their serum agglutinates human O erythrocytes at 4°C, frequently to very high titer, but not at 37°C. This transient cold agglutinin is an IgM antibody with cross-reactive specificity for the I antigen in erythrocyte glycophorin and membrane antigen(s) of M. pneumoniae.

Mycoplasma hominis. M. hominis in adults is a cause of prostatitis, pelvic inflammatory disease, as well as postpartum or postabortal sepsis. In newborns it is a cause of sepsis, lymphadentis, meningitis, pericarditis, and conjunctivitis. Diagnosis is difficult and mainly by exclusion of other sexually transmitted or neonatal diseases. There is a typical purulent infection with polymorphonuclear leukocytes in the cerebrospinal fluid and joint fluid. Treatment is with lincomycin or clindamycin.

Ureaplasma Urealyticum. *U. urealyticum* normally inhabits the oral and/or genitourinary tract and comprises eight serotypes (formerly referred to as T or "tiny" mycoplasma because of their small colony size). *U. urealyticum* infection is sexually transmitted and is an important cause of nonchlamydial, nongonococcal urethritis (NGU) in both sexes and of pelvic inflammatory disease. Antibodies to *U. urealyticum* rise during many pregnancies, suggesting that maternal infection with mycoplasma may contribute to perinatal morbidity. Under such circumstances, treatment with erythromycin during the third trimester has been reported to reduce the incidence of low-birthweight infants born to women colonized with genital mycoplasmas. Diagnosis is based on recovery and identification of urease-producing mycoplasma *(U. urealyticum)* on special media and metabolic inhibition with specific antibody. Tetracycline is the drug of choice in treatment.

L Forms of Bacteria. Many common gram-positive bacteria, cultivated in the presence of penicillin in media with increased osmotic pressure (*e.g.*, 3% sucrose), grow without their cell wall and are therefore called *protoplasts;* in many respects they are much like PPLO. Gram-negative bacteria retain the lipoprotein portions of their cell wall in the presence of penicillin and are therefore not wholly naked and are called *spheroplasts.* These cell-wall-less or cell-wall-defective forms are called L forms (from the Lister Institute, where they were first described) of the particular bacterium involved. Removed from the osmotically protective medium they undergo plasmolysis, that is, they are "osmotically fragile." With the removal of penicillin they revert to true bacteria. PPLO also not uncommonly revert to well-known species of bacteria, and vice versa. It is suggested that nonreverting PPLO are genetically stabilized bacterial L form mutants with decreased osmotic fragility. The possible development of L forms of pathogens *in vivo,* especially during penicillin therapy, with establishment of latent and antibiotic-resistant infections, is of obvious clinical importance.

A number of other species of PPLO, also bacterial L forms, are of importance in diagnostic work with viruses, since they can contaminate tissues used as sources of cell cultures for diagnostic virology as well as animal products used for cell culture. *Streptobacillus moniliformis* is a bacterial species, bacillary and streptobacilly in form, that produces minute PPLO called L_1 bodies, that revert in turn to *S. moniliformis*. Both forms may occur in the same culture. *Streptobacillus moniliformis* is related to one form of rat-bite fever and to Haverhill fever.

Minute Bacteria

FAMILY RICKETTSIACEAE

Rickettsia. Rickettsiae are pleomorphic cocci and rods, the latter often containing bipolar granules of unknown significance. The organisms can grow in cell cultures but are commonly propagated in cells of the yolk sac of embryonated hens' eggs. Machiavello's stain is commonly used. In spite of their minute size, rickettsiae do not pass through bacterial-retaining filters (but see *Coxiella* of Q fever, the exception). Their cell structure is prokaryotic, and their cell walls contain muramic acid, a substance found only in bacteria. They are obligate intracellular parasites and contain both DNA and RNA. Rickettsiae contain a potent endotoxin but produce no exotoxin. Cellular substances are antigenic and species specific, except the antigen that is shared with *Proteus* (see Weil-Felix reaction).

Habitat. Most rickettsiae are primarily parasites of insects and only secondarily of animals. They are transmitted from insects to humans and from person to person by the bites of insects or by being rubbed into scratches and cuts when infected insects are crushed on the skin.

Antibiotic Susceptibility. Rickettsiae possess bacterium-like, though limited, enzyme systems, including those of the Krebs cycle and those necessary to the synthesis of ATP, cell wall, and some proteins. Hence rickettsiae are susceptible to enzyme-inhibiting chemotherapeutic drugs, especially the tetracyclines and chloramphenicol, which are effective therapeutically. Relapses occur during therapy because the organisms survive intracellularly.

Diagnosis. Laboratory diagnosis of rickettsial disease is made by agglutination tests using purified yolk sac antigens to reveal group-specific antibodies in patient sera. Adult guinea pigs or white mice are inoculated with appropriate specimens (most often blood) and evaluated for febrile reactions; tissues from inoculated animals are examined at autopsy and put into cell culture for recovery of rickettsiae. Cell culture, however, is not appropriate for direct diagnostic inoculation of clinical specimens.

The **Weil–Felix test** depends on the differential agglutination of strains of *Proteus vulgaris* by the serum of patients with suspected rickettsiosis (Table 5-10). *Proteus* has no etiologic relationship to rickettsial diseases, but the O antigen in *Proteus* cross-reacts with a minor rickettsial antigen. Misleading positive reactions may occur in patients who are free of rickettsiae but who have urinary tract infections due to *Proteus* and a significant homologous antibody response.

Diseases Due to Rickettsiae. Three main groups of diseases are recognized as due to rickettsiae: (1) the ***typhus*** group, (2) the ***spotted fever*** group, and (3) the ***scrub typhus*** group. The first group includes European or "classic" epidemic typhus and Brill's disease (recrudescent typhus), in which the transmission is human–louse–human, the lice being killed by the infection, and murine or endemic typhus, in which transmission to humans is by the rat flea. Diseases of the second group are mainly tick-borne within animal reservoirs, the ticks maintaining infection transovarially and by sexual transmission and incidentally infecting humans. The one exception is rickettsialpox, transmitted by a mite from domestic murine reservoirs. Diseases of the third group are larval-mite borne. Q fever differs from all of the foregoing with respect to both etiology and clinical aspects.

Clinically, all rickettsial diseases (except Q fever, which resembles influenza, and rickettsialpox, which resembles chickenpox) have certain cardinal features in common: stupor and other neurological signs, rash, and invasion of reticuloendothelial cells by the rickettsiae. Usually there are both clinical and pathologic diagnostic differences between these rickettsioses, such as chronology, intensity, and distribution of the rash, development of eschar at site of arthropod bite, and so on.

In nature, epidemic typhus occurs only in humans, the other rickettsioses being primarily zoonoses (i.e., enzootic in lower animals, occurring only secondarily in humans). The rickettsiae of typhus and tsutsugamushi fevers remain in the cytoplasm of infected cells, while those of Rocky Mountain spotted fever and of rickettsialpox also invade the nucleus. In severe Rocky Mountain spotted fever the smooth muscles of peripheral vascular walls are destroyed. In rickettsialpox and tsutsugamushi there is a definite ulcer or eschar at the site of the infecting bite. Rickettsialpox is distinguished by its poxlike vesicles. Tsutsugamushi, Rocky Mountain spotted fever and epidemic typhus are generally more severe than murine typhus or rickettsialpox.

Brill-Zinsser disease is epidemic or classic typhus occurring sporadically in the total absence of body lice, as a relatively mild recrudescence of latent in-

fection years after the initial attack. In the febrile stage the disease is transmissible by body lice. Apparently the rickettsiae can remain viable but quiescent in the tissues for many years after initial infection. Occasionally, this disease appears in the United States, especially in immigrants from central Europe, Asia Minor, and eastern Mediterranean areas.

Coxiella. This genus contains only one species, *Coxiella burnetii*, named for H. L. Cox and F. M. Burnet, simultaneous discoverers. It is immunologically distinct from other rickettsiae. *C. Burnetii* causes Q fever (Q for "query") first observed and named by Derrick in Australia. *C. burnetii* has most of the properties of *Rickettsia* but differs in being (1) filterable; (2) quite resistant to environmental conditions (probably due to endospore-like forms) such as drying, diffuse sunlight, disinfectants, heating at 62°C for 30 minutes; (3) mode of transmission: improperly pasteurized contaminated milk; dust, from barns housing infected sheep, cattle, goats, rodents; tissues and parturition fluids from infectious animals; several species of ticks.

In **Q fever** the respiratory tract is most commonly affected. There is no rash. The disease clinically resembles influenza, often with interstitial pneumonitis. Mortality is low or nil. Q fever appears to be disseminated widely, especially among persons in the animal industries, having been reported from more than 31 states and 50 countries on 5 continents. The organisms may be isolated from the blood by animal inoculation. Diagnosis also may be made by serologic methods but *not* by the Weil-Felix test. Milk can be made safe only by pasteurization for 30 minutes at a temperature of 63°C (145°F). Tetracycline and chloramphenicol are the drugs of choice in treatment. An experimental Q fever vaccine for human and veterinary use has shown promise.

FAMILY CHLAMYDIACEAE

Chlamydia. Formerly classified with "filtrable viruses," *Chlamydia*, like *Rickettsia* and *Coxiella*, are bacteria modified to obligate intracellular parasitism due to their lack of certain protein-synthetic and oxidative enzyme systems. Chlamydiae are distinctive in lacking enzymes that synthesize ATP; they must use host-derived energy. These organisms exhibit a complex intracellular developmental cycle. Elementary bodies, the infectious units, attach to susceptible cells, penetrate by phagocytosis, and develop into reticulate bodies. The latter increase in number, some developing into intermediate forms, which end up as new infectious elementary bodies released by disruption of the cell.

The genus is divided into two main groups, *C. trachomatis* and *C. psittaci*. The first group (previously referred to as TRIC agents) is the most important because it includes classic ocular trachoma (serogroups A, B, and C), genital infections (particularly nongonococcal urethritis; NGU), inclusion conjunctivitis and pneumonitis of infants (serotypes D to M), and lymphogranuloma venereum (LGV serotypes I, II, and III). The second major group (*C. psittaci*) comprises the agents of psittacosis and ornithosis. *Chlamydia* possess a common group-specific antigen; individual serotypes can be distinguished by immunofluorescence using type-specific antisera. Members of both groups are readily isolated and propagated either in the yolk sac of chicken eggs or in cell culture systems (*e.g.,* McCoy cells treated with IUDR and cycloheximide to prevent cellular mitosis). The cytopathology induced by *C. trachomatis* is readily identified because of large intracytoplasmic inclusions. These are composed of glycogen and therefore stain readily with iodine (Lugol's solution) and autofluoresce in ultraviolet light without the addition of labeled antisera. Similar inclusions are diagnostic when discovered in tarsal scrapings from clinically suspected neonatal inclusion conjunctivitis. In adults, *C. trachomatis* is an important and frequent cause of sexually transmitted disease, manifest as NGU, proctitis and attendant complications in the male, and cervicitis and pelvic inflammatory disease in the female. In both sexes, it also occurs asymptomatically, but is still infectious. Chlamydial infection ranks with gonorrhea as a major cause of sexually transmitted disease and accordingly also accounts for a substantial number of cases of acute pharyngitis. The likelihood of coexistent chlamydial infection (estimated to occur in up to 20%) should therefore be kept in mind in the management of primary gonococcal infection. Rapid diagnosis of chlamydial infection is readily accomplished by direct immunofluorescence with monoclonal antibodies applied to smears of urethral or cervical secretions. In view of the possibility of dual infection, some form of combined therapy (*e.g.,* sulfamethoxazole-trimethoprim or penicillin, plus tetracycline, rather than penicillin alone with probenecid) should be considered in treating men with these infections. For women with probable combined infection, the current recommendation is to treat the gonococcal infection first (single dose of ampicillin, amoxicillin, or penicillin) and then give tetracycline for chlamydial infection, which may not be demonstrable but is probably present.

Lymphogranuloma venereum (LGV) (not to be confused with granuloma inguinale due to *Calymmatobacterium granulomatis*) is a sporadically occurring sexually transmitted disease, worldwide in distribution, commoner in blacks and males than in whites and females. Three serotypes of *C. trachomatis* (LCV I, II, and III, cross-reactive with serotypes D and E) are distinguished by microimmunofluorescence. Clinically, an initial painless superficial genital ulcer progresses to lymphadenopathy, draining bubo formation, and finally scarring of rectal mucosa and stricture. The diagnosis is made more often serologically (complement fixation tests on paired sera) than by isolation of the agent, which may be difficult. The Frei test, once the mainstay of diagnosis, is no longer much used. Treatment with tetracycline or sulfonamides is usually effective.

Chlamydia psittaci is the cause of psittacosis or parrot fever, named for psittacine birds that are the natural reservoirs of the organism. Domestic fowl and park pigeons may harbor the infection, and person-to-person transmission occurs. Human ornithosis, more frequent in occurrence than previously thought, is contracted by inhalation of dust harboring dried feces and respiratory secretions of infected birds. The disease occurs as a primary interstitial pneumonia with a patchy lobular distribution and is accompanied by variable constitutional signs and symptoms and normal leukocyte count. It must be distinguished from influenza, mycoplasmal pneumonia, legionellosis, and Q fever. *C. psittaci* can be isolated from the sputum in modified cell culture, as with *C. trachomatis;* however, no iodine-staining glycogen inclusions are formed. Diagnosis is made or confirmed retrospectively by complement fixation tests on paired sera. Tetracycline is considered to be effective in therapy.

VIRUSES

Viruses must be distinguished on the one hand from the smaller macromolecules of which they are constituted (DNA or RNA, proteins) and on the other hand from the larger bacteria or other parasitic microorganisms. Viruses are much smaller than bacteria or animal cells that they infect and can pass through filters that trap such cells.

General Concept of Viruses

A virus may be defined as a strictly particulate intracellular entity with an infectious phase, possessing only one type of nucleic acid (called the genome) and replicating or multiplying in the form of their genetic material, although in some virus families there may be an intermediate stage in nucleic acid replication involving another nucleic acid type. For example, retroviruses such as human immunodeficiency virus (HIV), the causative agent of acquired immune deficiency syndrome (AIDS), are RNA viruses that replicate through a DNA intermediate, and hepatitis B virus (HBV), a DNA virus, utilizes an RNA intermediate. Viruses are unable to grow by themselves or undergo binary fission, and finally, they are devoid of an energy-producing enzyme system.

Nomenclature and Structure

Animal viruses can be classified as either naked or enveloped: *Naked viruses* contain *only* RNA or DNA and a protein coat, while *enveloped viruses* contain *only* RNA or DNA + protein coat + lipid-containing membrane (also called an envelope).

The nucleic acid or *genome* as the hereditary material serves an absolutely necessary function; for some viruses, like poliovirus, the RNA after modification serves as mRNA on entry into the cell.

The *protein coat* protects the nucleic acid from nucleases. For naked viruses it also serves as an attachment vehicle to cells—the major determinant of host range. For enveloped viruses, glycoprotein spikes embedded in the envelope serve as the attachment site to specific host cell receptors. Thus, in AIDS, the HIV virus attaches by the gp120 spikes to cells with the OKT4+ receptors, such as T_h (helper) cells or certain monocytes.

In recent years, there have been breakthroughs made in the discovery of a smaller class of infectious agents than even viruses. These agents are called *viroids*. They are not viruses but appear to be covalently closed single-stranded RNA circles about 300 to 400 nucleotides in length, which are resistant to ultraviolet (UV) radiation, as well as to denaturing chemical agents. Viroids do not encode proteins. They replicate *in vitro* via the rolling circle model of replication. *In vivo* the pathogenesis caused by viroids may be a result of their interference with normal transcription inside host cells. Recently, the delta agent that causes a virulent form of hepatitis B disease ("fulminant hepatitis") has been isolated and characterized. It is a viroid RNA packaged into the hepatitis B virus capsid shell.

Terminology

Before undertaking a detailed discussion of viruses, it is important to define certain basic terms.

1. *Virion:* The complete virus particle
2. *Capsid:* The protein coat surrounding the nucleic acid or genome
3. *Capsomers:* The repeating protein subunits that make up the capsid
4. *Protomers:* The polypeptide chains that make up the capsomers. Note, noncovalent bonds between protomers are usually stronger than those between capsomers.
5. *Symmetry* of the virus, which can be:
   a. *Icosahedral:* A virus particle with 20 triangular faces, exhibiting 5 : 3 : 2 rotational symmetry, for example, adenovirus
   b. *Helical:* Exemplified by the measles virus, which contains a helical nucleocapsid inside the envelope
   c. *Bilateral:* A vaccinia virus is morphologically symmetrical when viewed by thin section electron microscopy.

The first known virus (tobacco mosaic) was discovered in 1892 by Iwanowski, regarded as a living contagious fluid (*contagium vivum fluidum*) by Beijerinck in 1898, and purified as protein in crystalline form by Stanley in 1935. The first known virus of vertebrates (foot-and-mouth disease) was discovered by Löffler and Frosch in 1898; the first known virus of humans (yellow fever), by Walter Reed and his associates in 1899. Studies of animal viruses were laborious, cumbersome, and expensive and progressed slowly until the discovery of bacteriophage (phage) by Twort in 1915 and d'Herelle in 1917. Because phage could be cultivated easily, quickly, safely, and inexpensively in test-tube cultures by allowing them to infect cells of a harmless bacterium (generally *Escherichia coli*), they became a principal experimental subject of virologists. Although bacteria are prokaryotes, studies of phage have yielded much information directly applicable to virology of animal cells. The development of practical means of cultivating animal tissue eliminated the drudgery and expense of using live animals and provided a relatively simple means, now widely used, of studying animal viruses.

Bacteriophage

Studies of phages have provided the foundation for studying mammalian viruses and are therefore discussed in some detail here.

Although phage have been found for many species of bacteria, blue–green algae, and some yeasts, the most studied phages are certain types that infect *Escherichia coli*, or *Bacillus subtilis*. They are identified by number(s) and letter(s), such as, the "T-even" phages: T2, T4, T6; the "T-odd" phages: T3, T7, etc., λ, φ X174, each with distinctive form, antigenic proteins, capsomers, and dimensions. Some have genomes of DNA, some of RNA, some single-stranded, some double. Some have 5-hydroxymethylcytosine in place of cytosine; some have uracil or 5-hydroxymethyluracil in place of thymine; some have tails, others do not. Small, tailless phages (24 to 60 nm, *e.g.*, φ X174, M12) are icosahedral in form; some (*e.g.*, fl, M13) are filamentous (800 nm long) with helical symmetry; larger phages (50 to 90 nm) have tails up to 210 nm long attached to the "head" or nucleocapsid. The tails of T-even phages are of very complex structure with terminal spikes and long thin fibers for attachment of the phage to its host cell. Other phage tails are relatively simple. Unlike animal viruses, few phages are enveloped. Small, RNA-containing phages are much like picornaviruses (animal) (see Table 5-13), though they contain RNA only equivalent to about five genes. The RNA of such viruses acts in the host cell as its own mRNA.

PHAGE ACTIVITY

Phages attach to specific receptors on susceptible cells, using structures such as tail fibers. By means of enzymic mechanisms located at the tip of the tail, an opening is made through the bacterial cell wall and cell membrane. Through this, the nucleic acid (NA) core from the head of the phage enters the cell. The capsid is now an empty shell that may remain attached to the exterior of the cell.

Some phages attach only to bacterial F pili and are therefore said to be male specific. Filamentous phages attach at the tip of the F pili, while male-specific icosahedral phages adsorb at various specific sites along the F-pilus. Once inside the bacterium, all phages, whether male specific or not, can no longer be demonstrable as phage *(eclipse phase)*. In some instances the phage NA becomes integrated with the genetic mechanism of the cell as though a part of the bacterial genome *(prophage)*, replicating with the bacterial chromosome. There it may remain there in a latent stage for many generations, doing no evident harm. Phage in this form is said to be *temperate*. The cell containing it is said to be *lysogenic*. The lysogenic cell is sometimes called a *lysogen*. The term lysogeny applies only to phage-

infected bacteria. However, analogous relationships are found between some transforming or oncogenic viruses and their animal host cells.

As a result of various chemical or physical stimuli (*e.g.*, ultraviolet or x irradiation) to the lysogenic bacterium, the prophage can be *induced* or *activated*. The temperate phage then multiplies vegetatively, injuring the host bacterium and takes control of the synthetic mechanisms of the cell to replicate itself.

In the active state (lytic or vegetative) the phage genome codes for enzymes that cause prompt disintegration of the host DNA to nucleotides, with resulting immediate cessation of cell synthesis, the synthesis of new DNA precursors and "early" replication of phage NA, as well as transcription of the phage genome. Functioning of host-specific mRNA stops, and "late" phage mRNA forms phage materials (NA, enzymes, capsids, etc.) using cell ribosomes. Similar events occur in animal cells infected by animal viruses, with modifications depending on the characteristics of each specific cell–virus system.

Once replicated, the new phage NA is *encapsidated;* nucleocapsids and the tails, if present, then combine and the intracellular virions are assembled as *mature* virions (end of the eclipse period). The bacterial cell wall is soon disintegrated by a phage-coded lysozyme *(lysis from within)*, liberating new virions. The various periods usually take about 30 minutes for phage and about 1 to 2 hours for analogous naked viruses.

A lysogenic cell containing prophage has *prophage immunity*, that is, it cannot be superinfected by another virion of that phage type 1, although NA of other lysogenic phage types may infect the cell.

When bacterial cells undergo phage lysis, they suddenly liberate many intact virions, producing a "one-step" increase in the number of virions or *plaque-forming units*. (Distinguish this type of growth curve from that of bacteria.)

Most nonlysogenic phages, on entering their susceptible bacterial host, proceed immediately to multiplication (vegetative activity) and destruction of the cell as described above. Such phages are said to be *lytic* or *virulent*.

PLAQUE FORMATION BY BACTERIOPHAGE

To demonstrate plaque formation with bacteriophage, a broth culture of bacteria is mixed with an appropriate number (50 to 500) of bacteriophage virions in semisolid agar. The mixture is spread over

(text continues on page 470)

TABLE 5-13. Classification of Viruses

FAMILY	VIRUSES	DISEASES
DNA Viruses:		
Naked (Unenveloped)		
Parvoviruses	Parvoviruses (Kilham rat virus, minute virus of mice, H viruses)	(Animals only)
ss positive strand; complementary (+ or –) in separate virions, icosahedral symmetry	Adenosatellite viruses (4 serotypes)	Indigenous, no recognized disease
	Densoviruses (insects)	
	Stem cell virus (12 + serotypes)	Bone marrow failure
Papovaviruses	Papillomavirus	Verruca vulgaris, condyloma accuminatum (?HPV16 precancerous)
ds, circular DNA naked, icosahedral symmetry	Simian virus 40 (SV40)	
	JC virus	Progressive multifocal leukoencephalopathy (PML)
	BK virus	
	Polyomavirus	(Multiple tumors in hamsters)
Adenoviruses	Adenoviruses (41 serotypes)	URTI
ds, icosahedral	Common CF antigen (hexon), type-specific antigens (penton), H	Gastroenteritis, conjunctivitis, lymphadenitis (certain types oncogenic in hamsters)
	(Animal adenoviruses)	
Hepatitis virus	Hepatitis B (HB) virus [Surface (s), core (c) and e antigens; Dane particle = virion]	Acute, chronic and inapparent infection ("long incubation," "serum"), ?hepatocellular carcinoma
ds		
Enveloped		
Herpesviruses	Herpes simplex, types 1, 2	Herpes labialis, herpes genitalis, encephalitis, keratoconjunctivitis
ds, icosahedral capsid		Latent, recurrent infection (oncogenic transformation in animals)
		Type 2: ?cervical carcinoma–associated, sexually transmitted
	Simian herpesvirus (herpes B)	Encephalitis
	Epstein-Barr (EB) virus	Infectious mononucleosis, (non-Forssman heterophile antibody)
		Burkitt lymphoma (lymphoma, malignant neurolymphomatosis), (?nasopharyngeal carcinoma), hepatitis
	Varicella-zoster (VZ) virus	Chickenpox–shingles; VZ pneumonia, postinfectious encephalitis (?Reye's syndrome)
	Cytomegalovirus (CMV)	Congenital, neonatal systemic infections; compromised host, hepatitis, mononucleosis (no heterophile antibody)
	Pseudorabies	(Equines)
	Variola virus	Smallpox (variola major, minor; alastrim)
Poxviruses	Vaccinia virus	Eczema vaccinatum, generalized vaccinia, postvaccinal encephalitis (rare complications of vaccination)
ds, complex, lateral bodies, separate HA		Cowpox
	Parapoxviruses	Milkers' nodes, Orf (sheep)
	Molluscum contagiosum	Multiple skin lesions
	Yaba virus	Localized skin lesions (monkeys)
RNA Viruses:		
Naked (Unenveloped)		
Picornaviruses	Enteroviruses [poliovirus (3 serotypes), echovirus and coxsackievirus (70 + serotypes), hepatitis A virus]	Meningitis, meningoencephalitis, poliomyelitis, inapparent infection (lower GI tract), herpangina, URTI, pleurodynia, myocarditis, exanthemata
ss, positive, icosahedral symmetry	Cardioviruses [encephalomyocarditis (EMC) virus]	
	Rhinoviruses (100 + serotypes)	URTI, CCS
Caliciviruses	Norwalk agent	Gastroenteritis in infants and children
Reoviruses	Reoviruses (3 serotypes), H	Lower gastrointestinal trace, ?disease
ds, segmented, linear icosahedral symmetry,	Orbiviruses (all are arboviruses)	Colorado tick fever, (various ungulates)
	Rotavirus (2 serotypes)	Infantile diarrhea (winter)

double shell capsid inner icosahedron

Enveloped		
Togaviruses ss, positive, icosahedral symmetry	Alphaviruses (formerly group A arboviruses), H Flaviviruses (formerly group B arboviruses), H Rubivirus (rubella), H	Encephalitis Hemorrhagic fever, yellow fever, dengue fever, encephalitis Rubella, with arthritis in adults, congenital rubella syndrome
Bunyaviruses helical symmetry, genome ss, 3 circular segments	Bunyamwera virus, H California encephalitis viruses Formerly group C arboviruses	Mild encephalitis, Crimean-Congo hemorrhagic fever, sandfly fever, Rift Valley fever
Orthomyxoviruses ss, segmented, negative, helical symmetry	Influenza viruses Serologic groups A, B (H–N types), C (H only)	Epidemic (group A) and sporadic influenza, CCS, (Reye's syndrome, group B)
Paramyxoviruses ss, unsegmented, negative, helical symmetry	Parainfluenza viruses (4 serotypes), HN Mumps virus, HN Respiratory syncytial virus (no H or N) Measles (rubeola) virus, H (no N)	URTI, croup, bronchiolitis, pneumonia Parotitis, orchitis, meningitis URTI, bronchiolitis, pneumonitis Measles, subacute sclerosing panencephalitis
Rhabdoviruses ss, helical symmetry, bullet shaped	(Vesicular stomatitis virus) (Kern Canyon [bat] virus) Rabies ?Marburg virus (simian) ?Ebola virus	Rabies Hemorrhagic fever (?nosocomial spread)
Retroviruses ss, RNA-dependent DNA polymerase (reverse transcriptase) in virion, inner icosahedral shell, helical core	Oncoviruses, leukoviruses (Foamy virus) (Maedi-Visna group of viruses) Human T-cell leukemia viruses (HTLV) HIV	Host-specific leukemias, sarcomas, mammary tumors (Persistent infection in different mammalian species) ("Slow" viral diseases in sheep: panleukoencephalitis, multiorgan involvement, non-oncogenic) Human T-cell leukemia (I, II), AIDS (HIV)
Arenaviruses Spherical virion, genome ss, 2 negative segments, host ribosomal particles	Lymphocytic choriomeningitis virus Lassa virus (?rats) Tacaribe complex (?rodents)	Choriomeningitis Lassa fever (nosocomial spread) Hemorrhagic fevers
Coronaviruses ss, enveloped, positive, helical symmetry	Coronavirus (3 serotypes) different animal species	Respiratory infections, CCS
Unclassified viruses Chronic infectious neuro-pathic agents		Kuru, Creutzfeldt-Jakob disease (CJD) (scrapie in sheep, mink encephalopathy)

Abbreviations

ss = single stranded; ds = double stranded; DNA = deoxyribonucleic acid; RNA = ribonucleic acid; URTI = upper respiratory tract infection; LRTI = lower respiratory tract infection; CCS = common cold syndrome; H = hemagglutinin; N = neuraminidase.

Definitions

Virion: The intact (infectious) viral particle.

Genome: Nucleic acid core, embodying genetic information required for viral replication.

Capsid: Protein associated with the genome in cubic or helical symmetry or in complex configuration. Capsids of unenveloped viruses contain protective antigens.

Capsomers: Structural subunits of the capsid.

Nucleocapsid: Viral nucleic acid combined with capsid protein. intact nucleocapsid of unenveloped viruses is the infectious unit.

Envelope: Lipoprotein coat that surrounds noninfectious nucleocapsid, contains virus-coded protective antigens, and is essential for infectivity.

the surface of nutrient agar in a Petri dish, which is then incubated. Small clear areas of lysis are seen that are called plaques. Each plaque is initiated by a single, infected bacterial cell in which phage has multiplied and from which progeny virions have been released to infect adjacent cells in the bacterial "lawn." Thus the infection spreads by diffusion from a single bacterium to involve many other adjacent cells. Several cycles of infection are required before a plaque becomes visible. A count of the plaques then gives an idea of the number of particles in the original phage suspension. The term plaque-forming unit (PFU) is used to describe the number of infective phage particles in the suspension.

Replication of Animal Viruses

In a manner similar to bacteriophage, animal viruses replicate in appropriately sensitive eukaryotic cells by a process in which separate components are synthesized in the infected cell and then are assembled into virions before release. To initiate the process, virions attach to susceptible cells by interaction of discrete components on the viral surface (e.g., H protein in orthomyxoviruses, fiber antigen on adenoviruses) with specific receptors on the cell. The virus then penetrates (either by viropexis or, in the case of enveloped viruses, by fusion of viral envelope with cell membrane) into the cytoplasm where the genome is uncoated and interacts with the synthetic apparatus of the cell. In most DNA viruses, the nucleic acid is double-stranded and, through mRNA, codes for synthesis of early proteins (enzymes required for synthesis of new viral DNA) and for later proteins (enzymes required for synthesis of viral structural proteins). Naked DNA viruses (e.g., adenoviruses) accumulate in the nucleus and are released by ultimate disintegration of the cell. Herpesviruses are enveloped, DNA viruses. They are also assembled in the nucleus; however, as they emerge the nucleocapsid acquires from the nuclear membrane a lipid-containing envelope into which virus-coded glycoproteins have been inserted. Poxviruses are synthesized and assembled in the cytoplasm. Parvoviruses contain only single-stranded DNA; some are defective such as adenoassociated virus (AAV) and require helper virus for replication. Certain DNA viruses (e.g., adenoviruses, herpesviruses) can transform nonpermissive cells (i.e., cells unable to support the complete viral replicative cycle), and viral DNA integrates into the host cell genome in a manner analogous to lysogeny by bacteriophage.

In RNA viruses with a single-stranded genome,

the RNA may be "positive" (i.e., have the same sequence of nucleotide bases as viral mRNA as in poliovirus) or "negative" (i.e., require an intravirion transcriptase–RNA polymerase to synthesize mRNA, utilizing virion RNA as a template, as in influenza or parainfluenza virions). It is particularly of interest to note that with influenza virus, there is a cannibalization of 5' caps (7-methyl inverted dGTP) from newly synthesized host mRNAs to serve as a primer for synthesis of the mRNA by the intravirion transcriptase. Also, note that the single-stranded RNA genome in orthomyxoviruses such as influenza is segmented, which accounts for the genetic reassortment of these viruses and hence the unique epidemiology of the disease influenza. In most other single-stranded RNA viruses (e.g., paramyxoviruses), the genome is unsegmented and therefore cannot undergo intratypic reassortment; such viruses are antigenically stable. Enveloped RNA viruses (including RNA tumor viruses) are released by budding through the cell membrane, which, at the sites of viral morphogenesis, acquires the proteins (e.g., H and N of influenza virus) subsequently found in the viral envelope. Newly synthesized surface components (e.g., H protein of orthomyxoviruses, capsid proteins of naked viruses) evoke antibodies that block attachment and penetration by subsequently introduced virus of the same type. Viral surface components therefore include the "protective" antigens that account for the efficacy of viral vaccines in stimulating specific antiviral immunity in susceptible individuals, and for the sustained immunity to reinfection following the primary disease (e.g., H antigen of measles virus, HN antigen of mumps virus). Antibody to internal antigens (e.g., nucleocapsid) does not neutralize infectivity, but is useful for classifying viruses, such as, influenza A or B. Some viruses have a double-stranded RNA genome (e.g., reoviruses, rotaviruses); their replication is even more complex.

Laboratory Cultivation and Analysis of Animal Viruses

A number of animal viruses, notably orthomyxoviruses, can be propagated in embryonated chicken eggs. For primary isolation, amniotic inoculation is best. Serial passage is done by chorioallantoic inoculation, virus being shed into the chorioallantoic fluid, from which it can be concentrated and purified (as for influenza vaccines). Cell and tissue culture is the mainstay of laboratory virology. Cells for culture are dissociated initially from tissue by digestion with trypsin and EDTA (versene), washed in balanced salt solution, and suspended in growth medium containing serum and necessary minerals, amino acids, vitamins, glucose, and a bicarbonate–CO_2 buffer system to equilibrate with ambient gases. Phenol red (phenolsulfonphthalein, PSP) is the usual indicator because its color change (alkaline to acid, red to yellow) is in the physiological range (around pH 6.8). Dissociated cells attach readily to the surface of glass or plastic and grow out in a spreading sheet one cell thick (monolayer). Cells derived from neoplastic tissue (aneuploid) can usually be serially passaged (i.e., trypsinized off the glass, divided and dispensed to new vessels) an indefinite number of times and are called cell lines. Cells derived from normal tissue (e.g., human foreskin, embryonic lung, kidney) are diploid and have a finite life in vitro, that is, they will survive only a few serial passages. However, certain diploid cell "strains" (e.g., WI 38 human embryonic lung cells) can be passaged many times before dying out and are therefore valuable for production of viruses in bulk for vaccine preparation.

The presence of virus in inoculated monolayers is signaled by the appearance of cytopathic effects (CPE) manifested as rounding, separation and necrosis of cells (e.g., enteroviruses), nuclear enlargement and clumping (e.g., adenoviruses), or cell-to-cell fusion with formation of syncytia or polykaryons (e.g., respiratory syncytial virus). These changes are usually visible in fresh unstained cultures when examined under low power with reduced light, or by phase-contrast microscopy. Monolayers prepared and infected on coverslips can be fixed and stained (Giemsa, H & E) to reveal so-called inclusion bodies, which are frequently pathognomonic of certain viruses. The site of these changes, whether cytoplasmic (e.g., respiratory syncytial virus, which, besides being syncytiogenic, produces large eosinophilic cytoplasmic inclusions) or nuclear (e.g., herpesviruses produce eosinophilic nuclear inclusions; adenoviruses produce Feulgen-positive nuclear inclusions, often in crystalline array), gives an indication of the class of infecting agent involved. DNA viruses, with the exception of poxviruses, mature in the nucleus; RNA viruses mature primarily in the cytoplasm. The composition of inclusions can be determined by cytochemical (e.g., Feulgen, acridine orange for NA, lipid stains) and immunochemical techniques (FAb, enzyme-labeled antibody) and by electron microscopy of ultrathin sections of infected cells. Inclusions are found to be aggregates of virions (mature and incomplete particles, as with herpesviruses) or

of viral subunits (e.g., paramyxoviral nucleocapsid).

Viral Hemagglutination (HA)

Many animal viruses, such as myxoviruses, paramyxoviruses, adenoviruses, some of the enteroviruses, agglutinate erythrocytes of different species in vitro, thereby providing a useful and relatively uncomplicated method for quantitating (titering) these viruses and for measuring antibody to them (hemagglutination inhibition, HI). In enveloped viruses, HA is mediated by an envelope glycoprotein (H in orthomyxoviruses, HN in paramyxoviruses). In orthomyxoviruses, a second glycoprotein (neuraminidase, N) is responsible for elution of the virus from the erythrocyte surface in vitro, as well as for the liberation of virions from the surface of infected cells. During elution from the erythrocyte, receptors for myxoviruses are destroyed with accompanying release of free N-acetylneuraminic acid (NANA). Cells in monolayer cultures infected with myxoviruses or paramyxoviruses adsorb erythrocytes (hemadsorption) owing to the presence of hemagglutinin glycoprotein in the cell membrane. This is a useful procedure to detect the presence of these viruses in diagnostic cell cultures. HA by poxviruses is mediated by a lipoprotein that is separate from the virion and is liberated into the medium during viral replication. Adenoviral HA is mediated by a capsid protein complex (penton fibers). Enteroviral HA is mediated by a specific capsid protein.

Viruses can be quantitated by plaque counts (in a manner analogous to bacteriophage). After inoculation of replicate monolayers with dilutions (usually decimal) of virus preparation, the cells are overlaid with semisolid agar containing nutrients and neutral red (a vital dye). The gel formed by the agar immobilizes any free virus remaining from the inoculum or progeny virus, thereby limiting subsequent cycles of infection to centrifugal spread from initially infected cells directly to others in immediate contact. After appropriate incubation, plaques are revealed as clear unstained areas of viral cytolysis. Intervening areas of remaining normal cells are stained. In plates inoculated with sufficiently dilute virus, each plaque represents the progeny of a single infectious unit. From the plaque count, the number of infectious viral particles (or more accurately, PFU) contained in the original preparation of virus can be estimated. With viruses that are not rapidly cytocidal, foci of infection can be revealed with special stains, immunofluorescence, or hemadsorption.

THE LABORATORY IN THE DIAGNOSIS OF VIRAL INFECTION

For the laboratory to be of maximal utility to the clinician, specimens submitted for diagnostic analysis must be accompanied by relevant clinical information regarding the patient's illness and what type of viral infection is suspected on the basis of signs, symptoms, and epidemiological data (*e.g.*, the type of infection "going around," age groups involved). The manner in which a specimen for primary isolation is handled will often depend on such data; specimens submitted with a request simply for "virus studies" are useless. For primary viral isolation, antibiotics are added (to suppress bacterial and/or fungal contaminants) and cell cultures are directly inoculated (primary human embryonic kidney and lung, WI 38 cells, HeLa, or other cell lines are those most frequently used) and subsequently observed periodically for CPE and/or hemadsorption. Detection of virus may be hastened by direct electron microscopic examination of culture fluid or of vesicular fluid (*e.g.*, herpes, vaccinia, varicella), of cells in urinary tract sediment or sputum (cytomegalovirus, measles virus) or of fecal samples (*e.g.*, rotaviruses). For direct electron microscopy, samples are stained with phosphotungstic acid ("negative" stain), which reveals the configuration and hence the identity of intact virions of each of the major groups. Specific agglutination with sera of known specificity or with patient sera is often demonstrable (immune-electron microscopy). Serologic diagnosis, even though of necessity retrospective, should always be undertaken whenever possible by submitting to the laboratory acute and convalescent serum samples to be tested concurrently (most frequently by complement fixation) with viral antigens of known specificity. The final identification of viruses isolated in cell culture or in embryonated eggs rests on neutralization tests (HI; neutralization of CPE) with antisera of known specificity. Recently developed monoclonal antibodies with greatly sharpened specificity will have increasing utility in serodiagnosis and identification of viral isolates.

Classification of Animal Viruses

The classification of animal viruses is based on (1) the morphology of the virion as revealed by negative staining and morphogenesis in infected cells; (2) the type and size of nucleic acid (NA), DNA or RNA, constituting the viral genome, whether single-stranded or double-stranded, and genetic relatedness (homology) among individual members of a group; (3) the presence or absence of a lipid envelope as reflected in morphology and by stability of viral infectivity to lipid solvents (ether, chloroform) or detergents; (4) configuration of nucleocapsid (cubic, helical, or complex); (5) the number and immunochemical identity of viral proteins (Table 5-13).

DNA VIRUSES

Parvoviruses. These are the smallest DNA-containing viruses known to infect vertebrate cells. The viral genome is a single strand of DNA, either + or −. Parvoviruses are pathogenic to many animals; in rodents they are oncogenic and immunosuppressive (*e.g.*, minute virus of mice). One genus of parvovirus requires a helper virus in order to undergo a complete replicative cycle (hence named **dependovirus**), and includes human adenoassociated virus.

The human parvovirus, B19, has been recently described as the probable cause of bone marrow failure due to a specific cytotoxic relationship with erythroid precursor cells resulting in a transient aplastic crisis for children with homozygous sickle-cell anemia.

Papovaviruses. The group name is derived from *pa*pilloma, *po*lyoma, and *va*cuolating viruses. Recently, the latter family has been condensed into the polyoma viruses. This group now includes rabbit or human papillomaviruses (HPV), mouse polyoma, and simian vacuolating virus 40 (SV40). The viruses can be lytic, where they undergo complete replication and kill their host (permissive) cell, in such cases as mouse polyoma (mouse fibroblast) and SV40 (African green monkey kidney cells), as well as exist in a transforming mode where they can cause tumor formation in their nonpermissive hosts (*e.g.*, newborn hamsters).

The molecular weight of the double-stranded, superhelical twisted DNA genomes of polyoma viruses is $3–5 \times 10^6$ daltons, and normally would be expected to have the coding potential for four polypeptides. However, it is known that the "transforming" gene of this virus (*e.g.*, T-antigen gene) alone codes for at least three different proteins. This is because of three potential reading frames and differential mRNA splicing. Polyoma viruses have been intensively studied as models for understanding the mechanisms of viral carcinogenesis and cellular transformation in tissue culture. The name polyoma refers to the fact that when large amounts of such virus are injected into newborn mice or hamsters, a wide variety of histologically different tumors is produced. However, in nature the virus is apparently not tumorigenic. Thus wild mice trapped in some (but not all) apartment buildings in New York City as well as on farms in Georgia were both found to be infected with mouse polyomaviruses; however the mice had no pathologic symptoms. SV40, a simian polyomavirus, can also be isolated from apparently normal cultures of rhesus monkey kidney cells, but only cause tumors (*e.g.,* usually sarcomas) in baby hamsters. Also, several human polyomaviruses related to SV40 have been isolated from patients with progressive multifocal leukoencephalopathy (SV40 PML and JC viruses) or from the urine of immunosuppressed patients (BK virus) and have been shown to induce brain tumors in newborn hamsters, although there is no evidence to indicate that they have a causative role in human tumor formation. As a sidelight it is of interest to note that millions of US residents were exposed to SV40 between 1955 and 1961 when they were immunized with contaminated polio vaccines, yet no SV40-related tumor has appeared. Thus, at this time the oncogenic potential of polyomaviruses appears of interest more in a laboratory than a clinical setting.

In contrast to polyoma, the family of papilloma viruses has become increasingly important in recent years because of their association with a number of human cancers. In general, though most of the 40 HPVs infect surface epithelia and cause benign rather than malignant epithelial tumors or warts at the site of entry (*e.g.,* on the skin or mucous membranes: genital and laryngeal papillomas). The virus is localized to the lesion and no viremia is observed.

Although virus particles can be seen in the electron microscopy of biopsy material, they have not yet been propagated in the lab. However, since papilloma viral DNA can be isolated, it has served as a useful diagnostic marker. The virus persists in the proliferating basal cell layer of the skin in the form of free DNA and matures into virions as tissue moves upwards and outward to form the keratinized layer at the surface. Degenerating cells and cell debris shed from the surface contain large amounts of virus particles. Virus can be transmitted from human to human by inoculation of a cell-free extract of wart tissue. Of the almost 40 different human papilloma viruses (HPV), most have been classified based on comparison of restriction DNA patterns or by the use of DNA hybridization techniques.

1. ***Verruca vulgaris:*** This most common family of warts has three known types (HPV-1, 2, 3) and may occur anywhere on the body but usually on fingers and hands. The warts are small (1 to 2 mm) epidermal tumors that are rough, elevated, firm to palpation, and occur in groups. They are stable for years or disappear spontaneously. Plantar wards ***(Verruca plantaris)*** are a clinical subvariety that occur in weight-bearing points of the body (usually beneath a callous), grow in depth, and cause acute pain (HPV-1) and (HPV-4).

2. ***Condyloma acuminatum*** or urogenital warts: Consists of two different papilloma viruses (HPV-6 and 11). These warts occur in warm, moist areas of the external genitalia. The lesions appear as large, soft, red masses that may coalesce and are transmitted as a venereal disease.

3. ***Verruca plana*** (juvenile warts): The flat, smooth lesions are always multiple, and occur on face, neck, dorsal surfaces of hands or arms. Lesions may remain unchanged for months or years, or disappear spontaneously.

4. ***Juvenile laryngeal papillomas*** (HPV-11): These occur predominantly in the 2 to 5-year age group, and mothers of these children frequently have a history of genital virus warts. By molecular cloning of HPV-11 DNA from laryngeal papilloma, partial (25%) identity was shown of HPV-11 with HPV-6.

5. ***Epidermodysplasia verruciformis*** (EV): HPV-5, HPV-8, and now HPV-38b lesions are seen in patients with the disease epidermodysplasia verruciformis (EV) and can become malignant (about 60% of the time). Malignant tumors of the skin develop at an early age in EV patients, predominantly in exposed areas of the skin. The time from onset of skin lesions to the onset of cancer suggests that interaction of HPV-38b with UV light and host factors are associated with development of the skin carcinoma.

6. ***Cervical cancer:*** HPV-16 and HPV-18 have recently been associated with a large proportion of squamous cell carcinomas of the uterine cervix. A probe utilizing fragments of these DNAs is being developed as a supplementary test to the Pap test.

As noted earlier, it is difficult to study viral growth and replication for papillomaviruses because there is no readily available tissue culture system (other than differentiating epithelial cells) for propagation of the viruses.

Adenoviruses. Their morphology is unique in that the icosahedral capsid comprises 240 ***hexons***

(one capsomer has six neighbors) and 12 *pentons* composed of one apical capsomer (with five neighbors) bearing a knobbed *fiber*. The penton fiber mediates attachment to cells and hemagglutination.

Adenoviruses have enabled researchers to recognize biological concepts of great significance, including splicing, viral hybridization, associated helper viruses, cell transformation, and viral oncogenesis. In terms of disease, those types most commonly associated with respiratory infections, such as types 1, 2, and 5, are nearly ubiquitous, infect most children very early in life (0 to 6 years), and their DNA may persist indefinitely in tonsillar tissues. Types 3, 4, 7, 14, and 21 are more likely to cause acute respiratory disease (ARD) in adults. Also, pharyngoconjunctival fever can be a major expression of infection with any of several types of adenovirus. However, in general, adenoviruses do not cause more than 5 to 8% of ARD in civilian populations. The highest attack rates (50 to 80%) are among military recruits.

At least 41 human adenovirus serotypes have been identified and classified into 4 different groups based on their oncogenic potential for newborn hamsters. In general, the virus reaches susceptible tissue, mostly by aerosol or direct skin contact, and multiplies there. Although there is no viremia, the virus multiplies in the GI tract and can be recovered from stool up to 18 months after infection. For most of the serotypes, adenoids may be latently infected for life after primary infection. In any case, a type-specific immunity remains for life, with no recurrent infection by the same serotype.

Most adenovirus infections are inapparent and result in a self-limited illness, followed by recovery and development of type-specific immunity. However, as indicated above certain types give a more serious illness.

1. ARD: types 3, 4, 7, 14, and sometimes 21; occurs in adults. Influenzalike fever, headache, chills, malaise, which last 2 to 4 days. Usually no complications. In young children, these viruses have been implicated in occasional cases of fatal nonbacterial pneumonia.
2. Pharyngoconjunctival fever: symptoms like ARD, with inflammation of throat and tonsils, and conjunctivitis. It is mostly associated with type 3, and sometimes with types 7, 14, and 21. The pharyngitis lasts 4 to 5 days; conjunctivitis can last as long as 3 weeks. No complications ensue.
3. Acute follicular conjunctivitis: caused mainly by type 3 or 7; can involve one or both eyes, with lacrimation and a serous exudate that lasts several weeks.
4. Epidemic keratoconjunctivitis: this is highly infectious; caused primarily by types 8 and 19. There is a sudden onset with edema of the conjunctiva accompanied by a mononuclear cell exudate, a low-grade fever, and periauricular lymphadenopathy. The keratitis consists of small opacities (0.01 to 0.3 mm) that may ulcerate. It may last weeks or months with no permanent damage.
5. Hemorrhagic cystitis and gastroenteritis without respiratory disease have also been seen in young children. Adenovirus types 40 and 41 have been isolated as the causative agents.

Herpesviruses. The human herpesviruses include herpes simplex virus (HSV) (types 1 and 2), varicella-zoster virus (VZV), cytomegalovirus (CMV) and Epstein-Barr virus (EBV). While the clinical manifestations of infection vary, all herpesviruses have the capacity to establish latent infection (*e.g., HSV* in trigeminal or presacral ganglia, VZV in dorsal root ganglia) from which endogenous recurrences emanate (*e.g.,* shingles is recrudescent varicella). Genital herpes (usually due to HSV-2) is sexually transmitted. Herpetiform genital lesions can also be caused by EBV or CMV. These two viruses, which can be found in semen and cervical secretions, must now be added to the list of sexually transmitted diseases (Table 5-14). Several of the herpesviruses have oncogenic properties (EBV apparently causes Burkitt's lymphoma, nasopharyngeal carcinoma, and lymphoproliferative disorders in immunodeficient hosts; HSV, CMV, and EBV transform cells *in vitro;* HSV-2 is associated with cervical carcinoma). A live attenuated varicella viral vaccine, first developed in Japan (Oka strain grown in human diploid fibroblasts), has been shown to be effective in preventing childhood varicella, even in leukemic children undergoing chemotherapy, and will doubtless become available. The potential for acquiring zoster from vaccine strains remains uncertain.

Poxviruses. These are the largest of the animal viruses (200 to 350 nm), the tightly structured lipoprotein enveloped virion having complex bilateral symmetry. The virus develops in the cytoplasm, where it produces characteristic eosinophilic inclusions (Guarnieri bodies). This family of DNA viruses is unique in that it replicates in the cytoplasm and carries its own transcriptase to make early mRNA. There is a two-stage uncoating process; after complete uncoating, viral DNA is replicated in

TABLE 5-14. Sexually Transmitted Diseases*

DISEASE	CAUSATIVE AGENTS	DIAGNOSIS	IMMUNE RESPONSE	TREATMENT
Gonorrhea	*Neisseria gonorrheae* (colony types 1,2)	Gram stain, culture, Fab	Antibody to pili	Penicillin (PPNG, CMRNG, spectinomycin)
Syphilis	*(N. meningitidis)* *Treponema pallidum*	Darkfield (1°,2°)	RPR, FTA-ABS	Penicillin
Vaginitis (nontrichomonal)	*Gardnerella vaginalis*	Gram stain, "clue cells"		Tetracycline (sulfonamide)
Chancroid (soft chancre)	*Hemophilus ducreyi*	Gram stain		Sulfonamide
Lymphogranuloma venereum (LGV)	*Chlamydia trachomatis* Immunotypes L₁,₂,₃	Smear and Giemsa stain, inclusions, Fab	CF antibody	Tetracycline (sulfonamide)
Cervicitis	Immunotypes D,E			
Nongonococcal urethritis (NGU)	D,E *Ureaplasma urealyticum* ("T" mycoplasma)	Culture	Mycoplasmacidal test (metabolic inhibition)	
Granuloma inguinale (donovanosis)	*Calymmatobacterium granulomatis*	CF antibody		
Pelvic inflammatory disease (PID)	Polymicrobial: *Bacteroides* and other anaerobes, Chlamydiae	Culture (endocerv.) & culdocentesis		Depends on cultures; penicillin
Herpes genitalis	Herpes simplex, type 2, (1) (CMV, EBV)	Primary isolation	Neutralizing antibody	
Anogenital warts (condyloma accuminatum)	Papovavirus (HPVG6,11)	EM of tissue cells		Podophyllin (fetal toxicity)
Genital molluscum contagiosum	Poxvirus (Molluscum contagiosum virus)	Giemsa stain, eosinophilic inclusions		
Hepatitis	Type A (B)	B: immunodiffusion RIA HBs ag, ab		
Intrauterine and Perinatal Infections	**T**oxoplasma (**O**ther–e.g., group B step. GC lues) **R**ubella **C**ytomegalovirus **H**erpes genitalis	Fab, CF test HI (IgM) Inclusion bodies	Primary vs. secondary	

*Also shigellosis, amebiasis, giardiasis in homosexual men; ectoparasites (lice, scabies); trichomoniasis (vaginitis, urethritis, balanitis).

excess (20,000 DNA/cell) with only 25% of the DNA used for progeny. Then late mRNA begins, with a switchoff of early mRNA, synthesis of capsid proteins, and of the transcriptase. Assembly then occurs in the cytoplasmic factories, which appear as inclusion bodies.

The following poxviruses affect humans.

1. *Variola (smallpox):* Humans are the only natural hosts; the last case as determined by the WHO was diagnosed about 20 years ago. Because of the tightly structured envelope, the virus is resistant to drying. It can persist in bedclothes and is airborne from skin lesions.
2. *Cowpox* (cattle, humans): Vaccination was discovered by Jenner in the 1700s, using serum from a cowpox lesion on a milkmaid. He inoculated the 8-year-old boy, who became resistant. Vaccinia virus, which is the current vaccine strain being used for recombinant DNA technology, is a variant of cowpox adapted to infect humans efficiently with a low-grade infection. Until 1971, all infants received vaccinia virus vaccine to provide variola immunity. This was discontinued because of the absence of endemic and imported disease, as well as concern about complications, for example, immunosuppressed patients or those with anti-IgG antibodies develop a progressive fatal vaccinia disease; infants scratching could get the virus in the eyes leading to keratitis; and patients with eczema were likely to develop diffuse vaccinial lesions over the skin.
3. *Paravaccinia* and *orf virus:* The cause of nodules on the hands of animal handlers.
4. *Molluscum contagiosum:* Causes the formation of benign epidermal tumors that ordinarily disappear within a few months.

RNA VIRUSES

Picornaviridae (L. pico + RNA). This group includes viruses of three genera pathogenic for humans: *Enterovirus, Rhinovirus,* and *Cardiovirus.*

Enterovirus. There are four categories of enteroviruses:

1. *Polioviruses* (three serotypes): These cause enteric infection, from which the viruses spread hematogenously to the central nervous system to cause poliomyelitis (infection of anterior horn cells, motor paralysis) or "nonparalytic poliomyelitis" (so-called aseptic meningitis); both syndromes are also occasionally due to other enteroviruses. True paralytic poliomyelitis is now a rarity thanks to effective vaccines.
2. *Coxsackievirus:* Group A viruses (23 serotypes) are distinguished from those of group B (six serotypes) on the basis of type-specific neutralization tests and selective tissue damage in suckling mice. These viruses cause a wide spectrum of disease: aseptic meningitis, encephalitis, pleurodynia (mostly group A), myocarditis (mostly group B), poliomyelitis.
3. *Echo viruses:* Originally called *enteric cytopathic human orphan* viruses. They are no longer "orphan" viruses; many agents of this group produce a wide spectrum of disease, including aseptic meningitis with neuronal injury and paralysis, acute respiratory disease, infantile diarrhea, summer febrile illness with rubeoliform exanthem.
4. *Hepatitis A:* This virus is type 72 enterovirus.

Rhinovirus. More than 100 serotypes of rhinovirus are known. Most are cultivable in human embryonic kidney cells, human diploid lung cells, or tracheal organ culture at 33°C. They are rarely found in the lower intestinal tract. Rhinoviruses are the most frequent causes of the afebrile common cold syndrome in adults; immunity to reinfection is type-specific.

Cardiovirus. This group includes pathogens for various animal species. *Encephalomyocarditis* (EMC) virus, the only human pathogen in the group, causes relatively undifferentiated mild febrile illness.

Caliciviridae. Members of this group differ from the picornaviruses because of their larger size and the fact that they possess but a single structural protein. The only human pathogen in the group (*Norwalk agent,* of which there may be at least four serogroups as determined by immune electron microscopy) has not yet been propagated in cell culture, but is readily seen by direct electron microscopy of negatively stained fecal extracts. The Norwalk agent is an important cause of acute epidemic gastroenteritis in all age groups.

Reoviridae. *Orthoreoviruses* (three serotypes) are widely distributed in humans and in lower animals, their role in human disease still not being clearly defined (*respiratory enteric orphan* viruses). Originally grouped with the echoviruses, they subsequently were found to differ significantly in being larger than picornaviruses and in having a double-stranded segmented RNA genome. Structurally similar but antigenically distinct viruses are *orbivirus,* the cause of Colorado tick fever (encephalitis) and therefore operationally an arbovirus, and *rotavirus*, the cause of acute infectious gastroenteritis in infants and young children. Two serotypes of rotavirus are distinguishable by immune electron microscopy of virions that appear in large quantity during active diarrheal disease. Efforts are under way to develop a vaccine against this important cause of enteric disease.

Togaviridae. These include viruses previously designated as *arboviruses* (*ar*thropod *bo*rne), four genera being distinguished primarily on the basis of antigenic analysis (CF, HI, N). Arboviruses typically infect mammals and avian species and are maintained in animal reservoirs by hematophagous arthropods. To become infectious, the arthropod vector must bite the animal during the viremic stage of infection. True arboviruses actually multiply in, or migrate from the stomach to the mouth parts of, the insect vector. The geographic distribution of arthropod-borne diseases depends on climate, which, in turn, determines the distribution of animal reservoirs and vectors. Human disease due to arboviruses takes many forms, including encephalitis as well as subclinical infection. *Alphaviruses* (formerly group A arboviruses) cause eastern, western, and Venezuelan equine encephalitides. *Flaviviruses* (formerly group B arboviruses) include viruses causing yellow fever, dengue (four serotypes), encephalitis, both mosquito-borne (Japanese B, St. Louis, Murray Valley, West Nile encephalitides) and tick-borne (Russian spring–summer and other animal encephalitides). *Rubeola* virus, the cause of German measles, is now classified in the Togaviridae as *rubivirus*. *Rubella* contracted during the first trimester of pregnancy causes severe fetal damage and results in the congenital rubella syndrome in surviving infants. Maternal HI antibody (resulting from prior infection or immunization with vaccine) connotes solid immunity to reinfection and hence fetal protection if exposure occurs during pregnancy. Although there is no evidence that the RA 27/3 vaccine can cause congenital rubella syndrome, the virus nevertheless can cross the placenta and infect the fetus. Pregnancy, therefore, remains a contraindication to vaccination. Inadvertent administration of rubella vaccine during pregnancy, however, should not be construed as a reason for artificial termination.

Bunyaviridae. This group (formerly group C arboviruses) includes the California encephalitis virus group, Rift valley and sandfly fevers, and Congo–Crimean hemorrhagic fever viruses.

Myxoviruses. The term is derived from the affinity of these agents for glycoproteins that are found in secretions and that are similar to if not identical with cell "receptors" for viral hemagglutinin and infection. Characteristically these viruses mature by budding at the cell surface where they are enclosed by a lipid-containing membrane (envelope) into which structural subunits (hemagglutinin, H, neuraminidase, N), are inserted. Viral glycoprotein and lipids are host-specific; the polypeptide portions and the enzymes required for glycosylation are virus-coded.

Orthomyxoviruses (influenza virus). These are smaller (80 to 100 nm) than the paramyxoviruses (100 to 150 nm) and are divisible into three major serogroups based on the specificity of the ribonucleoprotein (S) antigens with complement-fixing antibody that is not protective (the ribonucleoprotein is internal). Each group, particularly group A, is subdivisible into many serotypes based on the separate antigenic identities of H and N glycoproteins. The latter are subject to antigenic drift and shift resulting from complex genetic reassortments (the viral genome comprises eight segments) in response to immunologic pressures in the individual and herd environments. Group A viruses include swine, equine, and avian viruses; the human strains have hitherto been the cause of all epidemic influenza. Group B strains cause continuing sporadic incidence of influenza and are peculiarly related to the serious and often fatal complication of Reye's syndrome. Group C viruses are of apparently low intrinsic virulence and account for an unknown, but probably appreciable, proportion of minor respiratory illness, particularly in young children and the elderly. Antibodies to all the major groups are widespread in the adult population.

For diagnosis, orthomyxoviruses are readily recovered by the inoculation of throat washings into primary monkey kidney or human embryonic kidney cells. Hemadsorption indicates the presence of virus, which is then typed by hemagglutination inhibition with sera of known specificity.

Retrospective serodiagnosis is achieved by complement fixation with group-specific ribonucleoprotein antigens or with hemagglutination inhibition with standard viruses. Nonspecific inhibitors (nonimmunoglobulin sialoprotein receptor analogues) universally present in normal sera must be inactivated with receptor-destroying enzyme (RDE), which leaves specific antibody present to account for any HI activity in the serum.

Active immunization with killed virus vaccine is the single most important measure to prevent and/or attenuate the disease influenza. Vaccine currently in use is grown in chicken eggs (chorioallantoic fluid), inactivated with formalin, and partially purified to reduce the content of egg protein. When the virus in the vaccine has been disrupted by detergent (subunit, subvirion, or "split" vaccine), the content of H and N (protective antigens) is relatively enhanced, with correspondingly less total protein per dose. Split virus vaccine, reactions to which are less than to whole virus, should be used to immunize infants and children up to 12 years of age. H and N antigens of virus in the vaccine should match the antigens of strains prevalent in the community as closely as possible. No one with known allergy to egg protein should be immunized. Although pregnancy per se is *not* a contraindication to administration of influenza virus vaccine, immunization should be deferred until the second or third trimesters. The target groups with highest priority are (1) adults and children with chronic cardiopulmonary disorders, chronic metabolic diseases, renal dysfunction, anemia, immunosuppression, or asthma; (2) residents of chronic care facilities; (3) individuals over 65 years of age; (3) health care personnel who have extensive contact with high-risk patients. Amantadine hydrochloride (Symmetrel) is an alternative to active immunization. It is effective (by interfering with uncoating of virus during replication) in mollifying disease due to group A strains, but is *not* effective against group B strains. Amantadine is also effective prophylactically when influenza A outbreaks are anticipated.

Paramyxoviruses. These are large enveloped viruses in which the genome is a single strand of unsegmented RNA. This accounts for their antigenic stability. In parainfluenza, mumps, and Newcastle disease (of fowls) viruses, one glycoprotein in the envelope contains both H and N activities. Measles, canine distemper, and rinderpest (a disease of cattle) viruses, which are antigenically related to one another, lack N activity; respiratory syncytial virus has neither H nor N. A second separate glycoprotein (F) in the viral envelope accounts for the cell-fusing activity which characterizes the cytopathology of these viruses, particularly measles and respiratory syncytial viruses. Measles vaccine is an attenuated strain (Edmonston) of the virus grown in chicken embryo fibroblast culture.

Current efforts are being directed at developing a recombinant vaccinia virus vector to **human respiratory syncytial virus** (RSV), a major cause of viral lower respiratory tract illness in infants and young children worldwide. Previous attempts to develop a safe and effective RSV vaccine have met with failure. A formalin-inactivated vaccine tested 20 years ago not only failed to protect but also led to an enhancement of disease during infection by RSV.

The live recombinant vaccinia virus vector currently being developed expresses the glycoprotein fusion protein F, which mediates viral penetration and cell–cell spread by membrane fusion.

Rhabdoviridae. Viruses of this group are elongated, bullet-shaped particles (Gr. rhabdos, rod). The chief pathogen is rabies virus *(Lyssavirus)* and antigenically related viruses in various parts of the world. The virus has a lipoprotein–glycoprotein envelope containing a single (protective) antigen, and the helical nucleocapsid contains the genome as a single strand of negative (nonmessenger) RNA. The virion carries an RNA transcriptase and is cultivable in a variety of cells *in vitro*. The virus replicates in the cytoplasm, forming inclusions (Negri bodies), and matures by budding at the cell membrane. Virus grown in human diploid cells and inactivated constitutes the vaccine used for prophylaxis, in conjunction with human immune globulin from hyperimmunized individuals. Marburg and Ebola agents (hemorrhagic fevers transmissible from person to person without an intermediate vector) are probably in this biologic group; classification of these agents in the family *Filoviridae* has been proposed. Rabies in enzootic in rodents (bats, skunks, foxes, raccoons), which are the major sources of human infection. Infection of domestic animals is derived from infected endemic foci. Virus travels along nerve trunks from the sites of entry (usually an animal bite) and localizes in the central nervous system, salivary glands and, occasionally, viscera. Diagnosis is based on clinical and epidemiologic data and on demonstration of Negri bodies by immunofluorescence in smears of hippocampal tissue of the rabid animal.

Retroviruses. Retroviruses are enveloped icosahedral viruses with glycoprotein peplomers on their surface that contain two identical strands of RNA (~8,500 nucleotides) and the unique enzyme reverse transcriptase inside an icosahedral shell. Retrovirus replication, in brief, begins with adsorption of the virus by the spikes or peplomers to specific receptors on host cells, followed by uncoating of the icosahedral core in the cytoplasm, synthesis of a DNA intermediate by the reverse transcriptase, and subsequent integration of this double-stranded proviral DNA into cellular DNA. Transcription of this proviral DNA then provides both viral RNA (vRNA) and mRNA for the following three groups of viral proteins:

1. Group-specific antigens (*gag* proteins), which make up the icosahedral viral core and enclose the vRNA.
2. *pol* polyprotein includes the reverse transcrip-

tase, a viral specific protease, needed for cleavage of the *gag* polyprotein, and an integrase needed for integration of the viral DNA into cellular DNA.

3. *env* proteins are inserted at the membrane surface into the budding virus particle.

The *viral reverse transcriptase* (RT) is a unique enzyme in that vRNA is converted first to single-stranded DNA (minus strand) and then to double-stranded DNA (minus and plus strand). In the initial replication step, RT binds to a site at the 5' end of the genomic RNA where a specific cellular tRNA has also bound. Synthesis of the minus strand continues back through the tRNA binding site and, as this process occurs, RNase H activity of the RT degrades the vRNA. In the final stage, both a long terminal repeat (LTR) and double-stranded DNA are formed.

The retroviruses fall into two large families of viruses that cause serious disease in man and other vertebrates. One, the *oncogenic RNA viruses* or *RNA tumor viruses,* are the major cause of leukemias, lymphomas, and sometimes sarcomas in many species of animals, including chickens, mice, cats, cattle, and gibbon apes.

The principal morphology of the RNA tumor viruses is type C, in which an immature (uncleaved) particle is initially formed and then after cleavage of the *gag* and *pol* polyproteins, a mature (central dense nucleoid) infectious particle results. Among avian type C viruses are both nondefective leukosis viruses (low oncogenic potential), which cause lymphomas or leukemias in chickens, after 4 to 8 months, and the *Rous sarcoma virus* (RSV) family (high oncogenic activity because they contain the viral *src* gene).

The other family of retroviruses, the *lentiviruses,* which includes HIV, the causative agent of AIDS, has a different morphology, called type E. These viruses, such as visna (virus of sheep), are cytopathic rather than oncogenic. In a type E morphology, the particles have a ''C'' type budding or ''immature'' form of the particle, but once matured the particle develops a cylindrical or prolate nucleoid core.

For many years no retrovirus had been linked to a human disease; however, about 7 years ago, a human adult T-cell leukemia virus (HTLV-I) was isolated both in the U.S. and Japan from about 200 patients who had a rare type of T-cell lymphocytic leukemia called adult T-cell leukemia/lymphoma (ATL). Another human T-cell retrovirus was isolated from several patients with ''hairy'' cell leukemia and named HTLV-II. Antibodies to HTLV-I

are found in 10% to 12% of the population in villages of Southwest Japan. An increased positivity with age is consistent with sexual and/or blood transmission of the virus. Incidence of the disease ATL among HTLV-I seropositive individuals is relatively low (<0.1%) at this time, with an incubation period of more than 20 years. Recently, seropositive HTLV-I individuals are being detected among intravenous drug abusers in inner-city areas of New York. The link is thought to be through Caribbean area carriers. Both HTLV-I and HTLV-II were able to be isolated only because of the development of T-cell growth factors (interleukin-2) to keep T-cells from HTLV-infected patients growing in tissue culture for multiple generations.

In 1983 to 1984, the retrovirus HIV was isolated in France (LAV), as well as the U.S. (HTLV-III) and was shown to be the causative agent of AIDS. In contrast to HTLV-I and II, HIV is cytopathic. This is of interest, since early attempts to isolate the AIDS virus involved long-term culture of cells, anticipating that they were like other oncogenic retroviruses. Instead, it appears that HIV is cytotoxic for lymphocytes with OKT4+ on their surface and this specificity apparently explains the widespread damage to cell-mediated immunity in AIDS patients. The virus is transmitted through blood or other body fluids, such as semen. Direct physical contact appears to be required. Serologic tests have been developed to screen hospital blood supplies for the AIDS virus and vaccine developments using viral glycoprotein subunits are currently under development. At present there is no known cure for AIDS. As discussed above, HIV, although a retrovirus, does not belong to the same viral subfamily as the oncogenic retroviruses such as Rous sarcoma virus, or HTLV-I. Instead it shares homology with the *Lentivirus* subfamily, which are nononcogenic, but cytocidal for lymphocytes, such as Visna virus. Although HIV itself is not oncogenic, a large percentage of homosexuals who contract AIDS also have an unusual form of Kaposi's sarcoma (purple skin lesions). AIDS is discussed in greater detail in the section Immunodeficiencies and Gammopathies later in this chapter.

Arenaviruses. In this group of viruses, the virion contains characteristic electron-dense granules (L. *arena,* sand), which are now known to be host cell ribosomes. One of the group is the cause of lymphocytic choriomeningitis characterized by infiltration of meninges and choroid plexus, the first-recognized viral, aseptic meningitis. The symptoms are varied, and the disease is usually mild, rarely involving the central nervous system, being mainly referable to the respiratory and enteric tracts. The virus is enzoötic in domestic mice, the source of tangential human infection.

More serious diseases of the hemorrhagic fever type, with neurotropic involvement and hemorrhagic necrosis, and frequently fatal, involve the worldwide Tacaribe group of arenaviruses. Many are arthropod borne. Lassa fever virus is an arenavirus.

Coronaviruses. These agents are named for the "crown" of large, club-shaped projections from the envelope, which encloses a helical nucleocapsid. They are the cause of upper respiratory tract disease and common cold syndrome in adults. Coronaviruses grow poorly in anything but ciliated epithelial organ culture or in particularly sensitive human diploid cells. Twenty strains of coronavirus have been isolated, which by N and CF tests can be classified into three broad serogroups.

Hepatitis Viruses. Hepatitis A (HA) virus purified from human feces is a 27-nm particle that contains RNA and is now classified as a picornavirus (enterovirus 72). It is propagable in a variety of cells in culture, the way thus being opened toward development of an attenuated live viral vaccine. HA viruses are worldwide in distribution. Introduction of the virus is usually followed rapidly (15 to 45 days) by liver disease of varying severity, which is indistinguishable clinically from infection with hepatitis B virus or with so-called non-A, non-B viruses. Spread of HA is by the fecal–oral route and is related to socioeconomic status and crowded living conditions with poor sanitation. The most common age of incidence is childhood/young adulthood. Antibody is prevalent in a high percentage of most population groups. Percutaneous transmission of HA virus is infrequent. Diagnosis rests on the identification of A particles in feces and/or serodiagnosis with RIA. Specifically, IgM HAV appears after the onset of disease and can be detected by a modified competitive binding RIA. This is important since IgG anti-HAV has limited diagnostic value because it persists for life and it is difficult to see a fourfold rise over such a background. In patients diagnosed with HAV, a dose of 0.02 ml/kg pooled immune serum globulins (IgG) administered intramuscularly within two weeks after exposure can be 80% to 90% effective.

The complete hepatitis B (HB) virion is the Dane particle, surrounded by the surface (S) antigen (originally identified as Australia antigen) containing at least five antigenic specificities (a group antigen, two pairs of subtypic determinants, d/y, w/r, which are mutually exclusive). A variety of subtypes have been recognized. HBs antigen may ap-

pear free in the blood early after infection. The Dane particle contains a core that is circular and partially (60 to 85%) double-stranded DNA, as well as two additional antigens (c and e). HBV infection is acquired percutaneously (transfusions, blood-contaminated injection apparatus), or by contact with body effluvia (*e.g.,* semen, saliva). The disease has a relatively long incubation period (40 to 180 days) and insidious onset showing a prolonged elevation of liver enzymes, such as serum glutamic oxaloacetic transaminase (SGOT). Although the disease is most frequently self-limited (virus and HBs antigen disappear, antibody appears) in 5% to 10% of cases, it may evolve into persistent hepatitis (HBs antigen and/or Dane particles and/or HBc antigen persist, little or no antibody appears). Hepatic injury in persistent HB infection may be immunogenic, including both cell-mediated responses and antigen–antibody complex disease. Chronic HBV infection is implicated in the causation of hepatocellular carcinoma. Diagnosis of HB is by detection of HBs antigen and/or antibody and HBc antigen in the serum by radioimmunoassay. The Delta agent is a viroid (see earlier section) contained in an HBs coat. It was first described in Italy in 1977 and has since then been encountered worldwide. Superinfection with Delta or coprimary infection (HB + Delta) causes particularly fulminant disease. Since Delta never occurs in the absence of HB infection, immunization against the latter will protect against both agents. Pooled normal immunoglobulin affords effective postexposure or preexposure prophylaxis against both A and B viruses. Active immunization with HBs (hepatitis B surface antigen) purified from the plasma of persistently infected patients is noninfectious and is an effective prophylactic agent.

This vaccine was approved in 1981 by the FDA and is recommended for high-risk populations such as dialysis patients and health care professionals. Since there are about 100,000 new cases of HB disease each year in the U.S. with a 1% to 2% fatality rate, this vaccine or one with potentially fewer side effects that is being made by recombinant DNA technology (using yeast cells to produce HBs) is extremely important. The yeast vaccine is still being tested, and to date has been found effective in human volunteers.

No active immunization against other forms of hepatitis is available. Control measures are obvious from the known modes of transmission of both A and B viruses. Most (estimated at up to 80%) posttransfusion hepatitis is caused by so-called non-A, non-B virus(es), a diagnosis made by exclusion; that is, no IgM anti-HAV, no HBs, and no IgM anti-

HBc (in the absence of anti-HBs). It is very likely that there is more than one morphologic type of nonA, nonB virus.

Chronic Infectious Neuropathic Agents (CHINA Viruses). This group includes the agents (unconventional viruses) causing *kuru* and *Creutzfeldt-Jakob* disease (presenile dementia with myoclonus), both degenerative diseases of the central system (spongiform encephalopathies) with exceptionally long (months to years) incubation periods and usually a fatal outcome. Neither agent has been seen, let alone isolated, although both have been transmitted experimentally to primates. The agent of *scrapie,* a similar neuropathy of sheep, has similar properties. Recent evidence, based on resistance of infectivity to ionizing radiation, suggests that the scrapie agent (for which the term "prion" has been introduced), as well as the two human slow encephalopathy agents, may be classed with the smaller viruses rather than as agents "subviral" in size. No immune response develops to either human agent. These "slow virus diseases" are to be distinguished from those caused by conventional viruses, that is, subacute sclerosing panencephalitis (SSPE), associated with antecedent rubeola infection or congenital rubella syndrome, and progressive multifocal leukoencephalopathy (PML), caused by a papovavirus (JC virus).

Chemotherapy of Viral Infection

Each of the relatively few agents presently available for antiviral chemoprophylaxis and chemotherapy has restricted application. The amantanes, amantadine (Symmetrel) and rimantadine, by inhibiting uncoating and thereby primary transcription of virus, prevent infection with group A influenza viruses and mollify the disease once it has become clinically evident; these drugs are ineffective against infection with group B or C viruses. DNA analogues are effective in certain infections due to herpesviruses. Topical IUdR (5′-iododeoxyuridine), by blocking viral replication, inhibits the progression of early prestromal stages of keratitis caused by HSV, but cannot be used systemically. Trifluoridine (trifluorothymidine, TFT) is similarly active by topical administration. Adenosine arabinoside (ara-A, vidarabine) and 9-(2-hydroxyethoxymethyl)guanine (acycloguanosine, ACV, acyclovir) are useful in topical treatment of genital herpes simplex. ACV given by mouth markedly reduces, but does not prevent, recurrences of genital lesions; it is effective in systemic (intravenous) therapy of HSV encephalitis proven by brain biopsy as well as of severe herpetic

disease in the immunocompromised host. Both these nucleoside analogues are effective in limiting the spread of VZV in the immunocompromised host. Ribavirin (Virazole), an analogue of the purine precursor 5′-aminoimidazole-4-carboxamide, has a wider antiviral spectrum and is active against RNA- and DNA-containing viruses; it is currently undergoing clinical trials in herpesvirus 1 and 2 and VZV infections. Inosine pranobex (Immunovir), a new drug that acts by stimulating the immune system rather than by acting directly against the virus, significantly reduces genital shedding of HSV. Human interferons are receiving increasing attention as potential chemotherapeutic agents. Human leukocyte interferon (HUIFN α 1) has been found to limit systemic varicella infection in immunocompromised (lymphoma) patients. With recent advances in genetic engineering, large-scale production of interferon in cloned bacterial culture is now possible because interferon has been rigorously purified and the human genes coding for its synthesis have been isolated. Isatin-beta-thiosemicarbazone, one of the first antiviral drugs described, was found useful in prophylaxis of variola, which has now been eliminated globally.

PROTOZOA

These are eukaryotic unicellular microorganisms, a number of which are human pathogens, and some of which require insect vectors for transmission.

Blood and Tissue Protozoa

Developmental stages of these parasites occur in vertebrate hosts and in sanguivorous arthropod vectors; some are true zoonoses and cause tangential human infection.

TRYPANOSOMES (GENUS *TRYPANOSOMA*)

Protozoa of this genus may occur in one or more of four forms: *trypomastigote, epimastigote, promastigote,* and *amastigote,* depending on the species and whether in the arthropod vector or mammalian host. Mature trypanosomes are spindle-shaped, with an undulating, keel-like membrane, edged with an anteriorly projecting flagellum. They are from 15 to 30 nm in length and exhibit active lashing motility. The trypaniform stages occur in the blood, tissues, and spinal fluid of febrile victims of infection, thus furnishing a means of microscopic diagnosis.

The epimastigote form occurs in the arthropod vectors.

Trypanosoma brucei gambiense is endemic in west and central Africa; *T.b.rhodesiense* is enzootic in a number of wild and domestic animals. Both cause **African sleeping sickness** and are transmitted by infected tsetse flies of the genus *Glossina*. Although these infections occur primarily in Africa, the increasing intensity of world travel brings the heightened possibility of importation of these afflictions to other geographic areas. Infection with *T.b.gambiense* is a more protracted and chronic disease than infection with *T.b.rhodesiense,* which may be rapidly fatal without central nervous system involvement. Both go through three successive stages: parasitemia; lymphadenitis and invasion of the central nervous system, accompanied by increasing degrees of toxemia, wasting, and torpor; and ending in death. Trypomastigote forms are found in blood, lymph nodes, and, in protracted cases of encephalitis, spinal fluid. Trypanosomes evade the host's immune response by undergoing antigenic variation. FAb and ELISA provide useful diagnostic information, in conjunction with measurement of IgM levels. Intravenous suramin is the chemotherapeutic agent of choice, but its administration must be carefully monitored because of its major renal toxicity; in central nervous system involvement, melarsoprol (a toxic arsenical) is added to therapy.

American trypanosomiasis (Chagas' disease) is caused by *T. cruzi,* which differs from African trypanosomes in having an amastigotic intracellular (cells of the reticuloendothelial system [RES], myocardium and endocrine glands, and glial cells) phase. Trypomastigotes of *T. cruzi* bind specifically to surface "receptors" (identified as fibronectin) on the surface of cells which they subsequently penetrate. The predominant symptoms stem from myocardial failure, also the principal cause of death. Many species of triatomid (conenosed) bugs serve as vectors. Diagnosis is made in acute stages by blood smear, culture (both lifeless media and cell cultures), animal inoculation, and xenodiagnostic blood tests (using parasite-free triatomids). Limited therapeutic success is achieved with nifurtimox, which eliminates the trypomastigotes from the blood, but not tissue amastigotes; relapses therefore occur.

GENUS *LEISHMANIA*

These protozoa cause various forms of **leishmaniasis.** They are ovoid, about 3 by 1 nm in size, and occur circumterrestrially in warm, moist areas. The amastigote form (no free flagellum) occurs in macrophages of the mammalian host; the promastigote form, in the arthropod vector. Canines are the major animal reservoir, and bites of infected sand flies (50+ species of *Phlebotomus*) are the principal vectors. Laboratory diagnosis is by microscopic examination of ulcer scrapings, bone marrow, or blood smears, depending on the species. Striking polyclonal hypergammaglobulinemia (chiefly IgG) is frequent. Skin tests with leishmanin (killed promastigotes) reveal varying degrees of delayed-type hypersensitivity. Parasites may also be isolated in the promastigote stage in pure culture on special media at 20°C to 25°C. Serologic tests (*e.g.,* complement fixation, indirect fluorescent antibodies [IFA]) are of limited value in diagnosis because of cross-reactions with other parasites, notably trypanosomes. Although morphologically identical, species may be differentiated antigenically. Pentavalent antimony compounds (sodium stibogluconate [Pentostam] and *N*-methylglucamine antimonate [Glucantime]) have replaced trivalent antimonials in therapy. Amphotericin B is effective in dermal leishmaniasis refractory to antimonials. Secondary bacterial infections of leishmanial ulcers are frequent and call for appropriate antibacterial treatment. Variations within the following imprecise nosological classification of leishmaniasis depend on the species of infecting parasite, immunological reactions of the host, geographic location and animal reservoirs. Human-to-human transmission occurs (*e.g.,* kala-azar), especially in crowded urban settings.

Cutaneous leishmaniasis is caused by *Leishmania tropica, L. major* (oriental sore), *L. mexicana,* and *L. peruviana* (American leishmaniasis, uta, seen in Central and South America). The lesions are limited to the skin, where they evolve from initial maculopapular lesions to painless nodules which ulcerate. Macrophages laden with parasites are found at margins of ulcers. The ulceroglandular form of the disease mimics sporotrichosis.

Mucocutaneous leishmaniasis (espundia) is mostly associated with *L. brasiliensis.* Infections initiated in the skin metastasize to involve mucous membranes and ultimately cartilagenous nasal and tracheal structures in a destructive granulomatous process.

Visceral leishmaniasis (kala-azar) is caused mainly by *L. donovani* and results from hematogenous dissemination of parasites to cells of the RES in liver, spleen, lymph nodes, and bone marrow. Untreated kala-azar carries a high mortality rate.

GENUS *PLASMODIUM*

In nature the malarial parasites of humans are transmitted only by infected females of certain species of *Anopheles* mosquitoes. They can also be transmitted by blood transfusion or by the use of common injection apparatus, as occurs among drug addicts, who serve as a reservoir for mosquito-borne infections. The life cycle of *Plasmodium* sp. is complex and involves asexual phases in humans (*schizogony* and early *gametogony*) and sexual stages in the mosquito.

Asexual development in humans begins with the entrance of *sporozoites* from saliva in the proboscis of a mosquito. These first invade liver cells, undergoing replicative schizogony, the *exoerythrocytic stage.* In infections by *P. vivax* and *P. malariae* these may become latent and account for long-delayed relapses. Recrudescences may occur in inadequately treated *P. falciparum* infections. Many *merozoites* are liberated from the liver cells. The merozoites enter erythrocytes and become *trophozoites,* which undergo further schizogony. The erythrocytes rupture, liberating many new merozoites that either enter new erythrocytes to undergo further schizogony or develop into young *gametocytes* awaiting necessary maturation in an *Anopheles* mosquito. Massive destruction of erythrocytes produces anemia, pigmentation of phagocytic cells by *hemozoin* (iron-bearing malarial pigment), anoxia of tissues, and consequent difficulties. The cyclical destruction of erythrocytes during schizogony periodically releases pyrogens causing quartan, tertian (see below) chills, and fever. The cycles are often quite irregular. The time from the mosquito bite to the first febrile attack is called the *intrinsic incubation period.* Hepatomegaly and splenomegaly are typical of malaria.

The sexual cycle occurs only in the mosquito, and the period from infection of the mosquito to infectivity comprises the period of *extrinsic incubation* (10 to 14 days). As soon as blood enters the mosquito, male gametes exflagellate and fertilize female gametes, each pair producing a *zygote* that develops into a motile *ookinete.* This invades a cell of the stomach wall and forms an *oocyst* containing many sporozoites. These are liberated on rupture of the oocyst and migrate to the proboscis, ready to infect humans.

Laboratory diagnosis of malaria is most often based on Giemsa-stained blood smears (thick or thin or both) and recognition of the parasites.

Plasmodium falciparum (malignant tertian or estivoautumnal malaria).   Mainly tropical in distribution, and accounts for up to 85% of infections. The cycle of schizogony in humans varies in duration from 36 to 48 hours. Falciform gametocytes are diagnostic; schizonts are rarely seen. Clinically, this is the severest and most dangerous form of malaria, largely because the parasites invade erythrocytes of all ages, often in multiples, resulting in very extensive parasitemia. Marked capillary obstruction occurs, probably because of adherence of parasites to capillary endothelium. The resulting tissue edema when it involves the brain (cerebral malaria) is life-threatening.

Plasmodium malariae (quartan malaria).   This is mainly subtropical. The usual cycle of schizogony is 72 hours but is subject to variations in clinical effect. Morphologically, *P. malariae* resembles *P. vivax* and *P. ovale* (see below), except that no Schüffner's stippling is present, the erythrocyte is not enlarged, and the parasite is more compact. Pigment is darker and more conspicuous than that of *P. vivax*. There is very little ameboid activity. *P. malariae* attacks only mature erythrocytes, with consequent relatively mild parasitemias. Chronicity is frequent, and glomerulonephritis may occur.

Plasmodium vivax (tertian malaria).   This is found in temperate zones as well as in the tropics. The cycle of schizogony is 48 hours, but the clinical periodicity of chills and fever is quite variable. Active ameboid motion of the trophozoites and enlargement of the erythrocytes are diagnostic. Schüffner's stippling is conspicuous and may represent pits in the membrane. Gametocytes are large and appear early. *P. vivax* attacks only reticulocytes, with consequently limited parasitemias.

Plasmodium ovale.   Similar in most respects to *P. vivax,* but there is more Schüffner's stippling; erythrocytes are much enlarged and distorted; *P. ovale* infection is clinically milder than tertian malaria.

Treatment of malaria has been complicated by the emergence of drug-resistant strains of plasmodia in widely scattered geographic areas of the world. Choice of drugs will therefore be influenced by knowledge as to the source of infecting strains. Chloroquine is the drug of choice for infections by sensitive strains. In treating malaria originating in areas where chloroquine resistance is prevalent, quinine, pyrimethamine, and sulfisoxazole or sulfadiazine should be given. Mefloquine is a new antimalarial effective against chloroquine-resistant *P. falciparum*. Development of antimalarial vaccines is under active investigation. The most promising experimental approach is the elucidation of the structural gene encoding the immunodominant surface antigen (circumsporozoite protein) of *P. falciparum,* thereby paving the way toward development of a recombinant vaccine.

Intestinal Parasites

THE AMEBAE

The intestinal amebae multiply only by binary fission. The life cycles of many species alternate between very fragile, vegetative *trophozoites,* intermediate precysts and dormant cysts. Some do not form cysts. Many species are minor pathogens or commensals: *Entamoeba coli, Endolimax nana, Iodamoeba bütschlii, Dientamoeba fragilis.* These are of importance mainly because of possible confusion with *Entamoeba histolytica,* the only important pathogenic ameba of humans, during microscopic examination of stools.

Entamoeba histolytica causes amebiasis, including amebic dysentery. The fragile, pleomorphic, motile trophozoites, around 8 to 60 nm in size, are seen *only* (except when cultivated in special media) in acute diarrheic (or purged) stools and in invaded tissues. They sometimes contain ingested erythrocytes. The more resistant, diagnostically distinctive cysts (5 to 20 nm) are the forms most commonly seen in normal feces: round, quadrinucleate (when mature), with chromatoids (not always seen) and thick cyst membrane. Stained with iodine the nuclei are diagnostically distinctive in appearance.

The trophozoites secrete histolytic enzymes and penetrate the mucosa of cecum and colon, producing undermining ulcers and sometimes intestinal perforation. The amebae sometimes enter the portal venules or lymphatics, invading other tissues, notably liver and brain, with expanding abscess formation. There is rapid necrosis of liver parenchymal cells and lymphocytic infiltration of the abscesses. Symptoms then depend on the location of the lesion. Clinically, intestinal amebiasis ranges from subclinical (carriers) to severe dysentery characterized by bloody, mucoid stools, anemia, and dehydration. The so-called small-race of *E. histolytica* may or may not be pathogenic.

Transmission of amebiasis is only by cysts: fecal–sewage–food–oral; "hand-to-mouth."

Diagnosis is commonly by microscopic examination of stools for cysts. The **cysts** of the harmless *Entamoeba coli* are recognizable by their larger size and five or more distinctive nuclei (when mature). *Entamoeba coli* ingests few if any erythrocytes. Although it is a harmless commensal in the lower levels of the large intestine, its presence indicates that fecal material has been ingested.

GENERA TRICHOMONAS AND GIARDIA

Trichomonas hominis. The trophozoites of these pear-shaped flagellates are 7 to 15 nm by 5 to 15 nm with three to five anterior flagella and a keel-like, laterally attached, undulating membrane with marginal flagellum. A prominent axostyle extends from the anterior (large) end through the center and projects posteriorly as a spike. *T. hominis* occurs in the lumen of the cecum. Transmission is fecal–oral. Pathogenicity is debatable. Diagnosis is by microscopic examination of the stool for the trophozoites. No cysts are formed.

Giardia lamblia. This flagellate is endemic in most parts of the world, and infection occurs frequently as a water-borne common source epidemic. In children, it may cause illness resembling the celiac syndrome, with steatorrhea, anemia, marked weight loss, and retardation of growth. Giardiasis in individuals with immune deficiency (*e.g.,* AIDS) may be severely debilitating. The diagnosis rests on finding *G. lamblia* trophozoites and cysts in diarrheic stools. The trophozoites, which survive mainly in duodenal mucosal crypts, are flattened dorsoventrally and have two large, eyelike nuclei, eight active flagella, and a ventral sucking depression for attachment to intestinal epithelial cells. A number of drugs are effective in therapy: metronidazole (Flagyl), tinidazole, furazolidone, and quinacrine (mepacrine).

GENUS BALANTIDIUM

Balantidium coli is the largest of the protozoan parasites of humans. It is a pear-shaped ciliate about 75 to 55 nm, with a ciliated mouth **(cytostome),** anal opening, prominent pulsating vacuole and macronuclei and micronuclei. Multiplication is usually by transverse binary fission. There are many saprozoic and commensal ciliates that may be morphologically confused with *B. coli,* the only ciliate of importance as a human pathogen.

B. coli occurs in the large intestine, where it feeds on host cells, bacteria, and other nutrients. It produces dysentery, which can vary from a fatal one with profuse diarrhea to one that is very mild. *B. coli* also produces openings in the mucosa and can penetrate into the submucosa, causing the formation of ulcers that resemble, but are less penetrating than, those due to *Entamoeba histolytica.* Transmission is fecal–oral, chiefly among hogs, occasionally to humans. In humans, clinically, balantidiasis ranges from (usually) asymptomatic to (rarely) fulminating and fatal.

Genitourinary Parasites

Trichomonas vaginalis, a cause of vulvovaginitis, is slightly larger than *T. hominis,* but otherwise closely resembles it. No cysts are known. *T. vaginalis* occurs in the human vagina and prostate, occasionally in urine. Transmitted usually by coitus, trichomoniasis may also be transmitted by moist, freshly contaminated clothing, washcloths, and other agents.

Genitourinary trichomoniasis is usually asymptomatic in males and sometimes in females, but in the latter often causes mild to severe vulvovaginitis. Diagnosis is by microscopic examination of exudates for the trophozoites. Cysts have not been seen.

Toxoplasmosis

The worldwide protozoan that causes this disease was observed originally in North African rodents called gondi, hence its name, *Toxoplasma gondii.*

Toxoplasma gondii has a multiphasic life cycle, somewhat like that of the malaria parasites, to which it is distantly related. The sexual stage develops in the intestine of cats; the asexual stage, in the muscles and other tissues of numerous feline and nonfeline mammals, including humans. The crescentic, pear-shaped asexual trophozoite is motile by bending and gliding movements.

In the cat, the sexual stage of the parasites results in production of drought- and starvation-resistant infective oocysts that are passed in the cat's feces. The oocysts may be ingested by many different warm-blooded vertebrates. If ingested by a cat, new trophozoites develop, the sexual process is repeated, and more infective oocysts are produced. If ingested by humans or any animal other than cats, the oocysts develop into trophozoites. These multiply asexually by fission and invade the tissues, where they may produce an inflammatory reaction of greater or lesser severity, commonly subclinical. They may eventually form cysts (not sexually produced oocysts as in the cat) and remain encysted in the tissues, causing chronic toxoplasmosis, also usually subclinical, which remains chronic, probably for life. Animals eating them in any forms, cyst, oocyst, or trophozoite, may become infected. Humans become infected most often by ingestion of undercooked meat containing cysts.

A large proportion of persons (50% of adults in the United States) when tested show serologic evidence of having (had) subclinical toxoplasmosis.

Any mammal or bird eating raw or "rare" flesh containing the asexual cysts will contract the infection. Birds and mammals (except cats) do not pass infective oocysts so far as is known. Their flesh is infective but not their feces. Infected pregnant women can infect the fetus, sometimes with serious results: hydrocephalus, eye and brain damage. The disease appears to be worldwide in distribution and generally unnoticed.

Diagnosis of chronic toxoplasmosis is based on serology as well as on finding the pear-shaped parasites in tissues. Definitive identification of parasites can be made by indirect fluorescent antibody tests on biopsy material. Rising antibody titers, measured by ELISA or FAb, are suggestive. IgM antibody to *T. gondii* in cord blood establishes the presence of fetal (congenital) infection.

Cryptosporidiosis and *Pneumocystis Carinii*

Cryptosporidium (a coccidian parasite cultivable *in vitro* and related to *Toxoplasma*) was once thought to be a parasite primarily of bovine species. It has since been encountered in humans as the cause of explosive diarrhea, which in healthy individuals is self-limited; in immunologically compromised individuals, cryptosporidiosis may become chronic and debilitating and contribute to the lethal effects of other parasites, such as *Toxoplasma.* Cryptosporidiosis (for which there is no chemotherapy) and toxoplasmosis, along with infection with *Pneumocystis carinii,* have recently come into prominence as severe and often overwhelming opportunistic infections in persons with AIDS; *Pneumocystis* infection accounts for up to half of the fatalities among AIDS patients.

Pneumocystis carinii, while generally regarded as a protozoan, remains unclassified taxonomically. The organism is widespread in the animal kingdom; antibody is found in the majority of healthy adults, indicating that subclinical infection is almost universal. In immunocompromised individuals, particularly those with AIDS, it produces a massive generalized pulmonary infection in which large numbers of the organisms are found in needle aspirates or transbronchoscopic biopsies of the lung; when sufficiently numerous, they may be present in sputum. Pentamidine and trimethoprim–sulfamethoxazole are currently used as chemotherapeutic agents. Mortality may approach 50% and higher in AIDS patients. This is increased by the presence of other concurrent opportunistic infections.

HELMINTHS

The term **helminth** is commonly used to mean parasitic worms. There are two principal groups: phylum Platyhelminthes, or **flatworms,** which include class Cestodea (tapeworms) and Trematoda (flukes); and phylum Nemathelminthes, class Nematoda or **roundworms,** which includes hookworms, pinworms, etc.

Flukes (Class Trematoda)

The life cycles of all flukes parasitic in humans are complex, details varying with species. In general, fertilized eggs are produced by sexually mature adults in the definitive host, that is, the host that harbors the sexually mature stage of any parasite. All flukes are hermaphroditic except schistosomes, which are diecious.

Eggs are discharged in feces (in *Schistosoma haematobium,* mainly in urine). Eggs hatch in polluted fresh water, each liberating a free-swimming ciliated larva **(miracidium)** that penetrates an intermediate host, usually a species of snail, in which it becomes a sporocyst and (except in schistosomes) produces numerous **rediae** and daughter rediae or sporocysts. These finally become minute, tadpole-like **cercariae** (with forked tails in schistosomes) that penetrate the definitive host (see below), losing their tails and becoming **metacercariae** (incomplete in schistosomes). They enter the definitive host by (1) direct penetration of the skin of swimmers, waders, rice planters, and others (schistosomes); (2) encysting on aquatic plants such as, water cress, water chestnuts, and lotus, which are eaten raw (liver flukes: *Fasciolopsis buski; Fasciola hepatica*); (3) penetration of, and encystment in, tissues of aquatic animals (fish, crustacea) that are eaten raw (liver fluke *Clonorchis sinensis* and lung fluke *Paragonimus westermani*).

After ingestion by the definitive host and excystation (except schistosomes, which penetrate skin and do not form cysts), migration to specific organs occurs via blood and lymph channels and penetration through intestinal walls and other tissues. Diagnostically distinctive eggs of all species occur in stools, but those of *Schistosoma haematobium* appear mainly in urine and those of *Paragonimus westermani* also in sputum.

Pathogenesis by all flukes is due principally to obstruction of various vessels and ducts, to trauma due to tissue penetration and burrowing, to abscess formation around dead worms, to intense inflammatory reaction with fibrosis and stricture, and to more or less toxic action depending on species. Symptoms depend largely on tissue of localization.

BLOOD FLUKES (GENUS *SCHISTOSOMA*)

These are distinguished from other human flukes by their slender, cylindrical form, separate sexes, and the prominent, longitudinal, copulatory canal of males, which enfolds the female during copulation. Males range in length from 10 to 20 mm. Adults most commonly live in the mesenteric, the portal, or the vesical venules, whence eggs enter the intestine or the urinary bladder and appear in feces or urine, depending on species. Intradermal tests for specific allergy with schistosomal antigens are useful in diagnosis. Eggs are not operculate. Biopsy of intestinal mucosa may be necessary for definitive diagnosis if eggs are not found in fecal samples.

Schistosoma japonicum (Oriental blood fluke). This causes intestinal and hepatic schistosomiasis, chiefly in Japan, North China, and adjacent lands and islands. Eosinophilia is marked. This is the most dangerous form of schistosomiasis, as the worms are widely disseminated in the body. Distinctive eggs, with rudimentary lateral spikes covered with adherent fecal material, appear in the stools.

Schistosoma mansoni. This causes schistosomiasis mansoni or Manson's schistosomiasis in Africa and adjacent lands, the Caribbean islands, and Brazil. The diagnostically distinctive eggs are laterally spiked and appear mainly in stools.

Schistosoma haematobium (vesical blood fluke). This causes vesicle bilharziasis or urinary schistosomiasis in Africa and adjacent lands. Eggs with one polar spike appear mainly in urine.

Schistosomal dermatitis or swimmers' itch. This is due to preliminary penetration, into the skin only, by cercariae of various species of avian and mammalian flukes other than human. These do not develop further in humans. Swimmers' itch is annoying but self-limited.

Control of schistosomes involves elimination of vector snails: *Bulinus* and *Physopsis* for *S. haematobium; Biomphalaria glabrata* for *S. mansoni; Oncomelania* for *S. japonicum.* Praziquantel is the newest drug found to be effective in therapy.

Tapeworms (Class Cestodea)

Adult tapeworms are typically intestinal parasites of vertebrates. They are attached to the lining of the small intestine of the host by the worm's head or scolex, which is equipped with suckers, and by multiple hooklets in some species. The scolex narrows posteriorly to form a neck from which are produced, by budding, a series of new "segments" or flattened, roughly rectangular proglottids that remain attached to the neck and to each other to form a ribbon-like strobila, which may be millimeters to meters in length, depending on species.

Each proglottid later becomes a sexually mature, hermaphroditic, egg-producing parasite. The older (most distal, and gravid with eggs) proglottids break off and are carried out in feces along with ova (except *Taenia* sp. and *Dipylidium canium*). Most ova and proglottids have diagnostically distinctive morphology. The scolex remains attached to produce more proglottids. Neither flukes nor tapeworms have alimentary systems. Nutrition is osmotropic, that is, occurring by absorption through the surface structures. The life cycles and the intermediate hosts vary with species.

Taenia saginata. The beef tapeworm, 4 to 9 m in length, is found in peoples that eat raw beef, almost never in the United States. Herbivores acquire the embryonated eggs, each containing a six-hooked ***onchosphere,*** in sewage-polluted pasturage. The freed embryos invade the muscles and remain as encysted larvae (*Cysticercus bovis*) until eaten uncooked by humans. The scolex is about 3 mm in diameter and has four sucking disks but no hooklets (although hooklets are present in the egg). The eggs (*not* species distinctive) are found free by microscopic examination of human feces and in the proglottids that appear in the stools. Neurocysticercosis is a life-threatening complication of this infestation, for which praziquantel is effective when combined with steroids to reduce the inflammatory response.

Taenia solium. The pork tapeworm occurs in the encysted larval (cysticercus) stage in pork. Infection is rare in the United States. The distinctive scolex has four sucking disks and a ***rostellum*** with a double row of 26 to 28 hooklets. The species is recognized by counting the number of uterine branches, which in *T. saginata* range from 15 to 20 (average 18) on each side; *T. solium* has 7 to 13 (average 9) on each side. The ova are not distinguishable from those of *T. saginata*. The life history and human–pork relationship are analogus to the human–beef relationship of *T. saginata*. In addition, humans may ingest eggs via fecally polluted foods and develop cystercerci in the muscles. Hogs acquire eggs from foods polluted by human feces.

Hymenolepsis nana. The dwarf tapeworm (about 2 to 4 cm long and 1 mm wide) is the smallest and most common tapeworm affecting humans in

the United States, occurring most frequently in children. The head has a rostellum with 24 to 30 hooklets and four suckers. There are from 150 to 200 segments.

No intermediate host is necessary. The diagnostically distinctive eggs are passed in feces and are transmitted to the mouth of the same host ***(autoinfection)*** by soiled hands, underclothing and unclean habits in regard to feces. The ***cysticercoid*** larvae develop in the intestinal villi and the adults and then fasten to the duodenal or the jejunal mucosa and repeat the cycle. Personal cleanliness and sanitary disposal of feces are the best prevention.

Diagnosis depends on the discovery of ova in the feces.

Diphyllobothrium latum. The fish tapeworm may reach 12 m in length, with thousands of proglottids. The head, about 1 mm by 2 to 3 mm, has no hooklets but has two longitudinal sucking grooves. Each diagnostically distinctive egg has a small hinged lid or operculum at one end, suitable for hatching in water, and demonstrable by pressure on the coverglass on a slide.

Eggs from human feces in cool fresh water produce free-swimming embryos. These are swallowed by copepods ("water fleas" [*Cyclops* or *Diaptomus*]), where a larva forms. The copepod is eaten by a plankton-eating fish and forms a ***sparganum*** in the muscles. When the fish is eaten undercooked by a human host, the larval tapeworm matures and attaches in the proximal jejunum. Competition with the host for vitamin B_{12} may cause profound anemia. Eosinophilia is frequent.

Control involves avoidance of sewage pollution of waters in which the intermediate hosts breed and the cooking of all fish to be eaten.

Echinococcus granulosus and ***E. multilocularis.*** These cause unilocular and multilocular or alveolar echinococcosis respectively; hydatid disease. The definitive hosts of these tapeworms are not humans but other carnivorous mammals, especially canines. Cattle, sheep, swine, and people are intermediate hosts; these species harbor the larval cyst stage ***(hydatid cyst)*** that is analogous to the cysticerci of *Taenia* sp.

Adult *Echinococcus* tapeworms are 2 to 6 mm long. In dogs, they produce *Taenia*-like eggs that appear in the animal's feces and are swallowed with polluted fodder by a wide variety of intermediate hosts. In the case of humans, they are acquired from accidentally soiled hands, food, or both, especially among persons closely associated with dogs: Eskimos, sheep herders, and others.

The eggs produce larvae that penetrate through

venules to liver, brain, and other organs, where they usually slowly form either unilocular hydatid cysts *(E. granulosus),* often amenable to surgery, or alveolar or multilocular cysts *(E. multilocularis),* rarely amenable to surgery. The cysts may become very large and destructive and usually contain many infective daughter scolices that become adults when the cyst is ingested by a carnivore. In humans, a large proportion of the cysts of *E. multilocularis* are sterile: they do not have daughter cysts or scolices.

Diagnosis of echinococcosis or hydatid disease in humans may be made with hydatid-cyst-fluid antigen by complement-fixation or precipitin tests; cutaneous allergic reaction; or the finding of hooklets or scolices in the cyst fluid if surgical procedures are feasible.

Phylum Nematoda

Adult roundworms parasitic in humans generally attach to the intestinal mucosa except *Ascaris,* which remains free in the intestinal lumen, and filarial worms, which inhabit blood, tissues (especially skin), and lymph spaces. Female nematodes usually are larger than males.

Hookworms *(Necator americanus* and *Ancylostoma duodenale).* Male hookworms average around 8 by 0.4 mm. in size. Hookworm infection is widely endemic in the tropics and subtropics, especially in extraurban populations. Adults, attached to duodenal and jejunal mucosa by suckers and cutting plates, digest the mucosa and blood and produce diagnostically distinctive eggs that appear in feces. On warm, moist soil the eggs hatch and undergo 10 to 15 days of development through four larval stages. The last larvae are filariform and penetrate exposed skin of bare feet, causing ground itch.

The larvae migrate through blood vessels and lymphatics to the lungs with relatively little pneumonitis; thence, after further development, by the trachea, esophagus, and stomach to the intestine where, as adults, they attach and renew the cycle.

Pathogenesis involves continuous intestinal irritation and hemorrhage, with resultant anemia, and debilitation, both physical and mental.

Control is based mainly on sanitary disposal of feces and avoidance of direct contact with feces-polluted soil. As in any control program, elimination of sources of infection by treatment of infected persons is essential.

Giant roundworms *(Ascaris lumbricoides).* These are worldwide in distribution and among the most prevalent nematodes of humans, except in cold, dry climates.

Male *A. lumbricoides* may attain lengths of over 30 cm and diameters of 8 mm. Adults live mostly in the small intestine and may migrate *post mortem* into various parts of the gastrointestinal tract (bile and pancreatic ducts, stomach, *etc.).* They do not attach to the intestinal mucosa. They may perforate the intestinal wall or migrate out of anus, mouth, or nares. They die out after about a year but, in endemic areas, are replaced constantly.

Diagnostically distinctive eggs, passed in stools, mature in warm, moist soil in 2 to 3 weeks. Ingested, the mature eggs hatch in the small intestine. (Compare with hookworms, the eggs of which hatch on the soil, not in the intestine.) The larvae migrate actively to the lungs by way of blood, lymphatics, or both, with accompanying pneumonitis, possibly allergic, get into the alveoli and thence to pharynx and esophagus, where they are swallowed. In the small intestine they mature, produce eggs, and recommence the cycle. Large numbers can cause serious difficulties due to mechanical obstructions. General symptoms of gastrointestinal irritation and malnutrition are common. Severe infestations may require surgical intervention and are sometimes fatal.

Whipworms *(Trichuris trichiura).* Males are about 40 by 5 mm. Infection is circumterrestrial, mainly tropical. Adults attach to the cecal mucosa and produce diagnostically distinctive eggs in the feces. The eggs do not hatch, but on warm, moist soil the intraoval embryos become larvae. Under unsanitary conditions they are ingested by humans. The eggs hatch in the intestine, and the freed larvae migrate to the cecum, mature, and repeat the cycle. A heavy burden of worms causes mucosal inflammation and erosion, diarrhea, and hemorrhage, mostly in children. A light worm burden may not cause symptoms.

Diagnosis depends on recognizing the species-distinctive eggs in the stool.

Control is dependent on sanitary disposal of feces and avoidance of feces-polluted soil, food, or objects contaminated with such soil or feces and is potentiated by adequate treatment of infested patients.

Pinworms or seatworms *(Enterobius vermicularis).* Males are about 3 by 0.2 mm. The worms are circumterrestrial in temperate areas. Adults are attached in cecum and colon. Gravid females migrate to the anal and perianal area and deposit diagnostically distinctive eggs that are highly infectious and may be picked up for microscopic examination on clear adhesive tape. Sometimes the adult worms may be seen on the skin. Eggs are carried to the mouth on hands or on contaminated dust from clothing to the same *(autoinfection)* or another host. The eggs hatch in the intestine, and the freed worms attach and repeat the cycle.

Occurring mainly in children under unsanitary conditions, *E. vermicularis* causes perianal pruritus, local irritation, and scratching that invites transmission via hands and secondary bacterial infection. Eosinophilia is marked.

Control involves personal cleanliness and eradication of the worms by chemotherapy.

Trichina worm or pork worm *(Trichinella spiralis).* These worms cause trichinosis. Most carnivorous animals are susceptible, and the disease is enzootic in rats and swine. Both eat infected pork as municipal garbage or slaughter-house offal. Trichinosis occurs in humans as a result of eating undercooked pork containing live, encysted larvae.

Once ingested, the larvae excyst and mature in the crypts of duodenum and jejunum as small, slender worms about 1.5 mm long (males). After copulation the males die, and the females penetrate deeply into the mucous membranes where they produce large numbers of larvae (larviparous) that migrate through veins and lymphatics to the striated muscles. There the larvae grow and, about 3 weeks after ingestion of the infected meat, become encapsulated, coiled in the distinctive arrangement from which the species name is derived. In this condition they can remain viable for 12 years or more, although usually the cysts become entirely calcified in 10 to 12 months.

The early period of invasion by the newly ingested larvae is accompanied by local inflammation and gastroenteritis for several days and sometimes also by hemorrhage. The period (1 to 3 months) during which the newly produced ("second generation") larvae are migrating through the tissues and muscles is marked by fever, edema (especially of the face; periorbital), myositis or "muscular rheumatism," and general symptoms, including pain. Eosinophilia is marked. Severity depends on the numbers of larvae. Many mild, unrecognized cases occur; others may be fatal.

Diagnosis depends on finding the encapsulated larvae in bits of teased-out muscle after sectioning or digestion with trypsin. Immunologic tests are useful and include precipitin and complement-fixation tests using trichina extracts as antigen and the agglutination of antigen-coated latex particles. Intradermal tests for allergy with similar antigens are also valuable.

Control depends on cooking all garbage fed to swine, eliminating rats from garbage dumps and piggeries; adequate veterinary condemnation of infected swine (difficult); freezing of pork for at least 36 hours at $-27°C$ or thorough cooking or both; addition of thiabendazole to swine fodder.

Filarial Worms. Various species of these worms and their microscopic larvae *(microfilariae,* c. 275 by 7 μm) cause various forms of filariasis in tropical and some subtropical areas. Geographic distribution of the various species depends on distribution of the arthropod vectors (various mosquitoes, gnats, and biting flies) specific for each.

Although distinctive clinical features and epidemiology depend on the species of filarial worm involved, all forms of filariae and of filariasis have some basic similarities. In general, adult filariae inhabit fibrous subcutaneous or deep lymph nodules or other tissues of humans where they produce long, thin microfilariae. In some species these migrate into peripheral capillaries at hours (diurnal or nocturnal periodicity) when the arthropod vector specific for that species of worm bites.

After a series of maturation changes in the arthropod, the microfilariae migrate to the proboscis of the arthropod, ready to infect the next person bitten.

Active and extensive migrations of the microfilariae in the human host, their gathering together in large masses, and the allergic reactions consequent to chronic infection, result in pain, blindness *(Onchocerca volvulus),* and various distinctive types and locations of swellings.

Diagnosis before microfilariae appear in the peripheral blood is based on history of exposure, clinical picture, and intradermal sensitivity tests with filarial antigens. Later, microfilariae of some species are demonstrable microscopically in the peripheral blood during hours of periodicity or in "skin snips" macerated in saline solution *(O. volvulus). O. volvulus* does not circulate in the blood stream.

Chemotherapy against *O. volvulus* is not universally employed because of intense reactions that occur in the skin to the sudden release of large quantities of antigen. In Central America, nodules containing the adults are periodically removed as a means of control. Elimination of arthropod vectors is not always practicable, because the larvae grow in fast streams in which pesticides wash away quickly. Diversion of streams is often impossible, because coffee-growing areas are dependent on them.

Opportunistic Zoonotic Helminthic Infections

Toxocara canis, the canine ascarid, is the cause of a zoonotic disease in humans, **visceral larva migrans** (VLM), contracted by ingestion of developed eggs of the nematode, usually in soil contaminated by dog feces. The larvae are disseminated from the intestine to various tissues and organs, the number and distribution of larvae and the immune response to them determining to large extent the symptoms and severity of disease. Marked eosinophilia (over 50%) and hypergammaglobulinemia (IgM) are the rule, and eosinophilic granulomata around larvae are found in liver biopsies. Larvae do not return to the intestine through a pulmonary cycle and eggs are therefore not found in the stool. ELISA is useful in serodiagnosis; attempts at chemotherapy (with thiabendazole) have not been successful.

Ancylostoma braziliense and *A. caninum,* both hookworms of dogs, cause **cutaneous larva migrans** (CLM) or creeping eruption, another zoonotic opportunistic infection contracted by penetration of the skin (most often on the feet) by filariform larvae in soil contaminated with dog and cat feces. Intense pruritus, edema, and inflammation are seen at the sites of penetration, from which the larvae burrow through the layers of the skin causing linear raised inflammatory tracts and marked eosinophilic infiltration. Larvae do not mature in the human host, but survive for long periods in subcutaneous tissues. There are no serodiagnostic tests for CLM; skin lesions may heal with oral and/or topical thiabendazole.

FUNGI (EUMYCETES)

Fungi pathogenic for humans may cause one of three general types of fungal disease (mycosis):

1. Cutaneous mycoses *(dermatophytoses).* These are superficial and generally not dangerous per se. They involve only the skin, hair, and nails, alone or in combination. These mycoses are due to keratin-metabolizing, filamentous *dermatophytes* and sometimes to yeast-like *Candida albicans.*
2. Deep or *systemic mycoses.* These are usually serious, sometimes fatal.
3. *Subcutaneous mycoses.* These are usually chronic, localized infections of the skin, underlying dermis and occasionally the deep tissues, such as bones and muscles, principally of the extremities but also occasionally involving any exposed body surface. A variety of fungi, both dimorphic and monomorphic, are responsible.

Pathogenic fungi were previously grouped together under the term Fungi Imperfecti because a sexual or perfect mode of reproduction was not known. The discovery of a sexual reproductive cycle for many of these fungi prompted the adoption of Deuteromycetes (Gr. deutero, second) as their class name. Although identification of the sexual cycle resulted in a reclassification of the fungus according to the type of sexual spores produced, the name of the asexual form was retained and the organism in this form remained in the class Deuteromycetes. A sexual stage has been identified for several *Microsporum* species, assigned to the genus *Nannizzia,* several *Trichophyton* species, assigned to the genus *Arthroderma, Histoplasma capsulatum,* assigned the name *Emmonsiella capsulata, Blastomyces dermatitidis,* assigned the name *Ajellomyces dermatitidis,* and *Cryptococcus neoformans,* assigned the name *Filobasidiella neoformans.* Excepting *Filobasidiella neoformans,* which is placed in the class Basidiomycetes, all are grouped in the class Ascomycetes.

In general, diagnostic mycology is largely an exercise in morphology, supported secondarily by metabolic and immunochemical analysis (including the search for fungal polysaccharide antigens by CIE or ELISA). Infective agents are recovered in cultures of clinical material (scrapings, sputum, pus, tissue samples). The medium most widely used for general purposes of primary isolation and passage is Sabouraud's glucose (or maltose agar, *p*H 5.6), with added antibacterial drugs (usually chloramphenicol); in certain cases cycloheximide is also added to inhibit nonpathogenic fungi. Cultures are incubated for 1 to 4 weeks at 22°C and in special circumstances at 37°C. Pathogenic fungi are identified microscopically by characteristic mycelial formations (*e.g.,* spirals, favic chandeliers, racquet hyphae), distinctive asexual spores (*e.g.,* conidiospores, aleuriospores, chlamydospores), and color, texture and topography of colonies. For direct examination, scrapings, nail pairings, pus, and biopsy material can be macerated in 10% potassium hydroxide (KOH), or stained with lactophenol-cotton blue. Yeast cells are gram-positive; other structures do not stain well with Gram's stain. Periodic acid–Schiff stain is used to demonstrate fungal cell wall material in tissues (*e.g.,* hyphae, yeast cells). Although the primary immunologic defense against mycotic infection rests on cell-mediated mechanisms (indicated by delayed-type skin sensitivity), antibodies to fungal antigens are evoked, particularly in the deep-seated mycoses, and are useful diagnostically in certain instances. The serologic techniques used most widely are immunodiffusion and complement fixation. Skin tests with certain fungal antigens (notably histoplasmin) evoke specific antibody in persons already sensitive; anergy to fungal antigens suggests the presence of immunosuppression.

Cutaneous Mycoses

Dermatophytoses are caused principally by species of three closely related genera of keratin-metabolizing filamentous fungi called dermatophytes. Dermatomycoses are caused by a variety of yeasts and filamentous fungi, such as *Candida albicans* and *Pityrosporon furfur.*

Typically the dermatophytes grow in cutaneous tissues or in cultures in mold-like, branching, mycelial form. Asexual spores of dermatophytes, though little more thermostable than vegetative cells, survive for long periods in soil, shower-bath mats, floors, and hair brushes. Some dermatophytes *(Microsporum canis, Microsporum gypseum, Trichophyton mentagrophytes, Trichophyton verrucosum)* infect domestic animals and are directly transmissible to people. Some species can at times cause any of the conditions listed below subject only to restrictions as to skin, hair, or nails as noted. Person-to-person or animal-to-person transmission is common.

COMMON DERMATOPHYTES

1. Involve skin and hair; nails rarely.
   Microsporum audouini, M. canis, M. gypseum cause various forms of tinea (ringworm), especially in preadolescents; *M. canis* causes it in domestic animals also. The first two fluoresce yellow-green in ultraviolet light (Wood's light); *M. gypseum* fluoresces poorly or not at all. These species produce spores and hyphal elements outside the hair shaft, and hence are called **ectothrix infections.**
2. Involve skin and nails; not hair.
   Epidermophyton floccosum causes tinea pedis (athlete's foot), tinea cruris (jock itch), and tinea unguium.
3. Involve hair, skin, and nails.
   Trichophyton mentagrophytes, T. rubrum, T. tonsurans, T. schoenleini cause tinea pedis, favus sycosis, tinea unguium. The last two produce **endothrix infections** and the first two ectothrix infections of hair.

COMMON DERMATOMYCOSES

1. *Candidiasis*
   Candida albicans and other *Candida* species can cause otomycosis, onychomycosis, thrush, perlèche, vulvovaginitis, and skin lesions; *Candida* infections are among the most frequently encountered mycoses.
2. *Tinea versicolor*
   Pityrosporon furfur causes common superficial skin infection characterized by the formation of white-, brown-, or fawn-colored lesions.

Orally administered griseofulvin is effective against dermatophytoses. Topical agents such as miconazole nitrate, clotrimazole, and the nonprescription tolnaftate are effective against skin lesions, but less effective against nail infections. Nystatin (Mycostatin) is the drug of choice for dermatomycoses caused by *Candida* species. Keratinolytic ointments and scrupulous personal hygiene are recommended for tinea versicolor.

Deep or Systemic Mycoses

These diseases are caused chiefly by soil-inhabiting, dimorphic or **diphasic fungi,** that is, fungi capable of existing in two phenotypically distinct forms. In general, the free-living or **saprobic form** is a filamentous mold whereas the pathogenic, tissue-invading form is unicellular and yeastlike. Exceptions are *Candida albicans,* which is indigenous in humans and forms mycelia and pseudomycelia when it becomes invasive, *Coccidioides immitis,* which produces sporangiospores in mammalian tissues, and *Cryptococcus neoformans,* which is a monomorphic yeast. The two forms of each of these fungi may be reproduced on artificial media in the laboratory by manipulating environmental conditions such as pH, temperature, CO_2/O_2 ratios, humidity, and nutrients—amino acids, carbohydrates, and vitamins.

As would be expected in the case of soil-inhabiting organisms, infections are acquired by inhaling spores, resulting in primary pulmonary lesions, or by traumatically implanting spores into the skin, resulting in relatively localized infections involving the cutaneous and deeper tissues and occasionally the lymphatics of the affected areas. Systemic mycoses are slowly evolving, chronic diseases characterized by granulomatous reactions, abscess formation, necrosis, and the development of a cell-mediated immune response. Agglutinins, precipitins, and complement-fixing antibodies are formed and are useful in diagnostic and prognostic procedures, including latex aggutination, immunodiffusion, complement fixation and immunofluorescent staining techniques.

In contrast to dermatophytoses, person-to-person transmission of systemic mycoses is rare.

Systemic mycotic infections may also be caused by diverse, saprobic, monomorphic, filamentous fungi, such as, *Aspergillus* species, aspergillosis; *Mucor* and *Rhizopus* species, phycomycoses; and others less frequently encountered. Modern medical practice sometimes requires the use of immunosuppressants, antibiotics, hormones, and other drugs in conjunction with certain types of surgical and therapeutic procedures, thus compromising the patient and providing a target for these opportunistic fungal pathogens. In systemic pulmonary aspergillosis, early antigenemia is detectable by RIA.

CANDIDIASIS

Candida albicans, more frequently the etiologic agent of this mycosis than any other *Candida* species, is a common commensal of the human alimentary tract and vagina. Although *Candida* infections may involve any area of the body, those that involve the deep tissues and organs may be life-threatening and are therefore the most serious. Candidiasis is always endogenous.

Candida albicans is a nutritionally dependent dimorphic fungus growing as a yeast in its natural habitat or *in vitro* in the presence of glucose and as pseudomycelia and mycelia when it invades tissues and organs or in vitro in the presence of dextran, glycogen, or starch. Pathologically it is usually a secondary invader of injured, moist, superficial tissues, causing thrush (oral or vaginal), intertriginous dermatomycoses, perlèche, and paronychia. Rarely, deep invasions may occur producing pneumonias and meningitides. *C. albicans* may produce a serious enteritis as a result of suppression of the normally competitive intestinal bacterial flora by antibiotics following surgery. *C. albicans* is also a significant cause of endocarditis in surgical patients following cardiac valve replacement and in mainline drug addicts. Oral ketoconazole is effective in treating superficial candidiasis and other surface fungal infections.

COCCIDIODOMYCOSIS

Coccidioides immitis, the etiologic agent of this mycosis, reproduces in tissues as a sporangium, exhibiting endogenous sporulation, that is, a nucleus undergoes many divisions inside a thick-walled diagnostically distinct sporangium or spherule that ruptures in the tissues at maturity, liberating the spores to repeat the process. The soil-inhabiting, saprobic phase is truly mycelial, producing many highly infectious arthrospores on special hyphal branches from the vegetative mycelia. When disturbed, these arthrospores become airborne and, commingled with dust, are inhaled by animal and human hosts. *C. immitis* is common in hot arid areas of the United States and northern Mexico.

As in tuberculosis, most primary infections are short, asymptomatic, and pass unnoticed; however, they are both immunizing and sensitizing. Symptomatic pulmonary coccidioidomycosis with allergic hypersensitivity has been called **San Joaquin Valley fever** and **desert rheumatism.** Arrested pulmonary lesions seen in roentgenograms may be confused with those of tuberculosis. A generalized, chronic, progressive, and often fatal form of coccidioidomycosis called **coccidioidal granuloma** occurs, especially in dark-skinned peoples.

Coccidioidin, an antigen prepared from culture filtrates of *C. immitis,* is used in the coccidioidin skin test, which is analogous in all respects to the tuberculin test. A positive coccidioidin test in patients with significant shadows on chest roentgenograms is extremely suggestive, especially if they have been in the southwest United States or other endemic areas, if there is no clinical evidence of tuberculosis, and if the tuberculin test is negative. The presence of active disseminated disease is suggested by a rising complement fixation titer accompanied by a reversion of the skin test from positive to negative.

Primary pulmonary coccidioidomycosis, whether asymptomatic or symptomatic, has a high recovery rate, and therapy usually consists of bed rest or activity restriction and judiciously administered steroids to control the allergic manifestations of erythema multiforme and erythema nodosum. Amphotericin B is the drug of choice when antifungal therapy is indicated. There is no effective method of artificial immunization.

HISTOPLASMOSIS

The etiologic agent of this mycosis, *Histoplasma capsulatum,* is commonly found in the Ohio and Mississippi River valleys in soil of damp, fertile areas polluted by birds (especially chickens), bats, dogs, and skunks. This disease is unique among the systemic mycoses in that it primarily involves the reticuloendothelial system in which the yeastlike, oval parasite is found almost exclusively within macrophages and histiocytes. Parasitic phase cells may be grown *in vitro* under CO_2 at 36°C on artificial media enriched with blood, glucose, and cysteine. Diagnostically distinctive infective tuberculate macroconidiospores are produced in soil and in vitro on artificial media at 22°C. Inhaled spores give rise to primary pulmonary infections that, like coccidioidomycosis, are often silent, immunizing, and sensitizing. In overt or progressive disease, pneumonitis occurs, and lymphadenopathy may be generalized, with splenomegaly and skin lesions. Roentgenograms of arrested pulmonary lesions may be confused with those of tuberculosis and coccidioidomycosis. Progressive disease is severe and often fatal.

Dermal reactivity to histoplasmin is in all respects analogous to that seen with tuberculin and coccidiodin, indicating cell-mediated immunity to the respective agents. Diagnostically, the histoplasmin skin test is of relatively little value, because of the prevalence of inapparent infection. However, a negative reaction is consistent with deficiency in cell-mediated immunity and hence may indicate development of disseminated disease, especially in previously positive reactors.

Serologic tests with diagnostic and/or prognostic value are latex agglutination, immunodiffusion and complement-fixation, and counterimmunoelectrophoresis. The immunodiffusion test is particularly useful because the development and presence of certain precipitin bands, H and M, are indicative of active and chronic or healed histoplasmosis.

Most cases of primary pulmonary histoplasmosis heal uneventfully, with bed rest and supportive therapy prescribed for the moderately severe cases. Chronic, cavitary, or progressive systemic disease is treated with amphotericin B.

A clinically distinct form of histoplasmosis, **African histoplasmosis,** is caused by a large species of the genus *H. duboisii.* This mycosis is characterized by the development of granulomatous and suppurative lesions in the cutaneous, subcutaneous and osseous tissues. The lungs are rarely involved. Untreated cases can progress to cause death. Amphotericin B is the drug of choice.

There is a close antigenic relationship between the two *Histoplasma* species.

BLASTOMYCOSIS

Blastomyces dermatitidis, the etiologic agent of this mycosis, appears in lesions as large, ovoid to spherical, thick-walled, single budding, multinucleated, yeastlike cells. This organism is thermally dimorphic; therefore, the tissue phase may be obtained *in vitro* by inoculation onto most laboratory media and by incubation of the culture at 36°C. At 22°C in soil or on artificial media, the organism is filamentous. Infections are probably acquired by inhaling dust-borne spores.

Blastomycosis most often begins as a primary pulmonary infection and, unlike histoplasmosis and coccidioidomycosis, if untreated, progresses to a severe, disseminated, often fatal disease. Cutaneous lesions are common and probably result from the hematogenous metastasis of organisms from a pulmonary or abdominal site. These skin lesions begin as small papules and progress to confluent, granulomatous, verrucous ulcerations and swellings to abscesses. Rare primary cutaneous infections develop from indurated ulcers that necrotize into chancriform lesions accompanied by lymphangitis, lymphadenitis, and regional lymphadenopathy. In contrast to paracoccidioidomycosis, the mucocutaneous tissues and viscera are usually spared.

Dermal reactivity to blastomycin is not specific, and serologic tests are generally unsatisfactory for the same reason. Diagnosis is dependent upon finding the organism in a pathologic specimen and on clinical and roentgenographic evidence.

Blastomycosis responds quickly to therapy with amphotericin B, which is recommended for all forms of the disease. For those patients who cannot tolerate this drug, 2-hydroxystilbamidine has been used with some success.

CRYPTOCOCCOSIS

Cryptococcus neoformans, the etiologic agent of this mycosis, is a monomorphic, spherical, thin-walled, encapsulated yeast found in debris and accumulated guano in pigeon roosts. The yeasts, which are virtually unencapsulated in their saprobic existence, quickly acquire a demonstrable capsule following entry into a mammalian host; therefore, it appears that virulence is more closely associated with the potential for encapsulation than with the degree of encapsulation. Infections that progress to symptomatic diseases are most often seen in compromised patients.

It is well accepted that the primary lesions are probably pulmonary; however, these are usually silent and asymptomatic. Central nervous system cryptococcosis, particularly cryptococcal meningitis, is by far the most frequently diagnosed form of the disease, and *C. neoformans* exhibit a distinct predilection for this area. The yeasts elicit a feeble immune response in infected patients producing a histologic reaction consisting of numerous histiocytes, in which the organisms multiply profusely, and occasional giant cells, lymphocytes, and fibrosing stroma. Encapsulated organisms may be demonstrated by staining tissue preparations with muci-carmine or alcian blue stains.

C. neoformans may be detected in direct slide preparations of clinical specimens, especially spinal fluid, by mixing a drop of specimen with a drop of nigrosin, placing a cover glass over the preparation, and observing microscopically for encapsulated yeasts. When yeast cells are too few in number to be found readily, the spinal fluid is examined by CIE, ELISA, or latex agglutination (latex particles coated with antibody to cryptococcal polysaccharide) to detect the presence of free capsular polysaccharide. The organisms may be readily isolated from clinical specimens by inoculating Sabouraud's glucose agar or any good bacteriologic media incubated at 37°C. Because of the prevalence of nonpathogenic *Cryptococcus* species, isolates should be subjected to further identification procedures: mouse pathogenicity and urease production, and carbohydrate fermentation and utilization tests. Serologic tests are virtually valueless; immunofluorescent staining using rabbit antiserum to *C. neoformans* has a specificity paralleling that of the mucicarmine stains.

Amphotericin B, given parenterally, is the drug of choice for central nervous system cryptococcosis. Dermal or pulmonary disease may respond to the less toxic 5-fluorocytosine (flucytosine, 5 FC), administered by the oral route. Clinical studies indicate that optimal therapy may be a combination of these two antimycotics. Untreated cryptococcosis is often fatal.

PARACOCCIDIOIDOMYCOSIS

Paracoccidioides brasiliensis, the etiologic agent of this mycosis, is a thermally dimorphic fungus, appearing in tissues and *in vitro* at 37°C as a spherical, multiple-budding, yeastlike cell and in nature and on agar as a filamentous mold. The organism is endemic in Central and South America. Inhalation of dust-borne spores produces a mild, often asymptomatic pulmonary infection. Dissemination produces secondary lesions of the oronasal mucosa and skin, with lymphangitis of the involved area, and viscera, including liver, spleen, intestines, and lymphatics.

Untreated cases are often fatal. Amphotericin B and miconazole are recommended for all forms of the disease.

Subcutaneous Mycoses

SPOROTRICHOSIS

Lymphocutaneous sporotrichosis is the most common form of this disease, and the cutaneous form without lymphatic involvement is second in frequency for this reason. Sporotrichosis is sometimes grouped with chromomycosis, maduromycosis, and rhinosporidiosis as localized infections of the skin and subcutaneous tissues that rarely metastasize to distant sites. Primary pulmonary sporotrichosis, once extremely rare, is being reported with increasing frequency especially from large urban hospitals, probably because of increased awareness and improved diagnostic procedures. The rare disseminated form, which has a grave prognosis, involves multiorgan systems and is usually seen in compromised patients.

Typically, infection is initiated following the traumatic implantation into the skin of spores found on the bark and thorns of trees and shrubs and in garden mulches. An ulcerated, chancriform lesion develops at the inoculation site followed by the development along the lymphatic chain of multiple subcutaneous nodules that in turn become necrotic and ulcerate. The infection usually does not extend beyond the regional lymph nodes.

The etiologic agent, *Sporothrix schenckii,* is dimorphic, reproducing in tissues and *in vitro* at 36°C on blood agar enriched with glucose and cystine as oval, round, or elongated yeastlike cells and in nature and on agar at 22°C as a mold composed of septate mycelia bearing typical rosettes of small pyriform microconidiospores. There is usually a paucity of demonstrable organisms in biopsy material, even when special histologic stains are used; however, positive cultures of the same material are readily obtainable. Organisms have been demonstrated in tissues by immunofluorescent staining when none were seen using conventional techniques.

Infections are immunizing and sensitizing and elicit a cell-mediated immune response detectable by the intradermal sporotrichin test. Serologic tests using the yeast-cell antigen were found to be more specific than those in which sporotrichin was used; titers greater than 1:40 are considered significant.

Orally administered potassium iodide is used to treat lymphocutaneous and cutaneous forms of the disease. Local heat applications have been shown to promote healing. Amphotericin B is recommended for relapsed lymphocutaneous disease and disseminated sporotrichosis. 5-Fluorocytosine at a dosage of 100 mg/kg/day has been used with some success.

CHROMOMYCOSIS (CHROMOBLASTOMYCOSIS)

This mycosis, caused by a variety of dematiaceous, soil-inhabiting fungi belonging to the genera

Phialophora, Fonsecaea, and *Cladosporium,* is usually seen as an infection of the subcutaneous tissues, that is, verrucous dermatitis, but cases of cerebral chromomycosis (*i.e.,* cladosporiosis) have been reported.

Verrucous dermatitis is a chronic painless disease characterized by marked pseudoepitheliomatous hyperplasia. Granulomas with neutrophils, lymphocytes, plasma cells, and giant cells containing the sclerotic brown bodies of the tissue form of the fungus or strands of pigmented hyphae constitute the histologic picture. Secondary bacterial infection with resulting lymphostatis and elephantiasis is a complication.

Cerebral chromomycosis is characterized by single or multiple brain lesions, usually encapsulated abscesses formed around masses of brown pigmented hyphae. Symptoms are diverse, depending on the location of the lesions.

Surgical excision of lesions in the early stages of verrucous dermatitis is the most reliable treatment. However, most cases are not seen until the disease is well advanced and more refractory to antimycotics. Amphotericin B, used topically or by intralesion injection, thiabenzadole, used orally and topically, and 5-fluorocytosine have been used with varying degrees of success.

MADUROMYCOSIS

This disease, clinically identical to mycetoma caused by actinomycetes, is characterized by the development, usually on the extremities, of tumefactions, abscesses, fistulas, and sinuses that involve the deep tissues and bones. The lesions contain granules or grains composed of spores and hyphal strands of the offending fungus. A variety of fungi have been isolated as etiologic agents, among them *Madurella* species and *Allescheria boydii.* The disease is extremely refractory to antimycotic therapy; amphotericin B, griseofulvin, and nystatin have had limited success even in early cases (mycetoma, on the other hand, responds to sulfa drugs, penicillins, and tetracyclines). Excision of early localized lesions is recommended for those cases that do not respond to antimycotics. Amputation of the affected extremity may be necessary.

RHINOSPORIDIOSIS

Rhinosporidium seeberii, the etiologic agent of this infection, appears in tissues as large, thick-walled sporangia, producing, by successive nuclear divisions, endogenous sporangiospores that, at maturity, exit the sporangia through a "pore" (actually a thinned area of the sporangium wall). The organism has not been cultured *in vitro.* Rhinosporidiosis is a chronic granulomatous disease principally of the mucocutaneous tissues characterized by the formation of friable, sessile, and pedunculated polyps. As the name implies, the disease most often involves the nose. Obstruction of passages by large, unsightly polyps may be relieved by careful surgical excision. Superficial lesions may be removed completely; recurrence of surgically removed deep lesions is not uncommon. Local injection of amphotericin B is used as an adjunct to surgery to prevent spread. Other antimycotics are generally ineffective.

MECHANISMS OF RESISTANCE TO AND RECOVERY FROM INFECTION

Nonspecific factors that aid the human host in resisting invasion by pathogenic microorganisms include mechanical barriers (intact integument; hairs in anterior nares and auditory canal; secretions such as saliva, tears, respiratory, and vaginal mucus; ciliated epithelium in the lower respiratory tract); nonspecific chemical factors (gastric and vaginal acidity, lysozyme in tears; fatty acids in sweat, bile salts in the intestinal tract; alternate pathway of complement activation and secretory IgA) (see below).

Induction and Regulation of the Immune Response

The induction of both humoral and cell-mediated immune responses requires macrophages for "antigen processing" for optimal results. When small amounts of an antigen on the surface of macrophages are presented to T-helper cells that have receptors for that antigen, blastogenesis and clonal expansion occur. The release of soluble factors from these cells that are specific for this antigen induces a specific B-cell response to the same antigen (*i.e.,* clonal expansion). Both cells may or may not respond to the same antigenic determinant on the antigen molecule; however, if different antigenic determinants are involved, they must be located on the same molecule. In the case of a "hapten" conjugated to "carrier" protein, B cells may recognize the hapten, whereas T-helper cells may recognize an antigenic determinant on the carrier protein. Antigens that require this process are called T-dependent (Fig. 5-1 [1]). Most complex antigens fall into this category. Antigens that bear identical repeating antigenic determinants may

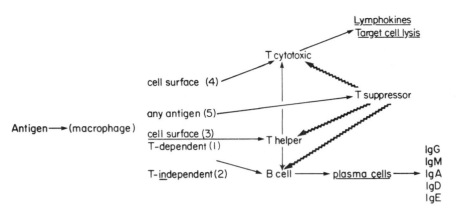

Fig. 5-1. Induction and regulation of the immune response.

stimulate B cells without T-helper cells (Fig. 5-1[2]). Examples of these T-*in*dependent antigens include gram-negative bacterial lipopolysaccharide, pneumococcal polysaccharide, and viral capsids (protein coats). Unlike the T-dependent process, only IgM immunoglobulins are formed without T-cell help. Cell surface antigens (*e.g.,* viral antigens, tumor-specific antigens, HLA-D alloantigens (Fig. 5-1 [3]) can induce T-helper cells to provide amplification of the T cytotoxic cell response (Fig. 5-1 [4]) to the same (viral, tumor) or other antigens on the cell surface (HLA-A,B,C alloantigens). T-cell helper factors may be both specific and nonspecific in this instance.

The character of the immune response to infection in the normal host is dictated in large measure by the nature of the parasite (used in the broadest sense) (Table 5-15). Microorganisms that are obligate extracellular parasites, that is, do not penetrate into normal cells and do not survive phagocytosis, evoke specific antibodies that are protective chiefly through neutralization of the pathogen (*e.g.,* enhancement of phagocytosis and intracellular killing, as in pneumococcal pneumonia, meningococcal meningitis). In acute and chronic infections with facultative intracellular parasites (*e.g.,* brucella, mycobacteria) cell-mediated immune (CMI) responses (evidenced in delayed-type hypersensitivity) come to the fore as important resistance and recovery mechanisms, although the humoral response plays a secondary role and is useful in serodiagnosis, particularly when the offending microorganism cannot be readily isolated. With obligate intracellular parasites (*e.g.,* all viruses, *Chlamydia*), CMI responses are the primary basis for containment of infection, the parasites being inaccessible to antibody except when transiently present in the blood stream (*e.g.,* spread of poliovirus from primary sites of infection in the gut to the central nervous system). The effec-

tiveness of vaccines is consistent with the foregoing concepts. Accordingly, killed antibacterial vaccines (*e.g.,* pneumococcal, pertussis) evoke protective antibody but no CMI against obligate extracellular parasites, and, by analogy, toxoids (*e.g.,* diphtheria, tetanus) evoke antitoxin that can neutralize toxin only when it is free in the blood stream. In contrast, living attenuated agents (*e.g.,* measles vaccine, BCG) must multiply in cells of the host in order to evoke both antibody and CMI, the latter being the chief mechanism of resistance and recovery. In certain infections, "abnormal" antibodies are elicited that have antigenic specificities distinct from those of the microbial agents involved (*e.g.,* Wassermann, heterophile antibodies) or that may relate to host autoimmune reactions (*e.g.,* rheumatic fever, mycoplasmal pneumonia).

The chief categories of **phagocytic cells,** which represent the first line of defense, particularly in acute bacterial infection, are:

1. **Polymorphonuclear leukocytes.** Neutrophils are a major component in acute inflammatory reactions, being actively phagocytic. They also have Fc and C3 receptors through which they mediate antibody-dependent cellular cytolysis (ADCC) (see below). Eosinophils are mobilized by eosinophil-chemotactic factor (ECF-A) from IgE-activated basophils and mast cells and are particularly associated with type I hypersensitivity and with helminthic infection (*e.g.,* direct antiparasitic effect of eosinophilic degranulation). Basophils and tissue mast cells, on binding IgE through specific surface receptors, are degranulated with concomitant release of vasoactive substances (histamine, slow-reacting substance A).

2. **Macrophages** (blood monocytes and fixed histiocytes) are central to the initiation of primary

TABLE 5-15. The Immune Response in Relation to Infection and Immunoprophylaxis

IMMUNOGEN	EXTRACELLULAR	INTRACELLULAR	IMMUNE RESPONSE:	
			Humoral	Cell-mediated
Parasites (active infection)	Obligate—acute Pyogens* Mycoplasma Facultative acute—chronic Brucella Francisella Mycobacteria Listeria Fungi		Protective antibody, opsonins Type III HS Agglutinins CF antibody, not (?) protective	Cellular immune mechanisms, T_c, NK, K (ADCC) Type IV HS
		Obligate acute—persistent Chlamydia Rickettsia* Viruses*	Neutralizing and CF antibody TYPE III HS	
Nonreplicating antigens	Toxins (toxoids)* Tetanus Diphtheria Botulinum Enterotoxins Anthrax		Antitoxin	
	Killed vaccines* Pertussis Influenza Rabies		Protective antibody	
Abnormal responses associated with infection	Enzymes Clostridial Streptococcal		Anti-enzymes	
	Autoimmune— crossreactive (?) Mycoplasma pneumoniae		Cold agglutinins	
	SSPE, ?PRP		Antiviral	Cellular immune mechanisms
	Infectious mononucleosis		Heterophilic antibody	
	Rheumatic fever			
	Lues and other (e.g., IM, malaria, SLE)		Wassermann, antibody, (BFP)	

*See Table 5-21 for immunoprophylactic reagents.

Abbreviations

ADCC = antibody-dependent cellular cytotoxicity.
BFP = biologic false-positive.
CF = complement-fixing.
HS = hypersensitivity.
IM = infectious mononucleosis.

K = killer cells.
NK = natural killer cells.
PRP = progressive rubella panencephalitis.
SSPE = subacute sclerosing panencephalitis.
T_c = cytotoxic T lymphocytes.

immune responses by B and T lymphocytes (see below) and also have Fc and C3 receptors important in ADCC. Macrophages are activated by lymphokines (*e.g.*, macrophage-arming factor) elaborated by the T lymphocytes mediating delayed-type hypersensitivity (T_{dth}). Macrophages are capable of supporting replication of some viruses and certain species of bacteria that are facultative (*e.g.*, mycobacteria) or obligate (viruses) intracellular parasites.

INTERFERON

Interferons (IFNs) are host-coded proteins synthesized by normal cells in response to various stimuli.

Alpha and beta IFNs are produced in leukocytes or fibroblasts, respectively, in response to viral infection or inactivated virus, isolated double-stranded RNA (not dsDNA), synthetic polyribonucleotides, or endotoxin. Gamma IFN is synthesized in unsensitized T lymphocytes in response to mitogens, and in sensitized T lymphocytes in response to specific antigen(s). Beta and gamma IFNs are glycoproteins; alpha IFN is not. The antiviral protective effect of IFNs is due to the induction, in normal cells, of new protein(s) with activity that inhibits replication (probably translation) of virus, thus aborting infection. IFNs are broadly species-specific, that is, mouse IFN is inactive in humans, but IFNs are nonspecific with respect to inducing viruses; human interferon may protect against several different viruses. For example, IFN limits the spread of VZV in immunocompromised hosts, and it has had extensive clinical trial (particularly gamma IFN) in treating certain neoplasms. The mechanism of observed antitumor effects is still wholly obscure. It is clear that IFNs are to be considered not only as antiviral agents but also to have profound cytoregulatory effects (*e.g.*, on cell growth and differentiation, on the immune system in modulating T-cell cytotoxicity and macrophage activity, on expression of histocompatibility antigens on cell surfaces). The antiviral activity of all three IFNs is comparable, but the anticellular activity of gamma IFN, in fact a lymphokine, is the most potent. Interleukin 2 (T-cell growth factor, IL 2) regulates the expression of its own receptors on T lymphocytes as well as the synthesis of gamma IFN by the same cells. The quantity of human interferons available for clinical trial has been limited by availability of human leukocytes and fibroblasts in which to produce it. With the advent of cloning techniques, production of IFNs in quantities large enough for adequate clinical trials can be realistically anticipated.

Specific Immunity

Specific immunity is the result of effector mechanisms directly involving antibodies and specific cellular elements of the lymphoid system. The immunologically specific host responses to infections as well as to stimulation by other chemical or biologic molecules involves two basic effector mechanisms: *humoral* (antibody) and *cell-mediated* (lymphocytes and macrophages). Both specific immune responses originate in the lymphoid system, each effector mechanism being primarily associated with a distinct subset of lymphocytes. For example, the production of antibody involves lymphocytes called B cells, whereas the cell-mediated response involves lymphocytes designated T cells.

ANTIGEN

Antigen may be any chemical or biologic molecule that under the proper circumstances is capable of inducing a humoral or cell-mediated response. The product of that response (antibody or T lymphocytes) will react specifically with the original antigen. Antigens may vary in their capacity to induce an immune response. This degree of effectiveness is called immunogenicity. The most immunogenic antigens are usually molecules that are completely "foreign" to the host such as microbial products or components. Tissue components from animals or another species (*xenoantigens*) are in turn much more immunogenic than equivalent components derived from members of the same species (*alloantigens*). An exception to the latter statement is the extremely strong cell-mediated allograft rejection observed in immunologically unrelated members of the same species. Under certain conditions, even one's own tissue components can be immunogenic (*autoantigens*). For example, individuals with collagen diseases may make a variety of antibodies to their own DNA (systemic *l*upus *e*rythematosus, SLE), immunoglobulins (rheumatoid factor), and various other components (smooth muscle).

Very low molecular weight substances (including chemicals) that are not immunogenic by themselves can induce an immune response if combined with immunogenic complex molecules (protein) of higher molecular weight. The low-molecular-weight substance or chemical compound is called a *hapten,* whereas the immunogenic complex molecule to which it is bound is called a *carrier.* Antibody made in response to a hapten–carrier complex binds specifically to the free hapten in the absence of the carrier. In a similar manner, certain small sequences of amino acids (proteins) or saccharides (carbohydrates) that are an innate part of complex immunogenic molecules can elicit an immune response to those specific areas of the molecule except that the remainder of the complex molecule acts as its own carrier. These integral small groupings of amino acids or saccharides are called *antigenic determinants* and, like haptens, determine the specificity of antibodies reacting with that particular antigen.

Some drugs, cosmetics, antibiotics, and industrial chemicals appear to act as haptens and utilize the host's own plasma or tissue proteins as carriers.

These combinations can give rise to specific allergic reactions involving IgE antibody in immediate-type hypersensitivity. These must be distinguished from drug idiosyncrasies that have no immunologic basis, but in which signs suggestive of hypersensitivity may appear (rash, arthralgias). In addition to the formation of antibody, other haptens (such as heavy metals and certain chemicals) when bound to host tissue elicit cell-mediated responses to the combined antigenic determinant of hapten and adjacent host amino acids. In this case, free haptens are *not* able to react specifically with T lymphocytes in the absence of host carrier proteins. Examples that can give rise to cell-mediated, delayed-type hypersensitivity reactions include contact dermatitis and poison ivy.

Heterophile antigens contain cross-reactivity or similar antigenic determinants occurring in certain tissues, organs, or erythrocytes, and shared by a wide variety of phylogenetically unrelated species of plants and animals: dogs, sheep, turtles, spinach, cell walls of gram-negative bacteria (*e.g., Salmonella*), guinea pigs, and hamsters. These Forssman heterophile antigens do not normally occur in pigs, frogs, or humans; antibodies to them are found in most human sera as agglutinins for sheep erythrocytes. Forssman heterophile antibodies can be absorbed out with guinea pig kidney tissue (rich in Forssman antigen). The heterophile antibody (sheep cell agglutinin) found in infectious mononucleosis (EBV) reacts with equine erythrocytes (Monospot test) and cannot be absorbed with guinea pig kidney tissue. The mononucleosis observed in CMV infection is not associated with a heterophile antibody response.

Soluble Factors in the Immune Response

ANTIBODY

In the electrophoretic analysis of serum, the major proteins are segregated into four principal portions: the alpha, beta, and gamma globulins, and albumin. Antibodies appear almost exclusively in the gamma portion and are commonly spoken of as gamma globulins or, more exactly, since they are not absolutely restricted to the gamma portion, as *immunoglobulins* (Ig). The immunoglobulins occur in five major molecular forms, designated as IgG, IgA, IgM, IgD, and IgE. There are several subclasses: $IgG_{1,2,3,4}$, $IgA_{1,2}$, $IgM_{1,2}$. The basic structure of IgG exemplifies the unit structure of all immunoglobulins (Fig. 5-2).

Each molecule of IgG is Y-shaped, consisting of

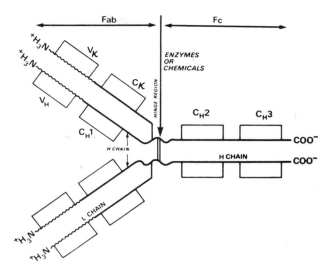

Fig. 5-2. A simplified model for an IgG1 (κ) human antibody molecule showing the 4-chain basic structure and domains. V indicates variable region; C, the constant region; and the vertical arrow, the hinge region. Thick line represents H and L chains; thin lines represent disulfide bonds. (Goodman JW, Wang A: Immunoglobulins: Structure and diversity. In Fudenberg HH, Sites DP, Caldwell JL, Wells JV (eds): Basic and Clinical Immunology, 2nd ed. Los Altos, CA, Lange Medical Publications, 1978)

part of a pair of identical polypeptide chains intertwined and held together by covalent disulfide bonds. Near the midlength, each chain bends away from the other to make the arms of the Y (hinge region). Each of these chains consists of about 440 amino-acid residues, whose sequence (primary structure) is determined genetically. The total molecular weight of each chain is from 53,000 to 75,000, depending on the class. These chains are called the **heavy** (H) **chains.** Attached to each of the divergent arms of the Y-shaped molecule is a shorter polypeptide chain of about 220 amino-acid residues, with a molecular weight of about 22,000 per chain. These are called the **light** (L) **chains** and are identical in any given molecule and may be of a κ or λ type. The entire structure (including tertiary) of each immunoglobulin molecule or unit is maintained by disulfide bonds.

On both L and H chains, the distal portion (N-terminal ends) is variable in amino acid sequence from one immunuglobulin to another, which enables it to conform to the antigenic determinant for which it is specific. Within the variable regions are primary sequences of amino acids that show even greater variability in sequence composition and that are called hypervariable regions. The primary structure of the rest of the L and H chains (COO⁻ terminal end) is constant except for differences between IgG, A, M, D, and E heavy chains or κ and λ light chains as well as some alloantigenic differences (Inv on light chains and Gm on IgG heavy chains). The "arms" of the molecule are flexible through a "hinge" region at the point of divergence of the arms to allow better binding for each antigen binding site. The hinge region is also vulnerable to enzymatic digestion with papain, which yields two Fab (ab for antigen binding) fragments and one Fc (c for crystalizable) portion. The Fc fragment binds to certain cells that have **receptors** for this portion of the immunoglobulin molecule such as mast cells (IgE), K cells (IgG), macrophages (IgG and IgM), and others. Components of serum **complement** are "fixed" or activated by regions in the Fc fragment. (Complement is discussed in more detail later.)

IgG as described previously is representative of the various classes of antibody molecules. It is a relatively small, bivalent monomer and is late in appearing in response to initial infection. It is the most plentiful immunoglobulin and is active in agglutination, precipitation, and complement activation. It is the only form of antibody that can pass the placenta. IgA occurs as a monomer or dimer of the IgG form, the units being held together at the C ends by covalent bonds of an extra component called J chain (Fig. 5-3). Secretory IgA is the primary defense against surface infections (*e.g.,* cholera, influenza, mycoplasmal disease). The molecule is equipped with a supplementary secretory piece that facilitates its transportation across membranes.

IgM is a pentamer of subunits linked together by covalent bonds initiated by interaction with J chain. Because of its polyvalency, IgM is especially effective in forming lattices with antigens. It is also active in complement activation and is the first to appear in response to infections. IgE is functional in antibody-mediated (anaphylactic type) of hypersensitivity reactions.

IgD on the surface of B cells is co-expressed with IgM, but appears later during ontogeny and is thought to be an indicator of the mature (*i.e.,* competent) but still uncommitted resting B cell. On pre-B lymphocytes, membrane IgD is required for antigen binding and has the same specificity toward antigen as IgM, but on antigenic stimulation, IgD is shut off and only IgM continues to be synthesized. IgD may be involved in interactions between T and B cells and in regulation of resting B-cell populations.

The reciprocal structural relationship between molecules of antigen and antibody is the basis of immunologic specificity. The antigenic determinant

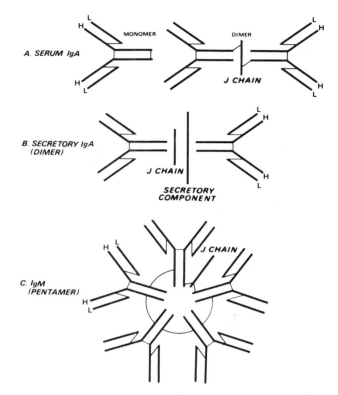

Fig. 5-3. Highly schematic illustration of polymeric human immunoglobulins. Polypeptide chains are represented by thick lines; disulfide bonds linking different polypeptide chains are represented by thin lines. (Goodman JW, Wang A: Immunoglobulins: Structure and diversity. In Fudenberg HH, Sites DP, Caldwell JL, Wells JV (eds): Basic and Clinical Immunology, 2nd ed. Los Altos, CA, Lange Medical Publications, 1978)

of a molecule and its corresponding specific antibody must "fit" accurately together in order for a specific and effective antigen–antibody reaction to occur. In effect, the better the "fit" is, the stronger are the bonds between antigen and antibody molecules. Antigen–antibody interactions do not involve covalent bonds but depend upon hydrogen bonds, ionic bonds, and Van der Waals forces, all influenced by ionic concentrations, pH, and temperature.

Since an antigen molecule may contain more than one type of antigenic determinant, an immune response directed against the antigen consists of a group of heterogeneous antibodies, each reacting with its own antigenic determinant on the antigen molecule. As previously discussed, antibody is at least bivalent, and now antigens (especially complex molecules) may also be polyvalent with multiples of the same antigenic determinant or an assortment of different antigenic determinants.

The recent introduction of *hybridoma techniques* has permitted the immunochemical dissection of polyvalent antigens (*e.g.,* cell membranes, viral proteins, *etc.*) at the molecular level. The basic technique calls for the fusion (originally with inactive Sendai virus, currently with polyethylene glycol) of dissociated splenocytes (from immunized animals) with mutant myeloma (plasmacytoma) cells deficient in hypoxanthine-guanine-phosphoribosyltransferase (HGPRT). After cell–cell fusion, remaining single plasmacytes die out in medium containing hypoxanthine, aminopterin, and thymidine (HAT medium); hybrid cells continue to multiply, using the HGPRT gene from the splenocyte moiety, which continues to synthesize its own brand of antibody (single isotype and idiotype) against a single antigenic determinant in the antigen used in the original immunization. The hybrid cells are *cloned* (*i.e.,* isolated as single cells and grown up in culture) and used to produce malignant ascites tumors (hybridomas) in mice, the resulting ascitic fluid providing a rich source of *monoclonal antibody.* "Monoclonal" in this context refers to the original single B lymphocyte represented in the hybridoma. Monoclonal antibody (mAb) is much more restricted in specificity (*i.e.,* single antigenic determinant) than the usual polyclonal antibody, even when the latter is directed against rigorously "purified" antigen. Hybridomas made with alloactivated normal T cells have been found to secrete functional lymphokines (*e.g.,* T-cell growth factor, allogeneic effect factor, macrophage arming factor).

Precipitation. This involves molecules of soluble antigen in optimal concentration in relation to concentration of antibody molecules (*i.e.,* neither in great excess of the other). A "lattice" is formed consisting of several molecules of polyvalent antibody, such as IgM or IgG, joined to several molecules of polyvalent antigen. Such complexes may form large, visible precipitates whose size and form depend in part on the relative concentrations of antigen and antibody, the ionic content, temperature, and other properties of the fluid in which the reaction occurs.

When antibody and antigen are present in ratios of 1:1 or slightly higher, for example, 3:1 or 3:2 ("optimal proportions"), aggregation of antigen and antibody is maximal and lattice formation is most rapid and copious.

Agglutination. This involves intact cells or antigen-coated particles (latex agglutination) and optimal electrolyte concentration. Agglutination is best achieved with IgM through multipoint binding of the pentameric antibody, but IgG and IgA can also agglutinate particles. Because of the large size of certain cellular antigens (*e.g.,* erythrocytes), IgM antibodies, being large and pentavalent, are most effective in their agglutination. IgG molecules, being small and only divalent, often fail to "bridge the gap" between large cells, and lattice formation therefore fails. However, they (IgG) may combine with receptors on the cells, preventing the combination of IgG antibodies, thus acting as "blocking" antibodies (see Coombs' test).

Neutralization. Neutralization of soluble toxins (and viruses) basically involves the blocking of reactive sites on the toxin (or virus) by antibody, thereby preventing expression of its toxic quality (or virus binding to host cells).

Opsonization. Microorganisms or foreign cells that have reacted with and retain specific antibody at their surfaces are said to have been *opsonized,* that is, rendered susceptible to phagocytosis by macrophages and polymorphonuclear leukocytes. The latter two cell types possess specific receptors for the Fc portion of immunoglobulins, particularly IgG, as well as for complement components (particularly C3) which, after binding to antigen–antibody complexes, contribute to opsonic activity by immune adherence (IA). Erythrocytes, neutrophils, lymphocytes, and monocytes possess receptors for IA, which is therefore important in clearing immune complexes from the circulation. This is also the basis for ADCC.

COMPLEMENT

Complement (C) is a system of 17 proteins in the serum. When activated by Ag–Ab reactions, it mediates such diverse biologic functions as cytolysis of mammalian cells and gram-negative bacteria, increased vascular permeability, release of chemotactic factors, and increased opsonization for phagocytosis. Binding of antibody to an antigenic determinant, whether on a cell surface or soluble molecule, causes distortion and unveiling of a site on the Fc portion of immunoglobulins (IgG, IgM); this event in turn starts the "classic" cascade effect with the binding of the first component (C1) (Fig. 5-4). The C cascade is in its simplest terms a series of enzyme precursors that are acted on in succession and converted to active enzymes. In addition to classic activation, C may be activated by aggregated IgA, lipopolysaccharides, and yeast cell walls (zymosan). This process is called "alternate" activation and includes the components properdin (P), B factor and D factor (Fig. 5-5). Both types of activation lead to the "effector" series of components

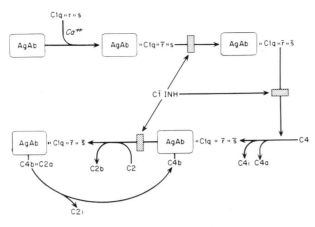

Fig. 5-4. Classic pathway of complement activation. This pathway is initiated by antigen–antibody (Ag-Ab) complexes and is controlled by the C1INH. (Austen KF: The classical and alternative complement sequence. In Benacerraf B, Unanue ER (eds): Textbook of Immunology. Baltimore, Williams & Wilkins, 1979)

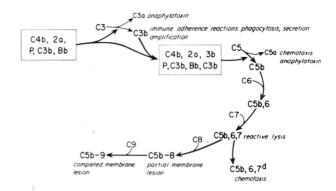

Fig. 5-6. The effector sequence of the complement system. The biologically active fragments and complexes are generated as a result of cleavage of C3 and C5 by the classic pathway and amplification of C3 and C5 convertases, respectively. (Austen KF: The classical and alternative complement sequence. In Benacerraf B, Unanue ER (eds): Textbook of Immunology. Baltimore, Williams & Wilkins, 1979)

C3 to C9. The split products of C3 to C7 with biologic activity are shown in Figure 5-6.

Cytolysis requires the interaction of C8 and C9, which cause lesions in the membranes. Complement is regulated by extrinsic inhibitors (C1 inhibitors) and by the intrinsic short half-life of the activated components. The absence of C1 esterase inhibitor is the cause of the disease, angioedema.

Deficiency of one or more components of complement (in the classic pathway all except C1a, C15 and C9) occurs in association with a number of disease processes (*e.g.,* systemic lupus erythemato-

sus). Lack of C3b inactivator is found in patients with recurrent pyogenic bacterial infection. Deficiency of C1 inhibitor is associated with hereditary angioneurotic edema. Some of these deficiencies are heritable.

C-REACTIVE PROTEIN (CRP)

Found in small quantities in normal serum, this beta globulin, which is not an antibody, is evoked in response to almost any acute inflammatory reaction (viral or bacterial infection, rheumatic fever). In these cases, increased serum levels of CRP have the same significance as other "acute phase reactants," for example, ESR. CRP in human serum is measured by immunoprecipitation with rabbit antibody to CRP, and the strength of the reaction is graded from 1+ to 4+; CIE and ELISA can also be used. CRP binds to phosphocholine determinants in C polysaccharide (group-specific pneumococcal antigen) thereby activating complement and enhancing phagocytosis. (See discussion of *Streptococcus pneumoniae*, previously).

Cells of the Immune Response

It is apparent that an individual has a diverse number of both T and B lymphocytes that are capable of recognizing a large number of antigenic determinants. In a modification of Burnet's original theory, Jerne has proposed that each cell has a limited number of genes that code for appropriate allotransplantation antigens including (one's own) antigens (germ line theory). Because we cannot tolerate cells that

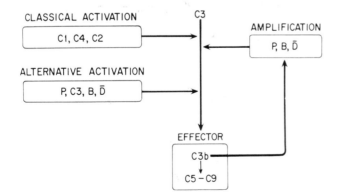

Fig. 5-5. Segregation of the complement proteins into four functional units: two pathways for initial cleavage of C3, the classic and alternative, the C3b-dependent amplification pathway for augmentation of C3 cleavage, and the effector sequence, from which are derived most of the biologic activities of the complement system. (Austen KF: The classical and alternative complement sequence. In Benacerraf B, Unanue ER: Textbook of Immunology. Baltimore, Williams & Wilkins, 1979)

would recognize our own antigens, these cells are suppressed as they appear by the overwhelming amount of our own antigens (immunologic tolerance). Diversification for recognition of all foreign antigens may come from somatic mutation of these cells so that mutant genes code for a variety of new antigenic determinants (somatic mutation theory). The combination of the two theories seems best to fit the evidence of immunologic tolerance, strong graft rejection, and that fact that cells are available that recognize synthetic antigens not involved in evolution. (This is considered to be an extreme oversimplification.) The interaction of a cell with its specific antigen leads to blastogenesis and replication (clonal expansion).

As indicated earlier, the specific immune re-sponse is mediated by lymphoid cells of two basic types, B and T lymphocytes. Precursor, immuno-logically uncommitted lymphocytes of both types originate from bone marrow stem cells (precursor stem cells, PSC) and migrate to either of two pri-mary lymphoid organs (Fig. 5-7). For B cells, the primary organ in mammalian species is the bone marrow and diffuse lymphoid structures of the gut (*i.e.*, Peyer's patches, appendix), which are func-tionally analogous to the bursa of Fabricius in avian species. In this microenvironment, lymphocytes are influenced to differentiate into immunologically competent B cells. In the earliest stage at which B cells can be recognized as such (pre-B cells), Ig is found in the cytoplasm. IgM then appears in the membrane and is soon joined by IgD. B lympho-

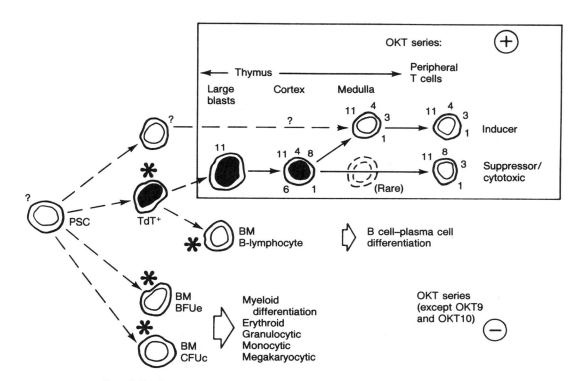

Fig. 5-7. The reactivity of OKT reagents and other corresponding monoclonal antibodies in relation to differentiation of blood cells. OKT1, 3, 4, 8, and 11 are restricted to T lineage cells. All identifiable bone marrow precursor cells tested (indicated by asterisks), and presumably also the human pluripotential stem cell (PSC), which cannot be tested *in vitro*, are unreactive with these reagents. The differentiation pathways are still hypothetical. (*BM*, bone marrow; *BFUe*, erythroid burst-forming unit *in vitro*; *CFUc*, granulocytic-monocytic colony-forming unit *in vitro*: *TdT*, terminal deoxynucleotidyl transferase present in the nucleus of pu-tative lymphoid precursors of BM and immature thymocytes [shown by black nucleus]) (Janossy G, Goldstein G, Cosimi AB: Monoclonal anti-human lymphocyte antibodies: Their potential value in immunosup-pression and bone marrow transplantation, Chap 4. In McMichael AJ, Fabre JW (eds): Monoclonal Antibodies in Clinical Medicine. New York, Academic Press, 1983)

cytes migrate to populate the secondary lymphoid tissue: germinal centers in lymph nodes and spleen, and more mature B cells then appear with surface Ig markers of single or multiple isotypes. IgG-producing cells may be derived from IgM-producing cells by a switch in genetic control of heavy-chain synthesis. Immature B cells without cytoplasmic IgM bear surface IgM and IgD markers. On stimulation by antigen recognized by the IgM, IgD is turned off, and these cells differentiate further into plasma cells, which synthesize any of the four classes of immunoglobulin, each cell producing a single class of antibody. "Memory" B cells bear surface Ig of the same class and differentiate to plasma cells on encountering homologous antigen. The class of immunoglobulin synthesized depends on the state of ontogeny, and the specificity of immunoglobulin

(variable region) is determined during exposure of the stem cell to the conditioning microenvironment (bursal equivalent).

The thymus gland is the other primary lymphoid organ serving as the microenvironment in which precursor stem cells differentiate into thymus-dependent lymphocytes, or T cells. The several subpopulations of T lymphocytes are identified by reactivity of surface markers with highly specific monoclonal antibodies (OKT series) and terminal deoxy-nucleotidyl transferase (TdT) (Fig. 5-8). Thymocytes differentiate into mature lymphocytes that have various biologic functions (T inducer/helper, T_i or T_h; T cytotoxic/suppressor, T_c; T delayed-type hypersensitivity, T_{dth}) and that populate the deep cortex of lymph nodes, and the periarterial sheaths of the spleen. T cells make up the major

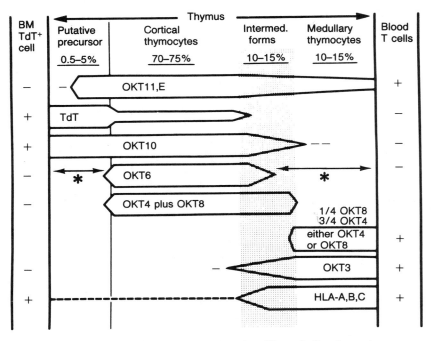

Fig. 5-8. Scheme of human lymphocyte differentiation based on reactions of monoclonal antibodies with membrane antigens and terminal deoxynucleotidyl transferase activity. Positivity of reactions among the cell populations is shown by horizontal bars; dotted lines indicate barely detectable or very weak positivity of a few cells. OKT6+ cells simultaneously express both OKT4 and OKT8, whereas OKT6− cells (asterisks) are heterogeneous; putative precursors are large TdT+ blasts (OKT11+, 10+) resembling bone marrow TdT+ cells (which are also OKT10+); medullary thymocytes have already been segregated into inducer/helper (OKT4+, OKT8−; majority) and suppressor/cytotoxic (OKT8+, OKT4−; minority) cell types. A number of forms (stippled area) are identifiable, which are intermediate between cortical and medullary thymocytes. (Data from Tidman N, Janossy G, Bodger M, et al: Clin Exp Immunol 45:437–467, 1981.) (Goldstein G, Lifter J, Mittler R: Immunoregulatory changes in human disease detected by monoclonal antibodies to T lymphocytes, Chap 3. In McMichael AJ, Fabre JW (eds): Monoclonal Antibodies in Clinical Medicine. New York, Academic Press, 1982)

cellular component of the lymph and are the most numerous lymphocyte normally found in the blood. T lymphocytes also have class I HLA antigens, an important fact in recognition of antigen by T_c cells. The normal ratio of T_h (OKT4+) to T_c (OKT8+) is about 2. The receptor on T_c cells for antigen and MHC is a heterodimeric structure (m.w. 90,000) deduced from cDNA sequences, comprising two glycosylated chains, alpha and beta, each with two extracellular Ig-like domains, an amino-terminal variable domain and a carboxy-terminal constant domain. Each of these domains is stabilized by an S–S bond between cysteine residues, and the two chains are held together by a single interchain S–S bond located close to the outer cellular membrane, in which the protein is anchored by one hydrophobic transmembranal peptide in each chain. The alpha chain may recognize primarily HLA molecules; the beta chain may react primarily with foreign antigens. Stimulation of T lymphocytes by specifically recognized antigen (or other mitogen) results in blastogenesis and elaboration of soluble factors (lymphokines), which modulate various aspects of the immune response, particularly interaction with B lymphocytes.

For many years it was thought that these factors were only specific to T lymphocytes; but now it appears that these "B-cell factors" influence a wide variety of cells. The original division was into two functional groups of B-cell growth factors (BCGF), involved in B-cell proliferation from early precursor B cells and B-cell differentiation factors (BCDF), needed for maturation of activated B cells into Ig-secreting cells. These factors are now renamed interleukins-4 through 6, and in some cases (IL-4) can have both BCGF and BCDF activities. These, as well as other lymphokines (IL-1 through 3 and γ-IFN), which were originally thought to work on target cells other than B cells, are all known to modulate B-cell functions at different developmental stages.

As noted above, the initial step in B-cell proliferation involves primary interaction of antigen with specific receptors on T lymphocytes; the lymphokines are wholly nonspecific with respect to antigen. These important lymphokines include gamma IFN, chemotactic factor, T-cell growth factor (interleukin 2), and macrophage inhibitory/activating factor (MIF/MAF). Interleukin 1 (Il 1) (previously known as lymphocyte-activating factor) is a protein (monokine) released by monocyte-macrophages undergoing an immune response. As indicated, IL 1 has a wide range of biological activities, all previously recognized on a functional basis, but now known to be due to this one macromolecule. IL 1

stimulates T cells, regulates B-lymphocyte differentiation (see below), controls growth of bone marrow cells and effects generation of cytotoxic T lymphocytes. Some of these properties are doubtless interconnected with release of IL 2 from T_h cells. IL 1 may be identical to macrophage endogenous pyrogen because *in vivo* it causes fever and an increase in circulating neutrophils and stimulates release of acute-phase reactants by liver cells, and *in vitro* IL 1 stimulates release of prostaglandin and collagenase from synovial cells as well as the growth of fibroblasts. There is evidence that symptoms of TSS appearing in connection with staphylococcal infection may be due to release of IL 1 in large quantities from cells of the immune system stimulated by staphylococcal "toxic shock protein" (see TSSE in section on TSS).

IL-1 is reactive to B-cell lymphocytes at two stages; the pre-B cell and activated mature B cell. IL-2, enhanced by IFN-γ in addition to its role in stimulating Th cells, also now appears to influence activated B cells. Considering the currently discovered pleiotropic nature of these as well as the other lymphokines, homeostasis likely will involve the multiple effects of these factors on other than hemopoietic cells.

The Major Histocompatibility Complex

The genetic control of graft rejection resides on the sixth chromosome in a complex of closely linked genes that is now called the major histocompatibility complex (HMC) (Fig. 5-9) coding for human leukocyte antigens (HLA). The known allelic forms for each locus in this extremely polymorphic system number at least 20 each for HLA-A, B and D, and 8

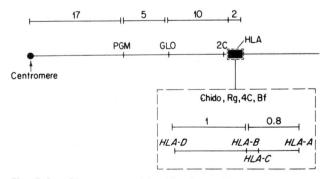

Fig. 5-9. Chromosomal localization of the human major histocompatibility complex (MHC). (Benacerraf B, Unanue ER: Transplantation immunology. In Benacerraf B, Unanue ER (eds): Textbook of Immunology. Baltimore, Williams & Wilkins, 1979)

for HLA-C. These genes are autosomal as well as codominant and segregate in progeny with one set of linked (on the same chromosome) alleles (haplotype) from each parent. HLA antigens resulting from class I genes (A, B, and C loci) are found on cells in every body tissue except brain. Products of class II genes (D and D-related, DR) are restricted to B lymphocytes, macrophages, sperm, epithelial, and myeloid precursor cells, and are collectively known as "Ia-like" antigens (*i.e.*, like murine B-cell antigens, referred to as Ia). HLA-A, B, and C locus antigens are detected by reacting alloantiserum (usually from multiparous women) with peripheral blood lymphocytes in the presence of complement. HLA-D and DR antigens are detected by mixing peripheral blood lymphocytes of one individual (containing some B lymphocytes) with those of another (mixed lymphocyte reaction). Differences at the HLA-D locus on stimulator B lymphocytes cause blastogenesis of responder T-"helper" lymphocytes. If the HLA-A, B, and C locus antigens are also different, responder T "cytotoxic" lymphocytes are induced that will lyse target cells bearing the same HLA-A, B, or C antigens as the stimulator cells. The induction of cytotoxic T lymphocytes is greater if HLA-D locus disparity occurs and T-"helper" lymphocytes are produced. These *in vitro* processes are the basis of primary graft rejection. The MHC also contains genes controlling B factor, the fourth component of complement (Bf,C4), certain "private" blood-group factors (*e.g.*, Chido, Roger) related to C4, immune response (Ir) genes (*e.g.*, ragweed atopic IgE antibody), and others.

The products of HLA-A,B and C genes consist of a transmembranal 44,000-dalton glycoprotein that binds noncovalently to beta-2-microglobulin. Products of the DR gene consist of a 34,000-dalton alpha-chain and 29,000-dalton beta-chain noncovalently bound to each other and inserted into the membrane with cytoplasmic carboxyl terminal ends. In both classes of antigen, alloantigenic specificity is contained in noncarbohydrate areas of the molecule, and not in the beta-2-microglobulin, which is the same in all members of a species.

Important linkage exists between disease states and specific HLA-B and HLA-D phenotypes. Some of the strongest linkage occurs between the allele HLA-B27 and ankylosing spondylitis, Reiter's syndrome and acute anterior uveitis. *Salmonella* and *Yersinia* enterocolitis, arthritis, and *Shigella* arthropathy have strong associations with HLA-B27. Several diseases have significant association with HLA-Dw3 including juvenile-onset diabetes, der-

matitis herpetiformis, and idiopathic Addison's disease. These strong associations are mostly limited to HLA-B and D loci (see Fig. 5-9), which may indicate the existence, in this area of the MHC, of numerous Ir genes controlling immune regulatory mechanisms.

Immunologic Tolerance

The acquired inability of an individual to express an immune response to a molecule that would normally evoke active cell-mediated or humoral responses is called "tolerance" or "immunologic unresponsiveness."

1. Antigens that stimulate an immune response in adults can induce a state of tolerance in newborns with undeveloped immunologic competence. In 1945, Owen observed that during fetal life of dizygotic (heterozygous) twin calves, blood and erythrocytes of each fetus circulated freely in both and, though nonself (foreign), were tolerated throughout adult life as if they were "self" (native); each twin was an erythrocyte chimera. This exemplifies permanent, antigen-specific immunologic tolerance under natural conditions. The studies of Burnet and Medawar extended Owen's work. They injected viable spleen cells of one strain of mice (A) into neonates of another strain of mice (B), thus artificially inducing in adult (B) mice complete, permanent and strain-specific immunologic tolerance to skin grafts from adult (A) mice.

2. T-*in*dependent antigens in extremely large doses can induce a state of "paralysis" or tolerance in an individual. Pneumococcal polysaccharide at 10 to 100 times the immunizing dose induces tolerance in animals. Challenge with immunizing doses does not induce an immunologic response. Because pneumococcal polysaccharide is a T-independent antigen, the tolerance is probably due to B-cell unresponsiveness.

3. T-dependent foreign protein antigens can be tolerogenic under the following circumstances: if the host is newborn or an immunosuppressed adult; if very low or very high doses of a low-molecular-weight molecule in soluble, monomeric physical form are used; if introduction is by the intravenous route; and if antigen is inherently a weak immunogen in its native form. High doses of antigen probably involve tolerance by both B and T cells. Low-dose toler-

ance apparently involves T-suppressor-cell induction in the absence of a response by T helper or B cells, which effectively prevents the induction of an immune response by excessive negative regulation.

4. Tolerance can be induced to new antigens if they are bound to the surface of the host's own cells. It has been demonstrated that haptens or glycoproteins covalently bound to the surface of autologous cells, when reintroduced into the host, can induce a state of functional tolerance with respect to the induction of the humoral response. T-suppressor-cell induction evidently is the main reason for unresponsiveness in this case, although T-helper tolerance may be involved under certain conditions.

Immunosuppression

This may be produced by various immunosuppressive measures, several of which are used in connection with organ "transplants" because there is as yet no generally acceptable and feasible means of inducing antigen-specific immunologic unresponsiveness to allografts. In general, they suppress proliferation and remove or destroy all clones of T and B lymphocytes nonspecifically and indiscriminately. Most of these measures have undesirable, often dangerous, side effects and also greatly enhance vulnerability to infection:

1. Whole body x-irradiation may be made specific under certain conditions and depends on injury to macrophages rather than to small lymphocytes.
2. Cannulization of the thoracic duct for mechanical removal of lymphocytes.
3. Beta-irradiation of blood; destruction of lymphocytes only.
4. Potent, equine, cytolytic, antihuman-lymphocyte globulins (ALG), especially in conjunction with thymectomy to delay regeneration of all antibody-producing lymphoid cells.
5. Drugs such as azathioprine, prednisone (and other corticosteroids), and cyclophosphamide.

Immunodeficiencies and Gammopathies

HUMAN IMMUNODEFICIENCY DISEASES

These are rare diseases, occurring at frequencies of 0.05% to 0.2%. The primary specific immunodeficiency diseases result from an absence or lack of maturation of T and/or B cells. A known familial predisposition or history of recurrent infections is a first sign that there may be an immunodeficiency. Upon further examination one finds for **B-cell defects** that there is low serum immunoglobulin present and no seroconversion to vaccines. For **T-cell defects** there is a reduced response to skin antigens and reduced response to viral or fungal infections as well as certain bacterial pathogens, such as *Mycobacteria tuberculosis*. A complete list of lymphocytic defects is shown in Table 5-16.

B-cell Deficiencies. An example is **X-linked agammaglobulinemia** (congenital agammaglobulinemia, Bruton's disease). There is a family history of brothers or maternal male relatives with recurring infections. Infants generally present with infections caused by encapsulated, pyogenic bacteria at 5 to 6 months of age: often pneumonia, otitis media, dermatitis, or meningitis-type diseases. Affected males have no B lymphocytes, no detectable IgM, IgA, IgD, IgE, and only 10% of normal IgG, as well as no response to immunization. There is little development of lymph-node germinal centers, and tonsils are abnormally small. These individuals do have a normal cell-mediated response with respect to delayed-type hypersensitivity and allograft rejection. Patients can be treated with gamma globulin. With increased age, patients are at increased risk of developing neoplasias and chronic sinopulmonary disease (due to lack of secretory IgA). The cause of the defect is not certain. Pre-B cells are present with cytoplasmic μ chains, but there is a severe decrease in the number of mature B cells possessing surface immunoglobulin. This suggests that there is a block in differentiation after B cells have undergone Ig heavy chain rearrangement, but before light chain expression.

Two other examples of B cell deficiencies showing reduced Ig levels are **transient hypogammaglobulinemia** and **selective IgA deficiency.** The former is similar to Bruton's disease in onset and features. However, in this disease patients who survive gradually develop significant antibody responses. In selective IgA deficiency, patients have reduced serum and secretory IgA levels but normal IgG, IgM, and cell-mediated immunity. This is the most common (1 : 500) immunodeficiency disorder known. Many individuals do not have overt disease and are healthy; others experience frequent respiratory infections or recurrent bronchitis and enteropathy. No IgA-producing plasma cells are found in the lamina propria, yet about 40% of patients have circulating anti-IgA Ab.

T-cell Deficiencies. An example is **congenital thymic aplasia** (DiGeorge syndrome). Thymic aplasia results from a congenital defect and is not hered-

TABLE 5-16. Lymphocyte Defects and Genetic Aspects of Selected Primary Immunodeficiency Syndromes

	AFFECTED LYMPHOCYTE POPULATIONS				
	T Cells		B cells		**MODE OF**
DISORDER	**STAGE 1***	**STAGE 2***	**STAGE 1**	**STAGE 2**	**INHERITANCE**
B-Cell Deficiencies					
Congenital hypogammaglobulinemia (Bruton type)	No	No	Yes	Yes§	X-linked
Congenital hypogammaglobulinemia	No	No	Yes	Yes	Autosomal recessive
Common variable immunodeficiency	No	(No)	No	Yes§	? Autosomal recessive
IgA deficiency	No	(No)	No	No§	Variable
IgM deficiency	No	No	No	?	Unknown
IgG subclass deficiency	No	No	No	?	X-linked
Immunodeficiency with elevated IgM	No	No	No	(Yes)	X-linked
X-linked immunodeficiency with normal globulin count or hyperglobulinemia	No	No	(No)	(Yes)	X-linked
Hypogammaglobulinemia with thymoma	No	No	No	Yes§	Unknown
T-Cell Deficiencies					
Thymus hypoplasia Nezelof's syndrome	Yes	Yes	(No)	(No)	Variable
DiGeorge syndrome	Yes	Yes	No	No	Variable
Purine nucleoside phosphorylase deficiency	Yes	Yes	No	No	? Autosomal recessive
Chronic mucocutaneous candidiasis (CMC) with endo-crinopathy	No	Yes	No	No	? Autosomal recessive
Combined B and T Cell Deficiencies					
Reticular dysgenesis	Yes	Yes	Yes	Yes	Unknown
SCID† (thymic alymphoplasia)	Yes	Yes	(Yes)‡	(Yes)	X-linked
SCID (Swiss type)	Yes	Yes	(Yes)	(Yes)	Autosomal recessive
SCID with ADA deficiency	Yes	Yes	(Yes)	(Yes)	Autosomal recessive
SCID with ectodermal dysplasia and dwarfism	Yes	Yes	Yes	Yes	? Autosomal recessive
SCID (sporadic)	Yes	Yes	Yes	Yes	Unknown
Wiskott-Aldrich syndrome	Yes	Yes	No	(Yes)	X-linked
Ataxia-telangiectasia	(Yes)	Yes	No	(No)	Autosomal recessive

* Indicates first or second stages of lymphoid cell differentiation.

† SCID = severe combined immunodeficiency.

‡ Statements enclosed in parentheses indicate defects that are variable in severity or expression

§ Recent evidence indicates the presence of excessive suppressor cell activity.

itary. Most patients present with intractable hypocalcemia or severe cardiac disease in the first few weeks of life. A classic facial appearance of notched or folded ears, and a small fishlike mouth is present at birth or will develop later. These individuals have no T cells and hence no delayed-type hypersensitivity or allograft rejection capability. Germinal centers are normal with normal numbers of plasma cells in lymphoid tissue. Serum immunoglobulins are normal, the result most likely of T-independent antigen stimulation from infectious agents. The lack of a cell-mediated response makes these individuals susceptible to fatal infections with viruses (measles and chickenpox), fungi, and acid-fast bacilli.

Two other T-cell deficiencies are *Nezelof's syndrome* and *purine nucleoside phosphorylase deficiency.* In the former a patient will have both a hypoplastic thymus and impaired cell-mediated immunity. Serum levels of antibody may be near normal, but the requirement for B–T cooperation means that some humoral immune responses will also be depressed. A number of bacterial, as well as viral infections occur in these individuals. In purine nucleoside phosphorylase deficiency, there is a defect in conversion of inosine and guanosine to hypoxanthine and guanine. The accumulation of deoxyguanosine and dGTP is selectively toxic for T cells. Thus, although serum immunoglobulin levels may be near normal, the decreased cell-mediated responses lead to viral and fungal infections, as well as increased tumor incidence. *Chronic mucocutaneous candidiasis* (CMC) is yet another cellular immunodeficiency characterized by chronic *Candida* infections of the skin, nails, and mucous membrane. It represents a highly specific disorder of T-cell function, since T-cell numbers are normal. Since these patients have antibodies that react with various endocrine tissues, this suggests that there is an autoimmune nature to the disease. Treatment involves use of ketoconazole as the drug of choice.

Combined B- and T-cell Deficiencies. An example is *severe combined immunodeficiency* (SCID) (Swiss-type agammaglobulinemia). This disease is characterized by a lack of both T and B lymphocytes. It is hereditary, being transmitted by X-linked or autosomal recessive genes. Individuals with SCID are agammaglobulinemic and are incapable of rejecting allografts or of developing delayed-type hypersensitivity. An absence of stem cells in the bone marrow is thought to be the cause of this disease. Without a bone marrow transplant, the disease is usually fatal. Thymopentin, a synthetic pentapeptide that corresponds to the active moiety of thymopoietin, has, in conjunction with bone marrow transplants, had limited success in treatment.

Adenosine Deaminase (ADA) Deficiency. About 50% of all individuals with this disease have acquired it as a sex-linked disorder. In the absence of the enzyme (which catalyzes conversion of adenosine to inosine) deoxyadenosine and dATP accumulate and are lethal to B and T cells, leading to a SCIDS-like condition. It is characterized by recurrent serious infections in infancy and bone abnormalities. If untreated, affected children die in early childhood. Transfusions with irradiated normal erythrocytes provide a source of enzyme and temporary improvement. Bone marrow transplants, if marrow from siblings or half-matched donors is used, is the preferred treatment. Most recently an experimental enzyme replacement therapy using the bovine ADA enzyme linked to polyethylene glycol (PEG) shows promise for patients who do not have bone marrow donors.

Other examples of combined immunodeficiencies are *ataxia–telangiectasia (AT)* and *Wiskott-Aldrich syndrome.* Both of these diseases are very rare, with AT having an incidence of 1:100,000. It is characterized by progressive cerebellar ataxia and oculocutaneous telangiectasia. The primary defect is one of DNA repair. At about 5 years of age, patients present with recurrent upper respiratory tract infections due to a depression in both humoral (IgA) and cell-mediated responses.

Wiskott-Aldrich Syndrome. This is an X-linked disorder characterized by thrombocytopenia with bleeding, eczema (in the first year), and immunodeficiency. Recurrent bacterial infection occurs leading to pneumonia and chronic otitis media, as well as viral (herpes family) and parasitic *(Pneumocystis carinii)* infections. Malignancy develops in more than 10% of patients. The mechanism of this disorder involves a defect in cell-mediated immunity and low IgM production. Poor response to polysaccharide (thymus-independent) antigens of pneumococci and cell membrane glycoprotein abnormalities suggest that the defect might involve the absence of specific glycoproteins on T-cell surfaces.

In addition to the primary immunodeficiencies described above, several secondary immunodeficiencies can result in severe recurrent infections. Among these are *chronic granulomatous disease* (CGD) and *Chediak-Higashi syndrome.* CGD is an X-linked recessive disease, characterized by a susceptibility in childhood to pyogenic infections by catalase-positive bacteria (*Staphylococcus aureus, Aerobacter aerogenes,* and enterobacteria) but not other bacteria, such as streptococci and pneumococci. This is because the latter provide the neutrophil with H_2O_2 (they are catalase-negative), which is then used to kill the microorganism, since myeloperoxidase can function normally in the neutrophil if it is provided with H_2O_2. The defect in this disease is both in neutrophil and macrophage phagocyte oxidative killing, apparently due to a deficiency of superoxide-forming enzymes (NADPH oxidase). In CGD bacterial infection leads to severe lesions that are slow to heal, followed by granuloma formation. The disease is often fatal, despite the use of antibiotics.

Chediak–Higashi syndrome is an autosomal recessive condition characterized by neutrophils and platelets with abnormally large lysosomes. There is an inability of neutrophils to kill both catalase-positive and negative bacteria (in contrast to CGD); chemotaxis in these lymphocytes is defective due to an inability to rearrange microfilaments. Bacterial infection and development of lymphoid neoplasms lead to an early death. Also, there are recurrent infections due to lowered phagocytic activity caused by a lack of opsonins (antibody or complement).

Acquired Immune Deficiency Syndrome (AIDS). Since 1981, this newly recognized syndrome has been encountered worldwide with increasing frequency, until at the present writing more than 76,000 cases with about 43,000 deaths have been reported in the United States, with the greatest concentrations in New York City, Los Angeles, San Francisco, and other major urban centers. What is even more frightening is the prospect that by the end of 1991, the Centers for Disease Control (CDC) project that there will be a cumulative 270,000 cases of clinical AIDS, with 179,000 persons having already died. The syndrome is characterized by lymphopenia and marked impairment of T-lymphocyte function due to profound depression in numbers of helper/inducer (Th, Ti, Leu3+, OKT4+) cells and consequent inversion of the ratio (normally about 1.7–2.0) of Th to cytotoxic/suppressor (Tc, Ts, Leu2+, OKT8+) cells. Clinically, there is generalized lymphadenopathy. A prodromal complex referred to as AIDS-related complex (ARC) may last many months and is characterized by fever, weight loss, leukopenia, and severe infection with opportunistic pathogens (bacterial, viral, fungal, parasitic). The most frequently fatal are *Pneumocystis carinii*, herpesviruses, cryptosporidium, *Cryptococcus, Toxoplasma gondii, Candida* (oral candidiasis may be a signal of impending AIDS), and various pyogenic bacteria. An unusual form of Kaposi's sarcoma (KS) with facial as well as lower trunk lesions is seen in AIDS patients. KS had only rarely been seen in North America or Europe but was known to occur endemically in equatorial Africa and among older Jewish men in some Mediterranean locales. Major groups at risk continue to be homosexual and bisexual men and intravenous drug users. Also, patients with hemophilia who rely on human blood products (Factor VIII) for survival are at high risk. Although a number of cases were caused by transfusions of whole blood prior to testing, the risk of contracting AIDS by this route is currently negligible. AIDS has also been documented in female sexual partners of AIDS patients, and in neonates born to IV drug users who were seropositive.

Asymptomatic virus-positive carriers continue to constitute a significant proportion of high-risk groups and are doubtless important in the dissemination of HIV through sexual contact. The mean interval between infection with HIV and the onset of AIDS is about 7 years for such high risk groups: homosexual and bisexual men, intravenous drug abusers, and hemophiliacs infected before the advent of serologic testing.

It appears that the overall prevalence of HIV antibody among Red Cross blood donors who have not previously been tested is about 0.04%. It is estimated that between 1 and 1.5 million Americans are infected with HIV. There is no evidence that the virus can be transmitted through casual contact; intimate sexual contact, sharing of contaminated needles, and transfusion of contaminated blood or blood products are the real hazards. Antibody to core protein (p24) declines late in infection. As noted earlier, AIDS-related complex (ARC) (lymphadenopathy, fever, weight loss) in which circulating immune complexes are prominent along with the aforementioned T-cell abnormalities, polyclonal hypergammaglobulinemia and autoantibodies, is a prodrome to the full-blown disease, capped by overwhelming opportunistic infections. A "wasting syndrome," characterized by weight loss and fatigue, but without recognized opportunistic infection or lymphadenopathy, is also seen. Non-Hodgkins' lymphoma, like KS, is a serious manifestation of AIDS and ARC in high-risk groups. As to the origin of HIV, current theory suggests that it may have appeared first in Africa (several thousand AIDS cases occur annually in Zaire alone) and thence have spread through migrant populations to Europe and the Caribbean area, and from the latter to the east and west coasts of the United States. Currently azidothymidine (AZT) is the drug used to prolong the life, albeit for only a relatively short period, of those AIDS patients who have *P. carinii* pneumonia. The drug appears specifically to block the HIV reverse transcriptase, but it also has side effects in damaging bone marrow cells. Other traditional drugs such as pentamidine are also used to treat *P. carinii*, until the occurrence of resistant organisms precludes its effectiveness.

Precautions to be taken by clinical and laboratory staffs should be as rigorous as those for hepatitis B. Any discussion of a vaccine for prevention of AIDS is premature, not only for ethical reasons, but also because of already evident variations among strains of HIV, which would pose significant problems. However, there may be some hope with several novel approaches. The most promising appears to be immunization with a form of the outer viral envelope glycoprotein gp120 obtained using recombinant DNA technology in one of several expression vector systems: *E. coli*, yeast, mammalian cells, or vaccinia virus. This is a reasonable approach, since AIDS patients uniformly possess antibodies against the *env* proteins at all stages of infection, whereas antibodies against other HIV proteins, such as *gag* diminish during the course of the disease. As noted, difficulties may arise with this vaccine, due to antigenic variation; however, there do appear to be a few regions on gp120, which are relatively constant. Also, vaccinia/AIDS recombinant viruses are currently being constructed to use as vaccines, since these viruses show evidence for shedding of gp120 from infected cells; if a variant gp120 arises, it can also be easily incorporated into the recombinant virus. Finally, another approach being tried is to synthesize peptides to constant regions of both gp120, as well as gp41 and utilize them in combination to elicit neutralizing antibodies. Studies are underway with all of these approaches in chimpanzees as well as, in some cases, human volunteers to test their efficacy.

GAMMOPATHIES

Gammopathies are the opposite of deficiencies, being characterized by the abnormal proliferation of cells involved in the humoral response. The result is that excessive amounts of immunoglobulin are produced. Table 5-17 shows the more important monoclonal gammopathies with their associated immunoglobulin classes.

Multiple Myeloma. This is a malignant proliferation of plasma cells with the following characteristics: cell-mass expansion; immunoglobulin protein elaboration; and the concomitant suppression of normal antibody synthesis. The whole immunoglobulin (M component) may be found in the serum with or without "free" light chains in the urine (Bence Jones proteins). The disease involves osteolytic lesions and pathologic fractures, anemia due to displacement of myeloid elements in the bone marrow by plasma cells, renal failure and nervous system involvement.

Macroglobulinemia (or Waldenström's Macroglobulinemia). This is characterized by the production of a homogeneous single immunoglobulin (IgM). Clinically, increased viscosity of the blood caused by large amounts of IgM results in thrombosis and bleeding (petechiae) in the skin, nasal mucosa, and gastrointestinal tract. Retinal hemorrhages may eventually cause blindness.

"Heavy Chain Disease". This was first described as being caused by the elaboration of a protein (55,000 daltons) apparently consisting of an incomplete IgG heavy chain and having the antigenic determinants of IgG, but no detectable light chains. Subsequently, IgA and IgM heavy chain diseases have been described. The syndrome is characterized clinically by frequent infections due to impairment of antibody production.

Allergy and Hypersensitivity

Allergy (Gr. allos, changed; ergon, action) or hypersensitivity is an altered state of reactivity of cells and tissues manifest through specific pathogenic immune reactions occurring in vivo (Table 5-18). Most of the manifestations of hypersensitivity are now explicable in terms of molecular and cellular interactions. The principal mechanisms underlying the clinical manifestations of allergy can be grouped conveniently under four principal headings.

Type I: anaphylactic atopic allergy, entirely mediated by IgE

Type II: cytotoxic type, dependent on antibody and complement

Type III: immune complex disease (serum sickness)

Type IV: cell-mediated immune reactions

Types I, II and III are all referred to as "immediate hypersensitivity," being mediated by specific antibody. Type IV hypersensitivity is essentially independent of antibody, all reactions being mediated by specifically sensitized T lymphocytes. Types I and IV are independent of complement. It will be evident that more than one of the four types may be operating in a given clinical situation. Moreover, implicit in each type of hypersensitive manifestation is a first experience with a given set of antigens constituting the primary immunization or sensitization. Subsequent exposure to the same or related sets of antigens evokes tissue reaction(s) in the previously "sensitized" host. The manner and route of primary sensitization are not always evident and may be respiratory (*e.g.,* hay fever), contact (poison ivy), or oral (food allergies). Atopic persons are those who inherit (MHC) a tendency to become allergic very easily to many different antigens by synthesizing abnormally high levels of IgE.

TYPE I HYPERSENSITIVITY

"Immediate"-type hypersensitivity refers to atopic allergy, manifested by a rapidly developing (minutes) wheal and flare (hives, urticaria) reaction in the skin in response to the intradermal injection of specific antigen(s), exemplified by hay fever (*e.g.,* ragweed allergy). There is no perceptible local cytotoxicity or leukocytic response. The same antigen given systemically (usually inadvertently) causes anaphylactic shock. IgE formed in response to primary (sensitizing) immune responses attaches, by the Fc portion, to specific Fc receptors on mast cells, basophils, and platelets, that is, become tissue-fixed and remain *in situ* for months or years. Reactions of homologous antigens with this fixed antibody trigger transmembranally the release of the vasoactive amines responsible for all of the manifestations of "immediate" hypersensitivity,

TABLE 5-17. Monoclonal Gammopathies

DISORDER	CLASS OF PROTEIN	LIGHT CHAIN
Multiple myeloma	IgG, IgA, IgD or IgE	κ or λ
Macroglobulinemia	IgM	κ or λ
Heavy-chain disease	IgG, IgA or IgM	None

TABLE 5-18. Hypersensitivity: Pathogenic Immune Reactions *in Vivo*

DESIGNATION, TYPE*	ROUTE OF PRIMARY ANTIGENIC STIMULATION	SPECIFICITY	SKIN TEST	CLINICAL EXAMPLES	MECHANISM	PREVENTION
I. Anaphylactic, "immediate"	Respiratory GI tract Subcutaneous	IgE (reaginic antibody; distinguish from Wassermann ab)	(Intradermal) "Immediate" wheal/flare sec.–min. Transferable with serum	Allergic rhinitis (hay fever); insect venom sensitivity (phospholipase A) DRUGS (e.g., penicillin). Hives (urticaria), asthma	Histamine SRS-A, ECF-A from sensitized mast cells, basophils, ?platelets. No tissue damage	"Blocking" IgG
II. Cytotoxic, ADCC	Parenteral, Infection, Drugs as haptens, Altered "self"	IgM, IgG (systemic)	(Systemic reaction, transferable with serum)	Transfusion reactions Hemolytic disease of the newborn (HDN) Hemolytic anemia (DRUGS) Viral infection (ADCC) Autoimmune diseases Thrombocytopenic purpura	C ("immune") lysis of sensitized cells (rbc, platelets) (tissue damage) Destruction of sensitized virus-infected cells by T_c lymphocytes (MHC restriction)	HDN: Rhogam prophylaxis against primary sensitization (not desensitization)
III. Antigen–Antibody complex disease, "Serum sickness"	Foreign protein, parenteral, infection	IgG, IgM ("Gatekeeper" IgE)	Arthus type (experimental passive)	Poststreptococcal AGN Rheumatoid arthritis SLE, hepatitis B Drugs, infections	Deposition of Ag/Ab/C in tissues evokes acute inflammatory reaction (pmn, platelets) Tissue damage	None specific
IV. "Delayed," tuberculin type, CMI	Persistent chronic intracellular infection (bacterial, fungal, viral, protozoal) Tumors Tissue grafts	T lymphocytes	(Intradermal) "Delayed" tuberculin type (PPD) 24–48 hours	Tuberculosis, other bacterial infections All mycoses, some viruses Contact dermatitis (e.g., drugs, poison ivy) Tumor and graft rejection	T lymphocytes specifically stimulated to release lymphokines (nonspecific) Transfer factor (specific) Tissue damage	None

*Types I, II, and III are all referred to as *Immediate-type hypersensitivity*, and all are mediated by specific antibody. Type IV is essentially independent of antibody, and all reactions are mediated by specifically sensitized T lymphocytes.

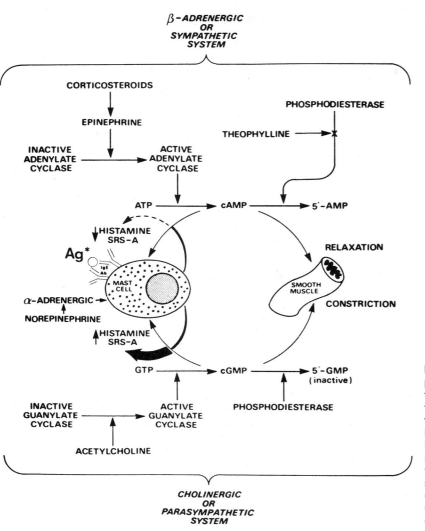

Fig. 5-10. The balance theory of sympathetic and parasympathetic regulation, indicating points of pharmacotherapeutic attack. (* Union of antigen with cell-fixed IgE antibody can be blocked by reaction with homologous IgG [blocking] antibody produced in response to "desensitization.") (Modified from Frick OL: Immediate hypersensitivity. In Fudenberg HH, Sites DP, Caldwell JL, Wells JV (eds): Basic and Clinical Immunology, 2nd ed. Los Altos, CA, Lange Medical Publications, 1978)

namely, histamine, bradykinin, slow-reacting-substance of allergy (SRS-A), all of which cause smooth-muscle contraction, vasodilatation, and increased capillary permeability. Increased coagulation time is due to heparin released from mast cells. Liver damage occurs, and cartilage and collagen tissues are affected. Edema and smooth-muscle contractions in large blood vessels, air passages, and elsewhere are frequently the immediate cause of death. Commonly, the active substances are quickly decomposed in the body and the manifestations of immediate allergy are therefore short-lived (2 to 48 hours). Fatal anaphylaxis, which is not unusual, can result from bee stings or from injection of avianized vaccines and antibiotics (especially penicillin), particularly in an atopic individual. Histamine release is under the control of AMP. Falling levels (blockade of adenylcyclase) promote hista-

mine release; promotion of cAMP synthesis by increased adenylcyclase activity (stimulated by epinephrine) reduces histamine release. Xanthines (used in therapy of type I hypersensitivity) block phosphodiesterase, which is responsible for the destruction of cAMP. Eosinophil-chemotactic factor A (ECF-A) is among the products released by basophil–mas cell activation. Eosinophils secrete their granular enzyme (arylsulfatase), which splits SRS-A, providing a feedback control mechanism. These reactions are summarized in Figure 5-10.

TYPE II HYPERSENSITIVITY

This type usually results from the cytotoxic or cytolytic action of complement on cells (tissue cells, erythrocytes) to which specific antibodies to cellular components (*e.g.,* blood group antigens) have attached. These cells are said to be "sensitized" to immune lysis, which is the mechanism underlying hemolytic disease of the newborn (HDN) (q.v.) and incompatible transfusion reactions. Some drugs (*e.g.*, Sedormid, penicillin) bind to tissue proteins and thereby become antigenic, the resulting antibody being specific for the drug (hapten). The same or related drugs adsorbed nonspecifically to cells make them the target for cytotoxic antibody (hemolytic anemia, thrombocytopenic purpura).

TYPE III HYPERSENSITIVITY

The term *"serum sickness"* refers to the older observation of anaphylactic and immediate allergic manifestations in persons receiving foreign serum therapeutically (*e.g.*, diphtheria antitoxin as horse serum). The term as now used connotes type I or III allergy caused by any foreign antigenic substances, which may include low-molecular-weight compounds (haptens) bound in the circulation to serum or to tissue proteins to become complete antigens. Classically, "serum sickness"-type hypersensitivity (type III) in a previously unsensitized individual follows 7 to 10 days after systemic injection of foreign antigen, that is, the period necessary to mount a primary antibody response. At a critical level of antigen, enough excess antigen–antibody complexes (IgM, IgG) are found deposited in the tissues, especially in the renal glomerular basement membrane, to cause accretion of complement and initiation of the complement cascade and inflammatory response, accompanied by release of anaphylatoxins (C3b, C5b), which activate directly (degranulate) basophils and mast cells to release vasoactive amines. Some IgE is inevitably formed in this primary immune response. This IgE sensitizes mast cells and basophils to react with circulating antigen with the same result. At its peak, serum sickness is a constellation of reactions resulting from the relatively protracted systemic release of vasoactive amines. Symptoms and signs subside as antibody appears in excess. Anaphylactic shock occurs in a person already sensitized (*e.g.*, to penicillin) who may or may not have had clinically evident serum sickness but in whom all basophils and mast cells have previously been sensitized (*i.e.*, IgE antibody may remain attached to basophils and mast cells for years following primary sensitization with the offending antigen). The sudden union of massive amounts of antigen with widely scattered sensitized mast cells effectively provides a sudden large systemic charge of histamine, with all of its consequences.

DESENSITIZATION

A severe immediate-type allergic reaction may be avoided in foreign serum injections (e.g., equine diphtherial antitoxin) if desensitization is carried out. This consists of a series of minute (0.001 to 0.01 ml) subcutaneous doses of the serum given at intervals of half an hour for several hours before the main dose. This, in effect, gradually saturates all IgE antibody already attached to mast cells, thus blocking access by antigen subsequently administered in therapeutic amounts. However, new IgE antibody eventually is formed and perpetuates the state of hypersensitivity so that there can be no permanent amelioration of the atopic state. By the subcutaneous administration of carefully graded doses of antigen (active desensitization), sufficient IgG and IgA antibody can be produced to compete with antigen for fixed IgE antibody and thereby prevent or reduce the triggering of histamine release (e.g., prophylactic treatment of hay fever allergy during the "off" season) (see Fig. 5-10).

Cell-Mediated Immune Response (CMIR) and Delayed Hypersensitivity

In the CMIR, "afferent" and "efferent" limbs serve, respectively, to bring the antigen(s) into the immunologic mechanism and to mediate the responses. When exposed to antigen processed by macrophages, a proportion of T lymphocytes in the afferent limb becomes sensitized, that is, has the potential to activate the efferent limb of the CMIR when reexposed to the same antigen. Antigens involved in the CMIR include certain microorganisms (*Mycobacteria, Listeria, Brucella, Chlamydia,* fungi, viruses) and tumor and transplantation cell-surface antigens; and simple chemicals (contact hypersensitivity). In the efferent limb of the CMIR, sensitized T lymphocytes reexposed to the sensitizing antigen may undergo blast transformation and then proliferate. The subsequent progeny of sensitized lymphocytes produce a variety of lymphokines that mediate the associated inflammatory response. The lymphokines themselves are nonspecific with respect to antigen, in contrast to antibody, which is antigen specific. These lymphokines include chemotactic factor, which attracts monocytes and macrophages to the scene of action, migration inhibition factor (MIF) and macrophage-activating factor (MAF), which hold and "activate" macrophages in the area, and lymphablastogenic factor, which stimulates nonspecifically other lymphocytes in the area to undergo blast transformation. The release of lymphokines from stimulated T lymphocytes is extremely important in "activating" macrophages toward enhanced microbicidal activity with those organisms resistant to intracellular killing (*i.e., M. tuberculosis*). Some of these specifically sensitized lymphocytes become long-term "memory" cells that circulate in blood and lymph, retaining reactivity for years. Sensitized T lymphocytes (T cytotoxic) exposed to the appropriate antigen may also produce certain lymphokines (*e.g., MIF or interferon*) without undergoing transformation or proliferation. These nontransforming cells may lyse target cells that have an appropriate antigen on their surface (*e.g., viral, transplantation*).

The prototypic "delayed" type CMIR is the positive reaction to the injection of tuberculin in patients or animals affected with *M. tuberculosis*. In response to the injection of antigen, there is an accumulation of T cells at the site of injection during the ensuing 24 to 48 hours, resulting in the formation of a palpable area of induration. This is in contrast to the "immediate" wheal and flare reaction caused by histamine release (type I) from IgE-sensitized tissue mast cells or basophils that follows within seconds or minutes the exposure to antigen. The tuberculin (type IV) CMIR accounts for the predominantly round-cell histologic appearance of tuberculous and other chronic infectious lesions (*e.g., mycoses*). Contact hypersensitivity results from constant exposure of the skin to simple chemicals or heavy metals. These materials form antigenic complexes with host proteins that evoke a delayed hypersensitivity reaction whenever the host is exposed to the chemical or metal.

IMMUNOHEMATOLOGY

Human erythrocytes (rbc) have at their surfaces a variety of genetically determined and usually dominant antigens (alloantigens, isoantigens, Table 5-19). Among the many clinically important rbc antigens are those discovered by Landsteiner in 1902 and called A and B. Numerous others (*e.g.*, A_1) have been discovered since. The A and B antigens are enzymically formed from a precursor antigenic substance that is cross-reactive with type XIV pneumococcal polysaccharide (SXIV). The basic antigenic structure is contained in a branched oligosaccharide. Addition of fucose to both branches confers H (heterogenetic) specificity. Addition of *N*-acetylgalactosamine (Gal-Nac) to the terminal galactose (Gal) of both branches confers A_1 specific-

ity. Addition of Gal only to the terminal Gal of branch II confers A_2 specificity. Alternatively, an additional Gal at the end of both branches confers B specificity (see diagram in Table 5-19). Inheritance of glycosyl transferases provides the basis for phenotypic expression of blood-group antigens. In the absence of A or B genes, H remains an unaltered antigen. Persons having both A and A_1 antigens are assigned to blood group A; those with A antigen only, to group A_2; those with B antigen, to group B; those with A, A_1 and B, to group AB; those with A and B antigens but not A_1, to group A_2B; those without A, A_1, or B but with H antigen, to group O (*i.e.*, cells are inagglutinable by anti-A or anti-B).

Rarely, persons originally found in Bombay, India, have none of the above antigens; they are assigned to the Bombay or Oh group. For preliminary and routine clinical purposes only the major groups of the ABO systems are determined, commonly by direct slide agglutination tests.

A or B antibodies (generally IgG) are continuously evoked by contact with specific A- or B-specific oligosaccharides from foods, and microorganisms and may be actively induced by transfusion with blood of the opposite group (A versus B; B versus A) or, in some cases, by pregnancy with a fetus of the opposite (incompatible) group.

Subdivisions (A_1, A_2, A_1B, A_2B and others) within each group account for unexpected occurrence of transfusion reactions. With specially prepared, adsorbed, monovalent sera containing *agglutinins* against group A or against group B erythrocytes, all four major groups may be identified.

In addition to A, B, and H antigens there are a score or more of other blood-group antigenic systems, some common, some very rare, all genetically and independently determined: Duffy, Kell, P, Kidd, Lutheran MNSs. Though occasionally involved in transfusion reactions and certain other conditions, most are of more importance in resolving problems of paternity and in genetic studies. The Lewis (a and b) antigens, when present, are found in plasma and in the saliva of secretors (SeSe, Sese) and are adsorbed to erythrocytes without contributing to the structure of the cell membrane.

Antigens of the ABO(H) system occur in soluble form in sputum, colostrum, secretions of the gastrointestinal tract, semen, tears, and sweat. They appear there in response to a secretor gene (Se) that is present in about 80% of persons and that is required for expression of the Le^b gene.

TABLE 5-19. Immunohematology

BLOOD GROUP SYSTEM (GENES)	GENOTYPE	PHENOTYPE		FREQUENCY (%)	ANTIBODY IN SERUM
		MAJOR BLOOD GROUPS			
ABO	O(H) O(H)	O(H)	*Ags on RBC membrane & secretions*	44	Anti-A, anti-B
	A₁A₁	A		42	Anti-B
	A₁A₂				
	A₁0				
	A₂0				
	BB	B		10	Anti-A
	BO				
	A₁B	AB		4	None
	A₂B				
Lewis		Leᵃ		22	
		Leᵇ*		78	
Se	SeSe	secretors		80	
	SeSe				
	sese	nonsecretors		20	
		Ags in RBC only			
MH	MM	M		27	
	NN	N		24	
	MN	MN		50	
S	SS	S		55	
	Ss				
	ss	s		45	
Rh†		DCe,DCE,DcE,Dce		85 ("Rh+")	
		dce,dCe,dcE,dCE		15 ("Rh−")	

Minor Blood Groups
Lutheran (Luᵃ, Luᵇ), Kell (K⁺, K⁻), Duffy (Fyᵃ, Fyᵇ)
Kidd (JKᵃ, Jkᵇ)
P (P₁,P₂,p) Paroxysmal cold hemoglobinuria (Donath-Landsteiner antibody, "cold" IgG)

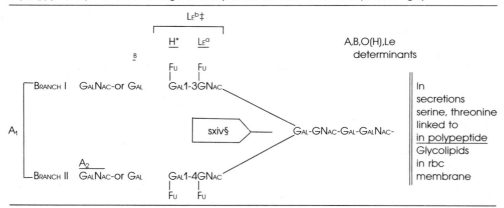

* Found in secretions and plasma of "secretors"; adsorbed to erythrocytes from plasma.
† Based on reactivity with 5 commonly available antisera: anti-D (anti-Rh 1), anti-C (anti-Rh 2), anti-E (anti-Rh 3), anti-c (anti-Rh 4), anti-e (anti-Rh 5)
‡ Se gene function required.
§ SXIV = type XIV pneumococcal polysaccharide cross-reactive with blood group substances because of the core common to both classes of antigen.

Rh Antigens: Erythroblastosis Fetalis

In 1940 Landsteiner and Wiener found agglutinogens on *Rhesus*-monkey red blood cells (RBC) that evoked agglutinins against RBC of about 87% of whites and about 95% of blacks, Native Americans, and Chinese. The same antigen was found in many human RBC and is known as Rh agglutinogen. Persons with such RBC antigens are said to be Rh positive (Rh+); those lacking it, Rh negative (Rh−). Unlike the "natural," exogenously stimulated agglutinins of the ABO system, agglutinins against Rh antigen occur only if an Rh− person is actively sensitized by transfusion with Rh+ blood or by pregnancy with an Rh+ fetus.

Fetal erythrocytes from the placental circulation may gain access to the maternal blood during the late stages of pregnancy and parturition and in a first heterospecific pregnancy thus sensitize the mother. On subsequent pregnancies, the mother produces IgG antibody that crosses the placenta to react with the homologous antigen in fetal erythrocytes. Maternal Rh antibodies cause extensive agglutination and hemolysis in the fetus or neonate, resulting in death due to erythroblastosis fetalis or hemolytic disease of the newborn (HDN).

Erythroblastosis fetalis occurs in an estimated 1% of all pregnancies. Of these about 66% are said to be due to ABO incompatibilities and are usually mild. About 30%, due to Rh incompatibility, are usually severe and are often fatal unless promptly treated by exchange transfusion. A small percentage is due to other incompatibilities. Rh erythroblastosis fetalis is entirely preventable by the administration of "Rhogam," which is obtained from Rh− males immunized with Rh+ erythrocytes. The globulins are given to Rh− mothers within 3 days after the birth of an Rh+ infant or fetus. The antibodies combine with and eliminate Rh+ erythrocytes of fetal origin that have passed into the maternal circulation, thus preventing the primary maternal immune response (sensitization). This must be done after each subsequent Rh+ pregnancy to avoid risk of maternal sensitization.

Two systems of nomenclature, each based on a different genetic interpretation, are used for the Rh antigens. One, the Wiener system, is based on the view that some 10 or more genes or gene complexes (multiple allelic genes) occupy a single locus (Rh locus), coding for some 28 or more antigen mosaics or complexes on RBC. Another system (Fisher and Race) assumes the existence of three linked loci with two alleles each, coding for six antigens (C, D, E, c, d, e). Numerous variants and "compound" antigens, e.g., $C^w dE$, $C^w DE$, $r y^w$, R^{zw}, also are found (Table 5-20). Rh_o and D are identical.

From a clinical standpoint the RH_o antigen and a variant of D, D^u ("weak D") are most important because, being both the most common and the most potent antigenically, they are most often involved in HDN. Administration of D^u cells should be restricted to D+ (RH+) recipients because D^u cells can evoke anti-D (Rh_o) antibodies. Conversely, D^u persons should receive only D− (Rh−) cells.

Because the complex Rh antigenic pattern is genetically controlled its determination has great significance in resolving questions concerning parentage and other relationships. For example, two Rh+ persons, one or both heterozygous, may have an Rh− child but two Rh− persons (always homozygous) cannot have an Rh+ child. Transfusions into Rh− females should always be with Rh− blood.

The Direct Coombs' Test

Immunoglobulin molecules evoked by RBC antigens are commonly IgG (relatively small, monomeric, bivalent); less commonly they are IgM (relatively large, pentameric, usually pentavalent).

TABLE 5-20. Relations of Wiener and Fisher Nomenclatures

ANTIGENS		GENES	
Wiener Blood Factors	Fisher Agglutinogens	Wiener Genes	Fisher Gene Linkages
rh′	C	Rz	CDE ⎫
Rh_o	D	R^1	CDe ⎬ D present = RH+
rh″	E	R^2	cDE ⎪
hr′	c	R^o	cDe ⎭
hr″	e	r^y	
		r′	CdE ⎫
		r	Cde ⎬ D absent = Rh−
		r″	cde ⎪
			cdE ⎭

Both, especially IgM, can cause agglutination. However, the IgM molecules are often present in low concentration. They are found in the fetal circulation only in response to fetal infection, and they do not pass the placental barrier in either direction. The relative ineffectiveness of IgG molecules in hemagglutination is due, in great part, to their small size; they have difficulty in attaching simultaneously in two RBC that are (as is commonly the case) widely separated by negatively charged ions (zeta potential) when suspended in saline. Direct agglutination by IgG antibody can sometimes be made to occur if the effect of the zeta potential is reduced by mechanical force (centrifugation) or by suspending the cells in high concentrations of salt or protein. These measures often bring the RBC sufficiently close together to permit lattice formation by the IgG molecules.

When IgG antibodies attach to erythrocytes without causing lattice formation, they occupy cell receptors (antigens) and block the action of agglutinating IgM or IgG. The attached, nonagglutinating antibodies are called "blocking" antibodies, because they interfere with agglutination and can be detected only with the Coombs test.

Immunoglobulins are antigenic in heterologous species, in which antibody to human immunoglobulin can be easily produced. Antiglobulin (Coombs' serum, named for R. R. A. Coombs, who first described the principle) agglutinates erythrocytes coated with blocking antibody that does not by itself agglutinate the cells. This is the direct Coombs' test used to detect sensitization of fetal (cord) erythrocytes by maternal antibody.

The Indirect Coombs' Test

Antibody to Rh and other minor blood group antigens can be detected by the indirect Coombs' test, in which the serum is mixed with erythrocytes of known antigenic specificity and then with antiglobulin. Agglutination indicates the presence, in the first serum, of antibody to the suspected blood group antigen. The test may be reversed by using "known" serum with "unknown" red blood cells.

It should be noted that in the foregoing discussion the term "sensitization" has been used in two distinct contexts. Erythrocytes to which antibodies are specifically adsorbed (e.g., Rh+ cells coated with anti-Rh) are said to be sensitized to the lytic action of complement, that is, immune cytolysis, the basis for HDN, or to agglutination by antiglobulin (Coombs' serum). Sensitization is also used as the functional equivalent of the primary IR, as in a first

untreated heterospecific pregnancy. In the latter instance, subsequent exposure of the maternal immune system to the same fetal (i.e., paternal) antigens evokes antibody in an anamnestic response, mostly IgG (type II hypersensitivity).

IMMUNOPROPHYLAXIS

I. Active immunization (Table 5-21)
   A. *Natural:* due to infection (clinically apparent as well as subclinical or inapparent) or exposure and sensitization to noninfectious "foreign" antigens (e.g., as in atopic allergy).
   B. *Artificial:* due to antigenic stimulation by vaccines
      1. Live attenuated microorganisms (e.g., oral poliomyelitis [Sabin] vaccine, measles, mumps, rubella vaccines, BCG) BCG is the only living bacterial vaccine used in the United States. The live vaccine used in veterinary medicine against Bang's disease (i.e., *Brucella abortus* strain 19) is a source of occasional accidental human infection. Vaccination (i.e., immunization against smallpox with vaccinia virus) is no longer required in the United States, because smallpox has been eliminated globally. However, thanks to advances in recombinant techniques, vaccinia virus is being actively investigated as a potential "vector" vaccine, in which discretely selected coding sequences for protective antigens (e.g., influenza viral hemagglutinin) are inserted into the vaccinia viral genome.
      2. Killed or inactivated microorganisms (e.g., pertussis and influenza vaccines, Salk poliomyelitis vaccine) or microbial fractions (e.g., pneumococcal, meningococcal polysaccharide vaccines)
      3. Toxoids (e.g., diphtheria and tetanus toxoids) or nonmicrobial antigens (as in "desensitization" to ragweed or other atopic allergens by injection of the offending antigen to produce IgG-blocking antibody). Toxoids are bacterial exotoxins that have been concentrated from culture fluids, treated with formalin under alkaline conditions to abolish toxicity but retain antigenicity, and precipitated on (i.e., adsorbed to) $Al(OH)_3$. When injected subcutaneously, the insoluble alum retains toxoid at the site, retarding its release and enhanc-

TABLE 5-21. Immunoprophylaxis of Infectious Diseases

ROUTINE UNIVERSAL IMMUNIZATION		INDICATIONS & AGE GROUP
Disease	Vaccine	
Active		
Diphtheria, tetanus, pertussis	DTP (APtoxoids, killed *B. pertussis* phase I)	Normal infants & children:
Poliomyelitis (paralytic)	Trivalent oral (Sabin) live attenuated viruses (human diploid cell culture) (oral polio vaccine, OPV)	DTP, OPV at 2, 4, 6, 18 months 4–6 years
German measles (rubella)	Live attenuated virus (RA 27/3, human diploid cell culture)	Over 1 year. Contraindicated in pregnancy even though risk to fetus minimal
Measles (rubeola)	Live attenuated virus (chicken embryo fibroblast culture)	Over 1 year
Mumps	Live attenuated virus (chicken embryo fibroblast culture)	Over 1 year
Active	RESTRICTED IMMUNIZATION	
Tuberculosis	BCG, attenuated *M. tuberculosis (bovis)*	Susceptible (tuberculin-negative) individuals at particular risk (e.g., medical personnel). Converts tuberculin reaction.
Poliomyelitis	Killed trivalent (Salk)	Adults at risk and without history of childhood immunization
Pneumonia	Multivalent pneumococcal polysaccharide	Individually assessed risk, compromised patients
Meningitis	Meningococcal A,C polysaccharides	Not effective under 2 years
Typhoid fever	Acetone–killed *S. typhi*	Special circumstances
Influenza	Influenza virus (groups A,B) of current H–N formulation grown in chicken embryos and formalin-inactivated	Infants (split virus) and 65 years and over; also compromised (e.g., immunosuppressed, metabolic-renal disease, asthma) patients and special-risk groups (whole or split virus, annually) (e.g., physicians, hospital personnel, chronic care facility residents)
Rabies	Rabies virus grown in human diploid cells, inactivated with tri-n-butyl phosphate, subunit	Individually assessed risk; combine with human hyperimmune globulin
Yellow fever	Attenuated 17D strain, grown in chicken embryos	Individually assessed risk of exposure
Smallpox (variola)	Live vaccinia virus (lyophilized)	Not required in United States (except armed forces, laboratory personnel at risk). Individually assessed risk of exposure
Hepatitis B	HB, antigen from pooled carrier plasma, cloned	Individually assessed risk of exposure
Anthrax	HB₅Ag, AP toxoid	Individually assessed risk of exposure
Passive	*Preparation*	
Hepatitis A,B	Pooled normal human immunuglobulin	Individually assessed risk of exposure
Tetanus	Tetanus tg (human)	Tetanus–prone injury in non-immunes
Diphtheria	Diphtheria AT ("despeciated" horse serum)	Early proven diphtheria
Varicella-zoster pneumonia	Zoster immune globulin (ZIG)	In severe proven infection in high-risk patients
Rabies	Human rabies hyperimmune globulin (RIG)	In conjunction with vaccine

AP = alum precipitated.
DTP = *Diphtheria, Tetanus* (toxoids), *Pertussis* bacterial (killed) vaccine.
OPV = Oral *Poliomyelitis* Vaccine.
  H = hemagglutinin.
  N = neuraminidase.
BCG = *Bacille Calmette-Guérin*

ing immunization (*i.e.*, adjuvant effect). Killed *Bordetella pertussis* in DTP has an additional adjuvant effect on production of tetanus and diphtheria antitoxins. Natural sensitization to products of commensal corynebacteria increases with age, with concomitant risk of severe hypersensitivity reactions (both immediate and delayed) to injection of DTP. This risk is lessened by use of adult-type diphtheria toxoid (Td contains less diphtherial protein than DTP) in susceptible (Shick-positive) individuals over 12 years of age, who should be skin tested with dilute Td (Moloney test) before being immunized.

II. Passive immunization: by acquisition of preformed antibodies contained in serum "gamma globulin" or immunoglobulin fraction(s).

A. *Natural:* transplacental passage of maternal IgG antibodies (e.g. protection of fetus against neonatal group B streptococcal infection; pathogenesis of HDN)

B. *Artificial:* administration of antibodies produced in another host (*e.g.,* diphtheria antitoxin is hyperimmune horse serum and its use incurs the risk of anaphylaxis and/or serum sickness; tetanus immune globulin is Ig fraction of human subjects hyperimmunized with tetanus toxoid; zoster immune globulin, [ZIG] is Ig from pooled sera of patients convalescing from varicella-zoster infection; anti-Rh, anti-D, Rhogam, is Ig from sera of men hyperimmunized with Rh+ erythrocytes). So-called normal human globulin (gamma globulin) is immunoglobulin from pooled sera containing high titers of naturally acquired antibodies against common infectious agents (*e.g.,* hepatitis viruses, poliovirus, measles virus). All human Ig fractions are free of hepatitis and other known viruses; use of human Ig avoids risk of heterospecific sensitization and reactions to animal sera.

QUESTIONS IN MICROBIOLOGY AND IMMUNOLOGY

The following questions are designed as a guide to reviewing microbiology and immunology. The student will have to consult additional sources in order to respond adequately to some of the items, which are for the most part designed to stimulate correlative thought rather than regurgitation of facts. As an additional aid, a list of suggested readings is appended to the end of this chapter.

Define and explain the mechanism of "serum sickness" as it relates to treatment of diphtheria, prophylaxis of tetanus, treatment with penicillin. How can potential serum sickness be avoided? Once manifest, how is it treated? What is its relation to atopic allergy? To acute poststreptococcal glomerulonephritis?

Define hemolytic disease of the newborn (HDN) and erythroblastosis fetalis in terms of (1) genetic predisposition; (2) risk to the fetus; (3) risk to the mother. How can HDN be prevented? What is the source of the prophylactic agent? When HDN is manifest at birth, how can the infant with HDN be treated? What, if any, may be the permanent residua in infants surviving HDN?

Explain immunological tolerance and the roles of T and B lymphocytes in induction and maintenance of tolerance.

Describe the cellular mechanisms, including biochemical sequences, involved in phagocytosis and intracellular killing of encapsulated bacteria; nonencapsulated bacteria; rickettsiae; viruses. By what immunological mechanisms is phatocytosis of pathogenic bacteria promoted? Inhibited?

Outline the mechanism of complement fixation (CF) as used, for example, in virologic serodiagnosis. How can CF be used to *identify* a viral agent isolated from a sample of sputum from a patient with bronchopneumonia? What is meant by "group-specific CF antigen" in adenoviruses? What is meant by the term "anticomplementary (AC) serum"?

Define *immune adherence,* and describe the mechanism involved and its relation to resistance to infection.

What is *anaphylaxis?* What is the immunological basis for anaphylactic reactions? Describe in detail how an anaphylactic reaction is brought about, using a specific antigen as an example (*e.g.,* bee venom).

What is the Coombs test and under what circumstances is it used? What reagents are required? Explain the difference between the "direct" and "indirect" Coombs test as the terms are used in blood-bank jargon.

Define the following terms: cestode, AP toxoid, endotoxin, exotoxin, virus, bacterium, *Rickettsia, Chlamydia,* zoonosis, enzootic, procaryotic cell, microaerophilic bacterium, virion, capsomer, nucleocapsid.

Discuss the role of plasmids in antibiotic resistance. What are resistance transfer factors (RTF) and how do they relate to the bacterial genome?

What is *lysogenic conversion* and how does it relate to the *virulence* of certain bacteria? Give specific examples.

List the principal structural features of bacteria (*e.g., Bacillus subtilis*) and indicate the function of each.

Define in molecular terms *lipopolysaccharide* (LPS) as found in gram-negative bacteria (*e.g., E.*

coli, N. meningitidis). What is the relation of LPS to pathogenicity? What *in vitro* tests are commonly used to detect LPS (*e.g.*, in solutions used for intravenous administration)?

Why are gram-positive bacteria commonly susceptible to penicillin and why are most gram-negative bacteria much less so? Explain the occurrence of resistance to penicillin in strains of gram-positive bacterial *pathogens*, citing specific examples. What measures have been successful in circumventing acquired bacterial resistance to therapeutic levels of penicillin G?

Why are viruses insusceptible to antibiotics commonly used to treat bacterial infections?

Compare and contrast SST (*e.g.*, VDRL) and FTA-ABS tests with respect to reagents, technique and specificity in the diagnosis of infection by *Treponema pallidum* (including, besides syphilis, yaws, bejel). What is the significance of the commonly used term "biological false-positive (BFP) test"? In what conditions may a BFP test occur?

Describe BCG vaccine, how it is administered, the reactions it evokes, and the principal indications or contraindications for its use in the United States.

List four diseases in which serum therapy or prophylaxis is of proven value. Name the species of animal in which each of the sera you mention is produced.

Discuss the initiation of an immune response in a normal individual to a protein antigen, a polysaccharide antigen. What is meant by an *anamnestic* response? What is the cellular basis for a "booster" response to tetanus toxoid?

Discuss present-day methods for isolation of anaerobic bacteria from clinical specimens, including the procedures used for identification of individual species. Indicate the molecular basis underlying the requirement of some species of bacteria for strict anaerobiosis.

List pathways involved in, and products of, glucose energy metabolism by strictly aerobic bacteria; by facultative bacteria; by strictly anaerobic bacteria. Draw comparison with analogous aspects of human muscle metabolism.

Describe the physical concepts underlying transmission (TEM) and scanning (SEM) microscopy, drawing comparisons with light microscopy. Include a consideration of resolving power and the limitations of the respective techniques. How does the preparation of specimens differ for each? How are antigen–antibody reactions recognized by TEM? How is TEM used in *rapid* diagnosis of viral infection?

Describe the principles underlying fluorescence microscopy and the use of antibody labeled with fluorescein. What other fluorescent labels can be used? How is fluorescence microscopy used in virological diagnosis? In bacteriological diagnosis? Cite specific examples. How does the use of antibody labeled with peroxidase or phosphatase differ from the use of fluorescent antibody? What are the advantages and disadvantages of each type of label?

Define the term *antibiotic*. What is the most common source of antibiotics? Outline the principal modes of action of several widely used antibiotics (*e.g.*, tetracycline, chloramphenicol, penicillin, streptomycin, polymyxin), as well as the mechanism(s) whereby certain species of bacteria *acquire* and *express* resistance to them. Indicate which antibiotics are mainly bactericidal and which are mainly bacteriostatic.

How does penicillin G differ from the semisynthetic penicillins? From cloxacilin? From oxacillin? From cephalosporins?

Discuss the indications for and limitations of sensitivity testing (antibiograms) of bacteria isolated from clinical specimens.

Outline the principal features of the major histocompatibility complex (MHC) and its role in allograft rejection, delayed hypersensitivity, and the activity of cytotoxic T lymphocytes. What is the relation of MHC to human disease(s)?

List three vaccines involving living attenuated microorganisms. How have recent discoveries in molecular biology greatly advanced the design of viral vaccines? Of bacterial vaccines? On what objective criteria are attenuated living viral and bacterial vaccines judged to be attenuated in virulence? What, if any, adverse reactions follow the use of any of the vaccines you have listed?

What are some of the factors that determine (1) whether or not infection occurs following exposure to a given agent; (2) the virulence of infectious agents. What is meant by the "carrier state"?

What is the role of histamine in allergic reactions? In which types of allergy are antihistamines likely to be of value? Why? What is SR-A? Where do histamine and SR-A originate? What is the role of eosinophils in allergy?

Outline the development of prophage, lysogeny, and bacterial lysis by phage. In the bacteriophage replicative cycle, what is the latent period? The eclipse period? The "burst size"?

What are viral plaques *(in vitro)*? What is the utility of plaque formation in animal virology?

Explain the mechanism(s) of viral hemagglutination and how it is used in diagnostic virology. Cite a specific example. What does the term "nonspecific serum inhibitor" mean when used in connection with viral serodiagnosis? Define and cite specific examples of the use of complement fixation and neutralization tests in diagnostic virology. What is ELISA? RIA? For what purposes are they used, and what are the mechanisms of each?

Explain the etymology of *picornavirus; myxovirus; arbovirus; echovirus; papovavirus; reovirus; rhabdovirus; coronavirus; arenavirus; parvovirus; calicivirus; togavirus; retrovirus.*

Name four species of pathogenic spore-forming bacteria. Explain how bacterial spores (not necessarily pathogenic) can be used to monitor the preparation of operating room sterile supplies and equipment.

What are bacterial capsules? What relation do they have to virulence? To immunologic specificity of the organism?

Define pathogenicity; virulence. Indicate the factors on which each depends. What is the role of the host in determining virulence? Give specific examples of microorganisms and the "virulence factors" of each.

Describe three pathogenic, strictly (obligate) anaerobic, nonsporulating bacteria; indicate how they cause disease, including sources of infection, prevention, and treatment. Under what circumstances do commensal organisms become pathogenic? Cite specific examples.

Give the minimal time and temperature for sterilization by compressed steam (autoclave); hot air oven. Explain the mechanisms of microbicidal or microbistatic action of cresols; $HgCl_2$; penicillin; trimethoprim–sulfamethoxazole.

Discuss viral cytopathology in relation to propagation of viruses *in vitro*. Give specific examples of viral cytopathology indicating the molecular basis of each.

List five diseases of viral etiology for which effective immunoprophylaxis is available. In each case, indicate the source of the immunizing agent, how and when it is administered, how susceptibility to the corresponding disease may be determined, and what if any adverse reactions to immunization should be expected.

List the immunizing agents presently available against diseases of bacterial etiology, indicating which of the vaccines are composed of bacterial component(s) rather than whole bacteria. What is the rationale for their use?

Discuss the biological, medicoepidemiological, and ethical problems attending the development and ultimate application of immunizing agent(s) against infection with herpesviruses; HIV.

Define interferons; indicate the principal categories of interferon, their induction and purification, and problems attending their use in clinical medicine.

Discuss hepatitis viruses and indicate the preventive measures, if any, which are available against each category of virus. Which is the most frequent cause of post-transfusion hepatitis? What diagnostic procedures are available for screening blood donors for hepatitis viruses? What prophylactic (active or passive) agents against hepatitis are available?

Discuss the molecular epidemiology of the disease influenza, with particular reference to current immunization practice and chemoprophylaxis.

Discuss immunoprophylaxis against rubella, including indications and contraindications for administration of vaccine.

List six sexually transmitted diseases in the order of current epidemiologic importance. Indicate what therapeutic agents, if any, are available for each. What diagnostic procedures are used for each disease you have mentioned?

Describe three mechanisms for the transfer of genetic information in bacteria, in each instance indicating the actual or potential clinical significance.

Name three diseases transmitted by the fecal–oral route, and for each name the etiologic agent and indicate the pathogenetic mechanism. How can each of the diseases you mention be prevented? Give two examples of bacterial food poisoning–infection, and outline the diagnostic procedures you would undertake to identify the causative agent.

Discuss the viridans (alpha-hemolytic) streptococci and the diseases they cause. Under what circumstances would you undertake antibacterial chemotherapy or chemoprophylaxis against organisms in this category?

What is "gram-negative sepsis"? What microorganisms are the most frequent cause, and how are they recognized? Explain the clinical manifestations of this condition. What therapeutic agents are used in proven cases? How would you monitor the course of therapy?

Discuss the spectrum of diseases caused by group A streptococci, and the measures you would take toward therapy and/or prevention of infection. Discuss infections caused by group B beta-hemolytic streptococci. On what bacterial component(s) is this group classification based? On what antigen(s) is the *type* specificity of group A streptococci based?

Define dimorphism as it applies to fungi. Give at least three examples of dimorphic fungi that are pathogenic in one form or the other. Define asexual reproduction in fungi and discuss its significance with respect to the mycoses. What chemotherapeutic agents are presently available for treatment of fungal infection? With each drug named, indicate its mode of action and the infections against which it is most effective.

List two pathogenic protozoa (one intestinal and one that invades the blood stream); pathogenic and opportunistic helminths; cestodes. For each outline the life cycle, vector (if any), pathogenesis, immune response, diagnostic methods, and epidemiology.

Describe the etiologic agents of filariasis and outline the usual clinical manifestations of the disease, including diagnostic methods and immune response. How do the clinical manifestations relate to the life cycle of the parasite?

Discuss toxoplasmosis with respect to pathogenesis, diagnosis, and treatment. What is the prevalence of toxoplasmosis?

Discuss infection caused by *Neisseria gonorrhoeae:* diagnosis in males and females, virulence factors, clinical picture including complications and sequelae, immune response, chemotherapy, and chemoprophylaxis. Discuss problems of drug-resistant *N. gonorrhoeae.* What is currently the leading sexually transmitted disease in the United States and how is it diagnosed? Treated?

Discuss infection caused by *Neisseria meningitidis,* including age incidence, epidemiology, clinical and laboratory diagnosis, treatment, immunoprophylaxis, and chemoprophylaxis. Include a consideration of resistance/sensitivity to available chemotherapeutic agents.

What is "undulant fever"? Name the specific cause(s) and outline the pathogenesis of the disease, and procedures for making the specific diagnosis. What chemotherapeutic agents are most effective?

Name the most frequent cause(s) of neonatal meningitis, and outline the diagnostic and therapeutic procedures most appropriate to each. What, if any, immunoprophylactic reagents are available?

On what basis would you suspect a diagnosis of botulism, and how would you arrive at the *specific* diagnosis? With respect to tetanus ("lockjaw"), is recovery of the organism in culture from any body source diagnostic? If so, why? If not, why not? Discuss both active and passive immunoprophylaxis against tetanus. For each, describe briefly the reagents used and what reactions (in the patient), if any, should be anticipated. Does one attack of tetanus in a previously unimmunized individual confer subsequent immunity?

Describe the "pertussis syndrome" and discuss the etiologic agent(s) and the epidemiology relative to each. What, if any, immunoprophylactic agents are available, how and when are they used, and what are the consequences of their use? What are some of the virulence factors in the organism(s) you mention?

Discuss the pathogenesis of diphtheria, including a description of the causative organism, possible factors related to a fatal outcome, immunoprophylactic (active as well as passive) measures to take against diphtheria, the role of antibiotics in treatment of the disease. Discuss problems attending immunization of adults.

Review the major sexually transmitted diseases against the panorama of current epidemiology, including socioeconomic factors that tend to perpetuate/increase the incidence of the diseases you mention.

Discuss the disease tuberculosis as opposed to infection with *Mycobacterium tuberculosis.* What are the species of microorganism that must be taken into consideration in the differential clinical diagnosis of pulmonary disease? What are the most important sites of extrapulmonary tuberculosis? Discuss chemotherapy of infection proven to be due to *M. tuberculosis.* Discuss the immunologic basis of diagnosis, and mechanisms of immune resistance to tuberculous infection. Outline the principles underlying immunoprophylaxis and chemoprophylaxis against infection with *M. tuberculosis.* Indicate the current problems of drug-resistant strains.

Discuss plague and plague-like illness with respect to etiology, epidemiology, diagnosis, and chemotherapy. What is the nature of the immune response to tularemia? To brucellosis?

Discuss the rickettsioses that may be encountered in the United States. For each one you name, indicate the vector (if any), the main clinical features and appropriate chemotherapy.

Discuss infection with nonsporulating anaerobic bacteria. Name principal species involved in the disease process, where they originate and how they are identified. What is "anaerobic cellulitis"?

Discuss anthrax with particular reference to sources of infection and microbial virulence factors and how the latter relate to pathogenesis and immunoprophylaxis. What antibiotics are effective in treatment?

Describe the rubella syndrome: causative agent, diagnosis, epidemiology, and prevention.

Outline the principal spirochetal diseases. For each, name the causative organism, indicate how the diagnosis is established, and what if any therapeutic agents are available. Discuss in detail the bacteriological and serological diagnosis of syphilis.

What are "L" forms of bacteria? How do they relate to pathogenesis of disease? Compare and contrast them to Mycoplasmatales. Name the known human pathogens in the latter group, and for each indicate the disease(s) caused, including epidemiology, specific diagnostic procedures, and appropriate therapy. What are "cold agglutinins"? Are they always due to infection? For what antigen(s) are they specific? Of what kinds of pathological processes are they a sign?

Discuss the immune response to the deep-seated mycoses (*e.g.*, histoplasmosis). Include a consideration of diagnostic problems, cross-reactions, resistance, and recovery. In what general type of immune deficiency do opportunistic mycotic infections occur? Give specific examples of immune deficiencies and opportunistic infections (of any type) to which they predispose. What antifungal antibiotics are currently available? List several mycoses which can be successfully treated with antibiotics.

What is *transfer factor?* Define its function in terms of the pathobiology of infection. Give specific examples. Is transfer factor of any use therapeutically? How is it prepared?

How is *Entamoeba histolytica* identified in diarrheal stools? in formed stools? How is amebic dysentery differentiated from bacillary dysentery both on clinical grounds and by laboratory methods?

Define the life cycle of a tapeworm commonly found in humans. Why is it necessary to recover the head of the worm in order to ensure a cure? What chemotherapy is available for this infestation?

Compare *Taenia saginata, Taenia solum, Echinococcus granulosus,* and *Diphyllobothrium latum* with respect to morphology, life cycle, diagnosis, and therapy.

What laboratory procedures are useful in the diagnosis of hydatid disease?

Describe the life cycle of *Necator americanus,* including the route taken by the parasite from the site of infection to its final location in the body. Briefly describe two laboratory procedures for diagnosis of this infection.

What is ancylostomiasis and how is it prevented?

What is the cause of trichinosis in humans? How may it be diagnosed? Prevented? Describe the life cycle of the parasite and the lesions it causes.

Describe the pathogenesis of filariasis, including epidemiology. What are the sequelae of chronic filariasis? How is it treated?

Outline the life cycle of the parasites that cause human malaria, distinguishing (if possible) their various developmental stages. Outline briefly what you know about cell receptors for malaria and how the parasite gains entrance into the erythrocyte. What factors predispose to resistance to malaria? Include a discussion of the vectors of malaria and current therapeutic practice. What approach would you consider potentially fruitful in developing a vaccine against malaria? Are there any good animal models? What is the global prevalence of malaria today?

Discuss the general principles underlying rapid diagnosis of viral infection, giving the most frequently used laboratory procedures and the interpretation of results.

Discuss the significance of bacterial pili with respect to morphology and function.

What is "smooth" to "rough" variation in bacteria and how is it recognized? Relate this phenomenon to problems of virulence and immunization against specific bacterial diseases.

What is bacterial recombination? Viral recombination? Viral genetic reassortment? Give specific examples. What are restriction enzymes and how are they used in classification of viruses? What are some of the practical applications of genetic mapping and restriction analysis?

Discuss the disease(s) caused by members of the family Legionellaceae, including the names of the species involved, laboratory diagnosis, and treatment of infection. What is the usual source of infection? Can legionellosis ever arise as a nosocomial infection? Is it directly transmissible from person to person?

Discuss the clinical manifestations, specific etiology, epidemiology, and treatment of Lyme disease.

Describe the molecular basis for the clinical manifestations of cholera. How is epidemic cholera treated? Prevented? What is the character of the immune response to cholera vaccine? How is cholera vaccine prepared?

Discuss the pathogenesis of rheumatic fever, including bacteriological and immunological aspects. Compare with the pathogenesis of acute glomerulonephritis, including epidemiology, treatment, and prevention.

What is "C-reactive protein"? What is its significance with respect to mechanisms of *resistance* to bacterial infection? What is the significance of CRP in the serum? How is it measured?

Discuss several clinical syndromes caused by exotoxins of coagulase-positive *Staphylococcus aureus.*

Describe the spectrum of disease caused by *Mycobacterium leprae,* including details of the immune response, both humoral and cellular, and any deficiencies that contribute to pathogenesis. What therapeutic agents are currently available and effective in combating leprosy? What is the current incidence of leprosy in the United States and what epidemiologic factors underlie the continuing importance of the disease?

Using specific examples, outline the main molecular events in the replication of RNA and DNA viruses. Indicate the points at which the clinically useful antiviral agents act, that is, inhibit viral replication. What are the currently available antiviral agents (besides interferon) and for which diseases are they used?

Discuss the rationale for the use of living, attenuated viral vaccines. Give several examples of diseases that are preventable with vaccines, how the vaccines are produced, and what the basis and criteria for attenuation are. What, if any, adverse reactions to immunization may be expected? What are the contraindications to using any of the presently available live attenuated viral vaccines?

Discuss the general properties of retroviruses, and indicate their significance to human disease.

Discuss the structure and function of each of the five classes of immunoglobulin.

What are the principal *sub*populations of T lymphocytes and how are they recognized *in vitro?* What is the function of each?

Outline the principles underlying the production of *monoclonal antibodies.* To what, specifically, does the "-clonal" refer? On what basis do monoclonal antibodies sharpen (*i.e.,* narrow) the specificity of immunological reactions? What are the advantages or disadvantages of such "sharpening" of specificity? Compare monoclonal antibodies to polyclonal antibodies in this respect, using a highly purified protein antigen (*e.g.,* crystalline serum albumin) as an example. How have monoclonal antibodies enhanced the precision of serodiagnosis? Give specific examples.

What is meant by "acute phase reactant"? Give several examples and indicate the clinical significance of each.

Define *antibody-dependent cellular cytotoxicity* and give several examples, citing the components of the reaction.

What does the term *heterophil antibody* signify? In what clinical conditions do heterophil antibodies appear and how are they measured? What is their clinical significance?

Discuss "slow viral disease" with respect to known agents, clinical course, analogous animal diseases, and diagnosis.

Make a list of agents known to be responsible for nosocomial infection; include viruses. Indicate how you would diagnose and treat each infection you have named.

What is the significance of circulating immune complexes (CIC)? Describe their molecular composition and how they are detected, citing specific laboratory tests. How are they removed from the circulation in the normal individual? In what diseases are CIC particularly indicative of active infection? In what tissues are they most often deposited and what reaction(s) do they evoke there?

Compare and contrast the human retroviruses, HTLV-I, HTLV-II, and HIV. What can be said about their morphology, replication, epidemiology, and pathogenesis?

MULTIPLE CHOICE QUESTIONS

Many of the following multiple-choice questions, all cast in formats used by the National Board of Medical Examiners, have been drawn from the computerized national *Microbiology and Immunology Test Item Bank,* through special arrangement with the Association of Medical School Microbiology Chairmen. The AMSMC, which owns and operates the MITIBANK, represents over 80 departments of microbiology and immunology throughout the United States and Canada. Questions submitted by participating departments for inclusion in the bank are accompanied by item analysis statistics and are subjected to rigorous initial review as well as periodic updating by the Editorial Committee of the AMSMC.

Section A

For each of the following (1 to 53), select the *single best answer* to the question or the *single item* that best *completes* the statement.

1. Cells specifically involved in cutaneous delayed hypersensitivity reactions:
   (a) Are B lymphocytes from germinal centers of the spleen white pulp
   (b) Probably recirculate from lymph nodes through the thoracic duct to the blood and back to the lymph nodes by the postcapillary venules
   (c) Migrate from germinal centers to the medullary cords of lymph nodes and red pulp cords of the spleen
   (d) Originate in the bone marrow and differ-

entiate in the "bursa equivalent" micro-environment

(e) Are derived from bone marrow precursors and reside in the germinal center caps

2. The immunologic mediator of type I (atopic hypersensitivity is:
   (a) Cytotropic IgG (IgG2) fixed to mast cells by the Fc portion
   (b) Cytotropic antibody of the autoimmune type (as in SLE) fixed to "self" antigens on leukocytes
   (c) IgE attached to mast cells and basophils, which fixes complement and triggers the complement cascade
   (d) IgE (reaginic) antibody fixed to tissue mast cells

3. Type I (atopic) allergy to ragweed antigens is passively transferable from a sensitive to a nonsensitive subject:
   (a) By either serum heated to 56°C for 30 minutes in order to destroy complement or peripheral lymphocytes
   (b) By serum and peripheral lymphocytes combined, but by neither alone
   (c) By serum alone
   (d) By washed peripheral blood lymphocytes in the absence of serum

4. In the pathogenesis of type III disease, the complexes that are most likely to be trapped in the renal glomerular basement membrane are:
   (a) Those formed in moderate antigen excess
   (b) Those formed in large antibody excess
   (c) Complexes of antibody (particularly IgM) with complement and no antigen
   (d) Those composed of antigen with IgE

5. In attempting to "desensitize" a person suffering from hay fever due to ragweed, graded injections of antigen are given subcutaneously over a period of weeks during the time of year in which the air is free of pollen. The mechanism underlying the amelioration of symptoms during the subsequent ragweed season is thought to be:
   (a) Elaboration of broadly specific IgE that "saturates" all potential binding sites, leaving none free to bind inhaled pollen
   (b) Stimulation of IgG antibody of the same specificity
   (c) Competitive suppression of the IgE locus of the Ir gene
   (d) Stimulation of IgM (primary immunization) that would bind to mucosal cells and act as blocking antibody

6. Mother is group O, Rh negative; father is group B, Rh positive; and the infant is group B, Rh positive. In this situation, the ABO incompatibility between the parents:
   (a) Enhances the chances of maternal elaboration of anti-D antibody
   (b) Lessens the chances of maternal iso(allo) immunization with Rh antigen(s)
   (c) Increases the changes of isoimmunization with minor blood-group antigens (e.g., Kell, Duffy)
   (d) Increases the risk of hemolytic disease of the newborn, particularly because there is also maternal–fetal Rh incompatibility

7. The "convertase" most closely resembling $\overline{C3bBb}$ of the alternate pathway is:
   (a) $\overline{C1}$
   (b) $\overline{C42}$
   (c) $\overline{C567}$
   (d) $\overline{C89}$
   (e) $\overline{C56789}$

8. Enhanced intracellular levels of cAMP, induced by agents such as prostaglandins, will:
   (a) Have no effect on phagocytic processes
   (b) Retard phagocytosis
   (c) Enhance phagocytosis

9. The antigenic determinants that define antibody class (isotype) would be best described as occurring:
   (a) In constant regions
   (b) In the variable region
   (c) In the hinge region
   (d) In Fab
   (e) In the carbohydrate moiety

10. Histamine, which is a vasoactive amine initially involved in immune complex disease tissue destruction, is released from:
    (a) Polymorphonuclear neutrophils
    (b) RBCs
    (c) Platelets
    (d) Lymphocytes
    (e) Macrophages

11. The presence of cryoglobulins in a patient's serum may indicate that the patient has:
    (a) Anemia
    (b) Circulating immune complexes
    (c) Hashimoto's thyroiditis
    (d) Pernicious anemia

12. A Coombs test is the most important laboratory aid for the diagnosis of:
    (a) Myasthenia gravis
    (b) Autoimmune hemolytic anemias
    (c) Waldenström's macroglobulinemia

(d) Rheumatoid arthritis

(e) Systemic lupus erythematosus

13. The most important antibody playing a role in the pathogenesis of systemic lupus erythematosus is:

(a) Antibody to thyroglobulin

(b) Antibody to DNA

(c) Antibody to mitochondria

(d) Rheumatoid factor

(e) Antibody to smooth muscle

14. The currently available vaccine pneumococcal infection contains:

(a) Heat-killed pneumococci of the 14 serotypes most frequently encountered

(b) Cell wall antigen(s), chiefly C substance

(c) Type-specific polysaccharide of 14 serotypes

(d) Attenuated pneumococci of the 14 serotypes most frequently encountered

15. In the syndrome of poststreptococcal glomerulonephritis:

(a) Streptococcal nucleases and streptolysin accumulate in the glomerular basement membrane.

(b) Streptococcal capsular antigen (hyaluronic acid) and glucuronic acid subunits precipitate with antibody and are deposited in the glomeruli in "lumpy" patterns.

(c) Immunoglobulin and complement localize in the glomerular basement membrane.

(d) Hematuria is due to the action of streptolysin O.

16. In group A beta-hemolytic streptococci, types are determined by the antigenic specificity of:

(a) The capsule

(b) The mucopeptide layer

(c) The M and/or T proteins

(d) The extracellular products, such as streptolysin O, which is produced only by group A streptococci

17. Prompt and adequate treatment of acute streptococcal pharyngitis constitutes prophylaxis of acute rheumatic fever because:

(a) The immune response is enhanced.

(b) The immune response to streptococcal antigens is aborted.

(c) Viable streptococci do not persist in the early rheumatic lesions.

(d) There is an antibody response to streptolysin and other streptococcal exoenzymes.

18. In the test for C-reactive protein (CRP) in patients' sera, the reagent used to precipitate the protein is:

(a) Group-specific cell wall antigen in *Streptococcus pneumoniae*

(b) Group-specific C antigen of beta-hemolytic streptococcus

(c) Factor C3 in the alternate complement pathway

(d) Rabbit antiserum

19. Recurrent staphylococcal infection in children with "chronic granulomatous disease" occurs because:

(a) The responsible organism almost always is found to produce penicillinase.

(b) No antibodies to staphylococcal teichoic acids are formed.

(c) There is a heritable defect in intraleukocytic killing of bacteria.

(d) These patients are prone to diabetes mellitus, which predisposes to bacterial infection.

20. The triple vaccine (DTP) routinely used in childhood immunization contains:

(a) Killed *Corynebacterium, diphtheriae, Bordetella pertussis* "toxoid," tetanus toxoid

(b) Diphtherial toxin exactly neutralized with antitoxin, *Bordetella pertussis*, tetanus toxoid

(c) Diphtherial toxoid, killed phase 1 *Bordetella pertussis*, tetanus toxoid

(d) Diphtherial toxoid, avirulent *Bordetella pertussis*, tetanus toxoid

21. Congenital rubella can be diagnosed in a week-old infant by:

(a) Demonstration of maternal IgM antibodies to rubella virus

(b) Testing for HI antibodies specific for the virus in the infant's serum

(c) Demonstration in the infant of circulating IgG antibodies to rubella virus

(d) Demonstration of rubella IgM antibodies in the infant

(e) The presence of infant IgA antibodies to rubella virus

22. Caesarian section has been found to eliminate neonatal complications due to which of the following viruses?

(a) Varicella-zoster

(b) Cytomegalovirus

(c) Poliovirus

(d) Echovirus

(e) Herpes simplex virus

23. To prevent hemolytic disease in a newborn

with an A-positive mother and an O-negative father, one would:

(a) Administer Rhogam to the mother after the birth of her first child
(b) Administer Rhogam to each of her subsequent children
(c) Administer Rhogam to the mother after her first A-positive daughter
(d) Administer Rhogam to her first O-negative child
(e) Do nothing—there is no danger to any of her children

24. Dermatophytes that infect special keratinized areas of the body, skin and nails only, are likely to belong to which genus?
(a) *Epidermophyton*
(b) *Trichophyton*
(c) *Microsporum*
(d) *Trichosporum*
(e) *Pitysporum*

25. In the currently accepted immunization schedule for children over the age of 6 years, one is advised to give "adult strength toxoid" instead of DTP. This is done:
(a) To prevent severe reactions to tetanus and/or pertussis antigens, to which children of that age already have developed antibody
(b) Only as a booster in children who have already had primary immunization with DTP at an earlier age
(c) To avoid hypersensitivity reactions to corynebacterial protein(s)
(d) Because susceptibility to diphtheria increases with age

26. In 1977, a U.S. Navy ship experienced a sudden outbreak of acute respiratory disease three days out of Manila, with 67% of the crew and 100% of those age 18 to 25 showing signs of respiratory disease in a 24-hour period. Armed forces epidemiologists flown to the scene isolated virus from transtracheal aspirates but not from the feces of those severely ill. The most likely agent of this outbreak was:
(a) Adenovirus, type 7
(b) Measles virus
(c) Respiratory syncytial virus
(d) Influenza of group A
(e) Influenza of group C

27. Most respiratory and intestinal infections by picornaviruses result in:
(a) Localized acute disease
(b) Latent infections

(c) Inapparent infections
(d) Recurrent infections
(e) Disseminated disease

28. Which one of the following is a binding site for amphotericin B?
(a) Cell wall mucopeptide
(b) 50s ribosomal subunit
(c) 30s ribosomal subunit
(d) Sterol-containing site in the membrane
(e) DNA

29. Rickettsiae differ from free-living bacteria in that the former:
(a) Contain DNA but no RNA
(b) Contain RNA but no DNA
(c) Are too small to be seen with the light microscope
(d) Customarily have arthropod vectors
(e) Cannot generate their metabolic energy requirements

30. The lipid envelop characteristic of some animal viruses:
(a) Contains proteins specified by the host-cell genome
(b) Contains lipids specified by the viral genome
(c) Is resistant to extractions by ether or detergents
(d) Contains lipids and carbohydrates determined by the host cell

31. Which of the following immunoglobulin classes are capable of complement fixation by the classical pathway?
(a) IgM and IgE
(b) IgM and IgA
(c) IgM and IgG
(d) IgM and IgD
(e) All of the above

32. The idiotype of an immunoglobulin molecule is determined by the amino acid sequence of the:
(a) Constant region of the H chain
(b) Constant region of the L chain
(c) Variable region of the H chain
(d) Variable region of the L chain
(e) Variable region of the H and L chain

33. A hapten is a substance that:
(a) Induces cellular immune responses but not antibody production
(b) Does not induce any immune response when given alone but does elicit an immune response when coupled to a larger molecule
(c) Induces tolerance when given alone
(d) When coupled to a larger molecule can be

recognized by B lymphocytes but not by T lymphocytes
    (e) Does none of the above
34. The antifungal activity of the polyene antibiotic amphotericin B is related to its:
    (a) Accumulation in keratinized tissue
    (b) Intercalation in mitochondrial DNA
    (c) Interaction with membrane sterols
    (d) Inhibiting cross-linking in fungal cell walls
    (e) Inhibition of DNA-dependent RNA polymerase
35. Which of the following are detected by mixed lymphocyte culture (MLC) reactivity?
    (a) HLA—A, B, C determinants
    (b) HLA—D determinants
    (c) HLA—Dr determinants
    (d) Immune response genes
    (e) All of the above
36. Abnormal neutrophil function is most often associated with recurrent infections caused by:
    (a) *Mycobacterium tuberculosis*
    (b) *Staphylococcus aureus*
    (c) *Legionella pneumophila*
    (d) *Streptococcus pneumoniae*
    (e) *Streptococcus pyogenes*
37. Rh-incompatible matings are not of concern where an ABO-incompatible situation also exists. This is based upon:
    (a) The fact that Rh antibodies are IgM
    (b) The fact that Rh antibodies cannot cross the placenta
    (c) The ability of the blood agglutinins to clear fetal RBCs rapidly before sensitization can occur
    (d) The fact that maternal antibodies, although in the fetus, will only cause minor agglutination but not lysis since complement levels are low in fetal circulation
    (e) The fact that fetal agglutinins will suppress maternal response to fetal RBC antigens
38. T (H) cells
    (a) Proliferate in response to free antigens
    (b) Bear OKT4 and OKT5 cell-surface markers
    (c) Help convert CTL precursors into active killer cells
    (d) Are restricted in their response to exogenous antigen by the requirement that they coordinately recognize HLA-A, B or C molecules
    (e) Are easily differentiated from T (DTH) cells

39. The MLR test can measure:
    (a) A proliferative response to OKT5+ cells
    (b) DNA synthesis in a population of cells which influence CTL precursors
    (c) Disparity of HLA-A, B, C antigens
    (d) The activity of CTLs
    (e) Capacity of the potential recipient of a marrow graft to mount a graft-versus-host response
40. In a sensitized subject, what cell specifically triggers delayed-type hypersensitivity?
    (a) Monocyte
    (b) OKT5+ T cell
    (c) OKT4+ T cell
    (d) Macrophage
    (e) Basophil
41. In a recombinant generated by generalized transduction, which of the following would be present?
    (a) DNA sequences of the virus
    (b) Proteins coded for by the virus
    (c) DNA sequences from the donor
    (d) Proteins coded for by the host cell
42. Actinomycin D inhibits DNA-dependent RNA synthesis. Which of the following viruses can replicate in the presence of actinomycin D?
    (a) Parainfluenzae (single-stranded RNA, antimessenger)
    (b) Poxvirus (double-stranded DNA)
    (c) Adeno-associated virus (single-stranded DNA)
    (d) Retrovirus (single-stranded RNA, messenger)
43. Which of the following is characteristic of "positive strand" RNA viruses?
    (a) A polymerase contained in the virion is necessary for replication.
    (b) The virion RNA can act as its own messenger RNA.
    (c) The virion RNA cannot be extracted in an infectious form.
    (d) Viral messenger RNAs are complementary to the virion RNA.
    (e) All of them are nonenveloped.
44. The end of the eclipse period is marked by:
    (a) The appearance of extracellular virions
    (b) Viral protein synthesis
    (c) Viral nucleic acid synthesis
    (d) Lysis of the cell
    (e) The appearance of complete virions
45. Reverse transcriptase:
    (a) Makes double-stranded RNA from single-stranded DNA template

(b) Is not required for cell transformation by RNA

(c) Is activated by sigma factor from host cell

(d) Is found in RNA oncogenic viruses

(e) Is found in DNA oncogenic virions

46. Respiratory–syncytial virus differs from other paramyxoviruses in that it:
    (a) Has a segmented genome
    (b) Lacks envelope fusion protein
    (c) Lacks envelope glycoprotein(s) with hemagglutinin and/or neuraminidase activity
    (d) Has icosahedral nucleocapsid symmetry
    (e) Replicates its genome in the cell nucleus

47. Which of the following components (viral antigens or specific antibodies) in the serum is most diagnostic of a past hepatitis B virus infection from which an individual has acquired immunity to subsequent hepatitis B virus infections?
    (a) HBsAg
    (b) HBcAg
    (c) HBeAg
    (d) Anti-HBsAg
    (e) Anti-HBcAg

48. In malaria, the infective stage is injected into human subjects by the mosquito is:
    (a) Sporozoite
    (b) Gametocyte
    (c) Cryptozoite
    (d) Merozoite
    (e) Oocyst

49. Antigenic shift within the influenza virus population:
    (a) Is associated with major changes in the amino acid sequence of the nucleocapsid (NP) antigen
    (b) Is the result of a mutation in the viral tRNA
    (c) Involves antigenic changes in the hemagglutinin or the neuraminidase
    (d) Results in a change in the amino acid sequence of the M protein of the virus
    (e) Does all of the above

50. Which ONE of the following statements concerning dental plaque and caries is true?
    (a) Bacteria form less than 10% of the total mass of dental plaque.
    (b) Mutants of *Streptococcus mutans* lacking the enzyme invertase are noncariogenic.
    (c) Gnotobiotic or germ-free rats fail to develop caries even when fed a cariogenic diet.
    (d) *Streptococcus sanguis* is a major component of subgingival plaque.

(e) *Streptococcus mutans* synthesizes a water-insoluble polypeptide that enables it to adhere to the enamel pellicle found on the surface of teeth.

51. Which one of the following antimicrobial agents inhibits bacterial cell wall synthesis at a step prior to the synthesis of UDP-MurNAc-pentapeptide?
    (a) Vancomycin
    (b) Bacitracin
    (c) Cycloserine
    (d) Penicillin G
    (e) Streptomycin

52. Antibiotic-associated colitis has been linked to a toxin produced by which one of the following organisms?
    (a) *Clostridium perfringens*
    (b) *Bacteroides fragilis*
    (c) *Bacteroides corrodens*
    (d) *Clostridium difficile*
    (e) *Campylobacter fetus*

53. One prokaryotic organism that is always resistant to penicillin is:
    (a) *Mycoplasma pneumoniae*
    (b) Group A streptococcus
    (c) *Treponema pallidum*
    (d) *Neisseria meningitidis*
    (e) *Histoplasma capsulatum*

Section B

Using the key shown below, answer questions 1 to 35 by selecting the best choice in each case according to the letters.

A: a, b, and c are correct.
B: a and c are correct.
C: b and d are correct.
D: d only is correct.
E: all are correct.

1. Virulence is attributable to the antiphagocytic properties of the capsules of:
    (a) *Neisseria meningitidis*, groups A and C
    (b) *Yersinia pestis* with V/W and F1 antigens
    (c) *Hemophilus influenzae*, type b
    (d) *Neisseria gonorrhoeae*, Arg⁻

2. Which of the following is/are true regarding the mode of action of diphtheria toxin?
    (a) The combined fragments of the toxin molecule act as an enzyme and bind to translocation factor EF-2.
    (b) NAD is required to split the toxin molecule into two fragments.

(c) Fragment A attaches to receptors on the cell membrane.

(d) Antibodies to fragment B block the action of the toxin.

3. Which of the following are characteristic(s) of *Nocardia asteroides?*

(a) The organism is normally found among the oral flora of humans.

(b) Benign pulmonary lesions often precede the development of metastatic brain abscess.

(c) Nocardiosis often manifests as a necrotizing infection of the extremities.

(d) Nocardiosis response best to treatment with sulfadiazine or sulfamerazine.

4. Characteristics of actinomycosis include which of the following?

(a) Infection may follow a tooth extraction.

(b) Abdominal infection may simulate appendicitis.

(c) Sulfur granules with peripheral clubbing may be present in exudates.

(d) Penicillin is the drug of choice.

5. The following are characteristics of the genus *Clostridium:*

(a) Ability to grow in the presence of oxygen ranges from aerotolerant to obligate anaerobes

(b) Ability to utilize a wide variety of carbohydrates for energy

(c) Production of large amounts of carbon dioxide (CO_2) by most species

(d) Production of some species of exotoxins that aid in the spread of organisms in tissue

6. Optimal recovery of anaerobic bacteria from clinical specimens may be promoted by:

(a) Addition of reducing agents and growth factors to media

(b) Addition of aminoglycosides to the media

(c) Prompt transport of specimens to the laboratory

(d) Use of candle jar to increase the level of CO_2 required for growth of obligate anaerobes

7. Anaerobic bacteria would *not* be expected to play a major role in which of the following?

(a) Nongonococcal pelvic infections

(b) Septic arthritis and osteomyelitis

(c) Lung abscess and empyema

(d) Urinary tract infections

8. Anaerobic bacteria should be considered in which of the following conditions?

(a) Myonecrosis

(b) Septic thrombophlebitis

(c) "Sterile pus" (no growth on blood agar in a candle jar)

(d) Debrided decubitus ulcer

9. Specimens that would be acceptable for culture of anaerobic organisms from infection of the female genital area are:

(a) Vaginal

(b) Cervical

(c) Urethral

(d) Culdocentesis aspirate

10. Which of the following apply to *Staphylococcus aureus?*

(a) Normal flora of nasal passages of most humans

(b) A frequent cause of nosocomial infections

(c) Usually susceptible to specific phage

(d) Twenty % or less of strains seen in family practice and outpatient populations are sensitive to penicillin G

11. Cytomegaloviruses are:

(a) Usually acquired before age 15

(b) Usually acquired as an inapparent infection

(c) Capable of causing fatal generalized infections in neonates

(d) Oncogenic in several animal hosts

12. "Nonspecific" effector mechanisms against infections (in contrast to the specific immune response) include:

(a) Interferon

(b) Lymphokines

(c) Lysozyme of tears and saliva

(d) Alternate complement pathway

13. Which of the following are associated with the immune response to a primary infection by *Mycobacerium tuberculosis?*

(a) Forty-eight to 72 hours after an intradermal injection of purified tuberculoproteins, an induration of 5 mm or more will appear at the inoculation site.

(b) A tubercle or granuloma will eventually form at the sites of bacillary proliferation.

(c) Tubercle bacilli survive and multiply within host macrophages.

(d) The host develops a relatively high antibody titer to tuberculoproteins.

14. The mode of action of diphtherial toxin on mammalian cells is analogous to the action of fusidic acid on bacterial cells at which of the following stages of macromolecular synthesis?

(a) Reversible inhibition of DNA synthesis

(b) Binding to the ribosome resulting in inhibition of mRNA synthesis

(c) Inhibition of membrane integrity

(d) Inhibition of mRNA translation mediated by inactivation of an elongation factor

15. A patient is diagnosed by the physician as having a deep abdominal abscess. The laboratory report identifies the causative agent as *Bacteroides fragilis*. Which of the following antibiotics could be used for therapy?
   (a) Chloramphenicol
   (b) Penicillin G
   (c) Clindamycin
   (d) Erythromycin

16. Chemotherapeutic agent(s) that is (are) safe and effective for systemic treatment of herpetic meningoencephalitis is (are):
   (a) Adenine arabinoside
   (b) Iododeoxyuridine
   (c) Acyclovir
   (d) Isatin-β-thiosemicarbazone

17. Cell-mediated immunity is most important in recovery from primary infections with:
   (a) Herpes simplex virus
   (b) *Streptococcus pyogenes*
   (c) *Mycobacterium tuberculosis*
   (d) *Corynebacterium diphtheriae*

18. Which of the following organisms exhibit a yeast-like form in infected tissues and in culture at 35°C and a mycelial form in the environment and in culture at 22°C?
   (a) *Blastomyces dermatitidis*
   (b) *Coccidioides immitis*
   (c) *Sporothrix schenckii*
   (d) *Cryptococcus neoformans*

19. The source of infection leading to a case of chickenpox may be:
   (a) Vesicular fluid from another child with chickenpox
   (b) Respiratory secretions from another child with chickenpox
   (c) Vesicular fluid from an elderly patient with herpes zoster
   (d) Respiratory secretions from an elderly patient with herpes zoster

20. Regarding hemolytic disease of the newborn:
   (a) It is a cytotoxic type II allergic reaction.
   (b) The mother forms Ab against fetal erythrocyte antigens which she lacks.
   (c) Anti-Rh globulin can suppress sensitization of Rh mothers soon after Rh-positive cell introduction into the mother.
   (d) The fetus forms Ab against maternal erythrocytes and destroys its own red blood cells.

21. Neutrophil membrane constituents that aid in phagocytosis include receptors for:
   (a) Endotoxin
   (b) C3b
   (c) Phytohemagglutinin
   (d) Fc

22. The assembly of human secretory IgA and its transport to secretions is thought to depend on:
   (a) Presence of J-chain in the IgA molecule
   (b) Existence of a disulfide-interchanging enzyme in the mucosal cells
   (c) Presence of secretory component on the surface of epithelial cells
   (d) Presence of secretory component in secretions

23. The major histocompatibility complex (MHC) has genes that code for:
   (a) Serologically detectable cell surface antigens
   (b) Antigens that cause rapid rejection of tissue grafts
   (c) Immune responsiveness
   (d) Blood-group antigens

24. Enzymes involved in the assimilation of ammonia (in the form of ammonia) include:
   (a) Transaminases
   (b) Glutamine synthetase
   (c) Glutamate synthetase
   (d) Glutamate dehydrogenase

25. Vaccines containing only capsular polysaccharide(s) are effective in inducing type- or group-specific immunity in humans against:
   (a) Acute rheumatic fever
   (b) Meningitis due to group C *Neisseria meningitidis*
   (c) Staphylococcal food poisoning
   (d) Pneumonia due to *Streptococcus pneumoniae*

26. Antibiotics that inhibit bacterial growth by interfering with protein synthesis include:
   (a) Streptomycin
   (b) Chloramphenicol
   (c) Erythromycin
   (d) Tetracycline

27. Which of the following mechanisms are known to account for the inactivation of aminoglycoside antibiotics?
   (a) Phosphorylation
   (b) Adenylation
   (c) Acetylation
   (d) Glycosylation

28. Ketoconazole is:
   (a) Antiprotozoal

(b) Useful in treatment of some *Bacteroides* infections

(c) Useful in treatment of trichomoniasis

(d) Antifungal

29. Segmented RNA genomes are characteristic of members of which of the following virus group?
    (a) Arenaviruses
    (b) Reoviruses
    (c) Bunyaviruses
    (d) Orthomyxoviruses

30. Interferon:
    (a) Is species specific
    (b) Reacts directly with virus particles to inactivate them
    (c) Reacts with cells, and the affected cells then become resistant to a number of different viruses
    (d) Is constitutively produced at high levels in cells but requires an inducer for activity

31. Which of the following viruses induce nuclear inclusions in infected cells?
    (a) Cytomegalovirus
    (b) Adenovirus
    (c) Papovaviruses
    (d) Smallpox virus

32. The life cycles of the following parasites include stages that normally pass through lung tissue:
    (a) *Ancylostoma duodenale*
    (b) *Giardia lamblia*
    (c) *Strongyloides stercoralis*
    (d) *Diphyllobothrium latum*

33. Which of the following statements is (are) true about the protozoan parasite *Pneumocystis carinii?*
    (a) It causes widespread disease of many organs in infants.
    (b) As many as two thirds of children have antibody evidence of infection by school age.
    (c) It has a narrow species host range.
    (d) It is pathogenic almost exclusively for immunosuppressed individuals or severely debilitated infants.

34. What immunologic mechanisms may be involved in killing virus-infected cells that display viral antigens on the cell surface?
    (a) Antibody-dependent cell-mediated cytotoxicity
    (b) Complement-dependent immune cytolysis
    (c) Specifically immune T cells
    (d) Secretory IgA

35. Activation of lymphocytes in type IV hypersensitivity (DTH) may result in the release of
    (a) Opsonins
    (b) Interleukins
    (c) Anaphylatoxins
    (d) Mitogenic factor

Section C

Select one (1) of the lettered items that best relates to each of the subsequent words or statements (1–65).

    (a) Mycoplasma
    (b) L forms
    (c) Spheroplast
    (d) Protoplast
    (e) All of the above

1. Can be described as insensitive to antibiotics affecting cell wall synthesis
2. Can be produced from gram-positive or gram-negative bacteria by β-lactam antibiotics
3. Cannot revert to a bacterium with a cell wall

    (a) *Klebsiella pneumoniae*
    (b) *Proteus mirabilis*
    (c) *Escherichia coli*
    (d) *Pseudomonas aeruginosa*

4. The leading cause of urinary tract infections among hospitalized patients
5. Kidney stones possibly induced by alkaline pH of urine associated with urinary tract infections
6. Responsible for respiratory infections in cystic fibrosis patients

    (a) *Shigella dysenteriae*
    (b) Enterotoxigenic *E. coli*
    (c) *Salmonella typhi*
    (d) *Salmonella enteritidis*
    (e) *Vibrio cholerae*

7. Infectious dose may be less than 500 bacteria
8. Often produces (ST) heat stable type of enterotoxin
9. Variations in O antigen produced by lysogenic conversion

    (a) Temperate phage
    (b) Virulent phage
    (c) Neither
    (d) Both

10. Produces enzymes mediating phage DNA insertion into the bacterial chromosome
11. Useful in phage typing of *Salmonella typhi* Vi antigen
12. Employable for gene isolation techniques

    (a) Mumps virus

(b) Rabies virus
(c) Measles virus
(d) Rubella virus
(e) Hepatitis B virus
13. Australia antigen
14. Koplik spots
15. Orchitis
16. Congenital cardiopathies

(a) Inhibition of viral DNA synthesis
(b) Inhibition of viral attachment
(c) Inhibition of viral RNA and/or protein synthesis
(d) None of the above
17. Iododeoxyuridine
18. Interferon
19. Acyclovir

(a) Penicillin V
(b) Cephalothin
(c) Oxacillin
(d) Carbenicillin
(e) Any of the above
20. Allergic reactions occur in less than 10% of individuals who are allergic to ampicillin.
21. Drug most likely to cure the "scalded-skin syndrome"
22. Drug most likely to cure conjunctivitis involving *Pseudomonas* or *Enterobacter*

(a) Spectinomycin
(b) Gentamicin
(c) Tetracycline
(d) All of the above
23. Binds to the 30S portion of the ribosome inhibiting the binding of tRNA to the ribosome–mRNA complex
24. Effect is more bacteriostatic than bactericidal
25. Employed for control of penicillinase-producing strains of *N. gonorrhoeae*
26. Capable of inducing an allergic state

(a) Sulfone
(b) Amphotericin
(c) Rifampicin
(d) Polymyxin
(e) Lincomycin
27. Drug that has a detergent-like action on bacterial membrane
28. Drug that has a detergent-like action on fungal membrane
29. Drug used for *M. leprae*
30. Drug that is used for treatment of *M. tuberculosis*

31. Inhibitor of protein synthesis used for gram-positive infections

---

(a) Penicillin V
(b) Ampicillin
(c) Carbenicillin
(d) Oxacillin
(e) Cephalosporin
32. Designed for use against penicillinase-producing staphylococci
33. Designed for use against gram-negative bacteria but sensitive to many β-lactamases
34. Designed for use against gram-negative bacteria that produce β-lactamase, such as *Pseudomonas*
35. Individuals allergic to penicillin G are not necessarily allergic to this drug

---

(a) *Chlamydia trachomatis*
(b) *Rickettsia rickettsii*
(c) *Coxiella burnettii*
(d) *Chlamydia psittaci*
(e) None of the above
36. Associated with eye infections
37. Associated with urethritis, thin discharge, and genital elephantiasis
38. Can cause high fever and rash with 90% mortality rate in untreated cases
39. Etiologic agent of ornithosis

(a) Reagin of syphilis
(b) Anti-*Treponema pallidum* antibodies
(c) Both
(d) Neither
40. Are present in the serum of patients with secondary syphylitic lesions
41. Decline in titer as the patient responds to treatment
42. Are identified in sera of patients with biologic false-positive reactions in screening tests for syphilis
43. Are measured by the VDRL and RPR screening tests
44. Are measured by the FTA-ABS test

(a) F(+) cell
(b) Hfr cell
(c) F′ cell
(d) F(−) cell
(e) None of the above
45. Transfers all bacterial genes more efficiently than plasmid genes
46. Efficiently transfers only plasmid genes
47. CanNOT transfer bacterial genes

48. Contains an integrated plasmid

    _____

    (a) IgE antibody
    (b) IgA antibody
    (c) IgM antibody
    (d) IgG antibody
    (e) IgD antibody

49. Associated with the release of histamine and slow-reacting substance of anaphylaxis (SRS-A)
50. Functions primarily as an opsonin
51. Most effective in the lysis of certain gram-negative bacteria when complement is present

    _____

    (a) Cell-mediated immunity
    (b) Humoral immunity
    (c) Both cell-mediated and humoral immunity
    (d) Neither cell-mediated nor humoral immunity

52. Demonstrates immunological memory
53. Memory cells may express surface IgD molecules
54. May be passively transferred from an immune to a native recipient
55. Responses may involve lysis of target cells
56. Most of the inflammatory cells at the site of this reaction exhibit specificity for the inducing antigen.

    _____

    (a) Permissive cells
    (b) Nonpermissive cells
    (c) Semipermissive cells
    (d) Resistant cells
    (e) Transformed cells

57. Transformed without virus production
58. Some cells transformed and some yield virus
59. Do not permit expression of any viral genes
60. Lose contact inhibition

    _____

    (a) *Bacteroides fragilis*
    (b) *Peptostreptococcus* species
    (c) *Clostridium tetani*
    (d) *Propionibacterium acnes*
    (e) *Clostridium perfringens*

61. A common anaerobic species usually resistant to penicillin G
62. Produces an enterotoxin as well as numerous toxic enzymes that contribute to its pathogenic potential as an exogenous causative agent of disease
63. A normal skin flora organism found as an invader in the production of endocarditis in patients following open heart surgery

64. A gram-negative rod that is the most common causative agent of anaerobic disease
65. Aerotolerant and/or microaerophilic gram-positive organism that is a common cause of disease frequently in association with other organisms in mixed infections

ANSWERS TO MULTIPLE CHOICE QUESTIONS

Section A

1. (b)	15. (c)	29. (d)	43. (b)
2. (d)	16. (c)	30. (d)	44. (e)
3. (c)	17. (b)	31. (c)	45. (d)
4. (a)	18. (d)	32. (e)	46. (c)
5. (b)	19. (c)	33. (b)	47. (d)
6. (b)	20. (c)	34. (c)	48. (a)
7. (b)	21. (d)	35. (b)	49. (c)
8. (b)	22. (e)	36. (b)	50. (c)
9. (a)	23. (e)	37. (c)	51. (c)
10. (c)	24. (a)	38. (c)	52. (d)
11. (b)	25. (c)	39. (b)	53. (a)
12. (b)	26. (d)	40. (c)	
13. (b)	27. (c)	41. (c)	
14. (c)	28. (d)	42. (a)	

Section B

1. (A)	10. (E)	19. (A)	28. (D)
2. (D)	11. (A)	20. (A)	29. (E)
3. (C)	12. (E)	21. (C)	30. (B)
4. (E)	13. (E)	22. (A)	31. (A)
5. (E)	14. (D)	23. (A)	32. (B)
6. (B)	15. (B)	24. (E)	33. (C)
7. (C)	16. (B)	25. (C)	34. (A)
8. (B)	17. (B)	26. (E)	35. (C)
9. (C)	18. (B)	27. (A)	

Section C

1. (e)	14. (c)	27. (d)	40. (c)
2. (b)	15. (a)	28. (b)	41. (a)
3. (a)	16. (d)	29. (a)	42. (a)
4. (c)	17. (a)	30. (c)	43. (a)
5. (b)	18. (c)	31. (c)	44. (b)
6. (d)	19. (a)	32. (d)	45. (b)
7. (a)	20. (b)	33. (b)	46. (d)
8. (b)	21. (b)	34. (c)	47. (d)
9. (d)	22. (c)	35. (e)	48. (b)
10. (a)	23. (d)	36. (a)	49. (a)
11. (b)	24. (c)	37. (a)	50. (d)
12. (a)	25. (a)	38. (b)	51. (c)
13. (e)	26. (d)	39. (d)	52. (c)

53. (b)	**57.** (b)	**61.** (a)	**65.** (b)
54. (c)	**58.** (c)	**62.** (e)	
55. (c)	**59.** (c)	**63.** (d)	
56. (d)	**60.** (e)	**64.** (a)	

SUGGESTED READINGS

Davis DD, Dulbecco R, Eisen HN, Ginsberg HS (eds): Microbiology, 3rd ed. Hagerstown, MD, Harper & Row, 1980

Rose NR, Barron AL (eds): Microbiology: Basic Principles and Clinical Applications. New York, Macmillan, 1983

Hoeprich PD (ed): Infectious Diseases, 4th ed. Philadelphia, JB Lippincott, 1989

Coonrod JD, Kunz LJ, Ferraro MJ (eds): The Direct Detection of Microorganisms in Clinical Samples. New York, Academic Press, 1983

Schwartz LM (ed): Compendium of Immunology, 2nd ed. Florence, KY, Van Nostrand Reinhold, 1983

Easmon CSF, Jeljaszewicz J (eds): Medical Microbiology, Vol 2: Immunization Against Bacterial Disease. New York, Academic Press, 1983

Warren KS, Mahmoud AAF (eds): Tropical and Geographical Medicine. New York, McGraw-Hill, 1984

Belshe RB (ed): Textbook of Human Virology. Littleton, MA, PSG Publishing, 1984

Notkins AL, Oldstone MBA (eds): Concepts in Viral Pathogenesis. New York, Springer-Verlag, 1984

Strickland GT (ed): Hunter's Tropical Medicine, 6th ed. Philadelphia, WB Saunders, 1984

Sikora K, Smedley HM: Monoclonal Antibodies. Oxford, Blackwell Scientific, 1984

6

Pathology

Jack P. Strong, M.D.
Boyd Professor and Head, Department of
Pathology, Louisiana State University School of
Medicine, New Orleans, Louisiana

This chapter is designed to assist the student or candidate in preparing for medical licensing examination in pathology. It was prepared with the assumption that the reader has completed an adequate course in pathology at some time in the past and has access to and is familiar with a good standard textbook of pathology. This review is therefore designed to emphasize those areas that would be most helpful in preparing for qualifying examinations.

Pathology is that branch of biology concerned with disease (Gr. *pathos,* disease). Disease can be taken to mean any departure from the normal condition of a living plant or animal. Thus, disease is an abnormal condition of a living thing, and pathology is that branch of biology that involves the study of living things in their abnormal forms and conditions.

The broadest definition of pathology is that it is the study of disease. Pathology is the science dealing with diseases: their essential nature, causes and development, and the structural and functional changes produced by them. Pathology is a biological discipline and a branch of the practice of medicine. In pathology as a scientific discipline, the pathologist investigates the causes, mechanisms, and effects of disease by observing tissues and organs in a postmortem examination and by correlating his observations with clinical findings; by examining tissues removed at surgery; by using animal experiments; and by using other methods in the laboratory. In practice, the pathologist acts as a consultant to other physicians in diagnosis of disease during life and after death of the patient by methods of the laboratory—chemistry, microbiology, serology, hematology, examination of surgically removed specimens, and autopsy or postmortem examination.

DISEASE AND ILLNESS

Illness is the reaction between the disease and the individual. In other words, individual plus disease equals illness. This is a useful consideration for the student of pathology: that he is *learning of disease,* as such. On the wards and in the clinics he learns about illness as he studies interaction of disease and patient. Obviously, one must know about disease to study and treat illness.

Disease, at least in its initial stages, is no more than a slight departure from the normal condition. While the student usually learns from study of advanced disease, he should always keep in mind that the disease process is a condition that arose from normal or healthy tissue and cells and that even in a severe disease—one with the greatest disruption of structure and deformity—many of the cells of the body or of the affected organ system are still within "normal" limits.

ETIOLOGY, PATHOGENESIS, AND LESIONS

In pathology, the terms etiology, pathogenesis, and lesions are used as key words to the study of disease.

Etiology refers to the cause of disease. There usually is a primary cause of a disease, but often there are many predisposing or contributing factors. For lobar pneumonia in a skid row alcoholic patient who is malnourished, has poor oral hygiene, and who was exposed to the elements while sleeping on a doorstep, the main etiologic agent is the pneumococcus organism, but the other factors have also contributed to the disease.

Pathogenesis refers to the mechanism of development of disease, or the stepwise development of disease.

A *lesion* is the result of disease, or the characteristic change in an organism produced by disease. From the viewpoint of recognition of disease, it is fortunate that constant and characteristic changes in the tissues and cells are frequently produced by disease. Many of them can be recognized grossly with the naked eye or microscopically. The electron microscope has greatly extended the ability to recognize the changes of disease. However, many diseases produce lesions at the level of the constituent metabolic units, the molecules. The classical example is sickle cell disease, which is due to an abnormal hemoglobin molecule with an abnormal pattern of amino acids in the protein. To encompass all of these changes, a lesion can be defined to be a tissue, cellular, or molecular alteration which develops as a result of disease-producing or pathogenic agents.

Some examples: Lobar pneumonia is a lesion. A myocardial infarct is a lesion. A mole is a lesion of the skin. A cataract is a lesion. A tumor of the lung is a lesion. A hemorrhoid is a lesion. A fractured rib is a lesion. An abrasion is a lesion. A boil is a lesion. A tumor of bone is a lesion. The hemoglobin molecule in a sickle cell disease is a lesion. The coating of an infant's red blood cells (RBCs) with antibody in hemolytic disease of the newborn is a lesion.

In a specimen of diseased tissue, whether obtained by surgery or at autopsy, one is examining an instant only—a piece in a continuous progression, a frozen section of time, a single frame of a motion picture. The student of disease must study disease processes at many different stages so that he can reconstruct the development of the disease.

GENERAL PATHOLOGY

The Cell

The human body is a vast, highly organized and complex accumulation of living cells. It is the condition of these cells that determines the state of health of the body or any of its parts. When the cells are normal and healthy, the body is healthy; when cells or specific groups of cells become disturbed or disorganized for any cause, then that part of the body, or under certain circumstances the entire body, is said to be the seat of disease. It seems wise, therefore, to start our discussion of pathology at the level of the cell.

THE NORMAL CELL

Every organ of the body consists of recognizable basic histologic patterns of cells of different types and the associated stroma. The cell is therefore regarded as the basic unit of multicellular organisms, including man. The basic structural and functional components of the cell can be divided into two groups: those that are essential for survival of the cell and those that serve specialized functions characteristic of the differentiated cell type. The former group, which can be regarded as basic components, consists of plasma membrane (maintenance of intracellular environment), the nucleus and nucleolus (site of genetic information and expression), mitochondria (energy production and storage through oxidative phosphorylation of compounds derived from nutrients), endoplasmic reticulum and ribosomes (protein synthesis), and centrioles (cell division). Soluble proteins of the cytoplasm, which contain the enzymes of the glycolytic pathway and other essential systems, also belong to this group. Although the Golgi bodies (transport of the products of protein synthesis) and lysosomes (storage of hydrolytic enzymes) are more specialized organelles, their widespread distribution in cells of different types justifies their inclusion in the group of basic cellular components. The group of specialized cell products includes striated and smooth myofilaments of skeletal and smooth muscle cells, zymogen granules of exocrine cells, neurofilaments of the nerve cell, hemoglobin of the erythroid cells, and others.

Although most cell organelles can be demonstrated by a battery of special methods in cytologic preparations used in light microscopy, detailed structural organization can be observed only with the electron microscope. Basic structural elements, seen at such high resolution, are the systems of membranes of molecular dimensions and well-defined particulate materials. The former, present in the plasma membrane, mitochondrial envelope, endoplasmic reticulum, Golgi vesicles, and nuclear membrane, consist of lamellae of lipid and protein molecules in fine distribution such that the macroscopically invisible substances do not segregate into larger droplets or vacuoles. The presence of large aggregations of lipids is therefore a sign of differentiation (cells of adipose reserve and the adrenal cortex) or of a disease process. The particular elements include chromatin material in the nucleus, nucleolus, and ribosomes, all of which contain nucleic acids.

To perform its specialized functions adequately, the normal cell must have sufficient basic structural and metabolic components to remain alive and to produce its specialized products. The numbers of different organelles and the amounts of soluble enzymes must vary according to the physiologic requirements as well as to the local environment. The normal state consists of a range of successful adaptive changes, rather than a rigid, idealized condition.

In routine histologic reactions used for light microscopy, the tissues are stained with a combination of an acidic and a basic dye. The cytoplasmic organelles are usually not demonstrable. Macromolecules with amphoteric properties stain differently according to the balance of the acidic and basic groups. Structures rich in acid groups of nucleic acids and certain mucopolysaccharides have strong affinity for the basic dye, while proteins are usually stained with the acid dye. The nucleus and ergastoplasms (large accumulations of ribosomes in rough endoplasmic reticulum) are thus basophilic, while the cytoplasm and many differentiated structures are acidophilic.

CELLULAR ADAPTATION

Cells adapt to alterations in their environment. The term cellular adaptation is applied to those changes which are intermediate between the normal unstressed cell and the overstressed injured cell. An example is the increase in muscle size in laborers or body builders in which there is an increase in size of individual muscle bundles as a response to increased work load. The most important changes of cellular adaptation include induction of endoplasmic reticulum or hypertrophy of endoplasmic reticulum, hypertrophy, atrophy, hyperplasia, and metaplasia. Three terms that are commonly considered in conjunction with these adaptive changes, even though they are not adaptive in nature, but are related to failure of an organ to develop—hypoplasia, aplasia, and agenesis—will also be considered in this section.

Induction of Endoplasmic Reticulum. The livers of patients who have received repeated administration of barbiturates over a period of time will develop more endoplasmic reticulum in response to

the drug administration. As a result they are able to detoxify a given amount of the barbiturate more rapidly. Once an increased amount of endoplasmic reticulum is present in the liver, the liver cells can also detoxify certain other drugs as well. This adaptive change is protective for the cell.

Atrophy. Atrophy is shrinkage of a cell by loss of cell substance, or decrease in the size of an organ due to decrease in the size of cells. The causes of atrophy include decreased work load, loss of innervation, diminished blood supply, inadequate nutrition, or loss of endocrine stimulation. Examples of atrophy are the muscles of a limb that has been immobilized in a cast, decrease in size of the testes or ovaries with old age, a decrease in the size of the thymus in the normal aging process. In atrophic tissue, in addition to the decrease in size apparent by gross inspection, microscopic changes are also apparent where autophagic vacuoles, or residual bodies, occur as a result of sequestration of cell organelles due to focal injury within the cells. The residual bodies are seen as lipofuscin granules under the light microscope. Lipofuscin is the so-called wear and tear pigment associated with aging and atrophy. It imparts a brown color to atrophic tissue such as the heart and liver.

Hypertrophy. Hypertrophy refers to increase in size of cells with resultant increase in the size of an organ. New cells are not formed in hypertrophy; there is enlargement of preexisting cells. The striated muscle cells hypertrophy in the muscles of a body builder. The myocardial muscle fibers increase in size in response to elevated blood pressure and increased peripheral resistance as well as to valvular disease that produces stenosis or insufficiency.

Hyperplasia. When stressed, cells capable of mitotic activity may respond by increasing in number. Hyperplasia is the increase in the number of cells in an organ or tissue, which usually results in increased size or volume. Hyperplasia and hypertrophy sometimes, but not always, develop concurrently. Hyperplasia may occur physiologically in response to changes in endocrine stimulation. The breast during puberty, pregnancy, and lactation is an example of an organ that undergoes hyperplasia of its component cells. In the gravid uterus there is both hyperplasia and hypertrophy of smooth muscle of the myometrium. Pathologic hyperplasia may follow excessive hormonal stimulation, for example, endometrial hyperplasia, thyroid hyperplasia, adrenal hyperplasia.

Hypoplasia, Aplasia, and Agenesis. The terms hypoplasia, aplasia, and agenesis are usually defined in conjunction with adaptive changes even though they are developmental abnormalities. Hypoplasia is failure of an organ to reach full adult size. Hypoplasia is a less severe developmental arrest than aplasia and agenesis. The organ, usually a lung or kidney, remains small rather than reaching full adult size. Aplasia and agenesis refer to total failure of an organ to develop.

Metaplasia. Metaplasia is a reversible change in which one adult cell type is replaced by another adult cell type usually as a result of chronic irritation. The change from normal pseudostratified ciliated columnar epithelium in the tracheobronchial tree to stratified squamous epithelium in the habitual cigarette smoker is an example of metaplasia. Change to stratified squamous epithelium from mucus-producing columnar epithelium in the endocervix is an example of metaplasia. Dysplastic and anaplastic changes representing a progression from normal adult cell types are covered in the section on neoplasia.

CELL INJURY AND RESPONSE

Because of our greatly increased knowledge of the structure and function of living cells, a consideration of the pathologic changes that result following injury and disease calls for more intensive study of disease processes at a deeper and more fundamental level. Since the cell is the basic functional unit of the organism, all abnormalities in the normal processes of the body that result from injury or disease must originate in the cell.

The causes of injury to cells may be grouped as follows:

1. Physical agents, such as trauma, heat, cold, electrical energy and radiant energy from different sources, may affect cells in a variety of ways—simple destruction of cells, burning or freezing of cells, or effects on the molecular structure of cell constituents such as water, enzymes, and proteins.
2. Chemical agents, such as acids, alkalies, and various poisons, may destroy cell membranes, alter cell functions, and even cause death of the entire organism.
3. Living agents such as bacteria, viruses, rickettsiae, and protozoan parasites of various kinds cause cell damage and death in a variety of ways. Viruses, for example, may actually compete for essential substances such as enzymes required for normal cell metabolism and convert them to their own use, thus indirectly destroying the cell.

4. Nutritional disturbances, especially the deprivation of protein or essential vitamins, but also nutritional excesses that may lead to obesity.
5. Genetic defects transmitted as hereditary diseases or resulting from mutations in the developing embryo.
6. Disturbances in arterial circulation leading to loss of blood supply and hypoxia.
7. Derangements in the immune mechanism based on exogenous or endogenous antigen stimuli.
8. Aging, with widespread regressive changes occurring in the brain, muscle, and gonads, sometimes suggesting a "genetic clock."

General Features of Cell Injury. Changes that occur following injury may affect both the cell cytoplasm and the nucleus, alterations in the latter being the more serious. It must be borne in mind, however, that, in the light of present knowledge, recognizable morphologic changes indicative of injury follow by a considerable time the first damaging effects that occur at the molecular level and are therefore not recognizable by any method yet available. The first recognizable changes are found in the cytoplasm, may be reversible, and are manifested by an increase in fluid content and swelling of the mitochondria. If the injury is more severe, the endoplasmic reticulum becomes swollen and vacuolated, and the ribosomes of the granular endoplasmic reticulum dissolve and disintegrate, leading to impaired protein synthesis. The lysosomes in the cells that contain them may rupture and undergo hydrolysis. Lipoprotein production is impaired, and lipid droplets may accumulate from cytoplasm degeneration or from damage to the cell membrane. Injured or damaged cytoplasmic organelles may become isolated in vacuoles or even digested by lysosomal enzymes.

Even if these changes appear severe in the cytoplasm, they may still be reversible if the nucleus remains relatively unimpaired and the injurious agent is removed or destroyed before nuclear damage is excessive. Irreparable damage to the nucleus is manifested by changes usually recognizable by light microscopy. These are the shrinkage in size of the nucleus and the accumulation of the chromatin into a dense homogeneous shrunken mass (*pyknosis*), the disintegration of the chromatin into fine granular fragments that are extruded through the ruptured nuclear membrane (*karyorrhexis*), and the swelling of the nucleus with disappearance of the chromatin (*karyolysis*). These nuclear changes are characteristic of cell death.

As the degenerative changes progress in the damaged cell the deoxyribonucleic acid (DNA) is impaired and the metabolic and synthetic activities of the cell, particularly the replication of DNA and the synthesis of ribonucleic acid (RNA) and protein, which are very sensitive to injury, are seriously interfered with and with cell death cease altogether. In spite of the fact that early and reversible, as well as late and irreversible, morphologic degenerative changes can be recognized in some cells by ordinary light microscopy, it is not possible, even with the elaborate methods of study that exist today, to follow stage by stage the biochemical alterations from slight to fatal cell injury. This is due to the fact that these changes take place at the molecular level where they are impossible to detect or observe.

Reversible Cell Injury and Degenerations. The most common reactions of the cell to injury are swelling, with or without the accumulation or appearance of abnormal substances in the cytoplasm and, later, changes of various kinds in the nucleus. Whether or not a change is reversible depends usually upon the severity of the injury to the nucleus.

Cloudy swelling, or *parenchymatous degeneration* or, still better, *cellular swelling,* since the first two designations refer especially to the gross appearance of the affected organ, is a reversible phenomenon observed most commonly in the parenchymal cells of the heart, the kidneys, and the liver. It occurs in these and other organs in most cases of acute infection or poisoning and is the most common type of acute degeneration. The affected organ is swollen, the capsule is tense, and the cut surface bulges. The tissue is opaque, pale, soft, and more friable than normal. The usual vascular markings may be retained. Microscopically the cells appear swollen, and their outlines may, or in some cases may not, be distinct. The swelling is due to the imbibition of water, and the granularity results from changes occurring in the finer cytoplasmic structures such as swelling, vesiculation or rupture of the endoplasmic reticulum, swelling, distortion and disruption of the mitochondria, and damage to the plasma membrane.

Hydropic degeneration is a more advanced, but still reversible, form of cellular swelling in which there is a greater degree of imbibition of water by the cell. In the gross, the general appearance resembles that of cellular swelling. Microscopically the parenchymal cells involved show fine and coarse vacuolization of the cytoplasm, due primarily to dilatation of the sacs of the endoplasmic reticulum and disaggregation of the ribosomal clusters. This form of degeneration may be seen as the result of any form of infection or poisoning, especially in the epithelial cells lining the convoluted tubules of the kidneys. The best examples of hydropic degeneration are seen in these cells after intravenous administration of hypertonic sucrose or ingestion of diethylene glycol or in patients with hypokalemia.

Fatty Change. Many terms have been used for abnormal accumulation of fat in the cytoplasm of parenchymal cells, including fatty degeneration, fatty metamorphosis, fatty phanerosis; however, fatty change is the most widely accepted term. There is general agreement about the following statements concerning fatty change. The appearance of fat vacuoles within cells represents an absolute increase in intracellular lipids. Fat accumulation in cells is not related to the type of injury but to an imbalance in production, utilization, or mobilization of fat. Many varied derangements lead to fatty change; thus, fatty change is a common expression of many types of cell injury or cell overload. Fatty change may be preceded by cellular swelling and imbibition of fluid. While reversible itself fatty change may be followed by cell death and is often seen in cells adjacent to necrotic cells.

Fatty change is seen most often in the liver, heart, and kidney. The liver enlarges and becomes yellow and greasy. Microscopically the process begins with development of small membrane-bound inclusions closely applied to the endoplasmic reticulum. As seen by light microscopy, small vacuoles occur first in the cytoplasm; they later coalesce to form large clear spaces on hematoxylin and eosin-stained sections. The vacuoles displace the nucleus to the periphery. In advanced cases the liver may almost resemble adipose tissue. Sometimes the cells rupture and fat globules coalesce to form larger fatty cysts.

After moderate but prolonged hypoxia such as may be seen in long-standing severe anemia, the heart may grossly have a "thrush breast" or "tabby cat" appearance with alternating bands of yellowish myocardium and darker red-brown myocardium. The yellow areas represent myocardium with fatty change and the darker areas are normal fibers. These changes are related to vascularization of the myocardium with the uninvolved area being closer to blood vessels and less subject to hypoxia. Histologically fat in the myocardial fibers is distributed in minute cytoplasmic vacuoles best seen after fat stains.

The kidneys also may be involved with fatty change. They become enlarged, pale, and yellow. The proximal convoluted tubules are most often affected with fat accumulation. Chemical poisonings and profound anemia are among the causes of fatty change of the kidneys.

Hyaline Degeneration. This is an unsatisfactory term usually applied to a variety of changes, some of which cannot be classed as true degenerations. The term *hyaline* is a descriptive term applied to any material that has a structureless, smooth, homogeneous, almost glassy appearance, and that stains pink by hematoxylin and eosin stains. The normal colloid of the thyroid gland is hyaline in appearance. Amyloid also appears hyaline, but it is not a true degeneration but rather an abnormal product of cell activity about which more will be said later. But there are changes that can be classified as degenerative or as the result of degeneration to which the term hyaline degeneration can be applied. Scar tissue anywhere, especially as it gets older, may become the seat of hyaline change, and a similar alteration can be found in the dense fibrous tissue of atherosclerotic plaques. Hyalinization of the walls of renal arterioles is typical of a severe form of chronic hypertension. Foci of hyaline degeneration can be found in neoplasms and, under certain conditions, for example, as a result of mercury poisoning, in the epithelial cells of the proximal convoluted tubules of the kidneys where the hyaline material occurs as droplets. Similar hyaline droplets can be seen in liver cells as a result of infection (yellow fever) or in the form of cirrhosis common in alcoholics. *Zenker's hyaline degeneration* is a special form that affects striated muscles and occurs as a complication of typhoid fever, influenza, and sometimes pneumonia. It is most common in the rectus muscle of the abdomen and may result in rupture of the fibers of this muscle. Microscopically, there is hyaline transformation of the affected muscle fibers with loss of their characteristic striations.

Amyloidosis. Amyloid is one of the hyalins that has certain more or less definite chemical properties and characteristic staining reactions with iodine, Congo red, and crystal violet. The chemical composition is not known; it is probably not a single substance but rather a group of related compounds that consists primarily of a protein polysaccharide complex. Amyloid is insoluble in water but soluble in strong alkalies and slightly soluble in strong acids. It is apparently an abnormal synthetic product of cells and begins as a deposit in the spaces between the cells. As it increases in amount, it causes pressure atrophy and sometimes disappearance of the adjacent cells and in some organs, especially the kidneys, may result in severe and even fatal injury.

Although amyloid appears to be a smooth, glassy, hyaline material when viewed through the light microscope, electron microscopic studies show it to be a complex accumulation of fine fibrils and rodlike structures, the fibrils predominating. The most common form appears as a complication of long-standing chronic infections, especially tuberculosis, leprosy, chronic osteomyelitis, and occasionally in other wasting disease. The condition may be focal or diffuse and microscopically appears in the form of an accumulation of a hyaline, structureless material in the region of the basement membrane of epithelial cells and surrounding capillaries or in the form of nodules replacing lymphoid tissue, as in the spleen. Most of the manifestations of amyloidosis are of this *secondary* type, occurring in parenchymatous organs or lymphoid tissue, mainly liver, kidneys, adrenals, or spleen. There is a form of *primary* amyloidosis, however, that occurs without any obvious cause. In this form the deposits are found in the mesenchymal tissue of the tongue, larynx, myocardium, or adipose tissue. A third form of amyloidosis may also occur in association with multiple myeloma. Localized amyloid tumors occur rarely.

Mucinous Degeneration. Mucin is structureless, clear, and viscid or slimy. It is composed of both carbohydrate and protein, is slightly acid and therefore stains faintly blue with basic stains. Mucinous degeneration occurs most commonly in association with catarrhal inflammation, and mucus is secreted in excess into the lumina of ducts. It is particularly common in mucinous carcinoma in various sites. An epithelial tumor cell filled with mucin in its cytoplasm, with the nucleus pushed aside, is another good example of a signet-ring cell.

Mucoid Degeneration. This is a change that occurs in connective tissue. It is found most commonly in subcutaneous regions in the myxedema of thyroid deficiency and in myxomatous neoplasms of bone, breast, and other organs. It differs significantly from mucin only in its higher sulfur content.

Irreversible Cell Injury (Necrosis). Necrosis is the term applied to cell or tissue death in the living body. It is difficult to determine exactly when death of a cell takes place for cells vary in their susceptibility to injury, and, as noted above, the earliest changes, being at the molecular level, are not detectable. Presumably certain powerful toxins or noxious agents can cause immediate cell death. Most probably, however, death comes more gradually, the cell first manifesting the cytoplasmic changes that characterize degenerations of various types and going on, with continuation of the injurious effect, to loss of cell structure, fragmentation of organelles and liquefaction of the cytoplasm, and the typical nuclear changes (pyknosis, karyolysis and karyorrhexis) that are indicative of actual cell death. Necrosis of tissue is merely the sum total of the necrosis of masses of cells. The causes of necrosis include injurious agents of many kinds: physical, chemical, bacterial, or viral, and so forth, as well as any cause of anoxia. From a morphologic standpoint necrosis may be of several types:

Coagulation necrosis, seen best in early infarction, is characterized by the general preservation of the architectural features of the organ, but with loss of cellular detail.

Liquefaction necrosis is characterized by the softening and eventual liquefaction of the dead tissue, such as is seen in infarcts of the brain or in the center of a furuncle or boil.

Caseous necrosis is characterized by its soft, cheesy gross appearance and is typical of tuberculous necrosis.

Gummatous necrosis resembles caseous necrosis; however, it is not soft, but rubbery and firm. It is typical of tertiary lesions of syphilis.

Fat necrosis is associated with pancreatic injuries or diseases such as the uncommon but serious condition known as acute hemorrhagic pancreatitis and is due to the liberation of pancreatic enzymes, notably lipases, amylases, and proteases, which act on the intraabdominal, mesenteric, omental, and even pancreatic fat, forming minute, circumscribed chalky white spots in these tissues. Microscopically these foci of recent necrosis usually are surrounded by extravasated red blood cells and polymorphonuclear leukocytes. Later, they may become the seat of deposition of calcium, with surrounding foreign-body type of inflammatory reaction.

Gangrene is massive death with putrefaction of a part of the body. *Moist gangrene* occurs in parts that are moist and congested. *Dry gangrene,* or mummification, develops in parts that are anemic or dry at the time of tissue death. It is most common in the extremities, in which, if caused by arteriosclerosis, it may develop slowly, but it may occur with great rapidity when a thrombus, forming on the roughened intima of an artery, or a large embolus from the left heart, cuts off the circulation suddenly. *Diabetic gangrene* results from arteriosclerosis. Gangrene in Raynaud's disease and ergot poisoning is caused by a spasm of the small arteries; that of thromboangiitis obliterans is due to endarteritis of toxic or infective origin and may be unilateral. Gangrene may also be caused by trauma, pressure, freezing, or infection, particularly infection caused by *Clostridium perfringens* in which it is associated with the formation of gas bubbles (hydrogen) within the tissues, producing the typical crepitus of this infection.

Zonal necrosis refers to conditions in which the injurious agent selectively affects a certain "zone" of a unit structure: for example, carbon tetrachloride causes necrosis of the efferent part of the lobule (centrilobular necrosis), yellow fever is reported to affect the middle zone of the lobules, and phosphorous poisoning affects the peripheral (efferent) portion of the lobule.

Focal necrosis consists of minute foci of dead tissue and is characteristic of lesions found typically in the liver in typhoid fever.

Sequelae of Necrosis. Inflammation occurs as a reaction to the injurious agent and to the components of necrotic tissue. Regeneration may occur particularly if the supportive stroma is not damaged irreversibly and if some parenchymal cells capable of regeneration survive. Repair with granulation tissue and subsequent scarring will fill a defect and replace necrotic tissue in many instances. Dissolution of tissue with cavity or cyst formation may occur as in pulmonary tuberculosis. Deposition of mineral salts (calcium and phosphorus) may occur if the necrotic tissue remains for an extended time leading to dystrophic calcification.

Calcification (Pathologic). In all sites where degenerated or necrotic tissues are found, especially following old infections such as tuberculosis, histoplasmosis or coccidioidomycosis, or almost any focus of old, chronic infection, calcification is referred to as dystrophic and is determined in great part by the local relative alkalinity of the tissue. The deposit is mainly calcium phosphate and carbonate. Dystrophic calcification is not caused by hypercalcemia. *Metastatic calcification* is a form in which previous degenerative or necrotizing changes in the tissues do not occur; it is associated with hypercalcemia from any cause, such as the destruction of bone and the solution of its deposit of calcium, hyperparathyroidism, hypervitaminosis D, or even excessive intake of calcium. The calcium is deposited wherever acid is being eliminated and there is relative alkalinity of tissues, such as in the kidney (phosphoric acid), the stomach (hydrochloric acid), and the lungs (carbonic acid).

Somatic death is death of the organism. In somatic death, rigor mortis refers to stiffening of skeletal muscles after death; algor mortis refers to gradual cooling of the body; and livor mortis refers to reddish discoloration of the dependent portions of the body due to gravitational sinking of the blood.

Inflammation, Regeneration, and Repair

Inflammation is the local reaction of the living body to any injury. Whether the tissues are bruised, cut, burned, invaded by pathogenic microorganisms, or in any other way hurt or damaged, a complicated and well-coordinated series of vascular and cellular reactions occurs at the site of injury. The object of these reactions is to destroy or remove the injurious agent if possible or to limit its spread, to neutralize toxins, to remove the remnants of destroyed tissues, and to prepare the area for the final repair of the damage that was done. The injurious agents may be physical, mechanical, chemical, bacterial, viral, toxic, or nutritional.

Repair, on the other hand, is the process whereby an attempt is made to restore to a normal, or approximately normal, state, the part of the body that has been injured. Cells that have been destroyed are either replaced by healthy cells of the same type growing in from adjacent living tissue *(regeneration)* or by the replacement of the dead cells by fibrous tissue and new blood vessels that also come from uninjured neighboring tissues (*granulation tissue* or *scar tissue* formation). There is a gradual merging from inflammation to repair. The repair process is one of the end stages of the inflammatory reaction just as it is for tissue necrosis.

FUNDAMENTAL MECHANISMS OF INFLAMMATION

Nearly 100 years ago Cohnheim gave such a clear and vivid account of the microscopic changes that occur at the site of acute inflammation that little can be added as a result of modern studies. He noted the dilatation of the local arterioles, venules and, ultimately, capillaries in the region of injury, the initial acceleration and later slowing of the blood flow, the escape of fluid from vessels into the surrounding tissue spaces, the margination of leukocytes along the endothelial linings followed by the emigration of these cells through the vessel walls into the region of injury. We can now attempt to explain these changes in some detail.

The main features of the acute inflammatory reaction can be divided into four broad headings: (1) active hyperemia; (2) increased microvascular permeability; (3) cellular exudation; and (4) reversal of these changes, resolution, regeneration, and repair.

INFLAMMATORY CELLS

The inflammatory cells are derived from leukocytes of the blood and certain tissue cells. The normal proportions of leukocytes of the blood are as follows: neutrophils 54% to 73%, eosinophils 2% to 4%, basophils 0% to 1%, monocytes 4% to 8%, and lymphocytes 21% to 35%. The proportion of these cells changes in disease states and with inflammatory conditions. The large variety of changes with

disease states is beyond the scope of this review. Only the basic characteristics of the inflammatory cells will be summarized.

A. Blood Cells
1. Polymorphonuclear leukocytes (granulocytes)
   a. Neutrophils—short-lived, end-stage cells remaining in the blood for 18 to 36 hours. They are mature when released from bone marrow with no further proliferation. Neutrophils are the first cells to accumulate in the acute inflammatory response. They are removed from the inflammatory site by phagocytic activity of macrophages or by dissolution and removal of lymph channels. They are actively motile and have directional mobility in the presence of chemotactic agents. They are actively phagocytic and are aided in phagocytosis by antibodies that coat the infectious organisms (opsonins). They contain receptors for IgG. They are the chief cells in pus and are sometimes called pus cells when found in tissues or urine. Neutrophils contain two types of granules, large azure granules containing acid hydrolases, neutral proteases, myeloperoxidase, cationic proteins and lysozyme (muramidase), and smaller specific granules that contain alkaline phosphatase, lactoferrin, and lysozyme.
   b. Eosinophils—short-lived cells with many functions in common with neutrophils, including motility and phagocytosis. They respond chemotactically to split products of C3 and C5 and to the trimolecular complex of C567. Eosinophils phagocytize antigens and antibody complexes. They are commonly seen in allergic responses and in the healing phase of inflammation. They also respond to eosinophil chemotactic factor of anaphylaxis (ECF-A), which is secreted by basophils. Ultrastructurally they contain characteristic crystalloid granules.
   c. Basophils—similar to tissue mast cells but less numerous. They have metachromatic granules that contain heparin and histamine in the preformed state (and in some species, not humans, serotonin).
2. Monocytes—the blood phase of the monocyte–macrophage system. They have a much longer life span than polymorphonuclear leukocytes, and they may progress in maturation

after liberation from the bone marrow. In some instances they may divide and proliferate. Most of the monocytes leave the blood stream to become tissue macrophages. Both monocytes and macrophages are vividly phagocytic, taking up both small and large particles, dead cells, cellular debris, and erythrocytes. They are markedly responsive to chemotactic agents $C3_a$ and $C5_a$ but are not responsive to C567. They also respond to certain lymphocyte products (lymphokines) and are modified by other lymphocyte products. Monocytes sometimes, but not always, kill the organisms they ingest.

3. Lymphocytes—small round cells that are less motile than neutrophils and monocytes and are not responsive to the usual chemotactic agents. They are related to the immune system and there are two basic types. The T-cells originate in the thymus and are related to cell-mediated immunity. The B-cells are related to plasma cells and are involved with immunoglobulin production and humoral immunity. The small or medium lymphocytes mediate antigen recognition and cellular immunity. The sensitized lymphocytes recognize and react with the antigens that stimulated their appearance.

B. Tissue cells
   1. Mast cells—similar to basophils. They contain heparin, histamine, and ECF-A. Mast cells also produce leukotrienes and platelet activating-factor (PAF).
   2. Tissue histiocyte or macrophage—the tissue counterpart of the blood monocyte and part of the reticuloendothelial system. These cells have great phagocytic activity especially when particulate matter is to be removed. Many macrophages are derived from monocytes, and some are derived from other tissue macrophages. They may become modified by what they have ingested. For example, hemosiderin-laden macrophages are seen in congestive heart failure secondary to mitral stenosis when they have ingested erythrocytes that have entered the alveolar spaces. They may contain carbon particles, parts of necrotic cells, and microorganisms, some of which can live symbiotically within the cells.
   3. Giant cells—multinucleated cells found in tissue formed by fusion of histiocytes. They may contain 50 or more nuclei.
   4. Plasma cells—not normally found in blood and not phagocytic. They are rich in endo-plasmic reticulum and active in protein synthesis. Plasma cells produce large quantities of immunoglobulins. They arise from B lymphocytes in the germinal center of lymph nodes, spleen, and the gastrointestinal (GI) tract.

SEQUENCE OF EVENTS IN ACUTE INFLAMMATION

The chronological sequence of events that occurs in acute inflammatory reactions from onset to termination with resolution is as follows:

Transient vasoconstriction
Dilatation of arterioles
Speeding of blood stream
Increase in permeability of venules and capillaries
Exudation of fluid rich in proteins—albumin and globulins, followed by fibrinogen (largest molecular weight)—between the junctions of endothelial cells of venules
Concentration and packing of erythrocytes
Slowing of blood stream, stasis, loss of laminar axial flow
Peripheral orientation of leukocytes (neutrophils) with margination and pavementing
Emigration of neutrophils first, monocytes second, and then other cells
Diapedesis of erythrocytes if injury is severe enough
Accumulation or aggregation of leukocytes and fluid in area of irritant
Phagocytosis of irritants by neutrophils and monocytes
Killing of microorganisms if present
Reversal of vascular changes
Neutrophils and monocytes carry off debris
Fluid reabsorbed by venules and by lymphatic drainage
Repair by ingrowth of capillaries and fibroblasts

This list of changes is essentially what Cohnheim saw and described those many years ago.

MEDIATORS OF INFLAMMATION

The two main classes of inflammatory mediators for acute inflammation are vasopermeability factors and leukotactic (chemotactic) factors. Vasopermeability factors have to do with increasing the permeability of the microvasculature, and leukotactic factors have to do with stimulating the unidirectional migration of white blood cells toward an attractant. Chemotaxis is the process in which inflammatory cells move toward a chemical attractant in a unidirectional manner with responsiveness to gradients.

Vasopermeability Factors. Vasopermeability is transient and temporary and only occurs when mediators are present. Increased permeability of the microvasculature begins in the venules and venular end of the capillary loops. Most investigators have concluded that it occurs because of changes in the endothelial cell junctions, which become open to the passage of fluid. Permeability factors apparently work by loosening endothelial cell junctions. All the vasopermeability factors that have been described cause smooth muscle cells to contract. They cause periendothelial cells (modified smooth muscle cells) and endothelial cells to contract, thus widening the endothelial cell junctions. Vasopermeability effects are temporary. They go away when the chemical mediators are no longer present. They do not lead to loss of erythrocytes and leukocytes from the vascular lumen.

There is a biphasic response for vasopermeability in the mild acute inflammatory response, an immediate and a delayed response. The first immediate phase of vasopermeability is histamine dependent and can be blocked by the administration of antihistamine drugs. Mast cells contain vasoactive amines (histamine). Several reactions can cause liberation of histamine from mast cells, including cytotoxic reaction and anaphylactic reaction. Certain products of the complement system, anaphylatoxins ($C3_a$, $C5_a$ cleavage products), can cause secretion of vasoactive amines by mast cells and increased vasopermeability.

The second or delayed phase of increased permeability is totally independent of the first. Antihistamines do not block the action. There is no clear single cause; probably multiple factors are involved. Those agents suspected of being involved in the delayed phase of vasopermeability include kinins, prostaglandins, and products of the complement system.

The common features of all vasopermeability factors are that they are reversible and temporary, acting only when present. They cause contraction of smooth muscle cells and opening of endothelial cell junctions.

The following is a list of suspected vasopermeability factors:

Vasoactive amines—histamine, serotonin
Kinins—bradykinin, a simple basic peptide generated by activation of the kinin system (involves Hageman factor XII, kallikrein, and kininogen). (Note: review kinin generating system and Hageman factor involvement in the coagulation cascade, kinin generating system, and fibrinolytic system.)
PF/dil—activated form of Hageman factor
Leukokinins—peptides generated by enzymes from leukocytes
Basic (cationic) peptides—preformed in lysosomal granules of leukocytes
Leukotrienes C_4, D_4, and E_4, formerly designated as slow-reacting substance of anaphylaxis (SRS-A)—substances generated in cell membranes from arachidonic acid by the lipoxygenase pathway
Prostaglandins and related compounds—substances generated from arachidonic acid by the cyclo-oxygenase pathway
Prostaglandins PGE, PGD_2, PGF_{2a}—vasodilation and edema
Prostacyclin in endothelium—inhibits platelet aggregation, potentiates edema, vasodilatation
Thromboxane A_2—vasoconstriction and platelet aggregation
Anaphylatoxins ($C3_a$, $C5_a$)—act by liberating histamine from mast cells and platelets

Leukotactic (Chemotactic) Mediators. The major substances that have been shown to attract white blood cells and which might play a role in acute inflammation include the following:

Leukotactic Factors of Host Origin

1. Complement derivatives (review complement cascade). Some chemotactic factors affect only neutrophils, some affect only monocytes, and others affect both. Fragments of C3 and C5 are chemotactic for both neutrophils and monocytes. The trimolecular complex of C567 is chemotactic for neutrophils but not for monocytes.
2. Leukotriene B_4. This leukotriene generated from arachidonic acid is a potent chemotactic agent and causes aggregation of leukocytes.
3. Cationic protein. Chemotactic for monocytes.
4. Activated plasma enzymes. Probably not very important to chemotactic factors.
5. Lymphocyte products—lymphokines. The most important of these is MIF (migration-inhibiting factor).
6. Tissue products—collagenase. Tissue enzymes that are capable of cleaving C3 and C5.

Leukotactic Factors of Microbial Origin

Soluble bacterial products from staphylococcus, streptococcus, and pneumococcus as well as certain other organisms.

Mediators with Potentially Multiple Functions

1. Oxygen-free radicals. Reactive oxygen metabolites produced by neutrophils and macrophages after exposure to chemotactic agents or immune complexes may cause endothelial cell damage with resultant increased vascular permeability; generation of chemotactic lipids nonenzymatically from arachidonic acid; and inactivation of antiproteases, such as α_1-antitrypsin. The effect on antiproteases if unopposed by antioxidant protective mechanisms may lead to tissue damage. The influence of oxygen-free radicals in any given inflammatory reaction is the balance between the production and inactivation of these metabolites.
2. Interleukin I. Interleukin I is a polypeptide macrophage product that activates lymphocytes, is chemotactic for neutrophils, produces fever, and stimulates specific protein synthesis by certain cells.
3. PAF. Also known as acetylated glycerol ether phosphocholine (AGEPC), PAF is a factor derived from antigen-stimulated, IgE-sensitized basophils, which causes aggregation of platelets and release of their constituents (such as histamine and serotonin). In addition to platelet stimulation, PAF causes vasoconstriction in high doses and at extremely low concentrations causes vasodilatation and increased vascular permeability. It also causes increased leukocyte adhesion *in vitro* and early leukocytic emigration. Basophils, neutrophils, and monocytes can elaborate PAF. PAF may act as a mediator *in vivo* directly or indirectly by releasing other mediators (*e.g.*, leukotrienes).

Leukotactic Factors by Inflammatory Cell Type

Chemotactic Factors for Neutrophils
1. Activated trimolecular complex of C567
2. A plasmin-split fragment of C3
3. Fragments of C3 that are found after cleavage by tissue proteases
4. A fragment of C5
5. Soluble bacterial factors from filtrates
6. Interleukin I

Chemotactic Factors for Monocytes
1. A plasmin-split fragment of C3
2. A fragment of C5
3. Soluble bacterial factors
4. A soluble factor derived from sensitized lymphocytes (a lymphokine)

5. Serum factor from serum treated with immune complexes
6. Cationic protein—basic peptides

Chemotactic Factors for Eosinophils
These are essentially the same as for neutrophils with an additional factor, ECF-A.

BACTERIAL KILLING BY INFLAMMATORY CELLS

Two mechanisms for killing bacteria after they are phagocytosed are (1) the oxygen-dependent mechanism involving NADPH and the H_2O_2-myeloperoxidase-halide system (chronic granulomatous disease of childhood being an example of a disease resulting when this system is genetically defective) and (2) oxygen-independent mechanisms such as low pH, lysozyme, phagocytin, or lactoferrin present in the inflammatory cells.

CLASSIFICATION OF INFLAMMATION

The process of inflammation may be classified based on duration (acute, subacute, chronic, healed), etiology (bacterial, viral, chemical, physical, and so forth), types of reaction produced (exudative, proliferative), and type of exudate produced. Types of inflammation based on types of exudate are:

Serous—extensive outpouring of watery inflammatory edema fluid

Fibrinous—containing large amounts of fibrinogen which precipitates

Catarrhal—containing large amounts of mucus

Purulent or suppurative—exudate characterized by large amounts of pus

Hemorrhagic—containing erythrocytes in addition to other elements of the exudate

Fibrinopurulent—a mixture of large amounts of fibrinogen and pus

Mucopurulent—a mixture of mucin and pus

PERTINENT DEFINITIONS

Pus—thick inflammatory fluid composed of living and dead polymorphonuclear leukocytes and necrotic debris.

Exudate—inflammatory edema fluid characterized by high protein content, high cell counts, specific gravity over 1.018, low glucose content, sometimes clots due to fibrinogen content. This is to be contrasted with:

Transudate—a noninflammatory edema fluid resembling an ultrafiltrate of plasma with certain characteristics: specific gravity about 1.010 (certainly less than 1.018), low protein content, low cell content, normal glucose content, clear, does not clot on standing. Transudates are related to circulatory disorders; exudates are related to inflammatory disorders.

Opsonins—a collective term for humoral factors, including antibacterial and antifungal antibodies, components of complement and other heat-labile substances that promote phagocytosis of bacteria.

MICROSCOPIC FEATURES OF ACUTE INFLAMMATION

Microscopically the acute inflammatory lesion shows varying proportions of (1) serous exudate, (2) fibrin, (3) polymorphonuclear leukocytes, and (4) large mononuclear cells. According to the character of the exudate, they are classified as follows:

1. *Acute serous or serofibrinous* inflammation occurs on serous membranes such as the pericardium, the pleura, or the peritoneum. The exudate is largely serous, with fibrin resulting from coagulation of plasma, and it may be absorbed completely or organized by the ingrowth of young connective tissue, often resulting in fibrous adhesion of visceral and parietal layers. In lobar pneumonia the pleural exudate is mainly serofibrinous. In this condition the exudate undergoes lysis and is either absorbed directly or, in part at least, removed by macrophages.
2. *Acute purulent, seropurulent, or fibrinopurulent* inflammation is characterized by the predominance of pus cells (polymorphonuclear leukocytes) and is the most frequent type outside of the serous membranes. It may be either (1) circumscribed or suppurative, to form an abscess, which heals by the walling off of fibrous tissue and scar formation; or (2) diffuse or phlegmonous, acute inflammation, often caused by streptococci, pneumococci, and so forth, that extends into the surrounding tissues and tends to invade the blood stream.
3. *Acute hemorrhagic* inflammation is characterized by intense capillary injury, with rupture, permitting large numbers of erythrocytes to escape into the tissues, as in hemorrhagic cystitis and some forms of glomerulonephritis.
4. *Acute catarrhal* inflammation is relatively mild; it is characterized by a seromucinous exudate on the mucous membrane, which later becomes mucopurulent, as in catarrhal inflammations of the upper respiratory and the alimentary tract.
5. *Pseudomembranous or diphtheritic* inflammation is formed by a fibrinous exudate over a necrotic layer of mucosa. It never organizes but is sloughed off or digested. This type of inflammation is seen in diphtheria and has been observed fairly frequently at autopsy in the alimentary tract of individuals who had been receiving large quantities of some antibiotics. A type of staphylococcus resistant to antibiotics is the usual cause in these cases.

Chronic inflammation differs from acute inflammation in that the cellular reaction consists primarily of lymphocytes, plasma cells, and macrophages together with newly formed collagenous fibers. This chronic process often follows an acute inflammatory one. When pus is associated with a chronic lesion, as in chronic suppurative osteomyelitis, it is termed chronic suppurative inflammation. When the formation of new connective tissue is prominent, the lesion is called chronic productive inflammation.

Granulomatous inflammation is a reaction to injury in which a proliferative response rather than an exudative response dominates the reaction. A small but important group of biological agents and physical and chemical agents characteristically induce the aggregation and proliferation of macrophages in addition to the usual changes of simple inflammation. Because macrophages have a strong tendency to arrange themselves in small nodules or granules, this group of conditions has come to be known as granulomatous inflammation. Some of the disorders that characteristically call forth a granulomatous response include tuberculosis, leprosy, syphilis, sarcoidosis, many mycotic infections including histoplasmosis, blastomycosis, coccidioidomycosis. Foreign bodies also call forth a granulomatous response. The most characteristic inflammatory cell of granulomatous inflammation is the epithelioid cell, which is a macrophage that has been altered in response to the inflammatory agent. Multinucleate giant cells sometimes but not always occur in the granulomatous reaction, and they are formed by macrophages becoming fused.

Some forms of granulomatous inflammation are influenced by cell-mediated immunity to the etiologic agent. Thus, T lymphocytes and their products have a role in granulomatous inflammation.

REPAIR

Repair consists of the replacement of dead or damaged cells by new healthy cells derived either from the parenchymal or connective tissue stromal elements of the injured tissue. Repair and healing are practically synonymous. Repair takes place through parenchymal regeneration and repair by connective tissue. Parenchymal regeneration can be remarkably complete when the preexisting stroma is not seriously damaged and when the residual cells have the capacity for active regeneration. When damage is severe and parenchymal regeneration cannot restore the organ, the repair process takes the form of connective tissue scarring. Scar tissue fills the defects and restores some of the bulk of the organ, but specialized functioning cells are replaced with non-functioning connective tissue. An example of this process is healing of a myocardial infarct in which contractile myocardial cells are replaced by non-functioning scar tissue.

Repair by regeneration is basically replacement of cells lost through injury or physiological wear and tear by cells of the same type. The ability to regenerate is greater in some cell types than in others. Cells of the body have been divided into three groups based on their capacity for regeneration: labile, stable, and permanent. Labile cells are cells that continue to multiply under normal conditions and that can respond rapidly by regenerating when damaged.

Labile cells include cells of the epithelial surfaces of the skin, oral cavities, the mucosa of the GI tract and genitourinary tract, and cells of the hematopoietic system. When these cells are lost, they are rapidly replaced by regeneration of adjacent cells. Stable cells do not normally replicate but have the ability to divide when injured. The stable cells include the parenchymal cells of most of the glandular organs (liver, tubular cells of the kidney, endocrine glands) and connective tissue cells such as fibroblasts, chondroblasts, and osteoblasts. The parenchymal cells can regenerate after damage has occurred and are most effective in replacing preexisting structure when the basic framework of the organ or tissue is unaffected.

Some muscle cells are capable of some degree of regeneration, but certainly not as much as other connective tissues. Regeneration of smooth muscle occurs in the wall of the intestine, urinary bladder, and uterus. Skeletal muscle makes some attempt at regeneration, although never complete. Cardiac muscle has no significant regenerative capacity.

Permanent cells are highly specialized cells that do not undergo mitotic division in postnatal life even after injury. The nerve cells in the central nervous system are permanent cells and are not replaced when irreversibly damaged. With regard to the peripheral nerves, when the cell body is destroyed, the entire nerve degenerates. If the peripheral axon is injured and the cell body is not damaged, regeneration may proceed from the cell body or from the proximal axonal segment. The distal segment degenerates entirely, and the proximal segment degenerates to the nearest node of Ranvier. The proximal segment then regenerates until it meets the distal channel, in which case the integrity of the nerve may be reestablished. Cardiac muscle fibers, since they do not regenerate, are also considered permanent cells.

Repair by fibrous tissue or scar formation is really the replacement of injured or destroyed tissue by a simpler form of tissue, namely, loose, vascular fibrous tissue, generally known as *granulation tissue* (fibroblasts and proliferating capillaries), which is at first very soft and delicate but which soon becomes more dense and compact, forming a fibrous patch or scar that takes the place of the original tissue destroyed as the result of injury. This form of repair commonly occurs following extensive damage with the loss of much of the original tissue. The healing of wounds illustrates these reparative processes admirably.

Healing by first intention is favored by apposition of the tissues in the absence of infection. There is slight exudate between the apposed surfaces. In 24 hours in the case of a tissue with an epithelial covering, there are mitoses in the epithelial cells and fibroblasts, and some leukocytes are present. In a few days the continuity of the epithelium is restored, and granulation tissue fills in from below the defect in the subepithelial tissue. The strength of the healing area is determined by the amount of collagen fiber that has formed.

Healing by second intention in noninfected wounds, in which tissue apposition cannot occur, begins with a thin surface exudate. In a few days the floor of the wound is covered by granulation tissue, consisting of capillary loops surrounded by fibroblasts and leukocytes, which gradually fills in from the side and the floor of the wound and is finally covered by epithelium. The exuberant granulation tissue in an open wound is called "proud flesh."

In *infected* open wounds there is a purulent exudate on the surface, and complete healing by granulation does not occur until the infection subsides.

Mechanisms of Repair. Several factors possibly play a role in parenchymal and connective tissue cell proliferation in the wound-healing process. Epidermal growth factor (EGF) produces epidermal proliferation and is mitogenic for fibroblasts. Platelet-derived growth factor (PDGF), stored in platelet granules and released upon platelet activation, is mitogenic for fibroblasts and smooth muscle cells. Fibroblast growth factor (FGF) also stimulates the proliferation of fibroblasts and smooth muscle cells. Macrophages may also produce products that stimulate connective tissue growth. Fibrin is associated with the formation of granulation tissue in wound healing. The exact roles of these factors in human wound healing have not been fully determined, but mediators obviously are active in the repair process just as they are earlier in the inflammatory reaction.

Abnormal Growth and Development

Many disease processes are initiated during embryonic life as the consequences of genetic, developmental, and intrauterine abnormalities. Some of these conditions become evident in early pregnancy, resulting in spontaneous abortions, while others do not manifest themselves until later pregnancy and postnatal periods. Of all live-born infants, the highest mortality rate occurs during the neonatal period (the first 4 weeks). Such mortality is closely correlated with prematurity of the infants at birth. In later infancy (up to 1 year), the survival rate increases sharply. The major causes of death are infections and their complications, congenital malformations, and sudden infant death syndrome. Accidental deaths, including those that occur in the home and the automobile, predominate during childhood. In the adult, developmental and genetic factors contribute significantly to a certain proportion of morbidity and mortality, although they may not be easily recognized by the attending physician.

NEONATAL DISEASES

The development of the fetus can be regarded as a preparation for extrauterine existence. There is a period in early gestation when the fetus is absolutely incapable of survival in the external environment. If pregnancy is spontaneously or artificially terminated during this stage of development, the result is an abortion. Later, the development is chronologically reflected by the growth of organs, which become progressively more adapted for independent life. For practical and statistical purposes, the birth weight of the infant is used as an estimate of the gestational age or the degree of developmental "maturity" with a fair degree of reliability. Infants born weighing less than 500 g (approximately 24 weeks of gestation age) are considered previable and are classified as abortuses. "Premature infants" are defined as those whose birth weights are

between 500 g and 2500 g. In this group, the survival rate increases progressively with birth weight. Although histologic evidence of immaturity can be discerned to some extent in infants weighing less than 1500 g., these features represent a stage of development, rather than conclusive evidence of the cause of death. The terminal air spaces are lined by cuboidal cells in the lungs of an immature infant. Infants of the same gestational age and birth weight that survive longer show a progressive flattening of the alveolar lining cells in the lungs, which reflects maturation of the lung. Although branching of the bronchial tree is completed by the eleventh week of gestation, additional terminal air spaces continue to form until at least the eighth year of life, according to quantitative studies made with the use of plastic casts of the airways. Immaturity is thus a problem determined by the number and structure of the alveoli and the need of the infant.

In a significant proportion of stillborn infants and in those that die during the first few days of life, autopsy findings consist mainly of petechial and, occasionally, ecchymotic hemorrhages in the visceral pleura, pericardium, and in the thymus. In some cases, petechiae are also demonstrated in the subependymal and subarachnoid spaces. In very severe cases, the immediate causes of death are massive hemorrhages in the pulmonary alveoli and in the subarachnoid and ventricular spaces of the brain. All these changes are ascribed to *intrauterine anoxia* (asphyxia neonatorum), which increases the permeability of the capillary endothelium and other membranes. Known causes of asphyxia include abruptio placentae, placenta previa, exposure to sedative or hypnotic drugs derived from the maternal blood stream, and umbilical cord compression during labor. It must also be noted that a prolonged uterine contraction, which is clinically associated with a marked drop in the fetal heart rate, is also an important cause of anoxia.

In some stillborn and newborn infants with a similar history, intrauterine aspiration of excessive amounts of amniotic fluid and its contents is demonstrated. In some cases, meconium is present in the fluid and in the lungs. In others, large numbers of squames, derived from vernix caseosa, fill the tracheobronchial tree and the terminal air spaces, preventing an adequate exchange of gases. Certain authors ascribed such *aspiration syndromes* to fetal anoxia, which, toward the end of prematurity and at full term, stimulates the respiratory center in the brain and relaxes the anal sphincter. The most common cause of death during the neonatal period is due to respiratory distress (respiratory distress syndrome of the newborn). Most of these cases correspond to pulmonary immaturity with hyaline membrane disease, although some represent cases of the aspiration syndrome, intrauterine pneumonia, and rare congenital anomalies of the lungs and heart.

Most commonly, hyaline membrane disease occurs in premature infants with immature lungs, but it is also significant in full-term infants of diabetic mothers and in those delivered by cesarean section. It is characterized by respiratory difficulty, beginning soon after birth, which becomes progressively worse with time. Clinically, there is progressive rise of P_{CO_2} and fall of P_{O_2}, which is unresponsive to 100% oxygen. Pulmonary function studies show a marked decrease of the residual volume of the lungs. At autopsy, the lungs are heavy, airless, reddish purple, and sink in the fixing fluid. Histologically, all the alveoli are collapsed, leaving no residual air spaces, while the alveolar ducts and terminal bronchioles are markedly dilated and are lined with eosinophilic, amorphous material, which is regarded as hyaline membrane. These membranes consist of fibrin, plasma proteins, and necrotic debris derived from necrotic alveolar lining cells. This injury to the alveolar lining cells is felt to represent oxygen toxicity, as most of these infants require high levels of inspired oxygen. These membranes are never found in stillborn infants who have never breathed.

The lungs of premature infants produce inadequate amounts of an alveolar surfactant, which is required to reduce the alveolar surface tension, which prevents alveolar collapse during exhalation. This substance has been shown to be lecithin, secreted by type II pneumocytes. It is also released into the amniotic fluid by the normal intrauterine respiratory movements. A lecithin–sphingomyelin ratio of greater than 2 : 1 in amniotic fluid has been used as an indicator of pulmonary maturity of the fetus before a cesarean section or an induced labor.

The most common complications of hyaline membrane disease are subependymal and intraventricular hemorrhages, which are occasionally massive. Hypoxic damage to the germinal matrix blood vessels is the postulated cause of these hemorrhages. In some series, these complications are found in about 50% of fatal cases. Necrotizing enterocolitis, where the bowel becomes necrotic, is also a common complication and is felt to be due to hypoxia.

The most common serious infection in the stillborn and newborn infants that die during the early neonatal period is *intrauterine pneumonia*. The disease is strongly associated with maternal acute chorioamnionitis. Microscopically, the terminal air spaces are filled with neutrophils, macrophages, and necrotic debris. The etiologic agents can be any organisms that reach the maternal genital tract. In the preantibiotic era, group A hemolytic streptococci were the most common cause. Subsequently, *Escherichia coli* became the most frequent agent causing the pneumonia. More recently, group B hemolytic streptococci are emerging as the most common causative organisms. Intrauterine pneumonia is frequently complicated by septicemia and meningitis.

Transplacental infections leading to a generalized disease with necrotic foci in various organs, including the liver, kidneys, adrenals and brain, are cytomegalic inclusion disease, herpes simplex, listeriosis, and toxoplasmosis. In congenital toxoplasmosis, foci of calcification can occasionally be observed in roentgenograms of the head, due to the presence of lesions in the brain.

Hemolytic disease of the newborn (erythroblastosis fetalis) is a group of diseases of considerable interest because of the immunologic mechanism of pathogenesis, which can be prevented by an appropriate measure. The most severe type is due to an Rh incompatibility between the maternal and fetal bloods. When the mother is Rh negative and the fetus is Rh positive, the fetal RBCs occasionally enter the maternal blood stream during birth, inducing an immunologic response. The first child is therefore usually unaffected by the disease because maternal sensitization occurs during birth. In subsequent pregnancies, however, IgG is produced in increasing quantities. Since this immunoglobin can readily enter the fetal circulation by passing through the placental barrier, the fetus develops a hemolytic anemia, which is variable in severity. In the most severe form, ***hydrops fetalis,*** the fetus manifests anasarca due to cardiac and liver failure, with consequent decrease of plasma albumin and osmotic disturbances. ***Icterus gravis,*** which is a slightly less severe variety, is characterized by a severe hemolytic anemia with a marked bilirubinemia, which must be treated promptly by a complete exchange transfusion. In fatal cases, the basal ganglia, cerebellum, and other areas of the brain are yellow, due to the passage of unconjugated bilirubin through the ineffective blood–brain barrier of the fetus. Such pathologic change, which is not found in the adult brain, is called kernicterus.

Hemolytic disease of the newborn due to ABO incompatibilities is more frequent but the manifestations are much milder than those of the Rh factors.

Traumatic injuries of the newborn are most commonly associated with molding of the head of the infant in its passage through the pelvic canal during delivery. These are usually insignificant, such as caput succedaneum and cephalhematoma, which are eventually resorbed. More severe consequences include subdural hemorrhages, due to tears of the dural sinuses, falx cerebri, and tentorium cerebelli, which can lead to a fatal outcome. Occasionally, subcapsular hematoma and rupture of such hematoma into the peritoneal cavity complicate the breech extraction procedure. Fractures of the clavicle and long bones during delivery are other complications.

DISEASES OF PREGNANCY

This review will be limited to diseases of pregnancy that are of general interest. More specialized topics are covered in the chapter on obstetrics and gynecology.

The most common complication of pregnancy is **spontaneous abortion,** which is defined as an expulsion of the fetus before it has developed sufficiently for extrauterine existence. It usually takes place in the first trimester, although an arbitrary dividing line between abortion and stillbirth has been set at 24 weeks of gestation. During the embryonic period (up to 8 weeks) more than 50% of the abortuses have severe chromosomal abnormalities, such as tetraploidy, triploidy, and aneuploidy of large chromosomes, which are usually incompatible with life. During the fetal period (9 weeks to term), infections, placental and uterine abnormalities, and maternal factors become more important factors that lead to pregnancy loss.

Extrauterine implantation of the fertilized ovum, or **ectopic pregnancy,** occurs most frequently in the fallopian tube (tubal pregnancy). It invariably terminates in a rupture of the tube and intra-abdominal hemorrhage, often before the patient realizes that she is pregnant. It is therefore an important consideration in the differential diagnosis of an acute abdominal emergency in the female of child-bearing age. In rare circumstances, ectopic pregnancy may occur in the abdominal cavity, which is compatible with a long survival of the fetus. The most common predisposing cause of ectopic pregnancy is chronic salpingitis.

Toxemia of pregnancy is a syndrome characterized by hypertension, massive proteinuria, and edema, usually initiated during the third trimester of pregnancy. In some cases, the condition terminates in episodic convulsions and coma, which is called **eclampsia.** The term **pre-eclampsia** is used when

toxemia of pregnancy is of such severity that eventual development into eclampsia can be justifiably suspected. It serves as an indication that an appropriate preventive measure must be taken. The maternal hypertension damages the delicate placental vascular bed, impairing transfer of maternal nutrients and oxygen to the fetus.

Eclampsia is frequently associated with **disseminated intravascular coagulation** (DIC), which is characterized by multiple fibrin thrombi in small blood vessels with a marked bleeding tendency. In the peripheral blood, fibrinogen, prothrombin, and many coagulation factors are markedly depleted. The appearance of fragmented erythrocytes (schistocytes) is also characteristic of the condition. In addition to hemorrhages in various organs, autopsy findings occasionally include peripheral necrosis of the liver and cortical necrosis of the kidneys.

In **hydatidiform mole,** the placental villi become large, cystlike structures that are readily recognized on gross inspection. Microscopically, there is a severe edema of the villus with a complete or partial absence of the fetal vascularization. Atypical changes in the trophoblasts of different degrees are the usual findings. In more atypical cases, trophoblasts can be demonstrated in the myometrium. Such a condition is called an **invasive mole (chorioadenoma destruens).** Malignant transformation of trophoblasts corresponds to a malignant neoplasm, **choriocarcinoma,** which is a vascular neoplasm with a strong tendency to spread hematogenously. It is sensitive to a chemotherapeutic regimen of methotrexate.

CONGENITAL MALFORMATIONS (TERATOLOGY)

It has been estimated that about 2% of fetuses and newborn infants are affected with significant malformations; many of these are compatible with life. Musculoskeletal anomalies, which are usually not fatal, are the most common. In those that die during the neonatal period, cardiovascular defects and multiple malformations predominate.

Many congenital anomalies are due to point mutations with typical mendelian distribution. These include multiple polyposis of the colon, polydactyly, albinism, ectodermal dysplasia, xanthoma tuberosum, and many others. Some congenital malformations are associated with chromosomal abnormalities (trisomy 21 of Down's syndrome, Klinefelter's and Turner's syndromes, trisomy 18 and 13). Most of these are consequences of mitotic errors. Environmentally induced malformations include the well-known rubella syndrome and phocomelia due to thalidomide, both acting during the critical period of morphogenesis (the first trimester). Other drugs and chemical or physical agents acting during this gestational period have also been strongly suspected as possible causes of congenital malformations, but they have not reached the epidemic proportions of the two agents mentioned. It must be noted that maternal rubella during the third trimester is occasionally followed by a generalized infection in the infant, rather than by congenital malformations.

AGING

Man and other animals have limited life spans. In man, many changes that are associated with aging are readily observable on external examination. These include the thinning and wrinkling of the skin, graying of hair, alterations of the general body form due to skeletal changes, and the frequent development of cataracts. Anatomically, atrophy of the heart and brain in older individuals is common. Microscopically, the accumulation of lipofuscin pigment in hepatocytes, myocardial fibers, and certain neurons with age has been observed since the beginning of the science of pathology. The apparent loss of neurons in the aging human brain has been corroborated by actual counting in the brains of aging rats. To this list must be added the increasing incidence of cardiovascular and neoplastic disease with age.

All the changes mentioned above, and the others that remain to be discovered, must depend on one basic mechanism which is responsible for the functional integrity of all the cells and tissues of the body. This mechanism is the regulated expression of gene activities in response to external and internal environments. Most modern theories of aging are based on this mechanism.

In one theory, the limited life span, and therefore the aging process, is programmed in the genetic constitution of the species and is therefore transmitted from one generation to the next. Other theories are based on somatic events in different cells of the body. Thus, one theory postulates somatic mutations, which may be spontaneous or environmentally induced, as the causes of differential alterations of the activities of some cells or tissues of the body. These alterations which reside in the DNA of different cells, account for the different manifestations in aging. Other theories are based on occasional failures of transcription and translation of the genetic information. The pathogenesis of cell aging must therefore reside in the synthesis of messenger

RNA (mRNA) and of the various proteins, including enzymes. It must be noted that these theories are not mutually exclusive. In the final analysis, it is highly probable that all of them may participate in the aging process.

Evidence in favor of these theories has been accumulating in the past few decades. First, extensive studies in a number of laboratories have shown that normal diploid cells of the species that have been investigated have limited life spans in culture. The life span is measured by the number of divisions that the cells can undergo. Thus, human cells have a replicative life span of approximately 50 generations, after which most of them fail to survive. Cells from other animals also have definite replicative capacity. Current data show that the number of divisions that cultured cells can undergo is correlated with the maximum life span of the species. Thus, cells of the turtle, which may live for more than 150 years, can survive 75 to 100 divisions, while those of the mouse, only 10 to 20 generations. In rare circumstances, certain cells in successive cultures become the so-called permanent cell lines, such as the HeLa cells, originally derived from a human source. Such permanent cell lines, however, are no longer normal diploid cells. Their chromosome constitution varies greatly even in the same culture; some may be tetraploid and others, octaploid. This phenomenon has been called heteroploidy.

Evidence for somatic mutation is more difficult to obtain because these cells are not readily amenable to conventional genetic analysis. That the phenomenon exists has been shown in certain traits in animals and man. Evidence for altered gene expressions in somatic cells is readily obtained in immunologic data related to the "clonal" responses of lymphoid cells to different antigens.

Neoplasms (Tumors)

PROCESSES OF NEOPLASIA

A neoplasm is an aberration of growth characterized by the abnormal, unregulated, excessive, and uncontrolled multiplication of cells with the formation of a mass. The mass that develops serves no useful purpose, grows at the expense of normal structures, may even destroy normal tissues and, with rare exceptions, is of unknown cause. The mass that forms as a result of this abnormal cell proliferation may be localized, as in benign tumors, or spreading and invasive, as in malignant tumors. While the terms "tumor" and "neoplasm" are sometimes used interchangeably, a tumor really refers to a swelling, while a neoplasm is specifically an autonomous new growth. Thus, a neoplasm gives rise to a tumor, but all tumors are not necessarily neoplasms.

GROWTH AND SPREAD OF TUMORS

Neoplasms receive their nutrition from the blood, but their growth is autonomous and not controlled by the normal regulatory mechanisms of the host's body. Moreover, because growth is uncontrolled, the tumor cells grow faster than the normal cells around them, and a mass forms that increases in size. In the benign tumors the mass grows slowly and centrifugally, that is, from the center outward, pressing the normal tissues about it and compressing them to form a kind of enveloping membrane or capsule, unless the tumor is on a surface, in which case the new growth projects from the surface in papillary fashion, without a capsule. Malignant tumors, on the contrary, invade and infiltrate the surrounding tissues, the neoplastic cells resembling the roots of a plant in that they insinuate themselves between the adjacent normal tissue cells, often causing their atrophy and destruction.

Malignant tumors may spread by direct extension or by metastasis. Direct extension may produce clinical signs and symptoms due to effects on adjacent structures, such as ureteral obstruction and uremia from advanced carcinoma of the cervix, a common cause of death from that malignancy. Metastasis is the distant spread of a tumor separate from the original or primary site and may occur by implantation or vascular dissemination. Implantation is often transcoelomic, for example, multiple peritoneal implants from an ovarian carcinoma, or it may occur by surgical inoculation along suture lines. Vascular dissemination may occur by lymphatics or blood vessels. Carcinomas tend to metastasize first by way of lymphatics but may also spread early by the blood stream. Sarcomas in general favor the blood stream for metastatic spread. Some malignancies tend to metastasize to certain organs because of their blood drainage or for unknown reasons. Thus, carcinoma of the stomach, intestine, and pancreas frequently metastasize to the liver. When bone metastases are first discovered, the most common tumors suspected are those from the lung, breast, prostate, kidney, and thyroid. Bone metastases are usually associated with a mixture of osteolytic and osteoblastic reactions, but prostatic carcinoma is noted for its dominant osteoblastic bone lesions. Multiple myeloma (plasmacytoma) is noted for its characteristic "punched out"

osteolytic lesions. Carcinomas of the lung frequently metastasize to the regional lymph nodes, brain, adrenals, bones, and liver.

Prevention of metastasis is a major objective of cancer therapy. Many factors are involved. The duration of the primary tumor is very important, and the earlier the treatment, the greater the chance that metastasis has not occurred. The type of tumor is significant; for example, basal cell carcinoma almost never metastasizes, while malignant melanoma may metastasize when the primary is so small that dermal invasion is no more than 1.0 mm. The size of the tumor embolus is important, single cells having less chance to survive in a pulmonary capillary than a large clump of several hundred thousand cells. The presence of surgical shock may cause small capillary thrombi that enhance the ability of smaller numbers of tumor cells to survive and produce a metastasis. Host resistance plays a major role, and when the immune system is compromised metastases are easily formed. This situation is seen particularly in patients on immunosuppressive drugs or with acquired immunologic deficiency. The role of trauma to the primary in the production of metastasis is controversial, but, nevertheless, clinical practice is designed to minimize trauma or excessive palpation that might dislodge tumor cells into the blood stream from the primary tumor. Malignancies cause death by various means, such as cachexia (a severe wasting away), intercurrent infections, loss of essential organ function by obstruction or replacement and massive hemorrhage.

BENIGN AND MALIGNANT NEOPLASMS

There is a succinct contrast between benign tumors and malignant tumors according to the criteria of differentiation, rate of growth, type of growth and tendency to metastasize. Benign tumors are well differentiated, and the neoplastic cells resemble their normal cell of origin. Malignant tumors have a range of differentiation from well-differentiated tissue resembling the tissue of origin to a poorly differentiated or almost completely undifferentiated appearance. Benign tumors grow slowly and may stop growing or regress. Evidence of cell division, such as mitosis, is scarce. In malignant tumors, growth is usually rapid, and mitotic figures may be frequent or abnormal. Malignant tumors are characterized by infiltrative growth, and encapsulation is rare. Benign tumors do not metastasize. Almost all malignant tumors metastasize; the presence of metastases is definite evidence of a tumor's malignancy. Those malignant tumors that do not usually metastasize, such as gliomas of the central nervous system and basal cell carcinoma of the skin, are invasive and locally destructive and may kill even though they do not metastasize. In general, tumors lose many of the specialized functions of their cell of origin, but some may continue such specialized functions, become hyperfunctional or acquire new functions. (See Table 6-1).

GRADING AND STAGING OF MALIGNANT NEOPLASMS

From a clinical standpoint, it is valuable to estimate the malignant potential and extent of spread at the time of first diagnosis of a tumor. *Grading* of a tumor is based on microscopic assessment of the differentiation of the tumor cells. Microscopically, malignant cells have enlarged, hyperchromatic nuclei that vary in size and shape; enlarged nucleoli; increased mitotic activity; and loss of expected nuclear polarity. When these dysplastic changes are extreme, the pattern is termed anaplasia. Anaplasia refers to the reversion of a tissue to an appearance of a more primitive, undifferentiated, or embryonic state. Carcinomas are usually graded on a scale of I to III or IV, depending upon accepted criteria for different primary sites. Sarcomas are often graded as low-grade, intermediate-grade, or high-grade malignancies.

In contrast, *staging* of malignancies is an important clinical process based on the size of the primary lesion and the extent of lymphatic spread or presence of distant metastases at the time of first diagnosis.

ETIOLOGY AND PATHOGENESIS

Many factors have been discovered relating to etiology and pathogenesis of neoplasia. There is general acceptance of the two-stage hypothesis of carcinogenesis, which holds that the process of neoplasia is first begun by an agent or event that *initiates* a change in the genome of the cell, followed by an essential period of latency during which other agents or events act as *promoters* that eventually may lead to the appearance of a neoplasia. Substances that act in the first stage are termed initiators, those in the second stage, promoters. Instantaneous neoplasms cannot be produced by an initiator, and a variable time period of latency always must occur. The process of initiation is an irreversible step that may or may not produce a neoplasm later, depending on future promoting factors. The process of promotion is reversible if the promoting agents are removed in time before the neoplasm develops. A carcinogen is any substance that will cause a cancer, and such substances may act as initiators, promoters, or both. Most known chemical carcinogens, oncogenic viruses, and ionizing radiations may act as both initiator and promoter. As such, these agents are termed complete carcinogens in contrast to incomplete carcinogens, which are defined as any pure initiating agent. Carcinogens may be complete at high dosages, but incomplete at lower dosages, losing their promoting ability. Thus, initiation lacks a dosage threshold level and may occur with a single exposure, whereas promotion has a dosage threshold that must be reached before the neoplasm will appear. Cigarette smoke appears to act as a promoter in that the risk of cancer increases significantly with the amount and duration of smoking and diminishes significantly if smoking is permanently stopped. Most pure promoting agents are substances that cause cell proliferation, such as croton oil, longstanding chronic irritation, and possibly hormones.

Some carcinogens are termed direct acting because they do not require metabolic chemical con-

TABLE 6-1. Common Tumors Associated with Functional Activity

TUMOR	SECRETION	FUNCTIONAL ACTIVITY
Carcinoid of intestine	Serotonin	Carcinoid syndrome
Renal cell carcinoma	Erythropoietin	Polycythemia
Anaplastic carcinoma of lung	ACTH	Cushing's syndrome
	Unknown	Hypercalcemia
T-cell lymphoma/leukemia	Lymphokine	Hypercalcemia
Thyroid medullary carcinoma	Calcitonin	Not significant
Islet cell carcinoma	Gastrin	Intractable peptic ulcers
Granulosa cell tumor of ovary	Estrogens	Feminization
Sertoli–Leydig cell tumor	Androgens	Masculinization
Thymoma	ACTH	Cushing's syndrome

versions to become active. A procarcinogen is a substance that must be metabolized in the body and converted to act as a carcinogen. An ultimate carcinogen is such a metabolic conversion product of a procarcinogen. For example, the aromatic amine 2-acetylaminofluorene (AAF) is a procarcinogen that is hydroxylated in the liver and in the presence of sulfotransferase becomes a highly active sulfate ester that reacts covalently with DNA. The male rat is most susceptible to AAF, developing hepatocellular carcinoma. In contrast, the guinea pig is resistant to neoplasia from AAF because he lacks the hepatic enzyme that hydroxylates AAF.

Of great interest is the recent identification of over 20 different oncogenes in man. Oncogenes are small DNA sequences that are capable of producing cellular transformation of tissue culture cells into a pattern of growth and nuclear change resembling that seen in neoplasms. These oncogenes may be normally present in cells and are referred to as "c-onc" genes, or they may be of viral origin, termed "v-onc." A number of studies seem to indicate that v-onc genes originated from normal (or c-onc genes). C-onc genes are widely preserved in the DNA of the vertebrate species and are probably necessary for cell growth and differentiation. Future research is directed toward answering the questions regarding if and how these oncogenes may be turned on or off and the role they play in carcinogenesis.

Chemical carcinogens are probably the most important cause of human cancer, especially in industrialized nations. The first example of chemical carcinogenesis was observed by Percival Pott in 1775 when he recognized that carcinoma in the scrotal area of chimney sweeps was due to irritation caused by the accumulation of soot in this area of the body.

Polycyclic hydrocarbons act as procarcinogens which are broken down to ultimate carcinogens that bind to DNA. Examples are 3,4-benzpyrene (in cigarette smoke), 9,10-dimethylbenzanthracene, cholanthrene and aromatic amines such as butter yellow (dimethylaminobenzene), and 2-naphthylamine. Alkylating agents such as nitrogen mustards, cyclophosphamide, and several other chemotherapeutic drugs are direct-acting carcinogens. Nitrosamines are potent direct-acting carcinogens that affect a variety of animal species. These may be formed when nitrites in the diet combine with proteins. Aflatoxins produced in stored peanuts by *Aspergillus* are potent carcinogens that act in several species. Exposure to metals such as chromium, uranium, and nickel has been associated with increased incidence of lung cancer. Exposure to asbestos, particularly in combination with habitual cigarette smoking, causes a greatly increased risk of lung cancer. Exposure to asbestos has also been associated with the development of mesothelioma of the pleura, a very rare tumor. Angiosarcoma of the liver is almost entirely due to exposure to vinyl chloride and is an occupational risk of some workers in the plastics industry.

Radiation carcinogenesis includes the effects of solar or ultraviolet radiation, as well as ionizing radiation from x-rays, nuclear fission, and radionuclides. Radiation injury is a well-documented carcinogen. Ultraviolet rays from the sun may lead to squamous cell carcinoma and basal cell carcinoma of the skin. Actinic keratosis (senile keratosis) is a recognized precursor of skin cancer. Light-complexioned individuals are more susceptible to the development of skin cancers than are dark-skinned individuals. These skin cancers obviously tend to occur on the exposed surfaces of the skin.

The carcinogenic effects of ionizing radiation have been known for many years. Ionizing radiation damages DNA and may produce mutations. Before proper precautions were observed, radiologists developed skin cancers on the hand when they personally positioned patients while roentgenograms were taken. Radioactive strontium, a product of nuclear fallout from atomic testing, is a source of ionizing radiation to humans, and strontium-irradiated animals will develop osteogenic sarcomas. Thorotrast, a radiopaque drug now banned in the United States and previously used in radiocontrast studies of the liver and spleen, is a low emitter of radioactivity and is suspected of causing hepatoma. The practice of treatment of enlarged thymus in children by irradiation during the 1950s has resulted in the development of papillary carcinoma of the thyroid in some of these patients. Individuals exposed to the Hiroshima atomic bomb have a higher rate of leukemia and carcinoma of the thyroid, breast, and lung as compared with unexposed individuals.

TUMOR VIRUSES

Most of the information concerning the action of tumor viruses is based on studies of animal tumor viruses. Oncogenic viruses act by integration of viral DNA into the host cell genome; DNA viruses act directly, and RNA viruses act indirectly through virally encoded reverse transcriptase. The RNA tumor viruses belong to a family known as retroviruses and may be exogenous (producing naturally occurring tumors) or endogenous (producing genetically transmitted tumors). Exogenous retroviruses account for most of the animal viral tumors so far and include those that cause cancers in chickens and leukemias or lymphomas in cats, cattle and other animals. DNA tumor viruses in animals include a herpes-type virus causing a T-cell lymphoma in chickens (Marek's disease) and a bovine papillomavirus that, along with ingestion of bracken fern, produces alimentary tract carcinoma in cattle.

The first virus that is gaining general acceptance as a cause of human cancer is the human T-cell lymphoma virus, type I, or HTLV-I, an RNA virus. Although a high incidence of human infection by this virus has been demonstrated in some geographic areas, only a relatively small number of lymphomas have occurred, indicating that other factors are also involved. The human immunodeficiency virus (HIV) causing acquired immunodeficiency syndrome (AIDS) is associated with the development of a vascular malignancy, Kaposi's sarcoma, and also malignant lymphomas.

The Epstein–Barr virus (EBV) is a herpesvirus (DNA) that has a strong association with a highly malignant lymphoma restricted to a tropical region of Africa where malaria is epidemic. Recently a chromosome abnormality was found in the lymphocytes of Burkitt's lymphoma in which a reciprocal translocation of the distal end of the long arm of chromosome 8 and either chromosome 14 (90%) or chromosome 2 or 22 has occurred. These chromosomes are known to carry the immunoglobulin genes. Also, the portion of chromosome 8 that is translocated carries the *myc* oncogene, a gene first isolated from chicken tumor cells and later found in the white blood cells of some human patients with leukemia or lymphoma. The EBV is also the cause of infectious mononucleosis, a benign disease. An association of EBV with nasopharyngeal carcinoma has also been demonstrated.

Patients with chronic hepatitis due to hepatitis B virus have been shown to be at high risk for the development of hepatocellular carcinoma.

An association has been shown but not proven that herpes simplex II virus and/or the human papilloma (condyloma) virus may be implicated in the causation of cancer of the uterine cervix.

Although viruses are proven carcinogens for some types of neoplasms, other cofactors as yet undefined appear to be necessary. Environmental agents, dietary habits, and genetic predisposition may have roles as cofactors.

Classification of Neoplasms

Tumors are generally classified on the basis of the type of cell or tissue from which they arise, as well as from their characteristic structure. (See Table 6-2.)

IMPORTANT TUMORS, MALIGNANT AND BENIGN, OF DIFFERENT ORGANS

Lip, Tongue, and Mouth. Carcinoma occurs frequently in these areas and can be highly malignant. About 75% of these cases are found in males and practically all are of squamous cell type. Fissures, ulcers, papillomas, and areas of leukoplakia should receive prompt attention because malignant growths not infrequently develop at the site of such lesions, and by the time the malignant nature of the process is recognized the lesion has metastasized to the deep cervical lymph nodes. Most of these tumors are associated with the use of tobacco in one form or another.

Esophagus. Esophageal carcinoma is of frequent occurrence, about 75% being found in males. It usually is squamous in type, frequently with cornification, though adenocarcinoma in the lower third is not uncommon. The tumor may perforate into the trachea, the larynx, or the mediastinum and metastasize to regional nodes, liver, and lung.

Stomach. Carcinoma of the stomach has diminished in incidence in the United States in recent years but is common in a number of other countries, for example, Japan, Chile, and Iceland, where the increased incidence may be related to dietary customs. Up to 30 years ago it was the most frequent cause of cancer mortality in males in this country but is now a less frequent cause of death than cancer of the lung, colon, and breast. The incidence of cancer of the stomach in females is about half that in males. Roughly 90% of these carcinomas occur after the age of 40. About 60% are in the distal third, causing stenosis and obstruction. Gastric carcinoma rarely may originate in a chronic peptic ulcer, but the vast majority appear to arise independently. The most common type is ulcerating adenocarcinoma, which invades the stomach wall and may extend into the lumen. Nearly as common is the fungating vegetative type that projects as a large cauliflowerlike mass into the gastric lumen. Somewhat less common is the diffusely infiltrating form that may spread superficially in the mucosa but more commonly invades the entire gastric wall, causing diffuse thickening and stiffness leading to the designation linitis plastica (leather-bottle stomach).

TABLE 6-2. Classification of Neoplasms

BENIGN	MALIGNANT COUNTERPART
I. Tumors of epithelial tissues	
Papilloma	Carcinoma
Squamous papilloma	Squamous cell carcinoma
. . .*	Basal cell carcinoma
Transitional cell	Transitional cell carcinoma
papilloma	Mucoepidermoid carcinoma
Adenoma	Adenocarcinoma
Cystadenoma	Cystadenocarcioma
. . .	Adenoacanthoma
Keratoacanthoma	. . .
Hydatidiform mole	Choriocarcinoma
II. Tumors of nonhematopoietic mesenchymal tissues	
A. Soft tissue	
Lipoma	Liposarcoma
Myxoma	Myxosarcoma
Fibroma	Fibrosarcoma
Fibrous histiocytoma	Malignant fibrous histiocytoma
Fibroxanthoma	Malignant fibroxanthoma
Desmoid fibromatosis	Fibrosarcoma
Leiomyoma	Leiomyosarcoma
Rhabdomyoma	Rhabdomyosarcoma
Hemangioma	Hemangiosarcoma
Lymphangioma	Lymphangiosarcoma
Hemangioendothelioma	Malignant hemangioendothe-lioma
Hemangiopericytoma	Malignant hemangiopericytoma
Synovioma	Synovial sarcoma
Parganglioma	Alveolar soft part sarcoma
. . .	Kaposi's sarcoma
B. Bone and cartilage	
Osteoma (exostosis)	Osteogenic sarcoma
Chondroma	Chondrosarcoma
Osteochondroma	Chondrosarcoma
	Osteogenic sarcoma
Chordoma	Malignant chordoma
Chondroblastoma	Chondrosarcoma
Giant cell tumor	Malignant giant cell tumor
	Ewing's sarcoma
III. Tumors of hematopoietic tissues	
Primary polycythemia	Leukemia
"Pseudolymphoma"	Malignant lyphoma
	Lymphoma, non-Hodgkin's type
	Hodgkin's disease
	Multiple myeloma
	Mycosis fungoides
	Plasmacytoma
IV. Tumors of neural tissues	
Neurilemoma	Malignant schwannoma
Neurofibroma	Neurofibrosarcoma
Ganglioneuroma	Ganglioneuroblastoma
Meningioma	Meningeal sarcoma
. . .	Neuroblastoma
. . .	Retinoblastoma
. . .	Astrocytoma
. . .	Oligodendroglioma
. . .	Glioblastoma multiforme
. . .	Medulloblastoma
. . .	Ependymoma
Pheochromocytoma	Malignant pheochromocytoma

(Continued)

TABLE 6-2. Classification of Neoplasms (*Continued*)

BENIGN	MALIGNANT COUNTERPART
V. Germ cell tumors	
. . .	Seminoma (dysgerminoma)
. . .	Embryonal carcinoma
. . .	Choriocarcinoma
Benign teratoma	Malignant teratoma
VI. Miscellaneous	
Mixed tumor	Malignant mixed tumor
Melanocytic nevus	Malignant melanoma
. . .	Carcinosarcoma
. . .	Wilms' tumor (nephroblastoma)

*. . . indicates category not applicable.

Gastric carcinoma spreads through the lymphatics to the peritoneal cavity, with secondary implants in the ovaries (Krukenberg tumors) or the rectovesical pouch (rectal shelf). Metastasis through the veins to the liver is very common, as well as extension to the transverse colon, the pancreas, and the spleen. The outcome is almost invariably fatal.

Small Intestine. Malignancies of the small intestines are not common; carcinomas (50%) and lymphomas (20%) are the more frequent types. Carcinoids (derived from Kulchitsky cells) also occur here and often metastasize to the liver and mesenteric nodes.

Appendix. Adenocarcinoma of the appendix is extremely rare, and carcinoid tumor is the more common type. The carcinoid is a low-grade malignancy but in the appendix is rarely associated with metastasis.

Carcinoid Syndrome. When a carcinoid arising in a site outside the appendix metastasizes to the liver or the lungs, or to both, a group of symptoms and pathologic changes termed the carcinoid syndrome may occur, that is, flushing of the skin, a peculiar type of cyanosis, bronchial constriction with asthmalike attacks, and diarrhea. For some time these symptoms were wholly attributed to the release by these tumors of serotonin (t-hydroxytryptamine), but other substances are also involved.

Large Intestine. Tumors of the large intestine now rank with the lung and the breast as one of the most common sites of malignant disease. The incidence is about equal in males and females. Although carcinoma of the large intestine occurs most often in older age groups, a number of cases of carcinoma of the rectum or colon have been reported in individuals from 3½ to 20 years of age. The majority of colon cancers occur in the sigmoid colon and rectum, the cecum being less often involved. These are adenocarcinomas, often producing much mucus. Some carcinomas arise from villous adenomas or polyps.

In the sigmoid colon the tumor often resembles a "napkin ring" and produces symptoms of obstruction. In the cecum and right colon the tumor is often bulky and fungating and may produce early symptoms of unexplained anemia. Bleeding from the rectum may be the first and most common early symptom of carcinoma of the colon from any site. Carcinoma of the anus may be squamous or basaloid. Both forms are highly malignant.

Pancreas, Gallbladder, and Liver. Of all visceral carcinomas, carcinoma of the pancreas forms about 1%; of the gallbladder, from 2% to 4%; and of the bile ducts and the liver, less than 1%. The carcinoma is usually in the head of the pancreas. In this site it may invade or compress the pancreatic ducts and the common bile duct, with the consequences of obstruction, digestive disturbance, and icterus. In contrast, carcinomas of the body and tail of the pancreas are not associated with jaundice and are often large and disseminated when first discovered. Metastasis to the lymph nodes occurs early, and metastasis to the liver is common.

Respiratory Tract. Carcinoma of the larynx is about ten times as common in males as in females and is usually found on the true vocal cords, although about one fourth of the cases are extrinsic, that is, involve laryngeal mucosa other than the true cords, and are potentially more serious. Most are squamous cell carcinomas and if superficial may be cured by conservative surgery and if invasive, by laryngectomy. Metastases involve the cervical and submaxillary lymph nodes. Direct extension to the esophagus may occur. The relative risk of developing carcinoma of the larynx is five times greater in cigarette smokers than in nonsmokers. Primary carcinoma of the trachea is rare.

Carcinoma of the lung is one of the most common and lethal of malignant diseases; it is the leading cause of death from cancer in men and approaches that in women. The disease occurs chiefly in the 40- to 60-year age group and is usually of bronchial origin, but may arise in bronchioles as well. One of the first clinical symptoms of bronchogenic carcinoma is the insidious development of a persistent hacking cough. Pleuritic pain, dyspnea, and sometimes pleural effusion may occur, but in some cases the disease develops so insidiously that the first signs are only loss of weight and appetite, yet by this time the disease could be widespread. Numerous statistical studies have confirmed that the single most important factor in the causation of lung cancer is cigarette smoking, accounting for over 75% of cases. It may be, too, that carcinogenic compounds that are present in air polluted by automobile exhaust fumes and other hydrocarbon-containing agents play an additive role, since lung cancer is more common in heavy-smoking city dwellers than in those who live in rural areas. Pipe and cigar smokers develop carcinoma of the bronchi less often probably because they rarely inhale the smoke, but even they, as well as cigarette smokers who have given up the habit, run a greater risk than those who have never smoked.

Bronchogenic carcinoma often can be demonstrated by gross and microscopic study to arise from the bronchial mucosa. The most frequent histologic type is squamous cell carcinoma, followed by adenocarcinoma and the highly undifferentiated forms such as small cell anaplastic carcinoma (including "oat cell type") and large cell carcinoma.

Mediastinal metastases may compress the thoracic viscera, and pleural effusion, pneumonia, lung abscess, and bronchiectasis are frequent complications. Metastases usually occur in the bronchial, mediastinal, and cervical nodes, the adrenals, the brain, and the bones.

Breast. For decades, carcinoma of the breast has been the most common cause of cancer death in women, but now in parts of the country lung cancer in women is the most common and this trend is increasing. Breast carcinoma is rare under the age of 25. Nulliparous women or women whose first full-term pregnancy occurs late in their reproductive life are at an increased risk. This fact suggests that prolonged estrogen activity unbroken by the hormonal changes that take place during pregnancy may play a significant role in the development of the disease. Extension to the axillary lymph nodes may occur early, often before the tumor is discovered or the axillary nodes are palpable. Axillary metastases are found in about two thirds of the patients at operation.

Trauma plays no part in the etiology of cancer of the breast. Some evidence supports the hypothesis that high-fat diet increases the risk, especially for postmenopausal tumors. Premenopausal tumors have a higher frequency of familial aggregation, the susceptibility being genetically transmitted by either of the two parents. The main morphologic types of breast carcinoma are the following:

1. *Infiltrating ductal carcinoma* is composed of solid cords of epithelial cells, probably of ductal origin, usually surrounded by dense collag-

enous bands (desmoplasia), which give the tumor a hard consistency (scirrhous) and often lead to nipple retraction and adhesions to the skin *(peau d'orange)* in more advanced cases.

2. *Infiltrating lobular carcinoma* is made up of smaller epithelial cells derived from mammary lobular epithelium that invade the stroma in characteristic single chains, or "Indian files." This tumor is associated with such a high incidence (25%) of a later or simultaneous primary in the opposite breast that contralateral prophylactic simple mastectomy has been advocated.

3. *Mucinous (colloid) carcinoma* is characterized by abundant mucous secretion and a better than average prognosis.

4. *Medullary carcinoma* is formed by solid masses of atypical epithelial cells that do not form ducts or glands and have abundant lymphoid stroma.

5. *Intraductal carcinoma* is the *in situ* stage of ductal carcinoma without stromal invasion. It most frequently has a papillary or "comedo" pattern, characterized by necrosis of the neoplastic cells at the center of each cystic duct.

6. *Lobular carcinoma in situ* is the precursor of invasive lobular carcinoma.

7. *Paget's disease* is seen clinically as a chronic "eczematoid" lesion of the nipple that is actually produced by invasion of the epidermis by large, clear cancer cells originating from the ducts deeper in the breast.

8. Less frequent types of breast neoplasms are the *cystosarcoma phyllodes,* which tend to metastasize by way of the blood stream; the *metaplastic carcinomas,* which may have squamous, cartilaginous, or osteoid components; *tubular carcinoma,* which carries a better prognosis; and *secretory carcinoma,* the predominant variety on the rare occasion that the tumor occurs in children. The so-called *inflammatory carcinoma,* clinically characterized by redness and pain, is due to massive permeation of lymphatic channels and carries a very poor prognosis.

Metastatic Breast Tumors.   In addition to the axillary lymph nodes, carcinoma of the breast may metastasize to the mediastinal and other distant lymph nodes, as well as to the lungs, liver, bones, adrenals, and brain. Widespread invasion of the skin of the thoracic wall also occurs. If biopsy reveals no metastasis in the axillary nodes, 65% are curable. With axillary metastasis, only approximately 20% are curable.

Uterus.   Carcinoma of the cervix uteri is less frequent than breast carcinoma and its incidence has been decreasing steadily during the last decade. Carcinoma *in situ* is more frequent in the 30s, while invasive carcinoma is more frequent after age 40. It mostly originates around the squamocolumnar junction and is preceded by dysplastic changes whose detection by vaginal cytology helps prevent invasive disease. The great majority of cervical carcinomas are of the squamous cell type. Endometrial adenocarcinoma, a postmenopausal neoplasm, is becoming the most common invasive carcinoma of the uterus. Choriocarcinoma is a rare tumor of the uterus derived from placental trophoblast. This tumor is highly malignant but may be completely cured by appropriate chemotherapy alone.

Ovary.   The most common and important tumors of the ovary are cystadenoma, dermoid cyst, fibroma, Brenner tumor, and dysgerminoma, which are nonfunctioning, and granulosa cell tumor, theca cell tumor (thecoma), and arrhenoblastoma, which have some functional properties.

The cystadenoma may be of serous or mucinous type, both of which may undergo malignant change.

The dermoid cyst is a benign teratoma, always cystic, containing a grayish yellow sebaceous material mixed with a variable amount of hair in the cavity. Skin and a variety of other tissues such as teeth, bone, thyroid, and brain may be found in at least a portion of this type of tumor. Because representatives of all three embryonic layers are present, it is a true teratoma. Solid teratomas may be benign or malignant. Choriocarcinoma of the ovary occurs very rarely and is similar to those occurring in the testis and uterus.

The fibroma of the ovary is a benign tumor of fibrous ovarian stroma that may be bilateral. The association of ascites, and especially of hydrothorax (Meigs' syndrome), with this type of tumor is an interesting but unexplained phenomenon. Removal of the tumor results in disappearance of the serous effusion.

The Brenner tumor usually is found after the menopause and has no endocrine function. The tumor is mainly fibrous, with islands or strands of epithelial cells throughout the stroma. The origin of this tumor is not established, but the epithelium strongly resembles that found in the Walthard rests near the ovary.

The dysgerminoma is a nonfunctioning tumor of germ cell origin that is analogous to the seminoma of the testis. It is found frequently in both ovaries.

Granulosa–theca cell tumors are composed of varying mixtures of granulosa and theca cells and are the most common of the functioning tumors of the ovary, producing excessive estrogenic hormone. In a child, this results in precocious sexual development, both anatomic and functional, that disappears when the tumor is removed. In adults there may be either amenorrhea or excessive menstruation. If it occurs after the menopause, resumption of menstruation is a characteristic feature, and there may be endometrial hyperplasia. Some of these tumors may be considered as low-grade malignancies, particularly the pure granulosa cell types, but the prognosis is usually very good following surgery in over 75% of them. When theca cell elements are the exclusive component of these tumors they are termed thecomas and are almost always benign. The theca cells have foamy cytoplasm and are rich in lipid.

The Sertoli–Leydig cell tumor is the masculinizing tumor producing amenorrhea, sterility, breast atrophy, hirsutism, deep voice, and hypertrophy of the clitoris. These effects also may be produced by adrenal cortical tumors. Sertoli–Leydig cell tumors vary from the well-differentiated type characterized by the presence of tubules lined by typical Sertoli cells to highly undifferentiated sarcomatous types.

For other tumors of the female genital tract, see the chapter on obstetrics and gynecology.

Testis. Tumors of the testis are almost all malignant and comprise less than 1% of the malignant tumors in males. They usually involve men in the 20s, 30s, or 40s.

Benign tumors of the testis are rare. The interstitial (Leydig) cell tumor in children may produce masculinization, and in adults gynecomastia. Both androgenic and estrogenic hormones may be produced. Less than 10% are malignant. The gonadal stromal tumor, or Sertoli cell tumor, is a rare tumor that may have variable endocrine effects, most commonly gynecomastia, but the type of hormonal production has not been well documented. Both Leydig cell tumor and gonadal stromal tumor have in common the presence of lipoid or lipochrome in the cytoplasm of some of the tumor cells. The cells are uniformly round or polygonal, with relatively clear cytoplasm and no mitoses or abnormal nuclear forms unless they undergo malignant change.

Malignant tumors of the testis are divided into well-differentiated teratoma, seminoma, embryonal carcinoma, and choriocarcinoma, all considered to be of germ cell origin.

Teratoma contains different types of tissue, varying from well-differentiated adult types to highly undifferentiated malignant types. Cartilage, bone, muscle, adenoid, myxomatous, and adipose tissue may be found. However, in many of these tumors, malignant foci of seminoma, embryonal carcinoma or even choriocarcinoma also may be discovered if sought for diligently.

Seminoma is composed of fairly uniform polygonal cells with a moderate amount of light-staining cytoplasm. The cytoplasm of these cells may be granular or chromophobic. There may be a considerable number of lymphoid cells between the large polygonal cells (seminoma with lymphoid stroma), and there may be foci of necrosis and hemorrhage throughout the tumor tissue. The analogous ovarian tumor is the dysgerminoma, which is less malignant than the seminoma.

Embryonal carcinoma is composed of many pseudoacinic structures, slits, or irregularly shaped spaces, all lined by one or more layers of high cuboidal epithelial cells suggesting glandular structures. Between these structures there may be large and small masses of polygonal and round cells, which vary in size and shape, with mitoses and abnormal nuclear forms. All of these epithelial structures are supported by a dense or a loosely arranged fibrous stroma. Occasionally there are syncytial masses of trophoblastic-type cells. Teratocarcinoma refers to a mixture of embryonal carcinoma and teratoma.

Choriocarcinoma is similar to that in the ovary or uterus, with syncytiotrophoblast and cytotrophoblast present as essential components of the tumor. The tumor is unusually vascular and at times shows only focal areas of highly atypical trophoblastic tissue in association with a teratoid tumor.

The blood and urine of some patients with the above malignant germ cell tumors may contain elevations of gonadotropic hormones that may be helpful in diagnosis and prognosis.

Prostate. Carcinoma of the prostate is the second most common malignant tumor in men and is described at length in the section on the male genital system.

Thyroid. Tumors of the thyroid gland are mainly the microfollicular (fetal) and macrofollicular (colloid), the papillary and the solid (Hürthle cell) adenomas and carcinoma. These are described at greater length in the section on the Endocrine System later in this chapter.

Pituitary Gland. Most neoplasms of the pituitary gland arise in the anterior lobe and are benign. They are traditionally classified according to light microscopic criteria as chromophobic, eosinophilic, or basophilic adenomas. Functional classifications according to endocrine activity as determined by clinical findings, measurement of hormone levels and response, histochemical studies of the tumor cells, and electron microscopy are under investigation. Most adenomas are inactive hormonally and are chromophobic, that is, the tumor cells contain no stainable granules. They cause symptoms of overgrowing and destroy normal pituitary tissue and the adjacent optic and hypothalamic structures. Hypopituitarism, blindness, and hypothalamic dysfunction may result. The tumor cells may be arranged in diffuse, sinusoidal, or pseudopapillary patterns. The cells tend to be uniform and polygonal with a richly vascular stroma. These neoplasms may expand the sella turcica, erode its walls, and escape from their confines to encroach on adjacent structures. They are gray red and encapsulated, sometimes undergoing cystic and hemorrhagic changes. They occur most commonly in middle-aged adults and affect both sexes.

Adenomas, producing gigantism and acromegaly, are usually composed of cells with acidophilic granules. They are usually smaller than chromophobic adenomas, and the cells are often pleomorphic. Prolactin-secreting adenomas may be acidophilic or chromophobic. Adenomas secreting adrenocorticotropic hormone (ACTH) are usually small and are composed, at least partly, of cells with basophilic granules that are PAS positive. These tumors are one of the causes of Cushing's syndrome. Thyrotropin-secreting adenomas may be chromophobic or basophilic.

Craniopharyngiomas are intimately related to the pituitary gland and its stalk. They are thought to be derived from remnants of Rathke's pouch and most commonly occur as suprasellar cystic lesions with calcified walls containing brown fluid rich in cholesterol. They appear in childhood, adolescence, and adult life. Endocrine disturbances may be produced by encroachment of the encapsulated lesion on the hypothalamus and pituitary gland, and the optic system may be damaged by gradually expansive growth of the lesion. Protrusion into the third ventricle may cause hydrocephalus. Microscopically these tumors are usually composed of nests of benign stratified squamous cells surrounded by basal cells in a loose fibrovascular stroma somewhat resembling the ameloblastoma of odontogenic origin.

MALIGNANT MELANOMA

This tumor, originating from melanoblasts, is one of the most malignant of neoplasms. The cutaneous form often develops from a flat, hairless melanocytic nevus that may be light or dark brown in color. Most melanocytic nevi are benign and remain so, but if such a lesion begins to darken, show unusual growth activity, or break down, ulcerate and bleed, malignant transformation should be suspected. In general, the hairy, elevated, papillary moles uncommonly become malignant. Malignant melanoma is uncommon before puberty.

Malignant melanoma of the skin may be of three general types: (1) lentigo maligna melanoma, (2) superficial spreading melanoma, and (3) nodular melanoma. These differ slightly in prognosis, but depth of invasion at the time of diagnosis is the most important prognostic indicator.

Dissemination occurs through the lymphatics and the blood stream as well as through the skin. The amount of pigment is no indication of malignancy, which is shown rather by an increase in nuclear size, chromatic staining and mitotic activity, especially abnormal ones. Metastasis may occur anywhere but is most frequent in the regional lymph nodes, skin, liver and lungs. The eye is sometimes a primary site, the growth developing in the choroid, the iris, or the ciliary body. Occasionally, melanomas are primary in the meninges or the anal or the rectal mucosa. The prognosis in these cases is grave.

CHLOROMA (GRANULOCYTIC SARCOMA)

A rare tumor, chloroma occurs primarily in association with myelocytic leukemia, usually the acute type. It is composed of cells of the lymphocytic, monocytic, or myelocytic types. In the gross, the striking feature of this tumor is light green color, which probably is caused by some breakdown product of hemoglobin, perhaps protoporphyrin.

MALIGNANT LYMPHOMAS

The classification of lymphomas is complex, and only a simplified scheme can be discussed here. Basically, there are two major groups, Hodgkin's disease and non-Hodgkin's lymphomas. Hodgkin's disease will be considered later in this chapter. Non-Hodgkin's lymphomas have been classified by the Rappaport system for many years, but more recently the new international formulation (NIF) is gaining acceptance. The NIF eliminates the confusing use of the term "histiocyte," used in the Rappaport classification for large cells that since have been proven to be of lymphoid origin, and uses the noncommital but descriptive term "large cell" in its place. In the NIF system lymphomas may be of low-grade, intermediate-grade, or high-grade malignancy. An example of a low-grade lymphoma is the small round lymphocytic type, which often develops into chronic lymphocytic leukemia later in the course of the disease. Intermediate-grade tumors comprise a variety of histologic types in which large, small, cleaved or noncleaved lymphoid types may be dominant. High-grade lymphomas comprise the large-cell immunoblastic tumors, lymphoblastic lymphoma, and Burkitt's lymphoma. Lymphomas are further subdivided histologically, an important distinction being whether or not the tumor has a follicular or diffuse pattern. The follicular patterns are often slower growing but more resistant to chemotherapeutic agents. The diffuse patterns are more rapid growers but may respond well to therapy, with many treated patients now living without evidence of disease. The majority of lymphomas possess immunologic markers characteristic of either B or T lymphocytes, and all are monoclonal in type. Benign reactive proliferations of lymphoid cells are polyclonal, a helpful feature in questionable cases. Southern blot analysis (DNA probes) may be used to demonstrate clonality as well as cell type. Rearrangements of immunoglobulin and T-cell receptor genes may be detected in virtually all B- and T-cell neoplasms, respectively.

Plasmacytoma (multiple myeloma) is a type of lymphoma in which the end stage of lymphocyte differentiation, the plasma cell, is the principal cell involved. This malignancy is a multicentric tumor of plasma cells that develops in the red bone marrow of many parts of the skeletal system. Any bone may be involved, but those most commonly affected are vertebrae, ribs, skull, pelvis, and femurs. The lesions in bone are multiple, soft, gelatinous, and pinkish red. They largely replace the marrow, and they destroy the bone, producing spontaneous fractures or characteristic "punched-out" osteolytic areas of bone destruction. Extension into adjacent soft tissue is not uncommon, and in the late stages of the disease widespread visceral metastases may develop. Histologically the neoplastic character of the growths is recognized by nuclear immaturity and abnormal multinucleate or giant plasma cells. Plasmacytomas are monoclonal and often produce large amounts of a single immunoglobulin, which may be measurable in the blood as a monoclonal peak or in the urine as light chains (Bence–Jones proteinuria). The kidney may be extensively damaged with subsequent renal failure.

Hodgkin's disease is also a malignant lymphoma, but its clinical behavior and pathologic features are so distinctive that it is important to consider it separately from the group of lymphomas as a whole. Clinically Hodgkin's disease may present similarly to other lymphomas, with lymphadenopathy being localized, regional, or generalized. Splenomegaly or involvement of the bone marrow or liver indicate

TABLE 6-3. Classification of Hodgkin's Disease

TYPE	RELATIVE FREQUENCY
Lymphocyte predominance	10%
Mixed cellularity	35%–60%
Nodular sclerosis	35%–60%
Lymphocyte depletion	5%–10%

progressively higher stages of the disease. Cut section of involved lymph nodes may show a soft, fish-flesh type of replacement or variable foci of necrosis and fibrosis. The hallmark for recognition of Hodgkin's disease is the microscopic presence of the Reed–Sternberg cell, a large cell with bilobed hyperchromatic nucleus, large acidophilic nucleolus, and perinuclear clearing of chromatin producing a "bull's eye" effect. Hodgkin's disease is classified in the Rye classification as shown in Table 6-3.

NEOPLASMS OF THE CENTRAL NERVOUS SYSTEM

Various neoplasms affect the central nervous system by arising from the nerve cells or glia of the brain and spinal cord, the meninges, or the nerve roots. Gliomas of astrocytic, ependymal, oligodendroglial, and microglial derivation occur in characteristic patterns, locations, and age groups. Neoplasms of nerve cells are rare. Meningiomas and neurilemomas are usually benign surface lesions indenting but not invading the parenchyma. Metastatic neoplasms involve the central nervous system much more commonly than primary neoplasms and may originate anywhere in the body. These will be discussed in greater detail in the section on the nervous system.

Immunopathology

The principles of immunity, the effectiveness of the immune system, and the normal immune response in man are described in detail in the chapter on microbiology and immunology. However, since disorders of this system are an important part of pathology, some of them will be considered briefly here with the main emphasis on immunologic tissue injury or hypersensitivity reactions, immunologic deficiency, and graft rejection. Immunoproliferative disorders are considered elsewhere in the section on neoplastic disease.

HYPERSENSITIVITY REACTIONS

Classification of immunologic tissue injury or hypersensitivity reactions includes anaphylactic hypersensitivity, cytotoxic hypersensitivity, immune complex hypersensitivity, and cell-mediated hypersensitivity.

Anaphylactic hypersensitivity is a rapidly developing immunologic reaction that occurs almost immediately after contact with an antigen to which an individual has been previously sensitized. The reaction may be systemic or local. Systemic reactions may produce vascular collapse and shock that may be fatal. Local reactions may be manifested as hives (urticaria), allergic rhinitis, or bronchial asthma. Anaphylactic hypersensitivity reactions are mediated by IgE antibodies, which are found in the serum and also are bound to mast cells and basophils. Mediators released in the anaphylactic reaction include histamine, ECF-A, SRS-A, and PAF. Histamine and ECF-A are preformed and stored in granules of mast cells and basophils, while SRS-A and PAFs are generated during the anaphylactic process. Mediator release follows a burst of intracellular cyclic adenosine monophosphate (cAMP) formation and can be modulated by either sympathetic or parasympathetic stimulation. (Refer to the chapter on pharmacology for the therapeutic intervention in anaphylactic disease.)

Cytotoxic hypersensitivity is mediated by complement and occurs when an antibody reacts with antigen on the surface of a cell and activates the complete sequence of the complement cascade, which results in direct membrane damage and lysis of the cells. This reaction is the type that occurs in transfusion reaction, erythroblastosis fetalis, and autoimmune hemolytic anemia, as well as in some adverse reaction to drugs.

Immune-complex hypersensitivity is a result of the localization of antigen–antibody complexes, which produce tissue damage by activating mediators in the complement system and with inflammation as the main feature. The immune-complex diseases include the generalized form, the classic example of which is acute serum sickness, as well as forms that may localize to the kidney, joints, or blood vessels. The mechanism of injury is similar once the complexes have been deposited and involves the activation of the complement cascade and the participation of polymorphonuclear leukocytes and monocytes, which release lysosomal enzymes capable of damaging tissue. One of the morphological features of this type of injury on light microscopy of hematoxylin and eosin-stained sec-

tions is a smudgy eosinophilic change in the blood vessel walls due to the presence of complement, immunoglobulins, and fibrinogen. This change is usually called "fibrinoid" necrosis but is not really true necrosis, nor is the morphologic appearance specific for an immunologic reaction. Immune-complex tissue injury is a common pathway for tissue injury in a diffuse collection of disorders.

Cell-mediated hypersensitivity is the result of lymphocytes that are sensitized to specific antigens. The sensitized lymphocytes cause delayed-type hypersensitivity such as that occurring in the tuberculin reaction. This reaction is mediated through the release of lymphokines, or the sensitized lymphocytes may have direct cytotoxic effects when they contact a target cell. This cytotoxic effect is a major mechanism responsible for acute allograft rejection. It also is involved in certain viral infections.

AUTOIMMUNE DISEASE

Autoimmune diseases are thought to occur when there is loss of tolerance to self-antigens, and the body mounts an immune reaction to these self-antigens. Defects in immunoregulation (*i.e.*, altered T-helper and suppressor subsets, and the idiotypic antibody network, genetic control of immunoregulation, hormonal factors, and other factors) also are currently thought to be important in the emergence of immune reactions to self-antigens. Diseases that are usually considered to be due to autoimmune mechanisms include systemic lupus erythematosus (SLE), progressive systemic sclerosis (scleroderma), rheumatoid arthritis, dermatomyositis, Sjögren's syndrome, mixed connective tissue disease, and polyarteritis nodosa. These disorders are systemic disorders with multisystem involvement. In addition, there are autoimmune disorders that affect primarily one system or one organ and these include autoimmune hemolytic anemia, idiopathic thrombocytopenic purpura (ITP) and neutropenia, Hashimoto's thyroiditis, pernicious anemia, myasthenia gravis, primary biliary cirrhosis, autoimmune Addison's disease of the adrenal gland, and others.

Basically autoimmunity is simply hypersensitivity tissue injury directed against antigens of "self." Both genetic factors and viruses seem to have a role in susceptibility or triggering of autoimmune reactions. Indirect immunomicroscopy is a valuable technique to screen for the presence of circulating autoantibodies.

SLE is the classic example of a systemic autoimmune disorder in which there is injury to the kidney, joints, skin, and serosal membranes. This disorder occurs predominantly in young women and involves the development of a number of autoantibodies that are involved in the pathogenesis of the disease and also are laboratory markers for diagnosing the disease. The autoantibodies include antinuclear antibodies against double-stranded and single-stranded DNA, RNA, deoxyribonucleoprotein, and antibodies against the Sm antigen. Some of these antibodies can be found in other systemic autoimmune disorders, but antibody to the Sm antigen and antibody to native double-stranded DNA are almost specific for the diagnosis of SLE. In fact, anti-Sm antigen, which is found in about 30% of patients with lupus, is considered to be almost pathognomonic of lupus when present. The morphologic features of SLE include characteristic changes in the skin, particularly in the butterfly area of the face, a variety of patterns of involvement of the kidneys including focal, diffuse, and mesangial changes, inflammation of the joints, pericardium and pleura, nonbacterial verrucous endocarditis of the heart valves and endocardium, and involvement of blood vessels in many of the organs throughout the body.

Progressive systemic sclerosis (scleroderma) is characterized by inflammation and fibrosis involving the skin, the GI tract, kidneys, heart, muscles, and lungs.

Sjögren's syndrome consists of dry eyes, dry mouth, and arthritis. It may occur by itself or in conjunction with another connective tissue disease such as rheumatoid arthritis.

Polymyositis is an autoimmune disorder characterized by myositis with degeneration of individual groups of muscle fibers and infiltration of chronic inflammatory cells. There is also involvement of the skin and connective tissue and of the organ systems. This disorder is associated with an increased risk of developing malignant tumors.

Mixed connective tissue disease, as the name implies, has features of several of the connective tissue diseases. The two most distinctive features are high titers of antibody to ribonucleoprotein (RNP) and lack of serious renal involvement. This disease has a better prognosis than SLE.

Polyarteritis nodosa, in its broadest definition, includes noninfectious necrotizing vasculitis involving vessels of any type. The broad definition includes the classical polyarteritis nodosa with macroscopic lesions of medium-sized and smaller arteries of differing ages and stages, as well as hypersensitivity angiitis that is detectable only microscopically. Hypersensitivity angiitis is frequently distinguished from polyarteritis nodosa because

smaller vessels are affected with all lesions appearing to be of the same age. Drugs such as penicillin and sulfonamides have been associated with the development of vasculitis, usually of the hypersensitivity small vessel type.

IMMUNOLOGIC DEFICIENCY DISORDERS

A number of primary immunodeficiency diseases that are genetically determined have now been described. Those disorders that best illustrate the different mechanisms of these immunodeficiencies include (1) X-linked agammaglobulinemia (Bruton's disease) in which B lymphocytes are absent or decreased and there is a resultant deficiency in immunoglobulins, T lymphocytes are normal in this disorder; (2) thymic hypoplasia (DiGeorge's syndrome) in which B lymphocytes and immunoglobulins are normal and T lymphocytes are deficient; (3) severe combined immunologic deficiency (Swiss type) in which B lymphocytes and immunoglobulins are absent or decreased, T lymphocytes are absent or decreased; and (4) combined variable immunodeficiencies, a poorly defined but common form of immunodeficiency in which there are abnormalities of B lymphocytes and immunoglobulins and sometimes abnormalities of T lymphocytes.

Secondary immunologic deficiencies may be caused by immunosuppression, irradiation, chemotherapy, malnutrition, and infections.

Inheritable defects in phagocytosis, chemotaxis, and complement components have also been described and are associated with significant clinical disease.

AIDS is a recently described entity of high morbidity and mortality due to infection by HIV. It is defined by the Centers for Disease Control (CDC) as " an illness characterized by one or more 'indicator' diseases, depending on the status of laboratory evidence of HIV infection." "Indicator diseases" include disorders such as disseminated candidiasis, extrapulmonary cryptococcosis, lymphoma of the brain, *Pneumocystis carinii* pneumonia, Kaposi's sarcoma, toxoplasmosis, and other unusual or opportunistic infections. The results of serologic screening and confirmation of the presence of antibodies to HIV are also key data to establish laboratory evidence of infection with HIV. Groups at highest risk for AIDS include promiscuous male homosexuals, intravenous drug abusers, and persons with hemophilia A. Heterosexual transmission has also been documented. Patients who are receiving immunosuppressive therapy (*e.g.,* corticosteroids), who have lymphoma with negative HIV serology, or who have congenital immunodeficiencies are excluded by the criteria. The cellular immune defect is manifested by lymphocytopenia, particularly T lymphocytes, and especially decreased numbers of the "helper" (T_4) subset of T lymphocytes. There is "inversion" of the normal ratio of T helper (T_4) to T suppressor (T_8) from approximately 2.0 to values of less than 1.0. Alpha$_1$-thymosin levels are also typically elevated in prodromal AIDS patients.

HIV is a retrovirus similar to HTLV. It has an affinity to infect the T_4 subset of lymphocytes. Vaccine prevention and a "cure" for this infection are not yet available.

GRAFT REJECTION

Among the most exciting surgical procedures of recent years have been tissue and organ transplantations, particularly of such organs as kidneys, heart, liver, lungs and certain important, and sometimes life-preserving, tissues like bone marrow. While the technical aspects of organ transplantation have reached a high state of perfection, a more subtle cause for failure of the procedure has been the development of tissue and organ rejection based upon the effectiveness of the immune system in bringing about the destruction of the transplant.

The causes of rejection have been subject to intensive study and cannot be dealt with in any detail here. Suffice it to say, however, that many elements enter into the matter of histoincompatability, especially the genetic makeup of the recipient and donor as far as tissue antigen components are concerned. Tissue grafts from one part of the body to another in the same individual are readily accomplished because no immune reaction is provoked. In similar fashion a tissue or organ can be successfully transplanted from one identical or monozygotic twin to the other. In those cases tissue compatibility can be taken for granted.

Rejection in humans occurs between individuals whose genetic backgrounds are different, and the process is generally most marked the more different these backgrounds are. Rejection is less marked, for example, between members of the same family, particularly between siblings or mother and offspring, but tends to be pronounced when the donor and recipient are totally foreign to each other. The rejection process is now known to involve both humoral and cellular mechanisms, and there is good evidence that complement may play a role. It is the effectiveness of these immune processes that one needs to suppress when organ or tissue grafts are contemplated.

The rejection of transplanted renal grafts is a very complex process in which both circulating antibodies and cell-mediated immunity are involved. The T lymphocytes are the cells causing injury to grafted tissue in the cell-mediated immune mechanism. The cytolytic T lymphocytes may be the major cause of tissue damage; specifically activated T lymphocytes may also cause damage by production of lymphokines that cause the attraction and activation of other cytotoxic cells such as macrophages and neutrophils. Humoral antibodies also may have a role in rejection of human kidney transplants. Circulating antibodies have a role in several types of rejection of human kidney transplants. In one instance, circulating antibodies have been preformed in the transplant recipients because they have encountered a particular foreign antigen before transplantation; this may occur as a result of previous blood transfusions, previous pregnancies, or certain infections. There may also be escape of antigens from the transplanted kidney after transplantation into the recipient's circulation so that the recipient then produces circulating antibodies. Circulating antibodies may lead to injury by several mechanisms, namely, the deposition of antigen–antibody complexes, complement-dependent cytotoxicity and antibody-dependent cell-mediated cytolysis. These antibodies appear to attack the graft vasculature as the initial point of attack.

There are three principal types of rejection reaction, the hyperacute rejection, the acute rejection, and the chronic rejection. The **hyperacute rejection** is the result of preformed circulating antibodies due to previous sensitization to some of the donor-specific antigens. It occurs almost immediately after transplantation. The histologic lesions are similar to those of the Arthus reaction with large numbers of neutrophils infiltrating the vasculature and with immunoglobulin and complement found in the vessel wall.

The **acute** type of rejection may be due to a combination of both cell-mediated immunity and humoral damage by circulating antibodies. This type of reaction may occur within a few days of transplantation if the patient is not given immunosuppressive therapy or may occur after immunosuppressive therapy has been used and then discontinued. At the microscopic level, in kidney transplants, acute rejection is characterized by mononuclear cell infiltration of the glomeruli and vasculature of the kidney. Acute rejection due to humoral mechanisms involves extensive vasculitis with neutrophilic infiltration, arterial necrosis, and deposition of complement, immunoglobulins, and fibrin. These changes lead to thrombosis of small vessels.

Chronic rejection may occur in patients in whom phenomena of the acute graft rejection are prevented by immunosuppressive treatment. In these renal transplant patients there is usually progressive renal failure over a period of months. Changes include intimal fibrosis of cortical arteries and ischemic manifestations in the glomeruli and tubules leading to atrophy of the kidney. In some cases there are changes of acute arteritis with presence of immunoglobulins and complement, and in other cases there are interstitial infiltrates of plasma cells and lymphocytes indicating a cell-mediated mechanism of rejection.

The use of bone marrow transplantation in the treatment of leukemia and other hematologic disorders in which immunologically competent cells are transplanted into the marrow of a diseased recipient gives rise to the possibility of two types of immunologic problems for rejection phenomena. The first is the rejection of the grafted bone marrow material by the host; such rejection follows the mechanisms previously described. In the other type of reaction, *graft-versus-host* (GVH) disease, T cells in the transplanted normal marrow can react against the recipient's tissue, leading to serious disease, susceptibility to infection, and, commonly, death. Mechanisms of rejection are similar in other organ transplants, such as the heart, liver, and so forth.

Circulatory Disorders

Edema is the accumulation of abnormal amounts of fluid in intercellular or interstitial spaces or body cavities, especially the natural mesothelium-lined cavities, such as the pleura, the pericardium, and peritoneum. Generalized edema, that is, accumulations of fluid in the subcutaneous tissues and the body cavities so that the body is literally waterlogged, is referred to as *anasarca*. In general, edema is found most commonly in association with cardiac failure, in which blood is dammed back into the venous system, thus increasing the hydrostatic pressure and forcing fluid through the capillary walls into the interstitial spaces, or in certain forms of renal disease in which protein loss through the kidneys lowers the plasma protein to a point that the plasma osmotic pressure drops, permitting the escape of fluid from the blood vessels into the tissues. This fluid is low in protein content and is a *transudate.* It differs from inflammatory edema, which is generally localized, is rich in inflammatory cells and protein, and is associated usually with infection. Its accumulation is due to the increased permeability of the endothelial lining of the capillaries and small venules brought about by direct injury to the vessel walls. This fluid is an *exudate.*

Nutritional edema results, in part at least, from a loss of plasma proteins following prolonged severe malnutrition or liver disease.

Hyperemia means an increased amount of blood in an organ or part, and it may be localized or generalized. It may be caused by active or passive dilatation of blood vessels, especially capillaries and the venules. *Active hyperemia* occurs physiologically in a muscle that is exercised and pathologically in acute inflammation as one of the first local responses to injury. *Passive hyperemia* or *congestion* results from obstruction of venous outflow of blood from a part. This may be brought about by venous thrombosis or any other condition that constricts or obstructs a vein. Passive congestion may be generalized when the venous return to the heart is impaired, as in cardiac failure. The cyanosis, the dyspnea, and the edema that occur in this condition are directly referable to the stasis. The "nutmeg" liver, with the congested central and midzonal regions of the lobules, and the enlarged red firm spleen that results from splenic vein obstruction are good examples of the chronic stasis in an organ. In the lung, the liver, and the spleen, as well as in other organs that may be the seat of chronic venous stasis, there may be a considerable deposit of hemosiderin in the interstitial tissue. In the lung small hemorrhages occur into the alveoli. The red cells are phagocytized, and the hemoglobin is converted into hemosiderin. These hemosiderin-containing macrophages are called *heart-failure cells.* In all organs that are the seat of chronic venous stasis or chronic passive congestion there also may be a considerable increase of fibrous tissue, which, in the liver, accumulates about the central veins of the lobules. This condition is called *cardiac cirrhosis.* In the lung such tissue leads to thickening of the alveolar walls, in which, as well as in the alveoli themselves, hemosiderin-containing macrophages (so-called brown induration) accumulate.

Ischemia is a decrease in the amount of blood flowing into a tissue. It may be the result of functional or organic arterial disease, such as spasm, arteriosclerosis or thromboangiitis obliterans, thrombosis, or even pressure on an artery from some external cause. Sudden deprivation of blood may result in infarction, with necrosis of the organ or part; a gradual reduction of the blood supply may result in atrophy of the parenchyma with replacement fibrosis.

A *thrombus* is a semisolid mass, composed of blood platelets, red and white cells, and fibrin, formed within the heart or the blood vessels during life. It is caused by (1) injury to the vascular endothelium; (2) slowing, stasis, or eddying of the blood flow; or (3) changes in the composition of the blood. A roughening of the endothelial lining caused by trauma or arteriosclerosis permits the adherence of platelets, to which red and white cells attach themselves. Fibrin is laid down sometimes, but not always. Sclerosis of the veins, malignant tumors penetrating their walls, and endocardial scars are common sites. Infection may cause thrombosis by the direct extension of a suppurative process, such as valvular and mural thrombi in the heart, or thrombophlebitis following typhoid or puerperal sepsis. Most common sites are in the veins, particularly in the lower extremities, in which the blood stream is slow. Substances that agglutinate red cells tend to form capillary thrombi. Some of the factors that have been shown to cause platelet aggregation include adenosine diphosphate (ADP), collagen fibers, and thromboxane A_2.

The fate of a thrombus varies. If it is a bland uninfected thrombus it may, after a few days, be lysed by enzyme activity. If resolution does not occur, fibroblasts and new capillaries invade the thrombus from the adjacent intima, not only attaching it firmly to the vessel wall but converting it to a fibrous scar—*organization* of the thrombus. If the thrombus is occlusive in type, that is, it completely obstructs the vessel lumen, newly formed vascular channels may pass through the fibrous tissue to form communications that serve to restore some degree of circulation in the vessel. Occasionally some venous thrombi become calcified and form phleboliths in the vessel lumen. If, on the other hand, bacteria are present, suppuration may occur, giving rise to bacteremia, in which minute, bacteria-laden embolic fragments of the thrombus circulate in the blood.

The other common sequelae of thrombosis include (1) embolism, (2) infarction, (3) edema, and (4) gangrene.

Embolism is the partial or complete obstruction of the lumen of a blood vessel by any mass that is carried to it in the circulating blood. The mass is called an *embolus*. Detached fragments of thrombi are the most common forms of emboli. If they originate in a noninfected thrombus their effects depend upon their size and the degree of vascular obstruction they cause. If they had their origin in an infected thrombus, however, they contain microorganisms and may cause inflammation, and even abscess formation and infarction, at the site of lodgment. In the pulmonary or renal capillaries they may form embolic abscesses without infarction. Emboli from a thrombus on the valves or mural endocardium of the left heart cause infarctions of the brain, kidney, spleen, intestines, and other organs. Those in the right heart may produce pulmonary infarcts, but these usually do not occur unless the lung is also the seat of passive congestion.

In *fat embolism* minute globules of fat may be liberated into the blood stream during an operation on an obese individual or following contusion or laceration of subcutaneous fat tissue. An important cause is trauma to bones, especially fractures of the long bones of the lower extremities. In the latter circumstance, emboli of actual bone marrow, as well as fat, may be found in the vessels of the lungs, brain, and kidneys.

Air embolism may occur as a result of the entrance of air by way of veins and may be of traumatic or surgical origin. Caisson disease, or the bends, occurs in divers and other individuals who work in atmospheres where the pressure is much higher than at sea level. If the pressure about them is lowered too quickly, bubbles of gas, chiefly nitrogen, develop in the blood, and they may coalesce to form larger bubbles that may cause vascular occlusion. In fatal cases of air embolism, frothy fluid may be found in the right side of the heart and in the larger veins.

An *infarct* is a localized focus of ischemic necrosis resulting from the occlusion of an artery or, less commonly, a vein. It may be caused by (1) embolism of the artery supplying the part, (2) thrombosis of the artery supplying the part, (3) thrombosis of a major vein, or (4) occlusion of the vessels supplying a part from external pressure. Grossly, infarcts are recognized by their conical or pyramidal shape, the base being at the surface of the organ. At first the region is red, but the center undergoes coagulation necrosis, and the infarct finally becomes pale, owing to depigmentation and to organization by fibrous tissue.

Infarcts of the spleen and the kidneys often are multiple and usually are caused by emboli from the left heart. Infarcts of the brain more commonly result from thrombosis of sclerotic cerebral arteries, causing *encephalomalacia*. Infarction of the lungs results from emboli from the systemic veins or the right heart but may be caused by thrombosis of the pulmonary vessels in a lung that is the seat of passive congestion. Intestinal infarcts are commonly the result of thrombosis of the mesenteric vessels. Infarction of the myocardium is almost always caused by thrombosis of a branch of the coronary arteries superimposed on an atherosclerotic plaque.

Infarcts of the myocardium, kidney, and spleen are "pale" infarcts because the organs are supplied by end arteries. Infarcts of the lungs and intestines are "red" infarcts because of collateral circulation.

SHOCK

An exact definition of shock has not been established, but shock basically is a decrease in effective blood volume with decreased perfusion of vital organs and tissues. Shock may affect the brain, heart, kidney, and lungs, as well as the endocrine system and GI tract. Because of decreased perfusion of these organs there is inadequate oxygen delivered to the cells and inadequate removal of metabolic products. One of the most characteristic morphologic findings of shock is tubular necrosis of the kidney.

Disseminated intravascular coagulation (DIC) is a condition that occurs in a variety of disorders in which there is activation of the intrinsic pathway of blood clotting. These disorders include eclampsia, abruptio placentae, amniotic fluid embolism, thrombotic thrombocytopenic purpura, septicemia, and widespread carcinomatosis. As a result of activation of the coagulation cascade, there is consumption of coagulation components and depletion of many of the clotting factors, including platelets, factor I (fibrinogen), factor II (prothrombin), and factors V, VIII, and X. The fibrinolytic system is also activated producing clot lysis, which aggravates the bleeding tendencies that occur because of the clotting factor deficiencies. The fact that there are small vessel thrombi in addition to bleeding can produce widespread and serious damage to the cardiovascular system, central nervous system, lungs, and kidney.

Processes of Infection and Infectious Disease

Infectious disease is caused by living microorganisms. The incidence of many of these infections has been greatly reduced in recent years as a result of the preventive administration of very effective vaccines or toxoid preparations and, in a few instances, the use of live but attenuated agents (vaccinia inoculations against smallpox and inoculations against poliomyelitis and rubella). Effective treatment is now also provided by the use of broad-spectrum antibiotics.

Pyogenic Infections

The most common pus-producing microorganisms are the staphylococci, pneumococci, and gonococci. All may produce local infections, as well as septicemia, and generalized, as well as localized, manifestations of acute suppurative inflammation in other parts of the body. *Klebsiella pneumoniae* and *Corynebacterium diphtheriae* also are capable of producing acute suppurative inflammation.

STAPHYLOCOCCAL INFECTION

This is the most common cause of furuncles or boils, which are localized abscesses of skin around hair follicles, and of carbuncles, which also are circumscribed but deep seated and of more extensive foci or suppurative inflammation in the skin and the subcutaneous tissue. Food poisoning frequently is caused by the toxin produced by the growth of *Staphylococcus aureus* in contaminated food. Osteomyelitis, bronchopneumonia, endocarditis, and meningitis are also some of the manifestations of staphylococcal bacteremia. Ninety percent of *Staphylococcus aureus* are resistant to penicillin G; however, most community-acquired strains remain sensitive to synthetic penicillins and other newer antibiotics. Resistance to the β-lactamase-resistant semisynthetic penicillins is a problem increasingly seen in hospital-acquired *Staphylococcus aureus* infection.

STREPTOCOCCAL INFECTION

The two main forms of pathogenic streptococci are *Streptococcus viridans* (a large group of α-hemolytic streptococci), the most common cause of subacute bacterial endocarditis, and *Streptococcus pyogenes* (β-hemolytic streptococcus, Lancefield group A), the cause of erysipelas, acute ulcerative endocarditis, and scarlet fever, to name only some of the conditions that result from this ubiquitous microorganism.

Erysipelas is a diffuse streptococcal infection of the skin characterized usually by large and small mononuclear cell infiltration, hyperemia, and edema of the corium, with suppuration a relatively uncommon complication.

Scarlet fever is also caused by streptococci capable of producing erythrogenic toxin. Sore throat, fever, and a widespread erythematous skin rash are the first manifestations of this condition. Acute interstitial glomerulonephritis and otitis media are complications. In this case, too, the inflammatory infiltrate is mainly lymphocytic. Suppuration is relatively uncommon.

MENINGOCOCCAL INFECTION

Disease due to *Neisseria meningitidis* probably always begins as a mild upper respiratory infection that is rarely recognized as such. In a small percentage of individuals, usually children or young adults, this leads to a bacteremia with localization of the infection in the central nervous system, resulting in purulent meningitis. In other individuals, the infection takes the course of rapidly fulminating meningococcemia with circulatory collapse and death.

Meningococcemia is accompanied by a rash, which is petechial, purpuric, or ecchymotic hemorrhages, scattered over the entire body surface. These hemorrhages are the result of microthrombi in the small vessels. There is a generalized Swartzmanlike reaction and disseminated intravascular coagulation due to endotoxemia. Bilateral adrenal hemorrhage, the Waterhouse–Friderichsen syndrome, occurs in some cases of acute meningococcemia.

PNEUMOCOCCAL INFECTION

Streptococcus pneumoniae is the most common cause of bacterial pneumonia. The organism is found as part of the normal flora in the upper respiratory tract. Infection of the lower respiratory tract occurs most often in children under 5 years of age and the elderly. Prior viral infection or alcoholism predispose to serious infection. Meningitis, sinusitis, and otitis media are also frequently caused by this organism. Pneumococcal disease of all kinds is common in persons with sickle cell anemia and in the asplenic. A commercial polyvalent vaccine composed of capsular polysaccharide from 23 pneumococcal serotypes is available.

GONOCOCCAL INFECTION

Gonorrhea, a venereal disease caused by *Neisseria gonorrhoeae,* usually is characterized by acute suppurative urethritis in the male and the female, and by acute cervicitis and bartholinitis in the female. In the male the condition may spread to the posterior urethra and involve the prostate, the seminal vesicles, and the epididymis. In the female it may spread to the fallopian tubes and to the peritoneum. The condition may become generalized and lead to local manifestations in other sites, especially acute suppurative arthritis, usually monoarticular. Acute, ulcerative, and vegetative endocarditis, usually on the right side of the heart, also may complicate the condition. The infection also occurs in newborns, as conjunctivitis, and in infants, as vaginitis. Blindness may result from involvement of the cornea, with resultant opacity.

Nonpyogenic Infections

DIPHTHERIA

The cause of diphtheria is *Corynebacterium diphtheriae,* a microorganism that produces acute membranous inflammation locally and serious generalized symptoms as the result of toxemia. The infection affects primarily the oropharynx, often with extension to the nose and larynx and occasionally the trachea, major bronchi, and even the esophagus. The typical local lesion is characterized by the presence on the affected mucous membrane of a dirty, whitish or grayish pseudomembrane composed primarily of a fibrin layer in which are enmeshed leukocytes, numerous microorganisms, and groups of necrotic epithelial cells. The underlying tissues are hyperemic, edematous, and inflamed, with numerous minute ulcerations, at which points the pseudomembrane is attached. If stripped from the mucosa, the fibrinous membrane leaves a focally bleeding, raw mucosal surface. The generalized symptoms of diphtheria are due to the profound toxemia caused by the toxin elaborated by the microorganisms that remain localized in the upper respiratory passage. The most serious effects of the toxin are found in the myocardium where they may be severe enough to lead to cardiac failure and death. Rarely, death may result from mechanical obstruction of the trachea or bronchi by the pseudomembrane. Upon the patient's recovery, the pseudomembrane disappears and the mucosa returns to normal.

RHEUMATIC FEVER

Rheumatic fever is an acute nonsuppurative inflammatory disease involving a variety of tissue structures and organs of the body, particularly the heart and joints, but the tendons, subcutaneous tissues, the larger arteries, and even parts of the central nervous system may also be affected. Although the pathogenesis of the disease is not yet fully understood, it is quite clear that it results from hypersensitivity associated with a prior infection due to group A β-hemolytic streptococci. The first symptoms develop usually from 2 to 4 weeks after the inciting hemolytic streptococcus infection, which occurs nearly always in the throat or pharynx. By this time the local lesions may have cleared completely, though serologic evidence of a recent hemolytic streptococcus infection is demonstrable in a great majority of cases. While the local lesions in the throat or pharynx, while active, actually harbor the streptococci, the systemic lesions of rheumatic fever are bacteria free. The characteristic lesions in the heart are described more at length in the section on the circulatory system.

TYPHOID FEVER

This is an infectious disease caused by a bacillus, *Salmonella typhi*. The microorganism gains entrance into the body by means of contaminated food or water, although the five Fs most related to the spread of the disease should be borne in mind: food, fingers, flies, fomites, and feces. The microorganism may be cultured from the blood, feces, the wall of the intestines, the spleen, and lesions in other organs that may complicate the disease. Pure cultures of the inciting agent may even be obtained from rose spots, the skin lesions characteristic of this disease. The important pathologic lesions are the ulcerations in the ileum, the severe mesenteric lymphadenitis, splenomegaly, and focal necroses in the liver and bone marrow. The lymphoid tissues in the lower ileum and the cecum are affected earliest and show the most severe changes. In Peyer's patches, the earliest changes are hyperemia and edema, soon replaced by the exudation and the infiltration of large numbers of mononuclear cells, which are characteristic of this condition. These cells exhibit phagocytosis of fragments of lymphocytes, of plasma cells, and even of typhoid bacilli. Necrosis then begins, with ulcers forming where the necrotic tissue near the surface sloughs off. These small foci of infection finally coalesce to form round or elliptical ulcers that coincide with a Peyer's patch, the long axis of the ulcer being in the direction of the long axis of the intestine. This is in contrast with the tuberculous ulcer, which tends to run transversely. The important complications of typhoid fever are severe intestinal hemorrhage from an eroded blood vessel in an ulcer, perforation of the intestinal wall as a result of deep extension of an ulcer, and rupture of the spleen. Death from severe hemorrhage or from peritonitis may occur. During healing, no stenosis occurs at the site of the ulcer, and in the mucosa, the region of the ulcer becomes covered with epithelium, but gland follicles do not reform at that site. Statistically, about 2% of patients who recover become carriers, that is, individuals who harbor the microorganisms at some site, usually the gallbladder, and who exhibit no signs of clinical disease.

PERTUSSIS (WHOOPING COUGH)

In the pathogenesis of pertussis, the microorganism *Bordetella pertussis* is transmitted from one individual to another by respiratory droplets. The droplets enter the respiratory tract, and there the bacilli proliferate, becoming enmeshed in the delicate cilia of the tracheal mucosa. Laryngitis, tracheitis, bronchitis, bronchiolitis, and interstitial pneumonitis may follow. The cough probably results from the irritative effects of the products of disintegration of the specific microorganisms, possibly aggravated by the presence of the bacilli on the mucosal surface.

Viral and Rickettsial Diseases

Details of viral and rickettsial diseases are covered in the Microbiology chapter; a few comments about pathologic findings in selected diseases will be covered here.

INFLUENZA

Influenza is the most common viral disease. It is caused by several antigenically different strains of influenza virus, including types A, B, and C, which may be identified by complement fixation and neutralization tests. The disease is characterized by acute inflammation of catarrhal type affecting the air passages, sometimes with necrosis and desquamation of the lining cells. In some cases interstitial pneumonitis may be present, and occasionally bacterial pneumonia may be a complication. No inclusion bodies have been demonstrated. In some cases localized alveolar or interstitial emphysema may be present. Resolution of the pulmonary lesions, if severe, may be by organization of the alveolar exudate.

TYPHUS FEVER

The cause of epidemic typhus fever is *Rickettsia prowazekii*, which is transmitted to man by the body louse. There is an endemic type, which is transmitted to man by the bite of the rat flea; it is characterized by immunologic differences from the epidemic, or louse-borne type. In the gross, hyperplasia of the spleen and cloudy swelling of the parenchymatous organs are present; microscopically, endothelial proliferation of the small blood vessels, with or without thrombosis, and perivascular infiltration of large and small mononuclear cells (typhus nodules) are characteristic of the disease. These lesions are most common in skin, brain, and heart muscle. In the heart there may be degeneration of the myocardial fibers, with diffuse interstitial infiltration of large and small mononuclear cells. Interstitial pneumonitis may occur, and in the brain there may be petechiae, perivascular infiltration of lymphocytes, and small foci of gliosis.

Other rickettsial diseases include Q fever, caused by *Coxiella burnetii*, probably tick-borne; the spotted fever group of which Rocky Mountain spotted fever is an example, caused by tick-borne *R. rickettsii*; tsutsugamushi disease caused by *R. orientalis*, transmitted by a tropical mite; and rickettsial pox caused by *R. akari*, transmitted by a rodent mite. The pathologic, and to a less extent the clinical, manifestations of all of these diseases resemble somewhat those of typhus fever.

Infectious Granulomata

TUBERCULOSIS

Tuberculosis is a chronic communicable disease caused by *Mycobacterium tuberculosis*. It most commonly involves the lungs but may occur in other organs. The incidence of the disease in this country has declined markedly in the past 50 years, but it still is a leading cause of death in other countries. Far more individuals may be infected with the microorganism than develop clinical disease, since only about 1 in 20 of those who have actually been infected come down with clinical tuberculosis.

The mode of infection of the lungs by the tubercle bacillus is usually by inhalation of droplets expelled from the mouth (coughing, sneezing, or even talking) of a patient with active lesions, or contained in particles of dust. Inhalation is the most important route. Direct infection of the skin or mucous membranes may also occur. In the case of the bovine tubercle bacillus, infections may occur through the alimentary tract from the ingestion of contaminated milk from infected cows. In this case the microorganism enters the body by way of either the cervical or the mesenteric lymph nodes.

The Tubercle. The peculiar character of the tissue reaction to *M. tuberculosis* in the newly infected host results in the formation of a *tubercle*. After a week or two, however, the host's body be-

comes sensitized, the reaction becomes intensified, and along with these changes partial immunity develops and persists.

The first reaction to the tubercle bacillus is the appearance of large mononuclear cells, histiocytes, which become the characteristic large epithelioid cells with vesicular nuclei and abundant cytoplasm, fusing to form multinucleated giant cells that ingest but often fail to destroy the microorganisms. The Langhans' type of multinucleate cell, with central eosinophilic zone and nuclei at the periphery, is most common in tuberculous inflammatory tissue. Surrounding these epithelioid and giant cells is a peripheral zone of lymphocytes. Soon, however, as hypersensitivity develops, the exudate becomes softer, central necrosis occurs, and the macrophages and giant cells become more effective in preventing proliferation of, or in actually destroying, phagocytized bacilli. In most cases of initial infection, healing of the tuberculous focus occurs with the infiltration of reticulin fibers, which become collagenous and finally surround the tubercle with scar tissue. The caseous center remains indefinitely, but after a long time it may become calcified. The bacilli may remain alive indefinitely in the necrotic and calcified center. From a clinical standpoint, however, the individual with these healed lesions does not suffer from clinical tuberculosis.

Because hypersensitivity and some degree of immunity develop as a result of the first infection with *M. tuberculosis*, later infection will provoke a very different response from that following the first. For this reason we speak of *primary infection* and *secondary infection* due to this microorganism.

Extension of tubercles may occur by several processes. In active lesions, the zone of peripheral epithelioid cells is killed by toxic substances, the caseous center enlarges, and a new zone of epithelioid cells is formed. This may be repeated until large masses are caseous. Extension also occurs through the lymphatics to the regional lymph nodes and thence to the blood stream through the thoracic duct, or by invasion of veins with the formation of infected thrombi, which form disseminating emboli. The coughing up of infected sputum from one bronchus and inhalation of it into another bronchus or the swallowing of tuberculous sputum may disseminate the lesions. Tuberculous sputum may cause lesions through skin abrasions.

Miliary tuberculosis may result from blood stream invasion, either direct or by way of the lymphatics. The primary source usually is the lungs or the bronchial lymph nodes. The miliary tubercles are found especially in the lungs, the spleen, the liver, and meninges. Miliary tuberculosis is most common in children, particularly miliary tuberculous meningitis. Tuberculosis of the kidney, the adrenal, the epididymis, or the fallopian tube usually arises as a hematogenous infection from the lung.

Pulmonary Tuberculosis. The *primary* type of pulmonary tuberculosis, once called "childhood" tuberculosis because it commonly developed in children, now may occur in young adults because, as a result of the greatly lowered incidence of the disease, the number of individuals in this age group who have never had contact with *M. tuberculosis* outnumbers those who have. Infection results from the aspiration of tubercle bacilli into the lung and the development of a primary focus, the Ghon lesion. This lesion, measuring about 1 cm to 3 cm in diameter, is usually situated in the subpleural region of almost any part of the lung except the apices. Small tubercles develop along the lymphatics to the bronchial lymph nodes draining the region infected. These show active caseation, and the process usually extends to other mediastinal lymph nodes. The lesion in the periphery of the lung, together with the involved tracheobronchial lymph nodes, is called the **Ghon complex.** In the great majority of cases, the Ghon complex heals and appears in later life as a calcified lesion in the lung and the regional bronchial nodes. Less commonly, the Ghon complex, instead of regressing and healing, may progress to tuberculous bronchopneumonia and, by dissemination of the microorganisms by way of the blood stream, to generalized miliary tuberculosis.

Secondary or adult-type pulmonary tuberculosis may be caused by reactivation of a primary focus, which is rare, or by endogenous or exogenous reinfection. It is much more serious than the primary type and differs from it anatomically and clinically. The primary infection, which occurs in the host who has never previously been infected, not only confers some degree of immunity in most cases but also sensitizes the body to the protein fractions of the microorganism. Thus the host's reaction to *M. tuberculosis* if it invades the body at some later time provokes a more intense reaction because of this hypersensitivity.

Secondary tuberculosis usually begins in the subapical portion of a lobe and extends downward from the apex; extension usually is from the coughing up and the inhalation of caseous material from one bronchus to another. The same lung simultaneously may show tuberculous pneumonia, nodular lesions with caseous necrosis, cavities, and scar tissue. The nodular lesions are the prevailing type and vary in size from miliary tubercles to massive lesions formed by the confluence of smaller ones. The larger nodules show much caseous necrosis, surrounded by the typical epithelioid and giant cells with small lymphocytes.

Cavities may arise from the sloughing of a tuberculous bronchus or extension of nodular lesions into a bronchus, with discharge of the caseous material by coughing. There usually is a secondary pyogenic infection that leads to suppuration and increased caseation. Erosion of blood vessels in the wall of a cavity causes hemorrhage, but this is not so common a complication as might be expected, because the local blood vessels, sometimes actually crossing the cavity, frequently are the seat of obliterative endarteritis. Cavities may undergo partial or complete arrest by the formation of fibrous tissue in their walls.

Healing of the pulmonary lesions, especially if cavitation is not present or is minimal, occurs slowly as a result of fibrosis and sometimes focal calcification. The presence of cavities complicates the healing process, and in some cases healing does not occur. If the tuberculous lesions extend to the pleural surface of the lungs, tuberculous pleuritis with or without effusion may occur, and healing results in fibrous adhesions.

Tuberculous Pneumonia. Whenever large numbers of tubercle bacilli are aspirated from a tuberculous cavity that is in direct communication with a bronchus, tuberculous bronchopneumonia may develop. This may be of the gelatinous, the caseous, or the mixed variety. The gelatinous type is characterized by edema of the interalveolar septa and fluid and large mononuclear cells in the alveoli and the bronchioles; the striking feature of the caseous type is the necrosis of the exudate and even of the pulmonary tissue.

Extrapulmonary Tuberculosis. The pleura is nearly always involved in pulmonary tuberculosis, with resultant adhesions or effusions. Many cases of fatal secondary pulmonary tuberculosis are limited to the lungs, but involvement of the intestine, the larynx, the adrenals, the meninges, and the kidneys is common.

The characteristic tubercle occurs in tuberculosis elsewhere in the body. Tuberculosis may invade practically any organ but is most common in the lungs, the pleura, the pericardium, the peritoneum, the larynx, the lymph nodes, the intestine, the epididymis, the seminal vesicles, the kidneys, the bladder, the skin, the fallopian tubes, the bones and joints, and the meninges.

SYPHILIS

Once one of the most important of diseases affecting man because of its protean and widespread manifestations, syphilis has shown a marked decline in incidence since the introduction of antibiotic therapy. Nevertheless, it still remains a major public health problem because of the marked upsurge in the number of cases, especially in the 15- to 24-year age group, in many parts of the United States.

Syphilis is certainly the most serious of the venereal diseases. It is caused by a spirochete, *Treponema pallidum*, which is present in the lesions it causes. Although the infection, once the incitant is in the body, is continuous, it manifests itself clinically in three stages: the initial infection, the chancre; a generalized secondary stage with a rash; and various tertiary manifestations that may occur years later.

Primary Chancre. The primary chancre develops, within 2 to 6 weeks after inoculation, from a macule into a papule with eroded or ulcerated surface, and from a few millimeters to several centimeters in diameter. The base of the single, circular ulcer is indurated but painless, and from the surface a nonpurulent serous fluid exudates. It usually is located on or near the genital organs, though extragenital chancres on the lips, the tongue and other parts of the body do occur. The treponemata are widely disseminated throughout the blood stream within 48 hours after inoculation (hence, before the appearance of the chancre). Shortly after the chancre appears, the regional lymph nodes become enlarged and firm, but not tender. Diagnosis is confirmed by darkfield examination of serum from the chancre or a bubo since the treponemata are usually abundant in these situations. Microscopically the chancre is a shallow ulcer with a dense accumulation of mononuclear cells in the corium and subcutaneous tissue, with perivascular infiltration of plasma cells and lymphocytes. The base of the ulcer is composed of well-vascularized, dense granulation tissue, also infiltrated with lymphocytes and plasma cells, with small numbers of granulocytes near the ulcerated surface. The histologic appearance is not specific or diagnostic. The necrosis and ulceration usually are superficial, unless the condition is complicated by secondary infection. Healing is complete in 2 months or less, and only a relatively small epithelialized scar remains to mark the site of the lesion.

Secondary Stage. The secondary stage results from the dissemination and proliferation of the treponemata throughout the body. The typical lesions occur on the average 6 or 7 weeks after the chancre and may be accompanied by the symptoms of acute infection. The characteristic secondary phenomena are (1) the eruption on the skin and (2) on the mucous membranes, (3) sore throat, and (4) lymphadenopathy. The cutaneous eruption is often inconspicuous but may be very marked. The most frequent lesion consists of generally distributed ham-colored macules, caused by perivascular and diffuse infiltration of the skin, which may be raised as papules. Pustules are uncommon, and vesicles are rare. All of these lesions contain numerous treponemata. Papules on hair surfaces cause loss of hair. Condylomata, or venereal warts, may appear on the genitals and the perineum or in the axilla. Histologically the secondary lesions are characterized by perivascular infiltration of lymphocytes and plasma cells. Unless there is secondary infection, there is no destruction of tissue, and healing occurs without scarring.

Sore throat, often severe and chronic, is common. Mucous patches are commonly found on the mucous membrane of the mouth, the tongue, the palate, and the tonsils, as well as between the labia, and correspond to the secondary skin lesions.

Localized periostitis, especially on the anterior surface of the tibia, sometimes occurs. There usually is moderate adenopathy of the inguinal, the posterior cervical, the occipital and epitrochlear lymph nodes, which show diffuse hyperplasia.

In the secondary stage, complement fixation, rapid plasma reagin (RPR), and Veneral Disease Research Laboratory (VDRL) tests are positive in almost 100% of cases. VDRL titers are generally low, 1 : 32 or less, in primary syphilis and increase to 1 : 32 or higher in secondary syphilis. Advanced tests include the treponemal immobilizing antibody (TPI) test, the fluorescent treponemal antibody absorption (FTA-ABS) test, and the *Treponema palladum* hemagglutination test. The FTA-ABS is the best confirmatory test for a patient with a positive VDRL result. Increase in the spinal fluid cell count and the globulin occurs in about 25%. Treponemata in the spinal fluid may be demonstrated by animal inoculation before these changes.

Tertiary Stage. Tertiary syphilis may occur from a few months to as long as 50 years after the chancre. The lesions involve the internal organs principally and are of two types: (1) the gumma and (2) diffuse chronic inflammatory lesions in which obliterative endarteritis with perivascular infiltration of inflammatory cells, chiefly plasma cells, predominates.

The *gumma* is the most characteristic but not the

most common lesion of tertiary syphilis. It may occur in any tissue, but its most frequent sites are skin, liver, testes, and bones. Gummata vary in size from the miliary gumma to those several centimeters in diameter. They usually are single but may be multiple and consist of a firm, elastic, central, necrotic portion surrounded by a dense fibrous or cellular zone. Microscopically, epithelioid cells are present, mixed with lymphocytes and some plasma cells, around the central focus of necrosis, but they are less conspicuous than in tubercles, and giant cells also are less common. In the necrotic zone, tissue structure may still be recognizable, at least in outline, and, in its center, especially in the later stages, fibroblasts may be present.

Diffuse chronic inflammatory lesions without necrosis and characterized by obliterative endarteritis, perivascular cuffing with plasma cells, and even local vascular proliferation are the most common type of tertiary reaction. They are found chiefly in the cardiovascular and the central nervous systems.

Cardiovascular syphilis affects the aorta more than the heart itself, the lesions occurring as endarteritis of the vasa vasorum, involving chiefly the region just above the aortic valve and the ascending portion of the arch. Necrosis of the media with secondary fibrosis follows, the inflammatory reaction frequently extending down to involve the aortic valve itself. The wall of the aorta is thicker than normal at first, because of lymphocytic infiltration and proliferation of fibrous tissue, chiefly in the adventitia but also involving the media. In the larger arteries of the adventitia there is likely to be obliterative fibrous proliferation of the intima. Later, the wall is weakened, thinned and dilated, and a typical syphilitic aneurysm may develop although such aneurysms are less common than they were some years ago. Other effects are (1) narrowing of the coronary orifices, causing angina pectoris, and (2) involvement of the aortic valves, with insufficiency, which may occur as a result of dilatation of the ring, thickening and shortening of the leaflets and fusion of the leaflets with the wall of the aorta at the site of their attachment, so that there is abnormal separation of the cusps at the commissures. Syphilis of the myocardium is rare.

Central nervous system syphilis manifests itself in several different ways, all of which are described in the section on the nervous system. One form, meningovascular syphilis, is characterized by the typical chronic inflammatory and vascular changes that resemble those in the aorta and coronary arteries, together with fibrous thickening of the meninges.

VDRL results are variable in tertiary syphilis and may be negative in one third of cases. FTA-ABS is the procedure of choice in tertiary syphilis.

Multiple gummata of the liver were relatively frequent before effective treatment was developed, and the scarred liver (hepar lobatum) is now also a comparative rarity.

Bones.   In the bones, syphilis may lead to perforations of the hard palate and destruction of the nasal septum, destruction of the calvaria and, in the long bones, gummata or diffuse destructive osteoperiostitis. In congenitally syphilitic children, osteochondritis used to be common, but this is less frequent since prenatal treatment of the mother has become almost the rule.

Congenital Syphilis.   Syphilis may be transmitted from the infected mother to the fetus. Infection of the fetus may occur at any time during intrauterine life.

The ***fetal type*** includes all stillborn syphilitic infants and all those who die soon after birth. The body is undersized, the skin macerated or covered with bullae, particularly on the palms and the soles. The chief gross findings are enlargement of the spleen and the liver, with disintegration of the hepatic cords, and portal fibrosis and infiltration of lymphocytes, plasma cells, and blood-forming cells. At the epiphyseal ends of the long bones, osteochondritis is common. In the liver, the pancreas, the kidneys, and the lungs, signs of delayed development are characteristic of congenital syphilis. An unusual amount of undifferentiated mesoblastic tissue is present. In the lungs the condition is known as pneumonia alba. In addition to the increase of interalveolar mesoblastic and fibrous tissue, the alveoli are small and lined by cuboidal epithelium.

The ***infantile type*** is a less severe manifestation of the infection, which is evidenced about the second month by snuffles, pemphigus, splenomegaly, and anemia. Often there are jaundice, rhagades, paronychiae, and alopecia.

The ***late type*** (lues tarda) is characterized by deafness, Hutchinsonian teeth (tapered or bulbous incisors, with a notch in the middle of the biting edge), saddle nose, periostitis, keratitis, splenomegaly, and neuroretinitis. Occasionally neurosyphilis may develop.

Serologic tests are not invariably positive in infants with congenital syphilis.

BRUCELLOSIS (UNDULANT FEVER)

This is an acute or remittent infectious disease caused by any species of *Brucella,* but most commonly by *Brucella abortus* or *Brucella suis*. The usual source of infection is occupational exposure to infected animal tissue in meat processing plants. Infection with *Brucella melitensis* has occurred following consumption of imported, unpasteurized goat-milk cheese. *Brucella* infection is characterized by invasion of the reticuloendothelial system with resultant hyperplasia and the formation of miliary granulomas resembling those found in tuberculosis, sarcoid, or tularemia.

TULAREMIA

Tularemia is a subacute infectious disease caused by *Francisella tularensis* in man. It is transmitted by the handling of infected rabbits, but the condition also occurs in ground squirrels, mice, and rats. The transfer of the infection between animals is effected by the wood tick. The condition may also be transferred to man by the bite of a blood-sucking insect, especially the wood tick and the deer fly. The most common type of the disease is the ulceroglandular, characterized by a primary lesion at the site of the inoculation and enlargement of regional lymph nodes. The results of the oculoglandular type are primary involvement of the conjunctiva and regional or distant lymph node enlargement. The acute type shows no identifiable primary lesion, and there is no obvious enlargement of lymph nodes. In man, the anatomic lesions are granulomatous foci characterized by a necrotic focus surrounded by large mononuclear cells. In the older lesions, fibrosis occurs around such a focus. These lesions are most common in the lymph nodes. They may be present also in the spleen and the lungs, in which there usually is also confluent bronchopneumonia.

LISTERIOSIS

Human infection with *Listeria monocytogenes* occurs most frequently in neonates or in adults who have some underlying debilitating disease or who are immunosuppressed. Infection in either group is usually manifest as septicemia and purulent meningoencephalitis. The mortality rate in debilitated adults is usually high, with focal abscesses being found in liver, spleen, lungs, and other organs. Infection occurring during the first trimester of pregnancy usually results in abortion, while colonization of the infant from the birth canal may lead to meningitis at 7 to 10 days of age. The organism is known to affect many animals and to survive in soil for long periods. The epidemiology of the infection in humans is still poorly understood.

ACTINOMYCOSIS

This is a chronic, granulomatous, inflammatory disease caused by any species of *Actinomyces,* but *Actinomyces israelii* is most frequently isolated from human infections. The disease manifests itself mainly in the face and the neck, the intestine or the lungs. The lesion is a granuloma. Microscopically, colonies of the organism (branching filaments) are present in the inflammatory and fibroblastic region surrounding the necrotic focus. In the gross, the granules appear yellow and are referred to as sulfur granules.

HISTOPLASMOSIS

The causative agent of histoplasmosis is *Histoplasma capsulatum,* a dimorphic fungus occurring in soil and animals. In the human body it is found in the reticuloendothelial cells. Fever, leukopenia, anemia, and loss of weight are the main symptoms, and it may be fatal. Granulomatous lesions are present in liver, spleen, lymph nodes, and lungs. The nodules become calcified when healing occurs, and can be confused roentgenographically and histologically with calcified tuberculous foci. The concentric lamination of the calcium deposits is characteristic of histoplasmosis.

COCCIDIOIDOMYCOSIS

Coccidioidomycosis results from infection with a fungus, *Coccidioides immitis.* Most cases occur in Texas, Arizona, and California. In warm dry climates the chlamydospores are carried in dust, and the infection occurs by inhalation. Entrance of the microorganism through the skin has been reported. The clinical manifestations may be slight or like those of influenza or pneumonia. A specific diagnosis may be made by detection of precipitins or by complement fixation test. In the progressive form (coccidioidal granuloma) the condition resembles tuberculosis or blastomycosis. The anatomic manifestations are similar to those of tuberculosis or blastomycosis, with the formation of granulomatous lesions, diffuse fibrosis, and even ulceration and cavitation. The differentiation from blastomycosis depends upon the study of the microorganism. *Coccidioides immitis* exhibits endosporulation, whereas Blastomyces reproduces by budding. The microorganisms may be found in giant cells or free.

CRYPTOCOCCOSIS

Cryptococcosis is caused by *Cryptococcus neoformans,* an encapsulated yeastlike fungus that reproduces by budding. The fungus has a worldwide distribution. While exposure to this ubiquitous fungus is common, disease is rare and generally is seen in individuals with decreased host resistance, including patients receiving corticosteroids, patients with lymphoreticular malignancies, and patients with AIDS. *Cryptococcus neoformans* may cause a diffuse meningoencephalitis. Respiratory, skin, and bone infections may also occur. Smears using India ink to define the capsule of this yeastlike organism are often performed for diagnosis.

OTHER FUNGAL DISEASES

Other fungal diseases beyond the scope of this section for detailed consideration are North American blastomycosis caused by *Blastomyces dermatitidis,* a thick-walled yeast form with a thick refractile wall, which reproduces by single budding; South American blastomycosis caused by *Paracoccidioides brasiliensis,* a double-contoured organism that produces multiple buds around the periphery; opportunistic fungus infections caused by *Candida albicans, Aspergillus fumigatus,* and the organisms causing mucormycosis (*Rhizopus, Mucor,* and *Absidia*).

LEPROSY

Leprosy (Hansen's disease) is a chronic, infectious granulomatous disease caused by the acid-fast bacillus *Mycobacterium leprae.* There are approximately 10,000,000 cases worldwide but only 2,000 to 3,000 cases in the United States. The acid-fast organism cannot be cultured *in vivo* but has been successfully grown in foot pads of mice. The organism has a low degree of infectiousness and usually is thought to require long periods of contact before transmission is possible from one person to another. Exposure to the organism in a normal individual frequently does not lead to progressive disease. In a susceptible host with decreased resistance, the disease may be progressive. It involves principally the skin, mucous membranes, and nerves. The two principal types of reaction in leprosy are the tuberculoid and lepromatous types. In tuberculoid leprosy, there are firm, raised, hypopigmented, sharply demarcated skin lesions. There is involvement of the nerves and sensory loss. A granulomatous inflammation occurs in the dermis, and perineural inflammation by epithelioid cells and lymphocytes is typical. Acid-fast bacilli may or may not be seen in sections of the nerves. In lepromatous leprosy there are macular, erythematous, nodular skin lesions with indistinct borders.

There is massive dermal infiltration by leprae cells, (vacuolated mononuclear cells containing acid-fast bacilli). There is also perineural inflammation. The main complications of leprosy are those caused by nerve damage, mucous membrane changes, and secondary effects of longstanding chronic infection. Amyloidosis is one of the complications of leprosy. In tuberculoid leprosy, T-lymphocyte function is normal. Lepromatous leprosy occurs in those patients with low host resistance due to impaired T cell function. While the prognosis of tuberculoid leprosy is good with adequate treatment, the prognosis of lepromatous leprosy is poor.

Noninfectious Granulomata

BOECK'S SARCOIDOSIS

Boeck's sarcoidosis is a systemic disease of unknown etiology with granulomatous manifestations in skin, lymph nodes, lungs, bone marrow of phalanges, liver, spleen, parotid, eyes, and other sites. The striking difference from tuberculosis is the absence of necrosis in the granulomatous nodules. Some multinucleated giant cells contain star-shaped crystalline rosettes, asteroid bodies, and rod-shaped elastic fibers encrusted with calcium and iron (Schaumann bodies), but these are not specific for this condition. Sarcoidosis is more common in young women than in men. Overall, the disease is ten times more common in blacks than in whites in the U.S. While the etiologic agent is unknown, it appears that patients who develop sarcoidosis respond in an abnormal manner due to an inherent immunologic defect.

Other Granulomatous Lesions

Granulomatous lesions similar to Boeck's sarcoid are produced by beryllium if it enters a wound. Magnesium silicate, present in talcum powder, can also produce similar lesions. The most common source of beryllium at one time was beryllium phosphor from fluorescent bulbs, but this source no longer exists. Inhalation of beryllium dust (usually the oxide) from ores may produce acute or chronic pulmonary berylliosis. Even powdered starch (from rubber surgical gloves) may induce the formation of granulomatous inflammation, especially of the peritoneum.

Genetic Disorders

Genetic disorders can be divided into three major groups: (1) those involving numerical or structural abnormalities of whole chromosomes, (2) those affecting individual genes and exhibiting mendelian transmission, and (3) those multifactorial disorders involving an interplay of multiple genes.

CHROMOSOMAL ABNORMALITIES

This group of genetic disorders is diagnosed by karyotype, which allows determination of chromosome number and morphology, as well as characterization of their specific banding patterns. Because of occasional artifacts, definitive diagnosis is usually reserved until a consistent result has been obtained by studying a number of metaphase plates.

Incidence. Among live-born infants, about 6 per 1000 have chromosomal defects with sufficient severity to cause some disability. About half of these abnormalities involve the sex chromosomes, in spite of the fact that there is only 1 pair of sex chromosomes to 22 pairs of autosomes. The highest frequency of chromosomal abnormalities is found among spontaneous abortuses, 40% to 50% of which have major chromosomal defects. In surviving adults, abnormalities are confined predominately to sex chromosomes.

Pathogenesis. Meiotic nondisjunction (movement of both homologous chromosomes to one daughter cell and none to the other) is the most common cause of abnormalities in chromosome number. The presence of an additional chromosome (trisomy) occurs fairly frequently, but the absence of an autosome (monosomy), as opposed to a sex chromosome, is practically never found among live-born individuals.

Abnormalities in the structure of individual chromosomes are usually the result of breakage and fusion of segments of chromosomes. The consequences are deletion, rearrangements, and translocation of those segments.

Autosomal Abnormalities. The most common abnormalities in the number of autosomes in live-born infants are trisomy 21 (Down's syndrome), trisomy 18 (Edward's syndrome), and trisomy 13 (Patau's syndrome). The general frequencies of these disorders are approximately 1 in 1,000, 11,000, and 15,000 live births, respectively. The incidence of each of the three autosomal abnormalities increases with the age of the mother. For example, Down's syndrome (mongolism), the most common autosomal disorder, occurs in about 1 in 3000 live births in mothers under 30 years of age, but in mothers over 45 years the incidence can be as high as 1 in 50.

Each of the three trisomy syndromes shows a fairly characteristic external appearance and multiple anomalies of internal organs. **Down's syndrome,** which is the only autosomal trisomy that is compatible with survival to maturity, is characterized by mental retardation, large forehead, flat nose, oblique palpebral fissures, and epicanthal folds. It is also associated with short stature and a predisposition to develop acute myelogenous leukemia. Individuals with trisomy 18 and trisomy 13 usually die in early infancy. **Trisomy 18 (Edward's syndrome)** is associated with severe growth failure, marked deformities of feet, and frequent malformations of internal organs. Cleft lip and palate, brain malformation, especially arrhinencephaly, small eyes, sloping forehead, and polydactyly are characteristic of **trisomy 13 (Patau's syndrome).**

More severe abnormalities in chromosome number, such as triploidy and tetraploidy (three and four complete sets of the entire chromosome complement) have been found in stillborn infants and abortuses. They are probably incompatible with intrauterine survival.

The most well-known structural abnormality of autosomes is the **cri du chat syndrome (partial 5p monosomy, cat-cry syndrome),** which leads to death in early infancy. This disorder is associated with deletion of a segment of p arm of **chromosome 5.** The syndrome is associated with growth retardation, underdevelopment of the central nervous system, and a small larynx (cause of the typical cry).

A variant of Down's syndrome, which is characterized by an attachment of the extra chromosome 21 to another chromosome by translocation, such as G/D or G/G translocation, can be classified as a structural abnormality. Because this condition can be transmitted through successive generations, it must be distinguished from the classic type. Unlike the latter, the incidence of translocation type of Down's syndrome is independent of the age of the mother.

Sex Chromosome Abnormalities. Most common abnormalities in sex chromosomes are numerical in nature. The normal female somatic cell contains two X chromosomes while the normal male contains an X and a Y. According to the **Lyon hypothesis,** one of the X chromosomes in the female is inactivated. Cytologically, this inactive chromosome is represented by the **Barr body,** condensed chromatin material in the nucleus of the somatic cell of the female. When more than one X chromosome is present in a cell of either sex, a Barr body will be formed. Thus, a normal female has a Barr body, and a normal male does not. If an extra X chromosome is present in a karyotype of a patient, regardless of the sex phenotype, an additional Barr body will be present.

The presence of only one X chromosome *(XO, Turner's syndrome)* occurs in a phenotypic female without Barr bodies. The syndrome is characterized by short stature, webbed neck, failure to develop secondary sex characteristics, and ovarian dysgenesis. The presence of an extra X chromosome *(XXX, the triple X syndrome)* is found in clinically normal females with or without certain behavioral abnormalities.

In *Klinefelter's syndrome* and its variants, there is one Y chromosome and at least two X chromosomes (XXY, XXXY, or XXXXY). The affected individual is phenotypically male with tall stature, poorly developed secondary sex characteristics, testicular atrophy, and occasional gynecomastia. His somatic cells are positive for Barr bodies.

ASSOCIATION BETWEEN CANCERS AND CHROMOSOMAL ABNORMALITIES

Many malignant neoplasms, especially those that are anaplastic, manifest chromosomal abnormalities. Although a majority of neoplasms do not show definite and predominant chromosomal anomalies, some neoplasms are associated with sex characteristic aberrations. These include (1) presence of the Philadelphia chromosome (Ph[1]) in about 85% of the patients with chronic myelogenous leukemia, (2) clonal karyotypic abnormalities involving chromosomes 5, 7, 8, and 21 (partial loss, monosomy, partial gain, or trisomy) in acute nonlymphoid leukemia, (3) association of 14q+ in Burkitt's lymphoma, (4) deletion of a segment of q arm of chromosome 13 in nonfamilial type of retinoblastoma, and (5) deletion of 11p13–14.1 in the sporadic aniridia-Wilms' tumors.

HEREDITARY AND FAMILIAL DISORDERS

Analyses of family pedigrees have shown that many diseases are transmitted from one generation to the next as simple mendelian traits. Each disease, however, manifests a combination of signs and symptoms that is fairly complex. It has been postulated that a single abnormal gene in these conditions can express a multiplicity of phenotypic traits. Such a phenotypic effect of a gene is called "pleiotropy."

In mendelian genetics, a gene is said to be dominant when it is phenotypically expressed in the heterozygote. A recessive gene, on the other hand, is that which is expressed phenotypically only in the homozygote. When both the normal and abnormal genes of a heterozygous pair are phenotypically expressed, the effect is said to be codominant.

Autosomal Dominant Disorders. In a pedigree analysis, an autosomal dominant trait is that which appears in some members of the family in every generation (a vertical distribution). Approximately 1400 well-established autosomal dominant disorders have been identified in man. These disorders are relatively mild. Some are manifested at birth, while others are not evident until later in life. *Huntington's chorea,* for example, rarely becomes manifest before the second decade. The degree of severity of dominant disorders may also be highly variable in the same family pedigree. For example, the extra digit in *polydactyly* may vary from a fully formed structure to a mere stump, consisting of a clump of connective tissue. Such a phenomenon is said to represent a variation in the *expressivity* of the gene. It is also conceivable that, even in the presence of the abnormal genes in the genome, the phenotype may not be observable at all. In that case, the gene is said to have *incomplete penetrance.* Relatively common autosomal disorders include familial hypercholesterolemia, Marfan's syndrome, multiple polyposis of the colon, hereditary hemorrhagic telangiectasia (Osler-Rendu-Weber disease), neurofibromatosis, osteogenesis imperfecta, von Willebrand's disease, and achondroplastic dwarfism.

Autosomal Recessive Disorders. In an autosomal recessive disorder, the mother and father of the affected individual are usually normal, as are more distant ancestors. Siblings of the patients are more frequently affected than normal. If the trait is rare, an increased consanguinity will often be observed among the parents. Relatively common autosomal recessive disorders include cystic fibrosis, deaf mutism, phenylketonuria and other aminoacidurias, Wilson's disease, albinism, emphysema due to α_1-antitrypsin deficiency, ataxia telangiectasia, and Friedreich's ataxia. Currently, more than 1100 well-established autosomal recessive disorders are known.

Sex-linked Dominant Disorders. This mode of inheritance is extremely uncommon. Heterozygous affected females will transmit the disease to both sexes with a frequency of 50%. Affected males will transmit the trait to all their daughters but to none of their sons. The erythrocyte antigen X_g^a and vitamin D-resistant rickets belong to this group of disorders.

Sex-linked Recessive Disorders. Recessive sex-linked traits are fairly common. On the average, half of the sons of normal heterozygous females will be normal and half will be affected. If the trait is not common, the affected individuals are usually males, while the females are carriers. This group of diseases includes the common red-green color blindness, hemophilia A, classic agammaglobulinemia (Bruton), glucose-6-phosphate dehydrogenase deficiency, Fabry's disease, and chronic granulomatous disease of childhood.

MULTIFACTORIAL DISORDERS

Some of the most frequently encountered diseases, including gout, hypertension, some forms of diabetes mellitus and congenital heart disease, spina bifida, cleft lip/palate, and many others are included within this category. These disorders have in common the interplay of both *genetic and environmental* influences. The genetic contribution is made up of at least two abnormal genes acting in concert to exert a dosage-type effect that, in turn, can be significantly influenced by numerous environmental factors. The result is *variable phenotypic expression* within the same family tree. Many diseases, including some malignancies, that have been described as "running in the family" are in truth multifactorial disorders.

CONTRIBUTIONS OF BIOCHEMICAL AND MOLECULAR GENETICS

The manifestations of hereditary disease are far removed from the primary site of gene expression and are often not defined precisely. The progress in medical genetics since the introduction of the concept of "inborn errors of metabolism" by Garrod has been to approach closer to the primary phenotypic defect of the abnormal gene as well as to elucidate the event at the level of the gene itself. The first major step was the demonstration that a large number of hereditary disorders are due to the deficiency of specific enzymes. The list of enzyme-deficiency disorders has grown considerably and is still growing. Some specific entities have already been described in the chapter on biochemistry. Most of these disorders are recessive traits. The deficiency of uroporphyrinogen I in acute intermittent porphyria is an example of autosomal dominant disorders in this group.

Application of the methods of protein chemistry and immunology has also added a long list of disorders that involve plasma proteins, coagulation factors, immunoglobulins, complements, and hemoglobins. In addition to providing very powerful diagnostic tools, these methods have modified our view of the recessivity of hereditary disorders. For example, sickle cell disease is considered to be a recessive trait because the heterozygous individual does not manifest the usual signs and symptoms in normal environment. Electrophoretic studies of hemoglobins have shown, however, that the heterozygote produces both **HbS** and **HbA,** the normal counterpart. As an hereditary trait, HbS must therefore be classified as being codominant. Recessivity of the trait is thus a phenotypic property, rather than an inherent property of the structural gene. This finding allows the use of more refined methods to identify carriers of clinically recessive disorders.

The success in the determination of the amino acid sequences of the polypeptide chains of certain protein molecules provides knowledge at the level of the primary products of structure genes. Since the discovery that HbS is associated with the substitution of valine for glutamic acid at position 6 of the β-chain, a large number of hereditary conditions has been shown to be due to abnormal amino acid sequences.

The methods of somatic cell hybridization and refined methods of chromosome identification have made assignment of specific loci to individual human chromosomes possible. Thus, 22 loci, 1 of which is the Rh locus, have already been mapped on chromosome 1. The histocompatibility complex (HLA), which consists of four closely linked and highly polymorphic loci, identified as HLA-A, HLA-C, HLA-B, and HLA-D, in that order, has been located on chromosome 6. In addition to its importance in organ transplantation, certain alleles within this complex are associated with certain diseases. The strongest association is between the HLA-B27 allele and ankylosing spondylitis. Further details on this topic can be found in the chapter on general microbiology and immunology.

More recently, the use of the methodology of recombinant DNA technology and somatic cell genetics have led to the identification of abnormal genes at the level of the nucleotide sequence of DNA. The most remarkable discovery is the identification of so-called oncogenes in man. These normal genes are widely dispersed in the genome and are very well conserved: they are not polymorphic. Two of the oncogenes from human bladder carcinoma lines have been extensively characterized. Both are variants of the normal oncogene, differing from it only at one nucleotide portion of its DNA sequence that codes for a protein. This raises the possibility that independent somatic mutations in the two tumors may have converted a normal DNA sequence into one that somehow causes malignant transformation.

Nongenetic Syndromes

CHEMICAL POISONS

In fatal *carbon monoxide poisoning* the blood and the tissues may have a striking "cherry red" color due to the carboxyhemoglobin. In the brain there may be symmetric foci of petechial hemorrhages and of encephalomalacia, most commonly in the basal ganglia, especially the lenticular nucleus and the globus pallidus. These are characteristic but nonspecific changes that are due to hypoxia.

Aside from the bright red color of the blood and the mucous membranes (in this case due to oxygenated hemoglobin), which at first might suggest carbon monoxide poisoning, there is no distinctive morphologic feature of *hydrocyanic acid* or *cyanide poisoning.* The peach kernel or bitter-almond odor of blood, vomitus, and tissues is characteristic.

In the later stages of *methyl alcohol poisoning,* atrophy of the optic nerves is the only anatomic feature characteristic of the disease.

In *acute ethyl alcohol poisoning,* cerebral edema and hyperemia, possibly with petechial hemorrhages of the gastric mucosa, are the only gross features. In *chronic alcoholism,* chronic catarrhal gastritis, fatty degeneration of the liver, and micronodular cirrhosis are the most common findings. Micronodular cirrhosis is considered by some to be due to the direct toxic effect of alcohol on the liver cells, but others attribute the liver damage primarily to deficiencies in the diet of the chronic alcoholic. There is much good evidence for both points of view.

In the acute case of *mercury poisoning,* in which the poison is taken by mouth, there is mucosal corrosion of the stomach and of the duodenum. The mucosa is white and opaque and shows a variable amount of erosion or ulceration. In the later stages, hemorrhagic membranous and ulcerative inflammation of the colon is common, while necrosis of the proximal convoluted tubules of the kidney is a characteristic and usually fatal feature.

In *chronic lead poisoning,* the so-called blue line of the gums is characteristic, and the coarse basophilic stippling of the red blood cells is another feature. Atrophy and fibrosis of muscles of the extremities, wrist drop, "lead colic," renal tubular abnormalities, and degeneration of the testes and of the anterior horn cells of the spinal cord are common. Lead usually can be demonstrated by chemical tests in the epiphysiodiaphyseal ends of the long bones, the kidneys, the liver, and the central nervous system. Elevated levels may be found in blood.

In *sulfonamide poisoning* the outstanding effects are acute nephrosis with interstitial edema and infiltration of lymphocytes between the tubules, showing the degenerative change and internal hydronephrosis that result from obstruction of some of the collecting tubules by the precipitation of crystals. In this type of nephrosis, the portion of the nephron that begins with the distal part of the loop of Henle shows the greatest degenerative change. This has been referred to as *lower nephron nephrosis,* although it is not limited to the distal portion of the nephron. Interstitial myocarditis with infiltration of leukocytes and eosinophils has been reported commonly. Panvasculitis, especially in the myocardium, and focal necrosis of the parenchymatous organs have been described. The changes in the bone marrow are characteristic of acute anemia and agranulocytosis. A rash, presumably on an allergic basis, may occur. Of the various sulfonamides, sulfathiazole is the most likely to injure the kidney.

Chronic fluoride poisoning occurs most commonly in the southern and the western sections of the United States but is also observed in all areas in which the drinking water contains excessive amounts of fluorides. Mottled tooth enamel, alternating patches of chalkwhite and gray enamel, caused by patchy hypoplasia of this tissue, is the earliest and the chief effect of this poison. The fluorine acts directly upon the ameloblasts. Osteosclerosis also occurs. Of interest and importance, however, is the fact that proper fluoridation of drinking water protects against dental caries.

Acute fluoride poisoning is rare and is usually the result of the accidental ingestion of sodium fluoride that has been mistaken for sugar, flour, or powdered milk. Less than 1 g can be fatal.

Acute mushroom poisoning, most commonly with *Amanita phalloides,* is characterized by acute gastroenteritis, acute nephrosis (with fatty degeneration of the kidney), and fatty degeneration of liver, heart, and skeletal muscles. Massive hepatic necrosis may occur. Foci of degeneration may occur in the brain if the condition is not immediately fatal. Mortality approaches 50%.

Food poisoning, usually caused by the contamination of food with microorganisms of the *Salmonella* group or with toxin-producing staphylococci, commonly causes acute enteritis. A special form of food poisoning is botulism, caused by exotoxin of *Clostridium botulinum,* an anaerobic bacillus that may grow and produce its toxin in certain canned or preserved foods that have been inadequately cooked and sterilized before sealing. The principal effects of the toxin are on the nervous system, and death, which occurs in a high percentage of cases, is usually the result of respiratory failure. There are no specific morphologic changes characteristic of this highly potent toxin.

VITAMIN DEFICIENCIES

The diseases or pathologic changes listed in Table 6-4 are known to be caused by vitamin deficiencies. Some of the pathologic conditions that have been attributed to vitamin deficiency in animals have not been observed in man.

RADIATION INJURY

Radiation injury may result from radiation therapy, exposure of personnel involved in diagnostic radiology and radiotherapy, and accidental exposure due to nuclear accidents. Extensive investigation of victims of the atom bomb explosions in World War II has significantly contributed to knowledge of radiation injury. Forms of radiation include α-particles containing two protons and two neutrons, the least penetrating of radiant energy forms; β-particles, electrons that may penetrate through only a few

millimeters of the body; gamma rays, emitted naturally from radium, uranium, and man-made radioisotopes, which penetrate deeply into tissue; and x-rays, machine-generated gamma rays, which may also have α- and β-particle effects as they penetrate tissues. Radiation injury is thought to occur either as a result of indirect action in which free radicals and peroxides are formed by ionization of tissue or by direct action with radiant energy directly damaging vital macromolecules in the cell. Tissues are sensitive to the effects of radiation approximately in order of their capacity for regeneration, with labile cells being most sensitive, stable cells being of medium sensitivity, and permanent cells being least sensitive.

Acute radiation injury, such as would occur with atom bomb explosions or accidental overexposure of the whole body to radiation, may produce: the cerebral syndrome, with coma setting in immediately and death following in a few hours; the GI syndrome, with necrosis of intestinal epithelium, nausea, vomiting, diarrhea and dehydration; and the hematopoietic syndrome, in which the white blood count begins dropping and different cell types are depleted in a characteristic fashion. Lympho-

TABLE 6-4. Vitamin Deficiency in Man

VITAMIN	DEFICIENCY STATE	CHARACTERISTIC PATHOLOGIC CHANGES
Fat-soluble		
A (retinol)	Night blindness; xerophthalmia; keratomalacia; epithelial keratinizing metaplasia; disturbances in bone growth	Xerophthalmia; hyperkeratosis of skin; deficient regeneration of visual purple; keratinizing squamous metaplasia of epithelium lining ducts and glands
D_2	Rickets (children)	Deficient calcification and endochondral ossification: Excess of osteoid tissue and of metaphyseal cartilage ("rachitic rosary")
Calciferol	Osteomalacia (adults)	Counterpart of rickets in the adult, except for absence of endochondral abnormality
K	Hypoprothrombinemia; hemorrhagic diathesis	Increased tendency to bleeding; prolonged coagulation time
Water-soluble		
C (ascorbic acid)	Scurvy	Hemorrhagic manifestation in various parts of the body; deficient osteogenesis and osteoporosis; intercellular cement substance deficient
B Complex B_1 (thiamine)	Beriberi	Degeneration of peripheral nerves; polyneuritis; edema; cardiac dilatation, especially of right side, with decompensation; Wernicke's encephalopathy; degeneration of mamillary bodies
B_2 (riboflavin)	Cheilosis; glossitis; dermatitis; ocular lesions	Cracks or fissures at corners of mouth; atrophy of tongue; scaly dermatitis; superficial interstitial keratitis
Nicotinic acid (niacin)	Pellagra	Dermatitis with redness, thickening, hyperkeratosis and scaling; glossitis; colitis with diarrhea; degenerative changes in central nervous system with dementia
Folic acid	Macrocytic anemia	Megaloblastic bone marrow changes
B_{12} (cobalamin)	Pernicious and other megaloblastic anemias; subacute combined degeneration	Pernicious anemia (B_{12} is extrinsic factor necessary, together with intrinsic factor from gastric mucosa, to prevent pernicious anemia); degeneration of posterior and lateral columns of the spinal cord

cytes are depleted within 24 to 36 hours, platelets within 2 to 3 days, neutrophils within 5 to 7 days, and anemia becomes evident in a matter of weeks or months if the patient survives. Damage to the hematopoietic tissue in the bone marrow may result in bleeding problems, immunologic deficiencies, and susceptibility to infection.

Chronic radiation injury may lead to radionecrosis of the skin and sloughing. Radium implants used to treat carcinoma of the cervix may lead to rectovaginal fistula because of radionecrosis. Thus, necrosis of normal tissue is a complication of radiotherapy of cancer. Some of the other complications of radiation are sterility, aplastic anemia, cataracts, developmental defects in fetuses exposed *in utero,* and an increased incidence of leukemia, thyroid cancer, and lung cancer.

SYSTEMIC PATHOLOGY

Cardiovascular System

Cardiovascular disease, which includes diseases of the heart as well as vascular lesions of the central nervous system, is the most important cause of morbidity and mortality in the United States and other highly developed countries. The disorders comprising cardiovascular diseases account for over half of all deaths in the U.S. Coronary heart disease is by far the most common cause of death. Vascular lesions of the central nervous system (stroke) are the third leading cause of death following cancer, which is second. Among diseases of the heart, coronary heart disease is the leading cause of death, hypertensive heart disease next, followed by the less frequent causes of rheumatic heart disease, congenital heart disease, syphilitic heart disease, and other primary and secondary types of heart disease. There is obvious overlap among coronary heart disease, vascular disease of the central nervous system, and hypertensive heart disease because of the interrelationships between atherosclerosis and hypertension.

CONGENITAL HEART DISEASE

This subject is also covered in the sections on internal medicine and pediatrics; only selected aspects will be presented here. The most important concept about etiology is that the injury producing congenital heart disease always occurs during the first trimester of pregnancy, because that is the period in which the development of the heart is completed.

Etiologic agents include maternal disease, such as rubella and possible other viruses, teratogenic agents, such as the antimetabolite drugs and the obsolete drug thalidomide, chromosomal defects, such as those that occur in Down's and Turner's syndromes, other single gene abnormalities which predispose to atrial septal defect, tetralogy of Fallot, and pregnancy at high altitude.

Congenital abnormalities of the heart are usually the result of abnormal communications or obstruction. The defects may result from abnormal septation, abnormal rotation, abnormal endocardial differentiation, and malformation of the aortic arch syndrome.

The major types of congenital heart disease are usually classified according to whether or not cyanosis (implying right-to-left shunt) is present. Those disorders with a left-to-right shunt and no cyanosis include: ventricular septal defect (the most common of *all* congenital heart malformations), atrial septal defect (including ostium primum defect, ostium secundum defect, and patent foramen ovale), common atrial ventricular canal or persistent ostium atrioventriculare, and patent ductus arteriosus. Those defects without shunt or cyanosis include pulmonary stenosis; coarctation of aorta (adult type with narrowing below the origin of the ductus, 95% of all cases of coarctation; infantile type with obstruction above the origin of the ductus, 5%); aortic stenosis; vascular rings from anomalies of aortic arch; and anomalous origin of the coronary arteries. Congenital heart defects with cyanosis and right-to-left shunt include tetralogy of Fallot (pulmonary stenosis, interventricular septal defect, overriding of aorta, and right ventricular hypertrophy), the most common form of *cyanotic* congenital heart disease; tricuspid atresia; transposition of great vessels; truncus arteriosus; Taussig–Bing heart; single ventricle; and hypoplastic left ventricle (underdevelopment of left side of heart or mitral and aortic atresia).

Congenital heart disease may also occur in which cyanosis develops only late in the course of the disease usually as the result of reversal of a left-to-right shunt. The term Eisenmenger's complex or syndrome, now obsolete, has been used to describe those cases in which left-to-right shunts from ventricular septal defects undergo reversal after pulmonary hypertension has developed.

RHEUMATIC HEART DISEASE

While rheumatic fever may cause arthritis, subcutaneous nodules, chorea, and other manifestations, the most serious sequelae of rheumatic fever result from involvement of the heart. Rheumatic fever causes pancarditis, involving all layers of the heart: pericardium, myocardium, and endocardium, especially the valves. Rheumatic fever and rheumatic carditis are not always fatal; however, patients who die during the first attack of rheumatic carditis usually die as a result of myocarditis with myocardial failure. Patients who die after repeated attacks of rheumatic carditis usually die from the complications of valvular disease. The most widely accepted theory concerning the etiology of rheumatic fever is that it is due to hypersensitivity to group A β-hemolytic streptococci. (See the section on infectious disease.)

The valves involved most often are the mitral and aortic with the tricuspid and particularly the pulmonary valves being less commonly affected. The mitral valve is involved in the vast majority of cases, and the aortic valve is affected with the mitral valve in about 50% of the cases.

Characteristically, multiple minute, firm, wartlike nodules are found on the atrial surface of the mitral valve and on the tricuspid valve when it is involved, situated about 1 mm to 3 mm from the free margins, and on the ventricular surface of the aortic valve. In the acute state the vegetations seldom are large enough to interfere with valvular function. The inflammatory process involves practically the entire thickness of the valve structure. In the early stages the valve is swollen and thick, with the verrucous nodules on its surface close to the line of closure. Microscopically the ground substance of the valve is increased and fibrinoid necrosis is present near or beneath the verrucous nodules. The inflammatory exudate is not abundant. About the zones of necrosis, palisades of inflammatory cells, often of Anitschkow myocyte type, are present, and sometimes monocytes or polymorphonuclear leukocytes or both may be present.

There are no bacteria in the verrucous nodules on the valve leaflets. In time they become organized and finally covered by a layer of endothelial cells that grow in from the intact endothelium surrounding them. Healing of the valvular inflammation occurs by fibrosis, which causes thickening, stiffening, and retraction of the leaflet. Recurrent inflammation of damaged valves is common. The chordae tendineae also are involved and, as organization proceeds, become thickened and shortened as well as fused. Retraction, deformity, and calcification of the scar tissue cause various degrees of valvular stenosis and insufficiency, with hypertrophy of the myocardial walls, the work of which is increased by these lesions. In mitral stenosis, the left atrium and the right ventricle become hypertrophic and dilated, but in aortic stenosis, there is hypertrophy of the left ventricle.

Aschoff bodies are found in the myocardium in about 80% of cases of acute rheumatic fever. These are localized, usually perivascular, foci of a proliferative inflammation that is composed of large mononuclear and multinuclear cells, with so-called owl-eyed vesicular nuclei and some lymphocytes surrounding a focus of collagenous degeneration or necrosis, especially in the early stage of the lesion. The lesion is specific for rheumatic inflammation in the myocardium or other tissues in which it has been observed.

In addition to the rheumatic lesions of the endocardium and myocardium, the pericardium in a majority of cases is also involved, particularly in the active phase. The characteristic lesion is a diffuse fibrinous or serofibrinous inflammation of nonspecific type.

BACTERIAL INFECTIVE ENDOCARDITIS

Anatomically, infective endocarditis is characterized by soft, friable vegetations on the affected valve, very different from the firm, granular verrucous nodules of rheumatic valvulitis. The course of the disease may be acute or subacute, but this method of classifying the disease is not as important as classifying by the etiologic agent. The morphologic findings in the heart are quite similar regardless of the etiologic agent or clinical course. About 50% of the cases that develop in a subacute fashion are caused by *Streptococcus viridans* and in many of these cases there has been previous damage to the heart by preexisting rheumatic heart disease or congenital heart disease. Many of the cases that develop rapidly are due to *Staphylococcus aureus*. A large number of infectious agents has been identified as causing infective endocarditis in addition to these two prototype organisms. They include large numbers of bacteria: other streptococcal species, gonococci, enterococci, coliform organisms, *Hemophilus influenzae, Proteus,* salmonellae, as well as mycotic organisms such as *Candida, Aspergillus,* and *Mucor.* Infective endocarditis is a serious risk in drug addition with intravascular injection of unsterile drugs, and it is also a serious complication of open heart surgery with valve replacement.

The typical lesion is a form of valvulitis, with large, soft, friable platelet and fibrin thrombi on the valve surface with numerous microorganisms both within and on the surface of the vegetations. Portions of this type of friable thrombus break off readily and, if on the mitral valve, may give rise to septic emboli that may be carried by the blood to other parts of the body. This type of endocarditis is extremely serious. Before antibiotics the mortality rate was high, close to 100%. Now a cure is possible in a majority of these cases as a result of intensive treatment with appropriate antibiotics.

SYPHILITIC HEART DISEASE

Syphilis of the heart affects primarily the aortic valve, resulting in dilatation of the valve ring with insufficiency and often causing narrowing of the orifices of the coronary arteries. The myocardium is occasionally involved, especially the smaller arteries, which may show low-grade endarteritis and periarteritis. The structure most commonly affected is the aortic arch, the wall of which, along with the distended aortic valve ring, shows inflammation of the vasa vasorum. Aortic stenosis is never found unless there is associated chronic rheumatic valvulitis or atherosclerotic calcification to account for it. The aortic insufficiency may be brought about by (1) separation of the valve cusps at the commissures, (2) thickening and retraction of the cusps themselves, and (3) stretching of the aortic ring. The cusps show diffuse proliferative inflammation, with thickening of the free margins that roll inward toward the ventricular chamber. Artificial valves made of plastic have been developed and now can be inserted in the aortic ring for correction of the insufficiency.

The inflammatory process may involve the coronary orifices in the aortic sinuses as well as the first portions of the arteries, causing narrowing of the lumina and producing myocardial ischemia, fibrosis, and angina pectoris.

In rare instances syphilis may cause gummata or diffuse exudative and proliferative inflammation within the myocardium, with consequent effects on conduction and muscular function.

CORONARY (ATHEROSCLEROTIC, ISCHEMIC) HEART DISEASE

This is the most common and the most important form of cardiac disease, being responsible for approximately 30% of deaths from all causes in the United States. Coronary atherosclerosis is the underlying cause of 95% to 99% of all cases of coronary heart disease, the rare exceptions being due to narrowing of the coronary ostia by aortic atherosclerotic plaques or syphilitic involvement or emboli to the coronary arteries. The clinical spectrum of coronary heart disease includes sudden death (presumably due to cardiac arrhythmias) as a result of coronary occlusion or severe coronary stenosis with ischemia, myocardial infarction as a result of coronary atherosclerosis with occlusion (usually due to thrombosis), and angina pectoris as a result of severe narrowing of the coronary arteries and intermittent ischemia resulting therefrom. Almost all patients with coronary heart disease have extensive involvement of the coronary arteries with advanced stages of the atherosclerotic process—fibrous plaques, calcified plaques, and complicated plaques with necrotic softening, hemorrhage, thrombosis, or ulceration. In the unusual case, coronary heart disease and even sudden death may result from an isolated but significantly placed atherosclerotic plaque with superimposed thrombus. This situation occurs in less than 1 in 20 cases.

The atherosclerotic lesions are scattered throughout the coronary system but occur most frequently in the more proximal portions of the major branches of the coronary arteries. The most common sites of significant atherosclerotic involvement are the first part of the anterior descending branch of the left coronary artery just after its bifurcation and the right coronary artery in the first few centimeters after its origin and another site in the right coronary artery just before it reaches the posterior interventricular septum.

Coronary atherosclerosis may lead to the ischemic complications listed above in the following ways in decreasing order of frequency: (1) slow buildup of atherosclerotic lesions over years and decades with a sudden occlusive event, usually thrombus, superimposed on a ruptured or ulcerated atherosclerotic plaque; (2) progressive narrowing of the coronary lumen by extensive atherosclerotic lesions until ischemia is produced; (3) ulceration of an atherosclerotic plaque producing atherosclerotic embolism in the distal coronary artery.

Risk Factors for Coronary Heart Disease. Epidemiologic studies have shown that there are markers or individual characteristics which are associated with an increased risk of developing coronary heart disease. Three strong and independent risk factors that have been shown to be related to increased risk of coronary heart disease are elevated serum lipids (serum cholesterol, especially cholesterol carried in low density lipoproteins), elevated blood pressure (either systolic, diastolic, or both), and cigarette smoking. Other significant risk factors include diabetes or glucose intolerance, hypothyroidism, obesity, a family history of coronary disease, and sedentary jobs or physical inactivity. Other suspected but somewhat controversial risk factors include "stress," use of oral contraceptives, and elevated uric acid levels.

MYOCARDIAL INFARCTION

The site of myocardial infarction is usually determined by which of the coronary arteries are involved and the portion of the vessel that is occluded. Occlusion of the anterior descending branch of the left coronary artery produces infarction in the anterior interventricular septum and anterior left ventricle. Occlusion of the circumflex branch of the left coronary artery produces infarction of the lateral wall of the left ventricle. Occlusion of the right coronary artery typically produces infarction of the posterior interventricular septum, the posterior portion of the left ventricle, and very rarely in a small portion of the right ventricle. The right ventricle is usually spared from myocardial infarction.

Complications of myocardial infarction include cardiac arrhythmias (the most severe being ventricular fibrillation), mural thrombi with distal embolism, myocardial failure, and myocardial rupture with hemopericardium and cardiac tamponade.

Myocardial scars, especially large scars greater than 1 cm in diameter, are nearly always the result of ischemia from coronary heart disease. They represent healing and replacement of necrotic muscle fibers by fibrous connective tissue. Any disease that produces myocardial necrosis followed by healing will obviously produce a scar, but coronary disease is by far the most common cause of such myocardial necrosis.

HYPERTENSIVE HEART DISEASE

This is a common form of cardiac disease that is the result of prolonged and continued systemic hypertension. Mortality from hypertensive heart disease and other hypertension-related diseases has declined in the United States in recent years. Nevertheless, more than 50,000 deaths occur annually as a result of hypertensive heart disease with cardiac failure, and there are many more deaths in which hypertension is an underlying or aggravating cause. Such conditions include two forms of stroke, hypertensive cerebral hemorrhage and cerebral infarction, coronary heart disease (because hypertension is one of the major risk factors), and renal failure from advanced arteriolar nephrosclerosis which occurs in conjunction with hypertension.

The typical findings at autopsy in a person who dies of hypertensive heart disease are a large heart and small kidneys. The heart in hypertension exhibits the major changes of extreme hypertrophy of the left ventricular myocardium (concentric hypertrophy) and an increase in the weight of the heart to 500 g or 750 g and in some cases even higher. The kidneys are small because of the associated arteriolar nephrosclerosis, which occurs with prolonged and sustained hypertension.

The only microscopic changes of note in the myocardium are marked hypertrophy of the muscle fibers as well as their nuclei. There may be foci of interstitial fibrosis as a result of sclerosis of small branches of the coronary arteries, or there may be some of the previously described changes from coronary atherosclerosis since hypertension aggravates coronary atherosclerosis. Cardiac hypertrophy is the result of increased total peripheral resistance resulting in increased work load for the heart over a long period of time. Once the increased demand of the heart cannot be met, there is cardiac dilatation and cardiac failure as a terminal event.

Endocardial fibroelastosis is a form of heart disease usually occurring in children in the first 2 years of life and characterized by marked thickening of the mural endocardium especially of the left side of the heart. While fibroelastic thickening sometimes occurs in conjunction with other forms of heart disease, particularly congenital anomalies, the condition in its primary form occurs typically in patients presenting with large globular hearts and cardiac failure and without evidence of valvular or other underlying disease. Theories of causation abound; however, the etiology is obscure.

The diagnosis of *primary cardiomyopathy* is made primarily by excluding known causes of myocardial disease. These cardiomyopathies are usually divided into three types: (1) congestive cardiomyopathy, characterized by marked enlargement of the heart, cardiac dilatation, and congestive heart failure; (2) hypertrophic cardiomyopathy, characterized by marked myocardial hypertrophy, which is frequently asymmetrical, most striking in the interventricular septum, and without significant dilatation; and (3) restrictive or constrictive cardiomyopathy with associated endocardial fibroelastosis or endomyocardial fibrosis. Cardiac abnormalities that mimic some of these primary cardiomyopathies may have been caused by a variety of etiologic agents, including alcohol, metabolic disorders, autoimmune connective tissue disease, amyloidosis, and others.

Myocarditis has been produced by almost all forms of microorganisms, including bacteria (both as a result of direct bacterial involvement and toxins produced by bacteria at distant sites), viruses, rickettsiae, and parasitic organisms. Worthy of special mention is diphtheritic myocarditis, one of the major complications of diphtheria and a result of toxin elaborated by the organisms, whether they be in the respiratory tract, genital tract, or elsewhere. Viral agents cited as frequent causes of myocarditis include the coxsackieviruses and echoviruses.

CONGESTIVE HEART FAILURE

The mechanisms and causes of congestive heart failure are discussed in the chapter on internal medicine. Basically, congestive heart failure occurs either because of a decreased myocardial capacity to contract or because of an increased pressure-volume load imposed on the heart. This section will include only the most significant pathologic findings in patients with congestive heart failure. In the heart there is dilatation of the affected chambers. The left ventricle and left atrium are dilated in left heart failure, and the right ventricle and right atrium are dilated in right heart failure. Failure of the left side of the heart also causes pulmonary congestion and pulmonary edema, and the histologic hallmark is the presence of hyperemic alveolar capillaries and granular precipitate in the alveoli. In chronic passive congestion, hemosiderin-laden macrophages are present in the alveoli. Failure of the right side of the heart leads to chronic passive congestion of the liver (giving it a nutmeg appearance), congestion of the spleen and other abdominal viscera, and peripheral edema and ascites.

PERICARDIAL DISEASE

Transudation of fluid into the pericardial sac, which may occur in cardiac failure or the nephrotic syndrome, is called *hydropericardium,* or pericardial effusion. *Hemopericardium,* blood in the pericardial sac, may be due to myocardial infarction with rupture, rupture of a saccular aneurysm of the aortic arch, or rupture of a dissecting aneurysm into the pericardium, penetrating wounds, and more rarely tuberculosis or malignant tumor involving the pericardium. Sudden massive hemorrhage into the pericardial sac from any of these causes can interfere with the action of the heart *(cardiac tamponade)* and is usually fatal.

Pericarditis. Acute pericarditis may be caused by both infectious and noninfectious agents. Organisms may involve the pericardium by direct extension from surrounding structures or by the blood stream. Among the bacteria that may cause pericar-ditis are staphylococci, pneumococci, streptococci, and many others. The pericardium may be involved in tuberculosis. A variety of viral agents also may involve the pericardium. Rheumatic fever characteristically produces fibrinous or serofibrinous pericarditis. Fibrinous pericarditis may be a result of uremia.

Chronic, or Healed, Pericarditis. Healed pericarditis may be the result of organization of previous involvement of suppurative or granulomatous inflammation. Significant healed pericarditis producing constrictive pericarditis most commonly occurs following infections with *Staphylococcus* and the tubercle bacillus. *Constrictive pericarditis* may prevent adequate filling of the heart during diastole and may cause marked congestion of the liver and spleen, as well as ascites. Another form of chronic pericarditis, *adhesive mediastinopericarditis,* leads to increased workload of the heart and cardiac hypertrophy and dilatation because of adhesions between the pericardium and surrounding mediastinal structures.

DISEASES OF THE BLOOD VESSELS

Aneurysm. A true aneurysm is a localized dilatation of an artery involving all coats of the vessel. Aneurysms are described according to their shape as saccular, fusiform or cylindrical. Three types of aortic aneurysms are *syphilitic aneurysms,* most commonly occurring in the aortic arch; *atherosclerotic aneurysms,* usually occurring in the abdominal aorta; and *dissecting aneurysms,* resulting from *idiopathic cystic medial necrosis.* Dissecting aneurysms usually begin in the arch of the aorta and may dissect throughout its length. The misnomer *mycotic aneurysm* refers to an aneurysm of an artery due to weakening of the wall by bacterial infection, frequently from an infected embolus. A *congenital* or *berry aneurysm* is the type that may form in the circle of Willis when the intravascular pressure causes bulging out from an area of congenital weakness at branching sites, especially at the junction of the internal carotid and middle cerebral artery. A false aneurysm is an extravascular hematoma communicating with the lumen of a blood vessel and is usually traumatic in origin.

Buerger's Disease (Thromboangiitis Obliterans). This is an obscure disease that characteristically involves arteries, veins, and nerves of the lower extremity with areas of inflammation and thrombosis. The upper extremities are also sometimes involved. It occurs almost exclusively in men who are heavy cigarette smokers. It causes intensive pain and may lead to gangrene. There is a close similarity of some of the features of Buerger's disease to other conditions such as peripheral atherosclerosis or embolization to the lower extremities, but it seems that the entity of Buerger's disease actually exists as a distinct condition.

Polyarteritis (Periarteritis) Nodosa. Because of the nature of the lesions, polyarteritis nodosa is now classed with the autoimmune diseases, involving primarily the smaller branches of the arterial system, especially in the internal organs, such as the heart, the kidneys, and even the brain, as well as in the skin and in striated muscle. The inflammatory reaction in the affected vessels is a violent one, and marked degeneration and necrosis are followed by intense leukocytic infiltration. Fibrinoid necrosis is usually marked. Polyarteritis nodosa is generally considered to be a response to autoimmune antigen–antibody complexes. In the later stages of the disease, perivascular inflammation is most pronounced, forming characteristic nodules or nodes. Thrombosis may complicate the lesions with obliteration of the vessel lumina, and aneurysmal dilatation may occur, sometimes with resulting hemorrhage.

Phlebitis. Phlebitis often results from an extension of a localized suppurative process, with the formation, in a local vein, of a thrombus that may extend into the larger veins. The vessel wall is infiltrated by leukocytes with thrombus formation at the sites where the intima is involved. Before the thrombus is completely organized, emboli may break off and lodge in the lungs and sometimes even in other organs. If infected, these emboli may set up new foci of inflammation, which may result in the formation of abscesses.

Arteriosclerosis. Arteriosclerosis, or "hardening of the arteries," is the term given to those changes that result in thickening, hardening, and loss of elasticity of arterial walls. There are three main morphologic types of arteriosclerosis: (1) atherosclerosis; (2) Mönckeberg's medial sclerosis, characterized by ringlike zones of calcification of the media in certain peripheral arteries, especially of the lower extremities; and (3) arteriolar sclerosis, characterized by proliferative fibromuscular or intimal thickening of the small arteries and arterioles.

Atherosclerosis. Atherosclerosis is of great interest because of its clinical significance in causing heart attacks and strokes. It is a specific form of arteriosclerosis. Atherosclerosis primarily involves the intima of large elastic arteries and the medium-sized muscular arteries with characteristic accumulation of lipid in the lesions. In addition to the accumulation of lipid, there is accumulation of connective tissues and various blood products. A number of complications can result from an atherosclerotic lesion, such as thrombosis, hemorrhage into a plaque, and ulceration. The hallmarks are that atherosclerosis is intimal and that it is characterized by the accumulation of fat. The importance of atherosclerosis is that it is the most prominent form of arteriosclerosis in causing clinically significant disease.

The principal lesions of atherosclerosis recognizable on gross examination of arteries are fatty streaks, fibrous plaques, complicated plaques with ulceration, hemorrhage or mural thrombi, and calcified plaques. Studies of the natural history of atherosclerosis have shown that fatty streaks begin in childhood as fat accumulation in a slightly thickened intima. Fibrous plaques develop early in adult life with connective tissue accumulation around the intimal fat. Complicated lesions leading to arterial occlusion and ischemia occur in later adult life, decades after the initial arterial lesions. Thus, the occlusive consequences of atherosclerosis (myocardial infarction, angina pectoris, cerebral infarction) indicate the end stage of a process usually active for 3 decades or more.

While the etiology and pathogenesis of atherosclerosis are not completely understood, the role of elevated plasma lipoproteins is well documented. The mesenchymal response with connective tissue accumulation in the arterial intima is also an important element. The two oldest theories of atherosclerosis are the encrustation theory of Rokitansky (incorporation of organized mural thrombi into the intima with development of atherosclerotic plaques) and the lipid infiltration theory of Virchow (imbibition of lipid from the plasma into a damaged intima). Some modern theories encompass aspects of both of these early hypotheses. For example, both plasma lipoproteins and platelet factors are thought to cause connective tissue proliferation in the atherosclerotic process.

Intimal fat in human and experimental atherosclerosis is both intracellular and extracellular. At least two cell types are important in atherosclerosis. Intimal smooth muscle cells accumulate lipid and may also elaborate collagen, elastin, and glycosaminoglycans. Lipid-containing macrophages (foam cells) are prominent features of atherosclerotic lesions and are quite distinct from the lipid-containing smooth muscle cells. While the exact role of endothelial cells (or endothelial damage) and elements of the coagulation system are not completely known, they may also have a role in the pathogenesis of atherosclerosis.

Clinical Significance of Atherosclerosis. Atherosclerosis is the main underlying cause of coronary heart disease, stroke, gangrene of the extremities, and aneurysms of the abdominal aorta. Atherosclerosis produces clinically significant disease by various mechanisms. First, it may narrow the lumen of arteries, thereby producing ischemia to some degree. This change occurs in angina pectoris, for example, in which the coronary arteries are stenotic or partially occluded, and the myocardium becomes ischemic under certain conditions. Second, atherosclerosis sets the stage for sudden complete occlusion with more severe ischemia and resultant death of tissue in an organ such as the heart (in which case, there is sudden death or myocardial infarction) or the brain (in which case, there is stroke) or the leg (in which case, there is infarction and gangrene). Third, atherosclerotic lesions in the aorta can be a source of emboli (thrombi or blood clots that break off from the vascular wall) to the extremities. Fourth, atherosclerosis can produce clinical sequelae by weakening the wall of the aorta. Even though atherosclerosis is primarily a disease of the intima, the media of the aorta may be secondarily weakened, and the result is an aneurysm or ballooning of the vessel wall.

Mönckeberg's Medial Sclerosis. In this form of sclerosis, which affects small- to medium-sized arteries, ringlike bands of calcification accumulate in the medial coats, particularly those of the arteries of the extremities. These changes usually are of relatively little clinical importance.

Arteriolar Sclerosis (Arteriolosclerosis). This change is limited primarily to the arterioles and sometimes the smaller arteries. It may be of hyaline or hyperplastic type. The former, when it affects the arterioles of the kidneys (and rarely other abdominal organs), may be associated with slowly rising blood pressure of moderate type; the latter, often referred to as the onion-skin type of vascular lesion, may be associated with acute and severe elevation of blood pressure such as occurs in rapidly progressing hypertension. Whether the arteriolar involvement in the kidneys precedes the development of hypertension and even whether the hemodynamic disturbance in the renal circulation bears a primary causative relationship to the production of the elevated blood pressure are still unsettled questions.

ANEMIA

Anemia is the condition in which there is a reduced number of erythrocytes per cubic millimeter or a reduced concentration of hemoglobin in blood, or both, with corresponding reduction in the oxygen-carrying capacity of the blood. The main causes are (1) blood loss due to hemorrhage, either external or internal; (2) excess erythrocyte destruction; and (3) diminished or defective red cell production.

Anemia from Blood Loss. With acute hemorrhage, depletion of the blood volume (hypovolemia) develops. The hemoglobin and hematocrit do not fall immediately but do so slowly over 24 hours as tissue fluids move into the circulation to compensate for the lost blood volume.

Anemia from Excess Erythrocyte Destruction. The hemolytic anemias resulting from excess destruction of red cells include those due to intracorpuscular defects in the erythrocytes. Laboratory evidence of hemolysis includes reticulocytosis ($>5\%$), elevated lactic dehydrogenase (particularly isoenzyme LDH-1), decreased serum haptoglobin, and the presence of methemalbumin, and plasma or urine hemoglobin. The direct antiglobulin test (DAT or Coombs' test) may be positive in immune hemolytic anemias.

The intrinsic (intracorpuscular) hemolytic anemias include abnormalities of the erythrocyte membrane, enzyme abnormalities, and abnormalities of hemoglobin structure (hemoglobinopathies) or hemoglobin synthesis (thalassemia syndromes).

Abnormalities of the erythrocyte membrane include those disorders in which the erythrocyte has an abnormal shape on peripheral blood smears. These include hereditary spherocytosis, hereditary elliptocytosis, hereditary stomatocytosis, and hereditary acanthocytosis. Hereditary spherocytosis, an autosomal dominant disorder, is characterized by an abnormal membrane permeability to sodium. The resulting spherical shape causes the cells to be more fragile than normal, to be vulnerable to splenic sequestration, and to have an increased osmotic fragility. Splenectomy results in clinical improvement but does not correct the basic abnormality.

Paroxysmal nocturnal hemoglobinuria (PNH) is unusual in that it is an acquired intrinsic erythrocyte defect in which the cells are unusually sensitive to complement lysis. The basic abnormality is thought to involve a progenitor stem cell since leukocytes and platelets may also be affected. Young adults are primarily affected, with pancytopenia a common presentation. Fifty percent of PNH patients have an abnormal clone arising spontaneously without evidence of bone marrow abnormality, while 20 percent to 30 percent have preexisting evidence of marrow abnormality (*e.g.,* aplastic anemia). Bone marrow transplantation may be used as treatment in some cases.

Enzyme abnormalities include glucose-6-phosphate dehydrogenase (G-6-PD) deficiency, a condition in which sex-linked inheritance of the mutant enzyme causes the production of red cells, which are vulnerable to episodic injury by oxidant compounds (*e.g.*, antimalarials, sulfonamides, aspirin, and phenacetin) and infection. Other enzyme deficiencies may predispose to hemolysis including the autosomal recessive one, pyruvate kinase deficiency.

Abnormalities of hemoglobin structure involve addition, substitution, or deletion of one or more amino acids of the globin chain. The prototype, sickle cell hemoglobin, results from the substitution of valine for glutamine at the sixth position on the β-chain. If both β-genes are affected, sickle cell anemia (disease) results; while one affected gene and one normal gene result in sickle cell trait. The abnormal hemoglobin is sensitive to oxygen tension and tends to form polymers (sickles) resulting in formation of rigid sickled erythrocytes that may cause vascular stasis and thrombosis as well as being susceptible to splenic destruction. Over time the spleen becomes small and fibrotic secondary to multiple episodes of infarction and healing.

Abnormalities of hemoglobin synthesis (the thalassemia syndromes) are a group of hereditary disorders characterized by a deficiency in the synthesis of one or another of the normal polypeptide (globin) chains; α- and β-thalassemia result from a decrease in synthesis of α- and β-chains, respectively. The disorders are heterogeneous in clinical severity and in distribution, although they are more frequent in populations of Mediterranean, African, or Asian ancestry.

Extrinsic hemolytic anemias (usually acquired) may be secondary to immune or nonimmune mechanisms. Nonimmune hemolysis may be induced by chemical agents (*e.g.*, drugs) and physical agents (burns, prosthetic cardiac valves, and so forth). The microangiopathic hemolytic anemias are secondary to physical damage to the erythrocytes caused by fibrin deposited in the microcirculation in a variety of conditions (*e.g.*, renal disease, collagen vascular diseases, infections, pregnancy, DIC, and thrombotic thrombocytopenia purpura). Infections (*e.g.*, malaria, bartonellosis, clostridia) may result in hemolysis due to infestation of the erythrocyte or production of lecithinases.

Immune hemolytic anemias may be due to auto- or isoantibodies. These may produce a positive DAT or Coombs' test. Isoimmune hemolytic anemias occur in hemolytic disease of the newborn and secondary to transfusions. Autoimmune hemolytic anemias may be due to "warm antibodies" (usually IgG) that are often directed against Rh system antigens. These may be idiopathic or occur secondary to SLE, lymphoma, or infections. "Cold antibodies" (usually IgM) are often directed against blood group antigens I or i. These also may be idiopathic or secondary to mycoplasma infections, infectious mononucleosis, or viral infections.

Diminished or Defective Erythrocyte Production. Iron deficiency anemia, perhaps the most common form of anemia, is due to inadequate supplies of iron in the marrow. Causes include defective absorption of iron, inadequate diet, and chronic blood loss, which is the most common cause in adults. In males the loss is most frequently due to GI bleeding, while in females the loss may be GI or menstrual. The resultant anemia is microcytic and hypochromic. It is characterized by decreased serum iron, ferritin, and transferrin saturation with an increased total iron-binding capacity (TIBC).

Deficiencies of vitamin B_{12} or folate may be produced by inadequate intake, defective absorption (defective production of intrinsic factor causing B_{12} malabsorption is the most common cause of B_{12} deficiency), or increased requirements. These deficiencies result in a macrocytic anemia and frequently pancytopenia. Hypersegmented neutrophils are characteristic. Neurologic symptoms may also occur with B_{12} deficiency.

Aplastic anemia is characterized by pancytopenia associated with hypocellularity of the bone marrow. The clinical course may be fulminant with profound pancytopenia or may follow a chronic insidious course. Approximately 50% of the cases are idiopathic, 33% are drug related, chemicals and toxins are implicated in 4%, and infections in 4%.

Myelophthisic anemia is characterized by marrow replacement by metastatic tumor, leukemia, lymphoma, multiple myeloma, or storage disease. The peripheral blood contains a varying number of normoblasts and immature granulocytes (leukoerythroblastic anemia). A similar peripheral blood picture is seen with myelofibrosis with myeloid metaplasia (one of the myeloproliferative disorders).

LEUKEMIA

Leukemia is a neoplastic proliferation of leukopoietic cells with or without involvement of the peripheral blood. Although the etiology remains unclear, a mutation in one cell is the most likely initial event. In the U.S. there are approximately seven new cases of leukemia per 100,000 population each year; of these, about 60% are acute, while 20% are chronic myelocytic leukemia (CML), and 20% are chronic lymphocytic leukemia (CLL). Leukemia, particularly CLL, is slightly more common in males. Acute leukemia has peak incidences below the age of 5 and between the ages of 15 and 20. The former are usually acute lymphocytic leukemia (ALL) and the latter primarily acute myelocytic leukemia (AML). Most cases of CML occur between the ages of 20 and 50, while CLL occurs with increasing frequency after age 45.

Acute leukemias may be myeloblastic, myelomonocytic, monocytic, or lymphoblastic. The onset is sudden, usually with fever, anemia, weakness, ulcerations of mucous membranes, and purpura. The peripheral leukocyte count may not be markedly elevated, as in the chronic form, and the spleen, liver, and superficial lymph nodes may not be enlarged. The acute leukemias may be classified according to the French-American-British (FAB) Classification utilizing cytochemical and Romanowsky stains.

In CML, weakness, splenomegaly, and anemia are prominent features. The leukocyte count is elevated (100,000–500,000) with a wide variety of granulocytes and their precursors present in the peripheral blood. These include blasts, promyelocytes, myelocytes, and usually an increased number of basophils. Nucleated red cells may occasionally be seen, and because the red cell–forming centers are invaded and destroyed by leukocytes, severe anemia is present at the time of diagnosis in over half of patients; 90% to 95% of patients with hematologically typical CML will have a Philadelphia chromosome (Ph[1]). Patients with a negative Ph[1] have a shortened life expectancy. The granulocytes in CML contain greatly decreased levels or no alkaline phosphatase in contrast to normal granulocytes. Leukemic infiltration of the kidneys and liver is common and may involve the skin, periosteum, intestines, and stomach.

CLL involves primarily the lymphatic system, including the peripheral lymph nodes as well as those in the mediastinum and abdomen. The spleen and liver are only slightly to moderately enlarged. The leukocytes in the blood are not abundant as in CML, varying between 20,000 and 200,000/mm^3. In general the lymphocytes tend to be morphologically similar in any given case. Varying numbers of large ("immature") lymphocytes occur, although the vast majority of cells are small lymphocytes. Most cases are of B-cell lineage. Often neither anemia nor thrombocytopenia is present at the time of diagno-

sis. The normal architecture of the spleen and lymph nodes is frequently obliterated with small lymphocytes. The bone marrow may be heavily infiltrated by lymphocytes late in the course, while early on only a slight to moderate lymphocytosis is present.

MYELOPROLIFERATIVE SYNDROME

The myeloproliferative syndrome provides a unifying concept for several abnormalities of the bone marrow involving one or more of the stem lines. It implies overlap and in some cases crossover from one of these conditions to another. For example, the rare case of polycythemia vera (an idiopathic condition characterized by greatly elevated red cell mass) may give rise to myeloid metaplasia, CML, or erythroleukemia (Di Guglielmo syndrome). Conditions that comprise the myeloproliferative syndrome include polycythemia vera, erythroleukemia, CML, megakaryocytic myelosis, megakaryocytic leukemia, and myelofibrosis (including myeloid metaplasia and agnogenic myeloid metaplasia). The final common pathway of many of these conditions is the terminal development of an acute "blastic" leukemia.

HEMOPHILIA AND VON WILLEBRAND'S DISEASE

Hemophilia A, the most common congenital disorder of the coagulation factors, is transmitted as an X-linked disorder with the resultant male hemizygotes primarily affected. Levels of factor VIII (factor VIII : C, clottable) are decreased to varying degrees in different individuals with lower levels associated with more severe clinical symptoms. Typically, bleeding occurs into joints, muscles, or postoperatively. The partial thromboplastin time (aPTT) is usually abnormal while the bleeding time, prothrombin time (PT), and platelet count are usually normal. Hemophilia is treated principally by factor VIII replacement therapy, either as cryoprecipitate or factor VIII concentrate. Approximately 10% to 15% of patients with severe hemophilia develop alloantibodies, which inhibit factor VIII : C.

Von Willebrand's disease, usually inherited as an autosomal dominant disorder, is characterized by easy bleeding from the mucous membranes, easy bruising, GI bleeding, and bleeding following dental extractions. The bleeding time in these patients is frequently abnormal, while the PT and PTT are usually normal. Factor VIII–related antigen, FVIII : C, and ristocetin cofactor activity (von Willebrand's factor [vWF]) are typically decreased. The vWF molecule circulates as a noncovalently linked complex (VIII/vWF); vWF appears to play a central role in the adhesion of platelets to subendothelial surfaces following vessel injury. Patients may be treated with either fresh frozen plasma or cryoprecipitate.

PURPURA

Purpura occurs in a group of diseases characterized by spontaneous hemorrhages into the skin and mucous membranes. It may occur secondary to conditions in which thrombocytopenia or increased fragility of the capillaries and smaller blood vessels occur, for example, leukemia, aplastic anemia, carcinomatosis of the bone marrow, or severe sepsis.

Henoch–Schönlein purpura is apparently the result of a form of hypersensitivity reaction in which small blood vessels are injured and focal and diffuse hemorrhages occur. Characteristically, purpuric skin lesions involving the extensor surfaces of the arms and legs, intestinal bleeding, nonmigratory arthralgia, and renal abnormalities are present. There is deposition of IgA, sometimes with IgG and C3 in the renal mesangium as well as in the small vessels of the dermis.

Idiopathic thrombocytopenic purpura (ITP) results from an accelerated platelet destruction attributable to an acquired immune process. It occurs in two forms: (1) an acute form, more common in children 2 to 6 years old without sex predilection with peak incidence in fall and winter paralleling the prevalence of upper respiratory tract infection; and (2) a chronic form, which may occur at any age and has a female to male ratio of 3 : 1. Epistaxis and uterine bleeding are very frequent; GI and urinary tract bleeding are less common. Platelets are greatly reduced during attacks but may be normal in the intervals. The PT and aPTT are normal, but the bleeding time is prolonged. The spleen is moderately enlarged, but the bone marrow is normal or shows increased megakaryocytes. Treatment includes corticosteroids, intravenous human immune globulin, and possible splenectomy.

Respiratory System

PNEUMOCONIOSES

The pneumoconioses are characterized by the deposition of dust particles (with or without fibrosis) in the lungs. This deposition is related to the concentration of the particle in the air; its size and shape; its chemical nature and solubility; and the duration of exposure.

Anthracosis. Carbon pigmentation of the lungs (anthracosis) is present to some degree in all city dwellers, especially cigarette smokers. In most cases, it is a relatively unimportant form of pneumoconiosis in that it does not stimulate the formation of fibrous tissue, and there is no correlation between the presence of anthracosis and any other pathologic process in the lung. The pigment is picked up by macrophages and primarily deposited in hilar lymph nodes, at the pleural surface, and around small bronchi and bronchioles. Anthracotic pigmentation is frequently significant in coal miners (black lung disease).

Silicosis. Silicosis is an occupational disease (sandblasting, stone cutting and polishing, glass manufacturing, and so forth) that is due to the inhalation of silica particles. The onset is insidious, and exposure for 10 to 15 years is usually necessary to produce severe disease. The affected lung contains fibrous nodules that tend to be located in the upper lobes and hilar regions. Eventually, a more diffuse fibrosis may occur and replace large areas of parenchyma. Hilar lymph node involvement is similar to that of the lung. Polariscopic examination of the nodules reveals birefringent particles of silicon dioxide. Serious complications of silicosis include tuberculosis, emphysema, right-sided heart failure (cor pulmonale), and pneumonia.

Asbestosis. Inhalation of asbestos fibers may not only stimulate diffuse interstitial fibrosis, but may also result in a markedly increased incidence of bronchogenic carcinoma and mesothelioma. Significant asbestos exposure is relatively common due to its widespread usage (*e.g.,* brake linings, insulation material, roofing shingles, acoustical products). In most cases, manifestations of the disease appear 10 to 20 years after exposure. The basal portions of the lower lobes and the pleura are particularly involved. Asbestos bodies (ferruginous bodies), consisting of asbestos fibers coated with iron, are identified microscopically. Emphysema, bronchiectasis, and cor pulmonale are additional complications.

PULMONARY EMBOLISM AND INFARCTION

Pulmonary embolism is common in situations requiring prolonged bed rest, immobilization of extremities, severe trauma, chronic congestive heart failure, and so forth. The majority of emboli arise in the deep leg veins and may result in hemorrhage, infarction, or sudden death depending on the size and location of the embolus and also on the cardiopulmonary status of the patient.

ADULT RESPIRATORY DISTRESS SYNDROME (ADULT HYALINE MEMBRANE DISEASE, SHOCK LUNG)

Adult respiratory distress syndrome occurs as a life-threatening complication of numerous conditions, including cardiac surgery, pulmonary infections, severe burns, oxygen toxicity, sepsis, narcotic overdose, and inhalation of irritants. The basic lesion is alveolar wall injury resulting in pulmonary edema, hyaline membrane formation, alveolar lining cell regeneration (type II pneumocytes) and hyperplasia. Interstitial fibrosis may result.

CHRONIC OBSTRUCTIVE LUNG DISEASE

This group of diseases is characterized by chronic obstruction to airflow within the lungs and consists of chronic bronchitis, emphysema, bronchial asthma, and bronchiectasis.

Chronic Bronchitis. Chronic bronchitis is a chronic respiratory disease characterized by persistent cough with sputum production, which is particularly common in habitual smokers and city dwellers exposed to pollutants. The most characteristic microscopic feature of chronic bronchitis is the increase in thickness of the submucosal mucous gland layer in the trachea and bronchi (Reid index). Increased numbers of goblet cells, chronic inflammation of the bronchial wall, and mucous plugs are additional features. Complications of long-standing disease include emphysema, cor pulmonale, and bacterial infections.

Emphysema. Emphysema is defined as an abnormal permanent enlargement of the air spaces distal to the terminal bronchiole, accompanied by destruction of their walls. Emphysema is more common and more severe in males, and the disease clearly is associated with heavy smoking. In the *centriacinar* type, the proximal portion of the acinus is involved and distal alveoli are spared. Centriacinar emphysema is most common in the upper lobes, especially in the apical segments. In *panacinar* emphysema, the entire acinus is involved. This type is more severe in the lower portions of the lobes and is the type of emphysema associated with α_1-antitrypsin deficiency. In advanced cases, adjacent alveoli fuse to produce large air-filled spaces and occasionally blebs or bullae. Severe emphysema frequently results in right-sided heart failure, respiratory acidosis, and pneumothorax. Peptic ulceration is found in up to 20% of emphysema patients.

Bronchial Asthma. Bronchial asthma is characterized by bronchial obstruction resulting from bronchospasm and tenacious mucous plugs. Most cases are considered to develop on an allergic basis but attacks may be produced by respiratory tract infection, chemicals, and so forth.

Grossly, the lungs are hyperinflated with occlusion of bronchi and bronchioles by thick, tenacious mucous plugs. Microscopic features include epithelial basement membrane thickening, infiltration of the bronchial walls by eosinophils, enlargement of the submucosal mucous glands, smooth muscle hypertrophy in bronchial walls, and mucous plugs containing numerous eosinophils.

Bronchiectasis. Bronchiectasis is a chronic necrotizing infection of bronchi and bronchioles that results in permanent abnormal dilatation of these structures. It usually develops as a result of bronchial obstruction and infection in conditions such as foreign body aspiration, bronchial tumors, scarring, asthma, chronic bronchitis, emphysema, and cystic fibrosis. Both lower lobes are usually involved, but the involvement may be segmental when resulting from tumors or foreign bodies. The affected bronchi and bronchioles are dilated and filled with purulent exudate. Bronchiectasis may be complicated by lung abscess, pneumonia, empyema, and amyloidosis.

BACTERIAL PNEUMONIA

Bronchopneumonia (lobular pneumonia) is characterized by patchy or focal consolidation of the lung and usually represents an extension of bronchitis or bronchiolitis. The disease is especially common in infancy and old age and may be produced by numerous pathogenic bacteria and occasionally fungi. Microscopically, the involved alveoli contain neutrophils, fibrin, and necrotic debris. Alveoli located in adjacent areas may be entirely normal. Bronchopneumonia may be complicated by abscesses, empyema, and bacteremia with possible abscess formation in other organs.

Lobar pneumonia is characterized by consolidation of a large portion of a lobe or of an entire lobe. This form of pneumonia is seen much less often now because of the effectiveness of antibiotic therapy. It occurs predominantly in chronic alcoholics, the elderly, and the debilitated. Most cases are due to pneumococci, but *Klebsiella* and other bacteria may also be responsible. Infection occurs by way of the bronchial tree, and spread occurs through the pores of Kohn.

Four stages of the disease are classically described: (1) congestion, in which the alveolar capillaries are distended and the alveoli are filled with a serous exudate containing numerous bacteria and few neutrophils; (2) red hepatization, in which the lung is solid and airless and the alveoli are filled with neutrophils, fibrin, and erythrocytes; (3) gray hepatization, in which the alveoli contain fibrin together with disintegrating neutrophils and erythrocytes; and (4) resolution, in which the exudate undergoes enzymatic digestion and resorption restoring the parenchyma to its normal state. Complications of lobar pneumonia include abscess formation, empyema, exudate organization (organizing pneumonia) resulting in scar formation, and bacteremia with possible abscess formation in other organs.

VIRAL AND MYCOPLASMA PNEUMONIA (PRIMARY ATYPICAL PNEUMONIA)

This disease is most frequently caused by *Mycoplasma pneumoniae,* but numerous viral agents also may be responsible. The characteristic pathologic features include interstitial mononuclear inflammation and intra-alveolar edema with hyaline membrane formation. Viral inclusions may be noted. Some cases are complicated by superimposed bacterial pneumonia.

PLASMA CELL (PNEUMOCYSTIS) PNEUMONIA

Pulmonary infection by the fungus *Pneumocystis carinii* usually occurs in debilitated or immunosuppressed patients (*e.g.,* leukemia, lymphoma, γ-globulin abnormalities, AIDS). Grossly, the lungs are homogeneously gray and airless. Microscopically, the alveoli are filled with a foamy, eosinophilic material, and there may be an interstitial mononuclear infiltration. The organisms that are present within the alveoli resemble *Histoplasma* and are best demonstrated by the Gomori methenamine silver (GMS) stain.

LUNG ABSCESS

Lung abscesses may be produced by virtually any pathogenic organism, aerobic or anaerobic. Abscesses may occur following aspiration of infected material, bacterial pneumonias, septic embolism, bronchial obstruction, and so forth. The characteristic feature is liquefaction necrosis of the underlying parenchyma with replacement by purulent exudate. Complications include empyema, brain abscesses or meningitis, and rarely amyloidosis.

INTERSTITIAL (RESTRICTIVE) LUNG DISEASE

This group of diseases is characterized by injury to alveolar walls frequently resulting in fibrous thickening that permanently impairs respiratory function. These diseases include sarcoidosis, which is characterized by interstitial noncaseating granulomas and nonspecific interstitial alveolitis; idiopathic pulmonary fibrosis (Hamman–Rich syndrome), which is characterized by a fibrosing alveolitis; Goodpasture's syndrome, which is characterized by a necrotizing interstitial pneumonitis combined with a proliferative glomerulonephritis; desquamative interstitial pneumonitis; idiopathic pulmonary hemosiderosis; and so forth. Other causes of interstitial lung disease (ILD) include the pneumoconioses, drugs (*e.g.,* busulfan, nitrofurantoin, penicillamine), and infections due to bacteria, fungi, viruses, and parasites.

TUBERCULOSIS AND CARCINOMA OF THE LUNG

Tuberculosis and carcinoma of the lung were discussed earlier in this chapter.

Gastrointestinal System

MOUTH AND SALIVARY GLANDS

Stomatitis has varied causes including aphthous ulcers, herpesvirus infections, erythema multiforme, pemphigus, and pemphigoid. It also may be associated with uremia, inflammatory bowel disease, malnutrition, advanced liver disease, lymphoma, agranulocytosis, and aplastic anemia. Opportunistic infection by *Candida* species may accompany or presage AIDS.

Dental caries, associated chiefly with *Streptococcus mutans* within a plaque of food and other microorganisms, produces cavitary destruction and loss of teeth. Gingivitis, also associated with dental plaque, progresses untreated to periodontitis with loss of ligamentous and bony support of roots, and migration, loosening, and exfoliation of the teeth. Gingival enlargement may be inflammatory, hereditary, drug-related (phenytoin [Dilantin] or nifedipine), or be due to a leukemic infiltrate.

The mouth is a source of microorganisms whose entrance into the blood is facilitated by inflammatory lesions, by mechanical movements such as chewing, and by surgical procedures. These microorganisms may produce infection elsewhere, particularly on previously damaged endocardium (*e.g.,* bacterial endocarditis).

Epithelial-lined cysts occur within the jaws, the

commonest being the apical periodontal (radicular, dental root end) cyst associated with carious or traumatized teeth. Next in frequency is the dentigerous cyst that develops around the crown of a non-erupted tooth. Ameloblastoma, typically a slow-growing but aggressive tumor of epithelium resembling that of the enamel organ, occurs in the jaws.

Mucoceles are cystic lesions of extravasated mucus attended by granulation tissue and inflammation. They are called ranulas when they occur in the floor of the mouth.

Most salivary gland tumors arise in the parotid gland, and most are pleomorphic adenomas. Mucoepidermoid carcinomas and adenoid cystic carcinomas are the most common malignant tumors of salivary gland origin. Within the mouth the posterior hard palate is a favored site for salivary gland tumors.

ESOPHAGUS

Common pathologic changes in the esophagus are atresia (almost 90% of cases are associated with tracheoesophageal fistula), varices, diverticula, both congenital and acquired (pulsion and traction types), esophagitis, and tumors. Reflux of gastric contents is the most common cause of esophagitis (reflux esophagitis) and is due to an incompetent lower esophageal sphincter.

The most common tumor of the esophagus is squamous cell carcinoma, which usually occurs in males over 50 years of age. The combination of excessive alcohol intake and heavy cigarette smoking increases the risk of developing esophageal carcinoma. The most frequent sites of this tumor are the lower and middle esophagus. When it occurs in the upper esophagus, it is often as a component of the Plummer–Vinson syndrome (i.e., proximal esophageal web, iron-deficiency anemia, atrophic glossitis, and hypochlorhydria), especially common in elderly females. This tumor extends to surrounding structures and causes obstruction of the lumen of the esophagus. Adenocarcinoma is rare, but it does occur in the lower end of the esophagus, where it can originate from the adjacent gastric mucosa or from the so-called Barrett's esophagus, characterized by the presence of gastric epithelium in the esophageal mucosa.

STOMACH

Hypertrophic Pyloric Stenosis. Stenosis occurs in the newborn infant and is the result of idiopathic hypertrophy of the circular layer of smooth muscle of the pylorus. The hypertrophic muscle and spasm together produce the stenosis and the obstruction. The onset of symptoms occurs 2 to 4 weeks after birth.

Gastritis. *Acute gastritis* is common, usually of minor import, caused by damage to the mucosal barrier, and often associated with local irritants as excess alcohol, certain drugs (notably aspirin, nonsteroidal anti-inflammatory agents, and steroids), and staphylococcal toxin in contaminated food. In the severe cases the gastric mucosa is hyperemic, edematous, and may even show slight to severe superficial mucosal erosions.

Chronic gastritis includes several clinicopathologic entities. *Chronic superficial gastritis* is a nonspecific inflammation limited to the upper portion of the lamina propria of the mucosa. *Chronic (atrophic) fundal gastritis* (type A gastritis) may be autoimmune in origin and often is associated with antibodies to intrinsic factor and gastric parietal cells and pernicious anemia. Individuals with pernicious anemia and atrophic gastritis are at increased risk of developing gastric carcinoma. *Chronic (atrophic) antral gastritis* (type B gastritis) may be associated with duodenal reflux or *Campylobacter pylori* infection and probably predisposes to gastric peptic ulcers. Atrophic gastritis is often accompanied by intestinal metaplasia.

Ulcers. Acute (stress) ulcers are most frequently hemorrhagic erosions, which may be found in all parts of the stomach, usually in association with acute gastritis, and may be caused by excessive alcohol, severe vomiting, infection, sensitivity to aspirin, steroid therapy, or ingestion of other noxious substances. These types of ulcers are also frequently terminal events in a variety of disease states. Severe burns may be associated with the so-called Curling's ulcers, which may be fatal due to uncontrolled hemorrhage or perforation. Hypothalamic syndromes, Cushing's disease, as well as severe stress or trauma also may be associated with similar ulcers.

True chronic peptic ulcer, by far the most important of the ulcers that occur in this part of the GI tract, develops in the lower stomach or the first part of the duodenum, being much more common in the latter situation. In the stomach it is located in the prepyloric region, on the posterior wall, within about 5 cm of the pyloric ring and near the lesser curvature. In the duodenum it is situated above the ampulla of Vater, in that portion bathed by acid fluids coming from the stomach. In general, acid production is greater in patients with duodenal ulcers than in those with gastric ulcers.

Typically the ulcer is round or oval, punched out, and deeply penetrating. It forms a sharply demarcated cavity or crater with indurated walls. These walls are covered on the surface by a layer of fibrin, beneath which is necrotic tissue resting on granulation tissue, which forms the deepest layer. The ulcer usually measures from 1 cm to 3 cm in greatest dimension and extends to the muscularis or—more usually—even deeper. Chronic peptic ulcers usually are solitary.

Peptic ulcers of the duodenum and the low pyloric channel frequently are associated with highly acidic gastric juice. Ulcers located high in the antrum (near the incisura angularis) frequently are associated with atrophic gastritis, which is thought to have antedated ulcer formation and perhaps to have contributed to its development.

Complications of chronic peptic ulcer include (1) hemorrhage from erosion of a large vessel, especially an artery; (2) perforation of the gastric or duodenal wall with consequent discharge of contents into the peritoneal cavity, which may result in peritonitis, or into the retroperitoneal tissues; (3) penetration of and adhesion to the liver or the pancreas; (4) pyloric stenosis with obstruction; and (5) malignant change in the chronic ulcer, which, on the basis of observed cases, occurs very rarely.

Gastric Polyps. These benign glandular proliferations fall into two main categories: hyperplastic and adenomatous. Hyperplastic polyps are composed of elongated, dilated, and tortuous glands that contain abundant mucin in the lumen. They are relatively common, randomly located, often multiple, and usually less than 2 cm in diameter. They are not considered premalignant lesions. Adenomatous polyps are composed of closely packed tubular glands with crowded elongated nuclei. They are uncommon, usually antral, solitary, and greater than 2 cm in diameter. They are important because they may give rise to adenocarcinomas.

Carcinoma of the Stomach. Once one of the most common tumors, especially in men, carcinoma of the stomach is now decreasing, especially in North America. It is still one of the most common types of cancer in Japan, Iceland, and some of the technologically underdeveloped countries of Latin America. Stomach cancer may differ in histologic and cytologic characteristics. A useful classification of the most typical forms is the following: (1) polypoid or fungating adenocarcinoma; (2) flat, superficially ulcerative adenocarcinoma; and (3) diffuse carcinoma (linitis plastica), which may, in its later stages, convert the stomach into a firm, thick-walled, hard, contracted structure sometimes called leather-bottle stomach. Spread of gastric cancer is by direct extension to adjacent structures and by metastasis to regional lymph nodes and liver and, rarely, to the left supraclavicular lymph nodes (Virchow's pilot node). Modern endoscopic techniques have made possible the diagnosis of dysplastic lesions and early carcinomas. When the tumor is localized to the mucosa of the stomach, the great majority of the patients are cured by gastrectomy.

SMALL INTESTINE

Meckel's diverticulum is a vestigial remnant of the omphalomesenteric duct usually located near the ileocecal valve. It may contain heterotopic rests of gastric mucosa and can present with bleeding or may mimic acute appendicitis.

Infective Enterocolitis. Acute viral gastroenteritis often is caused by Norwalklike viruses and rotaviruses. Herpes simplex virus and cytomegalovirus are important in immunosuppressed individuals. Bacterial enterocolitis may be due to a variety of agents, including *Salmonella, Shigella, Campylobacter, Escherichia coli, Yersinia, Vibrio,* and mycobacteria. In typhoid fever the specific lesions are found in Peyer's patches and solitary follicles of the distal ileum. Macrophages with phagocytized RBCs and debris are typical. Necrotic foci coalesce to form ulcers. The long axis of the typhoid ulcer lies parallel to the length of the intestine. Tuberculous ulceration also most frequently involves the distal ileum, but the long axis of the ulcer is transverse. Enterocolitis also may be due to fungal or parasitic organisms.

Regional Enteritis (Crohn's Disease). This involves the distal portion of the ileum, as a rule, often in segmental fashion with so-called skip areas of uninvolved normal mucosa between the involved portions, and the process may extend into the first part of the colon as well. In the gross, there is great thickening of the wall, mainly of the submucosa (ropy intestine), with stenosis of the lumen and ulceration of the mucosa. The neighboring lymph nodes are hyperplastic. Microscopically, there may be a granulomatous type of inflammation characterized by the infiltration of a variety of inflammatory cells but especially by the presence of foci of epithelioid cells and giant cells. Similar foci occur in the regional hyperplastic lymph nodes. The inflammation typically involves all layers of the bowel wall. The healing stage of regional ischemia of the small intestine from any cause (usually arterial thrombosis) may simulate regional enteritis. Extraintestinal manifestations include polyarthritis, uveitis, ankylosing spondylitis, hepatitis, pericholangitis, cholelithiasis, and skin lesions, such as pyoderma gangrenosum and erythema nodosum.

APPENDIX

Acute Appendicitis. Probably the most important cause of acute appendicitis is obstruction in some portion, usually the proximal part, of the lumen by a fecalith. Obstruction leads to interference with the circulation and local erosion of the mucosa with entrance of microorganisms that cause infection of the wall. The most common microorganisms are those normally found in the region, *Escherichia coli* or the enterococci, although streptococci may sometimes be found. Which of these processes, obstruction or infection, comes first is often not determinable.

COLON

Ulceration of the colon may be (1) bacillary, (2) amebic, or (3) idiopathic. In the bacillary type, the colon usually is involved throughout its entire course. The lesions are at first catarrhal or fibrinous in character, with necrosis beneath the exudate forming a false membrane that rubs off, leaving superficial or deep ulcers, the edges of which are not undermined. The mucosa may be hemorrhagic or gangrenous. Cicatrization follows severe ulceration, but perforation is rare.

Amebic Dysentery. This condition usually is confined to the upper colon but may involve the sigmoid and the rectum. The parasite *(Entamoeba histolytica)* that causes this disease is present mainly in the tunica propria of the mucosa. Nodules are produced from swelling and cellular infiltration in the mucosa and the submucosa, followed by the formation of ulcers with indurated, undermined edges that may become confluent. Suppuration may extend beneath the mucosa from ulcer to ulcer. Perforation may occur. Healing takes place by the formation of granulation tissue. The mesenteric lymph nodes may be enlarged, and the organisms pass through the lymphatics into the portal vein to form liver abscesses.

Idiopathic Nonspecific Ulcerative Colitis. This is a common and serious inflammatory condition that most frequently has its onset in adults in the second decade. Etiology is not clear, although bacteria, viruses, and parasites, as well as allergic states, nutritional deficiencies, and even psychogenic factors have been suspected. Recent studies would seem to imply a defect in immune body production since autoantibodies against colonic epithelial cells have been demonstrated in these patients. Whether these play an etiologic role or merely perpetuate the condition is not known. The affected colon, often the entire length, is contracted, and its mucosa is hyperemic, dark red and velvety, with irregular, coalescent ulcerations that are frequently undermined and have ragged margins. The underlying muscle is thickened and rigid. Remissions and exacerbations are common. In differentiating ulcerative colitis from Crohn's disease, it is helpful to remember that in ulcerative colitis the ulcerations rarely extend into muscularis, the inflammation is rarely granulomatous, and there are no "skip" lesions.

Pseudomembranous colitis frequently follows treatment with certain antibiotics (clindamycin) and is characterized by a marked dilatation of the crypts by mucin and polymorphonuclear leukocytes, covered by a fibrinopurulent exudate in the form of discrete pseudomembranes.

Tumors of the Colon and Rectum. *Nonneoplastic* colon polyps, which have virtually no malignant potential, include *hyperplastic polyps* and juvenile polyps (the latter is probably hamartomatous in origin). *Neoplastic* colon polyps include *adenomatous polyps* (tubular adenomas) and *villous adenomas.* The adenomatous polyp is common, especially after the age of 50, usually small, soft, and pedunculated. Histologically, the thickened mucosa consists of closely packed tubular glands lined by columnar to pseudostratified columnar epithelium with pencil-shaped, variably hyperchromatic nuclei. Variable degrees of atypia are seen. It rarely becomes malignant. The villous adenoma, on the other hand, is much less common but is larger than the pedunculated type, has a broad, sessile base and appears as a fungating, plantlike mass rising from the mucosa. Histologically, it is composed of villous glandular structures lined by epithelial cells similar to those lining adenomatous polyps. They often have associated carcinoma *in situ* or invasive adenocarcinoma. Three important neoplastic polyposis syndromes include *familial adenomatous polyposis, Gardner's syndrome,* and *Turcot's syndrome.* All are characterized by numerous adenomas of the colon (lesser numbers in small intestine and stomach) and a high malignant potential. Gardner's syndrome is distinguished by association of colon adenomas with osteomas, desmoid tumors, epidermoid cysts, and lipomas. Turcot's syndrome includes the association with malignant CNS neoplasms. *Nonneoplastic* polyposis syndromes include *Peutz–Jeghers syndrome* (hamartomatous polyps, mucocutaneous melanin pigmentation, and ovarian tumors), *juvenile polyposis* (probably hamartomatous polyps), and *Cronkite–Canada syndrome* (inflammatory polyps), all of which have a very low malignant potential.

Adenocarcinoma of the colon and rectum is one of the most common of all malignant neoplasms. In the United States, mortality for adenocarcinoma of the large intestine is second only to lung cancer in men and second only to breast cancer in women. It is found most often in the sigmoid colon and rectum—about 28% in the sigmoid and 40% in the rectum. In men only cancers of the skin and the lungs are more common, while in women only cancers of the breast and lung occur more frequently. In the sigmoid colon the neoplasms often encircle the colon in napkin-ring fashion, cause constriction and then obstruction of the lumen, and lead to obstipation, constipation, and narrow, stringy stools. In the rectum their gross appearance varies from round or oval ulcerated growths with raised edges to flattened, infiltrating lesions, both of which ulcerate easily and tend to bleed. Histologically these lesions are typical adenocarcinomas, often with much mucin production.

Adenocarcinoma also may occur less frequently in other parts of the colon. Of special interest is the right-sided lesion occurring in the cecum and ascending colon. It is a polypoid, fungating lesion that produces symptoms late and is difficult to diagnose; it is therefore more frequently fatal. The first suspicion of such tumors may be raised by iron deficiency anemia due to chronic blood loss.

Pancreas

CONGENITAL ANOMALIES

These are uncommon or of little significance. *Agenesis,* if it occurs, is associated with other malformations that are usually incompatible with life. *Aberrant* or *ectopic* pancreatic tissue is sometimes found in the stomach, in the duodenum, or in a Meckel's diverticulum.

ATROPHY OF THE PANCREAS

Atrophy may be caused by impaired circulation that results from arteriosclerosis. It affects both exocrine and endocrine structures, but generally is so slight that function is not significantly affected. More important is atrophy resulting from obstruction of the pancreatic duct. The effect of sudden obstruction of the main pancreatic duct may be

acute pancreatitis if infection of the intraductal pancreatic secretion and injury to the lining of the ducts are present. But if the obstruction develops slowly or lasts for a long time, atrophy and destruction of the parenchyma, interstitial fibrosis, and cyst formation may occur. Islet tissue usually remains well preserved. The main functional disturbance of such obstruction is interference with the exocrine secretions of the pancreas, the most important of which is trypsinogen.

CYSTIC FIBROSIS (FIBROCYSTIC DISEASE)

This is a hereditary disease transmitted as a mendelian recessive gene that may have serious consequences. Evidence of its presence may be apparent soon after birth with the development of meconium ileus, or later, when chronic bronchitis and upper respiratory infections, steatorrhea, and the secretion of sweat with a high concentration of sodium and chloride are discovered. The abnormality affects all mucous glands of the body, but especially of the pancreas, and the mucus produced is abnormal, being more thick and viscid than usual so that the pancreatic secretions do not reach the duodenum. The term *mucoviscidosis* has been given to the disease process. Histologically both the acini and the ducts of the pancreas are filled with mucus, the stroma is increased, and the exocrine glands are atrophied, but the islets of Langerhans are normal. The small intestine may be obstructed by inspissated meconium that results from the lack of pancreatic enzymes, and the intestinal glands are filled with thick mucoid secretion. The respiratory tract shows striking changes. Mucopurulent exudate is present in both trachea and bronchi, and bronchiectasis is often present. The mucus-secreting glands of the trachea and bronchi are dilated with inspissated mucus, and the bronchial and bronchiolar walls are acutely and chronically inflamed. Foci of emphysema, alternating with foci of atelectasis and even consolidation, are present in the lung tissue, apparently because of partial or complete obstruction of the bronchi and bronchioles by thick, viscid mucus complicated by secondary infection.

PANCREATITIS

Acute hemorrhagic pancreatitis, perhaps better known as *acute pancreatic necrosis,* because of the extensive hemorrhagic necrosis caused by liberated pancreatic enzymes, is so commonly associated with infection of the gallbladder and ducts that it is generally considered to be related to these conditions. It may be caused by regurgitation of infected bile into the pancreas when a gallstone lodges in the common opening of the bile and pancreatic ducts, the infected fluids injuring duct tissues and probably activating pancreatic enzymes. The condition sometimes follows an attack of acute alcoholism. The pancreas is enlarged, softened, and permeated with foci of hemorrhagic necrosis, not only of pancreatic parenchyma but also of peripancreatic fat, because of the digestive action of the pancreatic enzymes. The hemorrhage and the chalky white spots of fat necrosis are the most striking findings in this condition. Serofibrinous peritonitis also is present. Large portions of pancreatic tissue may become gangrenous. In the acute stage of the disease (within 48 hours following the onset of the process), the serum amylase usually is elevated greatly, and this is diagnostic.

Chronic suppurative pancreatitis occurs in pyemia but usually is secondary to primary carcinoma of the pancreas. Chronic interstitial pancreatitis is characterized by increase of fibrous tissue between or within the lobules and most commonly is associated with diabetes.

Carcinoma of the Pancreas. The most common site of carcinoma of the pancreas is in the head where approximately 60% to 70% occur. As the neoplasm grows larger, it gradually causes pressure upon the pancreatic ducts, with consequent interference with the entrance of the external pancreatic secretion into the intestine and with resultant digestive disturbances and inanition. It usually also causes obstruction of the common bile duct with resultant jaundice and its consequences. Pain is usually an early symptom, but its presence means invasion of, or pressure upon, adjacent structures.

Carcinoma of the body and tail of the pancreas is less common but is often more difficult to diagnose until weakness, weight loss, and cachexia have set in. It tends to be larger than carcinoma of the head because of the paucity of early signs and symptoms.

Practically all pancreatic cancers are adenocarcinomas of duct origin. They are hard, fibrous, gritty masses in which the epithelial cells grow in nests, cords, or atypical ducts embedded in dense stroma.

DIABETES MELLITUS

This is a disturbance in carbohydrate metabolism characterized clinically by an elevated blood glucose level and associated glycosuria. There are two typical forms: juvenile diabetes and adult diabetes, the first developing usually before the age of 15, the second after the age of 40 or 45. Juvenile diabetes begins acutely, is controlled with difficulty, and in many cases leads to blindness and to death in early adult life from cardiovascular complications. The adult type begins more slowly and responds better to treatment but may be associated with obesity and arteriosclerosis and its complications—not infrequently, impaired circulation to the lower extremities and gangrene.

The disease is the result of a deficiency, or lack of normal potency, of the hormone insulin, which is produced by the β-cells of the pancreatic islets of Langerhans, but the underlying cause of the condition is unknown. Because of this insufficiency of insulin, excess glucose accumulates in the blood, and much of the excess is eliminated in the urine. There is also incomplete oxidation of fat, so that ketone bodies are found in the blood, and acidosis results. Usually some evidence of damage to the β-cells can be demonstrated, but in about 20% of cases no recognizable pathologic changes are demonstrable in the islets.

In juvenile diabetes the number of islets is usually reduced, the β-cells contain few or no granules, and fibrosis of many islets may be present, together with evidence of mild, low-grade inflammation. In the adult diabetic the number of islets is about normal, the degree of granulation of the β-cells usually shows little variation from normal, but the islets exhibit varying degrees of hyalinization with compression atrophy of many islet cells. In some cases hydropic degeneration of the β-cells, shown recently to be caused by accumulation of glycogen within them, is prominent. Often there is no evident relationship between the severity of the clinical manifestations and the extent of the abnormal changes in the islets. Other changes in the pancreas are sometimes found, such as diffuse fibrosis and atrophy of the entire organ and evidence of chronic pancreatitis. Another condition, hemochromatosis, with diffuse fibrosis and hemosiderin deposition, may sometimes be associated with diabetes.

In other organs pathologic changes may also be found. Recent electron microscopic studies have disclosed rather widespread changes in the smaller blood vessels, especially the capillaries of the skin and skeletal muscles. The basement membranes of the capillary walls are irregularly thickened, sometimes by a homogeneous deposit and sometimes by a doubling of the membrane itself. Glycogen may be demonstrated in many tissues, particularly the kidneys, in which the epithelial cells of Henle's loops and some of the convoluted tubules may be distended with glycogen. Other manifestations of diabetes in the kidneys are nodular thickenings of the basement membranes of the glomerular capillaries (the glomerulosclerosis of Kimmelstiel and Wilson) and hyaline thickening of the walls of the afferent and efferent arterioles. In the liver the storage of glycogen is decreased within the cytoplasm of the liver cells, but the nuclei may have an increased amount and may appear vacuolated. Atherosclerosis is more marked in diabetics than in nondiabetics of the same age group and, in the heart and lower extremities especially, may lead, respectively, to coronary heart disease and diabetic gangrene of the toes and feet.

Liver

CONGENITAL LESIONS

Congenital anomalies are rare, but some may be of great consequence. Congenital hepatic fibrosis, characterized by a great increase of bile ducts in a fibrous stroma with linkage of portal areas, frequently eventuates in portal hypertension and its sequelae. Polycystic disease of the liver occurs with or without concomitant polycystic renal disease. The prognosis usually depends primarily on the severity of the renal disease. Choledochal cysts involving the extrahepatic biliary tree and segmental intrahepatic dilatation of bile ducts (Caroli's disease) may lead to cholestasis, choledocholithiasis, and cholangitis. Biliary atresia of both the intrahepatic and extrahepatic varieties have been thought to be congenital or developmental anomalies due to failure of formation or canalization of bile ducts. Recent evidence suggests that many cases represent acquired destruction of ducts associated with infectious, metabolic, or chromosomal abnormalities. The extrahepatic type is usually severe, leading to marked cholestasis, portal fibrosis and ductular proliferation, and eventual biliary cirrhosis. The liver in the intrahepatic variety shows cholestasis and an absence of bile ducts. Patients may survive many years before developing cirrhosis.

STORAGE AND PIGMENTATION

Storage of lipid in hepatocytes, designated fatty change, appears in conventional histologic sections as large cytoplasmic vacuoles that displace the nucleus to the periphery. Associated conditions include malnutrition, obesity, diabetes mellitus, alcoholism, malabsorption, some metabolic disorders, postjejunoileal bypass surgery, and exposure to some drugs (most commonly corticosteroids). Glycogen normally is stored in hepatocytes but is stored in excess in the glycogen storage diseases. A marked increase in copper content (frequently visible by special stains) characterizes Wilson's disease (hepatolenticular degeneration). Alpha$_1$-antitrypsin globules accumulate in periportal hepatocytes in alpha$_1$-antitrypsin deficiency. Severe cases are associated with the progressive development of periportal fibrosis and sometimes cirrhosis.

Lipofuscin pigment progressively accumulates with aging. An excess of pigment may follow chronic ingestion of some drugs. Hemosiderosis is the accumulation of hemosiderin (iron) in an organ. The term hemochromatosis usually refers to hemosiderosis plus tissue damage and fibrosis. Hemosiderin deposition results from blood transfusions, various hematologic disturbances, excessive dietary iron intake, and an inheritable condition, idiopathic (primary) hemochromatosis. The latter is most likely to be associated with hepatic fibrosis and even cirrhosis and tissue damage in other organs.

VASCULAR DISORDERS

Chronic passive congestion is a result of chronic congestive heart failure. The liver develops a "nutmeg" appearance, owing to the intense red brown color of the congested central zones, which contrasts with the tan peripheral lobular regions. Microscopically, the central zones show dilatation and congestion of sinusoids, atrophy of hepatocytes, and sometimes fatty change. Cases of long duration may show fibrous linkage of central veins, a pattern sometimes labeled "cardiac cirrhosis." Acute severe congestive heart failure or shock may produce centrilobular coagulation necrosis.

The Budd–Chiari syndrome results from obstruction of the major hepatic venous outflow (hepatic veins and inferior vena cava). Thrombi, tumors, congenital venous webs are responsible. Most cases are fatal. A related disorder, venoocclusive disease, follows restricted outflow from the central veins of the liver. The most common causes are ingestion of pyrollizidine alkaloids in various "bush teas" and radiation damage. The liver in venous outflow obstruction is enlarged, tense, and red purple. Rapidly accumulating ascites is common. Microscopic changes resemble those of severe congestive heart failure, except that changes in outflow veins (e.g., thrombi, intimal proliferation, fibrosis) are more likely found.

Hepatic infarcts are rare, since the organ possesses a dual blood supply. Occlusion of the hepatic artery or one of its branches by thrombi, inadvertent ligature, or polyarteritis nodosa is the most common cause.

HEPATOCELLULAR INJURY AND NECROSIS

Patterns of Necrosis.   Central necrosis (*i.e.*, necrosis chiefly localized about the central vein) is characteristic of injury associated with certain drugs and toxins. Carbon tetrachloride, acetaminophen in large doses, and the toxin associated with mushroom poisoning are the most notable examples. Midzonal necrosis, a rare phenomenon, is associated with yellow fever. Peripheral or periportal necrosis is found in eclampsia, DIC, and toxic injury associated with phosphorus or ferrous sulfate. Focal necrosis is seen in various infectious processes, such as typhoid fever. In diffuse necrosis, or massive hepatic necrosis, virtually the entire parenchyma is lost and the outcome is usually fatal. The collapsed, flabby parenchyma is red and is enclosed by a wrinkled capsule. Occasional islands of yellow to green regenerating parenchyma may be found. Less extensive involvement is termed submassive hepatic necrosis. The most common cause of massive and submassive necrosis is viral hepatitis, although a variety of other drugs and toxins may be at fault. The more usual form of viral hepatitis produces "panlobar injury" in which all zones of the lobule are affected but not all cells are necrotic. Some cells show degenerative changes such as ballooning degeneration, others regenerative changes, and others necrosis in the form of acidophilic bodies.

Viral Hepatitis.   Four types of viral hepatitis are currently recognized: A, B, non-A non-B, and delta hepatitis.

Hepatitis A (infectious hepatitis) is transmitted by the fecal–oral route. Infection usually results from close contact with infected individuals, ingestion of contaminated food or water, or swimming in contaminated waters. Following an incubation period of about 2 to 6 weeks, there is an abrupt onset of symptoms. Viral particles, 27 nm in diameter, have been identified in the stools of infected individuals by immunoelectron-microscopy, a technique too cumbersome for routine use. Antibodies to hepatitis A virus of the IgM class are indicative of acute viral hepatitis, type A; antibodies of the IgG class only indicate previous hepatitis A infection and are considered a sign of immunity. Microscopically, the usual case shows panlobular injury as described above. Cholestasis is sometimes present and may be marked. Fatty change is usually absent. An inflammatory infiltrate of predominantly lymphocytes is present in the lobules and in the portal tracts. Viral particles have been identified in the cytoplasm of hepatocytes by electron microscopy. The usual case resolves without sequelae. Rarely, submassive or massive hepatic necrosis, sometimes fatal, occurs. Chronic hepatitis or a chronic carrier state associated with hepatitis A is not recognized.

Hepatitis B (serum hepatitis) is classically transmitted by direct innoculation of blood or blood products (as by transfusion or by inadvertent injury with contaminated needles or instruments). More recent evidence indicates that transmission also occurs by the fecal, oral, and venereal routes. The incubation period is about 6 weeks to 6 months. A 42-nm spherical particle appears to represent the virus of hepatitis B (HB). It is composed of a 27-nm core (HB core antigen), which is produced in the nuclei of hepatocytes, and a 20-nm to 25-nm coat (hepatitis B surface antigen [HBsAG]), which is synthesized in the cytoplasm and added to the core. An excess of the surface antigen is released into the circulation during acute hepatitis and frequently in chronic hepatitis. Serologic tests for the surface antigen (formerly Australian antigen) have received widespread clinical application in diagnosis and in detection of potentially infectious blood donors. Tests for antibodies to the surface antigen and to the core antigen are frequently combined with surface antigen testing to yield a variety of patterns that indicate the stage of the disease. A related antigen, "e" antigen, indicates infectivity of a given host. The histologic findings in acute hepatitis are similar to those of hepatitis A. A small percentage of patients develop chronic hepatitis of variable severity. A benign form, chronic persistent hepatitis, is characterized by chronic inflammation in portal tracts and focal necrosis. Chronic active (aggressive) hepatitis has a worse prognosis and shows, in addition, periportal degeneration and necrosis of hepatocytes and periportal fibrosis. In some cases, the fibrosis is progressive and may eventuate in cirrhosis. Cirrhosis may also follow acute submassive necrosis in some instances. Patients with cirrhosis or with chronic hepatitis may have "ground-glass hepatocytes," a morphologic indicator of HB infection. The ground-glass appearance is accounted for by the presence of hyperplastic endoplasmic reticulum, which contains an excess of surface antigen. Special stains are available to confirm the presence of the antigen.

Non-A non-B hepatitis was recognized by the development of transfusion-associated hepatitis in patients without serologic evidence of hepatitis A or B. This type of hepatitis apparently accounts for approximately 90% of cases of post-transfusion hepatitis in the United States. The incubation period is approximately 2 to 15 weeks. Specific serologic tests have not been developed; the diagnosis remains one of exclusion. Lots of factor VIII, which were implicated in human disease, have been used to produce hepatitis in chimpanzees. Viral particles, 27 nm in diameter, were recovered from a homogenate of liver obtained from an infected animal. Further study is necessary to determine if such particles are the responsible agent. A morphologic spectrum of hepatic disease similar to that of type B hepatitis is observed in non-A non-B hepatitis.

Delta hepatitis is caused by a defective RNA virus requiring the presence of hepatitis B virus (HBV) as a helper. The infecting agent has a central core of delta antigen surrounded by a shell of HBsAG. Delta hepatitis may occur as an acute coinfection along with acute HB, or as an acute or chronic superinfection in a patient with chronic HBV infection.

A variety of other viruses may cause hepatitis that is not traditionally labeled "viral" hepatitis. Most notable are cytomegalovirus and herpesvirus.

Alcoholic Liver Disease. Fatty change may be caused by a short-term increase in alcohol consumption, but severe hepatocellular injury and cirrhosis follow many years of heavy intake. The precise role of nutritional deficiency in the production of injury is not established, but most investigators believe that alcohol itself is toxic to the liver. Some individuals are less susceptible to hepatic damage than others, but the protective factors are not known. Hepatocellular injury first develops in the central zones. Some hepatocytes show ballooning degeneration, and a neutrophilic infiltrate around degenerating cells and foci of necrosis are characteristic. Mallory's hyaline (alcoholic hyaline, Mallory bodies) is commonly found in degenerating hepatocytes; it consists of irregular cytoplasmic clumps of hyaline material. With continued damage, fibrosis appears around the central vein and extends radially into the lobule. Ductular proliferation and periportal fibrosis also develop, and fibrous linkage of the portal tracts and central veins eventually dissects the lobules into microunits resulting in a pattern of micronodular cirrhosis. Considerable parenchymal regenerative activity may be noted. Fatty change is commonly present during all active stages of this disease process.

Cirrhosis. Many classifications of cirrhosis have been devised, but none has received universal acceptance. This discussion will adhere to the classification of the World Health Organization. Cirrhosis is the extensive alteration of the hepatic architecture resulting from extensive fibrosis in areas of parenchymal degeneration and necrosis with the formation of "pseudolobules" of parenchyma bounded by fibrous septa. The pseudolobules frequently show evidence of hepatocellular regeneration. Three basic morphologic patterns have been defined: micronodular, macronodular, and mixed. In the micronodular variety, most of the pseudolobules are less than 3 mm in diameter. The macronodular type is characterized by a predominance of pseudolobules greater than 3 mm in diameter. The mixed type contains approximately equal numbers of micronodules and macronodules. A cirrhotic liver may be classified into one of the three basic categories and then subclassified according to etiology. Altered vascular relationships, impediment of blood flow through the microcirculation, and arteriovenous shunting are probably responsible for portal hypertension that accompanies many cases of cirrhosis. Portal hypertension may be followed by splenomegaly and collateral circulation between the portal and systemic circulation, the most important manifestation of which is esophageal varices. Such varices may rupture, producing serious hemorrhage.

The cirrhosis associated with alcoholic liver damage (formerly called Laennec's cirrhosis, portal cirrhosis, or nutritional cirrhosis) is the most common form of micronodular cirrhosis.

Biliary cirrhosis is also micronodular and follows prolonged obstruction of and/or infection of the biliary tree. In adults, tumors or calculi are the most common causes. Biliary atresia and choledochal cysts are the most likely etiologies in infants and children. Prominent cholestasis or cholangitis are the dominant morphologic manifestations of the obstruction in the liver. In time, there are prominent ductular proliferation and periportal fibrosis with linkage of adjacent portal tracts and formation of irregular micronodules. An idiopathic type of biliary cirrhosis (primary biliary cirrhosis) affects some middle-aged persons, usually women, and has some features of an autoimmune process. The disease is characterized morphologically by the gradual destruction of the intrahepatic bile ducts with eventual formation of micronodular cirrhosis and by the presence of antimitochondrial antibodies in the patient's serum.

The cirrhotic stage of hemochromatosis (pigment cirrhosis) is usually micronodular.

Cardiac cirrhosis is a very rare sequel of chronic congestive heart failure. Fibrous linkage of central veins results in a micronodular pattern.

The cirrhosis associated with viral hepatitis is typically macronodular. Usually the fibrous septa are thick and contain remnants of several collapsed adjacent lobules. The pattern has also been called "postnecrotic cirrhosis." In hepatitis B, ground-glass hepatocytes may be found in some pseudolobules.

Macronodular patterns are typically found in cirrhosis associated with Wilson's disease and α_1-antitrypsin deficiency. Mixed cirrhosis may sometimes be observed in those conditions that ordinarily produce a macronodular pattern and also in alcoholic liver disease.

Other infectious diseases, such as syphilis and schistosomiasis, may produce extensive hepatic fibrosis. Although formerly classified as cirrhosis, such disorders lack the diffuse architectural reorganization and pseudolobule formation characteristic of cirrhosis.

Tumors. The *hepatocellular adenoma,* although benign and rare, is receiving increasing attention because it may rupture and cause fatal hemorrhage and because of its apparent association with prolonged use of oral contraceptives in many cases. *Hepatoblastoma* is a malignant tumor of children. In addition to proliferation of immature hepatocytes, mesenchymal elements (*e.g.,* bone, cartilage) may be found. *Hepatocellular carcinoma* most commonly develops in livers with cirrhosis due to hemochromatosis, HB, or alcoholism.

Bile duct adenomas are rare and are usually of no clinical consequence. *Cholangiocarcinoma* (bile duct carcinoma) usually develops in noncirrhotic livers. The tumors resemble adenocarcinomas of other organs. Some cases in the Far East appear to be associated with clonorchiasis.

The *cavernous hemangioma* is the most common benign tumor of the liver. *Infantile hemangioendotheliomas* commonly produce congestive heart failure because of arteriovenous shunting. *Angiosarcoma* (malignant hemangioendothelioma) is a highly malignant neoplasm that may be produced by exposure to vinyl chloride, arsenic, or thorotrast in some cases. Other cases are idiopathic. Most hepatic tumors are metastatic. Tumors of the GI tract, biliary tract, and pancreas are common sources, but almost any organ may be a primary site.

Gallbladder

Cholecystitis, inflammation of the gallbladder, is usually associated with *Escherichia coli,* pyogenic cocci, or *Salmonella typhi* infection, but the route of infection is not definitely established. It may be hematogenous or ascending. Biliary calculi usually predispose to infection but may sometimes be secondary to it. Typhoid bacilli, if present, are usually residual from an old infection, and the host is considered to be a chronic carrier.

Acute cholecystitis may be catarrhal, phlegmonous, or gangrenous, with edema and leukocytic infiltration of the wall. Perforation may occur. In subacute and chronic cholecystitis, the wall is thickened, indurated and opaque, with chronic exudative and proliferative inflammation, restricted usually to the outer layers.

Cholesterolosis (strawberry gallbladder) results from the deposition of cholesterol in the hyperemic mucosa.

Empyema of the gallbladder is a form of acute or chronic suppurative cholecystitis in which the cavity is filled with pus and the duct is occluded.

Cholelithiasis is found in at least 75% of all forms of definitely diseased gallbladders. Obesity probably plays a predisposing role, as does pregnancy. Infection, stagnation, and supersaturation of the bile combine to determine the precipitation of cholesterol, bile salts, bile pigment, and calcium carbonate that accumulate around desquamated epithelial cells, bacteria, and organic detritus to form calculi. Some calculi may be primarily of pigment type, others of cholesterol, but the majority are of mixed type. The pigment type is composed of calcium bilirubinate and is usually associated with a hemolytic process. Biliary calculi may be present without producing symptoms, but occasionally, if caught in a duct through which they cannot pass, they may cause especially extreme pain (biliary colic). Biliary calculi that escape from the gallbladder and reach the common duct before being stopped may also cause severe icterus. The presence of calculi in the gallbladder may determine the presence of hydrops, empyema, fistula formation, cholecystitis (if not already present), and cholangitis. In some cases calculi have apparently played a role in inducing carcinoma of this organ.

Endocrine System

Some aspects of endocrinology are covered in the sections on biochemistry, physiology, internal medicine, pediatrics, and obstetrics and gynecology. Emphasis in this section will be on the pathologic changes in the endocrine system that are most frequent and most significant. Endocrine disorders are usually the result of increase or decrease of the hormone secretions of the endocrine glands, which may be the result of disease processes affecting the endocrine organs or from alteration of feedback and other mechanisms controlling hormone secretion. The endocrine organs may be affected by destructive lesions, neoplasms with varying degrees of autonomy, and changes reflecting altered control mechanisms. The decrease of hormone secretion can result from genetically determined enzyme defects, such as those that occur in cretinism and the adrenogenital syndromes, destructive lesions, such as those involving the adrenal, pituitary, and thyroid, and destructive lesions of the adenohypophysis and hypothalamus, which produce releasing and trophic factors. Increase in hormone secretion can result from autonomous tumors and hyperplasia of the endocrine organs, increased production of hypothalamic and adenohypophyseal trophic factors, secretion of trophic hormones from ectopic sites, such as tumors, and substances that compete for endocrine receptors. A description of selected endocrine disorders follows.

THYROID GLAND

This endocrine organ actively traps iodine from the blood and binds it to tyrosine residues to form mono- and diiodotyrosine (MIT and DIT) which are later coupled to form the thyroid hormones triiodothyronine (T_3) and thyroxine (T_4). These are incorporated to the thyroglobulin molecule and stored in the follicle. These hormones are released when needed by phagocytosis and proteolysis of thyroglobulin. When this process is interrupted, hypothyroidism results. In the adult, it is manifested as *myxedema,* a syndrome characterized by slowing of intellectual and motor performances, cold intolerance, peripheral edema, macroglossia, low basal metabolic rate, and low levels of T_3 and T_4 in the blood. *Primary myxedema* may occur after total thyroidectomy, radiotherapy, or severe chronic thyroiditis, or may be idiopathic. In such cases thyroid-stimulating hormone (TSH) levels are elevated. *Secondary myxedema* is usually associated with pituitary deficiency (Sheehan's syndrome or destructive tumors) and is accompanied by low blood levels of TSH and thyroid-releasing hormone (TRH). Severe iodine deficiency during pregnancy is believed to lead to *cretinism* in the offspring, characterized by mental and physical retardation, as well as deafness. Iodine deficiency in a community is associated with endemic goiter and sometimes, but not always, with *endemic cretinism. Sporadic cretinism* may be due to agenesis of the thyroid gland or to enzymatic defects which block

one or several of the steps required for thyroid hormone synthesis and release. In the latter cases multinodular goiter is observed, presumably due to unchecked continuous stimulus to cellular replication because of failure of the feedback mechanism which depends on the blood level of thyroid hormones.

Insufficient supply of iodine in a community results in *endemic goiter,* which used to be very prevalent in some areas of the United States, especially around the Great Lakes, but has practically disappeared since adequate iodine supply has been available. Several forms of goiter are observed in endemic areas. The most common is characterized by multiple solid nodules composed of proliferating follicular cells which compress the surrounding parenchyma and form a pseudocapsule. They may form follicular structures of different size or solid cellular cords. These nodules may attain a maximal size of 5 cm to 6 cm and usually involute because of central atrophy and fibrosis, intranodular hemorrhage, or cystic degeneration. This type is called *nodular parenchymatous goiter,* or NPG. The second type is characterized by excessive colloid accumulation diffusely distributed throughout the gland, so-called *diffuse colloid goiter,* or DCG. The third type, called *nodular colloid goiter,* or NCG, is characterized by excessive colloid accumulation present in all follicles but leading to pseudonodules, which compress each other but are not surrounded by a capsule. Mixed forms (parenchymatous and colloid nodules) are also frequent in endemic areas. After iodine supplementation, within the same generation, colloid goiter decreases in prevalence in children and diminishes in size in adults; the colloid component of mixed goiters is considerably reduced, but the NPG of adults does not decrease in frequency. The second generation with adequate iodine supply is free from endemic goiter and does not differ in this respect to people living in areas where iodine supply has always been plentiful. Goiter is still found in such populations at lower frequency (sporadic goiter), and the same basic histologic types are represented. The cause is unknown, but borderline enzymatic defects and goitrogenic substances in the environment are suspected. Nodules histologically identical with those of parenchymatous nodular goiter when found in populations free of endemic goiter are called adenomas or parenchymatous nodules. There is no proof that they are more or less premalignant than endemic goiter nodules. The majority of multinodular goiters cause no physiologic disturbances, although occasionally one nodule may become hyperfunctional and lead to mild hyperthyroidism, usually not accompanied by exophthalmos.

Exophthalmic goiter (diffuse hyperplastic goiter; Graves' disease or Basedow's disease) makes up about 75% of all cases of hyperthyroidism. It is four to five times as common in females as in males, occurs chiefly in young adults or in middle age, and is characterized by exophthalmos (the cause of which is not understood), tachycardia, increased metabolic rate, systolic hypertension, fine tremor, and moderate enlargement, usually symmetric, of the thyroid gland. The cause of Graves' disease has long been uncertain. An unusual finding in a large number of cases has been the presence of a long-acting stimulating substance, which may be responsible for the hyperactivity of the gland.

Microscopically there is hyperplasia, usually marked, of the parenchymatous tissues. The epithelial cells lining the acini are columnar, with deeply stained cytoplasm, and there are many papillary projections into the acinar spaces. The colloid is decreased in amount and shows peripheral vacuolation. Foci of lymphocytes frequently are present. If preoperative treatment with iodine is given, the excised gland may show only slight hyperplasia or even moderate degree of colloid involution.

Acute thyroiditis may develop in the course of infectious diseases. The gland is large and tender. There may be fever, and rapid enlargement of the gland, if it occurs, may cause dyspnea, dysphagia, and hoarseness.

Chronic thyroiditis is characterized by excessive lymphocytic infiltration and fibrosis. The gland may be larger or smaller and is usually firmer than normal. A common form of chronic thyroiditis is *Hashimoto's disease (struma lymphomatosa),* in which the gland is moderately but symmetrically enlarged, is markedly infiltrated by lymphocytes to the point of actual lymph follicle formation, and is usually moderately underactive, although in some cases function is normal. Fibrosis, while present, is not marked in the typical case. There may be varying degrees of atrophy of the acini, many of which are often embedded in broad fields of lymphoid cells and show deeply acidophilic cytoplasm. A sclerosing form of chronic thyroiditis with marked stony-hard fibrosis, sometimes mistaken for scirrhous carcinoma, has long been known as Riedel's struma.

Hashimoto's disease is one of the early diseases to be attributed to the effect of autoantibodies, and antibodies against colloid antigens, as well as epithelial cell elements, have been demonstrated in the blood of many patients.

Granulomatous thyroiditis (subacute or giant cell thyroiditis) is characterized by the presence of foreign body types of multinucleated giant cells and macrophages in addition to lymphocytes and plasma cells. The etiology is unknown and usually the disease resolves by itself without sequelae.

Tumors. The most common malignant thyroid tumor in the United States is the papillary carcinoma. It is more frequent in women and tends to occur at younger ages than other malignant neoplasms. Its clinical course is slower than most carcinomas and can be controlled by surgery in a large proportion of cases. It is composed of epithelial cells which tend to organize themselves in well-defined papilla but may also form well-structured follicles. The cells invade the thyroid gland and its neighboring structures by direct extension, penetrating lymphatic channels, and producing local lymph node metastasis. Follicular carcinomas are second in frequency and usually are found in glands previously affected by goiter or adenomas. The tumor cells form follicles or solid cords, grow by centrifugal expansion, and are surrounded by a capsule that usually contains numerous telangiectatic blood vessels, which are frequently invaded by tumor emboli. Spread is predominantly by blood-borne metastasis, but lymph node metastasis may also occur. Anaplastic carcinomas are characterized by rapid growth and aggressive local and distant spread. They are frequently found in older individuals of both sexes who usually have a long-standing goiter.

In addition to the thyroid hormone–producing cells, the thyroid gland harbors the parafollicular cells that secrete calcitonin, which lowers the level of calcium in the blood. These cells may give rise to a special type of tumor called medullary carcinoma with amyloid stroma, which belong to the family of the APUD (*a*mine *p*recursor *u*ptake [and] *d*ecarboxylation) tumors. There is a tendency for familial aggregation, and the patients frequently have pheochromocytomas, small cutaneous and mucosal neuromas, and parathyroid adenomas.

Exposure of the neck organs to irradiation, such as occurred in the past when irradiation of "enlarged" thymus in children was in vogue, is implicated in the development of cancer of the thyroid.

PARATHYROID GLAND

The chief pathologic changes exhibited by this organ are hyperplasia and adenoma or carcinoma, all of which frequently are accompanied by the clinical signs and symptoms of hyperparathyroidism. Hypercalcemia, osteitis fibrosa cystica, metastatic calcification, increased alkaline phosphatase in the blood, excessive excretion of calcium in the urine, and formation of urinary calculi are the most important changes that characterize this condition. The adenomas are composed most frequently of chief cells. The hyperplasia may be primary or secondary to renal excretory insufficiency, rickets, or osteomalacia. Destruction of the parathyroids from any cause including surgery results in symptoms of hypoparathyroidism.

THYMUS GLAND

At various times functional activities of various kinds have been attributed, without adequate evidence, to the thymus gland. However, a lymphopoietic function is generally recognized, and evidence of erythropoietic and myelopoietic activities has been noted during fetal life. As a result of studies carried out in thymectomized animals, there is good reason to believe that the thymus plays an important role in some immune reactions. The immunologic incompetence that follows extirpation of the thymus, especially in young animals, is accompanied by depletion of the small lymphocytes from the blood, spleen, and lymph nodes. Indeed, thymectomy has been advocated to aid in preventing the rejection of homotransplants. *Hyperplasia of the thymus* has been reported in nearly three fourths of the cases of myasthenia gravis and, in association with actual lymph follicle formation, with such autoimmune (collagen) diseases as SLE and rheumatoid arthritis as well as hypogammaglobulinemia, thrombocytopenia, and so forth. *Tumors of the thymus (thymoma)* are rare but may be of epithelial, spindle cell, and lymphoid types, though an occasional teratomatous variety has been reported. Thymomas may also be found in association with myasthenia gravis, and the latter condition appears to have an autoimmune origin, for autoantibodies against muscle tissue have been found in about one third of these patients. The indications, therefore, are that the thymus plays an important role in the body, and it is not surprising to find abnormalities of this gland associated with many of the diseases considered to be of autoimmune origin.

PITUITARY GLAND

This organ may exhibit a variety of pathologic changes, such as parenchymatous degeneration, atrophy, necrosis, infarction from embolism or thrombosis, inflammation, hyperplasia and neoplasia, some of which are associated with hypofunction and others with hyperfunction of the organ.

Hypopituitarism (Fröhlich's Syndrome; Dystrophia Adiposogenitalis). In the young, this is characterized by obesity, genital hypoplasia, and faulty skeletal growth. Because of deficiency of the anterior lobe hormone, which normally stimulates the growth of connective tissue, especially bone, there is bony underdevelopment; the head is small, the pelvis is broad, the teeth are flattened, the knees are knocked, the hair is scanty and of the female type, and there is general obesity of female distribution. The condition may be produced by invasive adenoma of the pituitary or by other pituitary tumors or by diseases injuring the base of the skull. *Pituitary dwarfism* of Lorain type, in which the stature is small but normal bodily proportions are maintained, may also result from the destruction of the anterior lobe in a child. Body form is thin and delicate, and secondary sex characteristics are usually defective. In some cases the cause of dwarfism is not destruction of the anterior lobe but rather a congenital deficiency of acidophil cells of the lobe. These latter patients are sexually and otherwise quite normal.

In the adult severe hypopituitarism is called *Simmonds' disease.* This occurs mostly in females and is characterized by profound cachexia (the result of fibrosis and atrophy in many other endocrine organs), loss of sexual function, weakness, low basal metabolic rate, loss of hair and of skin turgor, pigmentation of the skin, premature senility, low blood pressure, and hypoglycemia. When the disease is caused by postpartum necrosis of the pituitary from shock, it is called Sheehan's syndrome.

Hyperpituitarism. Overactivity of the pituitary gland before adolescence causes a symmetric overgrowth of the skeleton resulting in *giantism.* Hyperpituitarism after adolescence, when the epiphyseal junctions have fused, results in *acromegaly,* characterized by overgrowth of the orbital ridges, the lower jaw, the hands and the feet, and thickening of the nose and the lips. The sella turcica usually is enlarged. In mild cases there is only hyperplasia of the acidophil cells, but in severe progressive cases there is practically always an acidophil adenoma of the anterior lobe. Pressure on the optic chiasm may cause bitemporal hemianopsia and, later, complete blindness.

Tumors of the Pituitary Gland. These were described earlier in this chapter in the section on tumors.

ADRENAL GLANDS

Lesions of the adrenal glands may be divided into two categories, namely, those due to abnormal function of the cortical tissues, which are much more important, and those involving the medulla.

Adrenal Cortex—Hyperactivity (Hypercorticism). *Congenital adrenal hyperplasia* involves a number of distinctive clinical syndromes caused by complete or partial deficiency of a specific enzyme involved in the biosynthesis of adrenal steroids. The two most common forms are virilizing congenital adrenal hyperplasia, caused by partial deficiency of 21-hydroxylase, and salt-losing congenital adrenal hyperplasia, caused by complete deficiency of 21-hydroxylase. A less common type is a virilizing hypertensive type, due to deficiency of 11-hydroxylase. The hyperplasia in the congenital adrenal hyperplasia syndromes is bilaterally symmetrical and may be either diffuse or nodular. It is impossible to differentiate histologically congenital adrenal hyperplasia from some of the other forms of primary hyperplasia, such as seen in the other adrenal syndromes.

Cushing's syndrome, induced by excess elaboration of cortisol, is characterized in typical form by central buffalo-type obesity, affecting especially the face and trunk with prominent dorsal and supraclavicular back pads, thin legs, hypertension, osteoporosis, impotence or amenorrhea, muscular weakness, facial hirsutism, and virilism in women. There are four principal causes of the excessive elaboration of cortisol: (1) prolonged treatment with glucocorticoid drugs; (2) excess stimulation by pituitary ACTH only sometimes associated with a pituitary tumor; (3) a cortisol-producing tumor of the adrenal cortex (either malignant or benign); and (4) ectopic production of ACTH by a nonpituitary tumor, such as carcinoma of the lung, bronchial adenoma, thymoma, carcinoma, and others.

Hyperaldosteronism, most common in adults, especially women, in the fourth and fifth decades, may be primary or secondary. The symptoms include moderate hypertension, polyuria, some muscular weakness, hypokalemia with alkalosis, and sometimes parasthesias or even tetany. The primary form is usually produced by an aldosterone-producing adrenocortical adenoma (Conn's syndrome) or by hyperplasia of the zona glomerulosa of the adrenal. The secondary form is in reality an appropriate response of increased aldosterone as a result of renal ischemia, renin-producing neoplasms, or generalized edema.

Adrenal Cortex—Hypoactivity (Hypocorticism). *Addison's disease,* due to adrenal cortical deficiency, is characterized by asthenia, pigmentation of the skin and mucous membranes, anorexia, GI disturbances, hypotension, and nervous symptoms. It is due to the destruction of all, or almost all, of the cortical tissue of both adrenals; 30 or 40 years ago most cases were due to bilateral massive tuberculosis of the glands or, more rarely, replacement of the cortical tissues by amyloid deposits. Today most cases of Addison's disease are included with the autoimmune disorders, and the affected glands are extremely small, difficult to recognize grossly, and so contracted that the capsules seem to surround only the medullary portions which may still be recognized. Cortical tissue is usually not detectable. In significant numbers of these cases circulating autoantibodies against adrenal tissue have been demonstrated. In children *acute adrenal insufficiency* may be observed in the course of overwhelming septicemias, especially with meningococcal septicemia. The gland shows massive hemorrhagic necrosis (Waterhouse–Friderichsen syndrome).

Adrenal Medulla. The adrenal medulla is less important from a pathologic point of view than the cortex, and the only lesions of major significance are tumors. Of these the neuroblastoma and the pheochromocytoma are noteworthy.

Neuroblastoma. This is a highly malignant tumor occurring in infants and children. It is composed of vast numbers of small, dark, lymphocyte-like cells that sometimes exhibit a rosettelike arrangement about a network of fine neurofibrils. Widespread metastases usually occur early. Rarely *spontaneous regression* has been noted, or the neoplasm slows in growth and matures to form the more differentiated ganglioneuroma.

Pheochromocytoma. Composed of the cells that normally are found in the adrenal medulla, the pheochromocytoma (usually) is a benign functioning tumor that may occur in childhood or middle age. Usually unilateral, the tumor may reach a fairly large size—up to 10 cm or more in diameter. Symptoms are produced by the secretion of catecholamines, chiefly norepinephrine, and include paroxysmal or sustained hypertension, nervousness, tachycardia, sweating, trembling, and variations in pulse pressure. Catecholamines and their breakdown products are found in the urine.

Kidney and Urinary System

CONGENITAL MALFORMATIONS OF THE KIDNEY

Agenesis of the kidneys is rare. If bilateral, it is incompatible with life. *Hypoplasia* also is rare and usually unilateral. The hypoplastic kidney is smaller than normal, and the opposite kidney shows compensatory hypertrophy. *Horseshoe kidney* results from the fusion of the two organs across the midline, usually at the lower pole. This malformed organ generally functions normally.

Polycystic kidneys are a much more serious congenital defect. This may result in clinical disease or death at birth, or soon thereafter *(infantile polycystic disease),* if little or no functioning renal tissue is present. If functioning renal parenchyma is sufficient, the patient may live for some years *(adult polycystic disease).* However, usually before the fifth and sixth decade, hypertension and/or renal insufficiency appear and death may result from renal failure, either because of changes in the renovascular system or because of an increase in the size of the cysts, with resulting compression atrophy of functioning renal tissue. The adult form of polycystic disease is more common and is inherited as an autosomal dominant.

PYELONEPHRITIS

Pyelonephritis is characterized by inflammation of the renal pelvis, as well as the interstitial tissue of the kidney. It is caused by infection by one of several types of microorganisms, usually of the gram-negative variety. Infection may reach the kidneys by one of two ways. By the ascending route, in which case the bladder, ureter, and renal pelvis are infected first, and the process spreads in a retrograde fashion to involve the renal tubules and the interstitium; or by the hematogenous route, in which the microorganisms reach the kidneys by way of the blood stream. The former route is more common. It is often associated with vesicoureteral reflux of infected urine during micturition, or with obstruction, as in benign prostatic hypertrophy in males or cystitis and pregnancy in females. In both routes of infection, urinary obstruction may play an important role. Probably every case of pyelitis is accompanied by a certain amount of pyelonephritis.

In *acute pyelonephritis* the kidney is enlarged. Its surface is smooth. The capsule is nonadherent. In both cortex and medulla there may be obvious foci of suppuration even with abscess formation. Microscopically, the subepithelial portion of the mucosa of the pelvis is infiltrated by polymorphonuclear leukocytes, and there may be leukocytes infiltrating the epithelial cells lining the pelvis. Similar interstitial exudation may be present in the adjacent medullary pyramids, and frank necrosis of renal papillae (necrotizing papillitis) may occur. There is exudate in the lumens of the tubules. Obstruction of these tubules by the exudate may lead to dilation of the proximal portion of the tubules, some of which are filled with masses of homogeneous pink-staining material or exudate.

In *chronic pyelonephritis,* the characteristic changes are seen on gross rather than microscopic examination. The kidney is usually smaller than normal. The capsular surface is scarred with a variable number of rather flat, shallow depressions, some of which may be quite large. The organ is firm, cuts with resistance, and the incised surface characteristically shows distortion of the normal architecture, particularly the calyces. Small foci of suppuration may be seen in the cortex or medulla. The pelvis is thicker and rougher than normal, and its surface may be hyperemic or covered with exudate. Microscopically the most striking features are atrophic, dilated tubules filled with hyaline deposits, so-called colloid casts, especially in the proximal convoluted tubules of the cortex. In the collecting tubules, there may be some exudate consisting of polymorphonuclear leukocytes. Similar cells are also present between the tubules. Subepithelial lymphoid aggregates with germinal centers may be seen under the mucosa of the pelvis. A variable number of glomeruli show sclerotic changes. A common accompaniment of the condition is proliferative endarteritis, characterized by layers of fibroblasts and elastic fibers, the so-called onion-skin type of intima, in the larger intrarenal arteries. In "healed" pyelonephritis, the signs of active inflammation subside. When chronic pyelonephritis precedes the development of arteriolosclerosis or complicates existent nephrosclerosis, there is usually renal excecretory functional impairment, and the patient is predisposed to the development of the malignant phase of hypertension. Chronic pyelonephritis is an insidious disease, often mistaken clinically for chronic glomerulonephritis.

INTERSTITIAL NEPHRITIS

This is an interstitial inflammatory disease that may be morphologically indistinguishable from chronic pyelonephritis, but which is definitely not caused by bacterial infection. It has been related to the excessive intake of drugs, particularly analgesics (*e.g.,* phenacetin), which results in chronic interstitial inflammation, fibrosis, tubular atrophy, and medullary papillary necrosis. The papillae are affected bilaterally but irregularly. Interstial nephritis can also occur as a hypersensitivity reaction to some drugs (notably synthetic penicillins).

GLOMERULAR DISEASES

Glomerulonephritis. Glomerulonephritis may occur as a primary or secondary renal disease and may be either focal or diffuse. The characteristic lesion is an inflammatory reaction in the glomeruli with accompanying tubular injury. The glomerular changes vary with the etiology of the condition, but in all cases there will be varying degrees of swelling and proliferation of capillary endothelium, mesangial proliferation, leukocytic invasion, thickening of the glomerular capillary basement membrane, and proliferation of the glomerular capsular epithelium. The result of these reactions is a narrowing or closing of the glomerular capillaries that determines the resultant structural and functional changes.

The major clinical syndromes that result may either be **nephrotic** (proteinuria, hypoalbuminemia, hyperlipidemia, and generalized edema) or **nephritic** (hematuria, RBC casts, azotemia, hypertension, and oliguria).

Recent techniques have elucidated that immune mechanisms are implicated in the majority of glomerulopathies. Both circulating immune complexes, which may be trapped in glomerular capillaries or form *in situ,* and antibodies directed against glomerular basement membrane (GBM) antigens are responsible for activating secondary immune responses leading to glomerular injury. Further details of these immune mechanisms are beyond the scope of this review.

Nephrotic Syndromes. The hallmark features of these glomerulopathies is marked proteinuria, and this finding usually reflects changes in the GBM. **Membranous glomerulonephritis** is the major cause of nephrotic syndrome in adults and is characterized by the presence of numerous electron-dense immunoglobulin deposits in the subepithelial portion of the GBM, causing marked thickening and distortion of the GBM. The GBMs have a "spike and dome" appearance due to the visualization of the separate deposits and the distorted GBM. The etiology of membranous glomerulonephritis may be idiopathic or related to autoimmune disease, infec-

tion, or drugs. The precise pathogenesis remains obscure.

Lipoid nephrosis or **minimal change disease** is the major cause of nephrotic syndrome in children. The only morphologic alteration noted is fusion or effacement of the foot processes of the glomerular epithelial cells seen only by electron microscopy. The glomeruli otherwise appear normal. The etiology remains unknown, but a prominent clinical feature is the dramatic response of the disease to corticosteroid therapy. Prognosis is usually good with long-term remissions.

Focal and segmental glomerulosclerosis used to be considered a variant of minimal change disease but is now considered a distinct entity because of its markedly worse prognosis and failure to respond to steroid therapy. The morphologic lesions predominantly affect juxtamedullary glomeruli and are focal–segmental in distribution. Their distribution is spotty and sometimes affects only a portion of a tuft rather than the whole glomerulus. Progression to renal failure occurs at variable rates. This disease has been noted to recur in patients who receive renal allografts.

Membranoproliferative glomerulonephritis or **mesangiocapillary glomerulonephritis** describes a group of disorders that are characterized by alterations in the basement membrane and the proliferation of cells in the mesangium. The clinical manifestations are variable with two thirds of the patients being nephrotic and the remainder having elements of the nephrotic or nephritic syndromes. Serum complement levels are characteristically persistently decreased. The morphologic alterations include mesangial interposition into the capillary loops, giving the GBM a "double contour" or "train track" appearance. This is demonstrable by the presence of subendothelial immune deposits in the GBM, or by a uniform, ribbonlike deposition of immune deposits in the GBM (dense deposit disease) without a doubling of the GBM. Immune mechanisms including both circulating immune complexes as well as activation of the alternate complement pathway have been postulated to explain the mechanism of the glomerular injury. This disease has also been noted to recur in patients who receive renal allografts.

Nephritic Syndrome. The hallmark feature of these glomerulopathies is hematuria, and this usually reflects a proliferative-type lesion. The classic example of a primary nephritic glomerulopathy is **acute poststreptococcal glomerulonephritis.** The association of hemolytic streptococci of group A, particularly types 4, 12, 25, and Red Lake, as well as, though less commonly, pneumococci, staphylococci, and even certain viruses with acute glomerulonephritis, make it practically certain that these microorganisms, especially streptococci, must play some role, be it direct or indirect, in causing some cases of diffuse glomerulonephritis. The tissue lesions and urine are sterile, however. The disease is most common in children and young adults. In the majority of cases of acute glomerulonephritis, especially in the young, recovery is complete; a few die of uremia; and a smaller number, about 2%, progress to chronic glomerulonephritis.

It has been shown that soluble immune complexes of antibody and streptococcal-related antigen (exogenous antigen) circulating in the blood stream become trapped in glomerular capillary basement membranes and evoke an exudative inflammatory response. Immunofluorescent studies and electron microscopy visualize these subendothelial "humps" of immune deposits.

Goodpasture's syndrome (pulmonary hemorrhage with hemoptysis and associated renal failure with hematuria) is an example of a condition in which autoantibodies to basement membrane are present, and these antibodies react uniformly not only along the basement membranes of the glomeruli but also to the basement membranes of the pulmonary alveoli.

Another form of nephritic syndrome is *rapidly progressive glomerulonephritis* (RPGN), which is characterized by proliferation of glomerular epithelial cells that form crescents around glomeruli within Bowman's capsule and rapid deterioration of renal function leading to renal failure and possible death in uremia. This morphologic pattern does not describe a singular entity but can be a common pathway for several distinct etiologies, which may involve either deposition of circulating immune complexes or anti-GBM disease, or be idiopathic. Thus, RPGN can occur as a form of poststreptococcal glomerulonephritis, Goodpasture's syndrome, or in secondary glomerulopathies such as lupus nephritis, Henoch–Schönlein purpura, and others that are described below as secondary glomerulopathies.

Berger's disease (IgA nephropathy) is another hematuric syndrome that morphologically is unique because of mesangial hypercellularity and mesangial IgA containing immune complex deposits. There is usually little change in glomerular basement membranes initially, although there is progressive glomerular sclerosis, and the long-term prognosis is poor leading to chronic renal failure. IgA nephropathy also recurs in a significant proportion of patients who receive renal allografts.

SECONDARY GLOMERULAR DISEASES

Many systemic diseases are associated with renal lesions. The clinical manifestations and the morphologic lesions are varied and on pure morphologic grounds may be indistinguishable from primary glomerulopathies. Lupus nephritis (SLE) may cause glomerular changes that are focal or diffuse, membranous or mesangial. Diabetes mellitus may cause nodular or diffuse glomerulosclerosis. Likewise, amyloidosis, subacute bacterial endocarditis, polyarteritis nodosa, Henoch–Schönlein purpura, and various microangiopathic disorders all may cause renal disease, and their etiologies and manifestations are too varied to be considered here. They are distinguished from primary nephropathies by ancillary clinical and laboratory findings. Many secondary glomerulopathies may have a focal rather than diffuse distribution with glomerulonephritis as their initial morphologic pattern. The reason for the random distribution remains unclear, although immune mechanisms are thought to be involved.

CHRONIC GLOMERULONEPHRITIS

This is the end stage of glomerular disease and may have as an etiology any of the diseases listed above. Only occasionally is there a history of preceding definite acute glomerulonephritis. The urine in these cases contains albumin and casts in varying amounts. In the subacute stage, before the condition becomes truly chronic, oliguria may be present, but in chronic cases large amounts of urine with low specific gravity are passed. Edema may be present, and sometimes fluid collects in the serous cavities. Hypertension is common. Moderate left ventricular hypertrophy occurs, but rarely is there pronounced cardiac insufficiency. Diminished renal function is indicated by decreased clearance of the blood urea nitrogen and elevated creatinine. Later, there is the development of uremia and an ultimately fatal outcome. Secondary anemia may be pronounced. The kidneys are small, symmetrically contracted, firm, diffusely granular, and the glomeruli may show the residua of a primary disease progressing to global hyaline obliteration of glomeruli. Except for patients maintained on dialysis or who receive renal transplants, the outcome is invariably death.

HEMODYNAMIC DISTURBANCES

In addition to the diseases described above, hematuria or proteinuria may occur in association with other conditions which do not have the same consequences or sequelae. Orthostatic albuminuria may be caused by a marked fall in the pulse pressure in the upright position, by compression of the left renal vein in visceroptosis, or by kyphosis. It is of no clinical significance. Chronic passive congestion of the kidneys from heart failure may cause albuminuria and casts and sometimes diminished urea nitrogen excretion or clearance. These changes disappear when the heart becomes compensated. Furthermore, it is well known that transitory hematuria may result after vigorous exercise. None of these conditions are indicators of progressive renal disease.

VASCULAR DISEASE OF THE KIDNEYS

Acute Arteritis. This can be idiopathic or part of generalized polyarteritis nodosa. It also may be the result of lodgment of infected emboli or be secondary to acute suppurative inflammation in the kidney.

Renal Arterial Disease. In recent years, mainly as a result of arteriography, a stenotic lesion of the main renal artery, due to either fibromuscular dysplasia or atherosclerotic plaque of one or both kidneys, has been recognized with increasing frequency in patients with hypertension. In such patients, it is now generally admitted that hypertension is due to renal ischemia with secondary activation of the renin–angiotensin system, and corrective surgery has been performed. Favorable results are to be expected only in those individuals who have a stenotic lesion of one or both main renal arteries and who lack an intrarenal cause of ischemia in either kidney as determined by biopsy.

Arterial Nephrosclerosis. Arterial nephrosclerosis is caused by obliterative arteriosclerosis of the extrarenal or the larger intrarenal arteries. The kidney usually is roughly nodular, with irregularly shaped deep depressions of various sizes in the cortex that correspond to foci of atrophy of the parenchyma and replacement fibrosis. The visible arteries show obvious thickening of wall and reduction in the size of the lumen. The functional changes are usually minimal but may be significant if the degree of parenchymal atrophy is great.

Arteriolar (Benign) Nephrosclerosis. The kidney may be of normal size, but more commonly it is reduced in size and may be very small, especially if the larger intrarenal arteries are also involved. As a rule the capsule is not adherent. The outer surface is usually finely and uniformly granular with the small nodules of parenchyma projecting slightly above the reddish gray or gray network of connec-

tive tissue, which is usually depressed. The organ is firm and cuts with increased resistance, and the cut surface usually shows an atrophied cortex. If the larger vessels are also affected, and they usually are, the walls of these visible arteries may be thick and the lumens smaller than normal. Microscopically, there are the changes of ischemic atrophy. The walls of arterioles, particularly the preglomerular ones, and smaller arteries are thickened and hyalinized. In the arterioles the entire wall may be hyalinized; in the small arteries, the intima alone is involved. Special stains may reveal lipoid material in the hyalinized intima. The glomeruli vary from many that are normal to some that are transformed into completely fibrotic, hyalinized structures. Even in many of the glomeruli that appear normal, the basement membranes may be thickened and wrinkled. Focal glomerulitis or chronic pyelonephritis may complicate the picture and play an important part in the development of so-called malignant nephrosclerosis. Focal tubular atrophy and tubular epithelial degeneration are also common. Whole tubular units may be absent. Some of the tubules may be moderately or greatly dilated. There is usually an increase in interstitial fibrous tissue and mild focal interstitial chronic inflammation. Persistent hypertension is a frequent accompaniment of this condition, usually without associated significant disturbance of renal excretory function. In this type, called benign hypertension, the cause of death is usually either heart failure or apoplexy.

Malignant Nephrosclerosis. This condition may develop from the benign form of arteriolar nephrosclerosis, sometimes from chronic glomerulonephritis, chronic pyelonephritis, or it may arise, sometimes quite rapidly, without apparent previous clinical renal disease. It is extremely serious, being characterized by markedly elevated arterial pressure, azotemia, sometimes uremia, and characteristic vascular changes in the eyegrounds. Grossly the kidneys may show little, except for minute hemorrhages in the cortices, to account for the severity of the clinical symptoms. Histologically however, the changes are characteristic and marked. Most striking is the severe necrotizing arteriolitis affecting the interlobular and afferent arterioles. The walls are somewhat thickened and sometimes hyalinized. There is reduplication of the intima with concentric ring formation (onion skin). There are fibrinoid deposits and sometimes actual thrombi in the lumens, and occasionally extension of the degenerative process into some glomerular tufts. Otherwise the glomeruli show little and inflammatory cells are few.

URINARY CALCULI (UROLITHIASIS)

Calculi in the urinary system are relatively common, especially in the renal pelvis and calyces. The majority are calcium containing. They are composed of varying mixtures of calcium oxalate, calcium phosphate, ammonium phosphate, uric acid, and cystine that are precipitated from the urine under varying conditions, especially high concentrations of these substances. The most common calculi are mixtures of phosphates and oxalates, though pure phosphate and oxalate stones, as well as lesser numbers of calculi in which mixtures of these substances with uric acid and cystine are present, may also be found occasionally. Infection may play a role, and bacteria may even serve as the nidus on which the above elements are precipitated, particularly ammonium phosphate. Calculi may also cause hemorrhage, secondary infection, obstruction with hydronephrosis, or ureteral colic. In the renal pelvis, calculi tend to be irregular in shape and may form a cast of the pelvis called a *stag-horn calculus.* These are usually composed of ammonium phosphates.

Hypervitaminosis D also may be complicated by the formation of urinary calculi, and in both man and animals, hyperparathyroidism frequently is associated with the occurrence of urinary calculi. In both hypervitaminosis D and hyperparathyroidism, hypercalcemia occurs and is probably the determining factor.

BLADDER

Cystitis usually is secondary to diseases that cause obstruction and stagnation of urine, such as enlarged prostate, urethral stricture, tumors, calculi, or paralysis of the bladder. Bacteria that produce ammonia are particularly irritating to the mucosa. Less commonly cystitis results from a descending infection. In acute cases, the mucosa is edematous with a small amount of exudate but may become hemorrhagic or purulent. The inflammation may be ulcerative, gangrenous, or pseudomembranous. In chronic cystitis the lesion is less severe, but the walls are thickened by fibrosis and there is lymphocytic infiltration. In some cases of chronic cystitis not caused by infection with a virus or a fungus, histiocytic phagocytosis of fatty acids, polysaccharides, or both, with subsequent calcification, results in the development of granulomatous submucosal plaques referred to as *malacoplakia.*

Hypertrophy of the musculature of the bladder is caused by any obstruction of the urethra with the bulging of the hypertrophic musculature causing trabeculation of the mucosa.

Paralytic bladder may be caused by (1) tabes (tertiary syphilis) or (2) lesions of the lumbar cord (multiple sclerosis, tumors, myelitis, or trauma) that interrupt the reflex arc.

URETHRA

Gonorrheal urethritis is common in the male. It begins in the fossa navicularis and extends rapidly over the mucosa towards the bladder. The prostate usually is involved. The mucosa of the urethra is reddened and swollen with a rather profuse purulent exudate. Frequent complications include suppuration of the prostate, epididymis, seminal vesicles, and bladder. Rarely, gonorrheal arthritis or endocarditis results. Urethral stricture, usually in the membrane portion, is a late sequel that may occur as long as 20 years after infection.

Gonorrheal urethritis in the female usually is relatively mild. Infection with *Escherichia coli* is more frequent.

Noninfectious urethritis is very common and results from trauma or other forms of irritation.

TUMORS OF THE URINARY TRACT

Benign adenomas of the renal cortex are relatively common. The most important malignant tumors are renal cell (clear cell) carcinoma, carcinoma of the bladder and renal pelvis, and the relatively uncommon Wilms' tumor of childhood. Renal cell carcinoma is the most common, occurs chiefly in males of middle to late age, and usually is quite large when discovered because it can remain symptomless for a long time. Major symptoms are painless hematuria or a mass in the flank, or both, and even occasional low grade fever that is difficult to explain. Histologically most of these neoplasms are composed of "clear" or vacuolated epithelial cells that resemble cells of the adrenal cortex, a characteristic that has led to the inaccurate diagnosis of hypernephroma. The tumor has a tendency to invade the renal vein, and blood-borne metastases to the lungs and other sites, such as brain or bone, are common. Transitional cell papillomas may develop in the pelvis and other portions of the urinary tract, especially the bladder where they are most common and most dangerous, since some of these are actually early carcinomas when first discovered, or may become so. Indeed, the differentiation between benign and malignant bladder tumors is difficult and often depends on cellularity and the degree of invasion of the wall. Wilms' tumor, a massive malignant neoplasm reproducing primitive renal tissue embedded in fibromyxomatous stroma, is most common in children under 10 years of age. It is sometimes present in the newborn. Wilms' tumors currently respond well to combined surgical, radiotherapeutic, and chemotherapeutic treatment.

Genital System

MALE

Congenital anomalies of the urethra, such as **hypospadias,** in which the urethral opening is on the ventral surface of the penis, or **epispadias,** in which it is on the dorsal surface, are important since infertility and bladder infections are common complications. **Phimosis** is the condition in which the prepuce, because of a small and contracted orifice, will not retract normally to uncover the glans, so that an accumulation of smegma, secretions, desquamated epithelial cells, and so forth collect beneath, sometimes leading to infection that may at times be confused with gonorrhea. The most important infections of the penis are gonorrhea, syphilis, chancroid, and, sometimes, pyogenic infections of the glans and the prepuce that lead to ulcerative or gangrenous **balanoposthitis.**

Condyloma accuminata is a benign squamous papilloma of the penis caused by a virus. The most important malignant tumor is **squamous cell carcinoma** of the glans, a tumor that occurs in association with the accumulation of smegma or foci of infection or inflammation that have been present for a long time beneath the prepuce of men in older age groups (from 50 to 70 or more years). This form of cancer is extremely rare in Jewish men who practice circumcision, which effectively prevents accumulations of the secretion.

Testis and Epididymis. The most important anomaly of the testis is **cryptorchidism,** or undescended testis. Although opinions differ somewhat, the undescended testis is considered by some to be more susceptible to the development of malignant neoplasms.

Various forms of **orchitis** may occur. The most common are caused by gonorrhea, syphilis, and occur sometimes in adults who suffer from mumps. Mumps orchitis may be serious enough to lead to sterility.

Although testicular tumors are not very common, they are usually serious, and in young adult males between 25 and 35 they are almost the most common form of malignant disease. Among the more important types of malignant neoplasms are the **seminoma,** a fairly well-differentiated, relatively slowly growing malignant tumor; the **embryonal carcinoma** of high malignancy, with a varying but always poorly differentiated histologic pattern and poor prognosis; and the **teratoma** of immature or adult type. **Choriocarcinoma,** usually of high malignancy, rarely occurs. These tumors are described more at length in the section on neoplasms.

Epididymitis usually is caused by infection spread from the urethra. Abscesses may form, and the ducts may be occluded in the healing process. Bilateral epididymitis may result in sterility. Tuberculosis often involves the epididymis but seldom the testis. Syphilis, on the other hand, rarely affects the epididymis, but **gummas** of the testis may occur. The passage of spermatozoa into the interstitial tissue of the epididymis, most likely on a traumatic basis or following vasectomy, results in the formation of a granulomatous lesion in which degenerated spermatozoa, usually only the heads, are recognized.

Prostate Gland. Benign enlargement (hyperplasia) is by far the most common disease of the prostate gland, causing obstructive symptoms in about 8% of men over 60. The enlargement involves mainly the central and lateral areas of the gland. A nodule of the median lobe may project into the trigone of the bladder and cause obstruction of the internal urethral orifice. The nodules are composed chiefly of hyperplastic, hypertrophic, and cystic glands that may form adenomalike foci alternating with many small nodules composed mainly of smooth muscle and fibrous tissue.

Prostatitis in young men usually is caused by gonorrhea; in old men it frequently is caused by infection and injury from catheterization. The glands are filled with pus cells and desquamated epithelium, and abscesses may form that rupture into the urethra, the bladder, the rectum, or the pelvic connective tissues.

Carcinoma of the prostate is one of the most common malignant tumors occurring in men. Like benign hyperplasia, the incidence of cancer increases with age, although the two conditions appear to be independent and unrelated lesions. Carcinoma usually originates in the posterior lobe, is most often subcapsular in location, and may be present for a long time without being suspected. Histologically, carcinoma of the prostate can vary greatly. The simplest form is the latent type that grows slowly, causes no symptoms, and is usually found by chance at autopsy. A common form is also slowly growing but exhibits definite hyperplasia, sometimes atypical, and evidence of malignancy by invasion of perineural spaces. Finally, there is the very cellular, rapidly growing medullary anaplastic growth that replaces most of the gland. Metastases develop in the regional lymph nodes, the pelvic bones, and the spine. When metastases are present in the skeleton, the acid phosphatase level in the serum is usually increased.

FEMALE

Diseases of the female genital system are very common and will be considered in more detail in the chapter on obstetrics and gynecology.

The *vulva* may be the site of inflammations including ulcers that may be caused by a variety of infectious agents. There are a number of neoplasms of the vulva. Papillomas, inflammatory condylomas, leukoplakia, which must be considered at least a precancerous lesion, carcinoma-*in-situ,* and invasive squamous cell carcinomas are the most important examples.

The *vagina* in general is not commonly affected by primary disease, although moderate infections such as trichomonal or *Candida albicans* vaginitis not infrequently occur. Primary carcinoma is rare.

The *cervix* is perhaps the most important part of the female genital tract because of the fact that it is a very common site of malignant disease. Next to carcinoma of the breast and carcinoma of the colon and rectum, carcinoma of the cervix is the most common malignant disease in women. The disease may occur at almost any age, but is most frequent between the ages of 30 and 50, and married women are more frequently affected than are single women. The neoplasm is a form of squamous cell or epidermoid carcinoma, and from a pathologic point of view, it can be divided into five categories based upon the extent of the growth. It may vary from simple preinvasive or intraepithelial carcinoma (carcinoma-*in-situ*), to carcinoma confined to the cervix itself, and then to stages of invasion extending beyond the cervix to involve the vagina, the pelvic wall, the bladder or rectum, or both, and perhaps the ureters and even more distant organs.

In the *uterus* proper, endometrial inflammation is uncommon, but *endometriosis,* the presence of endometrial glands and stroma in abnormal locations, is a more important abnormality. Endometriosis may involve the myometrium (adenomyosis), but more important is "external" endometriosis in which foci of endometrial tissue are found in the pelvic peritoneum, in or on the surface of the fallopian tubes, and on the ovary.

Tumors of the uterus include the common leiomyoma, almost always benign, but often multiple and varying in size from a few millimeters to 15 cm to 20 cm, and the more serious endometrial adenocarcinoma. These tumors, too, are described in greater detail elsewhere.

The *ovaries* are the site of various types of tumors, the most important of which were described in the section on neoplasms. Of the diseases that occur in association with pregnancy, the most important are eclampsia, ectopic pregnancy, hydatidiform mole, and choriocarcinoma, all of which are described in more detail elsewhere.

Although the *breast* is not a part of the female genital tract, it is a closely related organ and a brief summary of the more important lesions may be given here. Supernumerary nipples and foci of breast tissue that develop in the mammary line are not infrequently seen. Of all breast lesions, *fibrocystic disease* or *mammary dysplasia* is perhaps the most common. It results from some abnormality of the cyclic changes that occur in association with the menstrual cycle. The breast tissues are more fibrous than normal and with varying numbers of cysts, small or large or a mixture, filled with yellowish, turbid, blood-tinged, or partly coagulated and gelatinous material. It is said that women who suffer from this condition and have epithelial hyperplasia are more susceptible to the development of breast carcinoma.

Benign tumors of the breast include—as the most common type in younger women—the *fibroadenoma,* a slowly growing, probably estrogen-induced fibroepithelial encapsulated nodule that is usually solitary but may be multiple and even bilateral. It rarely exceeds 4 cm in diameter. One typical manifestation of this tumor is the intracanalicular fibroadenoma in which the stroma is more actively growing than the epithelial element. A most unusual form is the giant intracanalicular fibromyxoma, more generally known as cystosarcoma phyllodes, which, in spite of its name, can be either malignant or benign. Intraductal papillomas may also occur in older women, and their relationship to the development of carcinoma has been suggested although not proven.

Malignant breast tumors are described in the section on neoplasms.

Nervous System

CONGENITAL MALFORMATIONS

Various harmful influences, genetic or environmental, acting at crucial times during embryonic development, can result in failure of normal formation of nervous system structures. Similar malformations can result from different causes, and a variety of malformations can be produced by a single cause. Anencephaly (absence of the brain) and amyelia (absence of the spinal cord) represent extreme degrees of arrested development. Failure of fusion of the neural tube can result in craniorachischisis with unfused central nervous system, meninges, skull, and spine or porencephaly (complete defect through brain tissue). Protrusion of nervous tissue and leptomeninges through a defect in bone and dura mater can involve the cranium (meningoencephalocele) or spine (meningomyelocele). Such defects may involve bone and meninges only (meningocele) or bone only (spina bifida occulta). Excessive fusion can result in such anomalies as cyclopia, arhinencephaly, and other failures of cleavage of nervous tissue into symmetrical paired structures. Aqueduct atresia is a common form of this process. The Chiari malformation includes a mixture of fusions and cleavages, displacements, and distortions, including dysplasia of the cerebral cortex, hydrocephalus, aqueduct atresia, malformation and caudal displacement of brain stem structures, cerebellar tonsillar caudal displacement, and meningomyelocele. Errors of migration lead to abnormal location of nerve cells (heterotopias), disarranged cerebral cortex (polymicrogyria, macrogyria, lissencephaly or agyria, and pachygyria). Nervous system anomalies are frequently accompanied by anomalies of other body structures.

A peculiar group of diseases having genetic and neoplastic features are included in the phakomatoses (tuberous sclerosis, von Hippel–Lindau disease, von Recklinghausen's disease, and Sturge–Weber disease). In addition to anatomic malformations, congenital abnormalities of nervous tissue metabolism leading to structural and functional changes may occur (phenylketonuria, lipid storage diseases, and leucodystrophies).

HYDROCEPHALUS

Most cases of hydrocephalus producing clinical manifestations are the result of obstruction of flow of the cerebrospinal fluid. When this obstruction is congenital it most frequently involves the aqueduct (stenosis or atresia), less commonly other areas such as the outlets of the fourth ventricle (Dandy–Walker syndrome), and results in enlargement of the head by separation of the cranial sutures. Brain damage is slowly progressive due to pressure and distortion. When the obstruction is acquired, it most frequently involves the subarachnoid space around the brain stem, where postmeningitic obliterative adhesions are most likely. Less commonly, the ventricular system may be obstructed by neoplasm. Rapidly progressive increased intracranial pressure and brain damage occur if the cranial sutures have closed.

Communicating hydrocephalus exists when the obstruction is between the outlets of the ventricular system and the arachnoid villi, allowing flow of cerebrospinal fluid from the ventricles into the lumbar subarachnoid space but preventing reabsorption. Noncommunicating hydrocephalus results from obstruction within the ventricular system.

CEREBRAL PALSY

Cerebral palsy is a broad term that refers to a heterogeneous group of nervous system disorders apparent from birth or early infancy characterized by diffuse, usually bilateral brain damage of variable severity associated clinically with various combinations of abnormal movements, spastic paralysis, and intellectual deficit. More than 2 per 1000 births are affected to some degree. Pathologic changes vary with the multitude of etiologic factors, including genetic abnormalities, intrauterine damage (hypoxia, infection, toxicity, deficiency, x-ray exposure), birth injury (hypoxia, trauma), kernicterus, and early infantile diseases (infection, seizures).

INFLAMMATORY DISEASES

Except for direct implantation through open skull fractures and during surgical procedures, microorganisms reach the central nervous system by spreading from a focus of infection elsewhere. Routes of infection are by continuity, blood stream, or along nerve roots. Infections may involve the meninges, the parenchyma, or the nerve roots. Almost any organism can be involved. Leptomeningitis is the most common type of central nervous system infection. It may be acute, subacute, or chronic. Most commonly it is due to bacterial infection. Coliform organisms are most frequently involved in newborn infants and in old and debilitated patients; *H. influenzae,* in infants; and *Neisseria meningitidis,* in children and young adults (epidemic meningitis). Other organisms are less influenced by age than by predisposing conditions such as lowered resistance, debilitating diseases, or loci of infection elsewhere in the body (pneumococcal, streptococcal, staphylococcal, tuberculous, mycotic, and parasitic). Gross pathologic changes consist of hyperemia of the pia–arachnoid membrane followed by purulent subarachnoid exudate. Microscopically the leptomeninges have acute inflammatory changes, and microorganisms can be detected by special techniques. Complications of bacterial meningitis may occur during active infection (cerebritis with herniation, arteritis with infarction, thrombophlebitis with venous infarction) or as postmeningitic sequelae (obstructive hydrocephalus, cranial nerve palsies, parenchymal destruction, and gliosis) leading to motor, sensory, and intellectual deficits and epilepsy. Tuberculous leptomeningitis is usually subacute, associated with pulmonary or miliary tuberculosis and tends to concentrate around the base of the brain as a fibrinous mononuclear exudate with severe vasculitis. Tuberculomas in the parenchyma are rare. Neurotuberculosis is more common in children than in adults. Fungus infections of leptomeninges tend to be chronic, occurring most often as opportunistic infections in debilitated patients. *Cryptococcus neoformans* is the most common organism, and causes mucinous exudate due to its thick capsule, and feeble inflammatory reaction. As in other, rarer, fungus infections (mucormycosis, histoplasmosis) the nervous system involvement is secondary to infection in other systems.

Brain abscess results from hematogenous dissemination of organisms usually from pulmonary suppuration or bacterial endocarditis or from contiguous spread from middle ear, mastoid, or paranasal sinus infections. The most common locations are frontal, temporal, or cerebellar.

Parasitic infections of the nervous system of greatest importance are malaria (capillary occlusions by parasitized erythrocytes), cysticercosis (parasitic cysts in the parenchyma, meninges, or ventricles), amebiasis (cerebritis, abscess), echinococcosis (cyst), and toxoplasmosis (granulomatous meningoencephalitis).

Viral infections of the central nervous system may be acute, subacute, or chronic and may affect the meninges or parenchyma. Various viruses tend to focus their damaging effect at particular levels in the central nervous system: nerve roots and ganglia, herpes zoster; spinal cord, poliomyelitis; brain stem, rabies; basal ganglia, encephalitis lethargica, Japanese B, St. Louis, equine encephalitis; cerebral cortex, Herpes simplex; leptomeninges, lymphocytic choriomeningitis, mumps, and infectious mononucleosis. The involved tissue is congested and swollen but usually intact. Intense inflammatory changes are evident. Distinctions between different types of infection may be possible on the basis of the location of major involvement, destructiveness, inclusion bodies, and by correlating pathologic changes with clinical manifestations. Subacute viral infections, such as those due to rubella, cytomegalovirus infection, progressive multifocal leucoencephalopathy, measles, and subacute sclerosing panencephalitis, may persist for months to years and produce extensive destruction of gray and white matter. Slow virus infection, in which a long latency period precedes the onset of clinical manifestations, is thought to be involved in kuru and Creutzfeldt–Jakob disease. Neurosyphilis may occur in meningitic or meningovascular forms or during tertiary stages as general paresis affecting the cerebral cortex or tabes dorsalis involving the spinal cord.

TRAUMATIC LESIONS

Concussion is a form of injury to nervous tissue due to physical force that causes temporary impairment of function without structural alteration. Contusion produces traumatic disruption of small blood vessels within the tissue of the brain or spinal cord at the site of injury. Brain contusions may be of the coup or contrecoup type. Lacerations of brain or spinal cord are often associated with fracture of overlying bones and are followed by scarring and permanent defects. Regeneration of nerve cell processes is possible only in the peripheral nervous system. Traumatic neuroma may result from improper healing. Focal subarachnoid hemorrhage is a frequent result of physical injury to the head or spine. Subdural hematoma results when head injury produces disruption of surface blood vessels, particularly veins. The hematoma may accumulate rapidly, causing acute displacement of brain tissue, or slowly, resulting in gradual encapsulation. Most subdural hematomas are traumatic, but occasional bleeding in this area results from ruptured arterial aneurysm, neoplastic infiltration of the dura, or blood dyscrasias.

Epidural hematoma, usually intracranial, is caused by laceration of the middle meningeal artery when the overlying bone is fractured. This most commonly occurs in the temporal region. The hemorrhage accumulates rapidly and must be evacuated promptly.

Posttraumatic syndromes result from combinations of these structural lesions with functional impairment frequently associated with subtle emotional factors.

PERIPHERAL NEUROPATHIES

Although peripheral nerve lesions may have different causes, the reactions are very limited and often nonspecific. Myelin sheaths or axis cylinders may be affected. Sensory, motor, or combined effects may result. Metabolic disorders (porphyria, diabetes mellitus), nutritional deficiencies (beriberi, pellagra, pernicious anemia), vascular diseases (polyarteritis nodosa, SLE), intoxications (heavy metals, diphtheria, drugs, and industrial poisons), infection (herpes zoster, leprosy), heredity (peroneal muscular atrophy, hypertrophic interstitial polyneuropathy, hereditary sensory radicular polyneuropathy), neoplasia (neurilemoma, neurofibroma), postinfectious, postvaccinal, acute infective polyneuropathy, paraneoplastic states, amyloidosis, and trauma (contusion, compression, avulsion) may be involved. Regeneration of peripheral nerve fibers is possible under optimal circumstances.

TOXIC AND NUTRITIONAL DISORDERS

The number of exogenous poisons capable of damaging the nervous system increases yearly and includes environmental, occupational, and medicinal substances. Carbon monoxide poisoning causes nervous system lesions by combining with hemoglobin and impairing oxygen transport. Widespread hypoxic nerve cell damage results. Symmetrical necrosis of the globus pallidus nuclei is characteristic. Lead intoxication results in encephalopathy (infants) or peripheral neuropathy (adults). Lead encephalopathy causes massive swelling and widespread damage in brain tissue. Peripheral neuropathy mainly involves motor nerves. In arsenic poisoning, acute encephalopathy with multiple petechiae in the white matter is mainly due to the toxic effect on small blood vessels. Peripheral neuropathy, associated with chronic intoxication, damages myelin sheaths and axis cylinders and affects predominantly sensory nerves. Manganese intoxication causes widespread neuronal damage concentrating in the basal ganglia and is associated with extrapyramidal signs. Mercury poisoning causes nerve cell loss characteristically severe in the granular layer of the cerebellum. Dementia, ataxia, and tremor are prominent clinical signs. Acute alcoholic intoxication causes reversible physiologic (depressant) effects on nerve cells often associated with congestion and edema. Chronic alcoholism may result in encephalopathy which is the effect of alcohol and nutritional deficiency. The cerebral cortex, periventricular gray matter, and particularly the mammillary bodies are characteristically involved by acute followed by chronic nerve cell changes. Korsakoff psychosis is the typical clinical manifestation of Wernicke's encephalopathy. Cerebellar cortical atrophy, central pontine myelinolysis, central necrosis of the corpus callosum, and peripheral neuropathy may be seen under these circumstances.

VASCULAR DISEASES

Vascular diseases of the central nervous system mainly concern atherosclerosis, which causes narrowing and occlusion of major arteries; hypertensive arteriolar sclerosis leading to hyperplasia, stenosis, occlusion with small infarcts, and necrosis with spontaneous hemorrhage; aneurysms; vascular malformations; venous occlusions; and rare inflammatory lesions of arteries and veins producing occlusions, ruptures, or focal dilatations, "mycotic aneurysms," due to inflammatory necrosis. Ischemic infarction is the most common parenchymal lesion of vascular type and is much more common in the brain than in the spinal cord. Following a sudden episode of total ischemia, there is a delay of several hours before characteristic nerve cell changes become apparent microscopically and the brain begins to swell. Maximal swelling is reached in 24 to 36 hours. As swelling subsides, liquefaction of the necrotic tissue occurs and is followed by phagocytic activity, shrinkage of the lesion, and gliosis leaving a permanent cavitated, indurated scar associated with atrophy of interrupted tracts. Thrombotic occlusion of arteries characteristically produces ischemic infarcts. Embolic occlusions, much less common, cause hemorrhagic infarcts. The emboli usually originate in the heart or major arteries supplying the brain. Saccular or berry aneurysms are outpouchings of the walls of intracranial arteries usually at bifurcations or branching sites near the circle of Willis. These usually measure less than 1 cm in diameter and occur in 2% to 3% of normal adults. They cause symptoms when they rupture or impinge on adjacent nerve roots or brain tissue. Multiple aneurysms are found in 10% to 12% of aneurysm patients. Venous occlusions characteristically cause hemorrhagic infarction of brain and spinal cord tissue and are most likely to occur during dehydration, hemoconcentration, and hypercoagulability in infants with diarrhea, postpartal women, women who smoke and take birth control pills, and patients with advanced debilitating disease. Vascular malformations are collections of abnormal arteries, veins, or capillaries in brain or spinal cord parenchyma that may produce clinical signs by rupturing or distorting nervous tissue. They may be asymptomatic or may cause recurrent bleeding and focal seizures.

DEMYELINATING DISORDERS

Demyelinating diseases are those in which myelin failure is the primary lesion, as opposed to the more common myelin destruction secondary to vascular, inflammatory, toxic, traumatic, or degenerative diseases. In demyelinating disorders there is selective deterioration of normally formed myelin or basically abnormal myelin. Oligodendroglia and myelin are the focus of the abnormality. Neurons and their processes are relatively spared. In multiple sclerosis, foci of myelin dissolution are scattered randomly through the brain, spinal cord, and optic nerves during recurrent clinical episodes. Evolving lesions usually contain lymphocytes. Old lesions are overgrown by astrocytes. All lesions are permanent because of their destructive effect on oligodendroglia, although clinical deficits may improve during remissions as inflammatory changes subside, some myelin is spared, and compensatory mechanisms are utilized. Lesions vary in size, shape, age, and completeness of demyelination, but tend to concentrate in periventricular white matter. The cause is unknown, but viral infection and immune mechanisms are suspected. Demyelination may occur after systemic viral infections or immunizations and may affect central and peripheral myelin, resulting in postinfectious, parainfectious, or postvaccinal encephalopathy, myelopathy, radiculopathy, or neuropathy. Sudden damage to myelin causes clinical manifestations that vary with the location of the lesions. The most common form of this process is polyradiculopathy resulting in ascending paralysis associated with increased cerebrospinal fluid protein and few inflammatory cells, Landry-Guillain-Barré syndrome with albuminocytologic dissociation. Rare forms of demyelination, mainly affecting children, also of unknown cause, involve large confluent areas of cerebral white matter and progress over months to years to involve the entire nervous system. Based on the age at onset, manner of progression, histologic and chemical features, and detectable enzymatic deficiencies, they may be divided into those that result from deterioration of formed myelin (diffuse sclerosis) and those due to abnormal myelin formation (leucodystrophy).

NEOPLASMS

Neoplasms involving the nervous system may be primary or metastatic. Primary neoplasms may arise in any of the cell types of the parenchyma or coverings. Metastatic neoplasms may arise in any tissue. Intracranial neoplasms most frequently involve the parenchyma, less often the meninges or nerve roots. Intraspinal neoplasms are most often extramedullary and usually involve the meninges or nerve roots. Neoplasms involving the central nervous system are more often malignant; those in the peripheral nervous system are usually benign. Of the primary neoplasms of the brain, astrocytomas are most common. They are usually malignant in adults (glioblastoma multiforme) and more benign in children. The malignant forms in adults usually involve the cerebral hemispheres; the benign forms in children usually involve the brain stem or cerebellum. Ependymomas involve the ventricular lining and are most frequent in the fourth ventricle. Oligodendrogliomas are most common in middle life in the white matter of the cerebral hemispheres, frequently extending to the surface. Characteristic calcification may be visible on x-ray examination. Medulloblastoma is a neoplasm of the midline cerebellum in childhood and is composed of primitive, undifferentiated, rapidly growing cells, which are sensitive to irradiation. Meningiomas are extrinsic lesions arising in the arachnoid membrane, usually benign and slow growing, and amenable to surgical cure. They become attached to the dura and indent the underlying parenchyma from which they are distinctly demarcated. They are typically composed of whorled and interlacing patterns of arachnoid cells. Malignant forms are rare. Nerve sheath tumors are common lesions of nerve roots and peripheral nerves and are usually benign. Intracranial forms usually arise in the acoustic nerve and produce hearing impairment. Intraspinal forms usually involve the posterior nerve roots. They are composed of spindle cells often arranged in palisades. Neurofibromatosis (von Recklinghausen's disease) is a familial disorder in which multiple neurofibromas are associated with pigmentation of the skin and sometimes with meningiomas and gliomas.

Intracranial metastatic neoplasms usually involve the parenchyma of the brain, are multiple, and come (hematogenously) from any primary site, commonly lung, breast, kidney, and skin (melanoma). Intraspinal metastatic neoplasms are usually epidural and come from similar carcinomatous or sarcomatous primary foci or as part of various lymphomas by lymphatic or blood–vascular routes, by direct extension, or by indirect extension from bone lesions.

EPILEPSY

Epilepsy is a clinical syndrome characterized by recurrent episodes of convulsive seizures or alterations of consciousness due to abnormal discharge of nerve cells within the gray matter of the brain. The pathologic substrate of epilepsy is twofold and consists of predisposing factors, about which little is known, and a brain lesion that may be of any type, generalized or focal, structural or functional. In symptomatic epilepsy a structural lesion may be demonstrated. In idiopathic epilepsy there is no such demonstrable lesion. Focal epilepsy with jacksonian seizures is usually associated with focal structural abnormality in an appropriate location. Temporal lobe epilepsy causing psychomotor seizures is usually produced by a lesion in or near the medial temporal cortex. Petit mal epilepsy is not associated with any known pathologic change in brain tissue.

DEGENERATIVE DISEASES AND AGING

During adult life there is gradual attrition of nerve cells even in healthy individuals. Advancing age is accompanied by atrophy of nervous tissue. This is most apparent in the brain where a slowly progressive loss of nerve cells and their processes results in shrinkage of gray and white matter and enlargement of the ventricular system. The frontal and parietal lobes are most affected. Microscopically the most characteristic change of aging is atrophy of nerve cells with the accumulation of lipochrome granules in their cytoplasm. Neurofibrillary degeneration and deposits of neurofibrillary debris, senile plaques, are expected after the sixth decade. Excessive degenerative changes of this type result in senile dementia. In Alzheimer's presenile dementia these changes begin early and progress at an excessive rate. Presenile dementia in Pick's disease is due to lobar sclerosis in the cerebrum with argyrophilic neuronal inclusions. Huntington's chorea is a heredofamilial disease which becomes manifest in middle life as dementia and chorea and is characterized by widespread degeneration of gray matter, particularly affecting the caudate nuclei, putamens, and cerebral cortex, accompanied by intense gliosis. The clinical syndrome of tremor, rigidity, and hypokinesis referred to as paralysis agitans or parkinsonism may be due to several causes. Usually idiopathic, this syndrome may be due to encephalitis, vascular disease, trauma, and poisoning. Pathologic changes are widespread but most constant in the substantia nigra and locus ceruleus, where pigmented neurons undergo degeneration and develop cytoplasmic inclusion bodies (Lewy bodies) and neurofibrillary tangles. Degenerative disease of motor neurons is of unknown cause and occurs in three main forms: amyotrophic lateral sclerosis, progressive bulbar palsy, and progressive spinal muscular atrophy. Motor neurons and their processes deteriorate selectively and result in atrophy of nerve cell processes and denervation of muscle.

Various combinations of degeneration of the cerebellum and spinal cord occur, most having a hereditary tendency. The most common form is the spinal type, Friedreich's ataxia, in which the predominant changes are atrophy of the posterior columns, corticospinal, and dorsal spinocerebellar tracts. Cystic cavitation of the spinal cord (syringomyelia) or of the brain stem (syringobulbia) is of unknown cause, most probably due to malformation or degeneration of the central parenchyma. In some cases there are neoplastic features. Dissociated anesthesia due to stretching of crossing nerve fibers is a characteristic clinical manifestation.

Osseous System

OSTEOMYELITIS

Pyogenic osteomyelitis is most commonly due to *Staphylococcus aureus,* which usually reaches the marrow cavity by hematogenous dissemination. The infection usually begins in the metaphysis and most commonly affects the long bones of the extremities. Acutely there is suppuration, which results in ischemic necrosis of bone fragments (sequestrum) and may penetrate the cortex forming sinus tracts, which sometime dissect to the skin surface. Chronic osteomyelitis is characterized by fibrosis and bony sclerosis. Amyloidosis is a potential complication.

Tuberculous osteomyelitis usually results from hematogenous dissemination of organisms from a focus of pulmonary tuberculosis and most commonly involves the long bones of the extremities and the spine (Pott's disease). This form of osteomyelitis is much more destructive and resistant to treatment than the pyogenic form. Both tuberculous and pyogenic osteomyelitis are more common in childhood.

OSTEITIS FIBROSA CYSTICA (VON RECKLINGHAUSEN'S DISEASE OF BONE)

This disease is caused by primary or secondary hyperparathyroidism and is characterized by osteoclastic resorption of bone resulting in thinning of cortical and cancellous bone and replacement of bone marrow by fibrous tissue. Focal areas of bone resorption may produce cysts (brown tumors) containing osteoclasts and hemosiderin-laden macrophages within a fibrous stroma (reparative giant cell granulomas). Bony deformities and fractures may occur in severe cases.

OSTEITIS DEFORMANS (PAGET'S DISEASE OF BONE)

This condition is characterized by osteoclastic bone resorption combined with formation of poorly mineralized bone demonstrating irregular osteoid seams (mosaic pattern) in both cortical and cancellous bone. The marrow cavity is eventually replaced by vascularized connective tissue. This disease most commonly affects the pelvis, skull, femur, and spine, resulting in bony deformity and fractures. The most ominous complication is the development of osteosarcoma in involved bones.

OSTEOPOROSIS

Osteoporosis is characterized by generalized or localized thinning of cortical and trabecular bone (unaccompanied by an increase in osteoid matrix) resulting in a reduction in bone mass. Osteoporosis occurs in a large variety of clinical situations including aging (senile osteoporosis), postmenopausal females (estrogen deficiency), Cushing's syndrome, hyperparathyroidism, immobilization, and so forth. The most common complications are compression vertebral fractures and fractures of the femoral neck.

TUMORS OF BONE

Osteoma. Composed of dense, normal-appearing bone, the osteoma is a benign tumor occurring most frequently in the skull and facial bones. They often protrude into one of the sinuses and have little clinical significance.

Giant Cell Tumor. Giant cell tumors usually arise in the epiphysis of long bones (distal femur, proximal tibia, proximal fibula) and result in a clublike deformity of the bone. These tumors are composed of numerous multinucleate giant cells scattered throughout a spindle cell stroma. The bio-logic behavior of these tumors is variable but frequently characterized by local recurrence and metastasis.

Osteosarcoma (Osteogenic Sarcoma). Osteosarcoma is the most common primary malignant tumor of bone. These tumors are usually rapidly growing and arise in the metaphysis of long bones (distal femur, proximal tibia, proximal humerus). The majority of these tumors occur between the ages of 10 and 25 years, but some occur in bones with underlying abnormalities (*e.g.,* Paget's disease, irradiation). Most invade the medullary cavity, penetrate the cortex (producing Codman's triangle by periosteal elevation) and extend into adjacent soft tissue. The anaplastic mesenchymal cells comprising the tumor form variable amounts of osteoid matrix and cartilage. Metastases occur early via the blood stream, most commonly to the lungs.

Chondrosarcoma. Most chondrosarcomas arise de novo, but some arise in preexisting benign cartilaginous lesions. These tumors usually occur in an older age group than osteosarcoma and most commonly involve the pelvic bones. They tend to grow slowly, forming large, bulky masses. The prognosis is closely related to the grade of lesion.

ARTHRITIS

Pyogenic Arthritis. This disease is most commonly produced by gonococci, staphylococci, streptococci, and pneumococci in adults and by *H. influenzae* in children. The bacteria usually reach the joint space by hematogenous dissemination, and large joints (knee, hip, ankle) are most frequently affected. An acute synovitis results that may involve the underlying cartilage and result in destruction of the joint.

Rheumatoid Arthritis. Rheumatoid arthritis is a chronic systemic inflammatory disease that primarily involves multiple joints (interphalangeal joints of the hands, wrists, and elbows) in symmetrical distribution. The characteristic lesion is a chronic synovitis resulting in synovial hyperplasia, vascularization of connective tissue, and chronic inflammatory infiltration (pannus). This pannus may erode into the articular cartilage and adjacent bone, eventually obliterating the joint space. The affected joints become increasingly stiff and eventually develop a fusiform appearance with atrophy of surrounding muscles. Skin nodules (rheumatoid nodules) are present in some patients and consist of a central focus of necrosis surrounded by proliferating connective tissue cells.

Osteoarthritis (Degenerative Arthritis). Osteoarthritis is probably a manifestation of aging that primarily affects hips, knees, vertebral column, and the distal interphalangeal joints of the fingers. The basic lesion consists of erosion of the articular cartilage with overgrowth of the underlying bone producing bone spurs. Unlike rheumatoid arthritis, ankylosis rarely develops, but joint deformity with limitation of motion is common. Nodules (Heberden's nodes) may occur at the base of the terminal phalanges, resulting from bone spur formation.

Gouty Arthritis. Gouty arthritis typically involves the joints of the great toe, foot, ankle, and knee. Monosodium urate crystals precipitate in the joint space and synovial membranes producing an acute inflammatory reaction. Following recurrent attacks of acute arthritis, the underlying articular cartilage may be destroyed by synovial proliferation and crystal deposition. Characteristic deposits of urates surrounded by foreign body giant cell reaction (tophi) occur in the periarticular tissue as well as in other sites (ear, bursae, kidney).

Eye

Only a few diseases of the eye of greatest general interest are briefly described in this review.

Cataracts result from opacification of the lens and typically occur in elderly persons, diabetics, and rarely at early ages (*e.g.,* in infants with rubella syndrome). *Diabetic retinopathy* is a serious complication of diabetes mellitus. *Glaucoma* is due to impeded outflow of aqueous humor, which, if untreated, leads to compression of blood vessels supplying the retina, atrophy of the retina, and blindness. *Malignant tumors* of the eye include *retinoblastoma* that occurs in childhood and *malignant melanoma,* which usually occurs in adults.

QUESTIONS IN PATHOLOGY

Choose the one best answer or completion in the following multiple choice questions. The answers are at the end of this chapter.

1. The edema of acute inflammation involves the exudation of protein-rich fluid:
   (a) Primarily through venules and capillaries
   (b) Primarily through arterioles
   (c) Only through capillaries
   (d) Through lymphatic vessels
   (e) Through all microvessels more or less equally

2. In inflammatory reactions, the presence of hemorrhage implies:
   (a) The action of chemotactic mediators
   (b) The action of vasopermeability mediators
   (c) The action of lymphocyte mediators (lymphokines)
   (d) Structural damage to blood vessels
   (e) None of the above

3. The principal chemical mediator of enhanced vessel permeability from neutrophils is:
   (a) A cationic protein
   (b) An acid phosphatase
   (c) Beta glucuronidase
   (d) Cholesteryl oleate
   (e) A mucopolysaccharide

4. All of the following are characterized by granulomatous inflammation *except:*
   (a) Sarcoidosis
   (b) Tuberculosis
   (c) Histoplasmosis
   (d) Diphtheria
   (e) Leprosy

5. The most characteristic feature of granulation tissue is the:
   (a) Resemblance to a granuloma
   (b) Growth of fibroblasts and new capillaries
   (c) Character of the exudate
   (d) Granular scar that results
   (e) Presence of monocytes and fibroblasts

6. Petechiae on pleural and pericardial surfaces and squames in alveoli of an autopsied neonatal infant suggest:
   (a) A transplacentally acquired viral infection
   (b) Intrauterine anoxia
   (c) A metaplastic epithelial response to oxygen therapy
   (d) A marked decrease in pulmonary surfactant
   (e) An inherent clotting defect

7. Spontaneous maturation of tumor cells and a more benign clinical course potential is occasionally observed in which of the following neoplasms of childhood?
   (a) Medulloblastoma
   (b) Osteogenic sarcoma
   (c) Nephroblastoma
   (d) Neuroblastoma
   (e) Retinoblastoma

8. The most common malignant neoplasm in women between the ages of 30 and 55 years occurs in the:
   (a) Breast
   (b) Colon
   (c) Lung

(d) Cervix

(e) Ovary

9. Which of the following combinations cause the greatest mortality from cancer in Americans?

(a) Carcinoma of lung and stomach

(b) Carcinoma of lung and large intestine

(c) Carcinoma of stomach and large intestine

(d) Carcinoma of breast and stomach

(e) Carcinoma of breast and kidney

10. The immunoglobulin class responsible for sensitization of man for local and systemic anaphylactic reactions is:

(a) IgA

(b) IgD

(c) IgE

(d) IgG

(e) IgM

11. Of the following, the earliest step in the formation of a thrombus is:

(a) Formation of fibrin

(b) Adherence of platelets to vascular intima

(c) Activation of Hageman's factor

(d) Trapping of erythrocytes

(e) None of the above

12. Which of the following statements about alcoholic liver disease is correct?

(a) It is rarely associated with fatty change.

(b) It invariably develops in individuals who consume large amounts of alcohol for more than three months.

(c) It produces extensive hepatic fibrosis rather than true cirrhosis.

(d) Mallory bodies and neutrophilic infiltrates are morphologic features of the early stages of the disease.

(e) It is not directly related to toxic effects of alcohol but rather to nutritional disturbances.

13. Autopsy of a 42-year-old white male found dead and suspected of suicide demonstrated numerous ulcerations of the mucosa of the stomach and ascending colon, along with marked coagulation necrosis of renal tubules. The most likely diagnosis is poisoning with:

(a) Bismuth

(b) Mercury

(c) Arsenic

(d) Phosphorus

(e) Inorganic acid or alkali

14. Chronic salpingitis is considered to be a significant condition predisposing to:

(a) Ectopic pregnancy

(b) Carcinoma of the cervix

(c) Leiomyomata

(d) Cystic hyperplasia of the endometrium

(e) Choriocarcinoma

15. All of the following statements regarding viral hepatitis are true *except*:

(a) Most cases resolve without clinical or morphologic sequelae.

(b) Hepatitis A, B, and non-A non-B may progress to chronic active hepatitis.

(c) "Ground-glass" hepatocytes are found in association with type B but not with types A and non-A non-B.

(d) Chronic active hepatitis is more likely to progress to cirrhosis than is chronic persistent hepatitis.

(e) In the United States, posttransfusion viral hepatitis is caused by type non-A non-B more frequently than by type B.

16. In the majority of cases of infectious hepatitis, 1 year after recovery the liver most often would appear:

(a) Coarsely nodular

(b) Finely nodular

(c) With residual fibrosis in the portal areas

(d) With only minimal pseudolobule formations and increased fibrous tissue in portal areas

(e) Histologically normal

17. Rickettsial diseases primarily affect:

(a) Endothelial cells

(b) Nerve cells

(c) Renal tubular cells

(d) Hepatocytes

(e) Fibroblasts

18. Most of the tissue damage evoked by fungi is due to:

(a) Exotoxins

(b) Their ability to modify the metabolic and reproductive activity of the cells of the host

(c) Progressive development of sensitization to the fungal antigens

(d) Endotoxins

(e) Obstruction of ducts, blood vessels, or lymphatics

19. The organ system that is most severely affected in *fatal* histoplasmosis is the:

(a) Central nervous system

(b) Genitourinary system

(c) Alimentary tract

(d) Respiratory system

(e) Reticuloendothelial system

20. Occlusion of the right coronary artery near its

origin by a thrombus would most likely result in:
(a) Infarction of lateral wall of right ventricle and the right atrium
(b) Infarction of the anterior left ventricle
(c) Infarction of lateral left ventricle
(d) Infarction of posterior left ventricular wall and the posterior septum
(e) Infarction of the anterior septum

21. A decrease in the number of granular leukocytes in the blood occurs most commonly following exposure to:
(a) Chlorine
(b) Salicyclic acid
(c) Benzene
(d) Cobalt
(e) Mercury

22. The type of Hodgkin's disease with the best prognosis is:
(a) Nodular sclerosis
(b) Mixed
(c) Reticular
(d) Lymphocyte depletion
(e) Lymphocyte predominant

23. Silicosis is most often complicated by:
(a) Asthma
(b) Carcinoma of lung
(c) Mesothelioma
(d) Tuberculosis
(e) Bronchioloalveolar carcinoma

24. The most common site of carcinoma of the colon is:
(a) Cecum
(b) Ascending colon
(c) Transverse colon
(d) Splenic flexure
(e) Rectosigmoid

25. The fate of acute poststreptococcal glomerulonephritis is usually:
(a) Development of chronic glomerulonephritis
(b) Development of membranous glomerulonephritis
(c) Development of lobular glomerulonephritis
(d) Development of subacute glomerulonephritis
(e) Complete recovery

26. Nodular hyperplasia (benign hypertrophy) of the prostate involves principally the:
(a) Anterior lobe
(b) Lateral lobes
(c) Posterior lobe
(d) Verumontanum
(e) Prostatic utricle

27. Bleeding from the nipple in a 45-year-old woman without a palpable breast mass should suggest:
(a) Fibroadenoma
(b) Sclerosing adenosis
(c) Intraductal papilloma
(d) Fat necrosis
(e) Medullary carcinoma

28. Spontaneous intracranial hemorrhage in hypertension is most closely related to:
(a) Rupture of venous structures in the subdural space
(b) Laceration of arterial vessels in the epidural space
(c) Fibrinoid necrosis of small penetrating arteries
(d) Inflammatory necrosis of small veins
(e) Atherosclerosis of medium-sized arteries

29. Cerebral infarcts most frequently occur in the:
(a) Amygdala
(b) Hypothalamus
(c) Corpus striatum and internal capsule
(d) Corpus callosum
(e) Nucleus subthalamicus

For each numbered item, select the one heading most closely associated with it. Each lettered heading may be selected once, more than once, or not at all.

(a) Neutrophils
(b) Eosinophils
(c) Basophils
(d) Monocytes
(e) Lymphocytes

30. Streptococcal cellulitis
31. Typhoid fever
32. Bronchial asthma
33. Pneumococcal pneumonia
34. Trichinosis

_____

(a) Retinoblastoma
(b) Squamous cell carcinoma of skin
(c) Basal cell carcinoma of skin
(d) Carcinoma of esophagus
(e) Renal cell carcinoma

35. Rarely metastasizes
36. Frequently occurs in siblings
37. Associated with alcoholism and smoking
38. Contains abundant lipid
39. Frequently spreads by invading veins

_____

(a) Rapidly progressive glomerulonephritis
(b) Minimal change disease
(c) Chronic glomerulonephritis
(d) Acute poststreptococcal glomerulonephritis
(e) Membranous glomerulonephritis

40. Increased mesangial and endothelial cells with neutrophilic infiltrate
41. Fusion of foot processes by electron microscopy
42. Epithelial crescents in Bowman's space
43. Thickened glomerular basement membranes with spike and dome immunofluorescence pattern

---

(a) Chancroid
(b) Chancre
(c) Granuloma inguinale
(d) Lymphogranuloma venereum
(e) Condyloma acuminatum

44. Donovan bodies
45. Spirochetes
46. *H. ducreyi*

(a) Amyotrophic lateral sclerosis
(b) Syringomyelia
(c) Multiple sclerosis
(d) Cervical spondylosis
(e) Diffuse sclerosis

47. Scattered foci of myelin damage with relative preservation of axons
48. Tubular cavitation of the spinal cord
49. Motor neuron degeneration

For each numbered item, indicate whether it is associated with:

(a) A only
(b) B only
(c) Both A and B
(d) Neither A nor B

(A) Rheumatoid arthritis
(B) Osteoarthritis

50. Proliferative synovitis
51. Immune complex deposition
52. Primarily an articular cartilage degeneration
53. Blood-borne infection of joint

(A) Healing by first intention (primary union)
(B) Healing by second intention (secondary union)

54. Granulation tissue
55. Re-epithelialization by 8 days

56. Proud flesh

(A) Squamous cell carcinoma of skin
(B) Basal cell carcinoma of skin

57. Predisposed to by chronic exposure to sunlight
58. Rarely, if ever, metastasizes

(A) Scurvy
(B) Rickets

59. Subperiosteal hematomas
60. Failure of osteoid mineralization

The gallbladder from a 26-year-old white female was found to contain multiple irregularly shaped black stones (nonfaceted) approximately 5 mm in diameter which cut easily with a knife and were uniformly black throughout.

61. The stones most likely are composed principally of:
(a) Cholesterol
(b) Calcium bilirubinate
(c) Calcium carbonate
(d) Mixed cholesterol and calcium bilirubinate
(e) Mixed cholesterol and calcium carbonate

62. A likely cause of these stones is:
(a) Chronic hemolytic processes
(b) Hypercholesterolemia
(c) Stasis of bile
(d) Infection of the gallbladder
(e) Typhoid fever

A 28-year-old man was admitted to the hospital because of severe shortness of breath and cyanosis. The patient died before treatment could be instituted. An autopsy was performed and the final pathologic diagnosis was as follows:

1. High interventricular septal defect in the heart (1.0 cm in diameter)
2. Bicuspid aortic valve
3. Bacterial (vegetative) endocarditis of the aortic valve (*Escherichia coli* was cultured from vegetations)
4. Hypertrophy and dilatation of right heart (severe)
5. Hypertrophy and dilatation of left heart (moderate)
6. Mural thrombi in right atrium of heart
7. Chronic passive congestion of liver (severe)
8. Chronic passive congestion of lungs (moderate)
9. Recent and old pulmonary infarcts

10. Septic infarcts in spleen and both kidneys
11. Atherosclerosis of coronary arteries and aorta

63. The most likely underlying cause of the bacterial endocarditis was:
    (a) Old rheumatic heart disease
    (b) Congenital cardiac anomalies
    (c) Transient *Escherichia coli* bacteremia
    (d) Probable dental manipulations prior to admission
    (e) Septic infarcts in the kidneys
64. Hypertrophy and dilatation of the right heart was most likely due to:
    (a) Chronic pulmonary congestion
    (b) Bicuspid aortic valve
    (c) Bacterial endocarditis of the aortic valve
    (d) Interventricular septal defect
    (e) Left ventricular hypertrophy and dilatation
65. Chronic passive congestion of the liver was most likely due to:
    (a) Failure of the right heart
    (b) Failure of the left heart
    (c) Septicemia
    (d) Chronic pulmonary congestion
    (e) None of the above
66. Which of the following is the most likely cause-effect relationship?
    (a) 8 → 4
    (b) 1 → 4
    (c) 2 → 4
    (d) 6 → 10
    (e) 2 → 8

A 45-year-old white male was a known alcoholic admitted with hematemesis and a shocklike state. He had a history of melena for 1 week prior to admission. He expired soon after admission. An autopsy was performed.

67. The liver was small, nodular, and yellowish brown in color, divided into small, uniform nodules on cut surfaces. The most likely diagnosis is:
    (a) Portal cirrhosis
    (b) Postnecrotic cirrhosis
    (c) Cardiac cirrhosis
    (d) Biliary cirrhosis
    (e) All of the above
68. Which of the following microscopic changes would you *not* expect to see in his liver?
    (a) Fatty change of parenchymal cells
    (b) Acute cholangitis
    (c) Alcoholic hyaline in parenchymal cells

(d) Pseudolobule formation
(e) Fine fibrous bands connecting the portal triads

69. Esophageal varices in this case are most likely the result of:
    (a) Increased blood flow to the liver
    (b) Right-sided heart failure
    (c) Decreased albumin in blood
    (d) Thrombosis of portal vein
    (e) Portal hypertension

Please answer questions 70 to 91 using (a) to (e) as follows:

    (a) Only *1, 2, and 3* are correct
    (b) Only *1 and 3* are correct
    (c) Only *2 and 4* are correct
    (d) Only *4* is correct
    (e) *All* are correct

70. Tissues highly sensitive to ionizing radiation include:
    (1) Brain
    (2) Intestinal mucosa
    (3) Liver
    (4) Lymphoid tissue
71. Vasopermeability factors that are generated by cleavage of plasma substrates include:
    (1) Histamine
    (2) Anaphylatoxins
    (3) Leukotrienes
    (4) Kinins
72. Significant chemotactic agents for neutrophils include:
    (1) Soluble bacterial products
    (2) Histamine
    (3) Components of the complement system
    (4) Bradykinin
73. Organisms that sometimes cause disseminated infections in the fetus include:
    (1) Cytomegalovirus
    (2) Herpes simplex virus
    (3) *Toxoplasma gondii*
    (4) *Treponema pallidum*
74. Viruses capable of including neoplasms in experimental animals include:
    (1) Polyoma virus
    (2) Measles virus
    (3) SV 40
    (4) Influenza B virus
75. Tumors that may produce substances with hormone activity include:
    (1) Oat cell carcinoma of the bronchus
    (2) Medullary thyroid carcinoma

(3) Granulosa–theca cell tumor of the ovary
(4) Renal cell carcinoma

76. In general, rickettsial infections are characterized by:
    (1) Obligate intracellular parasitism
    (2) Localization of organisms in endothelial cells
    (3) Transmission by arthropods
    (4) Phlegmonous inflammation

77. *Intranuclear* inclusion bodies occur in:
    (1) Smallpox
    (2) Chickenpox
    (3) Herpes simplex
    (4) Rabies

78. The Chédiak–Higashi syndrome is characterized by:
    (1) Hypopigmentation of skin, eyes, and hair
    (2) Large abnormal lysosomes in polymorphonuclear leukocytes
    (3) Predisposition to chronic infections
    (4) Abnormal response to delayed type of hypersensitivity

79. In patients with α_1-antitrypsin deficiency:
    (1) Symptoms appear at birth
    (2) Enzyme activity is decreased but not totally absent in persons with homozygous state
    (3) There is increased risk of developing bronchogenic carcinoma
    (4) Emphysema usually develops

80. Ostium primum defects:
    (1) Are commonly associated with a cleft mitral valve
    (2) Arise from abnormalities of rotation
    (3) Occur commonly in Down's syndrome
    (4) Occur at various locations in the intraatrial septum with approximately equal frequency

81. Cyanotic congenital heart diseases include:
    (1) Tetralogy of Fallot
    (2) Transposition of the great vessels
    (3) Total anomalous pulmonary venous return
    (4) Taussig–Bing anomaly

82. Hereditary spherocytosis is characterized by:
    (1) Decreased osmotic fragility
    (2) Autosomal recessive inheritance pattern
    (3) A small contracted spleen
    (4) A cell membrane defect

83. Features of ulcerative colitis include:
    (1) Superficial mucosal ulcers
    (2) Crypt abscesses
    (3) Pseudopolyps
    (4) Marked thickening of the gut wall

84. Hypertension may result from:
    (1) An adrenal medullary tumor
    (2) Addison's disease
    (3) An adrenal cortical tumor
    (4) Amyloidosis of adrenal gland

85. Papillary necrosis of the kidney may be associated with:
    (1) Acute pyelonephritis in combination with partial obstruction
    (2) Diabetes mellitus
    (3) Phenacetin abuse
    (4) Benign nephrosclerosis

86. Leiomyomata of the uterus:
    (1) Frequently undergo sarcomatous change
    (2) Are sharply circumscribed
    (3) Are encapsulated
    (4) Rarely arise after the menopause

87. Serous cystadenocarcinoma of the ovary:
    (1) Is bilateral in approximately 66% of cases
    (2) Frequently results in widespread abdominal implantation
    (3) Is commonly papillary with psammoma bodies
    (4) Is derived from the coelomic epithelium covering the ovary

88. Massive intracerebral hemorrhage characteristically:
    (1) Is preceded by longstanding hypertension
    (2) Occurs in the lenticulostriate region
    (3) Is due to rupture of small vessels
    (4) Is fatal more frequently than cerebral infarction

89. In a patient who dies with severe presenile dementia (Alzheimer's disease) the diagnostic histologic findings in the brain include:
    (1) Severe arteriolar sclerosis
    (2) Abundant senile plaques
    (3) Multiple cortical microinfarcts
    (4) Neurofibrillatory tangles in neurons

90. Organisms frequently responsible for meningitis in the newborn period include:
    (1) Group B streptococcus
    (2) *Neisseria meningitidis*
    (3) *Escherichia coli*
    (4) Pneumococcus

91. Characteristics of degenerative joint disease (osteoarthritis) include:
    (1) Pannus formation
    (2) Degeneration of articular cartilage
    (3) Ankylosis
    (4) Involvement of weight-bearing joints

ANSWERS TO MULTIPLE CHOICE QUESTIONS

1. (a)	**13.** (b)	**25.** (e)	**37.** (d)	**49.** (a)	**61.** (b)	**73.** (e)	**85.** (a)
2. (d)	**14.** (a)	**26.** (b)	**38.** (e)	**50.** (a)	**62.** (a)	**74.** (b)	**86.** (c)
3. (a)	**15.** (b)	**27.** (c)	**39.** (e)	**51.** (a)	**63.** (b)	**75.** (e)	**87.** (e)
4. (d)	**16.** (e)	**28.** (c)	**40.** (d)	**52.** (b)	**64.** (d)	**76.** (a)	**88.** (e)
5. (b)	**17.** (a)	**29.** (c)	**41.** (b)	**53.** (d)	**65.** (a)	**77.** (a)	**89.** (c)
6. (b)	**18.** (c)	**30.** (a)	**42.** (a)	**54.** (c)	**66.** (b)	**78.** (a)	**90.** (b)
7. (d)	**19.** (e)	**31.** (d)	**43.** (e)	**55.** (a)	**67.** (a)	**79.** (c)	**91.** (c)
8. (a)	**20.** (d)	**32.** (b)	**44.** (c)	**56.** (b)	**68.** (b)	**80.** (b)	
9. (b)	**21.** (c)	**33.** (a)	**45.** (b)	**57.** (c)	**69.** (e)	**81.** (e)	
10. (c)	**22.** (e)	**34.** (b)	**46.** (a)	**58.** (b)	**70.** (c)	**82.** (d)	
11. (b)	**23.** (d)	**35.** (c)	**47.** (c)	**59.** (a)	**71.** (c)	**83.** (a)	
12. (d)	**24.** (e)	**36.** (a)	**48.** (b)	**60.** (b)	**72.** (b)	**84.** (b)	

7

Pharmacology

Margaret A. Reilly, Ph.D.
Research Scientist, Nathan Kline Research Institute,
Orangeburg, New York

Adjunct Associate Professor, College of New
Rochelle School of Nursing, New Rochelle,
New York

Adjunct Assistant Professor, Pharmacology
Department, New York Medical College, Valhalla,
New York

John C. McGiff, M.D.
Chairman, Pharmacology Department, New York
Medical College, Valhalla, New York

With the assistance of the members of the New
York Medical College Pharmacology Department.

INTRODUCTION

Pharmacology is the study of the interactions of drugs with living systems. Drugs are substances that have the ability to influence the physiological or biochemical activity of cells. Included are substances used in the diagnosis, prevention, and treatment of disease, as well as substances used for nonmedical or "recreational" purposes, such as alcohol, heroin, and cocaine. Interactions of drugs with living systems are often complex, resulting not only in desired or therapeutic actions but also in unwanted and occasionally life-threatening effects. A full understanding of these actions requires a strong foundation in the principles of anatomy, physiology, and biochemistry.

Drug Names

Every drug is a chemical substance and thus will have a name that describes exactly its molecular structure. Chemical names are rarely encountered in clinical pharmacology; their major importance is in the area of drug development and production.

When a drug is ready for clinical testing, a generic or nonproprietary name will be selected after discussion by committees or representatives of the American Medical Association, the Food and Drug Administration (FDA), the United States Pharmacopeia, the World Health Organization (WHO), the National Formulary, and the commercial sponsor of the drug. Since 1961, the names finally selected have been known as United States Adopted Names (USAN), and they are intended to provide the features of brevity, easy recall, and some syllable or stem that indicates the group to which the drug belongs. International recognition of the USAN reduces the occasion for worldwide multiplicity of names.

The older nomenclature bodies that now participate in selection of the USAN continue to operate in their special areas. Since 1820, the U.S. Pharmacopeia (USP) has engaged in the selection of drugs based on therapeutic merit and has specified their standards of purity. The designation USP after a drug name is legal testimony on the part of the manufacturer that the product meets the published purity standards and that the drug has been considered to have therapeutic merit by revision committees acting every 5 years. The National Formulary designation NF is associated usually with older drugs and combinations of declining importance that are used sufficiently to satisfy an arbitrary standard. In 1975, the United States Pharmacopeial Convention acquired all rights to the National Formulary. As a result, the present USP and NF appear together in a single binding. Standards for essentially every chemical entity marketed as a drug in the United States, as well as many combination products, are found in that volume.

Proprietary or trademark names are selected by the commercial developer of the drug. These names become the property of the developer and cannot be used by other manufacturers unless permission is granted by the owner. Exclusive manufacturing and distributing rights may be held under patent for 17 years. However, trademarked drugs must also always be identified by their generic names.

Administration of Drugs

Drugs are given for a wide variety of purposes under many clinical situations. All drugs possess the potential to induce serious adverse reactions. To administer drugs safely and effectively, the physician must have extensive knowledge of pharmacology. This chapter serves merely as a review of some of that body of knowledge, and focuses mainly on drugs currently in frequent use. Other more comprehensive sources must be consulted before drugs are prescribed. One valuable publication is *AMA Drug Evaluations,* prepared by committees and consultants of the American Medical Association. It is particularly useful to determine available preparations and currently accepted therapeutic practises. The ubiquitous *Physicians' Desk Reference (PDR)* is a compilation of extensive drug information supplied by pharmaceutical manufacturers, much of it in the form of official package inserts that are in compliance with FDA regulations pertaining to drug labeling. Newly released drugs, newly recognized adverse effects, and other items of importance to the practicing physician are presented in publications such as the *FDA Drug Bulletin* and *The Medical Letter on Drugs and Therapeutics.*

Regulatory Control of Drugs

The Food and Drug Administration is charged with protection of the public interest insofar as it is affected by the sale and the distribution of drug products. This agency, founded in 1906 through the missionary-type efforts of Dr. Harvey Wiley, for many years was limited to the control of the sanitary state of manufacturing premises, the detection of adulteration, and the correction of minor features of labeling. Food and drug promotions with obvious fraudulent intent were liable to restraint or prosecution, but there was no authority to halt sales of disastrously dangerous drugs, and there were no governmental standards for proof of efficacy. In the Food, Drug and Cosmetic Act of 1938, Congress empowered the FDA to require demonstrations of reasonable safety at recommended drug doses, and, in 1962 (the Kefauver–Harris Amendment), to require proof of efficacy. In both instances, legislation followed disastrous incidents: in one case, the "elixir of sulfanilamide" tragedy, which cost over 100 lives because of unexpected toxicity of diethylene glycol, the solvent; in the other, the thalidomide experience, in which teratogenic effects of an apparently harmless sedative occurred in several thousand cases, almost all of them outside the United States.

In 1971, the FDA, in collaboration with the National Academy of Sciences and National Research Council, began rating the efficacy of drug products in an effort to provide the prescriber with the best possible clinical judgment in choosing drugs for patients. The efficacy ratings are commonly referred to as drug efficacy study implementation (DESI) ratings, and include "effective," "effective with restrictions or qualifications," "probably effective," "possibly effective," and "ineffective."

In 1952, the Durham–Humphrey Amendment to the Food, Drug and Cosmetic Act established specific regulations in regard to prescription practices. Distinction was made between drugs that may be dispensed on prescription only ("legend" drugs) and those that may be sold over the counter by any merchant. The first category bears the prescription legend "Caution: Federal law prohibits dispensing without prescription." Among the prescription-legend drugs, certain ones can be refilled for the time specified by the prescriber, as indicated by the "refill" instructions; however, it should be noted that such instructions as "refill prn" or "refill ad lib," or other notations that place no limit on the length of time in which the prescription may be refilled are not recognized by the FDA as valid refill authorizations. Persons receiving prescription drugs should be under continuous medical supervision, to detect changes in their clinical conditions or development of adverse effects.

The Comprehensive Drug Abuse Prevention and Control Act (Controlled Substances Act) of 1970, which supersedes the Harrison Narcotic Act, places further limitations on the prescribing and refilling of certain depressant, stimulant, and hallucinogenic drugs in five different "schedules." Those drugs that have no legal use (such as heroin and LSD) are all placed in schedule I. Those drugs in the remaining schedules (II through V) are rated according to their decreasing potential for addiction or habituation. Prescriptions for drugs in schedule II (morphine, cocaine, and methamphetamine, for example) cannot be refilled. Prescriptions for drugs in schedules III and IV may be refilled, if the prescriber authorizes, not more than five times nor for longer than 6 months after the prescription is issued. Drugs in schedule V (formerly referred to as "exempt narcotics") may be refilled according to the prescriber's instructions; if no refill instructions are supplied, the prescription may not be refilled.

When prescribing controlled substances, the prescriber must include the full name and address of the patient, must sign the prescription in ink, and must show his or her own address and Drug Enforcement Administration (DEA) registration number. It is illegal for a pharmacist to fill a prescription for a controlled substance unless all these requirements are met.

The Drug Regulation Reform Act of 1979 was the culmination of several years of effort on the part of members of Congress, the Administration, industry, academic researchers, and consumer activists. It is a major revision of the way in which new drugs are brought onto the market and includes provisions for their surveillance after marketing.

The Orphan Drug Act of 1983 was intended to foster development of agents useful in rare diseases. Economic incentives are provided to compensate for drug research that holds little potential for monetary return.

The Drug Price Competition and Patent Term Restoration Act passed in 1984 has simplified the requirements for approval of generic forms. The result has been a greatly increased number of such agents on the market. Although very few serious bioequivalence discrepancies have been reported, transfer of patients from one drug form to another always requires careful observation for variations in therapeutic response.

The Food and Drug Administration, first operated under the Department of Agriculture, is now part of the Department of Health and Human Services (formerly, Health, Education and Welfare), as a part of the Consumer Protection and Environmental Health Service. Other regulatory agencies include the National Microbiological Institute of the National Institutes of Health, which regulates vaccines, sera, and antitoxins under the broad class of "biologicals." The Drug Enforcement Administration operates under and is part of the U.S. Justice Department.

The Federal Trade Commission exercises control over direct public advertising of drug products that move in interstate commerce. Validity of advertising claims is judged in terms of possible direct injury and also of indirect hazard brought about by encouraging the use of ineffective remedies.

In addition to federal legislation, states, municipalities, institutions, and agencies often have regulations that will govern the dispensing and use of drugs.

Drug–Receptor Interactions

Many drugs appear to exert their effects by combining with structural components (or receptors) on cell membranes or within cells. Endogenous substances such as neurotransmitters and hormones also act by combining with these receptors. The kinetics of attachment and release are regulated by such chemical forces as covalent electron sharing, electrostatic charge, hydrogen bonding, and van der Waal bonding. Some attachments of drugs to receptors are stable and long-lasting, while others are relatively weak and easily reversible.

In interacting with receptors, some substances elicit physiological or biochemical responses from cells. These substances are called ***agonists*** and are said to have both affinity (the ability to bind to a receptor type) and intrinsic activity (the ability to provoke a cellular response). For example, the β-adrenergic agonists isoproterenol and epinephrine activate adenylate cyclase when they bind to beta receptors. The ensuing increase in intracellular levels of cyclic AMP (the "second messenger") sets into motion biochemical responses that are ultimately expressed as alterations in physiological activity of those cells that possess beta receptors.

Other substances bind to receptors but do not initiate cellular responses, that is, these substances have affinity but not intrinsic activity. Drugs called ***antagonists*** act in this manner, blocking the effects of endogenous substances as well as of other drugs by preventing their access to receptors. For example, the β-adrenergic antagonist propranolol can decrease the intensity of those physiological responses attributable to stimulation of (or agonist activity at) β receptors.

STRUCTURE–ACTIVITY RELATIONSHIPS

Drug–receptor interactions are specific or selective. Certain structural or spatial relationships must be present in a drug's molecular makeup in order for it to act as an agonist or antagonist at a receptor. Small molecular modifications can produce agonists or antagonists of varying potency, or convert agonist activity to antagonism. The pharmaceutical industry has utilized these structure–activity relationships in its efforts to develop drugs that will have greater therapeutic efficacy or lower incidence of adverse effects than prototype drugs. Narcotic antagonists and histamine H_2 receptor blockers were developed in this manner, as well as drugs with increased oral efficacy (e.g., the antiarrhythmic tocainide) and decreased susceptibility to hepatic or renal inactivation (e.g., the β blocker nadolol). Drugs with more selective actions have been discovered (e.g., β agonists and antagonists selective for β-1 or β-2 receptors). Completely new classes of drugs have evolved, for example, the sulfonylurea oral hypoglycemic drugs from the sulfonamide antiinfective agents. However, some agents thus developed do not represent major differences from related compounds, and merely contribute to the vast number of available drugs.

DOSE–RESPONSE CURVES

Physiological responses to drugs are usually related to the dose administered, up to a maximal limit. The dose–response curve (characteristically S-shaped or sigmoid) is a graphic representation of this observation. Greater potency will shift the dose–response curve to the left, that is, lower doses will produce the same effect as larger amounts of less potent analogues. Efficacy refers to the maximal limit of the response produced; the height of the dose–response curve is greater for drugs with increased efficacy.

Interactions between drugs also yield characteristic dose–response curves. Competitive or reversible inhibition results in a parallel shift of the curve to the right, with no change in height (or efficacy). This type of inhibitory effect can be overcome by administration of increasing amounts of agonist. A noncompetitive antagonist, or one that is not reversible by increasing dosages of agonist, will produce a dose–response curve in which the maximal height is diminished.

Pharmacokinetics

Pharmacokinetics describes the fate of a drug after it has been administered. Many factors influence absorption, distribution, biotransformation, and elimination of drugs. The onset, duration, and intensity of a drug's actions are in turn modified by these interactions with physiological and biochemical functions.

The movement of a drug through the human body depends upon its lipid solubility, which enables it to cross biological membranes with ease. Most drugs are, to some degree, lipid soluble. A solution of a drug that is a weak acid or a weak base will contain both nonionized (lipid soluble) and ionized (water soluble) molecules. Alterations in the pH of the solution will change the ratio of nonionized to ionized molecules. Alkalinization will enhance ionization of acids and reduce that of bases; acidification has the opposite influence. The pKa of a drug is that pH at which equal amounts of the molecules in solution are nonionized and ionized.

Absorption refers to the entry of drug molecules into the circulatory system. Drugs administered for systemic effects must be transported from the site of administration to the site of action. Intravenous administration places the drug directly into the circulatory system. Other routes, however, depend upon the ability of molecules to gain access to the blood by crossing biological membranes. Most drugs are passively absorbed down a concentration gradient. Lipid-soluble molecules are most readily absorbed, although capillary walls in many tissues are quite permeable to both lipid- and water-soluble molecules. The rate of blood flow through the site of administration affects the concentration gradient. Normal perfusion rapidly carries drug away and enhances entry of more molecules into the circulatory system. Sluggish flow, as might be encountered in shock or heart failure, will impede absorption from peripheral sites. Bioavailability refers to the fraction of an administered drug dose that reaches the circulatory system and thus becomes available for distribution to sites of action.

Distribution occurs when drug molecules leave the circulatory system and enter body tissues where sites of action, storage, or inactivation are located. Again, the importance of the ability of molecules to cross membranes is apparent. Drugs have relatively uniform access to most tissues, with the exception of brain. There, the blood–brain barrier formed by the tight junctions of capillary cells tends to exclude ionized, lipid-insoluble molecules.

Distribution of drug can be delayed by the binding of molecules to plasma proteins such as albumin and alpha-acid glycoprotein. These macromolecules normally are restricted to the circulatory system, and only the unbound portion of a drug dose will be distributed to body tissues. The binding of drug to plasma protein is reversible, and as molecules leave the circulatory system additional drug will dissociate from its binding sites. Drugs that bind extensively to plasma proteins will have prolonged plasma half-lives and durations of action. Physiological and pathological states (*e.g.,* very young or old age, or hepatic or renal disease) that induce changes in the amounts of plasma protein can influence characteristic patterns of protein binding.

Other tissues also will bind and accumulate certain drugs. For example, adipose tissue can sequester significant amounts of lipid soluble drugs. Perfusion of this tissue is low, thus drugs will accumulate and subsequently be released slowly.

Biotransformation, frequently accomplished by hepatic enzymes, involves the conversion of drugs to other substances. The action of many lipid-soluble drugs is terminated by transformation to molecules that are less lipid soluble and thus more readily excreted by the kidneys. Drug metabolites also are usually less pharmacologically active than the parent drug. However, some agents (*e.g.,* diazepam and procainamide) yield active metabolites that prolong the duration of pharmacological action. A few drugs are administered in inactive or prodrug form, and are biotransformed to active substances. Impairment of hepatic function (*e.g.,* in elderly persons or in the presence of hepatic disease) will reduce the effectiveness of biotransformation. Induction or enhancement of hepatic enzyme activity will increase the rate of drug metabolism. Some drugs are extensively extracted from the portal circulation by the liver. This "first-pass effect" greatly diminishes the effectiveness of drugs such as propranolol, and precludes the oral administration of drugs such as nitroglycerin and lidocaine.

The final factor in pharmacokinetics is excretion, which removes drugs and their metabolites from the body. The kidneys accomplish most excretion, although some drugs are eliminated by the lungs, in perspiration, or by secretion into bile and feces. Some drugs that are carried by bile into the gastrointestinal tract are reabsorbed in the intestine. This enterohepatic circulation contributes to the prolonged action of drugs such as the neuroleptics and digitoxin. Water-soluble drugs can be filtered and excreted as unmetabolized molecules. Changes in urinary pH will influence the ionization of drug molecules and alter rates of excretion. Some agents (*e.g.,* penicillins) are actively secreted by the neph-

ron. Renal impairment can markedly prolong the plasma half-life of drugs eliminated by renal excretion.

The rate of drug excretion is expressed as the biological half-life, which is the time interval required for the amount of drug in the body to decrease by one half. This is usually measured in clinical pharmacology as the plasma half-life, which can be influenced by many of the previously discussed pharmacokinetic factors. The total amount of drug in the body is difficult to ascertain, except immediately following an initial IV bolus. Drugs vary in distribution to and sequestration in body compartments. The volume of distribution (V_d), estimated by comparing the total amount of drug present to the concentration in plasma, indicates the ability of the drug to diffuse from the circulatory system and enter tissues and cells.

SPECIAL CONSIDERATIONS

Pharmacokinetic factors differ considerably among persons, allowing much interindividual variation in therapeutic responsiveness. Age, sex, nutrition, hydration, genetic traits, and pathological status all influence the fate of drugs in the human body. Special precautions are thus required when drugs are administered to certain groups of persons.

Geriatric Pharmacology. The elderly population (*i.e.,* those over 65 years of age) consumes a disproportionately large percentage of the drugs sold annually in the United States. Many elderly persons have multiple illnesses and are often receiving several drugs simultaneously. This age group is at greater risk of experiencing adverse drug reactions and interactions.

Alterations in certain pharmacokinetic factors predispose elderly persons to greater responsiveness to drugs.

Physiological functions, such as hepatic and renal activity, become less efficient. Drugs that are hepatically biotransformed (*e.g.,* sedatives and narcotic analgesics) or inactivated by renal excretion (*e.g.,* antibiotics) can have prolonged and intensified action in the elderly. Changes in patterns of blood flow may delay absorption and distribution of drugs and can also hinder their delivery to the liver and kidney for inactivation. An increase in the proportion of adipose tissue enhances the sequestration of lipid-soluble drugs.

Dehydration, occurring frequently in the elderly as renal water-conserving efficacy is lost, results in higher plasma levels of drugs, particularly those that are water soluble.

In addition to factors that affect many drugs in

general, some physiological changes in the elderly will have an impact particularly on individual types of drugs. For example, anticoagulants can be especially hazardous for several reasons. The elderly have fragile skin and blood vessels that increase the risk of hemorrhage following injury. In addition, decreased hepatic function will hinder the inactivation of these drugs, and also result in depletion of hepatically synthesized clotting factors and of plasma proteins to which these drugs avidly bind. Drugs that induce orthostatic hypotension can cause severe blood pressure fluctuations, since the vascular response to changes in position are reduced in the elderly. Drug-induced hypotension is believed to be a major cause of falls in older persons, who often have fragile bones (osteoporosis) that are easily fractured. Alterations in receptor sensitivity may occur at advanced age: this appears to underlie in part the increased responsiveness to benzodiazepines such as diazepam.

Despite the physiological changes that occur with age, many precautions can be taken to make drug administration safe and effective in the elderly. Only those drugs that are absolutely necessary should be given. Initial prescriptions should be written for smaller than normal amounts, and careful observation will reveal whether dosage adjustments are needed. Information can be provided to patients about anticipated adverse effects, in particular those that can warn of impending drug toxicity (e.g., anorexia caused by digitalis glycosides) and those that endanger personal safety (e.g., drowsiness or orthostatic hypotension). Attention can also be paid to possible drug interactions, especially those involving foods, alcohol, or over-the-counter preparations. If the patient's clinical condition deteriorates, or new symptoms appear, consider the very real possibility that these effects may be drug related. Occasionally, some elderly individuals may need larger doses than younger adults in order to attain therapeutic blood levels. This usually has a genetic basis associated with rapid metabolism of the drug. These considerations can pertain to drug administration in patients of any age group.

Pediatric Pharmacology. Very young persons respond to drugs differently than adults. Most drugs are not specifically studied for their safety and efficacy in children. Instead, retrospective observation provides a body of knowledge that skilled physicians can use to administer drugs appropriately to pediatric patients. Several mathematical formulas, based on age, body weight, and surface area, can be used to proportion adult doses to suitable amounts for children. Drug prescriptions may also be based on body weight (e.g., mg/kg) to provide for a child's smaller size.

Several physiological factors can alter drug pharmacokinetics in children. Neonates, in particular those born prematurely, are most at risk of heightened drug effects. Their hepatic enzyme systems that inactivate drugs are immature. Suboptimal renal blood flow and function result in inefficient excretion of drugs and metabolites. The blood–brain barrier is not fully developed, allowing entry of water-soluble drugs into the central nervous system. Levels of plasma proteins are reduced and are frequently bound with endogenous substances such as bilirubin. The neonate has higher body water volume and a lower proportion of adipose tissue than older infants, thus distribution of drugs may be altered. Many substances are easily absorbed across the neonate's permeable skin. Differences in gastrointestinal pH, motility, and bacterial population can affect absorption of drugs following oral administration.

Physiological systems gradually attain the maturity found in adults. However, development occurs at varying rates, and drug responses may be quite different among children of the same age and size. Close observation and careful adjustment of doses can help to make pediatric drug administration safe and effective.

Drugs During Pregnancy. Drugs administered during pregnancy gain access to the fetus via the placental circulation. Lipophilic drugs cross the placenta most readily, but it must be considered that almost any chronically administered drug can reach the fetus. Drugs can exert a variety of adverse effects on the developing fetus, which, like the neonate, has little ability to inactive these substances. During the first trimester, some drugs interfere with the early establishment of organs and systems. At birth, the infant may have major anatomical malformations. Called teratogens, these drugs include the sedative thalidomide, several antineoplastic agents, and alcohol.

In later pregnancy, drugs can retard mental and physical development of the fetus, or can produce effects identical to those observed in the mother. For example, β-adrenergic antagonists can markedly depress fetal cardiac function, and oral anticoagulants can induce severe fetal or neonatal hemorrhage even though the mother's prothrombin time is within acceptable limits. Women who are physiologically dependent on drugs such as opiates and barbiturates during their pregnancy will often give birth to an "addicted" infant who will exhibit abstinence signs during the first hours or days of life.

Smoking of cigarettes during pregnancy results in fetal damage and low birthweight. Drugs administered during labor and delivery (*e.g.,* anesthetic and analgesic agents) can evoke respiratory depression in the neonate.

Pregnancy must be considered a contraindication to the administration of all drugs. However, maternal diabetes, hypertension, convulsive disorders, or pre-eclampsia must be controlled for the safety of both mother and infant. Required drugs should be administered in the lowest possible doses, and under close medical supervision. Breast-feeding is also a contraindication for drug administration, although there is controversy regarding which agents reach sufficient levels in breast milk to be harmful to the nursing infant.

DRUG INTERACTIONS

Drugs administered concurrently or sequentially can enhance or diminish each others' actions. Some drug interactions are beneficial, such as the potassium-retaining effects of angiotensin converting enzyme inhibitors offsetting the potassium-losing effects of thiazides. Enhancement of effect can be due to simple addition of the similar actions of two drugs, for example, severe suppression of the cholinergic nervous system when two drugs with anticholinergic efficacy are given simultaneously. *Potentiation* (occasionally referred to as synergism) refers to the marked intensification of a drug's action by another, so that the combined effect is greater than the sum of the two drugs acting independently. For example, very small amounts of alcohol and benzodiazepines combined can produce central nervous system depression of greater severity than anticipated.

Drug interactions can be pharmacokinetic or pharmacodynamic. *Pharmacokinetic interactions* involve alterations in drug absorption, distribution, biotransformation, or excretion. Bile acid sequestrants will bind many orally administered drugs, including digoxin and warfarin, in the gastrointestinal tract and impede their absorption. Probenecid prolongs the action of the penicillins by inhibiting their renal secretion. Tricyclic antidepressants reduce the efficacy of guanethidine by hindering its entry into presynaptic nerve terminals. *Pharmacodynamic interactions* generally occur at the site of drug action. The dopamine-blocking action of neuroleptic drugs will antagonize dopamine agonists such as levodopa and bromocriptine, used in the treatment of Parkinson's disease.

Chemical or physical interactions can occur *in vitro.* Combining sodium bicarbonate and epinephrine in the same solution will inactivate the latter. Diazepam is precipitated from solution by several drugs. Many such incompatibilities exist and will preclude the combination of drugs in one syringe or infusion.

In addition to its interaction with central nervous system depressants, alcohol can react adversely with many other drugs. It will enhance gastric irritation of salicylates and other nonsteroidal anti-inflammatory drugs. It potentiates the hepatotoxicity of methotrexate and acetaminophen. Severe vasodilatation and hypotension can occur when alcohol and antianginal nitrates are concurrently administered. Because of the widespread use of alcohol, patients should always be advised when its consumption may be hazardous.

Drugs can also interact with components of foods. Wines, cheeses, and other foods containing tyramine can provoke hypertensive emergencies in persons receiving monoamine oxidase inhibitors. Pyridoxine (vitamin B_6) is a cofactor for the decarboxylase that inactivates levodopa, and will reduce the efficacy of this antiparkinsonian agent. Bile acid resins such as cholestyramine will bind fat-soluble vitamins and prevent their intestinal absorption.

Beneficial interactions have prompted the use of drug combinations to treat some diseases. For example, hypertension is frequently managed with two or three agents that provide a good therapeutic response in patients refractory to single drugs. Cancer also is often treated with carefully selected combinations of drugs.

The incidence of undesirable drug interactions can be decreased by health care personnel who are familiar with the pharmacology and the recognized interactions of the drugs they administer. A thorough medical history will reveal other drugs (including over-the-counter) that the patient is taking, and any clinical condition that might enhance interactions. Patients can be given information regarding potential drug or food interactions.

AUTONOMIC DRUGS

The autonomic nervous system, consisting of sympathetic (adrenergic) and parasympathetic (cholinergic) branches, modulates a vast variety of physiological activities. Thus it is not surprising that drugs that either stimulate (agonists) or inhibit (antagonists) these systems are frequently used in the management of many disorders. Some agonists have a direct effect on receptors, while others enhance the release of neurotransmitters or block their enzymatic degradation. Norepinephrine, the "chemical messenger" in the sympathetic system, acts upon both α- and β-adrenergic receptors. Acetylcholine stimulates muscarinic receptors at the autonomic effector sites, and also nicotinic receptors in the autonomic ganglia and at the neuromuscular junctions of the somatic nervous system. Both of these acetylcholine receptor types appear to be present in the central nervous system. Antagonists of the effects of the autonomic nervous system are relatively selective for only one type of receptor. Because of the diffuse distribution of the autonomic nervous system, and its considerable influence on physiological activity, drugs that alter its activity will have many side effect that occasionally limit their usefulness.

Parasympathomimetic Drugs

Acetylcholine is synthesized in the nerve terminal by the enzyme choline acetyltransferase and is stored in synaptic vesicles for release subsequent to action potentials transmitted along the neuron. Acetylcholine is inactivated in the synaptic cleft by the enzyme acetylcholinesterase, and choline is transported back into the terminal for resynthesis to acetylcholine. Among the numerous autonomic effects of this neurotransmitter are miosis, ciliary muscle spasm, salivation, lacrimation, sweating, negative chronotropy, peripheral vasodilation, and stimulation of smooth muscle contraction and secretion in the respiratory, gastrointestinal, and urinary tracts.

Acetylcholine itself is not a useful pharmacologic agent because it is too rapidly metabolized and not orally active. Several synthetic analogues that directly stimulate muscarinic receptors have proved to be effective (Table 7-1). These drugs can be given subcutaneously (SC) or orally (PO) but should not be administered IV or IM since subsequent extreme bradycardia, bronchospasm, and bronchial secretion may be fatal. Fortunately, the toxic effects of these cholinergic agonists can be reversed by atropine-like drugs (see below). *Bethanechol* stimulates in particular the urinary and gastrointestinal smooth muscle, thus is administered to alleviate neurogenic, postsurgical, and postpartum nonobstructive urinary retention, bladder atony, and abdominal distention. It has a prolonged duration and relatively little influence on cardiovascular activity. Carbachol and pilocarpine are used mainly as topical agents to reduce intraocular pressure in glaucoma and to induce miosis during ocular surgery. *Pilocarpine* may be administered systemically (PO, SC) to restore flow of saliva. *Methacholine* is seldom used, although it will terminate paroxysmal atrial tachycardia, and its stimulation of catecholamine release can be diagnostic in pheochromocytoma.

Side effects of the acetylcholine agonists in general include gastrointestinal distress, involuntary urination and defecation, salivation, marked bradycardia, postural hypotension, syncope, and dyspnea. These drugs are contraindicated in patients with peptic ulcer, asthma, obstruction or weakness of the gastrointestinal or urinary tract, pregnancy, and many cardiovascular disorders. Hypertensive patients may experience a profound reduction in blood pressure.

Muscarine is a cholinergic agonist of toxicologic importance, since it is the substance in *Amanita muscaria* responsible for poisoning when this mushroom is ingested.

ANTICHOLINESTERASES

Some parasympathomimetics are reversible inhibitors of the enzyme acetylcholinesterase. By slowing inactivation of endogenous acetylcholine, these anticholinesterases (Table 7-1) increase the intensity and duration of cholinergic actions. In contrast to direct-acting cholinergic agents, these drugs can affect ganglionic and neuromuscular junction transmission because they will inhibit acetylcholine degradation at these sites also. The anticholinesterases have been especially useful in the management of glaucoma and myasthenia gravis.

Physostigmine (Antilirium) is a naturally occurring alkaloid with a relatively short duration of action. It is frequently used to reverse both central and peripheral effects of anticholinergic drug overdose. Children are especially sensitive to this drug;

TABLE 7-1. Cholinergic Drugs

GENERIC NAME	TRADE NAME
Direct-acting Stimulants	
Bethanechol	Urecholine
Carbechol	Carbacel
Pilocarpine	Pilocar
Anticholinesterases	
Ambenonium	Mytelase
Echothiophate	Phospholine iodide
Edrophonium	Tensilon
Neostigmine	Prostigmin
Physostigmine	Eserine
Pyridostigmine	Mestinon

thus its pediatric use is limited to life-threatening episodes of anticholinergic poisoning.

The longer acting agents *neostigmine* (Prostigmin), pyridostigmine (Mestinon), and ambenonium (Mytelase) are used in the management of myasthenia gravis. This neuromuscular deficit in acetylcholine transmission causes extreme skeletal muscle weakness. In addition to cholinesterase inhibition, neostigmine appears to have a direct effect on nicotinic receptors. Although usually given orally, these drugs can be administered parenterally in myasthenic crisis or to patients who cannot swallow. Edrophonium (Tensilon) has a very short duration of action, making it especially useful in the diagnosis of myasthenia gravis and in differentiating myasthenic from cholinergic crises. Both of these emergencies are characterized by extreme muscular weakness that can lead to respiratory failure. However, while anticholinesterases alleviate myasthenic crisis, they will exacerbate cholinergic crisis.

The anticholinesterases are also used to reverse muscle paralysis induced by nondepolarizing neuromuscular junction blockers such as curare derivatives and gallamine. However, they will intensify the effects of the depolarizing muscle relaxant succinylcholine.

The adverse effects of the anticholinesterases include all the symptoms of excessive parasympathetic action: increased gastrointestinal and respiratory secretion, intestinal and urinary tract hypermotility, bronchoconstriction, convulsions, bradycardia, and hypotension. In addition, nicotinic symptoms such as fasciculations, weakness, and respiratory paralysis can occur. Atropine will reverse the muscarinic actions of these drugs but will not alter neuromuscular effects. Drug tolerance, or "anticholinesterase insensitivity," may develop with chronic use. Drugs must then be withheld and patients provided with respiratory assistance as needed until cholinergic responsiveness returns.

Irreversible inhibition of cholinesterases is achieved by the use of several organophosphates. Topical preparations containing demecarium (Humorsol), isoflurophate (Floropryl), and echothiophate (Phospholine) are used in the management of glaucoma and strabismus. Diisopropyl fluorophosphate (DFP) and parathion are contained in commercial insecticides. Organophosphates phosphorylate the cholinesterase enzyme, rendering it incapable of hydrolyzing acetylcholine. Recovery of neurotransmitter inactivation may take up to 3 months, since new cholinesterase molecules must be synthesized.

The highly lipid soluble insecticides can be absorbed through the skin as well as by inhalation and ingestion. Poisoning provokes both peripheral and central manifestations of excessive acetylcholine levels. Bronchoconstriction, bradycardia, and hypotension are autonomic in origin, while somatic nicotinic activity causes fasciculations and weakness of skeletal and respiratory muscles. Central nervous system symptoms include restlessness, tremors, convulsions, respiratory depression and paralysis, and circulatory collapse. Atropine will ameliorate central and peripheral muscarinic effects, but mechanical ventilation may be required to sustain respiration. Measurement of plasma cholinesterase levels can indicate the extent of insecticide poisoning.

Pralidoxime (Protopam) reverses organophosphate toxicity by reactivating the cholinesterases. Its greatest effect is upon skeletal and respiratory muscle paralysis; it does not enter the central nervous system. Usually given IV, pralidoxime is relatively short-lived and can be readministered if needed. However, it has some cholinergic depolarizing action and can induce muscular weakness, vision disturbances, and hyperventilation. The action of atropine may be accelerated, and barbiturates (used to alleviate convulsions of organophosphate toxicity) are potentiated by pralidoxime.

CHOLINERGIC ANTAGONISTS

Drugs that reverse the effects of acetylcholine are relatively specific for the autonomic nervous system, for ganglionic transmission, or for the neuromuscular junction. This selectivity becomes somewhat obscured at high drug doses. The first type of drug is considered in this section; the latter two are discussed subsequently.

Atropine, a belladonna derivative that competitively blocks the postganglionic effects of parasympathetic stimulation, is the prototype anticholinergic drug. (In large doses, atropine has some nicotinic blocking action also.) There are naturally occurring and synthetic analogues (Table 7-2) that have much the same characteristics and uses as atropine. Some are quaternary rather than tertiary amines, thus having less central nervous system activity but greater potential to alter ganglionic transmission. Atropine will reverse all the effects of parasympathetic stimulation. Low doses inhibit perspiration and salivation; gradually higher doses will exert cardiac actions and suppression of gastrointestinal and urinary smooth muscle. Quite large amounts are required to reduce gastric secretion.

TABLE 7-2. Anticholinergic Drugs

GENERIC NAME	TRADE NAME
Antimuscarinics	
Atropine	Atropisol, Dey-Dose, others
Hyoscyamine	Levsin, Bellaspaz, others
Scopolamine	Transderm-Scōp, others
Antispasmodics	
Clidinium	Quarzan
Dicyclomine	Bentyl
Glycopyrrolate	Robinul
Oxybutynin	Ditropan
Propantheline	ProBanthine
Antiparkinsonian Agents	
Benztropine	Cogentin
Biperiden	Akineton
Ethopropazine	Parsidol
Procyclidine	Kemadrin
Trihexyphenidyl	Artane

The anticholinergics are used in the treatment of spastic and inflammatory bowel and biliary disorders, and as adjunctive peptic ulcer therapy to reduce gastric acidity. As presurgical medication (atropine and scopolamine in particular), these agents reduce respiratory tract secretions and prevent bradycardia, bronchospasm, and laryngospasm. Asthmatic bronchoconstriction can be alleviated, as can urinary tract irritability. Ipratropium is administered by inhalation to alleviate chronic obstructive respiratory difficulty. Cold medications may contain an anticholinergic to reduce nasal secretions. Some anticholinergics are used to alleviate symptoms of parkinsonism and are discussed under that topic. *Scopolamine* in transdermal patches (Transderm Scōp) has provided a new route of administration for a time-honored remedy for motion sickness. Atropine will reverse digitalis suppression of atrioventricular conduction and vagally induced bradycardias such as those encountered in acute myocardial infarction. (However, it must be noted that low doses of this drug can further slow heart rate, and high doses can induce tachyarrhythmias and postural hypotension.) Scopolamine combined with a narcotic analgesic such as morphine or meperidine produces a particular kind of analgesia called "twilight sleep" that was once used frequently in obstetrics. Anticholinergics are included in some over-the-counter sleeping aids, and brief-acting agents, such as homatropine and eucatropine, are topical mydriatics and cycloplegics that facilitate ocular examination. Anticholinergic drugs are also used to manage overdose or exaggerated response to parasympathomimetic agents.

Because the anticholinergics have a wide variety of effects, those actions that are therapeutic in some instances can become unwanted side effects in others. For example, the increase in heart rate that is beneficial when bradycardia accompanies acute myocardial infarction may be undesirable when anticholinergics are used as gastrointestinal antispasmodics. Additional side effects include dry mouth, constipation, urinary retention, blurred vision, elevated intracranial pressure, intestinal paralysis, suppression of perspiration, nervousness, and insomnia. In hot environments, normal doses of anticholinergics may induce fatal hyperthermia. Low doses of anticholinergics can depress central nervous system activity, while higher doses cause stimulation. Elderly persons, who are especially sensitive to anticholinergics, may experience marked mental confusion or excitation.

Anticholinergic overdose induces cutaneous vasodilation and flushing (hot, dry skin), hyperthermia, respiratory stimulation followed by depression, tachycardia, dilated pupils, changes in blood pressure, muscular incoordination, confusion, delirium, and coma. The anticholinesterase physostigmine is the drug of choice to control anticholinergic overdose; benzodiazepines may also be given to reduce central nervous system stimulation. Pressor agents such as norepinephrine or metaraminol will alleviate hypotension.

Anticholinergics are contraindicated in glaucoma, prostatic hypertrophy, some types of cardiovascular disease, gastrointestinal atony or obstruction, ulcerative colitis, and myasthenia gravis. Caution must be used in patients with renal or hepatic disease or hyperthyroidism. In addition to the elderly, young children also are especially sensitive to anticholinergic effects. Many types of drugs (*e.g.*, tricyclic antidepressants, neuroleptics, antihistamines) can significantly suppress cholinergic function; thus, they are subject to all the precautions and contraindications relevant to anticholinergics.

Concomitant administration of two drugs that reduce parasympathetic activity requires great caution to ensure that excessive suppression does not occur. Monoamine oxidase inhibitors block the hepatic biotransformation of cholinergic antagonists, thus intensifying their effects. Anticholinergics administered IV to persons receiving cyclopropane anesthesia can precipitate ventricular arrhythmias. Absorption of orally administered drugs can be enhanced by the prolonged gastrointestinal transit time induced by cholinergic antagonists.

Sympathomimetic Drugs

There are at least four distinct receptor types in the adrenergic nervous system. α-1 Receptors, found postsynaptically, mediate in particular contraction of blood vessels, gastrointestinal and urinary sphincters, and the radial muscle of the eye. Presynaptic α-2 receptors, so-called "autoreceptors," exert negative feedback inhibition of norepinephrine release. Postsynaptic α-2 binding sites appear to influence intestinal secretion and glucose-induced insulin release. Lipolysis and cardiostimulant actions of the adrenergic system are mediated through β-1 receptors, while β-2 receptor stimulation induces relaxation of smooth muscle resulting in vasodilation, uterine relaxation, decreased gastrointestinal motility, and bronchodilation. Muscle glycogenolysis is also a β-2 function.

The existence of multiple receptors has been demonstrated by the selective effects of drugs on adrenergic action. Norepinephrine, the adrenergic neurotransmitter, stimulates the vascular α-1 receptors (thus inducing vasoconstriction and an increase in blood pressure) and the cardiac β-receptors (causing positive inotropy and chronontropy). Epinephrine, released from the adrenal medulla in response to various stressors, stimulates both α and β receptors.

The synthetic β agonists isoproterenol, albuterol, and terbutaline are especially useful as bronchodilators. Isoproterenol in addition is a powerful β-1 receptor stimulant. Beta antagonists may block both β-1 and β-2 receptors (*e.g.,* propranolol) or may be somewhat selective (*e.g.,* metoprolol and atenolol) for the cardiac β-1 sites, except at higher doses where β-2 activity also becomes apparent (*e.g.,* metoprolol). Clonidine, a centrally acting antihypertensive, is an α-2 agonist that reduces sympathetic stimulation apparently by inhibition of norepinephrine release.

Some sympathomimetics work by direct stimulation of receptors (*e.g.,* isoproterenol) while others act indirectly by releasing endogenous catecholamines (*e.g.,* amphetamines). Still others have both direct and indirect effects (*e.g.,* metaraminol). Tachyphylaxis can develop to the effects of indirect acting agents, as norepinephrine is depleted from nerve terminals.

The catecholamines (norepinephrine, epinephrine, dopamine, and isoproterenol) must be admin-

istered parenterally. All are rapidly inactivated, norepinephrine and epinephrine by presynaptic reuptake as well as by the catechol-o-methyltransferase and monoamine oxidase enzyme systems. 3-Methoxy-4-hydroxy mandelic acid, the final metabolite, is occasionally measured as an indicator of catecholamine synthesis and turnover.

Norepinephrine, in the form of the synthetically prepared levo isomer levarternol bitartrate (Levophed), is used in the management of acute hypotensive states (*e.g.,* those accompanying spinal anesthesia or cord damage). Blood volume deficits must be replaced before or concurrently with pressor amine administration. Norepinephrine returns blood pressure toward normal levels by vasoconstriction (mediated by α-1 receptors) and cardiac stimulation (mediated by β-1 receptors). Cardiac output and venous return increase, and systemic blood flow and coronary artery perfusion improve. Heart rate, often reflexly increased in hypotension, will slow as blood pressure rises.

Administered intravenously, the rate of infusion of norepinephrine must be carefully and constantly adjusted to the patient's response. Severe hypertension and reflex bradycardia can develop; cardiac output can fall as a result of extreme elevations in total peripheral resistance. Headache can be a symptom of elevated blood pressure due to excessive α stimulation. A large vein in the upper body should be selected as the infusion site, which must be constantly observed for signs of extravasation. The intense vasoconstrictor action of norepinephrine will deprive subcutaneous tissue of its blood supply, and cause necrosis and sloughing. If extravasation occurs, infiltration of the α antagonist phentolamine can help to limit subcutaneous tissue damage. Termination of drug administration should be accomplished gradually, with frequent monitoring of blood pressure. Norepinephrine administration requires caution in persons with vascular disease or heart failure.

Epinephrine's actions differ somewhat from those of norepinephrine. Vascular beds possessing β receptors (*e.g.,* skeletal muscle and coronary artery) will dilate in response to low doses of epinephrine. A decrease in peripheral resistance and diastolic pressure can induce reflex tachycardia. However, both epinephrine and norepinephrine increase cardiac irritability and force of contraction as well as myocardial oxygen consumption. Epinephrine, acting on extracardiac β receptors, induces glycogenolysis and release of fatty acids from adipose tissue. Blood glucose and lactic acid concentrations increase. By its action on pulmonary β-2 receptors, epinephrine is a powerful bronchodilator.

Solutions of epinephrine ranging from 1 mg/ml to 0.01 mg/ml are available for IV, IM, or SC administration. Direct intracardiac injection may be used to restore heart beat in cardiac arrest. Epinephrine can also be administered by endotracheal tube in an aerosol. Epinephrine is the drug of choice in anaphylaxis and other life-threatening allergic reactions; it rapidly alleviates shock and asthmatic bronchoconstriction. It is available as a spray for nasal decongestion, and also as an ophthalmic vasoconstrictor and mydriatic. Epinephrine is frequently combined with local or intraspinal anesthetics to induce vasoconstriction and retard systemic absorption. Inadvertent IV administration can cause marked central nervous system and cardiovascular stimulation.

Isoproterenol (Isuprel) is a synthetic, purely β-adrenergic agonist. It is administered IV, sublingually (although absorption is inconsistent), by rectal suppository, and by inhalation. It may reverse atrioventricular heart block and can assist in the reversal of cardiac arrest. It is contraindicated in tachyarrhythmias, except for those dysrhythmias that may be ameliorated by its marked action on the sinoatrial node. Isoproterenol is a highly effective bronchodilator. However, it has caused sudden death (often attributable to excessive use); propellants contained in aerosol forms may sensitize myocardial cells to the arrhythmogenic action of the catecholamines. Isoproterenol can increase myocardial oxygen consumption and may exacerbate situations in which coronary perfusion is compromised (*e.g.*, acute myocardial infarction).

Dopamine (Intropin), the precursor of epinephrine and norepinephrine, is used in the treatment of shock subsequent to myocardial infarction, congestive heart failure, renal failure, septicemia, and trauma. In low doses (2 to 5 μg/kg/min) dopamine acts at dopaminergic receptors to dilate renal and splanchnic blood vessels. Glomerular filtration rate and sodium excretion are increased. Doses in the range of 5 to 10 μg/kg/min stimulate cardiac β receptors and also release norepinephrine from sympathetic nerve terminals, thus improving myocardial function. Alpha receptors are responsive at higher doses (10 to 20 μg/kg/min) of dopamine, and vasoconstriction will occur. Dopamine can exert significant positive inotropy with less increase in myocardial oxygen requirement than isoproterenol. Dopamine is administered only by IV infusion, carefully adjusted to the patient's response. Ex-

travasation should be avoided. Dopamine is also a central nervous system neurotransmitter.

Dobutamine (Dobutrex), similar in structure to dopamine, is indicated in the short-term management of cardiac decompensation subsequent to cardiac surgery or refractory heart failure. Its main action is direct β-1 receptor stimulation, producing a marked increase in contractile force with less effect on heart rate and myocardial oxygen demand. In contrast to norepinephrine's vasoconstrictive effects, renal and splanchnic vessels are dilated by dobutamine. It has a short plasma half-life and is administered by IV infusion.

Many of the responses to adrenergic β stimulation have been linked to activation of adenylate cyclase. Catecholamines and other sympathomimetics are considered "first messengers," which activate this enzyme that catalyzes the conversion of ATP to cyclic AMP. The latter "second messenger" then activates other enzyme systems that alter cellular activity and produce characteristic adrenergic actions.

Among the many adverse effects of catecholamines and other adrenergic agonists are anxiety (epinephrine in particular induces apprehension), restlessness, tremor, convulsions, vertigo, headache, nausea, urinary retention, palpitations, severe changes in blood pressure, arrhythmias, anginal pain, and cardiac or respiratory arrest. Sympathomimetics are contraindicated in severe hypertension, certain cardiovascular disorders, hyperthyroidism, narrow angle glaucoma, and in persons receiving monoamine oxidase inhibitors or anesthesia with halothane or cyclopropane. The effects of direct-acting agents can be potentiated by tricyclic antidepressants, while those of indirect-acting amines that require entry into presynaptic terminals is reduced. Reserpine also will reduce the effectiveness of indirect acting agents since this drug depletes synaptic stores of norepinephrine. Risk of arrhythmias is increased by concomitant administration of digitalis or thyroid hormones.

Amphetamines (Table 7-3) appear to act indirectly by releasing endogenous catecholamines. They are powerful central nervous system stimulants (see discussion under that topic), and also pos-

TABLE 7-3. Amphetamines

GENERIC NAME	TRADE NAME
Amphetamine	—
Benzphetamine	Didrex
Dextroamphetamine	Dexedrine
Methamphetamine	Desoxyn

sess vasoconstrictor and cardiac stimulant properties. Because of their euphoriant and energizing actions, the amphetamines are subject to abuse. Both psychological and physiological dependence can develop to these schedule II controlled substances. Amphetamines have a brief anorexient action (2 to 3 weeks) that has occasioned their use in initiating weight reduction or intermittently sustaining such programs. They should be used only when other dietary and nondrug measures have failed. A large number of anorexients (Table 7-4) related to amphetamines are available, but all are subject to rapidly developing tolerance and drug dependence. Phenylpropanolamine (PPA) is available over the counter, although occasionally marked cardiovascular stimulation contraindicates the use of this drug.

Amphetamines also have some value in the management of childhood attention-deficit disorders (minimal brain dysfunction), and narcolepsy. Methylphenidate (Ritalin) is used similarly to amphetamines in attention-deficit disorders, and as an antidepressant: elderly women with refractory depression can be especially responsive to this latter action.

Metaraminol (Aramine) and *methoxamine* (Vasoxyl), direct-acting α-receptor agonists, have been used to correct hypotensive states. By producing reflex bradycardia, these agents can terminate paroxysmal atrial tachycardia. These drugs are administered parenterally and have a longer duration of action than the catecholamines. Many α-adrenergic drugs are utilized as nasal decongestants (Table 7-5; see also Respiratory Pharmacology).

Ephedrine is an indirect-acting sympathomimetic that can be administered orally. It has a relatively long duration of action, and is an effective bronchodilator, mydriatic, and decongestant. Acting on skeletal muscle, ephedrine can relieve the weakness characteristic of myasthenia gravis. Significant central nervous system stimulation induced by ephedrine can be reversed by concomitant administration of a barbiturate.

The β agonists metaproterenol (Alupent), terbutaline (Bricanyl, Brethine) and albuterol (Ventolin,

TABLE 7-4. Anorexients

GENERIC NAME	TRADE NAME
Fenfluramine	Pondomin
Mazindol	Mazanor, Sanorex
Phendimetrazine	Bontril
Phenmetrazine	Preludin
Phenylpropanolamine	Acutrim, Dexatrim

TABLE 7-5. Adrenergic Decongestants

GENERIC NAME	TRADE NAME
Ephedrine	Efedron
Epinephrine	—
Naphazoline	Privine
Oxymetazoline	Dristan
Phenylephrine	Neo-Synephrine
Prophylhexedrine	Benzedrex
Tetrahydrozoline	Tyzine
Xylometazoline	Otrivin

Proventil) can be administered orally, SC, or by inhalation to prevent or alleviate bronchoconstriction (see Respiratory Pharmacology).

Ritodrine (Yutopar) is a β agonist that relaxes uterine smooth muscle and will reverse premature labor that occurs *after the twentieth week of pregnancy*. Intravenous infusion can terminate acute episodes, then oral administration is instituted to prevent recurrence. This drug is not used when postponement of delivery may threaten the survival of either the mother or the fetus (*e.g.,* in the presence of uncontrolled maternal diabetes mellitus, eclampsia, or intrauterine fetal death). Because of its β-stimulating properties, ritodrine is also contraindicated by tachyarrhythmias and hypertension. Intravenous administration can elevate serum free fatty acid, glucose, and insulin levels, and decrease potassium levels. Diabetic patients and those receiving diuretics that promote potassium loss require close observation. Adverse effects that occur most frequently following IV infusion include alterations in heart rate (both maternal and fetal) and blood pressure, pulmonary edema, palpitations, nausea, tremor, and anxiety. Sudden significant changes in maternal or fetal heart rate or blood pressure, or signs of circulatory overload, require that IV infusion of ritodrine be slowed or terminated. In the neonate, hypoglycemia, hypocalcemia, hypotension, and paralytic ileus may be present.

ADRENERGIC ANTAGONISTS

Adrenergic blocking agents are generally selective for either α or β receptors. Most are competitive antagonists at postsynaptic sites. Alpha antagonists, which reduce sympathetically induced vasoconstriction, are administered in vasospastic diseases such as Reynaud's syndrome, and in the management of pheochromocytoma. They are investigational in the treatment of shock, since a marked vasoconstrictive component may occur before the final vasodilatory response characteristic of circulatory failure.

α-Adrenergic Blocking Agents. *Phenoxybenzamine* (Dibenzyline) binds to both α-1 and α-2 receptors. It produces a gradually developing (4 to 6 hours) but long-lasting (1 to 4 days) "nonequilibrium" blockade by forming with the receptor a stable complex that is reversible only in the early stages of interaction. This drug is administered orally in the management of pheochromocytoma. Because of its slow onset, doses must be increased cautiously. Phenoxybenzamine is hazardous in the presence of marked cerebral or coronary arteriosclerosis, when a fall in blood pressure can further compromise perfusion of vital organs. Nasal congestion, reflex tachycardia, miosis, and postural hypotension can occur. Severe hypotension may follow concomitant administration of β-adrenergic agonists, which will induce unopposed vasodilation.

Phentolamine (Regitine) has a more rapid onset and shorter duration of action than phenoxybenzamine. Administered either orally or parenterally, it also blocks both types of α receptors and also has a direct vasodilatory action. Phentolamine will control hypertensive episodes before and during surgical removal of pheochromocytoma, and has been used in hypertensive emergencies induced by abrupt termination of antihypertensive medication and by drug interactions with monoamine oxidase (MAO) inhibitors. Vasoconstriction and tissue damage resulting from extravasation of norepinephrine or dopamine can be minimized by administration of phentolamine. Contraindicated in coronary artery disease, this drug can cause coronary and cerebral artery occlusion following IV administration. Its side effects are similar to those of phenoxybenzamine. Reflex tachycardia can be alleviated with a β-antagonist, and excessive hypotension can be treated with norepinephrine or a purely α agonist to reverse the competitive alpha blockade. Epinephrine is contraindicated in the presence of an α blocker; the beta vasodilatory action of epinephrine predominates and will further decrease blood pressure. This effect has been termed "epinephrine reversal."

Tolazoline (Priscoline) is similar to phentolamine, and has the ability to stimulate the myocardium, gastric secretion, and gastrointestinal motility. It is "possibly effective" in the management of peripheral vascular disease, and is used investigationally to reduce elevated pulmonary vascular resistance in infants.

In contrast to phenoxybenzamine and phentolamine, which can enhance norepinephrine release by their blockade of presynaptic α-2 receptors, *prazosin* (Minipress) and *terazosin* (Hytrin) are selective antagonists at postsynaptic α-1 receptors. These drugs do not potentiate sympathetic stimulation of cardiac β receptors, and are effective antihypertensive agents (see discussion under that topic).

β-Adrenergic Blocking Agents. Indications for the "β blockers" include many cardiovascular disorders that are alleviated by reduction of β-receptor-mediated positive inotropic (contractile force) and chronotropic (heart rate) effects. *Propranolol* (Inderal), one of the most widely prescribed drugs in the United States, alleviates symptoms of angina pectoris and hypertrophic subaortic stenosis. It can control arrhythmias induced by excessive β-receptor activation; its membrane-stabilizing or local anesthetic effect enhances its antiarrhythmic efficacy. It is administered prophylactically to patients who experience frequent and severe migraine headaches. Propranolol appears to prevent the vasodilatory initiation of this disorder but will not reverse acute migraine attacks. β blockers are effective in preventing recurrence of myocardial infarction and sudden death. Once considered contraindicated in congestive heart failure, these drugs may be cautiously administered to reduce excessive sympathetic stimulation that has become detrimental to cardiac activity.

Perhaps the most common indication for β blockers is in the management of hypertension. These drugs appear to have both central (reduction of sympathetic outflow from the central nervous system) and peripheral (decreased inotropy and chronotropy, and suppression of renin release) hypotensive actions, and will also block reflex tachycardia induced by many other antihypertensive agents such as diuretics and vasodilators. The β blockers are discussed further under such topics as "Antihypertensive Agents" and "Antianginal Agents."

The clinically available β-receptor blockers (Table 7-6) have many similarities, although some possess special characteristics. While most are inactivated hepatically, atenolol and nadolol are excreted renally. These two agents have a longer duration of action, which allows for once-daily oral administration. Because of their lower lipid solubility, they are less able to cross the blood–brain barrier. Some "cardioselective" agents (*e.g.*, *metoprolol* and *atenolol*) are more selective for β1 receptors and can be administered cautiously to persons with asthma. However, these drugs may cause β2 medi-

TABLE 7-6. β-Adrenergic Antagonists

GENERIC NAME	TRADE NAME
Nonselective	
Nadolol	Corgard
Propranolol	Inderal
Timolol	Blocadren
Cardioselective	
Acebutolol	Sectral
Atenolol	Tenormin
Esmolol	Brevibloc
Metoprolol	Lopressor
Intrinsic Activity	
Pindolol	Visken
α Blockade	
Labetalol	Normodyne, Trandate
Ophthalmic	
Betaxolol	Betoptic
Levobunolol	Betagan
Timolol	Timoptic

ated bronchoconstriction at higher doses or in sensitive individuals.

Acebutolol (Sectral) and *pindolol* (Visken) have some intrinsic activity at β-adrenergic receptors, and may cause less reduction in heart rate and cardiac output than other β blockers. However, this action has not been demonstrated to be of significant advantage in any of the indications for these drugs. Acebutolol yields a pharmacologically active metabolite with a long plasma half-life. This may be of possible benefit in some indications, although once-daily dosing with any of the beta blockers often appears to be effective in the treatment of hypertension. *Labetalol* (Normodyne, Trandate) blocks both α and β receptors, and is reported to produce a greater incidence of orthostatic hypotension and sexual dysfunction. This agent can be effective in hypertensive emergencies (see discussion under that topic).

Timolol (Timoptic), *levobunolol* (Betagan), and *betaxolol* (Betoptic) are used topically on the conjunctivae to decrease intraocular pressure in chronic open angle glaucoma. In contrast to the cholinergic agonists, β blockers cause little vision disturbance. Sufficient amounts of drug can be absorbed to produce characteristic systemic adverse reactions; thus these agents are subject to all the usual precautions for β blockers (see below). Betaxolol is a selective β-1 receptor antagonist, while timolol and levobunolol are nonselective.

Esmolol (Brevibloc), administered only by IV in-

fusion, is a cardioselective agent with rapid onset and brief duration of action. Extensively inactivated by an esterase found in erythrocytes, it is used for rapid short-term control of supraventricular tachycardias.

Since the β blockers will suppress all physiological functions mediated by β receptors, they have numerous side effects. Bradycardia, atrioventricular heart block, hypotension, heart failure and pulmonary edema may develop. Caution is required in the presence of congestive heart failure, in which a high degree of β stimulation can be essential to maintaining circulation. β Blockers, except for those that are cardioselective, are contraindicated in persons susceptible to asthma since bronchoconstriction can occur. In persons with diabetes, β blockers will suppress the signs and symptoms (tachycardia, tremor) of hypoglycemia. Agents that block β-2 receptors can enhance insulin-induced hypoglycemia and inhibit insulin release in response to hyperglycemia. Blockade of cardiac β receptors can exacerbate bradycardia or atrioventricular (AV) heart block. The manifestations of thyrotoxicosis may be suppressed. Abrupt discontinuance of β blockers can precipitate arrhythmias, angina pectoris, rebound hypertension, and myocardial infarction. β blockers can induce mental depression and may be contraindicated in persons with a history of this disorder.

β blockers interact with several types of drugs. Additional suppression of AV conduction occurs with digitalis, and of cardiac activity with catecholamine depletors (*e.g.*, reserpine), calcium channel blockers (*e.g.*, nifedipine), and other cardiac depressants. The actions of β agonists are blocked. Administration of MAO inhibitors (MAOI) must be terminated 2 weeks before β antagonist therapy. Hepatic enzyme induction shortens the half-life of lipid soluble β blockers, while cimetidine (Tagamet) prolongs their action.

Ganglionic Antagonists

Although ganglionic blocking agents will interrupt transmission through both parasympathetic and sympathetic ganglia, they are used most frequently to reduce blood pressure by suppressing the sympathetic branch of the autonomic nervous system. *Mecamylamine* (Inversine) is occasionally administered orally in the management of severe hypertension. *Trimethaphan* is a short-acting agent infused IV to produce controlled hypotension during surgery or to alleviate hypertensive emergencies. Blood pressure must be monitored, and drug administration is reduced gradually to prevent rebound hypertension. Preexisting cardiovascular disorders, especially those exacerbated by decreased tissue perfusion, mandate the use of caution when ganglionic blockers are used. Orthostatic hypotension is a prominent side effect; others are manifestations of parasympathetic blockade: decreased gastrointestinal and urinary tract tone, pupillary dilation, dry mouth, and exacerbation of glaucoma. Trimethaphan releases histamine from tissue storage sites such as mast cells. Mecamylamine crosses the blood–brain barrier and may induce hallucinations, tremor, and convulsions through central nervous system stimulation. Renal impairment increases mecamylamine toxicity. The hypotensive action of the ganglionic blockers is enhanced by concomitant administration of other drugs that cause a fall in blood pressure. Vasopressor agents such as the α-adrenergic agonists phenylephrine and mephenteramine can reverse excessive hypotension.

Other ganglionic blockers include pempidine (Perolysen), pentolinium (Ansolysen), and chlorisondamine (Ecolid). Nicotine will stimulate and then block ganglionic nicotinic receptors.

DRUGS AFFECTING SKELETAL MUSCLE

Neuromuscular Junction Blockers

Neuromuscular junction (NMJ) blockers interact with nicotinic receptors to interrupt the flow of impulses from the somatic nervous system to the motor end plate of skeletal and respiratory muscle. Two types of blockers are available. Nondepolarizing or competitive blockers can be reversed by agents that increase or mimic acetylcholine at the receptors. Depolarizing blockers produce sustained nonresponsiveness of muscle fibers that is intensified by acetylcholine or its analogues. Both types of agents produce flaccid paralysis and can cause respiratory arrest. Facial muscles are affected at low doses of drug, then the extremities, and, finally, at high doses, the diaphragm ceases to function.

d-Tubocurarine and dimethyl tubocurarine (metocurine, Metubine) are nondepolarizing analogues of the alkaloid curare. Metocurine has a shorter onset and greater effect than *d*-tubocurarine. These agents have some blocking action at the ganglionic nicotinic receptors, and also cause histamine release that will result in bronchoconstriction and hypotension. Pancuronium (Pavulon) is more potent than the alkaloid derivatives, has a more rapid onset of action, and is relatively free of histamine-releas-

ing properties. Its vagolytic actions may result in significant tachycardia and hypertension. Gallamine (Flaxedil) also does not release histamine, and has a shorter duration of action. It also has vagolytic effects and can induce tachycardia that may be hazardous in cardiovascular disorders. Vecuronium (Norcuron) and atracurium (Tracrium) are relatively short acting blockers with low incidence of side effects. The half-life of atracurium (approximately 20 minutes) is primarily a function of the intrinsic instability of the molecule in aqueous solution.

Succinylcholine (Anectine) is the most frequently used depolarizing NMJ blocker. Initial depolarization of the motor end plate will cause fasciculations. Subsequent nonresponsiveness of the receptors yields irreversible paralysis. Decamethonium, because of its marked depression of respiratory muscles, is seldom used.

NMJ blockers are used during surgery to provide deep muscle relaxation to accompany those general anesthetics that do not have this capability. Short-acting NMJ paralysis facilitates endotracheal intubation, and will protect patients from injury during electroconvulsive shock therapy. These agents may also be used in the management of patients on mechanical ventilation. Administration is usually by the IV route, although IM injection can be used if it is more appropriate.

Except for atracurium, which is inactivated in plasma, the nondepolarizing agents are excreted renally and thus will have a prolonged plasma half-life in the presence of kidney dysfunction. Succinylcholine is usually rapidly inactivated by a plasma cholinesterase level that is genetically defective in some persons, who will experience intense and persistent muscle paralysis. Dehydration and electrolyte imbalance (*e.g.*, potassium depletion, acidosis) can alter responsiveness to NMJ blockers. These drugs are usually contraindicated in patients with myasthenia gravis and respiratory depression. The intensity of NMJ blockade is enhanced by calcium, magnesium, general anesthetics, antibiotics (*e.g.*, aminoglycosides, polymixins, tetracyclines) that depress myoneuronal transmission, and drugs having a membrane-stabilizing or local anesthetic effect. Preadministration of nondepolarizing blockers will prevent the effects of succinylcholine, probably by blocking its interaction with receptors. On the other hand, nondepolarizing blockers given after succinylcholine will intensify paralysis. Patients who have received NMJ blockers can be completely paralyzed and unable to communicate yet be fully aware of their surroundings. Means for mechanical respiration must be immediately available when these drugs are used. Succinylcholine may cause malignant hyperthermia that can usually be controlled with dantrolene (Dantrium). Succinylcholine is contraindicated in open eye injuries and glaucoma. Administration during labor and delivery may cause apnea and muscle flaccidity in the neonate.

Skeletal Muscle Relaxants

Skeletal muscle relaxants will alleviate painful spasm induced by injury and by musculoskeletal disorders such as cerebral palsy, multiple sclerosis, and inflammation. These agents are often used in conjunction with rest, heat, physical therapy, and analgesics. Some have sedative and anxiolytic properties that possibly contribute to reduction in muscle tension. A placebo effect may also be involved.

Baclofen (Lioresal) is an analog of *gamma aminobutyric acid (GABA),* an inhibitory neurotransmitter in the central nervous system. Although its mechanism of action is uncertain, it crosses the blood–brain barrier and appears to reduce reflex efferent motor stimuli. Baclofen is especially useful in alleviating the spasticity of multiple sclerosis and spinal cord injury. It is well absorbed from the oral route and is excreted renally largely as unchanged drug. The seizure threshold in persons with convulsive disorders may be lowered. Side effects that can be minimized by cautious drug administration include drowsiness, confusion, mood alterations, hypotension, and nausea.

Chlorzoxazone (Paraflex), and carisoprodal (Rela, Soma), which is structurally related to the antianxiety drug meprobamate, may induce muscle relaxation due to their sedative actions. Drug dependence can develop to carisoprodal, which has also been reported to induce an idiosyncratic reaction characterized by extreme muscle weakness, confusion, and ataxia. Chlorzoxazone can be hepatotoxic, and both drugs may provoke allergic responses.

Benzodiazepines such as diazepam, chlordiazepoxide, and clonazepam are used as skeletal muscle relaxants. These agents are sedative and anxiolytic, and also appear to inhibit polysynaptic reflexes in the spinal cord. The pharmacology of these drugs is discussed under "Antianxiety Agents."

Dantrolene (Dantrium) is a peripherally acting skeletal muscle relaxant that blocks calcium availability and utilization and thus "uncouples" muscle contraction from stimulation. Intravenous adminis-

tration of dantrolene is an important adjunct to supportive measures in malignant hyperthermia induced by neuroleptic or general anesthetic agents, and can be given orally to prevent this medical emergency in susceptible persons. It is hepatotoxic and thus contraindicated in persons with liver disorders. Drowsiness, weakness, and diarrhea that can be severe are frequent adverse effects. Respiratory impairment can be exacerbated. Dantrolene has a long (up to 9 hours) plasma half-life, binds to plasma proteins, and is metabolized hepatically.

Administration of central nervous system depressants, including alcohol, concurrently with the skeletal muscle relaxants is generally contraindicated. Caution is also advised in patients who are dependent upon some degree of muscle rigidity to walk or perform other daily activities.

PSYCHOTHERAPEUTIC AGENTS

Major psychiatric disturbances are categorized into psychotic (*e.g.*, schizophrenic) and affective (*e.g.*, depressive) disorders. A significant number of psychiatric patients will respond to neuroleptic and antidepressant drugs, although many require long-term treatment to keep symptoms under control. The causes of psychiatric disorders are not fully understood. The observation that specific central nervous system neurotransmitter systems are altered by psychotherapeutic agents has generated biochemical theories for the evolution of these disorders.

Antidepressants

Tricyclic antidepressants (TCA) and *monoamine oxidase inhibitors* (MAOI) are the major drugs used in the treatment of depression. Although the exact mechanism of action of these agents is not known, most will suppress the inactivation of central nervous system neurotransmitters, norepinephrine and serotonin in particular. The original "amine hypothesis" of depression proposed that a deficit in these neurotransmitters resulted in depressed mood. However, the inhibition of transmitter inactivation occurs rapidly, while clinical effects develop over several weeks. More recent studies have indicated that most if not all antidepressant agents, including electroconvulsive therapy, cause a slowly evolving decrease or down-regulation in β-adrenergic receptor density that may be related to their therapeutic efficacy.

TRICYCLIC ANTIDEPRESSANTS

The TCA (Table 7-7) inhibit presynaptic reuptake of norepinephrine or serotonin, or both. The onset of therapeutic effectiveness is delayed for 3 weeks or longer, and patients may need encouragement to continue taking a drug when they are experiencing no apparent benefit. Severely depressed patients may require hospitalization during this time. Electroconvulsive therapy can provide a more rapid antidepressant effect that can then be sustained by pharmacotherapy. If necessary, drug doses can be gradually increased, with time allowed for a therapeutic response. Studies have suggested that treatment of depression is often abandoned before adequate dosages and time intervals are achieved.

The therapeutic usefulness of the TCA is limited at times by their adverse effects. The intensity of anticholinergic activity varies among these agents. Most can cause the characteristic side effects discussed earlier in this chapter, and are subject to the usual precautions and contraindications for anticholinergic drugs. High drug doses can induce central nervous system symptoms such as confusion, convulsions, delirium, and coma. The anticholinesterase physostigmine will reverse many of these effects, and diazepam can be given IV to terminate convulsions. Elderly persons in particular are at risk of TCA-induced anticholinergic toxicity.

The α-adrenergic blocking action of the TCA probably accounts for their ability to cause orthostatic hypotension and nasal congestion. Sedation is a prominent adverse effect, although the degree of drowsiness produced differs among the TCA. Since these drugs have a long duration of action (up to 72 hours), this effect can often be minimized or used to advantage by giving most or all of the daily dose at bedtime.

Cardiac toxicity is most likely to appear after TCA overdose or in persons with preexisting cardiovascular disease. TCA depress cardiac conduction in a manner similar to the antiarrhythmic agent quinidine. A widening of the QRS interval is characteristic of TCA toxicity. Severe bradycardia or tachycardia as well as cardiac failure can develop. Lidocaine or propranolol may control rhythm disturbances. Small doses of TCA can induce lethal cardiotoxicity in children.

Therapeutic doses of TCA can provoke seizures, especially in persons with convulsive disorders. Other central nervous system effects include panic reactions, mania, hostility, insomnia, and exacerbation of psychosis. Extrapyramidal disorders such as parkinsonism and tardive dyskinesia can develop. Increased appetite, endocrine changes, and gastrointestinal discomfort are additional adverse effects.

The TCA are hepatically biotransformed, some to metabolites that also possess antidepressant activity. Extensive binding to plasma proteins occurs.

Drug interactions are numerous. Central nervous system depressants, including alcohol, will enhance the sedative action of TCA. Other anticholinergic drugs will add to the suppression of the parasympathetic nervous system. Sympathomimetic amines that are transported by the presynaptic reuptake mechanism will be potentiated, while peripherally acting antihypertensive agents such as guanethidine and guanadrel will be less effective. Elevated serum levels of thyroid hormones (either endogenous or exogenous) can increase the risk of cardiac arrhythmias. Although the combination of TCA and MAOI can be hazardous, skillful concomitant administration of these two types of antidepressants is often effective in persons with refractory illness. Both drugs may be instituted simultaneously, although greater safety is probably ensured if the TCA is begun first, followed by careful administration of an MAOI. Cardiovascular responses must be monitored, and dietary restrictions relative to MAOI therapy (see below) must be observed.

The so-called "second-generation" antidepressants (Table 7-7), although related to the TCA, do differ in some important aspects. Trazodone, which interacts with serotonin receptors, causes less cardiotoxic and anticholinergic action. Maprotiline has a marked tendency to provoke seizures. Amoxapine, structurally related to the neuroleptic loxapine, has antipsychotic efficacy and may be especially useful when agitation or psychosis coexists

TABLE 7-7. Antidepressant Drugs

GENERIC NAME	TRADE NAME
Tricyclic Antidepressants	
Amitriptyline	Elavil
Desipramine	Norpramine, Pertofrane
Doxepin	Adapin, Sinequan
Imipramine	Tofranil
Nortriptyline	Aventyl, Pamelor
Protriptyline	Vivactil
Trimipramine	Surmontil
Second-Generation Antidepressants	
Amoxapine	Asendin
Maprotiline	Ludiomil
Trazodone	Desyrel
Monoamine Oxidase Inhibitors	
Isocarboxazid	Marplan
Phenelzine	Nardil
Tranylcypromine	Parnate

with depression. It can, however, cause characteristic neuroleptic effects such as malignant hyperthermia and extrapyramidal disturbances.

MONOAMINE OXIDASE INHIBITORS

Although the MAOI are effective antidepressants, they have been consigned to second-line status by their characteristic potential for provoking hypertensive episodes when certain foods or drugs are ingested concurrently. The MAOI irreversibly inhibit the enzymatic deamination of many amines, including the catecholamines. Thus they, like the TCA, enhance the availability of norepinephrine and serotonin at the synapse. Because new enzyme synthesis is required to overcome the action of MAOI, their effects can persist up to 14 days.

Common adverse effects include orthostatic hypotension, confusion, insomnia, dry mouth, blurred vision, mania, and alterations in cardiac rhythm. Severe hepatotoxicity can occur. The MAOI are usually not administered in the presence of hypertension, cerebrovascular disorders, or renal or hepatic dysfunction. Drug overdose can induce muscular hyperexcitability, hyperthermia, convulsions, marked changes in blood pressure and heart rate, and cardiovascular collapse.

Ingestion of pressor amines when MAO is inhibited can result in hypertensive crisis. Many over-the-counter cold remedies and appetite suppressants contain α-adrenergic stimulants, and many foods (Table 7-8) contain tyramine. Catecholamines or their precursors, or substances that release these agents or sensitize the myocardium to their effects can be hazardous. Meperidine (Demerol) is contraindicated, since it may trigger potentially fatal hyperpyrexic reactions in the presence of MAOI. Dosages of other narcotic analgesics should be reduced, since MAOI potentiate their actions. MAOI are he-

TABLE 7-8. Foods Contraindicated by Administration of Monoamine Oxidase Inhibitors

Aged cheese
Beer
Wines (e.g., Chianti)
Chicken liver
Bananas
Avocados
Soy products
Preserved meats
Meat tenderizers
Chocolate
Caffeine (in excess)

patically inactivated and will interfere with the metabolism of many drugs. Concomitant use of hypotensive agents such as diuretics and spinal anesthesia may induce a marked fall in blood pressure.

ADDITIONAL AGENTS

Lithium carbonate is effective in preventing and ameliorating the manic aspects of bipolar affective disorder. It is also reported to have antidepressant action and to enhance the efficacy of TCA and MAOI. The mechanism of lithium's action appears to be linked to an ability to decrease phosphoinositide turnover, which is an important biochemical pathway involved in transmembrane signaling by neurotransmitter receptors.

Lithium is excreted renally, in direct proportion to levels of filtered sodium. Thus, sodium depletion (e.g., that induced by chronic diuretic administration) will promote retention of lithium. The plasma half-life of lithium is also prolonged in the elderly and in persons with renal dysfunction. Large amounts of lithium may be required to control manic behavior. Dosages should then be reduced to maintenance levels.

Lithium has a low therapeutic index. Optimal plasma concentrations measured 8 to 10 hours after the last drug dose range from 0.9 to 1.4 mEq/liter. Elderly persons in particular may experience toxicity at levels as low as 0.4 mEq/liter. Adverse effects include nausea, severe diarrhea, weakness, tremor, ataxia, fatigue, thirst, frequent urination (polyuria), cardiac arrhythmias, circulatory failure, seizures, and changes in thyroid function.

Carbamazepine (Tegretol) is an anticonvulsant reported to alleviate severe refractory manic and depressive episodes. It should be administered only when other drugs have been ineffective. Several weeks usually are required for a significant therapeutic response. Carbamazepine can provoke fatal hepatitis and blood abnormalities, and drug-induced skin rashes can progress to severe exfoliative dermatitis. Toxicity is potentiated by erythromycin and isoniazid.

Neuroleptics

Antipsychotic or neuroleptic agents will alleviate both the mood and thought disturbances of schizophrenic disorders, and will calm aggressive and agitated behavior. Although these drugs do not cure psychoses, they often reduce the need for institutional care and enable patients to maintain relatively stable lives. The observation that clinically effective neuroleptics are dopamine receptor antagonists has yielded the hypothesis that enhanced dopaminergic activity in the central nervous system underlies schizophrenic behavior. Amphetamines, which stimulate dopamine receptors, can induce psychotic behavior that closely resembles schizophrenia.

Neuroleptics are classified mainly into three chemical groups (Table 7-9). Antipsychotic activity was first recognized in the phenothiazines; chlorpromazine is the prototype drug against which other neuroleptic agents are compared. The exact site of antipsychotic action is not known. However, the limbic system of the central nervous system has been proposed as the site of action because of its participation in emotional responsiveness and its rich dopaminergic innervation. Chronic administration of neuroleptics is often required to prevent recurrence of symptoms.

Side effects of the **phenothiazines** are numerous. Marked sedation is characteristic of many agents in this group, although tolerance can develop to this effect. Their anticholinergic action makes the neuroleptics subject to all the precautions and contraindications that pertain to drugs with parasympatholytic action. Blockade of α-adrenergic receptors induces nasal congestion and orthostatic hypotension. Severe reduction in blood pressure can occur in elderly or debilitated persons. Tachy-

cardia, bradycardia, electrocardiographic (ECG) changes, and cardiac arrest have been reported.

The phenothiazines exert an antiemetic effect via suppression of the central chemoreceptor trigger zone. They are used in particular to suppress vomiting induced by antineoplastic and general anesthetic agents. Paradoxically, they do not suppress vestibular emesis (*e.g.*, motion sickness) despite their antihistaminic action.

Extrapyramidal disturbances believed to result from dopamine receptor blockade or subsequent hypersensitivity occur frequently with neuroleptics. Parkinsonism, acute dystonias, and motor restlessness (akathisia) may develop early in treatment and can usually be controlled by reduction or termination of neuroleptic, or by administration of antiparkinsonian drugs. The most troublesome extrapyramidal response is tardive dyskinesia: choreiform movements usually involving facial muscles. Characteristic of chronic administration of neuroleptics, this syndrome is usually irreversible and does not respond to antiparkinsonian drugs. Tardive dyskinesia may not appear until drug administration is terminated, and can be precipitated or exacerbated by abrupt discontinuance of a neuroleptic. Simultaneous administration of antiparkinsonian drugs may mask the early symptoms that should prompt gradual drug withdrawal.

The ability of neuroleptics to alter temperature regulatory control can be especially hazardous in elderly persons. Fatal hyperthermia has been reported at normal and elevated ambient temperatures. Bone marrow depression, lowering of seizure threshold, obstructive jaundice, hyperprolactinemia, and other endocrine changes are additional adverse effects. Neuroleptic agents can add to the effects of anticholinergic and central nervous system depressant drugs. Because they are dopamine receptor antagonists, neuroleptics counteract antiparkinsonian agents and are contraindicated in this neurological disorder. Neuroleptics administered simultaneously with drugs such as lithium and digitalis may mask the nausea that warns of impending toxicity. The major site of neuroleptic inactivation is the liver, where several enzymatic pathways produce water-soluble metabolites.

The **thioxanthenes** are quite similar in structure and have much the same pharmacology as the phenothiazines. The butyrophenone haloperidol does not differ markedly, although sedation and adrenergic and cholinergic antagonism may be less than that occurring with other neuroleptics. **Haloperidol** will suppress the manifestations of Tourette's syndrome. Molindone and loxapine are

TABLE 7-9. Neuroleptic Drugs

GENERIC NAME	TRADE NAME
Phenothiazines	
Acetophenazine	Tindal
Carphenazine	Proketazine
Chlorpromazine	Thorazine
Fluphenazine	Permitil, Prolixin
Mesoridazine	Serentil
Perphenazine	Trilafon
Prochlorperazine	Compazine
Promazine	Sparine
Thioridazine	Mellaril
Trifluorperazine	Stelazine
Triflupromazine	Vesprin
Thioxanthenes	
Chlorprothixene	Taractan
Thiothixene	Navane
Butyrophenone	
Haloperidol	Haldol
Additional Agents	
Loxapine	Loxitane
Molindone	Moban
Pimozide	Orap

additional agents used in the treatment of schizophrenia; their actions are quite similar to other neuroleptics. Loxapine appears to pose considerable risk for convulsive episodes.

Anxianxiety Agents

Benzodiazepines (Table 7-10) are frequently prescribed to alleviate emotional and somatic symptoms of overwhelming anxieties. They are best utilized only for brief periods of time, since chronic administration of high doses can lead to psychological and physiological dependence. Patients should be encouraged to resolve anxiety-provoking situations, or to investigate nondrug modalities for coping with those that cannot be eliminated. Prior to the development of the benzodiazepines, the barbiturates were used as antianxiety agents and day-time sedatives, but frequently produced an unacceptable degree of drowsiness. The benzodiazepines have a more favorable therapeutic index, producing less general central nervous system depression when used in recommended doses and not combined with other depressants. Benzodiazepines are also used clinically as skeletal muscle relaxants, hypnotics, anticonvulsants, and as presurgical sedatives. The benzodiazepine mechanism of action may involve the ability to enhance the affinity of GABA for its central nervous system binding sites. This inhibitory neurotransmitter increases the influx of chloride ions through cell membrane channels and thus inhibits membrane depolarization.

Benzodiazepines are well absorbed from the gastrointestinal tract but less so from IM sites. The onset of therapeutic action is gradual; several days may be required to attain good anxiolytic effect.

TABLE 7-10. Benzodiazepines

GENERIC NAME	TRADE NAME
Antianxiety Agents	
Alprazolam	Xanax
Chlorazepate	Tranxene
Chlordiazepoxide	Librium
Diazepam	Valium
Halazepam	Paxipam
Lorazepam	Ativan
Oxazepam	Serax
Prazepam	Centrax
Sedatives	
Flurazepam	Dalmane
Midazolam	Versed
Temazepam	Restoril
Triazolam	Halcion

Intravenous forms are available, although changes in blood pressure, respiration, and heart rate may occur when this route is used. Respiratory and cardiac arrest have been reported following IV diazepam. Extensive hepatic metabolism converts benzodiazepines to a variety of metabolites including *n*-desalkylated and hydroxylated compounds and glucuronide conjugates. Several of these metabolites are pharmacologically active and serve to prolong the duration of action. In persons with decreased hepatic function (*e.g.*, the elderly) drugs such as diazepam and halazepam will produce extended periods of sedation.

Benzodiazepines appear to exert their greatest depressant action in the limbic system. However, these agents can elicit a significant degree of sedation, especially at the initiation of therapy. Driving a car or operating machinery can be hazardous activities for persons taking benzodiazepines. Concomitant use of other central nervous system depressants, including alcohol, can markedly potentiate central nervous system suppression to produce coma, respiratory failure, and death. Cross-tolerance in the mechanism of physiological dependence to alcohol and benzodiazepines enables the latter drugs to alleviate symptoms of the alcohol withdrawal syndrome. Long-acting agents such as diazepam and chlordiazepoxide are most useful in this context. Paradoxically, benzodiazepines have occasionally caused central nervous system stimulation resulting in confusion, delirium, and aggressive behavior.

Three benzodiazepines are valuable for the alleviation of insomnia. Flurazepam rapidly induces sleep but rapid eye movement (REM) time is suppressed, and daytime drowsiness can persist. Temazepam has a slower onset and a longer duration, making it advantageous for persons who have difficulty maintaining adequate sleep time. Triazolam has a short duration and is especially useful in patients whose difficulty is in falling asleep. However, early morning awakening can occur. Abrupt discontinuance of these hypnotics may occasionally induce "rebound" REM sleep, nightmares, and anxiety.

Midazolam is a rapid-acting parenteral benzodiazepine that provides sedation for brief diagnostic procedures and before surgery, and induction for general anesthesia. It can be mixed in solution with perioperative opiates and anticholinergics. (Diazepam is incompatible with most drugs.) Respiratory depression and occasional failure can occur. Hypotension can be especially severe when the opiate fentanyl (Sublimaze) is administered concurrently.

Alprazolam is unique among benzodiazepines in its reported antidepressant action. Other benzodiazepines are not recommended for patients with notable depression or psychosis.

Meprobamate (Equanil, Miltown), introduced as a skeletal muscle relaxant, was the first of the "modern" antianxiety agents but has subsequently been largely replaced by the benzodiazepines. This drug causes drowsiness, hypotension, and occasional hematological disturbances. REM sleep is suppressed. Tolerance and physical dependence can develop. Drug overdose produces respiratory depression, shock, and pulmonary edema.

Buspirone (BuSpar) is a nonbenzodiazepine reported to have anxiolytic properties. Sedation and impairment of motor skills are not induced by this drug, nor is the depressant action of alcohol enhanced. Dizziness, headache, restlessness, and dysphoria have been reported. Buspirone interacts with serotonin and dopamine receptors in the central nervous system. Persons who have used benzodiazepines may not respond to buspirone: its lack of sedative action may serve to dissuade patients of its benefit. Buspirone is rapidly extracted from the portal circulation and inactivated hepatically. It binds extensively to plasma proteins and may displace digoxin.

Sedatives and Hypnotics

Insomnia, or difficulty in falling asleep or maintaining adequate sleep, is a not uncommon disorder that can severely compromise physiological and psychological well-being. Attempts must be made to determine the cause(s) for sleep disturbance, and to alleviate problems through nonpharmacological measures. Drugs should be used only when other means are unsuccessful, and only for brief periods of time. Tolerance rapidly develops to the sleep-inducing action of sedatives and hypnotics, and chronic use may lead to psychological and physiological drug dependence.

A variety of drugs are used for promoting sleep. Ideally, such drugs should have a rapid onset of action, a duration of 7 to 8 hours (to sustain a full night's sleep), and no adverse effects that persist into the following day. Unfortunately, no single agent possesses all of these characteristics. Many sedatives produce a daytime lethargy or "hangover." As central nervous system depressants, these drugs interact with other depressants including alcohol, and many can induce marked respiratory depression and cardiovascular insufficiency when used at high doses. When taken in overdose,

either by accident or with suicidal intent, many of these agents are lethal. The benzodiazepines are the exception to this: overdoses can produce marked lethargy and somnolence, but are not reported to be fatal unless a second central nervous system depressant has been ingested concomitantly. For this reason, the benzodiazpines have largely replaced other hypnotic agents.

The benzodiazepines include several drugs administered for a variety of clinical indications. All will produce some degree of drowsiness and sedation, and three (flurazepam, Dalmane; triazolam, Halcion; and temazepam, Restoril) have been approved for the alleviation of insomnia. These are discussed under "Antianxiety Agents."

Before the advent of the benzodiazepines, the "short to intermediate acting" barbiturates (*e.g.*, pentobarbital, Nembutal; secobarbital, Seconal; butabarbital, Butisol; talbutal, Lotusate) were the most commonly used sedatives and hypnotics, and some are still available for the management of insomnia. In contrast to the benzodiazepines, which appear to suppress discrete brain areas selectively, the barbiturates are general central nervous system depressants. However, the reticular activating system is particularly sensitive to the latter group of drugs. Both classes of sedatives appear to exert their effects through interaction with the inhibitory neurotransmitter GABA.

The *barbiturates* are controlled substances; their continual use induces psychological and physiological drug dependence similar to that of alcohol. Withdrawal can be severe; symptoms include delirium, hyperthermia, convulsions, hypotension, and cardiovascular failure. Deaths have been reported to occur during uncontrolled barbiturate withdrawal. Detoxification of dependent persons can be most safely accomplished by substituting gradually diminishing doses of a long-acting barbiturate such as phenobarbital. This is usually done in hospital under close observation. The dose of barbiturate can be increased slightly if withdrawal symptoms appear, and seizures can be controlled with IV diazepam.

The barbiturates, like many other hypnotic agents, suppress REM sleep. Although the exact physiological function of this aspect of sleep in which dreams take place has not been determined, REM deprivation results in sleep that is not restful, and in rebound REM once use of the suppressive agent is discontinued. Consequent unpleasant dreams or nightmares may cause patients to resume drug use.

The barbiturates have many additional adverse

effects. Paradoxical excitation, confusion, and anxiety may occur, especially in children and the elderly. Gastrointestinal disturbances and suppression of respiration and cardiovascular function develop. Hypersensitivity reactions, in particular skin rashes that may be severe, are likely to occur in persons with allergies. Rarely, hematological abnormalities appear. Barbiturates can heighten the awareness of pain, although in combination with analgesics they ameliorate the apprehension provoked by pain and help to promote rest. Barbiturates are teratogenic, and can cause neonatal hemorrhage. Habitual use during later pregnancy results in neonatal drug dependency with an abstinence syndrome appearing shortly after birth. Administration of barbiturates during labor can suppress uterine contractions, and lead to central nervous system and respiratory depression in the neonate. Nursing mothers who use barbiturates may find their infants excessively lethargic.

Overdose of barbiturates causes severe respiratory depression; supportive measures must be instituted rapidly to prevent fatalities. Symptoms include markedly depressed respiration, Cheyne-Stokes syndrome, hypotension, tachycardia, hypothermia, renal failure, and loss of consciousness. Maintenance of respiration with supplemental oxygen may minimize hypoxic tissue damage. Attempts should be made to retrieve any unabsorbed drug from the stomach. Intravenous fluids may ameliorate hypotension and shock. Mannitol diuresis or alkalinization of the urine will promote barbiturate excretion, unless renal failure has developed. Hemodialysis can assist in the removal of drug. Patients who survive intentional overdose of barbiturates (or other substances) must be offered psychological as well as physiological assistance. The abuse of these drugs is further discussed under that topic.

The barbiturates are metabolized in the liver, and are capable of inducing enzyme activity. This is the basis for the decreased effectiveness of many drugs (*e.g.*, oral anticoagulants, digitoxin, corticosteroids, tricyclic antidepressants, and estrogens including those contained in oral contraceptives) administered concurrently. When barbiturates are discontinued, patients receiving other hepatically inactivated drugs must be observed for signs of overdose. The MAOI enhance barbiturate action by delaying their biotransformation. Barbiturate effects are also potentiated by concomitant administration of other respiratory or central nervous system depressants; respiratory arrest can occur. Administration of narcotics should be well-spaced

between doses of barbiturates if both types of drugs are required.

Porphyria, severe hepatic dysfunction, or previous drug dependence contraindicates the use of barbiturates. Extreme caution is required in patients with respiratory depression or renal impairment. Abrupt termination of barbiturate administration may provoke status epilepticus or other severe withdrawal symptoms. Injectable solutions of barbiturates are usually prepared at alkaline pH to promote ionization and water solubility of the drugs. Given IM or SC, these preparations can produce considerable local irritation, occasionally with abscess formation. Sodium phenobarbital is the least irritating of these agents.

Several drugs with pharmacological action similar to the barbiturates have been used as sedatives and hypnotics; these also are now largely replaced by the benzodiazepines. Glutethimide (Doriden) has marked anticholinergic activity in addition to its barbiturate-like central nervous system depression and suppression of REM sleep. Ethchlorvynol (Placidyl) may interact with tricyclic antidepressants to induce delirium. These agents, along with methyprylon and ethinamate, are controlled substances, capable of producing psychological and physiological drug dependence. Methaqualone (Quaalude) became so widely abused that it was taken off the market in the United States.

Relatively little respiratory depression is caused by *chloral hydrate* and triclofos, both of which are metabolized to the pharmacologically active trichloroethanol. Used as sleeping aids and for presurgical sedation, these agents are gastric irritants. Arrhythmias may develop, particularly in persons with cardiac disease. *Paraldehyde* (Paral) is a liquid with unpleasant taste and odor. It can be administered enterally or parenterally in the emergency management of convulsions (*e.g.*, in eclampsia, status epilepticus, and intoxication with central nervous system stimulants) and of hyperexcitable psychiatric episodes. The use of paraldehyde has been largely replaced by benzodiazepines, chlordiazepoxide in particular. Drug inactivation is largely by way of hepatic enzymes although up to 20% of a dose is eliminated from the pulmonary capillaries. Impairment of either of these systems can delay paraldehyde removal. Intramuscular injections are usually painful, and sites traversed by major nerve trunks must be avoided since paraldehyde can damage nerves. Intravenous injection, used only in extreme emergencies, can induce coughing. *Disulfiram* (Antabuse) interferes with paraldehyde metabolism, resulting in the characteristic reaction observed when alcohol and this aldehyde dehydrogenase inhibitor are ingested concurrently. Overdose of paraldehyde, although rare because of its disagreeable physical properties, can elicit respiratory and cardiovascular depression, hypotension, pulmonary edema, metabolic acidosis, renal failure, and prolonged coma.

Central Nervous System Stimulants

Central nervous system stimulants vary considerably in their pattern of effects, some acting most intensely at the cerebrum, others in the pons–medulla or the spinal cord. All have the potential to cause seizures, many are also cardiovascular stimulants. These drugs have few clinical indications, since other supportive measures are generally more effective and more easily titrated to the patient's response.

Doxapram (Dopram) and *nikethamide* (Coramine), which act in the brain stem, are occasionally administered to stimulate respiration (see "Respiratory Pharmacology"). Pentylenetetrazol (Metrazol) may be used in the diagnosis of seizure disorders. These analeptic agents appear to interact with GABA-mediated movement of chloride ions in the central nervous system. The possible occurrence of convulsions and severe cardiovascular and respiratory stimulation makes their administration hazardous. Barbiturates can terminate such seizures but will also produce return of respiratory depression.

Amphetamines and related agents (discussed under "Autonomic Drugs") are psychomotor stimulants that interact with sympathetic transmission. Amphetamines and methylphenidate (Ritalin) reverse the central nervous system depression that induces the sleep and cataplexy characteristic of narcolepsy. Methylphenidate and pemoline (Cylert) alleviate the symptoms of childhood minimal brain dysfunction (hyperkinetic syndrome). Suppression of nutrition and growth, and interference with sleep are adverse effects. Amphetamines have very limited use as anorexients, since tolerance and drug dependence (both physiological and psychological) develop rapidly.

Xanthines (discussed under "Respiratory Pharmacology") produce varying degrees of central nervous system stimulation. Caffeine, found in coffee, tea, chocolate, and cola, produces wakefulness and mild euphoria. This substance is available in combination with sodium benzoate to alleviate alcohol- and drug-induced respiratory depression, and in over-the-counter preparations to ward off drowsiness. The latter use is hazardous, since profound fatigue can develop. Excessive caffeine consumption induces insomnia, nervousness, palpitations, and other symptoms of central nervous system and cardiovascular hyperactivity. A mild form of dependence can develop, so that abrupt discontinuance of consumption causes headache and fatigue. Caffeine is combined with aspirin or ergot alkaloids, as it may be somewhat effective in ameliorating headaches.

Many drugs produce unwanted central nervous system stimulation, as do many illegal abused substances. The latter are discussed under "Drug Abuse."

ANTICONVULSANTS

Seizures arise from aberrant electrical activity in the central nervous system that is manifested in involuntary motor activity and changes in level of consciousness. Generalized seizures include general convulsions and absence seizures as well as akinetic and atonic episodes in which muscle tone is reduced. In partial seizures, limited areas of the body are affected, and consciousness may be lost. Convulsions have many causes, including epilepsy, brain tumors, head injury, hypoglycemia, eclampsia, childhood fever, drug overdose, and withdrawal from drug dependence. Astute diagnosis is required before chronic drug therapy is instituted.

Several drugs (Table 7-11) are available for the management of seizure disorders. Although these drugs represent several classes of chemical compounds, similarities are conferred by various combinations of five- and six-membered ring structures. Most anticonvulsants are effective for either generalized convulsions or absence seizures, and may exacerbate the type of seizure that they do not control. Termination of any anticonvulsant medication must be accomplished by a gradual reduction in dosage, since abrupt termination can precipitate seizures. Some patients respond inadequately to drugs; trials of several single agents should precede a decision to use multiple-drug regimens.

Phenobarbital has long been used in the control of generalized convulsions and partial seizures. Its mechanism of action may include potentiation of the inhibitory action of the neurotransmitter GABA. The most frequent adverse effect of this long acting barbiturate is sedation. Tolerance may develop, although some patients continue to report an unacceptable level of daytime drowsiness. Ataxia and allergic rashes can occur.

TABLE 7-11. Anticonvulsants

GENERIC NAME	TRADE NAME
Barbiturates and Related Agents	
Phenobarbital	Luminal
Mephobarbital	Mebaral
Primidone	Mysoline
Hydantoins	
Phenytoin	Dilantin
Mephenytoin	Mesantoin
Succinimides	
Ethosuximide	Zarontin
Methsuximide	Celontin
Oxazolidinediones	
Trimethadione	Tridione
Paramethadione	Mysoline
Benzodiazepines	
Clonazepam	Klonopin
Diazepam	Valium
Additional Agents	
Carbamazepine	Tegretol
Valproic acid	Depakene
Acetazolamide	Diamox
Phenacemide	Phenurone

Phenobarbital is biotransformed by the hepatic enzymes that are also induced by the presence of this drug. An initial reduction in the inactivation of concurrently administered drugs will often progress to more rapid metabolism and decreased efficacy. Drug doses that have been increased to compensate for this interaction must subsequently be reduced when use of phenobarbital is terminated. The coumarin anticoagulants in particular have been involved in this type of interaction. Phenobarbital can enhance the action of central nervous system depressants.

Phenobarbital is also excreted renally as unchanged drug; up to 25% may be inactivated by this mechanism. Alkalinization of the urine promotes drug ionization and enhanced excretion.

Other anticonvulsant barbiturates that are occasionally used are metharbital and mephobarbital, which is metabolized to phenobarbital.

Phenytoin, or diphenylhydantoin, is used extensively in the treatment of general and partial seizures. The hydantoins mephenytoin and ethotoin have no advantage over phenytoin and are seldom used. By decreasing intracellular sodium and calcium, phenytoin appears to suppress the spread of abnormal electrical activity in the central nervous system. A major advantage of phenytoin is its lack of sedative action. However, numerous other adverse effects can limit the use of this drug. Ataxia,

visual disturbances, dizziness, behavioral changes, gingival hyperplasia, teratogenicity, and hirsutism are characteristic reactions. Since phenytoin is a myocardial depressant, IV administration can induce cardiovascular collapse. This drug has some use in the management of cardiac arrhythmias.

Many drugs affect the hepatic metabolism of phenytoin. Inhibition of hepatic inactivation of phenytoin occurs with concomitant use of diazepam, cimetidine, dicoumarol, and disulfiram. Inactivation is accelerated by carbamazepine and theophylline. Phenobarbital and alcohol may either increase or decrease the hepatic metabolism of phenytoin.

Carbamazepine may be more effective than phenytoin in the treatment of generalized convulsions and partial seizures. Although these agents appear to work by similar mechanisms, they can have additive effects that provide control of seizures that are refractory to each drug alone. Carbamazepine is metabolized hepatically and induces enzyme activity. Its biological half-life can extend to 60 hours. Common adverse effects include gastrointestinal and vision disturbances. More serious reactions such as jaundice, hematological disturbances, hallucinations, hypotension, congestive heart failure, and rashes progressing to Stevens-Johnson syndrome are reported.

Valproic acid is effective in absence seizures, occasionally in cases that are refractory to other drugs. This agent will also suppress generalized convulsions and partial seizures. Valproate potentiates the inhibitory action of GABA in the central nervous system. It is well absorbed following oral administration, and is highly bound to plasma proteins. Adverse effects include gastrointestinal disturbances, hair loss (alopecia), headache, insomnia, weight gain or loss, and suppression of platelet function. Valproate can produce potentially fatal hepatotoxicity.

Valproic acid may be combined therapeutically with other anticonvulsants. It can elevate plasma levels of phenobarbital and primidone, and reduce those of phenytoin. Close observation is required, and adjustment of dosages may be necessary. Valproic acid can enhance the effects of central nervous system depressants.

Ethosuximide is a succinimide used very effectively in the management of absence seizures. Other drugs in this chemical group are methsuximide and phensuximide. Ethosuximide has a long plasma half-life; it is both metabolized hepatically and excreted as unchanged drug. Hepatic and renal function should be monitored in patients receiving these agents. Gastrointestinal disturbances occur frequently. Psychological aberrations, hematological disorders, a lupuslike reaction, and skin rashes including Stevens-Johnson syndrome may develop. The succinimides can induce generalized seizures in susceptible patients; they may be administered concurrently with other anticonvulsants to persons who experience other types of seizures in addition to absence seizures. Methsuximide is occasionally effective in refractory patients.

Trimethadione and *paramethadione* are oxazolidinediones that can induce serious adverse effects; thus, they are administered only when other drugs have proven unsatisfactory. Hematological disturbances, hepatitis, nephrosis, a lupuslike syndrome, and severe skin rashes occur. Patients must be closely monitored, and the drug should be discontinued if symptoms of adverse responses appear.

The *benzodiazepines* clonazepam and diazepam administered IV are especially effective in terminating status epilepticus. Clonazepam can reduce the incidence of atonic and akinetic seizures. Central nervous system depression and drug dependence are adverse effects of the benzodiazepines, which are discussed under "Antianxiety Agents." Intravenous phenobarbital and phenytoin are alternative drugs for treatment of status epilepticus.

The carbonic anhydrase inhibitor acetazolamide may be administered in several forms of epilepsy, often in combination with other drugs. The mechanism of action for its weak anticonvulsant action is not known, but may be related to its ability to decrease the formation of cerebrospinal fluid. Tolerance develops as this drug induces mild acidosis; efficacy may be restored by administration of sodium bicarbonate, or by intermittent drug administration. Acetazolamide is also used as a diuretic and in the management of glaucoma.

Phenacemide is used to treat refractory cases of partial seizures, especially those originating in the temporal lobe. Phenacemide has a high incidence of adverse effects such as psychosis, depression and other behavioral changes, hepatotoxicity, leukopenia, anemia, and nephritis. Treatment with phenacemide should be initiated in the hospital to allow for close observation.

Magnesium is occasionally administered parenterally to control convulsions in eclampsia, glomerulonephritis, and hypothyroidism, conditions in which hypomagnesemia may contribute to seizure activity. Adequate renal function is required, since this ion is inactivated solely by renal excretion. Magnesium is a uterine relaxant that can inhibit labor. Marked depression of the central nervous system and of cardiac and respiratory function can occur. Calcium salts (chloride or gluconate) administered IV can reverse the toxic effects of magnesium.

A characteristic shared by many of the anticonvulsants is their potential teratogenic action. These agents should be administered with caution in women of child-bearing age. However, therapy must be continued during pregnancy; the possible adverse effects must be weighed against the benefit of preventing seizures and possible fetal hypoxia. Phenobarbital in later pregnancy may cause a neonatal coagulation deficit.

While anticonvulsants do not "cure" seizure disorders, medication can occasionally be withdrawn from persons who have been seizure-free for a considerable time interval. Careful reduction of dosage with close observation is required.

Pharmacotherapy of Parkinson's Disease

Degeneration of dopaminergic neurons traveling from the substantia nigra to the basal ganglia (caudate nucleus, pallidus, and putamen) underlies the gradually developing tremor, rigidity, and bradykinesia characteristic of Parkinson's disease. This disorder can be induced by exposure to manganese, carbon monoxide, and other neurotoxins such as 1-methyl-4-phenyl-1,2,5,6-tetrahydropyridine (MPTP). Arteriosclerosis, and some forms of encephalitis, may also be causative factors in some forms of parkinsonism. In most instances, however, the cause of this movement disorder is not known. Reversible states of "parkinsonism" can be induced by administration of dopamine receptor antagonist drugs such as the neuroleptics.

Levodopa was the first effective drug available for Parkinson's disease. In modern practice, its use is often delayed until resistance to other therapies has occurred. Levodopa (L-dopa) is the precursor of dopamine but differs from the latter substance in its ability to cross the blood–brain barrier. Once in the central nervous system, levodopa enters dopaminergic neurons, is metabolized to dopamine, and released in the same manner as endogenous neurotransmitter. L-Aromatic amino acid decarboxylase, the enzyme that converts L-dopa to dopamine, is found in tissues outside the central nervous system, most notably the gastrointestinal tract, liver, and kidneys. To prevent breakdown of levodopa before it reaches the brain, a decarboxylase inhibitor is frequently administered concurrently. Agents such as carbidopa do not cross the blood–brain barrier, thus will selectively block peripheral decarboxylation. Lower doses of levodopa become effective, and side effects due to peripheral actions of dopamine can be alleviated. Sinemet combines levodopa and carbidopa, although the inhibitor alone is also available as Lodosyn to facilitate dosage adjustment for each drug.

Levodopa can effect marked improvement in parkinsonian symptoms, with tremor more slowly and incompletely resolved than rigidity and bradykinesia. However, levodopa often gradually loses its effectiveness, apparently as the loss of nigrostriatal neurons progresses. Rapid variations in effectiveness may develop during treatment with levodopa. Fluctuations in the plasma level of drug may be related to this "on–off" phenomenon, which is occasionally relieved by more frequent administration of levodopa or by the addition of bromocriptine.

Adverse effects attributable to levodopa include nausea and vomiting, orthostatic hypotension, dyskinesias, psychoses, and cardiac arrhythmias. Many of these will respond to reduction in dosage, and tolerance will develop to some. Nausea may be alleviated by taking the drug with meals, although food can delay the absorption of levodopa, and amino acids derived from dietary proteins can compete with levodopa for transport into the central nervous system.

Levodopa is contraindicated in persons with narrow-angle glaucoma or with a risk or history of melanoma. Extreme caution is required in the presence of asthma, peptic ulcer, or cardiovascular disease. Levodopa is not administered concurrently with monoamine oxidase inhibitors. Cautious use of tricyclic agents may alleviate the depression that often accompanies parkinsonism. The anticholinergic action of the latter drugs can be beneficial to parkinsonian symptoms, but may also exacerbate orthostatic hypotension induced by levodopa or the disease itself. Levodopa can potentiate the actions of adrenergic agonists. Neuroleptics and other agents that block dopamine receptors are contraindicated in parkinsonian patients regardless of drug treatment, since antagonism will further aggravate the striatal dopamine deficit. Pyridoxine (vitamin B_6), a cofactor for the decarboxylase enzyme, will enhance peripheral conversion of L-dopa to dopamine. This action of pyridoxine is suppressed in the presence of decarboxylase inhibition.

Bromocriptine (Parlodel) is a dopamine receptor agonist that works in much the same manner as dopamine. Its adverse effects, attributable to receptor activation, are similar to those of levodopa. Bromocriptine augments the action of levodopa, and can be effective when levodopa's usefulness is waning or unstable. Since dopamine exerts inhibitory influence over prolactin release, bromocriptine will suppress hyperprolactinemia and postpartum lactation. Chronic administration occasionally induces pleural effusion and pulmonary infiltrates.

Amantidine (Symmetrel) is a moderately effective agent that can enhance the action of levodopa. Its mechanism may involve release of dopamine from striatal nerve terminals, thus its action would be expected to decrease as neuronal degeneration progresses. Tolerance does develop to the beneficial effects but can often be reversed by interrupting therapy. Adverse effects similar to those of levodopa can occur. Congestive heart failure and a lowering of seizure threshold also are reported. Characteristic is livedo reticularis, a bluish discoloration of the skin, particularly at the ankles where edema may also develop. Abrupt termination of amantidine may exacerbate parkinsonian symptoms.

The efficacy of anticholinergic agents (see Table 7-2) in alleviating symptoms of parkinsonism appears to arise from a reciprocal inhibitory relationship between dopamine and acetylcholine in the striatum. As dopaminergic influence wanes, that of acetylcholine increases. Anticholinergics are especially effective in alleviating tremor early in the course of disease, and like other drugs, can add to the effectiveness of levodopa. Histamine H_1 receptor blockers that possess anticholinergic activity are also used; diphenhydramine is the most notable among these.

ANESTHETICS

General Anesthetics

The basic mechanisms by which drugs depress the central nervous system to produce general anesthesia are not clear. Theories based upon alterations in membrane permeability, depression of cellular respiration, and formation of crystal hydrates have been proposed to explain the effects of these agents, which represent several diverse chemical groups. The Meyer-Overton correlation relates their oil–water partition coefficient to their ability to act, or to reach their sites of action. The most potent anesthetics are those with the greatest lipid solubility. Agents with low blood solubility but high lipophilicity will rapidly leave the circulatory system and cross the blood–brain barrier. Drugs with a higher capacity to remain in the vascular compartment will require greater plasma concentrations to attain equilibrium and reach anesthetic levels in the central nervous system. However, there are many substances with comparable oil–water partition co-efficients that do not induce general anesthesia.

The major site of action of general anesthetics is thought to be the reticular activating system of the brain stem. This multisynaptic pathway has been shown to be primarily responsible for the control of sleep and waking patterns, as well as the integration of prolonged behavioral response to sensory perception. Anesthetic action at this level serves the dual purpose of producing sleep and decreasing sensory perception by reducing neural transmission to the cortex.

The objectives of general anesthesia are to produce unconsciousness, analgesia, amnesia, and muscular relaxation. Ether is virtually the only agent that can induce all of these responses. Other anesthetics must be combined with each other or with nonanesthetic drugs to achieve an adequate response. This is referred to as balanced anesthesia.

STAGES OF ANESTHESIA

The classic stages of anesthesia are most apparent when ether is utilized. Because this agent is quite soluble in blood and body tissues, effective concentrations are slowly achieved in the central nervous system and characteristic changes in levels of consciousness and involuntary activity are prominent. While many general anesthetics produce a somewhat similar sequence of events, some stages are minimized. Simultaneous administration of other drugs (e.g., in balanced anesthesia) can obscure these classic hallmarks that indicate the level of anesthesia.

Stage I, or induction of anesthesia, begins with drug administration and ends when consciousness is lost. If analgesia is provided, minor surgical procedures can be performed in this state.

Stage II, reduced with the use of many modern anesthetics, begins with loss of consciousness, and is characterized by central nervous system excitation, rapid, possibly irregular respiration, dilated but reactive pupils, and delirium. Involuntary movement and vocalization may occur; patients should be restrained to prevent injury. Salivation and vomiting present the risk of aspiration; thus general anesthesia is best preceded by several hours of restricted oral intake. Myocardial stimulation, evidenced by increases in heart rate and blood pressure that occur during this stage, can seriously compromise the safety of persons with cardiovascular disease.

Stage III begins with the return of rhythmic respiration, and is divided into four planes of deepening surgical anesthesia and muscular relaxation. In plane 1, the swallowing and pharyngeal (gag) reflexes disappear, as do spontaneous and reflex eyelid closure. The eyes are generally wandering and off-center. When the eyes become centrally fixed, plane 2 has begun. Most surgery is performed at this level, which is characterized by marked skeletal muscle relaxation when ether is the anesthetizing agent. Other anesthetics frequently must be supplemented with skeletal muscle relaxants to prevent reflex responses to painful stimuli. Increasing suppression of intercostal muscles, and greater diaphragmatic maintenance of respiration signal the beginning of plane 3. Skeletal muscle becomes profoundly relaxed, and certain types of surgery may require this degree of anesthesia. However, respiration can be seriously impaired. Paralysis of intercostal muscle activity marks plane 4, which is dangerously close to stage IV and complete diaphragmatic and respiratory arrest. Obviously, heroic measures must be rapidly instituted to prevent cardiovascular failure and death. Plane 4 and stage IV should be avoided, through careful administration of the anesthetic agent and close observation of patient response.

When drug administration is terminated, the patient will go through the stages of anesthesia in reverse order. Those agents that produce a characteristically slow induction will have a prolonged recovery period. Vomiting may again occur, and patients should not be left unattended until they have emerged from the delirium stage.

General anesthetics include both inhalation and intravenous agents, all having characteristic advantages and hazards. The choice of agent (or combinations of agents) is based upon many factors, including the physiological condition of the patient and the type of surgery to be performed.

INHALATION ANESTHETICS

Inhalation anesthetics include gases and volatile liquids that are absorbed from the alveoli. Their lipid solubility enables these agents to cross biological membranes, including the blood–brain barrier, and partial pressure gradients govern their pharmacokinetics to a large extent. Anesthetics are drawn into the lungs by either spontaneous or assisted respiration. Inspired gases contain a high concentration of the anesthetic, which will travel across the alveolar wall and into the pulmonary capillaries. A large fraction of cardiac output is delivered to the brain; thus, this tissue is exposed to a high concentration (or partial pressure) of anesthetic. Those agents that are less water soluble (*e.g.*, nitrous oxide) will leave the systemic circulation rapidly, entering the central nervous system as well as other tissues. Anesthetics with greater water solubility (*e.g.*, ether) will remain longer in the vascular compartment and have an extended onset of action. These agents are also sequestered in adipose tissue, although accumulation of drug occurs gradually because of the low rate of perfusion of this tissue. When anesthesia is terminated, the partial pressure of the agent in inspired gases is low, and promotes the removal of drug from the circulatory system and body tissues. Anesthetic in adipose tissue is gradually released, and can contribute to slow emergence from anesthesia.

Inhalation anesthetics are generally administered with "anesthesia machines." Completely open systems, in which liquids were dropped onto gauze or cloth face coverings, are obsolete. Current practice utilizes semiclosed and closed systems of administration. In both types of systems, anesthetic gas or vapor (the latter from heated volatile liquids) is mixed with oxygen and administered through a close-fitting face mask. Respiration may be spontaneous or assisted with a rebreathing bag. In a semiclosed system, exhaled gases are released to the environment. In a closed system, gases are circulated through a chamber that adsorbs carbon dioxide, and are remixed with oxygen and additional anesthetic and readministered to the patient. The latter system greatly reduces the exposure of operating room personnel to anesthetic, but does not allow precise control over the amount of drug in the inspired mixture.

The most frequently used inhalation anesthetics are the halogenated volatile liquids such as halothane, isoflurane, enflurane, and, to a lesser extent, methoxyflurane. Although these agents are similar in structure, their individual properties give them characteristic advantages and disadvantages. Because these drugs are nonflammable, they have largely replaced the use of ether and cyclopropane.

Halothane (Fluothane), relatively insoluble in blood, provides a rapid onset and termination of action. Because anesthesia is accomplished rapidly, close observation is necessary to prevent lethal overdose. Respiration is significantly depressed by halothane; ventilatory assistance is often required, especially at deeper levels of anesthesia. Hypotension, due in part to vasodilation, and myocardial depression occur. In the presence of halothane, catecholamines (including those exogenously released)

can induce severe cardiac arrhythmias. The risk of hepatitis and liver necrosis is reported to be increased in halothane administration, although many factors can contribute to this reaction. Biliary surgery and history of hepatic disease may contraindicate use of this anesthetic agent. Several months should be allowed between halothane administrations, since drug-induced hepatitis may represent a hypersensitivity response. Halothane, which produces little analgesia or skeletal muscle relaxation, is usually combined with other agents in balanced anesthesia. Halothane is partially metabolized by hepatic enzymes.

Isoflurane (Forane) produces less myocardial depression and sensitization to catecholamines than halothane. Pressor amines can be coadministered with caution. A greater degree of skeletal muscle relaxation is achieved, thus lower doses of neuromuscular blockers are required. Isoflurance undergoes less biotransformation than halothane, and appears less likely to cause hepatic changes. A major disadvantage of this agent is its unpleasant odor.

Enflurane (Enthrane) shares many characteristics with halothane, including rapid induction and emergence and suppression of cardiovascular and respiratory function. Myocardial sensitization to catecholamines and the incidence of hepatitis are reported to be less pronounced. An increase in respiratory secretions may occur. Compared to halothane, enflurane achieves a greater degree of skeletal muscle relaxation. However, at deeper levels of anesthesia, paradoxical muscle contraction may occur.

Methoxyflurane (Penthrane) produces slow induction and prolonged recovery; the latter may be shortened by discontinuing drug administration approximately 30 minutes before the completion of surgery. Its effects on the cardiovascular and respiratory systems are similar to those of halothane, except that myocardial sensitization is less marked. Methoxyflurane has significant analgesic activity. The use of this agent, however, has been greatly curtailed by its characteristic nephrotoxicity. Hepatic metabolism produces free fluoride ions that irreversibly damage tissue and result in high-output renal failure, hypernatremia, and elevated blood urea nitrogen levels.

Ether, once widely used, has generally been discontinued. Although it is one of the few agents that provides all the characteristics of general anesthesia with relatively little respiratory depression, it is highly explosive and flammable. Induction and emergence are prolonged and characterized by significant risk of emesis.

Nitrous oxide is a widely used anesthetic gas that induces analgesia and loss of consciousness but little skeletal muscle relaxation. It may be used alone for brief procedures, and is often a component of balanced anesthesia since it provides rapid induction and potentiates the effects of other agents. Nitrous oxide is administered in fairly high concentrations and must be mixed with oxygen to prevent hypoxia and subsequent tissue damage. This combination of gases is hazardous as it readily supports combustion; the addition of ether results in an explosive mixture. Central nervous system excitation and nausea may occur during nitrous oxide administration. Respiratory and cardiovascular function are relatively unchanged by nitrous oxide. The actions of central nervous system depressants such as barbiturates and opiates may be potentiated. Hypotension caused by halothane may be ameliorated by concomitant administration of nitrous oxide, in part by a reduction in the amount of the halogenated agent required.

Cyclopropane is seldom used, because of its explosive nature and its sensitization of the myocardium to catecholamine-induced arrhythmias. Induction is rapid, with good skeletal muscle relaxation achieved at levels of surgical anesthesia. Respiration and cardiovascular function are usually well maintained.

INTRAVENOUS ANESTHETICS

Similarly to the inhalation anesthetics, the IV agents are often used as components of balanced anesthesia. These are quite lipid soluble and are rapidly delivered to the central nervous system, quickly inducing loss of consciousness. The inactivation of (or emergence from) IV agents depends upon redistribution of drug to tissues such as skeletal muscle, and ultimately upon hepatic biotransformation. This is in contrast to the inhalation agents, which are relatively rapidly excreted by the lungs once the flow of anesthetic vapors is terminated. Thus the IV agents are not suitable for prolonged administration, since recovery would require an excessive period of time. Intravenous anesthetics generally do not enhance myocardial responsiveness to catecholamines, and they rarely produce emesis during induction and emergence.

The barbiturates include several drugs with varying durations of action that make them suitable for a variety of clinical purposes (*e.g.,* see ''Sedatives'' and ''Anticonvulsants''). Those barbiturates that are ''ultrashort-acting'' can be used as IV anesthetic agents. Rapid loss of consciousness and sub-sequent amnesia are achieved, but neither analgesia nor skeletal muscle relaxation is provided by the barbiturates.

Thiopental (Pentothal) is frequently used to produce rapid and comfortable induction of anesthesia that is then maintained with inhalation agents. Occasionally, brief procedures are accomplished under thiopental supplemented with nitrous oxide for analgesia. Characteristic of all barbiturates, the ultrashort-acting agents can induce respiratory depression and laryngospasm. Consequent elevation of plasma CO_2 may cause cerebral vasodilation and an increase in intracranial pressure. Myocardial depression and peripheral vasodilation, with subsequent changes in heart rate, can be hazardous in patients with cardiovascular disease or blood volume depletion. Allergic reactions to the barbiturates can occur. Drug-induced changes in hepatic enzyme activity exacerbate acute intermittent porphyria; these agents are contraindicated in persons with this disorder. Hepatic impairment prolongs the actions of barbiturates.

Methohexital (Brevital) has a shorter duration of action (5 to 7 minutes) and is used in a manner similar to thiopental. *Thioamylal* (Surital) is reported to cause fewer adverse effects than thiopental; both can be given to obtain control of status epilepticus. Thiopental can be administered by rectal suspension for preanesthetic sedation. These agents are sequestered in adipose tissue, from which gradual release prolongs their plasma half-life. Barbiturates are prepared in alkaline solutions (pH 11) and may precipitate in the circulatory system following rapid administration. Since methohexital is more potent, it is administered in smaller doses and is less likely to separate out of solution. Barbiturates should not be added to IV solutions containing acid drugs.

Etomidate (Amidate, Hypnomidate) is a rapid-acting nonbarbiturate used for the induction of anesthesia and to supplement agents such as nitrous oxide for brief surgical procedures. This drug does not provide analgesia. It has less pronounced effects on cardiovascular and respiratory functions than the barbiturates. Pain may occur at the site of injection; this can be reduced by slow administration into a large vein. Involuntary movement of skeletal muscles, and occasional changes in blood pressure and heart rate, are reported. Hypersensitivity reactions occur less frequently than with barbiturates. Etomidate may suppress stress-induced adrenal release of corticosteroids. This agent is not recommended for children under 10 years of age, nor for obstetric patients.

Ketamine (Ketaject, Ketalar) produces a dissociative anesthesia in which patients appear to be conscious but do not respond to external stimuli. In contrast to other IV anesthetics, ketamine produces profound analgesia. It can be used alone in subanesthetic doses for brief painful procedures. Cardiovascular and respiratory stimulation commonly occur, although suppression of these systems resulting in bradycardia, hypotension, and apnea are also possible. Persons with cardiovascular insufficiency or blood volume depletion may experience a marked reduction in blood pressure. Skeletal muscle tone increases. Elevations in intracranial and intraocular pressures may occur, making ketamine hazardous in head or eye injury or surgery. Emergence from ketamine anesthesia can be characterized by confusion, hallucinations, vivid unpleasant dreams, delirium, and vomiting. Patients should be kept in a quiet environment under close observation for 24 hours following ketamine administration. Severe reactions can be ameliorated with diazepam. Ketamine can be given IM, and is safe for cautious administration to children. It is inactivated hepatically.

Droperidol (Inapsine), a butyrophenone similar to the neuroleptic haloperidol, and the narcotic analgesic fentanyl (Sublimaze) are combined in the IV formulation known as Innovar that induces a state of marked analgesia and reduced motor activity. In this neuroleptanalgesia, patients appear somewhat detached from reality but are able to respond to verbal communication. Nitrous oxide may be administered concurrently to provide loss of consciousness. Cardiovascular function is usually not markedly altered, although changes in heart rate and blood pressure can occur. The opiate component can induce respiratory depression and emesis; these effects can be rapidly reversed by narcotic antagonists. Laryngospasm and bronchospasm have been reported, as well as extrapyramidal symptoms. Innovar can be administered also for presurgical sedation.

Opiates such as fentanyl, sufentanil (Sufenta), alfentanil (Alfenta), and morphine can be used as sole agents for some types of surgery. Because these drugs have little effect on myocardial activity, they can be especially useful to anesthetize persons with cardiac disorders. The drug doses required to induce anesthesia can severely depress respiration, frequently necessitating mechanical ventilation. Hypotension can occur, particularly with the use of morphine. This effect may be in response to opiate-induced release of histamine, since it can be ameliorated by concomitant administration of H_1- and H_2- receptor antihistamines. Excessive muscle rigidity may require the addition of neuromuscular blocking agents that will further compromise respiration. Close observation of the patient is necessary to ensure that an adequate level of anesthesia is maintained. Once surgery is completed, the effects of the opiate can be rapidly reversed by administration of a narcotic antagonist. Additional doses of antagonist may be required as the opiate is gradually biotransformed and eliminated.

ADJUNCTS TO GENERAL ANESTHESIA

Several types of agents are used in conjunction with general anesthesia to supplement or counteract drug effects. Since apprehension and anxiety can significantly interfere with induction of anesthesia, presurgical medication often includes a phenothiazine or a benzodiazepine. The latter group of drugs also induces amnesia, while the antiemetic action of the neuroleptic agents can suppress nausea during induction and emergence. Anticholinergics may be administered to reduce laryngospasm, bronchospasm, vagally induced bradycardia, or respiratory secretions, although most contemporary anesthetic agents are less irritating to the respiratory tract than ether. To provide skeletal muscle relaxation, neuromuscular blocking agents such as tubocurarine, pancuronium, and vecuronium are given. The action of these drugs is enhanced by nitrous oxide and the halogenated hydrocarbons, and respiratory arrest may occur. Succinylcholine, with its brief duration of action, facilitates endotracheal intubation.

Postsurgically, narcotic analgesics may be administered to alleviate intense pain. Patient-controlled intravenous administration of opiates is reported to provide satisfactory pain reduction with minimal adverse reactions.

Local Anesthetics

A number of agents (Table 7-12) are used to provide local and regional suppression of peripheral nerve function. Sensory nerves, with their smaller fiber size and relatively more surface area for drug action, are paralyzed more rapidly and at lower concentrations than motor nerves. Local anesthetics are thought to work at the neuronal membrane surface, suppressing depolarization and subsequent propagation of the action potential. Temporary stabilization of the membrane, apparently achieved as local anesthetics compete with calcium ions at neuronal membrane sites, prevents the influx of sodium that normally occurs during depolarization. Cal-

TABLE 7-12. Local Anesthetics

GENERIC NAME	TRADE NAME
Benzocaine	Ambesol, Solarcaine, Unguentine, Americaine, others
Butacaine	—
Butamben	Butesin
Bupivacaine	Marcaine
Cocaine	—
Chlorprocaine	Nesacaine
Dibucaine	Nupercainal
Etidocaine	Duranest
Lidocaine	Xylocaine, others
Mepivacaine	Carbocaine, Isocaine
Prilocaine	Citanest
Procaine	Novocain
Tetracaine	Pontocaine

cium binding sites may regulate sodium entry into nerve cells; reinforcement of calcium ion concentrations will reduce the efficacy of local anesthetics.

Two chemical classes, esters and amides, are represented among the local anesthetics. Both types of agents possess a lipophilic and a hydrophilic region. Esters are inactivated by plasma pseudocholinesterase; amides are biotransformed hepatically. Additional differences among these agents include onset and duration of action, local irritation, passage across mucous membranes, and incidence of systemic toxicity.

Cocaine, the oldest of the local anesthetics, currently is limited to topical application. This drug induces vasoconstriction, which tends to slow systemic absorption from skin. Absorption from mucous membranes, particularly of the urinary tract where its use is contraindicated, can be quite extensive. Cocaine inhibits presynaptic neuronal uptake of norepinephrine, and thus can exert sympathomimetic actions. This drug is discussed further under "Drug Abuse."

Procaine (Novocain) is regarded as one of the safest of the local anesthetic agents; it induces serious toxicity much less often than other drugs in this group. The duration of action (usually 1 hour) can be extended by the inclusion of epinephrine in injectable preparations. The vasoconstrictor action of the catecholamine slows systemic absorption of the anesthetic. Although the quantity of epinephrine is small, inadvertent IV administration of this powerful adrenergic stimulant can elicit marked cardiovascular responses. A major limitation of procaine is its inadequate penetration through skin and mucosal surfaces. Chloroprocaine is similar in action to procaine, although its duration of effect is shorter.

Lidocaine is a widely used agent that is highly effective following injection or topical application. Lidocaine's amide structure is biotransformed hepatically, in part to metabolites that retain pharmacological activity and appear to contribute to this drug's central nervous system toxicity. Epinephrine is frequently combined with lidocaine to intensify its local action. The use of lidocaine as an antiarrhythmic agent is discussed under that topic. Mepivacaine, quite similar to lidocaine, has a longer duration of action.

Tetracaine has a greater potency than procaine or lidocaine; its longer onset of action is coupled with a more prolonged duration. Dibucaine and bupivacaine also have greater potency and duration of action. Most of these agents are effective both topically and when given by injection.

Some agents (*e.g.*, benzocaine, butamben) are used only for surface anesthesia to alleviate discomforts of skin or mucous membrane disorders and injuries. Since these drugs are so poorly absorbed, systemic reactions rarely occur when they are used. Their most prominent adverse effects are dermatological in nature.

TOXIC EFFECTS

Topical application or injection of local anesthetics can result in sufficient quantities entering systemic circulation to induce serious side effects. The considerable lipid solubility of many of these agents promotes central nervous system reactions that may be excitatory or depressant. Toxic responses can include characteristics of both types of reactions; stimulation may be followed by depression. Central excitation elicits restlessness, anxiety, tremor, hyperpyrexia, and convulsions. Sedation, coma, and respiratory difficulty and arrest can also occur. Cardiovascular effects of local anesthetics include changes in blood pressure and heart rate, myocardial depression, and cardiac arrest. Upon injection, local anesthetics must not be inadvertently delivered into blood vessels. Means for resuscitation must be immediately available when these agents are used. Vasopressor amines and IV fluids may alleviate drug-induced hypotension; seizures can be controlled with diazepam or a short-acting barbiturate. Persons receiving MAO inhibitors or tricyclic antidepressants may develop severe hypertension following administration of local anesthetic formulations that contain a vasoconstrictor.

ADMINISTRATION

Anesthesia is accomplished by infiltration of a large volume of a weak solution (*e.g.,* procaine 0.5%) into the operative area, or by conduction block or regional block, in which small volumes of a more concentrated solution (procaine 1 to 2%) are injected around nerve trunks supplying the operative area.

Spinal anesthesia is a form of block anesthesia in which the drug is injected into the subdural space. Puncture usually is made just below the level of the second and third lumbar vertebrae, and the anesthetic is directed to the desired level by varying the injected volume, by barbotage, or by the position of the patient. Sensory and sympathetic nerve structures are paralyzed for a longer time and at lower concentrations than are motor nerve roots.

Tetracaine is currently the most frequently used agent for spinal procedures; lidocaine, dibucaine, and procaine are also used in this manner. Formulations that contain preservatives are not intended for spinal or epidural use.

Spinal anesthesia provides good muscular relaxation with a minimum of metabolic disturbances and no pulmonary irritation. Postoperative distention is less than with general anesthetics, since vagal tone is not affected. Disadvantages of this route include postpuncture headache (presumably due to meningeal leakage) and occasional paralysis of bladder function (due chiefly to paralysis of sacral autonomics supplying the detrusor muscle of the bladder).

Deaths from spinal anesthesia rarely are attributed to a rise of anesthetic in the spinal canal, causing corresponding paralysis of nerve structures regulating respiration and circulation. Patients must be closely monitored for indications of cardiovascular or respiratory difficulty, and resuscitative measures must be promptly instituted as necessary.

The disadvantages of meningeal puncture are avoided by the use of epidural or peridural anesthesia, in which the anesthetic is injected into the peridural space to travel out with the nerve trunks through the intervertebral foramina. Since relatively large amounts of anesthetic are needed, there is increased danger of systemic drug absorption.

Continuous caudal anesthesia is a special form of extradural block used chiefly in obstetrics. The anesthesia is delivered incrementally through a needle or a catheter inserted into the caudal canal through the sacral hiatus.

ANALGESICS

Analgesics provide relief from pain. Those used clinically can be classified into narcotic analgesics, which will alleviate severe pain, and nonnarcotic agents, generally effective only for ''mild to moderate'' pain. Since pain is symptomatic of an underlying disorder, the cause for persistent pain must be investigated.

Both types of analgesics have other therapeutic indications. Many nonnarcotic agents are also antipyretic and anti-inflammatory. Narcotic or opiate drugs are used as antitussive and antidiarrheal agents and for presurgical sedation and anesthesia.

Nonnarcotic Analgesics

Aspirin (acetylsalicylic acid) is the most effective and widely used salicylate, although others (*e.g.,* sodium salicylate) are available. Diflunisol is a derivative of salicyclic acid that retains many of the characteristic salicylate effects. Aspirin is analgesic, antipyretic, and anti-inflammatory. Its actions appear to involve both central and peripheral mechanisms. At the hypothalamus, aspirin interferes with the transmission of pain impulses, and restores the heat-dissipating efficacy of the thermoregulatory centers. Aspirin also inhibits the enzymatic synthesis of prostaglandins, the biochemical mediators involved in the production of pain, fever, and inflammation.

Aspirin (325 mg daily) is recommended for the prevention of myocardial infarction in persons with unstable angina pectoris or history of previous myocardial infarction, and also for the prevention of transient ischemic attacks and strokes in men. Suppression of the synthesis of thromboxane A_2, a vasoconstrictor and platelet aggregating factor, appears to be the mechanism by which aspirin exerts its protective action. Because of its effect on platelet aggregation, aspirin can significantly prolong blood clotting time. Anemia or spontaneous gastrointestinal bleeding may develop. Salicylates generally are contraindicated after surgery or concomitantly with anticoagulant medications.

Salicylates are gastric irritants that can induce stomach pain, nausea, vomiting, and erosion of the gastric lining. Additive effects of alcohol, corticosteroids and the nonsteroidal anti-inflammatory drugs will increase the risk of peptic ulceration. Other adverse effects, seen particularly in persons maintained on chronic high doses of salicylates, include dizziness, confusion, and tinnitus. Allergic reactions may take the form of rashes, angioedema, asthma, or anaphylaxis. Children who are prone to asthma often are hypersensitive to aspirin; the appearance of bronchospasm shortly after administration of a salicylate suggests that nonsalicylate agents be substituted.

Controversy persists over the relationship of aspirin administration during chicken pox (varicella) and influenza infections and subsequent appearance of Reye's syndrome in children. Many authorities recommend that acetaminophen be used if antipyretic or analgesic action is necessary in the course of these diseases. Children who must receive salicylates for the chronic management of inflammatory disorders should be inoculated annually against the prevailing strains of influenza.

Salicylates depress tubular secretion of uric acid, and in high doses block its reabsorption, exerting a uricosuric effect. The ability of probenecid and sulfinpyrazone to promote uric acid secretion is reduced by salicylates. Aspirin is contraindicated in persons receiving methotrexate since the renal excretion of the latter drug can be suppressed. The toxicity of drugs that bind to plasma proteins (*e.g.,* thyroid hormones, nonsteroidal anti-inflammatory drugs, penicillins, oral anticoagulants) can be enhanced as the salicylates compete for available binding sites.

Salicylates are well absorbed from the acid environment of the stomach. Because they are largely nonionized at normal urinary pH, these drugs are reabsorbed from the renal tubules. Alkalinization of the urine promotes ionization and excretion, and can be used to aid in the management of aspirin overdose. Hepatic enzymes biotransform the salicylates to inactive water-soluble metabolites.

Aspirin overdose can be lethal, especially in children. Acid–base imbalances occur as a consequence of respiratory stimulation, renal excretion of bicarbonate ion, uncoupling of oxidative phosphorylation, and accumulation of pyruvic and lactic acid. Hyperthermia, hypoglycemia, convulsions, circulatory collapse, and coma can occur. Extensive supportive measures are required to prevent death.

Diflunisol has a long (8 to 12 hours) duration of action. It is a less effective antipyretic, but its analgesic and anti-inflammatory actions are comparable to aspirin. A lower incidence of platelet dysfunction and gastrointestinal bleeding are reported.

TABLE 7-13. Nonsteroidal Anti-inflammatory Drugs

GENERIC NAME	TRADE NAME
Fenoprofen	Nalfon
Ibuprofen	Motrin, Advil, Nuprin
Indomethacin	Indocin
Ketoprofen	Orudis
Meclofenamate	Meclomen
Mefenamic acid	Ponstel
Naproxen	Anaprox, Naprosyn
Phenylbutazone	Butazolidin
Piroxicam	Feldene
Sulindac	Clinoril
Tolmetin	Tolectin

The nonsteroidal anti-inflammatory drugs (NSAID, Table 7-13) are a rapidly expanding group of agents closely related to aspirin and sharing many of its therapeutic and adverse actions. These prostaglandin synthetase inhibitors are useful in the treatment of rheumatoid arthritis and other inflammatory disorders in persons who do not respond to or cannot tolerate the side effects of aspirin. It must be emphasized that while aspirin and NSAID relieve the symptoms of arthritis, they do not prevent progression of the disease. *Ibuprofen* (Motrin, Nuprin, Advil) and *naproxen* are intermittently administered for relief of dysmenorrhea; their suppression of prostaglandin synthesis is thought to be the mechanism by which they alleviate menstrual discomfort. *Indomethacin* is investigational for inducing closure of neonatal patent ductus arteriosus. *Phenylbutazone,* among the original NSAIDs, is seldom used now because of its potentially severe toxicity that includes hematological disorders. *Piroxicam* is reported to have a longer duration of action than other NSAIDs and can be effective in single daily doses.

Although reported to be less severe than those induced by aspirin, gastrointestinal disturbances are a frequent effect of NSAIDs. Gastric ulcer and severe hemorrhage can develop. Preexisting peptic ulcer contraindicates the use of NSAIDs, indomethacin in particular. Severe diarrhea induced by mefenamic acid requires dosage reduction or termination.

Changes in renal function, including azotemia and anuria, occur. Preexisting renal impairment increases the risk of this adverse action; kidney function should be monitored in persons receiving NSAID. Sodium and fluid retention can exacerbate cardiovascular disorders. Hematological disturbances are reported. Inhibition of platelet aggregation is less pronounced with NSAID therapy, although these drugs require caution when administered to persons with coagulation abnormalities. Changes in vision and liver function can develop; monitoring of ophthalmic and hepatic activity may be necessary. Chronic administration of fenoprofen may cause hearing impairment. Persons who are allergic to aspirin are frequently also hypersensitive to NSAIDs.

These agents bind avidly to plasma proteins and may displace other bound drugs. The effect of anticoagulant agents can be enhanced. Indomethacin has been reported to reverse the antihypertensive efficacy of thiazide diuretics and β-adrenergic blockers, and to inhibit renal clearance of lithium.

Aniline derivatives have analgesic and antipyretic efficacy similar to that of aspirin, but are not anti-inflammatory. Their action appears to occur mainly in the central nervous system; they are weak prostaglandin synthetase inhibitors in peripheral tissues. Phenacetin is seldom used, except in combinations with aspirin and caffeine. *Acetaminophen* (Tylenol and other over-the-counter and prescription preparations) is a widely used analgesic that is generally a suitable substitute for aspirin. It causes minimal changes in gastrointestinal or platelet function. Cross-allergenicity with aspirin does not occur. Chronic administration can induce methemoglobinemia and hemolytic anemia. Acetaminophen overdose provokes slowly developing irreversible hepatic damage, and has been used by persons intent upon suicide. Administration of sulfhydryl donors such as acetylcysteine (Mucomyst) within 12 hours (possibly up to 18 hours) following acetaminophen overdose can prevent fatal hepatic damage. Chronic alcohol ingestion potentiates acetaminophen hepatotoxicity.

Additional nonanalgesic agents are used in the management of gout, rheumatoid arthritis, and other painful disorders. *Colchicine* appears to reduce migration of neutrophils to areas of uric-acid-induced inflammation. It provides rapid relief and can prevent recurrence of acute attacks. Gastrointestinal disturbances occur in a large portion of patients. Uricosuric drugs such as probenecid and sulfinpyrazone inhibit renal tubular reabsorption of uric acid. Allopurinol inhibits xanthine oxidase, which catalyzes the formation of uric acid from xanthine and hypoxanthine. Since the antineoplastic agents mercaptopurine and azathioprine are inactivated by xanthine oxidase, their toxicity is markedly potentiated by allopurinol.

Gold salts appear to interact with the immune system to prevent or retard the progressive deterio-ration of function in rheumatoid arthritis. These agents can induce severe toxicity, and are reserved for refractory patients. However, the greatest benefit is derived when gold salts are administered before significant damage to joints has occurred. Other anti-inflammatory agents can be administered concurrently. Gold is retained in body tissues for a prolonged period of time, although its removal can be facilitated with penicillamine or dimercaprol (BAL). Gold salts are administered orally (auranofin, Ridaura) or IM, and occasionally IV (Myochrysine, Solganol).

Penicillamine (Cuprimine) can alleviate the symptoms of arthritis; its onset of action, like that of gold salts, is gradual. Gastrointestinal, renal, and hematological disturbances may necessitate drug termination. *Antimalarials* (chloroquine, Aralen; hydrochloroquine, Plaquenil), which interact with several aspects of immune responsiveness, can ameliorate the symptoms of arthritis, as can the corticosteroids. Cytotoxic immunosuppressant agents such as azathioprine, cyclophosphamide, and methotrexate may be administered in severe degenerative refractory arthritis. Their use is limited, however, by their potentially lethal adverse effects.

The anticonvulsants phenytoin and carbamazepine can alleviate the discomfort of trigeminal neuralgia, while the tricyclic antidepressants are occasionally effective in diabetic neuropathy.

The alkaloid ergotamine is effective in aborting impending migraine headaches. However, the potent vasoconstrictor action of this drug can lead to gangrenous fingers and toes. Methysergide, a related substance, is a serotonin receptor antagonist that may prevent migraine. Its chronic use is limited by the development of pulmonary and retroperitoneal fibrosis. β-Adrenergic blockers also can reduce the incidence of migraine but are not effective in acute attacks.

Narcotic Analgesics

The narcotic analgesics differ from others in their ability to alleviate severe pain, in particular sustained dull visceral pain. In addition, the narcotics are neither antipyretic nor anti-inflammatory. These analgesics work via opiate receptors in specific areas of the central nervous system. Both the perception of pain and the emotional response to pain are altered by the opioid drugs. Endorphins are endogenous substances that interact with opiate receptors and appear to modulate transmission of information relating to pain, emotional behavior, and other physiological processes.

The usefulness of the opiates is limited by their adverse effects. Both drug tolerance and dependence develop to these agents, rendering them unsuitable for the management of chronic pain. Administration for more than a few days is advisable only in instances of severe pain accompanying terminal illness. Should the patient survive, drug dependence can be reversed. Tolerance will develop, thus drug doses should be just sufficient to reduce pain to an acceptable level. The euphoriant effect of these drugs makes pain less noxious; patients will experience pain but its anxiety-provoking aspect is ameliorated.

Opiate analgesics are respiratory depressants at therapeutic doses. Action at the respiratory control centers in the brain stem produces slow, shallow, irregular breathing. These drugs are contraindicated in persons with depressed respiration; they can progress to respiratory failure. Mechanical respiratory assistance must be available when opiates are administered. Because a reduction in pulmonary gas exchange will elevate Pco_2 and induce cerebral vasodilation, these agents must not be administered when intracranial pressure is or may become elevated. Furthermore, the central nervous system depression produced by the opiates can obscure the characteristic signs of neurological deterioration.

Although sedation usually results from narcotic administration, restlessness, dysphoria, and excitation may also occur. Loss of mental acuity ("mental clouding") is characteristic. Diagnostic of opiate use is marked miosis ("pinpoint pupils"), unless cerebral hypoxia and dysfunction have become sufficiently severe to produce pupillary dilation.

Nausea and orthostatic hypotension following narcotic administration can be reduced by encouraging the patient to remain recumbent. Tolerance rapidly develops to nausea, and higher doses have an antiemetic effect. Through their action on opiate receptors within the gastrointestinal tract, the narcotics increase smooth muscle tone, decreasing motility and prolonging transit time through the stomach and intestines. Constipation is a frequent consequence, to which little tolerance develops. Opiates are contraindicated in some gastrointestinal disorders; thus the cause for abdominal pain must be determined before these analgesics are administered.

Biotransformation of the opiates occurs in the liver, and doses must be reduced in the presence of hepatic dysfunction. Opiates potentiate the action of other central nervous system depressants.

Morphine is generally administered parenterally since its rapid hepatic extraction from portal circulation reduces its oral efficacy. It is used particularly to alleviate severe pain of brief duration. Often administered during acute myocardial infarction, it reduces pain and allays the accompanying apprehension that heightens sympathetic stimulation and increases myocardial oxygen demand. The labored breathing resulting from pulmonary edema is converted by morphine to slower, more efficient respiration. Presurgical sedation can include morphine, although low doses of this drug can enhance the emetic action of some general anesthetics. Morphine is antitussive and antidiarrheal; however, oral medications are usually preferred for these indications. Morphine can release histamine that will cause bronchoconstriction. Extreme caution is necessary when this drug is administered to asthmatic persons. Morphine also promotes release of antidiuretic hormone and of epinephrine from the adrenal medulla, which in turn causes mild hyperglycemia.

Codeine, like morphine, is a naturally occurring substance. It is a less potent analgesic but a highly effective antitussive. Codeine, which is orally active, is often combined with nonnarcotic analgesics such as aspirin (*e.g.*, in Emcodeine and Percodan) or acetaminophen (*e.g.*, Percocet, Tylenol w/codeine). Adverse effects occasionally observed with codeine include central nervous system stimulation and seizures.

As a result of efforts to develop potent analgesics free of opiate toxicity, many semisynthetic and synthetic narcotic agents have become available. Although they vary in potency and duration of action, their side effects do not differ significantly from each other nor from morphine.

Meperidine (Demerol) is administered orally or parenterally. Its duration of action is shorter than morphine, but it produces less intense spasm of the gastrointestinal tract. It is less potent both for analgesic and adverse effects. Like codeine, meperidine can stimulate the central nervous system; lethargy and seizures may occur simultaneously. This drug should not be administered concomitantly with MAO inhibitors due to the danger of fatal hyperpyrexic reactions.

Methadone is an orally active analgesic that has a prolonged duration of effect. This opiate is also used in the detoxification and maintenance of persons physiologically dependent upon opiates. Detoxification involves administration of methadone in amounts just sufficient to suppress the abstinence (withdrawal) syndrome; doses are then gradually reduced over several days until the patient is drug-free. Methadone maintenance substitutes this opiate for morphine, heroin, and other opiates. A well-managed methadone program should enable former "addicts" to return to a stable life-style although their opiate dependency is maintained. Unfortunately, diversion of methadone from treatment programs has created many addicts. Withdrawal symptoms develop more slowly in methadone dependence because of its prolonged plasma half-life.

Propoxyphene (Darvon) is structurally similar to methadone but its actions bear closer resemblance to those of codeine. It is a moderately effective analgesic frequently combined with aspirin (Darvon w/acetylsalicylic acid) and acetaminophen (Wygesic, Darvocet). In large doses, propoxyphene can induce seizures. *Levorphanol* (Levo-Dromoran) is effective orally and parenterally and produces less nausea than morphine. *Dextromethorphan,* the d-isomer of levorphanol, has considerable antitussive effect but a negligible degree of other characteristic opioid actions. *Hydromorphone* (Dilaudid) and *oxycodone* (Hycodan) are semisynthetic analgesics with activity similar to morphine and codeine.

Fentanyl (Sublimaze) is a potent short-acting opiate used as a component of balanced anesthesia. Innovar combines fentanyl with droperidol to induce a sedated analgesic state known as neuroleptanalgesia. General anesthesia produced with large doses of opiates such as morphine, fentanyl, and the related sufentanil (Sufenta) and alfentanil (Alfenta) can be used for surgery in high risk myocardial patients (see discussion under "General Anesthetics").

Natural opium alkaloids are available in several forms (Pantopon, paregoric, opium tincture) that have the indications and adverse effects common to all opiates. Heroin, or diacetylated morphine, has no approved use in the United States but is used in some countries as a component of Brompton's mixture and for the maintenance of persons dependent upon opiates. All of the opiates are controlled substances.

Agonist–Antagonist Analgesics

The search for nonaddicting potent analgesics has yielded several agents that have both agonist and antagonist action at opiate receptors. *Pentazocine* (Talwin) produces the characteristic analgesia, respiratory depression, and sedation of the opiates, although gastrointestinal effects such as nausea and constipation are milder. In higher doses its euphoriant effect is replaced with dysphoria, and hallucinations can occur. Caution is required in its use during acute myocardial infarction, since pentazocine can

elevate heart rate and blood pressure. Parenteral administration can cause subcutaneous tissue damage. Tolerance and physiological opiate dependence develop with chronic administration. Talwin Nx reduces the abuse potential of pentazocine by combining it with naloxone (see "Narcotic Antagonists" below), which is not absorbed from the gastrointestinal tract and will not interfere with analgesia when tablets are ingested orally. However, if this form of pentazocine is injected, naloxone will block the opiate receptor binding of the agonist. "Ts and blues" is a street drug combination of pentazocine and the histamine H_1-antagonist tripelennamine, which frequently induces pulmonary disturbances, vascular obstruction, and seizures.

Nalbuphine (Nubain) is a potent rapidly acting antagonist–analgesic that in high doses produces less dysphoria and respiratory depression than pentazocine. Its abuse potential is reported to be low. *Butorphanol* (Stadol) shares characteristics of both pentazocine and nalbuphine. These analgesics are administered parenterally and have a relatively short duration of action (3 to 4 hours). They can produce sufficient respiratory depression to cause elevations in intracranial pressure.

Because of their weak narcotic antagonist activity, the agonist–antagonist analgesics can precipitate an abstinence syndrome in persons who are physiologically dependent on opiates.

NARCOTIC ANTAGONISTS

Narcotic antagonists are classified as "mixed" or "pure." Mixed (or agonist–antagonist) agents exert both stimulating and blocking action at the opiate receptors, and include levallorphan (Lorphan), nalorphine (Nalline), and the agonist–antagonist analgesics discussed above. Pure antagonists have no agonist activity, they merely block the access of opiates to the receptors. Naloxone (Narcan) and naltrexone (Trexan) are in the latter category.

Narcotic antagonists reverse the effects of the opiates only; the actions of other central nervous system depressants are not ameliorated by these agents. A highly specific interaction of drugs and receptors appears to be the basis for the effects of the opiates and their antagonists. The latter drugs have greater affinity for opiate receptors, and will reverse the effects of agonists by displacing them from cellular binding sites. Thus, antagonists can rapidly reverse the symptoms of opiate overdose, and can just as rapidly induce (or "precipitate") the abstinence syndrome in persons who are physiologically dependent upon opiates. This type of withdrawal is not easily reversed by administration of opiates, since their access to the receptors is blocked until the antagonist is inactivated. Observations of the interactions of these opposing drug types led to the first investigations of drug receptors. Subsequent studies suggest that at least four distinct types of opiate receptors mediate various effects of these agents.

The mixed antagonists cause characteristic respiratory depression, although with a lower maximal intensity than that of opiate agonists. For this reason, mixed antagonists are contraindicated in respiratory depression unless it is severe and known to be caused by opiates. Mixed antagonists can exacerbate respiratory depression from other origins. In contrast to the euphoria usually induced by opiate agonists, the response to mixed antagonists can include dysphoria, anxiety, and hallucinations.

The pure antagonist naloxone is the drug of choice for reversing opiate overdose. Intravenous administration rapidly alleviates sedation and respiratory depression. However, this drug has a relatively short half-life, and central nervous system depression can recur if sufficient amounts of opiate remain after the antagonist is metabolized. Patients must be observed for returning signs of overdose, and additional doses of naloxone may be required.

Naltrexone is an orally active analogue of naloxone that has a considerably longer half-life. Chronic alternate-day administration of this antagonist may assist former addicts to remain drug-free, since it will prevent the euphoriant effect of opiates and obviate this positive reinforcing aspect of drug abuse.

CARDIOVASCULAR PHARMACOLOGY

Inotropic Agents

Inotropic agents are used in congestive heart failure (CHF) to improve cardiovascular hemodynamics. CHF is characterized by decreased cardiac contractility resulting in underperfusion of tissues. As blood pressure falls, peripheral vascular resistance increases reflexly, adding to afterload and further reducing cardiac output. Preload also is increased, due to increases in venous return and end-diastolic volume. As the diameter of the heart enlarges, cardiac efficiency declines further. Inadequate renal perfusion mobilizes responses that enhance vasoconstriction and sodium and fluid retention. As hydrostatic pressure builds in capillaries, fluid leaks out of the circulatory system and becomes evi-

dent as ascites and pulmonary and peripheral edema. Sympathetic stimulation is often increased in CHF, provoking a rapid but ineffective rate of contraction.

Inotropic agents are effective in CHF because they increase the contractile force of the heart. Cardiac output increases, blood pressure normalizes, renal perfusion improves, sodium and fluid are excreted, sympathetic activity abates, venous return falls, and cardiac dilation is alleviated. Myocardial efficiency improves while oxygen consumption remains the same or decreases.

Digitalis has long been used as an inotropic agent. Several substances derived from plants such as foxglove and strophanthus are commonly utilized: these are known as the digitalis glycosides (Table 7-14).

The basic digitalis structure is a steroid nucleus with a lactone ring at C-17 (together called the aglycone or genin) and one to four sugar residues attached at C-3. Removal of the sugars reduces the potency and duration of action of the drug. Saturating or removing the lactone ring nullifies inotropic activity. All of the digitalis glycosides exhibit the same pharmacology and toxicity. They differ in potency, degree of binding to plasma protein, route of inactivation, gastrointestinal absorption, and plasma half-life.

An important characteristic of the digitalis glycosides is their narrow therapeutic index. The dose required to achieve beneficial effects is close to the dose that can provoke serious cardiac arrhythmias such as paroxysmal tachycardia with block, premature ventricular complexes, nodal rhythms, bigeminy, multifocal ventricular ectopic tachycardias, and ventricular fibrillation. Persons receiving digitalis must be observed for signs and symptoms of impending drug toxicity: anorexia, nausea and vomiting, visual disturbances, weakness and fatigue, mental confusion and depression (especially in elderly patients), and psychotic behavior.

The toxic cardiac effects, and possibly the therapeutic actions, of digitalis appear to occur through inhibition of myocardial cell membrane sodium–potassium ATPase. This "sodium pump" normally extrudes sodium that enters the cell during depolarization, and transports potassium back into the

TABLE 7-14. Digitalis Glycosides

GENERIC NAME	TRADE NAME	ROUTE	INACTIVATION
Deslanoside	Cedilanid-D	IM, IV	Renal
Digitoxin	Crystodigin	IM, IV, PO	Hepatic
Digoxin	Lanoxin	IV, PO	Renal

cell. Na^+-K^+ ATPase has been proposed as the "digitalis receptor site." By influencing myocardial electrolyte concentration, digitalis alters cardiac electrophysiology. Increased amounts of free intracellular calcium enhance the force of contraction of the heart. Digitalis also has marked effects on myocardial conduction velocity. Atrioventricular (AV) node conduction and refractory periods are prolonged, predisposing to varying degrees of heart block. A pulse lower than 60 beats/minute (50 beats for some patients) in persons receiving digitalis can be a warning of approaching toxicity. In the ventricles, particularly in Purkinje fibers, digitalis shortens the action potential and decreases the refractory period. Automaticity is enhanced, giving rise to ectopic pacemakers and ventricular escape rhythms. The ability of ventricular cells to assume control of heart rate is enhanced by digitalis-induced AV block that hinders sinus rhythm.

In addition to its direct effects on the heart, digitalis also exerts cholinergic or "vagal" effects on cardiac activity. These actions, which can be reversed by atropine, include slowing of AV conduction at low digitalis doses, and shortening of the atrial refractory period. The vagal action of digitalis may help to slow cardiac rate in the failing heart, although the improvement in hemodynamics (*i.e.*, increased stroke volume, increased ejection fraction, decreased end-diastolic volume, decreased central venous pressure) and subsequent reduction in sympathetic stimulation also contribute to this effect.

The toxic effects of digitalis on the myocardium are enhanced by hypokalemia, hypomagnesemia, and hypercalcemia. While diuretics such as the thiazides and organic acid ("loop") agents promote renal excretion of potassium, these drugs are often administered concurrently with digitalis in the management of CHF. Patients' serum electrolyte levels must be monitored and consumption of foods rich in potassium (*e.g.*, fresh orange juice, bananas) should be encouraged. Vomiting and diarrhea, which often occur in digitalis overdose, can exacerbate K+ loss and further enhance toxicity. Potassium supplements may be required. In persons receiving digitalis, calcium salts (especially when given parenterally) are hazardous and usually contraindicated.

Several agents are used in the management of digitalis-induced arrhythmias. The antiarrhythmics phenytoin and lidocaine can be effective. Use of a beta blocker such as propranolol must be carefully monitored since these drugs can enhance AV heart block. Administration of potassium salts may alleviate ventricular arrhythmias, particularly if hypokalemia is present. However, elevated levels of potassium also can slow AV conduction, and the blocking action of digitalis on entry of K+ into cells will promote hyperkalemia. A specific antidote is now available for toxicity induced by digitoxin and digoxin. Digoxin immune fab (Digibind) utilizes drug-specific antibodies (similar to those used for radioimmunoassay of blood levels of digitalis) to bind the drug in the circulatory system and promote its removal from body tissues. The agent is usually reserved for severe life-threatening digitalis intoxication that is unresponsive to other therapy.

Additional drug interactions can enhance the toxicity of digitalis. Concurrent administration of quinidine, amiodarone, and calcium channel blockers will elevate serum digoxin levels, apparently through a decrease in renal clearance. Severe bradycardia may develop when digitalis and beta blockers are administered concomitantly. Sympathomimetic agents enhance ventricular responsiveness to digitalis, and anticholinergics, erythromycin, and tetracycline promote its gastrointestinal absorption. On the other hand, the efficacy of digitoxin is reduced by bile sequestrants such as cholestyramine that bind the drug following oral administration, and by hepatic enzyme inducers (*e.g.*, barbiturates) that accelerate its biotransformation. The plasma half-life of digitoxin is prolonged in hepatic impairment, and that of digoxin by renal insufficiency.

In persons who are seriously ill, therapeutic serum levels of digitalis may be achieved rapidly by administering large loading or digitalizing doses of drug. Lower maintenance doses are then substituted. The use of radioimmunoassay to monitor serum drug levels can be helpful in selecting drug doses that are therapeutic but not toxic. Therapeutic levels usually range between 0.5 and 2.5 ng/ml serum. However, individual characteristics influence responsiveness to digitalis. Hyperthyroid states, or administration of thyroid hormone, make digitalis less effective while hypothyroidism enhances its actions. Infants, especially premature, and the elderly are sensitive to the actions of digitalis.

In addition to CHF, the therapeutic indications for digitalis include certain atrial arrhythmias. Through its prolongation of AV conduction, digitalis will slow the ventricular rate in response to atrial flutter or fibrillation. Digitalis can convert flutter to fibrillation, which may revert to sinus rhythm once drug administration is stopped. In paroxysmal atrial tachycardia, the vagal action of digitalis can help to slow atrial rate.

Amrinone (Inocor), a nondigitalis cardiotonic agent, often alleviates CHF refractory to conventional therapy. A phosphodiesterase inhibitor, this drug elevates intracellular cAMP, decreasing Ca^{2+} utilization and inducing vasodilation. Amrinone improves myocardial efficiency with little change in heart rate or blood pressure. However, adverse central nervous system and gastrointestinal reactions limit the use of this agent to short-term IV administration. Milrinone, a derivative of amrinone currently under investigation, may have a more favorable side effect profile.

Other drugs that dilate blood vessels and thus reduce cardiac preload and afterload are used to ameliorate the workload of the failing myocardium. Captopril, prazosin, nitroprusside, and nitroglycerin have been used with varying degrees of success. However, all have characteristic actions that limit their effectiveness and that can exacerbate suboptimal hemodynamic functioning.

Antiarrhythmic Drugs

Several types of drugs have the ability to suppress myocardial action and alleviate abnormal patterns of contraction. A classification based on electrophysiological effects (Table 7-15) has been estab-

TABLE 7-15. Antiarrhythmic Drugs

GENERIC NAME	TRADE NAME
Class Ia	
Procainamide	Pronestyl
Quinidine	Quinaglute, Cardioquin
Disopyramide	Norpace
Class Ib	
Lidocaine	Xylocaine
Mexiletine	Mexitil
Tocainide	Tonocard
Phenytoin	Dilantin
Class Ic	
Encainide	Enkaid
Flecainide	Tambocor
Class II*	
Acebutolol	Sectral
Esmolol	Brevibloc
Propranolol	Inderal
Class III	
Bretylium	Bretylol
Amiodarone	Cordarone
Class IV	
Verapamil	Calan, Isoptin
Diltiazem	Cardizem

*For additional β-adrenergic blockers, see Table 7-6.

lished, although some drugs may have multiple antiarrhythmic actions. The class I agents reduce myocardial automaticity and excitability, slow the rate of depolarization, and prolong the effective refractory period. They depress ventricular automaticity to a greater degree than that of the sinoatrial node. Class IB agents have less effect on the rate of depolarization than those in IA, while IC drugs cause a profound slowing of depolarization. Class II antiarrhythmics are β-adrenergic antagonists ("β blockers") and will suppress the arrhythmogenic influence of sympathetic stimulation. Some of these agents (e.g., propranolol) also possess membrane-stabilizing activity. The major action of the class III agents is a prolongation of the myocardial action potential that can reverse refractory ventricular tachycardia and prevent fibrillation. Class IV drugs, the calcium channel antagonists, reduce the entry of calcium into cells during myocardial depolarization and recovery. Activity in the sinus and AV nodes is most influenced, making these agents especially effective against supraventricular arrhythmias.

Characteristic of class IA antiarrhythmics, **quinidine** depresses activity in atria and ventricles. Its action at the AV node can be influenced by the dose and by the degree of parasympathetic tone. In small amounts, quinidine is anticholinergic and will enhance AV conduction and sinus node depolarization rate. In higher doses, the direct depressant effect of the drug will prolong AV conduction time. Quinidine markedly prolongs the P–R, QRS, and Q–T intervals of the electrocardiogram.

The indications for quinidine include ventricular tachycardias and premature ectopic beats arising in the atria, AV node, or ventricles. It can convert atrial flutter and fibrillation to normal sinus rhythm, although digitalis is usually administered first to slow AV conduction and reduce the ventricular rate. Reentrant tachyarrhythmias (e.g., Wolff-Parkinson-White syndrome) can be controlled with quinidine. This drug is usually given orally, often to prevent recurrence of arrhythmias. IV administration is hazardous since the cardiodepressant action of quinidine combined with its direct vasodilatory effect can produce a profound fall in blood pressure. Extensive binding to plasma proteins occurs. Quinidine is inactivated by the liver, although a small amount is also excreted renally. Alkalinization of the urine reduces the degree of ionization of this basic drug and enhances its renal reabsorption. Hepatic dysfunction or congestive heart failure also prolongs its plasma half-life.

Like all antiarrhythmics, quinidine is also arrhythmogenic. Prolongation of the Q–T interval facilitates the occurrence of ventricular rhythms such as torsade de pointes. Quinidine can induce or exacerbate AV heart block and may depress ectopic pacemakers, leading to cardiac arrest. Sudden death due to ventricular tachycardia or fibrillation has occurred in persons taking normal doses and in those on maintenance quinidine ("quinidine syncope"). Quinidine reduces the renal clearance of digoxin, and in higher doses may add to the block of AV conduction. Additional adverse effects of this drug include gastrointestinal disturbances, blood dyscrasias, and cinchonism.

Procainamide has many characteristics similar to, and is used in much the same way as, quinidine. However, its vasodilatory and cardiosuppressant actions are less intense and thus it is more appropriate for IV administration. Procainamide is both inactivated hepatically and excreted renally. Renal impairment shifts biotransformation to the liver, and also causes increased plasma levels of the *n*-acetyl metabolite that also has antiarrhythmic action. Procainamide has a short plasma half-life, making it less suitable than quinidine for chronic prophylactic administration.

Procainamide can elicit hypotension, AV heart block, and ventricular arrhythmias, especially following rapid infusion. Chronic administration elevates serum levels of antinuclear antibodies and may induce a lupuslike syndrome that is usually alleviated by discontinuing use of the drug. Cross-allergenicity between procainamide and the local anesthetic procaine occurs frequently.

Because of their cardiodepressant action, both quinidine and procainamide require extreme caution in the presence of impaired AV node or ventricular conduction. Actions of other cardiosuppressants are additive, and congestive heart failure can be exacerbated. Hyperkalemia enhances responsiveness to these agents while hypokalemia reduces their efficacy. Because of their membrane-stabilizing effect, these drugs are contraindicated in patients with myasthenia gravis.

Disopyramide is administered orally and has a longer duration of action than other class IA agents. Its effects, both direct and via cholinergic antagonism, resemble those of quinidine and procainamide. It is used in particular for ventricular arrhythmias. Disopyramide is reported to have a lower incidence of adverse effects, although it can induce hypotension, congestive heart failure, and arrhythmias. Either renal or hepatic impairment may require a reduction in dosage.

Lidocaine has long been the prototype class IB antiarrhythmic. Its major disadvantage is its lack of effectiveness following oral administration, caused by extensive first-pass hepatic extraction that prevents attainment of therapeutic blood levels. Its short plasma half-life necessitates continuous IV infusion (often preceded by a bolus dose) and is lengthened by impairment of hepatic function or perfusion. Lidocaine's greatest effect is on ventricular conduction, with minimal actions in supraventricular areas. The P–R, QRS, and Q–T intervals usually are unaffected. Lidocaine is often the drug of choice to terminate or prevent ventricular arrhythmias subsequent to acute myocardial infarction or digitalis toxicity. Neurotoxic metabolites of lidocaine can cause drowsiness, disorientation, respiratory depression, and convulsions. A single IM dose of lidocaine may be administered in certain emergency situations to control or prevent arrhythmias. Concurrent propranolol administration can prolong lidocaine's action.

Mexiletine and *tocainide* are orally active analogues of lidocaine. Their effectiveness and pharmacokinetics are similar to lidocaine, with the exception that hepatic metabolism occurs more slowly and sustained ventricular tachycardia is less responsive. Adverse effects of these agents include gastrointestinal disturbances (foods or antacids may alleviate these symptoms) and central nervous system toxicity. Tocainide can induce agranulocytosis. Changes in urinary pH can significantly influence renal clearance.

Phenytoin has electrophysiological actions quite similar to lidocaine. It can be given orally or IV, although rapid administration by the latter route can cause cardiac arrest. Absorption after oral administration is slow; hepatic metabolism of this drug shows great variability among patients. Phenytoin is most effective in ventricular arrhythmias that result from acute myocardial infarction and digitalis toxicity. Hypotension following phenytoin administration is due partly to its vasodilatory action. Hyperglycemia, hematologic abnormalities, and severe skin rashes may occur. Other characteristics of phenytoin are discussed under "Anticonvulsants."

Class IC drugs such as *flecainide* and *encainide* markedly suppress myocardial conduction and prolong the ventricular refractory period. Ventricular arrhythmias are especially responsive to these agents. They can, however, provoke or intensify rhythm disturbances. Flecainide can induce AV heart block and may exacerbate sinus node and left ventricular dysfunction. The extent of biotransformation of encainide to a pharmacologically active metabolite varies among individuals. Flecainide, inactivated by both hepatic and renal mechanisms, has a long plasma half-life (13 to 16 hours) that may be extended in the presence of cardiovascular disease. Concurrent administration of other antiarrhythmics or cardiac suppressants is usually contraindicated.

Those β-blockers with membrane-stabilizing action (e.g., propranolol and acebutolol) are the most effective class II antiarrhythmics. Suppression of sympathetic stimulation also contributes to control of rhythm disturbances but can be hazardous in patients with compensated heart failure sustained by increased adrenergic tone. β-Blockers suppress activity in all cardiac regions. Sinoatrial node depolarization and AV node conduction are slowed, atrial excitability and conductivity and ventricular automaticity are reduced. β-Blockers have negative inotropic and chronotropic effects. They are especially useful in suppressing arrhythmias enhanced by prolongation of the Q–T interval as well as those induced by excessive catecholamine activity, such as in thyrotoxicosis and halothane or cyclopropane anesthesia. β-Blockers can elicit hypotension, hypoglycemia, and bronchospasm that is resistant to β-agonists. Likewise, congestive heart failure exacerbated or induced by β-blockers can be unresponsive to catecholamines. However, glucagon or amrinone can stimulate cardiac activity in the presence of β-receptor blockade. Other cardiac depressants can add to that effect of the β-blockers. Acebutolol is somewhat β-1-receptor-selective and has less intense metabolic and respiratory effects than propranolol. It also has partial agonist activity and thus causes less slowing of atrial rate. The β blockers are discussed further under "Sympathomimetic Drugs."

The class III antiarrhythmic agents prolong the duration of the myocardial action potential and are especially effective in controlling refractory ventricular tachyarrhythmias and in preventing ventricular fibrillation. **Bretylium** is administered IV to patients who have not responded to other first-line antiarrhythmics. An initial release of catecholamines from sympathetic nerve terminals can elicit a brief exacerbation of tachycardia and vasoconstriction. Then sympathetic block ensues due to depletion of norepinephrine stores. Duration of therapy is usually limited to 5 days. Hypotension is the major adverse reaction. Bretylium enhances myocardial responsiveness to electrical defibrillation.

Amiodarone is administered orally to control severe refractory ventricular arrhythmias. It prolongs the myocardial refractory period and the P–R, QRS, and Q–T intervals. A large percentage of persons treated with this drug experience a variety of adverse effects. Hepatotoxicity, nephrotoxicity, pulmonary alveolitis, congestive heart failure, and exacerbation of arrhythmias are among the most serious. Nausea, corneal microdeposits, central nervous system dysfunction, changes in thyroid activity, photosensitivity, and skin discoloration also occur. Amiodarone is excreted in the bile and has a remarkably long (from 10 to 50 days) plasma half-life. The inactivation of many drugs, including digoxin, oral anticoagulants, and other antiarrhythmics, is inhibited.

Verapamil is the calcium channel blocker most frequently used for treatment and prevention of supraventricular tachycardias. It causes marked depression of AV conduction and slowing of sinus node depolarization may occur. Verapamil binds extensively to plasma proteins and is inactivated hepatically. IV administration produces a rapid onset of action. Combination with a β antagonist can elicit extreme bradycardia, while concurrent disopyramide can precipitate congestive heart failure. Verapamil administered in the presence of Wolff-Parkinson-White syndrome is hazardous. The calcium channel blockers are used also as antihypertensive and antianginal agents and are discussed under those headings.

Hypolipemic Agents

The complexes of lipid and protein (lipoproteins) found in the circulatory system are of several types. Chylomicrons are the least dense. They are composed mainly of dietary triglycerides and are present in the greatest amounts shortly after eating. Very low density lipoproteins (VLDL) or prebeta lipoproteins carry triglycerides and cholesterol within the circulatory system. Low-density lipoproteins (LDL) contain large amounts of cholesterol; elevated levels of LDL have been found to correlate with increased risk of coronary heart disease (CHD). High-density lipoproteins (HDL) contain small amounts of triglycerides and cholesterol and appear to transport the latter from body tissues to the liver. Elevated levels of these lipoproteins are associated with reduced risk of CHD.

Hyperlipidemia, or elevated blood levels of lipoproteins, occurs in various forms (Table 7-16). Although there is still some controversy over the relationship between elevated serum lipid levels and the development of CHD, attempts are usually made to correct hyperlipidemia. Dietary changes such as decreased calorie and saturated fat ingestion are used first in the management of elevated lipid levels. If these measures are not effective after a trial of at

TABLE 7-16. Hyperlipidemias

TYPE	LIPIDS ELEVATED
I	Chylomicrons, Triglycerides
IIa	LDL, Cholesterol, Triglycerides
IIb	LDL, VLDL
III	Cholesterol, Triglycerides
IV	VLDL, Triglycerides
V	Chylomicrons, VLDL, Cholesterol, Triglycerides

least 6 months, drugs may have to be administered. Dietary modifications must be continued to enhance the efficacy of pharmacotherapy.

Several types of hypolipemic agents are available. Clofibrate (Atromid S), most useful for types III, IV, and V hyperlipidemias, appears to inhibit synthesis and/or secretion of hepatic cholesterol and release of VLDL into plasma. It also reduces serum levels of VLDL by enhancing the activity of lipoprotein lipase. Biliary and fecal excretion of cholesterol are increased. The most common side effects of this drug are gastrointestinal disturbances. Cardiac arrhythmias and reactivation of peptic ulcer have been reported. Clofibrate may be teratogenic and carcinogenic. It potentiates the effects of oral anticoagulants.

Gemfibrozil (Lopid), which is similar to clofibrate in its actions, is occasionally administered in refractory hyperlipidemia. Both drugs have been associated with the development of gallstones. Persons receiving hypoglycemic drugs may require increased doses when gemfibrozil is administered concurrently.

The anion-exchange resins cholestyramine (Questran) and colestipol (Colestid), which bind bile acids in the intestine and promote their excretion in the feces, are used in the management of type II hyperlipidemia. Cholesterol metabolism is increased, while its serum levels and those of LDL are lowered. The resins are suspended in water or juice and are consumed at mealtimes. Gastrointestinal distress is the most frequent adverse effect. Since fat-soluble vitamins (A, D, and K) also bind to these resins, deficiencies can develop. The gastrointestinal absorption of many drugs (e.g., digoxin, warfarin, antibiotics, and thiazide diuretics) is reduced by concomitant resin administration. Cholestyramine is also used to alleviate pruritus associated with biliary tract obstruction.

Nicotinic acid lowers plasma levels of VLDL and LDL and elevates HDL levels. Its administration has been associated with decreased risk of CHD. The prominent side effect of cutaneous flushing can be alleviated with inhibitors of prostaglandin syn-

thesis. Nicotinic acid is hepatotoxic, can decrease glucose tolerance, and can activate peptic ulcer. Because of its relaxant effect on blood vessels, it should not be administered to persons with marked hypotension. It can add to the effects of antihypertensive agents. In the treatment of hyperlipidemia, nicotinic acid used concurrently with bile-acid binding resins is an effective regimen for achieving maximal reductions in LDL cholesterol.

Probucol (Lorelco) is a second-line hypolipemic agent that reduces plasma levels of both LDL and HDL. The mechanism of action of probucol is not completely understood. It has been reported to increase LDL catabolism and the biliary excretion of cholesterol. Since this drug is cardiotoxic, it is contraindicated in patients with cardiac arrhythmias or Q-T interval prolongation. The most frequent adverse effects are gastrointestinal disturbances and headache.

The observation that premenopausal women have a low incidence of CHD led to the investigation of female hormones as antilipemic agents. While estrogens lower serum cholesterol levels, they elevate triglyceride levels and have not been proven effective. They produce feminizing side effects, and are contraindicated in the presence of thromboembolic disorders, pregnancy, and estrogen-dependent breast carcinoma.

Thyroid hormones serve to normalize serum cholesterol levels, and dextrothyroxine (Choloxin) has some use in treatment of type II hyperlipemia. The turnover and excretion of cholesterol appear to increase, resulting in lowered serum levels of LDL. Dextrothyroxine is contraindicated in persons with cardiovascular disease.

Lovastatin (Mevacor), useful in the treatment of type II hyperlipidemia, interferes with cholesterol formation by inhibiting the rate-limiting enzyme for cholesterol synthesis, HMG CoA reductase. Reductions in plasma LDL cholesterol levels of 35% to 38% have been reported and greater than 50% reductions have been achieved when this drug is administered in combination with either nicotinic acid or cholestyramine. Myositis, renal failure, headache, gastrointestinal distress, lens opacities, and elevation of serum aminotransferase levels have been reported. Visual acuity and hepatic function should be monitored. The long-term safety of lovastatin is yet to be established.

Pharmacotherapy of Angina Pectoris

Angina pectoris is chest pain that occurs when the myocardial oxygen supply becomes inadequate. Effort-induced or classic angina develops when atherosclerotic deposits encroach upon the coronary blood supply and compromise the ability of coronary vessels to dilate. An increased cardiac workload fails to elicit an increase in blood flow, and oxygen demands are not satisfied. Variant or Prinzmetal's angina, which appears to result from coronary artery vasospasm, can occur even in the absence of physical or psychological stress. Myocardial infarction can occur if periods of ischemia are prolonged. Drugs that increase coronary perfusion or decrease the myocardial workload can alleviate ischemic pain. Some antianginal drugs exert both effects. Reduction in the incidence and severity of anginal attacks, and increased exercise tolerance, are the goals of antianginal therapy.

Nitroglycerin and related nitrates continue to be the primary drugs used in the prevention and alleviation of angina. Nitroglycerin is inactive when given orally but its marked lipid solubility allows rapid absorption and onset of action following sublingual administration. Transdermal and transmucosal forms of this nitrate are also available (Table 7-17). The efficacy of the transdermal patches has been questioned. Intravenous nitroglycerin (Tridil, Nitro-Bid IV, Nitrostat IV) can be used to maintain consistent plasma levels of drug. Isosorbide dinitrate, erythrityl tetranitrate (Peritrate) and pentaerythrityl tetranitrate are administered orally and sublingually. Amyl nitrate is inhaled to alleviate anginal pain. Sustained-release forms can prolong the duration of action of these drugs, which are rapidly inactivated in the liver.

The nitrates relax smooth muscle of arteries and veins. Arteriolar dilation decreases the resistance to cardial outflow (afterload), while dilation of veins reduces venous return to the right atrium (preload). Both of these effects reduce myocardial oxygen demand. The nitrates can elicit marked hypotension with reflex tachycardia that may intensify myocardial ischemia. Postural hypotension frequently occurs, and dilation of cerebral vessels can induce

headaches. Tolerance may develop to side effects and also to the beneficial effects of the nitrates; this can be minimized by administering doses that are just effective and by alternating therapy with other antianginal agents. Sublingual nitroglycerin tablets should provide rapid relief from pain. Failure of two or three tablets administered 5 minutes apart may indicate acute myocardial infarction. Nitroglycerin tablets must be stored properly to prevent spontaneous decomposition. Termination of nitrate administration must be accomplished gradually to avoid angina recurrence or myocardial infarction. Persons exposed to industrial sources of nitroglycerin may experience these consequences when removed from their work environment. Methemoglobinemia can occur with overdose of nitrates. Individual sensitivity or concomitant alcohol consumption can provoke profound hypotension characterized by nausea, weakness, anxiety, and loss of consciousness.

β-Adrenergic antagonists such as propranolol and nadolol are also used to prevent the occurrence of angina. By reducing sympathetic stimulation of the heart, these drugs have negative inotropic and chronotropic effects that reduce myocardial oxygen demand. When given with nitrates, the β-antagonists suppress the reflex tachycardia induced by the vasodilators. Propranolol is rapidly biotransformed in the liver in contrast to nadolol, which is less lipophilic, is excreted renally, and has a longer plasma half-life. The pharmacology of these drugs is discussed under "Adrenergic Antagonists."

The calcium antagonists (or slow channel calcium entry blockers) are a relatively new group of drugs that are effective in preventing both effort-induced and variant angina. The entry of calcium ions through specialized membrane channels is altered by these agents. Reduced intracellular calcium causes slowing of sinus nodal depolarization and prolonged AV conduction time. Relaxation of vascular smooth muscle, particularly in the coronary and cerebral vessels, also occurs. The sensitivity of various tissues to the calcium antagonists is not uniform. Cardiac cells are most responsive to verapamil and diltiazem, while vascular smooth muscle is most affected by nifedipine. Vasodilation can, in turn, provoke reflex increase in sympathetic activity.

Calcium antagonists are most effective in alleviating angina produced by vasospasm. Nifedipine and diltiazem have slightly greater efficacy than verapamil. These drugs can be combined with nitrates and also with beta antagonists, although the latter combination may precipitate heart failure or AV

TABLE 7-17. Nitrate Vasodilators

GENERIC NAME	TRADE NAME
Amyl nitrate	—
Erythrityl tetranitrate	Cardilate
Isosorbide dinitrate	Isordil, Sorbitrate
Nitroglycerin	Nitrostat, Nitrogard, Deponit, Nitrodisc, Transderm-Nitro, Tridil, Nitrostat IV, Nitrospan, Nitrol
Pentaerythritol tetranitrate	Peritrate, Duotrate, Naptrate, others

conduction block. Concomitant IV administration of a beta blocker and verapamil is contraindicated. Side effects such as dizziness, headaches, and tachycardia that result from vasodilation occur most frequently with nifedipine. Verapamil is most likely to cause negative inotropy, chronotropy, and gastrointestinal complaints. Peripheral edema can occur. The calcium antagonists are inactivated in the liver.

Antianxiety agents are occasionally useful adjuncts in the treatment of angina. Benzodiazepines (*e.g.*, diazepam) appear to have an additional vasodilatory action on coronary vessels.

Antihypertensive Agents

Hypertension (persistent elevation of systolic and diastolic pressure) is broadly defined as essential (primary) or secondary. The latter results from some identifiable disease process such as nephritis, renal artery obstruction, arteriosclerosis, or toxemia of pregnancy. When the underlying cause is corrected, secondary hypertension is resolved.

The cause of essential hypertension, which accounts for 90% of patients with elevated blood pressure, is not known. Hyperactivity of the sympathetic nervous system may contribute to the development of hypertension. Regardless of its origin, chronic high blood pressure produces end-organ damage chiefly of the vasculature of the kidney, heart, and brain, resulting in myocardial infarction, stroke, renal failure, and premature death. Reduction of elevated pressure, through diet (weight loss and decreased sodium intake), reduction in smoking, alterations in life-style, or the use of antihypertensive drugs when other modalities fail, can prevent potential adverse sequelae. Essential hypertension can remain asymptomatic for many years; thus periodic measurement of blood pressure is important.

A considerable number of drugs have been used in the management of essential hypertension (Table 7-18). Several different mechanisms of action are represented, and persons refractory to one type of agent often respond to another. In addition, combinations of two or three types of drugs are frequently used, with the advantage that low doses can be given, thus reducing the incidence of side effects while maintaining an adequate therapeutic response. "Stepped therapy" for hypertension refers to initiating treatment with a single agent (a thiazide, β-blocker, angiotensin-converting enzyme inhibitor, or calcium antagonist) then adding in a stepwise manner additional drug(s) as necessary.

TABLE 7-18. Antihypertensive Drugs

GENERIC NAME	TRADE NAME
Centrally Acting Agents	
Clonidine	Catapres
Methyldopa	Aldomet
Guanabenz	Wytensin
Guanfacine	Tenex
Peripheral Amine Depletors	
Reserpine	Serpasil, Reserfia, others
Guanethidine	Ismelin
Guanadrel	Hylorel
Direct Acting Smooth Muscle Vasodilators	
Hydralazine	Apresoline
Minoxidil	Loniten
Prazosin	Minipress
Terazosin	Vasocard
Angiotensin Converting Enzyme Inhibitors	
Captopril	Capoten
Enalapril	Vasotec
Lisinopril	Prinivil, Zestril
Calcium Channel Blockers	
Diltiazem	Cardizem
Nifedipine	Procardia
Verapamil	Calan, Isoptin
Diuretics (see Table 7-22)	
β-Adrenergic Antagonists (see Table 7-6)	

Essential hypertension will frequently require life-long therapy. Compliance with drug regimens can be problematic: annoying side effects experienced by a previously asymptomatic patient may elicit a decision to abandon drug treatment. Patients must be told of the possible severe consequences of untreated hypertension, and must be encouraged to take measures to reduce blood pressure. Often, a different type of drug with more tolerable side effects can be substituted.

The thiazide diuretics (see Table 7-22) are among the most frequently used antihypertensive drugs, both as single agents and as components of combination therapy. Their mechanisms of action include sodium depletion and reduction of plasma volume. In addition, there is evidence that the thiazides have a direct relaxant effect on arteriolar smooth muscle and may reduce vascular responsiveness to endogenous constrictors. The "potassium-sparing" diuretics such as spironolactone and triamterene may be combined with the thiazides to minimize potassium loss. Metolazone (Zaroxolyn) is an antihypertensive diuretic with actions very similar to the thiazides. The loop diuretics such as furosemide are occasionally used in treating hypertension, although their greater diuretic action can result in increased incidence and severity of adverse effects. The diuretics are discussed further elsewhere in this chapter.

The β-adrenergic antagonists such as propranolol, atenolol, or metoprolol also are used widely in the management of hypertension, frequently in combination with thiazides and other agents. Their mechanism of antihypertensive efficacy may include reduction in sympathetic outflow from the central nervous system, suppression of response to sympathetic stimulation of cardiac β-1 receptors, and inhibition of renin release. Because β blockers will reduce many aspects of sympathetic stimulation, they cause a wide range of side effects. Metoprolol (Lopressor) and atenolol (Tenormin) represent a selective generation of β antagonists that preferentially block β-1 receptors in cardiac tissue rather than the β-2 receptors in bronchial and vascular tissues. This selective action confers advantages over earlier β blockers such as propranolol. There is relatively less danger of provoking undesirable bronchoconstriction in patients with asthma and other forms of chronic obstructive pulmonary disease. A temporary rise in peripheral resistance at the start of therapy, and sudden pronounced rises in blood pressure after physical exertion and emotional stress, are less likely to occur. The most common adverse reactions are tiredness and dizziness, depression, diarrhea, and shortness of breath with bradycardia. As with other β blockers, there have been reports of exacerbation of angina pectoris and occasional myocardial infarction following abrupt cessation of therapy. Like the nonselective β blockers, metoprolol and atenolol are contraindicated in sinus bradycardia, heart block greater than first degree, and cardiogenic shock. The β blockers are discussed further under "Adrenergic Antagonists."

Other antihypertensive agents that appear to work by reducing sympathetic outflow from the central nervous system are methyldopa (Aldomet), clonidine (Catapres), and guanabenz (Wytensin). Several theories have been proposed to explain the action of *methyldopa*. It is now generally accepted that α-methylnorepinephrine, a metabolite of this drug, activates presynaptic α-2 receptors (autoreceptors) that in turn inhibit release of the neurotransmitter norepinephrine. Methyldopa also reduces plasma renin levels. Common adverse effects are sedation, dry mouth, nasal congestion, and postural hypotension. Similarly to β blockers and vasodilators, methyldopa causes sodium and fluid retention; thus a diuretic is usually given concurrently. Methyldopa can induce autoimmune reactions in the form of elevated antiglobulin antibodies (positive Coombs' test), hemolytic anemia, thrombocytopenia, and leukopenia. Fever and hepatitis may develop, making this drug contraindicated in patients with hepatic disease.

Clonidine acts by direct stimulation of central α-2-adrenergic receptors and may also stimulate the baroreceptor reflex pathway, inducing a fall in blood pressure. The greatest effect of clonidine occurs when the patient is in the upright position. The most commonly encountered side effects are drowsiness and dry mouth. Constipation may occur and, rarely, orthostatic hypotension. Administration of clonidine (like propranolol) must not be terminated abruptly, since rapid withdrawal can provoke restlessness, tachycardia, and rebound hypertension. A diuretic is usually given concurrently to enhance hypotensive action. Tricyclic antidepressants can reverse the therapeutic effects of clonidine. Investigational uses for this drug include treatment of migraine and of the symptoms of opiate withdrawal. Clonidine is available in a transdermal form (Catapres TTS) that is applied once weekly. Guanabenz and guanfacine (Tenex) work in much the same manner as clonidine to reduce blood pressure. Guanfacine is reported to cause milder side effects than other agents in this class.

Some drugs reduce blood pressure by decreasing sympathetic activity at the peripheral nerve terminals. Reserpine, one of the earliest antihypertensive agents, depletes neuronal norepinephrine, dopamine, and serotonin. Numerous adverse effects are reported for this drug. Its suppression of sympathetic activity allows parasympathetic predominance that leads to bradycardia, increased gastrointestinal motility and diarrhea, and exacerbation of peptic ulcer. A most troublesome aspect of reserpine is its ability to elicit profound mental depression; a history of affective disorder contraindicates this drug. The onset of action of reserpine is slow, requiring several days to produce a full antihypertensive effect. β-Adrenergic blockers add to the sympatholytic action of reserpine; if these drugs are combined, severe hypotension and bradycardia can occur. Patients taking reserpine may experience marked hypotension under general anesthesia. Once used in the management of psychiatric disorders, reserpine has largely been replaced by phenothiazines and other neuroleptics.

Guanethidine (Ismelin) depletes adrenergic neuronal norepinephrine and also inhibits its release in response to sympathetic stimulation. Its onset of action is several days. Guanethidine has a long plasma half-life (5 days) that may be extended in persons with renal impairment. To exert an antihypertensive action, guanethidine must enter the adrenergic nerve terminal. Thus, tricyclic antidepressants and other drugs that inhibit the neuronal membrane uptake system can reverse the actions of this drug. Side effects include diarrhea, bradycardia, retrograde ejaculation, postural hypotension, and sodium and fluid retention that is managed with concurrent diuretic administration. In the presence of pheochromocytoma, guanethidine may elicit hypertension as it suppresses neuronal reuptake of catecholamines. Extreme caution is required when this drug is administered to persons with peptic ulcer, asthma, coronary insufficiency, cerebral vascular disease, severe cardiac failure, or recent myocardial infarction. Use of MAOIs must be terminated at least 1 week prior to guanethidine administration. Drugs or other factors (*e.g.*, warm environment) that cause vasodilation can exacerbate postural hypotension of this agent. Guanadrel (Hylorel) works in a manner similar to guanethidine but has a shorter duration of action. Bretylium also has a similar mechanism but is no longer used extensively for the treatment of hypertension.

Prazosin (Minipress) and terazoxin (Hytrin) blocks postsynaptic α-1-adrenergic receptors, thus reducing sympathetic vasoconstriction. It dilates arterioles and veins, resulting in a reduction in both preload and afterload. Because of these effects, prazosin may be used to ameliorate congestive heart failure refractory to digitalis and diuretics. Prazosin rarely causes tachycardia. A ''first-dose phenomenon'' is marked postural hypotension and syncope 30 to 90 minutes after the initial administration or a rapid increment in dose. This may be prevented by instituting treatment with a low dose that is gradually increased as required.

Hydralazine (Apresoline) and minoxidil (Loniten) are direct-acting arteriolar dilators. Hydralazine reduces diastolic pressure more than systolic. A diuretic is usually given concurrently to prevent sodium and fluid retention, and a β blocker is given to minimize reflex tachycardia. Chronic administration of doses in excess of 200 mg/day can provoke development of a lupuslike syndrome. Other adverse effects include headache, tachycardia, angina pectoris, nausea, vomiting, and diarrhea. These may be alleviated by reducing the dosage. The presence of cardiovascular disease requires caution in the use of hydralazine. This drug appears to increase renal blood flow, in contrast to many antihypertensives that reduce renal perfusion.

Minoxidil, which can cause marked fluid retention and occasional pericardial effusion that may progress to tamponade, is usually reserved for severe hypertension that is refractory to other drugs. Congestive heart failure can occur; concomitant administration of a diuretic (frequently furosemide) is advised. Tachycardia can be suppressed with a β blocker or other sympatholytic agent. Guanethidine should not be used concurrently with minoxidil because severe hypotension may occur. Hypertrichosis is a frequent side effect, and topical preparations of minoxidil are being tested as a treatment for baldness.

The *angiotension converting enzyme (ACE) inhibitors* captopril (Capoten), enalapril (Vasotec), and lisinopril (Prinivil, Zestril) reduce blood pressure primarily by suppressing the renin–angiotensin–aldosterone system. Angiotensin II is a powerful endogenous vasoconstrictor. Persons with elevated plasma levels of renin (*e.g.*, those with renovascular hypotension or who are volume depleted) are most responsive to these agents and may experience severe hypotension. Proteinuria may develop, especially in persons with preexisting renal impairment. Hematological changes and altered taste perception are characteristic side effects; myelosuppressive drugs can exacerbate agranulocytosis. Because they result in decreased aldosterone secretion, the ACE inhibitors may cause potassium retention. Potassium supplements or potassium-sparing diuretics are contraindicated when a converting-enzyme inhibitor is used. A diuretic may be given concurrently to enhance the action of the ACE inhibitors. The nonsteroidal anti-inflammatory drugs may reverse or attenuate the antihypertensive effect of these drugs. Captopril added to digitalis/diuretic therapy can be beneficial in refractory congestive heart failure.

Saralasin (Sarenin) is a competitive inhibitor of angiotensin II that can act as an agonist when angiotensin II levels are very low. It has been used to diagnose renovascular or angiotensin-II-sensitive hypertension. (The agent is at present unavailable commercially.) In the presence of high levels of angiotensin II, saralasin displaces this substance, causing less vasoconstriction and a fall in blood pressure. However, as noted above, when plasma levels of angiotensin II are low, saralasin's agonist activity will elicit an increase in blood pressure.

The MAOI were among the earliest antihypertensive agents but have largely been replaced by newer drugs. *Pargyline* (Eutonyl) is occasionally used in the management of moderate to severe hypertension. Common side effects include gastrointestinal disturbances, dry mouth, fluid retention, and postural hypotension. A major disadvantage of the MAOI is the number of potentially severe drug interactions that can occur. Sympathomimetic amines, or drugs that can release or block uptake of catecholamines, may cause hypertensive crisis in the presence of MAOI. Foods that contain tyramine (*e.g.*, certain wines and cheeses) can provoke the same type of occasionally fatal response (the so-called "cheese reaction"). The hepatic biotransformation of many drugs (*e.g.*, sedatives and opiates) is suppressed. Meperidine (Demerol) is contraindicated in persons receiving MAOI. These drugs can exacerbate parkinsonian symptoms as well as the adverse effects of antiparkinsonian drugs. Diabetic patients may experience severe hypoglycemia. MAOI are used also in the management of depression, and are discussed further under that topic.

The calcium entry blockers (or calcium antagonists) such as verapamil, nifedipine, and diltiazem are used as antianginal and hypertensive agents (see discussions under these topics), and verapamil has been used for the treatment of certain dysrhythmias (*e.g.*, tachycardia). These drugs reduce the entry of calcium ions into vascular and cardiac muscle, thereby reducing contractility. Vasodilation occurs and blood pressure falls. Nifedipine can induce a reflex increase in heart rate, while verapamil and diltiazem prolong A-V conduction time. Because of their cardiac suppressant action, the calcium entry blockers can exacerbate congestive heart failure.

MANAGEMENT OF HYPERTENSIVE EMERGENCIES

Hypertensive emergencies occur when extreme risk of vascular or organ damage coexists with markedly elevated blood pressure. Clinical episodes including aortic dissection, excessive adrenergic stimulation, severe hypertension accompanying vascular surgery, intracranial hemorrhage or pulmonary edema, and malignant hypertension with evidence of organ damage require lowering of blood pressure to a safer level in a relatively rapid but carefully controlled manner. Excessive fall in pressure can adversely affect renal, cerebral, or coronary perfusion and function and may induce vomiting. Persons who are elderly or have vascular disorders are especially at risk of such adverse consequences. In some acute hypertensive situations, more gradual (*i.e.*, over several hours) reduction of pressure is appropriate.

Several types of drugs (Table 7-19) are used in the management of hypertensive episodes. Although the choice of drug can be influenced by the cause of the crisis, therapeutic measures often must be instituted before a diagnosis is definitive. Intravenous

TABLE 7-19. Drugs Used in the Management of Hypertensive Emergencies

GENERIC NAME	TRADE NAME
Nitroprusside	Nipride
Diazoxide	Hyperstat
Hydralazine	Apresoline
Nitroglycerin	Several
Trimethaphan	Arfonad
Labetalol	Normodyne, Trandate
Verapamil	Calan, Isoptin
Nifedipine	Procardia
Phentolamine	Regitine

administration is required in true emergencies; other routes can be effective in less urgent cases.

Nitroprusside, is the drug of choice for certain hypertensive emergencies; it dilates veins and arterioles. Its rapid onset is coupled with a brief duration of action that necessitates continuous IV infusion but allows fine control of patients' response. Since a marked reduction in blood pressure may occur rapidly, close observation of patients is required. Elderly and hypertensive persons are especially sensitive to the effects of this and other hypotensive agents. Nausea, headache, psychotic behavior, palpitations, tachycardia, and anxiety can accompany nitroprusside administration. Biotransformation of this drug yields cyanide and thiocyanate. Hepatic and renal impairment, and administration for longer than 24 hours, increase the risk of toxic accumulations of these substances. Metabolic acidosis or tolerance to drug effects often presage this toxicity. Nitroprusside is rapidly decomposed; infusion solutions should be protected from light with aluminum foil wrapping, and darkly discolored solutions should be discarded. A β blocker such as propranolol may be used to suppress reflex tachycardia and to minimize additional damage in aortic dissection.

The arteriolar vasodilator diazoxide, administered by IV bolus, has a rapid onset (within minutes) but an extended duration (several hours) of action. Severe prolonged hypotension may be avoided by the use of small doses (miniboluses or pulse injections) and close observation. Diazoxide is contraindicated in patients with aortic dissection, coronary artery disease, and myocardial infarction. Reflex tachycardia can be reduced by concomitant administration of a β-adrenergic antagonist. Diazoxide promotes sodium and fluid retention, and extended use may require the administration of a diuretic. Similarly to the related thiazide diuretics, this drug can induce hyperglycemia that necessitates adjustment in dosage of antidiabetic medication. Phlebitis and myocardial and cerebrel ischemia can occur following diazoxide administration. Since diazoxide relaxes uterine muscle, it can terminate contractions during labor.

Hydralazine, also an arteriolar dilator, is considered by many to be the drug of choice to ameliorate hypertension that accompanies eclampsia. The IM or IV route provides a prompt onset of effect, although patients' responses are variable. Reflex tachycardia and an increase in myocardial oxygen demand can induce angina. Additional adverse effects include those that frequently accompany rapid lowering of blood pressure: nausea, dizziness, and palpitations. Sodium and fluid retention can be avoided by concurrent administration of a diuretic, and β-blockers can reduce excessive cardiac stimulation.

Nitroglycerin, administered by IV infusion provides a rapid reduction in blood pressure that can be titrated to the patient's response. Dilation of veins and of coronary blood vessels occurs, and at higher drug doses arterioles also are affected. The resultant hemodynamic changes usually will decrease myocardial oxygen demand. Glyceryl trinitrate should be considered for use in hypertensive patients with coronary insufficiency. Adverse effects can include nausea and vomiting, headache, bradycardia, and marked hypotension.

The ganglionic blocker trimethaphan, especially useful in the management of aortic dissection, dilates both veins and arterioles. Elevation of the patient's head potentiates the hypotensive action of trimethaphan, which is administered by continuous IV infusion. Trimethaphan releases histamine from mast cells and thus can be hazardous in persons sensitive to this amine. The development of coronary and cerebral ischemia can be relieved by cautious administration of sympathomimetic pressor agents such as phenylephrine. Respiratory arrest has been reported following rapid infusion rates. Pupillary dilation induced by the anticholinergic action of trimethaphan can hinder detection of cerebral anoxia. Since tolerance develops to this drug, hypertension may recur during administration.

Labetalol is an α- and β-adrenergic antagonist that appears to have additional direct vasodilator action. It will rapidly lower blood pressure while its β-component prevents reflex tachycardia. Severe hypotension may develop. Persons with coronary insufficiency or myocardial infarction often respond favorably to this drug. Continuous IV infusion of intermittent low-dose bolus injections with close

monitoring provides the most satisfactory responses. The usual contraindications to β blockers apply also to labetalol; bradycardia, bronchial asthma, congestive heart failure, or heart block greater than first degree preclude the use of this drug. The α-blocking efficacy of labetalol can induce orthostatic hypotension.

Calcium channel blockers cause vasodilation and provide rapid lowering of elevated blood pressure. Verapamil is available for IV administration; both bolus and infusion are reported useful in hypertensive emergencies. Verapamil's negative inotropic action may exacerbate heart failure, and heart block may develop. Nifedipine capsules can be pierced to administer the drug sublingually and elicit a fall in blood pressure within 5 to 10 minutes. However, excessive hypotension may be difficult to manage since this drug has prolonged action. Calcium channel blockers can elicit either bradycardia or tachycardia. Concomitant administration of β blockers, however, can be hazardous since both types of drugs have a depressant effect on cardiac conduction. Preexisting conduction deficits may contraindicate the use of calcium channel blockers.

Phentolamine possesses α-adrenergic blocking efficacy that is particularly advantageous in hypertensive emergencies induced by excessive sympathomimetic activity. Abrupt termination of antihypertensive drugs such as clonidine and propranolol or MAO inhibitors can predispose to "rebound" hypertension. In addition to the usual hypotensive adverse responses, phentolamine can induce severe arrhythmias or myocardial infarction.

Certain oral antihypertensive agents (see previous section of this chapter) are used to induce more gradual reduction in blood pressure when hypertensive episodes are not so likely to produce immediate life-threatening consequences. Minoxidil will produce prompt reduction in blood pressure. However, marked hypotension and reflex tachycardia can occur. β-Blockers and diuretics are frequently administered concomitantly.

The angiotension converting enzyme inhibitor captopril is well absorbed from the gastrointestinal tract and can reduce blood pressure within 30 to 60 minutes. Precipitous hypotension may occur in persons who are receiving diuretics or are otherwise hypovolemic. These agents may be particularly useful in patients with cardiac failure, and some may be available for intravenous administration.

Nifedipine, given orally or sublingually, and oral labetalol can be useful in hypertensive emergencies. Clonidine can lower pressure within 2 to 3 hours, usually without altering cardiac output or rate of contraction or causing severe hypotension.

Precautions and contraindications relevant to each of these drugs must be considered when emergency antihypertensive therapy is selected. Once the hypertensive episode is controlled, steps must be taken to determine its cause and to prevent its recurrence. Transition from IV to oral drug administration must be accomplished carefully to avoid return of hypertension.

DRUGS AFFECTING BLOOD COAGULATION AND COMPOSITION

Anticoagulants

Intravascular coagulation of blood is rare, unless the endothelial lining of the vessels is damaged and platelets come into contact with the subendothelial surface. Formation of thrombi can impede local circulation, and may be the source of emboli that cause ischemia in distant vital organs. The risk of thromboembolism is increased by blood flow stasis during prolonged immobilization in persons with atrial fibrillation, rheumatic heart–valvular disease, and implanted artificial valves. Controversy over use of anticoagulants in management of acute myocardial infarction continues. Some studies suggest that administration of anticoagulants for 2 to 4 weeks following infarction provides significant benefit to certain patients.

Anticoagulants are of two types: heparin, which must be given parenterally (SC or IV), and the coumarin-type or orally active agents. The major toxic effect of both is excessive suppression of clotting mechanisms, resulting in severe spontaneous or accidental hemorrhage. Conditions that predispose to risk of bleeding (*e.g.*, thrombocytopenia, gastrointestinal ulceration, severe hypertension, spinal anesthesia) generally preclude the administration of anticoagulants. Caution is required in elderly patients who frequently have fragile skin, blood vessels that are easily damaged, and reduced plasma levels of hepatically synthesized clotting factors.

Heparin sodium USP (Liquaemin), a large, highly charged sulfated polymer of paired units of acetylated glucosamine and glucuronic acid, is inactivated in the gastrointestinal tract and must be administered parenterally. Preparations ranging from 1,000 to 40,000 units/ml are derived from bovine lung and porcine intestinal mucosa. "Low-dose" heparin (5,000 units SC every 8 to 12 hours) is fre-

quently adequate to prevent thrombosis. When there is overt thromboembolism, high doses of up to 30,000 units IV per day may be required. Continuous infusion rather than intermittent bolus injection best maintains consistent therapeutic plasma levels and reduces the danger of severely compromised coagulation. Careful monitoring of the partial thromboplastin time (PTT) will assist in the selection of properly individualized drug doses. The PTT should be maintained at 1.5 to 2.5 times the control value.

Heparin interacts primarily with the "intrinsic" pathway of coagulation by inactivating several factors that are essential to the complex process of clot formation. Heparin enhances the action of a required plasma cofactor, antithrombin III, which chiefly inactivates thrombin. Because of its direct interference in clot formation, the onset of heparin's effect is rapid (almost immediate with IV administration; within 2 hours after SC injection). The plasma half-life of this drug is 1 to 2 hours. Inactivation is by both hepatic metabolism and renal excretion of unchanged drug; renal impairment delays its removal from blood. Because of the risk of hematoma, heparin should not be administered IM.

The use of heparin to treat disseminated intravascular coagulation (DIC) is controversial. This condition is characterized by excessive activity in both the fibrinogenic and fibrinolytic systems; thrombi may occlude small vessels at the same time that severe hemorrhage is occurring. Close monitoring of patients is required since many do not respond to heparin. Therapy should be discontinued after 4 to 8 hours if no significant benefit is derived. Indeed, all forms of treatment, including fresh plasma, may be hazardous. Aminocaproic acid may be administered concomitantly.

Intravenous heparin has the ability to produce rapid clearance of dietary lipids from plasma. It appears to release from various tissues a lipase that catalyzes the hydrolysis of triglycerides in chylomicrons. β-Lipoproteins of high molecular weight and low density are converted into low-molecular-weight, high-density lipids.

In addition to an increased risk of hemorrhage, heparin can suppress aldosterone synthesis, resulting in increased sodium and fluid excretion. Paradoxically, heparin can cause thrombocytopenia by inducing platelet aggregation and thromboembolism (white clot syndrome). Chronic high doses of heparin have caused osteoporosis. Hypersensitivity reactions, often to the animal protein contaminating the drug, have occurred. Other drugs that prolong coagulation, such as dextran, aspirin, and other

TABLE 7-20. Oral Anticoagulants

GENERIC NAME	TRADE NAME
Anisindione	Miradon
Dicumarol	—
Phenprocoumin	Liquamar
Warfarin	Coumadin, Antithrombin-K

nonsteroidal anti-inflammatory drugs, are usually contraindicated in heparinized patients.

Positively charged protamine sulfate, administered by slow IV infusion, binds to negatively charged heparin in the circulating blood and prevents its anticoagulant action. One mg will neutralize approximately 100 units of heparin; the time interval between the last dose of heparin and protamine administration must be considered in estimating the dose of the latter drug. Protamine also is anticoagulant (this effect becomes apparent when protamine is in excess of heparin) and has a longer plasma half-life than heparin. Adverse effects include hypotension, bradycardia, anaphylaxis in previously sensitized subjects, and exacerbation of DIC.

Oral anticoagulant therapy, which has a more prolonged onset of action, may be initiated concomitantly with heparin. The mechanism of action of these drugs (Table 7-20) differs from heparin in that they decrease hepatic synthesis of clotting factors II, VII, IX, and X by preventing reduction of vitamin K epoxide to the active reduced form necessary for coupled gamma carboxylation of the precursors of these factors. Those factors already present in circulating blood must be depleted (over 3 to 5 days) before the full anticoagulant effect of the oral drugs becomes apparent. **Warfarin** is used most frequently because it is well absorbed from the gastrointestinal tract. The action of the oral anticoagulants affects in particular the "extrinsic" clotting pathway and is monitored through the prothrombin time (PT). One-stage PT should be maintained at 1.5 to 2.5 times greater than control value. When heparin is administered concurrently, blood for prothrombin testing should be drawn at least 4 to 5 hours after the last IV dose or 12 to 24 hours after SC injection.

As with heparin, the major adverse effect of oral anticoagulant therapy is hemorrhage. Gastrointestinal bleeding, widespread petechiae, prolonged hemorrhage from open wounds, hematuria, and excessive bruising can occur. Adrenal hemorrhage and resultant insufficiency (which can occur also with heparin) may require glucocorticoid replacement therapy.

The hemorrhagic action of oral anticoagulants can be reversed by vitamin K preparations (menadiol, Synkayvite; menadione; and phytonadione, Mephyton) that stimulate hepatic synthesis of clotting factors. Control of hemorrhage can usually be achieved within 3 to 6 hours following parenteral phytonadione, with prothrombin attaining normal levels after 14 hours. Oral phytonadione is effective in 6 to 12 hours, while parenteral menadiol requires 8 to 24 hours. Because of this long onset of action, significant bleeding may necessitate emergency administration of plasma, whole blood, or factor IX complex (Konyne, Proplex). The efficacy of vitamin K is dependent upon functioning hepatocytes. The action of heparin is not reversed by these drugs. Administration of vitamin K can reduce the effectiveness of subsequent doses of oral anticoagulant for several weeks.

Additional adverse reactions observed with the oral anticoagulants include diarrhea, depressed levels of formed elements of blood, hepatitis, renal damage, and dermatological symptoms. Lack of bioequivalence among warfarin preparations from various manufacturers has been reported. Anticoagulant therapy should be interrupted several days before anticipated surgery. Patients should wear or carry medical identification noting their use of anticoagulants and must be observant of signs of hemorrhage.

Many drugs, including over-the-counter preparations, interact with the oral anticoagulants to either enhance or reduce their actions (Table 7-21). The PT must be closely monitored whenever drug doses are increased or decreased, or when drugs are added to or withdrawn from the patient's regimen.

TABLE 7-21. Drug Interactions Affecting Oral Anticoagulant Activity

Drugs That Enhance Anticoagulant Effect
Cimetidine
Clofibrate
Dipyridamole
Gemfibrozil
Quinidine
Salicylates, other nonsteroidal anti-inflammatory drugs
Sulfinpyrazone
Sulfonylureas
Many antibiotics

Drugs That Reduce Anticoagulant Effect
Barbiturates
Bile sequestrants
Carbamazapine
Estrogens
Phenytoin
Vitamin K

The oral anticoagulants are hepatically inactivated and induction of drug-metabolizing enzymes will decrease their effectiveness. Patients should not concomitantly use aspirin, which has its own anticoagulant effect and also displaces the coumarin-type drugs from plasma protein binding sites. Alcohol should be avoided, as well as activities that increase the risk of injury. Consumption of large amounts of leafy green vegetables that contain vitamin K can suppress anticoagulant action. Impaired renal or hepatic function can prolong the plasma half-life of the these drugs. Discoloration of urine by indandiones may mimic hematuria.

Thrombolytics

Although anticoagulants prevent additional clot formation, they do not generally dissolve those already present. Thrombolytic or fibrinolytic agents (streptokinase, Streptase; urokinase, Abbokinase; tissue plasminogen activator [tPA] Activase) are used for this purpose. Disruption of clots is desirable in the management of thrombosis and pulmonary embolism, and the maintenance of access shunts and intravascular catheters. Several studies have indicated that thrombolytic agents, administered early in the course of evolving myocardial infarction, can restore blood flow through occluded coronary arteries and may limit myocardial damage.

Circulating blood contains a fibrinolytic system that dissolves intravascular fibrin aggregates as they form. Fibrinolysin (or plasmin), the major component of this system, is a proteolytic enzyme that disrupts fibrinogen and fibrin. Plasminogen is the inactive circulating precursor of fibrinolysin. Thrombolytic drugs convert plasminogen to plasmin, thereby setting into motion the fibrinolytic mechanism.

Streptokinase is derived from streptococcal bacteria strains. Its action is suppressed by antistreptococcal antibodies, commonly found in patients' blood in response to prior streptococcal exposure. Large loading doses may be required. Streptokinase itself can induce antibody formation. Readministration of this drug can result in allergic responses or in inadequate thrombolytic action. *Urokinase* is derived from human urine or from cultures of human embryonic renal cells. Its actions are similar to those of streptokinase. It is less likely to induce antibody production but is more costly. Tissue plasminogen activator (alteplase) is an endogenous activator of the fibrinolytic system. It can be produced by recombinant DNA technology and is used as a thrombolytic agent in treatment of myocardial infarction. Several analogs of tPA are under investigation.

Since these drugs (particularly streptokinase and urokinase) may also lyse fibrinogen and other blood clotting factors, a major disadvantage is the risk of severe hemorrhage. Active internal bleeding, or significant potential for cerebral hemorrhage, contraindicate their use. Streptokinase and urokinase have a more widespread effect on blood clotting throughout the circulatory system. The action of tPA occurs more selectively at the surface of thrombi, although this agent is not completely free of systemic anticoagulant action. However, tPA also has a relatively short plasma half-life (6 to 8 minutes). In the management of acute myocardial infarction, tPA given IV may be more effective than streptokinase unless the latter drug is administered by the hazardous, costly, and time-consuming procedure of intracoronary injection. To be effective in limiting myocardial damage, thrombolytic drugs must be given early (usually within 6 hours) in the course of vessel occlusion. Patients receiving thrombolytic therapy must have some measure of clotting time or fibrinogen content monitored, and must be protected from activities or procedures that may evoke bleeding. Observation for signs of spontaneous bleeding (e.g., nausea, abdominal pain, or change in neurological status) is necessary. Cardiac arrhythmias often develop as perfusion of myocardial cells is reestablished. Heparin and/or oral anticoagulants may be administered subsequently to reduce the risk of additional thrombosis.

Debriding Agents

Streptokinase–streptodornase (Varidase) is a debriding agent used topically to remove blood clots and purulent material from wounds. Sufficient enzyme may be absorbed to produce systemic anticoagulation. This agent is contraindicated in active hemorrhage. Other enzymatic debriding preparations include fibrinolysin and desoxyribonuclease (Elase), trypsin and chymotrypsin, papain, and bromelains (Ananase). When applied topically, these agents remove necrotic debris and promote healing of dermatological ulcers, severe burns, and other wounds. Collagenase (Biozyme-C, Santyl) removes necrotic tissue and attached strands of collagen and may induce more rapid healing. Dextranomer (Debrisan) hydrophilic beads are applied to draining wounds to remove exudates and bacteria that can hinder tissue repair.

Agents that Restore Plasma Volume

Circulating plasma volume is maintained largely by the oncotic influence of plasma proteins such as albumin. When plasma volume becomes inadequate (*e.g.,* following severe hemorrhage, generalized vasodilation, trauma, or extensive burns) survival may depend upon a rapid replenishment of circulating fluid. Solutions such as dextrose and saline have limited capacity to maintain vascular volume, since their components of relatively small molecular size readily diffuse across capillary walls. Much more effective in restoring plasma volume are the nondiffusable colloids such as dextran (Gentran, Macrodex) and hetastarch (Hespan). These substances are relatively stable and inexpensive, and do not present the risk of infection or incompatibility that may be encountered when blood products from natural sources are used. However, colloids can provoke allergic or anaphylactoid reactions, and in persons who are dehydrated they may severely deplete extravascular volume by attracting interstitial fluid into the vascular compartment. The latter hazard can be reduced by concomitant IV infusion of fluids. Observation for circulatory overload and signs of pulmonary edema or congestive heart failure is necessary. Colloidal solutions do not enhance the oxygen-transporting capacity of blood; erythrocyte replacement is required to correct this deficit.

Dextran is a polymer produced by the action of *Leuconostoc mesenteroides* on sucrose solutions. The large, extensively branched colloids are modified by acid hydrolysis to molecular weights averaging 40,000 and 75,000. Preparations containing predominantly one size of molecule are available. The lower-molecular-weight solution (dextran 40) is used as a volume expander, and as a hemodiluent for pump–oxygenators during extracorporeal circulation. Since dextran suppresses platelet agglutination, it is used to prevent venous thromboembolism following orthopedic surgery. Because it can prolong bleeding time, dextran is contraindicated in persons with coagulation deficits including those induced by anticoagulant drugs. Active hemorrhage can be exacerbated as blood volume and perfusion pressure increase. Renal failure, probably due to viscous obstruction of renal tubular flow, has occurred in persons receiving dextran.

Dextran 70, consisting of larger-molecular-weight particles, is more efficient in maintaining plasma volume because it remains longer (24 hours or more) within the vascular compartment. However, it produces a higher incidence of adverse effects including histamine release from mast cells, increased bleeding time, and alteration of erythrocyte sedimentation and aggregation. An osmotic diuretic such as mannitol may be coadministered with dextran to maintain urinary output.

Hetastarch is used as a volume expander, and also in leukapheresis where it improves the recovery of granulocytes. This colloid, prepared by ethylene oxide treatment of waxy sorghum starch, has many of the same properties and adverse effects of dextran. It may be somewhat less allergenic.

Plasma protein fractions (Buminate, Plasminate) are albumin and protein preparations derived from human blood. These are administered to correct volume depletion and are useful adjuncts in the management of hypoproteinemia that may occur in premature infants or consequent to renal or hepatic disease. Because these substances are of human origin, the incidence of adverse effects such as anaphylaxis is low. Changes in blood pressure may occur. The possibility of hepatitis transmission has been obviated by heating these solutions for 10 hours at 60°C, which destroys the virus but does not denature plasma proteins.

Antiplatelet Drugs

Platelet aggregation is a contributing factor to thrombus formation that can result in coronary and cerebral artery occlusion. Platelet interaction with collagen may also enhance the development of arteriosclerotic deposits on blood vessel walls. Drugs that reduce platelet adhesion may prove to be effective inhibitors of these cardiovascular disorders.

Thromboxanes and prostacyclin, synthesized by the cyclo-oxygenase pathway, have been implicated in platelet function. Aspirin, which blocks the action of this enzyme, is reported to reduce the incidence of transient ischemic attacks and the risk of myocardial infarction in men with unstable angina. Low doses (as low as 20 mg/day) are most effective, possibly because they do not affect vascular endothelial prostacyclin production, which itself has antiplatelet activity.

The coronary vasodilator *dipyridamole* (Persantine), occasionally used to alleviate angina pectoris, suppresses *in vitro* platelet interaction with damaged blood vessel endothelium. Inhibition of phosphodiesterase and accumulation of cyclic AMP within platelets may account for the antiplatelet effects of dipyridamole. However, this drug alone has not been shown to reduce recurrence of myocardial infarction. The efficacy of anticoagulants or other antiplatelet agents may be enhanced by dipyridamole; drug combinations are used following cardiac valve implantation. Adverse effects of this drug are generally mild and transient; gastrointestinal disturbances, nausea, and syncope may occur, and angina can be exacerbated.

Sulfinpyrazone (Anturane), usually used as a uricosuric, has a platelet inhibitory action that may be beneficial in persons with coronary artery disease or implanted cardiac valves. Persons receiving this drug may develop hematological deficits; close monitoring of blood counts is required. Sulfinpyrazone can precipitate gout, renal stone formation, and possibly renal failure. Adequate hydration and urinary alkalinization can reduce the precipitation of uric acid in the urinary tract. Aspirin may be given concurrently with sulfinpyrazone to reduce deep venous thrombosis following hip surgery.

Pentoxyfylline (Trental) is a methylxanthine phosphodiesterase inhibitor that decreases serum levels of fibrinogen and reduces aggregation of platelets. Its greatest action, however, appears to be promotion of capillary blood flow by enhancing erythrocyte flexibility. Pentoxyfylline alleviates symptoms of intermittent claudication in some patients. Adverse effects of this drug, which is metabolized by erythrocytes and hepatocytes, include headaches, dizziness, and nausea. Clinical response may require up to 8 weeks of drug administration.

Hemostatic Agents

Local application of a variety of substances will retard bleeding from small vessels such as capillaries. *Thrombin* (Thrombostat) helps to control bleeding during surgery or in easily accessible sites, for example, nose and dental socket bleeding, in hemophiliac and other patients. Administration of this substance, which catalyzes the conversion of fibrinogen to fibrin, is limited to body surfaces since its entry into large blood vessels can result in potentially lethal intravascular clotting. Oxidized cellulose (Oxycel, Surgicel) reacts physically with blood to form a clotlike complex. It can be used to control surgical or mucous membrane bleeding. Epithelialization and bone regeneration are suppressed by prolonged topical application to denuded areas and fracture sites.

Absorbable gelatin hemostatics (Gelfoam, Gelfilm) need not be removed when surgical incisions are closed. The film can be used to "patch" dural or pleural injuries. Healing of skin incisions may be inhibited, although leg and decubitus ulcers are treated with these agents. Infection usually contraindicates their use.

Antihemophilic factor VIII will replace the factor absent in classic hemophilia (type A) and help to control bleeding in persons with this deficit. Administration is by the IV route, and doses are closely individualized to patients' needs. Factor VIII inhibitors can develop. Since this substance is derived from human plasma, transmission of hepatitis and AIDS has occurred. The presence of blood-group-specific antibodies in this product derived from plasma can elicit hemolytic anemia.

Factor IX complex (Konyne, Proplex), containing several vitamin-K-dependent clotting factors, can prevent or alleviate hemorrhagic episodes in Christmas disease (hemophilia B). Risk of hepatitis usually precludes the use of this plasma-derived product in persons with preexisting liver disease. Intravascular coagulation can be exacerbated by administration of factor IX complex. Rapid infusion rates cause hypotension and tachycardia that necessitate temporary termination of drug administration.

Vitamin K (discussed under "Vitamins") is beneficial in deficiencies of vitamin-K-dependent factors, provided that hepatocytes are functional.

Aminocaproic acid (Amicar) inhibits fibrinolysis and is useful in bleeding states caused by excessive fibrinolytic activity, such as open heart surgery, bleeding of the urinary tract, neoplastic diseases, hepatic cirrhosis, and abruptio placentae. This amino acid, which is related to lysine, inhibits the conversion of plasminogen to plasmin and also, to a lesser degree, directly inhibits the action of plasmin, the active fibrinolytic enzyme. In severe hemorrhagic emergencies, concomitant administration of fibrinogen and fresh whole blood may be necessary. Aminocaproic acid is contraindicated in DIC, since thrombus formation can be enhanced. Hyperfibrinolysis should be established before this drug is administered.

Tranexamic acid (Cyklokapron), similar to aminocaproic acid, is administered (PO or IV) concomitantly with coagulation factors (VIII or IX) to reduce the risk of hemorrhage following dental extraction in hemophiliac patients. Preexisting hematuria or subarachnoid hemorrhage preclude the use of tranexamic acid and, like aminocaproic acid, this drug is contraindicated in DIC. Vision aberrations, including changes in color discrimination, have been reported.

Drugs That Correct Hemoglobin Deficits

Iron is required for the synthesis of hemoglobin. Deficiency of this essential element, resulting from malabsorption of dietary iron or excessive blood loss (e.g., menstrual or occult gastrointestinal bleeding) will cause anemia. Iron deficiency attributed to inadequate dietary intake is not unusual in children aged 6 to 24 months, teenagers, and pregnant women.

Several preparations (including many over-the-counter) are available for the reversal of negative iron balance. Oral administration is preferred, although iron dextran (Imferon) can be given IM or by slow IV infusion to persons with inadequate gastrointestinal absorption or intolerance to the oral route. The ferrous form of iron is most readily absorbed, chiefly in the duodenum. Vitamin C promotes this action. In the circulatory system, iron is bound to a plasma protein (transferrin) that transports it to tissue sites of storage and utilization. Normally, only a small proportion of dietary iron is absorbed. However, when iron stores are depleted, the capacity of the intestinal mucosa to transport iron into the circulatory system increases. Certain malabsorption diseases will interfere with absorption of iron, and loss of blood interrupts the physiological cycle that captures used iron from the spleen and other tissues and transports it back to bone marrow for further use in hemoglobin, or to sites (e.g., the liver) for storage.

Oral administration of iron salts (e.g., ferrous fumarate, gluconate, and sulfate) can cause nausea, diarrhea, constipation, abdominal cramps, and changes in fecal pigmentation. Gastrointestinal symptoms can be reduced by taking these preparations with meals. However, simultaneous ingestion of eggs, milk, antacids, and tetracycline antibiotics suppress the intestinal absorption of iron. Supplements should be used only by persons with true iron deficiency. Excessive amounts of this metal can be hazardous. Acute overdose causes severe gastrointestinal irritation and mucosal injury, which further enhances iron absorption. Lethargy, dyspnea, shock, and metabolic acidosis can develop. Chronic overdose induces iron storage excess (hemosiderosis and hemochromatosis). Parenteral administration of chelating agents such as deferoxamine (Desferal) will promote renal excretion of iron. Dimercaprol should not be administered in cases of iron excess.

Peptic ulcer and inflammatory disorders of the intestines usually contraindicate oral administration of iron. Parenteral administration requires extreme caution. Intramuscular injections may be painful; leakage of iron solutions can discolor the skin; IV infusion can induce phlebitis. Patients must be closely observed for allergic responses including anaphylaxis; a test dose of drug followed by 1 hour of observation may be given initially. The required parenteral dose should be calculated based upon measurement of the patient's hematocrit. Oral and parenteral administration must *not* be used concurrently.

Megaloblastic anemias occur when insufficient amounts of vitamin B_{12} (cyanocobalamin) and folic acid are available for production of formed elements of blood. These substances are discussed under "Vitamins." In pernicious anemia, gastric mucosal cells fail to secrete intrinsic factor that is required for vitamin B_{12} absorption. Pernicious anemia may be accompanied by glossitis and specific neurological deficits (loss of vibratory sensation, paresthesias of hands and feet, ataxia) due to degenerative changes in dorsal and lateral columns of the spinal cord.

DIURETICS

Diuretics are used extensively in the management of cardiovascular disorders. In congestive heart failure, increased capillary pressure forces body water out of the vascular compartment and into body tissues and cavities, resulting in edema and ascites. Diuretics ameliorate hypertension, an action related to reduction in blood volume. Edema accompanying renal dysfunction, hepatic cirrhosis, and administration of drugs such as estrogens and corticosteroids also can be alleviated by diuretics. In addition, some diuretic agents are used for specific conditions: mannitol to relieve cerebral edema, and the carbonic anhydrase inhibitor acetazolamide (Diamox) to reduce elevated intraocular pressure in glaucoma.

The mechanism of action of most diuretics appears to involve reduction of active sodium and/or chloride reabsorption at the basal surface of the tubular epithelial cells. Sodium in the tubular filtrate enters the epithelial cells and is then transported out into the interstitial space through the activity of an ATPase-dependent sodium–potassium exchange. Water is reabsorbed passively along an osmotic gradient in those regions of the nephron that are water permeable, chiefly the collecting ducts.

Several types of drugs (Table 7-22) have the ability to induce diuresis. Their sites of action in the renal tubule vary and can influence the net effect of the drug. The mercurial and organic acid ("loop") diuretics, such as furosemide, exert their greatest effect in the ascending limb of the loop of Henle, where active transport of sodium and chloride contributes to the countercurrent gradient that pro-

TABLE 7-22. Diuretics

GENERIC NAME	TRADE NAME
Mercurial	
Mercaptomerin	Thiomerin
Thiazides	
Benzthiazide	Hydrex, others
Chlorothiazide	Diuril
Hydrochlorothiazide	Hydrodiuril, others
Trichlormethiazide	Diurese
Carbonic Anhydrase Inhibitors	
Acetazolamide	Diamox
Dichlorphenamide	Daranide
Methazolamide	Neptazane
Organic Acids (Loop Diuretics)	
Bumetanide	Bumex
Ethacrynic acid	Edecrin
Furosemide	Lasix
Potassium-sparing	
Amiloride	Midamor
Spironolactone	Aldactone
Triamterene	Dyrenium
Osmotic Diuretics	
Mannitol	Osmitrol
Urea	Ureaphil
Additional Diuretics	
Chlorthalidone	Hygroton
Metolazone	Zaroxolyn
Indapamide	Lozol

motes passive reabsorption of water in the collecting tubules. The carbonic anhydrase inhibitors and the thiazides impede sodium reabsorption in the proximal and distal tubules of the nephron, respectively. Potassium-sparing diuretics reduce the distal tubule exchange of sodium for potassium and hydrogen ions. They may act by inhibiting the action of aldosterone (*i.e.*, spironolactone) or the sodium-for-potassium pump mechanism (*e.g.*, amiloride or triamterene). Osmotic agents, filtered by the glomeruli but not reabsorbed, promote the excretion of an osmotically equivalent amount of water. Drugs such as the xanthines (*e.g.*, theophylline and caffeine) and agents that affect secretion of antidiuretic hormone (ADH) also have a diuretic action.

Although they are a varied group of drugs, causing varied degrees of diuresis and effects on electrolyte excretion, these agents share some noteworthy characteristics. Most have the potential to induce severe electrolyte depletion and imbalance; preexisting electrolyte disturbances should be corrected before diuretics are administered. Several diuretics can provoke severe dehydration with attendant hypovolemia, progressing to circulatory collapse and

predisposing to thrombosis and embolism. The thiazides appear to reduce vascular responsiveness to the neurotransmitter norepinephrine, which may account in part for their antihypertensive efficacy. Diuretics suppress renal excretion and enhance the toxicity of lithium; thus concomitant administration is usually contraindicated. Corticosteroids enhance the potassium loss that occurs with most diuretics. Although digitalis and diuretics are often given simultaneously, the hypokalemia induced by the latter will enhance the risk of toxicity of the cardiac glycosides. Concurrent administration of potassium salts or potassium-sparing diuretics can ameliorate this interaction.

Mercurial Diuretics

Among the earliest available diuretics, these drugs have been replaced by newer, safer, and more easily administered agents. However, *mercaptomerin* (Thiomerin) is still available and can be effective in alleviating edema that is refractory to other treatment. The exact mechanism of action is not known, but may involve inhibition of sulfhydryl-catalyzed transport of chloride and sodium in the ascending limit of Henle's loop. Substances that replenish -SH groups will reduce the diuretic action of the mercurials. Significant amounts of sodium, chloride, and water are excreted. Hypochloremic alkalosis may occur as a result of the extensive loss of chloride ions.

The mercurials are most frequently administered IM. They are ineffective when given orally, can induce fatal cardiac arrhythmias when given IV, and may cause sloughing and abscess when given by the SC route. The maximum effect develops in 2 hours, and action may continue up to 36 to 48 hours. A major disadvantage of the mercurials is their severe nephrotoxicity. They are contraindicated in most forms of renal disease. Dimercaprol (BAL) may provide some protection against renal damage. The mercurials are most effective in an acid urine and are inhibited by the development of alkalosis.

Thiazides (Benzothiodiazides)

The thiazide or sulfonamide diuretics are currently among the most widely used drugs in the United States. Their action appears to involve alteration of sodium and chloride reabsorption in the distal tubule as well as inhibition of carbonic anhydrase, which promotes excretion of sodium and bicarbonate (see carbonic anhydrase inhibitors below). The onset of action of most thiazides is 2 hours after oral administration, with a duration up to 12 or more hours. Chlorthalidone and indapamide, closely related diuretics, are effective up to 36 and 72 hours, respectively. The action of the thiazides, unlike carbonic anhydrase inhibitors and organomercurials, is little influenced by variations in pH of body fluids. Since thiazides are secreted by the same tubular transport mechanism that excretes uric acid, hyperuricemia and exacerbation of gout are side effects. Hyperglycemia (probably via inhibition of pancreatic insulin release) also may occur, predisposing to diabetes or necessitating increased dosage of insulin or oral hypoglycemics.

Thiazides are often combined with digitalis in the management of congestive heart failure. Their use as antihypertensives is discussed in that section. Paradoxically, thiazides are used to decrease urine volume in diabetes insipidus, particularly the nephrogenic form. Thiazides affect calcium absorption; their ability to ameliorate hypercalciuria enables them to inhibit formation of calcium stones in the kidneys.

Caution is required when thiazides are administered in the presence of renal impairment because azotemia may occur. In persons with hepatic disease, alterations in fluid or electrolyte balance can precipitate hepatic coma. Thiazides administered during pregnancy can induce neonatal jaundice and aberrant carbohydrate metabolism. However, these drugs are used cautiously in the management of eclampsia.

Like most diuretics, the thiazides promote excessive potassium excretion and increase the risk of digitalis toxicity. Thiazides can reduce the excretion of quinidine (by urinary alkalinization) and may induce hypercalcemia when calcium salts are given concurrently. Thiazides potentiate the action of most antihypertensive agents, and will produce severe postural hypotension in combination with opiates, barbiturates, and alcohol.

Acetazolamide (Diamox) causes diuresis through its action on carbonic anhydrase. Inhibition of this enzyme, which catalyzes the reaction of CO_2 + H_2O to yield H^+ and CO_3^-, reduces tubular reabsorption of sodium in exchange for hydrogen ions and results in alkalinization of the urine. Metabolic hyperchloremic acidosis develops and hinders the efficacy of the carbonic anhydrase inhibitors, probably by inhibiting hydrogen–sodium ion exchange. Intermittent drug administration allows normalization of plasma pH by facilitating natural correction of the metabolic acidosis.

Carbonic anhydrase inhibitors alleviate elevated intraocular pressure in glaucoma by decreasing the formation of aqueous humor. Their effectiveness in some forms of epilepsy may be due to decreased formation of cerebrospinal fluid with reduction in intracranial pressure. Acetazolamide is used investigationally to ameliorate high-altitude hypoxia. Analogues of acetazolamide include dichlorphenamide (Daranide) and methazolamide (Naptazane). These drugs, like the thiazides, are sulfonamide derivatives and are contraindicated in persons allergic to this chemical class.

Organic Acid Diuretics

Furosemide (Lasix), *ethacrynic acid* (Edecrin), and *bumetanide* (Bumex) work primarily in the loop of Henle, thus their designation as "loop" diuretics. This portion of the nephron extends down into the medullary region of the kidney where much of the sodium, chloride, and urea (but not water) are reabsorbed in the thick ascending limb of the loop. Urine entering the distal tubule is hypotonic, while the medullary interstitium is hypertonic. This osmotic gradient (or countercurrent multiplier) becomes important in the collecting ducts that traverse the medullary region and that, under the influence of ADH, are rendered permeable to water. The greater the osmolarity of the medulla the greater the water reabsorption, resulting in a concentrated urine. The loop diuretics reduce medullary osmolarity, and cause intense diuresis with significant excretion of sodium, chloride, and potassium. These drugs have greater efficacy than most other agents including the thiazides, and are often referred to as "high ceiling" diuretics. Refractory edema often will respond to the loop diuretics, which can be given orally or IV and have a rapid onset of action.

These agents are highly bound to plasma proteins, and are secreted into the proximal tubules by the same system that transports thiazides and uric acid. This transport appears to be necessary for their effects, since they work at the luminal side of the nephron.

Because of their intense diuresis, the loop diuretics produce excessive dehydration and marked depletion of electrolytes. Elderly persons, in whom renal function usually is less than optimal, are especially at risk and require close observation when these drugs are given. Some physicians recommend that loop diuretics not be administered to the elderly, preferring instead to use thiazides. Loop diuretics can cause hyperuricemia, hearing impairment, and glucose intolerance. Toxicity is enhanced in patients with renal disease.

Characteristic drug interactions of the loop diuretics include inhibition of salicylate excretion and potentiation of theophylline and succinylcholine. Indomethacin (and possibly other nonsteroidal anti-inflammatory drugs) reduce the efficacy of furosemide. The ototoxicity of the aminoglycoside antibiotics may be enhanced.

Potassium-Sparing Agents

The potassium-sparing diuretics are unique in their propensity to cause hyperkalemia rather than potassium depletion. Their site of action is the distal convoluted tubule, where the hormone aldosterone mediates sodium reabsorption in exchange for potassium and hydrogen ions. *Spironolactone* (Aldactone) is a specific competitive aldosterone antagonist, while *triamterene* (Dyrenium) and *amiloride* (Midamor) inhibit sodium entry into the collecting tubular cell. Spironolactone is most effective in the presence of high levels of renin and aldosterone, and is used in the management of hyperaldosteronism.

Most diuretics result in delivery of increased amounts of sodium to the distal tubule. As the nephron exerts a final attempt to reabsorb this ion, much potassium can be lost. The greatest use of the potassium-sparing agents, which alone produce only mild diuresis, is in combination with other diuretics to reduce this potassium wasting. Excessive potassium intake, either dietary or in the form of supplemental salts, must be avoided, particularly in the presence of renal disease, which might produce dangerous elevations of potassium when a potassium-sparing agent is given.

Osmotic Diuretics

As their name implies, the osmotic diuretics carry fluid through the circulatory system and the renal tubules by elevating oncotic pressure. Administered IV, these substances are restricted to the vascular compartment and attract considerable amounts of extravascular fluid. *Mannitol* (Osmitrol), the most frequently used in this class of drugs, is completely filtered at the glomeruli but is neither secreted nor reabsorbed by the nephron. Osmotic diuretics usually have minimal effects on electrolyte excretion, and are used mainly to alleviate intracranial edema and to prevent renal failure by maintaining urine flow. Refractory elevation of intraocular pressure may respond to osmotic agents. Urinary output must be maintained during administration of these drugs; renal failure or severe dehydration contraindicate their use. Persons with cardiovascular disease may tolerate poorly a sudden increase in intravascular volume produced by the osmotic diuretic agent.

Corticosteroids may be coadministered with mannitol in the management of elevated intracranial pressure. However, both types of drugs promote potassium excretion, and marked hypokalemia may develop.

RESPIRATORY PHARMACOLOGY

Pharmacotherapy of Asthma

Asthma, or difficulty in breathing attributable to reversible airway obstruction, is a frequent component of allergic reactions and may also result from psychological stress, respiratory infections, or exposure to irritant environmental chemicals. Bronchioles become constricted and edematous, and viscous secretions are trapped within the airways. Several types of drugs will alleviate this potentially life-threatening condition.

Bronchodilators reduce obstruction to airflow by relaxing bronchial smooth muscle. β-Adrenergic agonists are especially effective, since stimulation of β-2 receptors in airways induces bronchodilation. *Epinephrine* and *isoproterenol* can be administered by injection (SC in particular) or by inhalation. Metaproterenol is active orally and by inhalation. Although hazardous, isoproterenol can be administered IV to control refractory status asthmaticus, especially in children.

Several relatively β-2 receptor-selective agonists (Table 7-23) available in aerosol and oral forms have a longer duration of action than epinephrine and isoproterenol, and cause less cardiac (β-1 receptor) stimulation. Terbutaline can be administered SC. These agents are used to alleviate acute attacks and also to reduce the recurrence of bronchospasm.

Tremor is a major adverse effect of the sympathomimetic bronchodilators, induced by stimulation of β-2 receptors in skeletal muscle. Anxiety, cardiac arrhythmias, and pulmonary edema may occur particularly following use of nonselective β agonists. β-2-Selective antagonists can stimulate β-1 receptors in high doses or in sensitive persons. Inhalation of drugs usually provides prompt relief of symptoms with a lower incidence and severity of adverse effects than is observed following systemic routes. Tolerance to the therapeutic actions of β-agonists can develop. Other characteristics of these agents are discussed under "Autonomic Drugs."

TABLE 7-23. Bronchodilators

GENERIC NAME	TRADE NAME
β-Adrenergic Agonists	
Epinephrine	Bronkaid, Medihaler
Isoproterenol	Isuprel
Metaproterenol	Alupent
Albuterol	Proventil, Ventolin
Bitolterol	Tornalate
Ephedrine	Efedron
Isoetharine	Bronkometer
Terbutaline	Brethine
Methylxanthines	
Theophylline	Theo-Dur, Bronkodyl, Slo-Phyllin, others
Dyphylline	Dylline, Lufyllin
Aminophylline	Amoline, Somophyllin, others
Oxtriphylline	Brondecon, Choledyl
Corticosteroids	
Beclomethasone	Beclovent, Vanceril
Flunisolide	AeroBid
Triamcinolone	Azmacort
Anticholinergic	
Ipratropium	Atrovent

Theophylline and aminophylline are effective bronchodilators that can be administered by slow IV infusion to reverse acute asthma. Several oral and rectal formulations are used in chronic asthma to reduce the incidence and severity of symptoms. Rates of inactivation of theophylline vary extensively among patients and doses must be adjusted to each person's response. Cardiac, hepatic, or pulmonary disease, fever, cigarette smoking, age, and the presence of other drugs will influence hepatic metabolism of theophylline. Concomitant food ingestion has variable effects on absorption of oral preparations. Adverse effects include restlessness, nausea, and insomnia. The therapeutic index of theophylline is low, and overdose can result in seizures and fatal cardiac arrhythmias. Plasma concentrations of drug should be monitored; optimal levels range from 5 to 20 μg/ml.

Corticosteroids (Table 7-23) can be combined with other drugs in the management of refractory asthma. By alleviating airway inflammation, they enhance bronchodilation and reduce the required doses of other drugs. Administered orally or by inhalation, they have a gradual onset but prolonged duration of action. Prednisone may be administered on alternate days as a single oral dose taken shortly after awakening. The numerous adverse effects of the corticosteroids are discussed under "Adrenal Pharmacology." Asthmatics receiving systemic corticosteroids should not be switched abruptly to inhaled corticosteroids without tapering the systemic dosage to allow recovery from adrenal cortical suppression. Following inhalation, sufficient drug may be systemically absorbed to suppress the hypothalamic–pituitary–adrenal axis and result in severe adrenal deficiency in times of stress, or when drug doses are reduced or terminated. Administration of corticosteroids should be discontinued gradually rather than abruptly. Oral infections with *Monilia* (candidiasis) may occur with inhalation of these drugs. The propellants utilized in some aerosol formulations have been implicated in sudden deaths among asthmatics. There are two types of inhaled corticosteroid preparations: those absorbed systemically, which suppress adrenal cortical function (*e.g.*, dexamethasone, triamcinolone, flunisolide); and (2) those that are essentially not absorbed from airway surfaces (beclomethasone).

Cromolyn sodium (Intal), an inhaled powder that prevents release of histamine from mast cells, is used prophylactically to reduce the occurrence of allergic or exercise-induced asthma. It is of no use and is contraindicated during asthmatic episodes. Adverse effects are relatively infrequent, although pharyngeal irritation and nausea do occur.

Ipratropium (Atrovent) is available as an inhaled, poorly absorbed, atropinelike bronchodilator with a slower but more prolonged action than the β-agonists. Blood levels are very low and inhalation is usually free of adverse effects. Ipratropium does not cross the blood–brain barrier. It apparently does not increase the viscosity of respiratory secretions or interfere with their expectoration.

Nasal Decongestants

Several α-adrenergic agonists (***ephedrine, epinephrine, naphazoline, oxymetazoline, phenylephrine, tetrahydrozoline,*** and ***xylomethazoline***) are applied locally in sprays and drops to alleviate nasal "stuffiness" that accompanies upper respiratory tract infections and allergic reactions. Otic congestion of middle ear infections may also respond to these drugs. Stimulation of α receptors constricts blood vessels and reduces capillary leakage that causes swelling and excessive secretion. Systemic adverse effects that can occur if sufficient drug is systemically absorbed include anxiety, psychotic disturbances, arrhythmias, and changes in blood pressure. These agents are contraindicated in persons with hyperthyroidism, hypertension, and other cardiovascular disorders. Young children and the elderly are particularly sensitive to the effects of α

agonists. Concomitant administration of MAO inhibitors is contraindicated. The effectiveness of some antihypertensive drugs that utilize neuronal amine pump uptake mechanisms may be reduced. Excessive use of decongestants can result in rebound congestion, leading to the need for a further increase in dosage.

For nasal congestion that is refractory to decongestants, topical preparations of corticosteroids (*betamethasone, dexamethasone,* and *flunisolide*) are available, and cromolyn may be helpful. Administration of topical corticosteroids should not be continued beyond 3 weeks unless definite symptomatic relief is obtained. Systemic absorption of corticosteroids may alter adrenal function. Local responses include nasal dryness, irritation, epistaxis, sneezing, and infection.

Antitussives

The cough reflex is a protective mechanism that clears obstructive substances from the respiratory tract. A dry nonproductive cough that interferes with proper rest is ameliorated by antitussives. Opiates and related drugs that suppress the central cough reflex are most effective. *Codeine* and *hydrocodone* can induce characteristic opiate effects such as respiratory depression and drug dependence. *Dextromethorphan* and *noscapine* have antitussive but not analgesic activity, and cause relatively few adverse reactions. *Diphenhydramine,* an antihistamine that mildly suppresses the cough center, characteristically causes sedation. *Benzonatate* is a nonnarcotic that decreases responsiveness of stretch receptors and central cough mechanisms. Locally acting agents such as glycerin or honey help to alleviate pharyngeal irritation. Expectorants (*e.g.,* *glyceryl guaiacolate,* and *potassium iodide*) may increase fluidity of respiratory secretions so that they may be expectorated more easily. Sufficient hydration and humidified air can ameliorate respiratory irritation and reduce the viscosity of secretions.

Acetylcysteine (Mucomyst) administered by inhalation reduces the viscosity of mucus by depolymerizing mucopolysaccharides.

Respiratory Stimulants

Respiratory stimulants (analeptics) are seldom used, since mechanical ventilatory assistance is generally a more effective and safer mode of supporting respiration. *Doxapram* (Dopram) and *nikethamide* (Coramine) may alleviate drug-induced respiratory depression (*e.g.,* following general anesthesia) and may enhance ventilation in persons with chronic pulmonary disorders. The major adverse effect of these drugs is central nervous system stimulation including convulsions. Patients must be closely observed for untoward reactions and also to ensure that ventilation is adequate.

The carbonic anhydrase inhibitor acetazolamide is investigational in the treatment of high-altitude hypoxia or "mountain sickness." It induces a mild degree of acidosis that stimulates respiration but also reverses the efficacy of the drug. Intermittent administration, or addition of bicarbonate, can prevent drug tolerance.

Therapeutic Gases

Oxygen, essential to many forms of life including mammalian, normally constitutes 20% of inspired air. This gas is frequently administered in clinical conditions that foster hypoxia (reduction in tissue oxygenation) or anoxia (absence of tissue oxygenation). Oxygen deficit occurs by several mechanisms. In anoxic anoxia, entry of oxygen into the lungs or the pulmonary capillaries is reduced. Such anoxia, frequently encountered in pulmonary disease and general anesthesia, is most amenable to oxygen administration. Stagnant anoxia occurs in disorders such as myocardial infarction, congestive heart failure, and shock, when systemic circulation fails to supply adequate blood flow to tissues including the lungs. An enhanced oxygen supply may be of some benefit in these situations. The value of oxygen administration is lower in anemic anoxia, characterized by a deficient oxygen-transporting capacity of blood, and in histotoxic anoxia, caused by substances that suppress cellular utilization of oxygen.

Oxygen is supplied in tanks, commonly color-coded green in the United States. Several devices, capable of delivering varied amounts of oxygen, are available. The rate of flow of oxygen will determine the final concentrations in inspired air. Nasal cannulae or nasopharyngeal catheters, which allow considerable concomitant inspiration of ambient air, can provide 25% to 50% oxygen. Face masks, dependent upon tightness of fit and type of valve (rebreathing or nonrebreathing) can deliver up to 100% oxygen. When spontaneous respiration is absent, mechanical ventilation is required to achieve movement of gases into and out of the lungs. Arterial blood gases (*i.e.,* oxygen and carbon dioxide) must be monitored to determine the actual extent of pulmonary gas exchange.

Oxygen administration should be limited to as

brief a time as possible. Oropharyngeal and pulmonary irritation induce coughing and respiratory difficulty. Prolonged exposure to oxygen alters normal patterns of pulmonary gas exchange by provoking edema, fibrosis, hemorrhage, and formation of a hyaline membrane. This adult respiratory distress syndrome occurs most frequently at high oxygen tension, and may become irreversible. Seizures have been reported to occur with oxygen administration. Premature infants given oxygen are at marked risk of retrolental fibroplasia and blindness. If required, extended periods of oxygen therapy in such infants should utilize oxygen concentrations lower than 40% of inspired air. Commercially prepared oxygen is anhydrous and will dehydrate mucous membranes and cause increased viscosity of respiratory secretions. Since oxygen supports combustion, its use always requires strict precautions to avoid explosion or fire. Smoking, use of open flame, and sparks from electrical appliances must be avoided.

Administration of oxygen is especially hazardous in persons with chronic obstructive pulmonary diseases, as it may aggravate hypoxemia and hypercapnea. Prolonged hypoxia alters the sensitivity of carotid and aortic chemoreceptors, and spontaneous respiration becomes dependent upon low plasma oxygen tension. Increased oxygenation of arterial blood can cause respiratory arrest, necessitating mechanical assistance to breathing. Ventricular arrhythmias may occur with rapid reduction of chronically elevated arterial carbon dioxide levels.

Hyperbaric chambers can provide an atmosphere of increased oxygen pressure. Their use may be of value in the treatment of obstructive lung disease, gas gangrene, decompression sickness, severe and extensive burns, and carbon monoxide poisoning. The usefulness of oxygen in carbon monoxide poisoning is limited by the impaired oxygen-transport capacity of hemoglobin. Oxygen is somewhat soluble in plasma, and inspiration of 100% oxygen can provide small increases in delivery to tissues via this route. The potential adverse effects of oxygen administration can be decreased by keeping chamber pressures at or below three atmospheres.

Oxygen is added to perfusing fluids for excised organs being readied for transplantation, and is used to oxygenate blood during extracorporeal circulation (i.e., in cardiopulmonary bypass). Carbon dioxide is added to pump oxygenators to maintain optimal gas concentrations. The latter is a powerful stimulant to respiration, but excessive amounts in the circulatory system induce respiratory acidosis. Although carbon dioxide dilates cerebral blood vessels, it has been used with little success to alleviate cerebrovascular insufficiency. Carbon dioxide should not be administered to persons with cerebral edema, head injury, or any other source of increased intracranial pressure.

Histamine and Antagonists

Histamine is endogenous to many mammalian cell types, most notably mast cells in the skin and lungs, parietal cells of the gastric mucosa, and basophils. Histamine is also found in the central nervous system, where it appears to be a neurotransmitter. Secretion of gastric acid is markedly influenced by histamine. Antigen–antibody interactions, as well as several drugs (e.g., morphine, trimethaphan) stimulate release of histamine from mast cells. Allergy symptoms such as urticaria, nasal congestion, asthma, and anaphylactic shock are attributable at least in part to this amine.

Histamine exerts its effects by interacting with two distinct types of binding sites, designated H_1 and H_2 histamine receptors. H_1 receptors are most responsible for allergy responses, while H_2 receptors mediate gastric secretion. Both types of receptors are found in brain, and both receptor types probably mediate cardiovascular actions of histamine.

Histamine was administered in the past as a test for gastric secretion when pernicious anemia was suspected. Betazole, a relatively H_1-receptor-specific analogue of histamine, was used in a similar manner. However, side effects that can be life-threatening have made this use obsolete. Prostaglandin has now replaced histamine as a test for gastric-acid secretory responses. Histamine use as a provocative test in the diagnosis of pheochromocytoma is also obsolete. Histamine stimulation of the cells of the adrenal medulla, coupled with an exaggerated reflex response to histamine-induced hypotension, results in massive release of catecholamines in these individuals. Chemical assays of catecholamines are now used. Administration of histamine can provoke all the symptoms of allergy, including asthma and anaphylactic shock. Persons who have allergies are especially responsive to histamine. Additional adverse reactions are headache, dizziness, hypotension, tachycardia, and exacerbation of peptic ulcer symptoms. Betazole causes fewer and less intense side effects.

The conventional or "classic" antihistamines are H_1-receptor antagonists (Table 7-24). They are used extensively in the prevention and control of allergic reactions. Several are available over the counter for this purpose. The most prominent side effect of

TABLE 7-24. Antihistamines

GENERIC NAME	TRADE NAME
H_1-Receptor Antagonists	
Azatadine	Optimine
Brompheniramine	Dimetane
Chlorpheniramine	Chlor-Trimeton, others
Clemastine	Tavist
Cyproheptadine	Periactin
Diphenhydramine	Benadryl, others
Terfenadine	Seldane
Tripelennamine	Pyribenzamine
Triprolidine	Actidil
H_2-Receptor Antagonists	
Cimetidine	Tagamet
Famotidine	Pepcid
Ranitidine	Zantac
Nizatidine	Axid

these drugs is sedation, although recently developed agents such as terfenadine (Seldane) are reported not to cross the blood–brain barrier. H_2-antihistamines are also anticholinergic and will produce dry mouth, urinary retention, thickening of bronchial secretions, and exacerbation of glaucoma. Over-the-counter sleeping aids and motion sickness preventatives often contain antihistamines.

H_2-receptor antagonists (Table 7-24) are used clinically for their ability to suppress both daytime and nocturnal gastric acid secretion in response to a variety of stimuli (*e.g.,* pentagastrin, insulin, histamine, and food ingestion). Treatment and prevention of peptic ulcers, including those that can occur with stress or with Zollinger-Ellison syndrome, are the major indications for these drugs. During clinical development, *cimetidine* (Tagamet) appeared remarkably free of adverse effects. However, postmarket surveillance revealed an inhibition of hepatic metabolism that can result in elevated serum levels of such drugs as diazepam, warfarin, theophylline, and propranolol. Although the H_2-receptor antagonists do not readily cross the blood–brain barrier, cimeditine can cause mental confusion particularly in patients who are elderly or have impaired renal function. Agranulocytosis and thrombocytopenia can occur. *Ranitidine* and *famotidine* have fewer adverse CNS effects because they cross the blood–brain barrier poorly. A longer period of time on the market is needed before their side effects can be fully established.

Prostaglandins

Most tissues can synthesize prostaglandins from free arachidonic acid, which is usually stored in phospholipids and released by phospholipases. The nonsteroidal anti-inflammatory drugs, including aspirin, inhibit the enzyme cyclo-oxygenase, the first step in the formation of prostaglandins. These substances, which have a relatively short biological half-life, exert local actions frequently via activation of adenyl cyclase. Prostaglandins have varied and occasionally opposing action on physiological functions. For example, prostaglandin E_2 (PGE_2) dilates bronchioles while $PGF_{2\alpha}$ is a bronchoconstrictor. PGE_2 and $PGF_{2\alpha}$ both stimulate the pregnant uterus but have opposite effects on the nonpregnant uterus and on blood pressure.

The actions of the prostaglandins have prompted research into possible clinical uses for these substances. Prostaglandins and their analogue have been used as second-trimester abortifacients. Clinical studies on prostaglandin analogues for the alleviation of peptic ulcer and asthma are ongoing. Prostaglandins are involved in inflammation, dysmenorrhea, patent ductus arteriosus in the neonate, and other disease processes. PGE_2 appears to have an important role in renal function.

Additional members of the prostaglandin family are thromboxane A_2 (TxA_2), a potent vasoconstrictor and platelet-aggregating agent, and prostacyclin (PGI_2), which is a vasodilator and antiaggregant. PGI_2 is synthesized in the vascular endothelium and Tx in platelets. The balance between PGI_2 and TxA_2 contributes to the aggregability of platelets.

Another pathway of arachidonic acid metabolism is via lipoxygenase, which gives rise to the leukotrienes. These products, which constrict airways and most blood vessels, have been implicated in the pathogenesis of allergic reactions. A mixture of leukotrienes including C_4 and D_4 account for the activity of slow-reacting substance of anaphylaxis (SRS-A).

GASTROINTESTINAL PHARMACOLOGY

Antacids

Mildly alkaline salts are used to relieve gastric discomfort arising from hyperacidity or peptic ulcer. Healing of the latter may be promoted by the addition of antacids to other regimens of treatment. Antacids can also be administered to achieve alkalinization of the urine, which can be of value in combatting urinary infections and in preventing precipitation of uric acid and various types of drugs.

Antacids contain aluminum, calcium, magnesium, and sodium ions in varying combinations and concentrations. Aluminum and calcium salts have a constipating effect while magnesium salts cause diarrhea, thus antacids are often combined or alternated to promote normal lower intestinal function. Antacid preparations that contain sodium can be deleterious in persons who must restrict their intake of this ion. Magnesium ion in particular can accumulate to toxic levels in the presence of renal impairment. Antacids consumed for an extended time may induce systemic alkalosis; this occurs especially with the water-soluble sodium bicarbonate. Some antacids contribute to the formation of renal stones. Many antacids are available over-the-counter; persons receiving drugs such as digitalis and tetracyclines must be advised of possible interference with drug absorption.

Sucralfate (Carafate), a complex of aluminum hydroxide and sulfated sucrose, promotes healing of duodenal ulcers by forming a local barrier that is protective against pepsin activity. Constipation is the major adverse effect of this drug, which is poorly absorbed. Possible interference with gastrointestinal absorption of digoxin, cimetidine, warfarin, phenytoin, or tetracycline antibiotics can be avoided by administering these drugs at least 2 hours before or after sucralfate.

H_2 histamine receptor antagonists and anticholinergic agents, also used in the management of peptic ulcer and Zollinger-Ellison syndrome, are discussed elsewhere in this chapter.

Emetics

Emetics can be useful in evacuating some toxic substances from the stomach if gastric lavage is unavailable. It must be noted, however, that induction of vomiting is contraindicated following ingestion of corrosive substances that may further damage the esophagus. Guidance from a poison control center can be useful in determining proper treatment of some poisonings. Emetics should not be administered to persons who are lethargic or unconscious. Patients should be monitored until vomiting has ceased.

Drugs that induce vomiting may act through nonspecific gastric irritation, or may stimulate the chemoreceptor trigger zone or the vomiting center in the central nervous system. *Apomorphine* has a central site of action, producing vomiting within 15 minutes following SC administration. A single dose only is given. Apomorphine can induce characteristic opiate central nervous system depression and cardiovascular failure.

Ipecac syrup appears to act through local irrita-

tion of the gastric mucosa and stimulation of central control areas. This drug is administered orally. If vomiting does not ensue, ipecac *must* be evacuated from the stomach by other means. Systemic absorption of this drug is hazardous because of its marked cardiovascular effects. The more highly concentrated ipecac fluid extract should not be confused with ipecac syrup.

Antiemetics

Suppression of vomiting may be desirable to reduce the risk of malnutrition, dehydration, and electrolyte depletion. Emesis itself is a sign of local or central irritation, and the cause for persistent vomiting must be investigated.

Antihistamines such as dimenhydrinate, hydroxyzine, and meclizine are most effective in alleviating emesis of vestibular origin. Several motion sickness remedies containing these drugs are available over-the-counter. The anticholinergic *scopolamine* is incorporated into a transdermal form (Transderm-Scōp) for this indication. Phenothiazines and other drugs such as *metoclopramide* (Reglan), which block central dopaminergic receptors, can be used to alleviate vomiting following general anesthesia, and may be somewhat effective in reducing the severe emesis that often accompanies antineoplastic therapy. *Diphenidol* (Vontrol) and *benzquinamide* (emete-Con) can alleviate moderate nausea and vomiting. Caution must be exercised in the use of drugs with antiemetic action because they can suppress this manifestation of drug toxicity or organic disease. Tetrahydrocannabinal (THC) (only sold in a few states at this writing) or its synthetic analogue nabilone can be used to treat the vomiting associated with cancer chemotherapy.

Laxatives

Laxatives are used to facilitate evacuation of contents from the lower intestinal tract. The irritant action of laxatives including *bisacodyl, cascara, castor oil,* and *phenolphthalein* promotes peristalsis. They also affect water content by increasing secretion by PGE_2, cAMP and inhibition of Na^+-K^+-ATPase. Other laxatives add moisture and bulk to fecal material, softening the stool and enhancing passage through the bowel. Nonabsorbed, bulk-forming laxatives include *methylcellulose* and *psyllium.* Saline or osmotic laxatives (*e.g.,* glycerin, lactulose, magnesium salts, and sodium phosphates) draw fluid into the intestinal tract. Calcium *polycarbophil* can act as a bulk-forming laxative, or can alleviate diarrhea by drawing excess water out of loose fecal matter.

Surface-acting or wetting agents such as the docusates do not relieve constipation but will counteract further formation of hard dry feces. Persons with cardiovascular disease or hernia, in whom straining to defecate can be hazardous, benefit from the use of these drugs.

Abdominal pain, nausea, or other indications of gastrointestinal obstruction or acute abdomen contraindicate the administration of laxatives. Persons who experience frequent constipation should be encouraged to increase their intake of fluids and fiber-rich foods. Regular exercise also can promote normal intestinal function. Chronic use of laxatives, many of which are available without prescription, can induce dehydration, electrolyte imbalance, and dependence upon these agents for bowel function. The use of laxatives can reduce the absorption of orally administered drugs by shortening their transit time through the intestine.

ENDOCRINE PHARMACOLOGY

Anterior Pituitary Hormones

Under the regulation of stimulatory and inhibitory factors released by the hypothalamus, the anterior pituitary synthesizes and releases several hormones that affect growth and development, often through actions on other endocrine organs. Somatostatin, which inhibits release of growth hormone, is found also in the gastrointestinal tract and pancreas, where it reduces secretion of insulin, glucagon, and digestive fluids.

Adrenocorticotropic hormone (ACTH) promotes synthesis and release of hormones such as cortisol from the adrenal cortex and is in turn subject to negative feedback control by plasma levels of these hormones. It is used clinically to differentiate between primary and secondary adrenocortical insufficiency. In persons with functional adrenals, administration of ACTH provokes secretion of corticosteroids that is reflected in elevated plasma and urinary levels of 17-hydroxycorticosteroid and 17-ketosteroid metabolites. ACTH is seldom used to treat adrenal insufficiency, since administration of corticosteroids provides more consistent and reliable hormone replacement. Symptoms of multiple sclerosis, myasthenia gravis, and hypercalcemia resulting from carcinoma may be alleviated with ACTH. This hormone is derived from animal pituitary and must be administered parenterally. Adverse effects are similar to those observed with adrenocortical hyperactivity or administration of corticosteroids. Allergic reactions, some provoked by contaminating porcine protein, can develop. Sustained action forms of ACTH that contain zinc hydroxide and gelatin must not be administered I.V. Contraindications to the use of ACTH include osteoporosis, congestive heart failure, and hypertension.

Cosyntropin (Cortrosyn) is a synthetic analogue containing the first 24 amino acids in the ACTH sequence. It is a diagnostic agent for adrenocortical responsiveness, and is less likely than ACTH to provoke allergic reactions.

Metyrapone (Metopirone), an agent diagnostic for anterior pituitary function, inhibits the enzymatic biosynthesis of the corticosteroids. This reduces negative feedback control and increases the release of ACTH if pituitary function is adequate. Subsequent synthesis of corticosteroid precursors will be reflected in elevated urinary levels of 17-hydroxy and 11-deoxy metabolites. Responsiveness of the adrenals should be determined before metyrapone is administered. Phenytoin, cyproheptadine, exogenous estrogen, and pregnancy may alter the results of metyrapone testing.

Thyroid-stimulating hormone (TSH, thyrotropin) induces iodine uptake and hormone synthesis in the thyroid gland. Similarly to ACTH, TSH is used to diagnose primary and secondary hypothyroidism. Because it provokes release of triiodothyronine (T_3) and thyroxine (T_4), inappropriate administration of TSH can elicit symptoms similar to hyperthyroidism and thyrotoxicosis; tachycardia, angina pectoris, and congestive heart failure may develop or be exacerbated. The long onset (up to 8 hours) and duration (24 to 48 hours or more) of action necessitate persistent observation of patients. Secretion of TSH is stimulated by the hypothalamic thyrotropin-releasing hormone (TRH), and is under negative feedback control relative to plasma levels of thyroid hormones.

The gonadotropic hormones of the anterior pituitary promote and maintain sexual development and function. *Follicle-stimulating hormone* (FSH) induces maturation of ovarian follicles and secretion of estrogen. *Luteinizing hormone* (LH) causes rupture of the follicle (ovulation) and supports secretion of progesterone by the corpus luteum. LH also induces synthesis and release of testosterone from testicular Leydig cells. *Menotropins* (human menopausal gonadotropins, Pergonal) are derived from urine of postmenopausal women and contain large amounts of FSH and LH. Anovulatory women with functional ovaries can be given menotropins to induce follicular development, and subsequent administration of **human chorionic gonadotropin** (HCG, Follutein, which has pronounced LH-like activity) will elicit ovulation. This treatment for infertility presents the risk of ovarian hyperstimulation resulting in rupture of cysts and severe intraperitonal hemorrhage. The incidence of multiple fetuses is increased, and pregnancies often terminate with the premature birth of high-risk infants. Spermatogenesis also can be stimulated by menotropins, and HCG is used to induce testicular descent in prepubertal boys.

Human growth hormone (HGH, somatotropin, Asellacrin) will stimulate growth and development in children with growth hormone deficiency. Treatment must be given before epiphyseal closure, and concomitant or induced hypothyroidism must be corrected. HGH is diabetogenic and influences protein, fat, and electrolyte metabolism. Recombinant DNA technology has made available a more abundant supply of HGH (somatrem, Protropin; somatropin, Humatrope) free of the risk of transmitting Creutzfeldt-Jakob disease.

Prolactin, normally elevated only during pregnancy and lactation, stimulates the mammary glands to produce milk. Release of this anterior pituitary hormone is under inhibitory control of the neurotransmitter dopamine. The dopamine agonist bromocriptine (Parlodel) is administered to reverse hyperprolactinemia that is not GH-dependent and to suppress unwanted postpartum lactation. Pharmacological agents that deplete dopamine (*e.g.,* alpha methyldopa) or which block dopamine receptors (*e.g.,* the neuroleptics) will promote prolactin release.

Posterior Pituitary Hormones

Vasopressin (antidiuretic hormone, ADH) and oxytocin are secreted by the posterior pituitary (neurohypophysis). Vasopressin influences renal reabsorption of water by altering membrane permeability in the distal tubule and collecting duct of the nephron. Vasopressin (Pitressin) and the synthetic analogue desmopressin (DDAVP) and lypressin (Diapid) will alleviate diabetes insipidus caused by endogenous ADH deficiency. (Nephrogenic diabetes insipidus, characterized by renal unresponsiveness to ADH, is treated with thiazide diuretics.) Fluid intake and output must be monitored, because water intoxication can occur. Like many hormone preparations, vasopressin must be administered parenterally. Desmopressin and lypressin are given intranasally. Vascular constriction caused by vasopressin can induce hypertension, angina pectoris, and myocardial infarction; persons with cardiovascular disease are at greatest risk. Oxytocic-like activity, apparent at high doses, makes this drug hazardous during pregnancy. The synthetic analogues cause less stimulation of vascular and uterine smooth muscle and are, therefore, preferable to ADH in pregnancy. Vasopressin is also used to alleviate postsurgical abdominal distention. Desmopressin induces a temporary increase in plasma levels of clotting factors that can help to control abnormal bleeding in some types of Von Willebrand's disease and hemophilia.

Oxytocin secreted by the posterior pituitary appears to have an important physiological role in parturition and lactation. Responsiveness of the uterine muscle to oxytocin gradually intensifies during pregnancy. Increased amounts of this hormone are released at the time of labor and delivery, possibly in response to dilation of the cervix and vagina.

Exogenous **oxytocin** (Pitocin) is occasionally administered to enhance uterine activity in carefully selected patients in whom pregnancy or labor is not progressing normally. It is too hazardous for use in routine deliveries since powerful sustained contractions can result in fetal hypoxia or uterine rupture. Fetal or maternal arrhythmias and water intoxication (oxytocin has some ADH activity) can be severe. There are many contraindications to the use of oxytocin, such as malpositioning of the fetus, maternal history of cervical or uterine surgery (including cesarean section), placenta previa, and umbilical cord prolapse. Oxytocin is administered by slow IV infusion carefully titrated to produce contraction patterns similar to those of normal labor. Patients must be under continual observation, and drug administration is terminated if fetal distress, uterine hyperactivity, or significant changes in maternal vital signs occur. After the infant and placenta have been delivered, oxytocin can be given to control uterine atony and hemorrhage. The sustained uterine contractions help to seal off bleeding from arterioles. Oxytocin is an abortifacient, especially in later pregnancy (during the first trimester, the uterus is relatively unresponsive to oxytocin). Flow of milk ("milk letdown") is stimulated by this hormone, which is available in a nasal spray to be used by lactating women. Oxytocin can potentiate the pressor effect of sympathomimetic drugs.

The ergot alkaloids (ergonovine and methylergonovine) are oxytocics that are used to control postpartum atony and hemorrhage of the uterus. Vasoconstriction can occur and occasionally produces severe hypertension or circulatory stasis in the extremities.

Thyroid Hormones

The thyroid gland synthesizes *thyroxine* (T_4) as well as small amounts of *triiodothyronine* (T_3). Many tissues in the human body convert T_4 to T_3, which is the more active form of thyroid hormone. In the circulatory system, most T_4 and T_3 is bound to thyroid hormone-binding globulin and to albumin.

Thyroid hormone is essential for proper growth and metabolism. Its absence is especially severe in infants and very young children, in whom arrested physical and mental development known as cretinism can occur. Thyroid deficiency is treated with hormone-replacement therapy. Thyroid USP and thyroid extract (Proloid) are prepared from animal thyroid. *Levothyroxine* (Synthroid) and *liothyronine* (Cytomel) are synthetic sodium salts of T_4 and T_3 that can be administered either orally or intravenously. *Liotrix* (Euthyroid, Thyrolar) combines levothyroxine and liothyronine in a 4:1 ratio that approximates the endogenous levels of thyroid hormones. Thyroid preparations have a gradual onset and long duration of action due in part to their extensive binding to circulatory proteins. (Levels of thyroid hormone-binding globulin can be decreased by corticosteroid administration and increased in pregnancy). Thyroid hormones are used clinically to suppress excessive release of TSH.

The replacement dosage of thyroid hormone must be individualized to produce the desired response in each patient. Many drugs (*e.g.*, aspirin, lithium, propranolol, and estrogens) can alter the results of thyroid function tests. Excessive amounts of hormone will produce symptoms similar to those of hyperthyroidism (*e.g.*, tachycardia, angina pectoris, irritability, insomnia, and heat intolerance). Hormone administration is contraindicated in persons with cardiovascular disease unless hypothyroidism coexists. Thyroid hormones appear to increase the number of myocardial β-adrenergic receptors, producing increased responsiveness to catecholamines and to sympathetic stimulation. The action of the oral anticoagulants can be increased by concomitant thyroid hormone administration, while the effectiveness of antidiabetic therapy is decreased.

Hyperactivity of the thyroid can be alleviated by surgical removal of the gland, or by pharmacological treatment. The antithyroid drugs *propylthiouracil* (PTU) and *methimazole* (Tapazole) inhibit the synthesis of thyroid hormones. They do not block the actions of the hormones, which are occasionally administered concurrently (*e.g.*, during pregnancy) to maintain a desirable level of thyroid influence. Because antithyroid drugs deplete circulating amounts of T_4 and T_3, the negative feedback control of TSH release is reduced. The resulting increase in TSH can induce enlargement and vascularization of the thyroid. Bone marrow suppression, which increases susceptibility to infections and severe hemorrhage, is a major adverse effect of antithyroid agents. Oral anticoagulant activity can be potentiated. Fatal hepatitis can be induced by administration of these drugs. Their use is contraindicated in nursing mothers because of the danger of inducing cretinism in the infant.

High doses of iodides (sodium and potassium iodides, and "strong iodine" or Lugol's solution) are given to suppress thyroid hormone synthesis and release. They may be combined with antithyroid drugs in the presurgical treatment of thyroidectomy patients. Intravenous administration is indicated for the management of thyrotoxicosis (thyroid crisis or storm). These agents have a slow onset and prolonged duration of action. Marked sensitivity to iodides may cause laryngeal edema and suffocation. Pretesting for reactivity is advisable, especially if the parenteral route is to be used.

Radioactive iodine (^{131}I) is used to assess thyroid function and to treat hyperthyroidism and thyroid carcinoma. This cytotoxic isotope is concentrated by the thyroid. ^{131}I is contraindicated in pregnancy and lactation, and is rarely administered for hyperthyroidism in persons younger than 30 years of age. Treatment with ^{131}I can cause sore throat, bone marrow suppression, radiation sickness, and eventual hypothyroidism as the gland is destroyed. Antithyroid drugs will hinder uptake of ^{131}I, thus administration of such agents must cease 3 to 4 days before isotope therapy. Radiation safety precautions may be instituted to protect patient, staff, and visitors from injury.

Parathyroid Hormones

Parathyroid hormone (PTH) strongly influences plasma calcium levels by increasing bone resorption, enhancing renal reabsorption of calcium and excretion of phosphate, promoting intestinal uptake of dietary calcium, and stimulating the activation of vitamin D. Secretion of this hormone is regulated by plasma calcium levels. PTH is rarely used in the management of hypocalcemia since it rapidly provokes formation of antibodies. Administration of PTH is diagnostic for hypoparathyroidism, provoking an excessive increase in urinary phosphorus excretion in persons with hormone deficiency.

Hypocalcemia can be alleviated by administration of vitamin D, which is converted to its active forms, calcitriol and dihydrotachysterol, in the kidneys and liver. Vitamin D promotes intestinal absorption of calcium; thus adequate dietary intake is essential for the efficacy of this treatment. Calcium salts (*e.g.,* chloride, gluconate, and glucepate) can be administered IV to alleviate severe hypocalcemia manifested as tetany or marked prolongation of the myocardial Q–T interval. Calcium enhances responsiveness to defibrillation, and may help to restore cardiac rhythm. Extreme caution is required in patients receiving digitalis because calcium potentiates both the inotropic and toxic effects of the cardiac glycosides. Sodium bicarbonate will precipitate calcium salts from solution. The use of oral calcium to alleviate osteoporosis in women after menopause is controversial: studies indicate that concomitant estrogen replacement is required for adequate use of this ion.

Excessive amounts of vitamin D can produce hypercalcemia. Symptoms include muscle weakness, nausea, and diarrhea. Significant demineralization of bone can occur, and renal stones and soft-tissue calcium deposits may develop.

Calcitonin, a hormone synthesized by the thyroid, has actions opposite to those of PTH (*i.e.,* inhibition of bone resorption and enhancement of renal excretion of calcium and phosphate). Hypercalcemia induces the release of calcitonin. This hormone is used in the treatment of osteoporosis, hypercalcemia, and Paget's disease, which is characterized by abnormal osteoclastic and osteoblastic activity. Salmon calcitonin (Calcimar) provokes antibody formation and allergic responses. Synthetic hormone (Cibacalcin) identical to human calcitonin is also available.

Etidronate (Didronel), a diphosphatase that suppresses bone formation and resorption, also is used to manage Paget's disease and to reduce aberrant ossification following hip replacement or spinal cord injury. Etidronate is administered only for a limited time (6 months for Paget's disease, 3 months following surgery or injury). The onset of action is gradual, and the dosage should be increased cautiously. Adequate calcium and vitamin D intake must be maintained.

Adrenocortical Hormones

Adrenocortical hormones are essential for human survival. Addison's disease and other forms of ad-

renal insufficiency necessitate chronic corticosteroid replacement therapy. Endogenous cortical secretions are of two types: the *glucocorticoids,* which serve mainly to regulate carbohydrate and protein metabolism and resistance to stress; and the *mineralocorticoids,* which influence sodium and water balance. Synthesis of *hydrocortisone* (cortisol), the principal glucocorticoid in humans, is stimulated by ACTH. Plasma levels of glucocorticoids follow a pattern of circadian variation, with highest amounts just after awakening. Administration of exogenous cortisol in a similar pattern (*i.e.,* once daily or on alternate days early in the waking period), often provides a good therapeutic response with lower incidence of adverse effects. An increase in dosage may be necessary in times of increased stress (*e.g.,* illness or surgery).

Secretion of the mineralocorticoids (desoxycorticosterone and aldosterone) is regulated by circulating blood volume. A decrease in volume activates the juxtaglomerular apparatus and the renin–angiotensin system, which in turn stimulates aldosterone release. This hormone acts in the distal tubule of the nephron, promoting sodium reabsorption in exchange for potassium and hydrogen ion. The naturally occurring glucocorticoids possess some mineralocorticoid activity, and some persons with adrenal insufficiency can be maintained solely on hydrocortisone plus adequate dietary sodium chloride. *Fludrocortisone* (Florinef) is an orally active synthetic steroid possessing glucocorticoid and mineralocorticoid activities and is useful in patients with Addison's disease who need greater assistance in maintaining water and electrolyte balance. *Desoxycorticosterone* (Percorten) can be administered when the parenteral route is preferred. In Addison's disease, response to the mineralocorticoids may be heightened, resulting in edema, hypokalemia, hypertension, and cardiac arrhythmias. Increased aldosterone secretion can occur in adrenal hyperplasia or malignancy, toxemia of pregnancy, renal hypertension, and hepatic cirrhosis with ascites. The potassium-sparing diuretic spironolactone (Aldactone) is an aldosterone antagonist.

In addition to their use in replacement therapy, the naturally occurring glucocorticoids and their synthetic analogs (Table 7-25) are administered in pharmacologic doses in the management of many illnesses including rheumatoid arthritis, rheumatic fever with carditis, acute leukemia, exfoliative dermatitis, pulmonary fibrosis, ulcerative colitis, nephrotic syndrome, systemic lupus erythematosus, and other inflammatory and autoimmune diseases. Cerebral edema and anaphylactic shock are indica-

TABLE 7-25. Glucocorticoids

GENERIC NAME	TRADE NAME
Cortisone	Cortisan, others
Hydrocortisone	Cortef, Hydrocortone, others
Beclomethasone	Beclovent, Vanceril
Betamethasone	Celestone
Dexamethasone	Decadron, others
Flunisolide	AeroBid
Methylprednisolone	Medrol
Prednisone	Meticorten, others
Prednisolone	Delta-Cortef, Cortalone
Triamcinolone	Aristocort, Azmacort, others

tions for the glucocorticoids. The use of prednisone in particular to suppress immunity aids the survival of organ transplants.

The adverse effects of these drugs are numerous and can be serious, even life-threatening. Suppression of the hypothalamic–pituitary–adrenal axis falls into the latter category. Prolonged administration of glucocorticoids inhibits release of corticotropin (CRF) and ACTH, allowing the adrenal cortex to atrophy. If administration of hormone is abruptly terminated, the individual is left in a state of adrenal insufficiency. For this reason, glucocorticoid dosages must always be tapered gradually, with careful observation for signs of hypoadrenalism. Once daily or alternate-day dosing is reported to affect ACTH release minimally.

Administration of glucocorticoids suppresses immune responsiveness, predisposing to the development or exacerbation of infections. Bone demineralization (osteoporosis), diabetes, weight gain, edema, hypertension, weakening of blood vessel walls, peptic ulcer, electrolyte imbalance, mental changes, cataracts, glaucoma, impaired wound healing, menstrual irregularities, muscle weakness, and protein wasting are a few of the many additional adverse reactions to the glucocorticoids. Administration during pregnancy may cause cleft palate and pituitary–adrenal suppression in the fetus. Glucocorticoids are contraindicated in active tuberculosis, malignant hypertension, uremia, psychoses, active peptic ulcer, and in nursing mothers. Both types of adrenal hormones are biotransformed in the liver to a variety of metabolites such as sulfates and glucoronides, which are renally excreted.

Many of the synthetic corticosteroids (*e.g.*, prednisone, prednisolone and dexamethasone) have greater anti-inflammatory potency with lower mineralocorticoid activity than cortisone and cortisol. Synthetic glucocorticoids also have a longer duration of action than the natural substances. Predni-

sone acts for 18 to 36 hours while dexamethasone's effects may persist up to 48 hours.

Because glucocorticoids influence carbohydrate metabolism, they can increase the requirement for insulin or oral hypoglycemics in diabetic patients. Drugs that induce hepatic enzymes can enhance the biotransformation of corticosteroids, while oral contraceptives may inhibit their inactivation. Corticosteroids can alter blood coagulation; concomitant administration of aspirin or coumarin-type drugs requires observation for abnormal bleeding tendencies. Mineralocorticoid-induced potassium loss will add to diuretic-induced hypokalemia, and can enhance digitalis toxicity.

Beclomethasone (Beclovent, Vanceril), **flunisolide** (AeroBid), and **triamcinolone** (Azmacort) are corticosteroids in aerosolized form used in the management of asthma that is inadequately controlled by other drug regimens. Drug amounts systemically absorbed from the lungs can be sufficient to suppress the hypothalamic–pituitary–adrenal axis, yet insufficient to substitute for systemically administered corticosteroids. Any alteration in drug regimen requires close observation for adrenal deficiency.

Nasal aerosols of beclomethasone and dexamethasone will alleviate inflammatory nasal conditions (see "Respiratory Pharmacology"). A variety of ocular inflammatory disorders are treated with ophthalmic ointments and solutions of dexamethasone and prednisolone. Topical corticosteroid creams and ointments, some available over-the-counter, will relieve pruritic and inflammatory dermatoses such as eczema; poison ivy, oak, or sumac; insect bites; and allergic reactions. **Betamethasone** (Diprolene) and **clobetasol** (Temovate) are the most potent of these agents, and present the greatest risk of adrenal suppression due to systemic absorption.

Aminoglutethimide (Cytadren) blocks the conversion of cholesterol to pregnenolone, thus reducing adrenal synthesis of steroids. This agent is occasionally used in the control of Cushing's syndrome, and may be palliative in some patients with advanced breast cancer or metastatic carcinoma of the prostate.

Insulin

The pancreas secretes insulin (from β cells in the islets of Langerhans) and glucagon (from α cells), both important for proper metabolism. Insulin is essential for the entry of glucose into many human tissues (exceptions to this are brain, liver, red blood cells, β-cells, and kidney tubules). This hormone appears to work by interacting with receptors on cell membranes. Release of insulin is stimulated by elevated blood levels of glucose, and by gastrin, secretin, ketone bodies, and glucagon. Epinephrine and norepinephrine, acting at β-adrenergic receptors, suppress insulin release. Many of the actions of insulin are opposed by glucagon, which promotes ketogenesis, glycogenolysis and hyperglycemia. Glucagon release is promoted by amino acids and suppressed by glucose, ketones, and free fatty acids.

In diabetes mellitus, insulin is lacking (type I, insulin-dependent, or juvenile-onset diabetes) or fails to function adequately (type II, non-insulin-dependent, or maturity-onset diabetes). Failure of the pancreas to synthesize insulin requires that this hormone be administered throughout the lifetime of the patient. Diet and exercise must be properly balanced against insulin intake to maintain blood glucose within relatively safe levels. Persons who have diabetes are at greater than normal risk for cardiovascular disease, renal disease, and degenerative ocular changes. Hyperglycemia can cause brain damage, coma, and death, and can be fetotoxic.

Several forms of insulin are available for the management of diabetes mellitus. Most are derived from animal sources; all must be administered parenterally. Crystalline zinc insulin or *regular insulin* is a clear solution that can be administered by either the SC or IV route. It has a rapid onset and short duration (6 to 8 hours) of action. All other forms of insulin can be given only by the SC route.

Ultralente insulin is crystalline insulin with an onset of 4 to 6 hours and a duration of action up to 18 hours. *Semilente* or *amorphous insulin,* with an onset of 2 to 4 hours and duration of 12 to 16 hours, can be mixed with ultralente to provide an intermediate-acting lente insulin. Protamine insulin suspensions are gradually absorbed from the SC site and provide a long duration of action. *Neutral protamine Hagedorn* (NPH) insulin or isophane insulin is a crystalline modification of protamine zinc insulin. Regular insulin can be added to NPH insulin without losing its rapid, intense action. Protamine zinc insulin will retard the absorption of regular insulin.

Insulins can be combined to provide both immediate and sustained control of blood glucose. Three concentrations of insulin are currently available: U100 (or 100 units per ml) is most commonly used, U40 is available for administration of small doses, and U500 is used by persons who have developed insulin resistance and must receive large doses.

Hypersensitivity can develop to contaminants such as glucagon and somatostatin found in insulin. Highly purified insulin preparations (*e.g.,* single-component and purified porcine insulin) are available but are more expensive and limited in supply. Recombinant DNA technology has produced a biosynthetic human insulin (Humulin) that is expected to be less allergenic than that derived from animals.

Since chronic SC injection of insulin can cause atrophy or hypertrophy of subcutaneous tissue, injection sites should be rotated. Administration of insulin carries the risk of overdose or underdose and subsequent hypoglycemia or hyperglycemia. Changes in exercise or eating habits, or increased physiological or psychological stress, alter insulin requirements. Persons who are diabetic must be aware of all factors that can affect their well-being. Regular testing of the blood or urine for glucose is essential to diabetic control. Patients must also be alert to symptoms of hypoglycemia (hunger, nausea, irritability, tremor, mental confusion, tachycardia, ataxia), which can be alleviated by administration of some source of glucose. Severe hypoglycemia, which can result in convulsions, coma, and irreversible brain damage, can be treated with IV dextrose or SC or IM glucagon. Since β-adrenergic blockers can mask the symptoms of hypoglycemia, these drugs are hazardous in diabetic persons.

Persistent hypoinsulinemia leads to elevated plasma levels of glucagon, epinephrine, and growth hormone, which mobilize free fatty acids and eventually produce ketoacidosis or diabetic coma. Administration of insulin will reverse these effects by normalizing glucose utilization. Hydration with normal saline and infusion of dextrose may also be necessary. Marked depletion of body stores of potassium can accompany ketoacidosis, although plasma levels of this electrolyte may be normal. Administration of insulin promotes reentry of potassium into cells with subsequent hypokalemia. However, potassium supplements are given only when plasma levels persistently fail to normalize, and renal function is adequate.

Type II diabetes can often be ameliorated by administration of the sulfonylurea or oral hypoglycemic agents (Table 7-26). These drugs are ineffective in the total absence of endogenous insulin. The exact mechanism of action of the oral hypoglycemics is not known. Studies have suggested that they may enhance release of insulin from the pancreas or promote the utilization of insulin by body tissues. Control of type II diabetes should initially be attempted through diet, exercise, and weight loss where appropriate. Patients receiving oral hypoglycemics

TABLE 7-26. Oral Hypoglycemic Drugs

GENERIC NAME	TRADE NAME
First Generation	
Acetohexamide	Dymelor
Chlorpropamide	Diabinese
Tolazamide	Tolinase
Tolbutamide	Orinase
Second Generation	
Glipizide	Glucotrol
Glyburide	Diabeta, Micronase

must balance food intake, physical activity, and stress with their drug regimen. Failure to do so can cause hypoglycemia or hyperglycemia.

Side effects of the oral hypoglycemics include dermatological allergic reactions and gastrointestinal disturbances. Chlorpropamide may cause sodium and fluid retention, while the newer agents, glyburide and glipizide, have a mild diuretic effect. Tolerance can develop to the hypoglycemic action of these drugs. Controversial results of the University Group Diabetes Program study suggested that these drugs may increase the risk of cardiovascular disease.

Some of the oral hypoglycemics, chlorpropamide in particular, can induce a disulfiram-like reaction following alcohol ingestion. Extensive plasma protein binding of these drugs may alter the actions of other drugs. Many drugs can affect blood glucose levels (*e.g.*, thiazide diuretics and sympathomimetics elevate while β-adrenergic blockers lower glucose levels) and may thus alter insulin or oral hypoglycemic requirements.

Female Hormones

Estrogens and *progesterone* are endogenous steroid hormones synthesized principally in the ovary and the placenta. In addition, small amounts of these substances are formed in adipose tissue, adrenal cortex, liver, kidney, and other organs; these remain a source of female hormones in postmenopausal women. Naturally occurring estrogens include *estradiol, estriol,* and *estrone.* Salts and esters of these hormones, as well as synthetic analogues, are available (Table 7-27). In general, the naturally occurring estrogens must be administered parenterally, although *conjugated estrogens* (Premarin, sodium salts of sulfate esters) and *esterified estrogens* (Amnestrogen) are active when given by the oral route. Many topical preparations, and estradiol in a

transdermal system, are also used. Estrogens are extensively metabolized in the liver.

The estrogenic substances have many physiologic actions: *e.g.*, the primary effects of stimulation of the development of female reproductive organs, proliferation of the endometrium during the menstrual cycle, and maintenance of pregnancy. Secondary sex characteristics such as skin texture, adipose tissue distribution, and skeletal growth are influenced by estrogens. Adverse effects caused by these hormones include nausea, menstrual changes, headache, depression, sodium and fluid retention, thromboembolism, hypertension, hyperglycemia, and closure of epiphyses when administered before completion of skeletal development. Estrogens may increase the risk of endometrial carcinoma; concomitant administration of progestogens has a protective effect.

A major clinical use for estrogens is in combination with progestogens in oral contraceptives (discussed below). Estrogen can help to slow bone demineralization in osteoporosis; it is most effective when administration is begun before extensive bone loss has occurred. The effectiveness of calcium salts in osteoporosis is greatly enhanced by concomitant estrogen administration. Estrogens will alleviate menopausal symptoms, including urogenital atrophy, and are used as replacement therapy in endogenous hormone deficiency. Treatment of inoperable breast or prostate cancer often includes estrogenic substances.

Progesterone is secreted principally by the corpus luteum. This hormone converts endometrial proliferation to the secretory phase of the menstrual cycle, prepares the uterus for ovum implantation, and subsequently maintains pregnancy. Progesterone is not active when taken orally, but several synthetic progestogens (Table 7-27) are effectively absorbed from the gastrointestinal tract. Inactivation of these substances is accomplished mainly by hepatic enzymes.

Progestogens are widely used in oral contraceptives, for regulation of menstrual abnormalities, and in endometrial and renal carcinoma. Progesterone may occasionally be effective in relieving symptoms of premenstrual syndrome. Progestogens induce many of the same adverse effects attributable to estrogens. Both types of hormones are contraindicated during pregnancy since the risk of subsequent cancer and of fetal damage resulting in congenital defects is considerable.

Many of the oral contraceptives combine an estrogen and a progestogen. The mechanism of action of these preparations is thought to be suppression of

TABLE 7-27. Estrogens and Progestogens

GENERIC NAME	TRADE NAME
Estrogens	
Chlorotrianisene	Tace
Conjugated estrogens	Premarin
Diethylstilbestrol	Stilphostrol
Estradiol	Estrase, Estraderm, others
Estrone	Theelin
Ethinylestradiol	Estinyl
Quinestrol	Estrovis
Progestogens	
Hydroxyprogesterone	Delalutin
Medroxyprogesterone	Depo-Provera
Norethindrone	Norlutin
Norgestrel	Ovrette
Progesterone	Femotrone, Progestaject

ovulation by inhibiting the release of pituitary gonadotropins in a negative feedback manner. However, there is evidence that they are effective in doses lower than those necessary to suppress gonadotropins, and there may also be a direct effect on the ovary or interference with transport of ova or with fertilization or implantation. Oral contraceptives are a unique pharmacological entity, as they are used for substantial intervals of time by large numbers of relatively healthy young women to alter normal physiological functions. Although the incidence of serious side effects is low, the potential for thrombophlebitis, embolism, and hypertension must be recognized. Cigarette smoking greatly increases the risk of serious cardiovascular sequelae, particularly in women older than 35 years. Coexistence of both of these conditions should contraindicate the use of oral contraceptives. More frequent adverse reactions include nausea, sodium and fluid retention, breast tenderness, and breakthrough bleeding. Because of possible adverse effects on the fetus, pregnancy must be absolutely ruled out before oral contraceptive therapy is begun, and drug administration must be terminated if pregnancy is suspected. Cardiovascular disease, including hypertension and thrombotic tendency, and certain types of cancer contraindicate the use of oral contraceptives.

Combination contraceptives consist of 21 daily doses of an estrogen plus a progestogen, followed by 7 drug-free days. (Placebos frequently are substituted for this interval, to maintain the daily pattern of taking one tablet.) *Ethinyl estradiol* or *mestranol* provides the estrogen component; the progestogen may be *norgestrel, levonorgestrel,* or *norethindrone.* Recent formulations contain the lowest effective doses and correspondingly produce minimal adverse effects. A second type of oral contraceptive, the "minipill," which contains progestogen only, has a lower efficacy than combination drugs. Sequential formulations, in which 16 days of estrogen-only administration was followed by 5 days of estrogen plus progestogen have been discontinued because of an apparent risk of endometrial carcinoma. Drugs that induce hepatic enzymes can enhance the inactivation of these hormones and reduce the efficacy of contraception.

The antiestrogen *clomiphene* (Clomid) enhances pituitary release of gonadotropins, which in turn induces ovulation. Used as a fertility agent, this drug frequently results in multiple fetuses. Blurring or other visual disturbances occasionally develop, and can impair the ability to drive or operate machinery.

The antiestrogen *tamoxifen* (Nolvadex) is discussed under "Chemotherapy of Malignant Disease."

Male Hormones

Testosterone is the principal endogenous androgen. Like the female hormones, it is metabolized in the liver and is ineffective when given orally. Several synthetic analogs (Table 7-28) can be administered PO. These hormones stimulate the maturation of male reproductive organs and sexual characteristics. Androgens are also potent anabolic substances, promoting skeletal muscle development.

Androgens are administered as replacement therapy when endogenous testosterone is deficient. Several nortestosterone derivatives are used particularly for their anabolic action, which may be of value in severely debilitated or burned patients who are experiencing negative nitrogen balance. The use of such steroids to enhance athletic ability is of

TABLE 7-28. Androgenic Drugs

GENERIC NAME	TRADE NAME
Androgens	
Testosterone (several forms)	Several
Danazol	Danocrine
Fluoxymesterone	Halotestin
Methyltestosterone	Metandren, others
Testolactone	Teslac
Anabolic Steroids	
Ethylestrenol	Maxibolin
Nandrolone	Anabolin, Durabolin
Oxandrolone	Anavar
Oxymetholone	Androyd
Stanazolol	Winstrol

questionable efficacy but considerable hazard. Androgens may be administered to suppress unwanted lactation, and to ameliorate endometriosis, fibrocystic breast disease, and advanced breast cancer.

Adverse effects of androgens include hypercalcemia, psychological aberrations, sodium and fluid retention with exacerbation of congestive heart failure, and increased plasma levels of low-density lipoproteins, which may promote coronary artery disease and changes in hepatic function. Negative feedback inhibition of pituitary-gonadotropin release can induce sexual dysfunction. Hypertension, hepatic impairment, hormone-sensitive carcinomas, and pregnancy contraindicate the administration of androgens.

CHEMOTHERAPEUTIC DRUGS

Antineoplastic Agents

Antineoplastic drugs have effected cures in some forms of cancer, and can produce remissions and alleviation of symptoms in other forms. Hodgkin's and non-Hodgkin's lymphomas, myelogenous and acute lymphocytic leukemia, testicular, and breast cancers all respond exceptionally well to treatment, particularly when instituted early in the course of neoplasia.

Unfortunately, antineoplastic agents are cytotoxic also to normal cells and can provoke severe, even life-threatening adverse responses. Cells that are rapidly replicating are most affected by these drugs. Suppression of bone marrow synthesis of formed blood elements results in anemia, thrombocytopenia, and leukopenia; severe hemorrhage or infections can prove to be lethal. Another rapidly proliferating tissue that can be severely damaged is the gastrointestinal mucosa; ulceration may develop at any location along that tract, including the oral cavity. Germinal epithelium is suppressed, resulting in amenorrhea and decreased spermatogenesis. Interaction with fetal growth, which involves rapid cell division, can cause fetal damage or death. Perhaps the most innocuous effect in terms of physiological damage is suppression of follicular activity resulting in alopecia (hair loss); however, this response can have marked psychological impact in persons who are already coping with a severe disease. Many antineoplastic agents have additional characteristic organ toxicities that produce damage to the liver, kidneys, lungs, and myocardium. Hyperuricemia, resulting from tumor cell metabolism or destruction, may be alleviated with urinary alka-

linization, proper hydration, and the xanthine oxidase inhibitor allopurinol. Anaphylaxis and other allergic symptoms can occur following administration of antineoplastic drugs.

One of the most prominent adverse reactions characteristic of many antineoplastics is nausea and vomiting. Physiological sequelae include dehydration, malnutrition, and electrolyte imbalance; psychological responses include psychogenic nausea and reluctance or refusal to undergo subsequent courses of drug treatment. The exact mechanism of antineoplastic induction of vomiting is not understood. Stimulation of central mechanisms, formation of toxic products during cell destruction, and direct gastric irritation have all been proposed. A degree of relief is afforded to some persons by the concomitant administration of antiemetic agents such as phenothiazines, metoclopramide (Reglan), and corticosteroids. Nabilone (Cesemet) and dronabinol (Marinol), derivatives of the active marijuana component tetrahydrocannabinol, seem to have some usefulness in young adult patients.

A variety of chemotherapeutic agents (Table 7-29) is used. Alkylating agents and antibiotics suppress cell growth by interacting with DNA replication. Antimetabolites, analogues of essential naturally occurring substances, enter into and disrupt cellular metabolic functions. Alkaloids interfere with mitotic spindle integrity. Hormones and the antiestrogen, tamoxifen, are effective in hormone-responsive neoplasms, and some will alleviate the symptoms of other cancers.

Despite this chemotherapeutic arsenal, many types of neoplasms continue to be especially refractory to treatment. Some cancers respond initially, then become resistant to further drug treatment. The search for substances with antineoplastic potential involves laboratory screening models such as protozoal culture systems, tissue cultures of human carcinoma cells, tumors grown in embryonated eggs, transplanted rodent tumors, and leukemias either of spontaneous origin or induced by viruses, radiation, or carcinogens (e.g., polycyclic hydrocarbons, aromatic amines and amides, azo dyes, and a variety of miscellaneous agents such as urethane, podophyllin, and dimethylnitrosamine). For some agents, one oral dose will dependably produce tumors in rats in a few weeks, while others require prolonged feeding or special strains of animals. Laboratory screening tests for sensitivity of human tumors to antineoplastic agents include autoradiographic determination of the rate of incorporation of tritiated thymidine or deoxyuridine into DNA in tumor slices.

TABLE 7-29. Antineoplastic Drugs

GENERIC NAME	TRADE NAME
Alkylating Agents	
Busulfan	Myleran
Mechlorethamine	Mustargen
Chlorambucil	Leukeran
Melphalan	Alkeran
Cyclophosphamide	Cytoxan
Dacarbazine	DTIC
Nitrosoureas	
Carmustine	BiCNU
Lomustine	CeeNU
Semustine	
Antimetabolites	
Methotrexate	Mexate, Folex
Mercaptopurine	Purinethol
Thioguanine	Lanvis
5-Fluorouracil	5-FU, Adrucil
Cytarabine	Cytosar
Antibiotics	
Doxorubicin	Adriamycin
Daunorubicin	Cerubidine
Dactinomycin	Cosmegen
Bleomycin	Blenoxane
Plicamycin	Mithracin
Mitomycin	Mutamycin
Vinca Alkaloids	
Vinblastine	Velban
Vincristine	Oncovin
Additional Antineoplastics	
Tamoxifen	Nolvadex
Megestrol	Megace
Mitotane	Lysodren
Leuprolide	Lupron
Cisplatin	Platinol
Etoposide	VePesid
Streptozocin	Zanosar
Procarbazine	Matulane
Hydroxyurea	Hydrea
L-asparaginase	Elspar
Estramustine	Emcyt
α-Interferon	Intron, Roferon

Alkylating Agents

Alkylating agents interfere with strand separation of DNA chains. Suppression of this requisite for cell division imparts antineoplastic activity, but also gives these drugs mutagenic and carcinogenic potential. Alkylation of other cell constituents is the probable basis for many of their less specific cytotoxic actions.

Nitrogen mustard (mechlorethamine, Mustargen) was among the earliest antineoplastics. Its current use is relatively limited to the treatment of Hodgkin's disease and other lymphatic cancers, often as a component of the MOPP combination (Table 7-30). Rapid inactivation of mechlorethamine gives it a characteristically brief (approximately 10 minutes) half-life. Adverse reactions include marked myelosuppression, nausea and vomiting, diarrhea, stomatitis, hyperuricemia, and alopecia. Herpes zoster infections may be activated. Concurrent radiation therapy can potentiate bone marrow suppression. Persistent infertility in men and women has followed mechlorethamine therapy. This drug is also reported to be teratogenic.

Because of its vesicant action, thrombophlebitis can be a complication of the IV administration of mechlorethamine. Dilution into a rapidly flowing infusion, and administration into a large vein can reduce the incidence of this effect. Extravasation into subcutaneous tissues can cause marked irritation and sloughing that may be prevented by immediate local infiltration with isotonic sodium thiosulfate. Health care personnel must take precautions to avoid inhalation or skin or eye exposure to mechlorethamine. Accidental contact necessitates immediate irrigation of accessible sites.

Mechlorethamine is given in short courses of IV therapy, allowing for sufficient recovery of bone marrow function before subsequent drug administration. Intracavity instillation may reduce pleural or peritoneal effusion; analgesics may be required to alleviate accompanying discomfort.

Chlorambucil (Leukeran), used in the management of lymphomas, is administered orally and produces less severe adverse reactions than mechlorethamine. Myelosuppression is its prominent toxic effect. Frequent monitoring of formed blood elements is required; radiation therapy generally is not utilized concomitantly. This drug has teratogenic and carcinogenic potential.

Melphalan (Alkeran) is similar to chlorambucil in its route of administration and toxicity. Sustained myelosuppression may occur. Pulmonary toxicity has been reported with both of these drugs.

Cyclophosphamide (Cytoxan) is a nitrogen mustard derivative that is biotransformed hepatically into antineoplastic metabolites. It is administered PO, IM, or IV, and is active against a wider range of cancers than other mustard compounds. Several chemotherapy combinations include cyclophosphamide (Table 7-30). Renal function should be monitored to forestall toxic accumulations of this drug and its metabolites. Adverse effects include myelosuppression, nausea and vomiting, pulmonary fibrosis, and induction of bladder carcinoma and other secondary cancers. Adequate hydration

TABLE 7-30. Frequently Employed Chemotherapy Combinations

NAME	DRUGS	NEOPLASM
ABDV	Doxorubicin, Bleomycin, Vinblastine, Dacarbazine	Hodgkin's disease
BACOP	Bleomycin, Doxorubicin, Cyclophosphamide, Vincristine, Prednisone	Diffuse histiocytic lymphoma
BEP	Bleomycin, Etoposide, Cisplatin	Testicular
BCVPP	Carmustine, Cyclophosphamide, Vinblastine, Procarbazine, Prednisone	Hodgkin's disease
CAF	Cyclophosphamide, Doxorubicin, 5-Fluorouracil	Breast
CAMP	Cyclophosphamide, Doxorubicin, Methotrexate, Procarbazine	Lung
CAP	Melphalan, Cisplatin, Doxorubicin	Ovarian
CAV	Cyclophosphamide, Doxorubicin, Vincristine	Ewing's sarcoma
CHAP	Cyclophosphamide, Hexamethylmelamine, Doxorubicin, Cisplatin	Ovarian
CMFP	Cyclophosphamide, Methotrexate, 5-Fluorouracil, Prednisone	Breast
COMLA	Cyclophosphamide, Vincristine, Methotrexate–leucovorin, Cytarabine	Diffuse histiocytic lymphoma
CVPP	Chlorambucil, Vinblastine, Procarbazine, Prednisone	Hodgkin's disease
FAM	5-Fluorouracil, Doxorubicin, Mitomycin	Gastric
M-2 Protocol	Vincristine, Carmustine, Cyclophosphamide, Melphalan, Prednisone	Multiple myeloma
M-Bacop	Bleomycin, Doxorubicin, Cyclophosphamide, Vincristine, Prednisone, Methotrexate–Leucovorin	Diffuse histiocytic lymphoma
MOPP	Mechlorethamine, Vincristine, Procarbazine, Prednisone	Hodgkin's disease
POCC	Procarbazine, Vincristine, Cyclophosphamide, Lomustine	Lung
PVB	Cisplatin, Vinblastine, Bleomycin	Testicular
VP	Vincristine, Prednisone	Acute lymphocytic leukemia

can reduce the risk of hemorrhagic cystitis, apparently due to bladder irritation, that is characteristic of cyclophosphamide therapy. Early detection of hematuria and termination of drug can minimize urinary tract damage. Cyclophosphamide has additional clinical use as an immunosuppressant agent in severe refractory autoimmune disorders (see "Immunosuppressant Drugs").

Dacarbazine has the characteristic actions of alkylating agents, and can cause hepatic necrosis. Extravasation will damage subcutaneous tissue. *Busulfan* is relatively selective; it has virtually no pharmacological action other than myelosuppression and is useful in the induction of remission in chronic granulocytic leukemia. *Thio-tepa* and *uracil mustard* are additional alkylating agents used in the treatment of neoplasms.

The *nitrosourea* compounds (*carmustine, lomustine,* and *semustine*) are lipid soluble and will cross the blood–brain barrier. They are used in the treatment of brain tumors as well as other types of neo-plasms. Their toxicity is similar to that of other alkylating agents. Myelosuppression may be delayed and severe. Sustained courses of treatment can induce pulmonary fibrosis. Streptozocin, a water-soluble nitrosourea, is administered IV or intra-arterially in carcinoid and pancreatic tumors. Release of insulin as malignant pancreatic cells are destroyed may result in marked hypoglycemia. Nausea, vomiting, and nephrotoxicity are frequent. Renal function must be monitored, and the use of other nephrotoxic drugs is to be avoided.

Antimetabolites

FOLIC ACID ANTAGONISTS

Methotrexate is the major folate antimetabolite currently in use. Amelioration and maintenance of remission in choriocarcinoma and childhood leukemia can be achieved with PO or IV administration. The intrathecal route is used in meningeal neoplasia.

Methotrexate blocks the enzymatic conversion of folic acid to tetrahydrofolate, an intermediary in the synthesis of DNA, by covalently binding to dihydrofolate reductase. Tumor cells can develop resistance to methotrexate, resulting in termination of remission and unresponsiveness to folic acid analogues.

Methotrexate has numerous adverse effects, some of which can be lethal. Blood counts must be monitored; marked myelosuppression requires that drug administration be stopped. Nausea and vomiting, stomatitis, and gastrointestinal ulceration can occur. Characteristic is renal damage caused by precipitation of drug in the nephrons. Renal function must be monitored, since this is also the route of elimination of this highly toxic drug. Renal dysfunction contraindicates its use. Salicylates and probenecid reduce renal excretion and enhance toxicity, as do drugs that compete for plasma protein binding sites. Hepatic toxicity can occur; alcohol and other hepatotoxic drugs should be avoided. Methotrexate is tetratogenic and abortifacient. Folinic acid (leucovorin or citrovorum factor) can minimize some of the toxic effects of this drug.

The immunosuppressant action of methotrexate has been utilized in the management of severe, refractory psoriasis and rheumatoid arthritis. However, the extremely hazardous nature of this drug must be considered against the relatively nonlethal course of these diseases. Close and persistent monitoring of patients for early indications of toxicity is necessary.

PURINE ANALOGUES

Mercaptopurine, among the earliest effective antineoplastics, is most useful against leukemias. The action of this drug evolves from its ability to disrupt the synthesis of nucleic acid and other substances that contain the purines adenine and guanine. Myelosuppression, stomatitis, gastrointestinal ulceration, nausea, and vomiting are anticipated adverse effects. Leukocyte counts should be monitored. Potentially lethal hepatitis can develop; monitoring of liver function can detect early changes that require termination of drug use.

Allopurinol, which may be concomitantly administered to alleviate hyperuricemia, inhibits the xanthine oxidase enzyme necessary for inactivation of mercaptopurine. To avoid serious toxicity, the dosage of the latter drug should be reduced to one third and often as low as one quarter of the usual dose.

Thioguanine is a guanine analogue that acts in a manner similar to mercaptopurine. Its toxicity is generally less severe than that of mercaptopurine. However, myelosuppression and hyperuricemia can occur. Dosage reduction is not required in concomitant allopurinol administration since thioguanine is not inactivated by xanthine oxidase. This drug is administered orally, although its absorption is slow and incomplete. Cellular resistance to the actions of purine analogues can arise through an acquired reduction in the enzyme (hypoxanthine–guanine phosphoribosyltransferase) necessary for their activation.

Azathioprine is a purine analogue immunosuppressant. It is metabolized to mercaptopurine, thus its actions are potentiated by allopurinol.

PYRIMIDINE ANALOGUES

5-Fluorouracil is a pyrimidine analogue that must be enzymatically activated in order to disrupt DNA synthesis. Intravenous administration achieves the most favorable response from this drug, which undergoes rapid hepatic inactivation. The considerable potential for toxicity with 5-fluorouracil mandates close patient monitoring and termination of drug administration if stomatitis, severe diarrhea or vomiting, or hemorrhage or precipitous changes in formed-blood elements occur. Myelosuppression can be severe. Since this drug crosses the blood–brain barrier, it can produce central nervous system symptoms such as lethargy, weakness, and ataxia. It is catabolized as uracil and is more effective with allopurinol support. Topical preparations of 5-fluorouracil are used in the treatment of keratoses and superficial basal cell carcinoma.

Floxuridine, an analogue of 5-fluorouracil with similar toxicity, is infused intra-arterially in patients with inoperable hepatic metastases.

Cytarabine (cytosine arabinoside), an analogue of the pyrimidine cytidine, is activated by tumor cells and subsequently inhibits DNA synthesis. It is used particularly in the treatment of leukemias. Because it is rapidly metabolized by several body tissues, cytarabine is most effective when administered by continuous IV infusion. This drug crosses the blood–brain barrier, and can be administered directly into the cerebrospinal fluid. Myelosuppression, particularly of white cell production that may continue to fall 2 to 3 weeks after drug therapy is stopped, is a frequent consequence of cytarabine. Drug therapy may be interrupted to allow recovery of leukocyte and platelet counts. Nausea and vomiting can be severe; slow IV infusion rates reduce the incidence of this response. Stomatitis and hyperuricemia also occur.

Antibiotics

Numerous antibiotics are useful cancer chemotherapeutic agents. **Doxorubicin** is effective against many types of neoplasms and is a component in many combination chemotherapy regimens (Table 7-30). It intercalates by hydrogen bonds into the DNA double helical structure, thus suppressing the synthesis of nucleic acids. Cardiotoxicity is uniquely characteristic of this drug; preexisting cardiovascular disease may increase the risk of potentially lethal myocardial changes. At total doses greater than 550 mg/m^2, doxorubicin can induce congestive heart failure that is refractory to cardiotonic drugs. Monitoring of ECG and observation for signs of myocardial deterioration may reveal early cardiomyopathy, although severe arrhythmias can develop rapidly. Myelosuppression also occurs with doxorubicin; preexisting bone marrow dysfunction contraindicates initiation of therapy with this drug. Biliary excretion is the major route of inactivation; hepatic insufficiency increases the risk of toxicity. The IV route of administration is utilized, and extravasation can destroy subcutaneous tissue. Infiltration with a corticosteroid may minimize damage.

Daunorubicin is structurally and pharmacologically similar to doxorubicin, but its use is limited mainly to treatment of leukemias. It too is myelosuppressant and cardiotoxic, and both drugs can cause red discoloration of the urine that may be mistaken for hematuria.

Actinomycin D (dactinomycin), useful for a variety of tumors, is a frequent component of drug combinations. On a molar basis, it is one of the most potent antitumor agents. Major adverse effects are nausea and vomiting, myelosuppression, stomatitis, and a synergistic effect with exposure to radiation. Like many antineoplastics, it disrupts DNA function. Its plasma half-life averages 36 hours; unchanged drug is excreted in bile and urine.

Bleomycin appears to damage DNA by liberating free oxygen radicals such as superoxide. The characteristic toxic effects of this drug are pneumonitis and pulmonary fibrosis. Renal impairment enhances the risk of toxicity. An idiosyncratic reaction of fever, hypotension, and wheezing has been reported; volume expansion or pressor amines may be required to support blood pressure.

Plicamycin is used to ameliorate elevated plasma and urine levels of calcium that accompany advanced cancers. It can be severely toxic; patients require close (preferably in-hospital) observation. Life-threatening hemorrhage can occur; platelet counts should be monitored. Preexisting coagulation deficits contraindicate use of this drug. Electrolyte imbalance (depletion of plasma calcium, potassium, and phosphate), nausea and vomiting, and changes in hepatic and renal function should be anticipated. Thrombophlebitis and tissue damage upon extravasation indicate the irritant nature of plicamycin.

Mitomycin is usually a second-line or combination drug for gastric or pancreatic carcinoma. Because myelosuppression frequently occurs, intermittent therapy must allow adequate recovery of thrombocyte and leukocyte counts. Renal and pulmonary toxicity and nausea and vomiting are other adverse effects. Extravasation may damage subcutaneous tissue.

Vinca Alkaloids

Vinblastine and vincristine, alkaloids from the periwinkle plant, interrupt the function of the mitotic spindle. These drugs are useful in the treatment of several types of tumors, including lymphatic cancers. However, they are not identical in either therapeutic or adverse actions. **Vinblastine** markedly suppresses bone marrow function; severe leukocyte depletion places patients at considerable risk of secondary infection.

Vincristine is a component of many chemotherapy combinations. The characteristic toxicity is neurological. Muscular weakness, loss of sensation and deep-tendon reflexes, ataxia, and suppression of gastrointestinal and urinary tract function are usually reversible upon termination of drug. Paralytic ileus may lead to upper colon fecal impaction. In contrast to vinblastine, there is little myelosuppression. Both drugs are potent vesicants; extravasation can damage subcutaneous tissue. Infiltration of hyaluronidase may be beneficial.

Hormones

Corticosteroids (cortisone, prednisone, and prednisolone) have some antileukemic action, and will alleviate symptoms of these disorders. Dexamethasone, a synthetic glucocorticoid, may reduce the severity or the psychological impact of chemotherapy-induced vomiting.

Estrogen can effect some degree of regression in prostatic carcinoma, probably by suppression of androgen release and subsequent remission of hormone-dependent cellular growth. **Estramustine** is a combination of estradiol and nitrogen mustard. Estrogens may alleviate symptoms of breast cancer, but may also promote development of endometrial and mammary carcinoma. Conflicting reports have made this a controversial topic. Bone metastasis of breast cancer is an indication for the administration of androgens, particularly in postmenopausal patients. The characteristics of these hormones are discussed under "Endocrine Pharmacology."

Tamoxifen is an antiestrogen useful in breast cancer, particularly in postmenopausal women. Estrogen-sensitive neoplasia, evidenced by the presence of estrogen receptors in tumor tissue, is most responsive to tamoxifen, although some studies have indicated that estrogen-receptor-negative tissue can also be suppressed by this drug. Metastatic cells are responsive; transient bone pain and increase in the size of soft-tissue lesions appear to be indicative of therapeutic drug action.

Tamoxifen is slowly absorbed from the gastrointestinal tract and metabolized in the liver to active metabolites. Excretion into bile and subsequent enterohepatic circulation probably contribute to its long (7 days) plasma half-life. Doses should be evenly spaced 12 hours apart to maintain consistent therapeutic plasma concentrations. Side effects are generally mild: nausea, hot flashes, edema, vaginal discharge or bleeding, and hypercalcemia in patients with significant bone metastases. Long-term administration of high doses has occasionally induced deterioration in vision.

Mitotane is an adrenocortical suppressant that may afford symptomatic relief in inoperable adrenal cortex carcinoma. Adrenal insufficiency can develop, necessitating steroid replacement. Nausea, vomiting, or diarrhea occurs in a large percentage of patients; depression, lethargy, and dizziness also occur frequently. Large doses and long-term administration may be required for clinical response. The appearance of adverse effects should guide the upper limits of dose as long as beneficial effects are apparent, although a 3 month (occasionally longer) interval of drug administration may be necessary to induce the latter.

Leuprolide, an analog of LHRH, can suppress pituitary release of LH, diminishing hormone synthesis in the ovaries and testes. Amelioration of mammary and prostatic cancers can be obtained. Sexual hypofunction can occur.

Additional Antineoplastic Agents

Cisplatin is especially effective both alone and in drug combinations against ovarian, testicular, and bladder tumors, although it is also used in the treatment of various other cancers. Disruption of DNA function appears to be its mechanism of action. Severe vomiting that is often refractory to antiemetics occurs in almost all patients treated with cisplatin. Metoclopramide or dexamethasone may partially alleviate this response. Renal toxicity, also a prominent adverse effect, may be reduced by maintaining sufficient hydration. Intravenous fluids can be initiated 8 hours before and continued throughout drug administration. Mannitol administered concurrently with the drug will promote rapid elimination from the renal tubules. Dehydration subsequent to vomiting may enhance nephrotoxicity. Renal damage is cumulative, and function should return to normal levels before subsequent drug doses are given. Simultaneous use of other nephrotoxic agents is contraindicated. Cisplatin is ototoxic; loop diuretics and aminoglycoside antibiotics should not be given concurrently. Myelosuppression, neurotoxicity, and hyperuricemia are additional adverse reactions. Infusion equipment that contains aluminum will inactivate cisplatin.

Etoposide induces bone marrow dysfunction in a large percentage of patients, and causes other adverse effects common to antineoplastics. It is generally used in combination therapy of refractory testicular cancer. Hypotension can occur with rapid IV infusion.

Procarbazine is a component of several drug combinations. Myelosuppression, nausea, and vomiting occur frequently. The drug readily enters cerebrospinal fluid and can cause central nervous system symptoms such as depression, anxiety, ataxia, tremors, and confusion. An MAO inhibitor, procarbazine may provoke hypertensive emergencies when drugs or foods containing sympathomimetics are ingested. Effects of other central nervous system depressants and of some antihypertensives can be potentiated. Consumption of alcohol may induce a disulfiram-like reaction.

Hydroxyurea can reduce leukocyte levels in chronic myelocytic leukemia. Preexisting bone marrow depression or renal insufficiency contraindicates use of this drug. Hyperuricemia is a frequent adverse effect.

L-asparaginase, an enzyme that deaminates asparagine, exploits the asparagine-dependent characteristic of certain tumor cells. Its use in acute lymphoblastic leukemia is associated with a significant number of hypersensitivity reactions as well as induction of diabetes mellitus. Depletion of clotting factors can lead to hemorrhage. Renal failure and central nervous system symptoms occur.

α-Interferon is one of the most recent additions to antineoplastic pharmacology. Its use is currently limited to hairy-cell leukemia, although other leukemias and malignancies may prove to be responsive. This naturally occurring component of the immune system can be produced in *E. coli* by recombinant DNA technology. Its proposed mechanism of action is inhibition of DNA and protein synthesis. Fatigue and a flulike syndrome of chills and fever, malaise, and headache are the most common adverse reactions. Antipyretics and analgesics can alleviate patient discomfort. Myelosuppression and cardiovascular and central nervous system disturbances can occur. Extreme caution is recommended in persons with preexisting cardiac, hepatic, or renal disease or with seizure or other central nervous system disorders. Interferon must be administered parenterally (SC, IM).

Combination Therapies

The use of several antineoplastic drugs simultaneously has been remarkably effective in suppressing some types of cancers. Mechlorethamine, vincristine, procarbazine, and prednisolone (MOPP) and other combined chemotherapies have effected cures of Hodgkin's disease; other frequently used combinations are listed in Table 7-30.

Combinations of drugs must be carefully chosen, using agents that have varied antineoplastic mechanisms and do not duplicate each other's toxicities. Drugs may be administered intermittently for several cycles to achieve complete eradication of malignant cells.

Antineoplastic drugs are also used in conjunction with surgery or radiation therapy. This adjuvant chemotherapy can delay or prevent the recurrence of neoplasia. Since treatment may continue for months or years, drugs with minimal adverse effects are the most appropriate.

RADIOISOTOPIC AGENTS

Radioisotopes are useful in clinical medicine as diagnostic agents because their selective localization to specific body tissues can be easily measured. They are also useful as antineoplastic agents because of their cytotoxicity. However, many of these substances can be administered only by physicians licensed by the Nuclear Regulatory Commission. Elements commonly used include ^{125}I and ^{131}I, ^{32}P, ^{51}Cr, and ^{14}C-labeled carbohydrates. Generally, small doses are used for diagnostic purposes, while larger amounts of isotope are required to destroy tissue. Doses are often expressed as curies or fractions of this unit, such as the millicurie or microcurie. Energy is emitted in the form of α, β, or γ radiation. A fixed percentage of atoms disintegrate per unit of time; therefore these substances have a predictable radioactive half-life.

Radiolabeled iodine is particularly useful in the diagnosis of thyroid dysfunction or in the management of hyperactivity or carcinoma of this gland. Iodine concentrates within the thyroid; persons with overactivity of the gland will exhibit increased accumulation of isotope in the region of the thyroid, increased serum protein-bound isotope, and slower than normal urinary excretion of radioactive material. The objective of the treatment of hyperthyroidism or carcinoma is destruction of thyroid cells. This can be facilitated by coadministration of thyroid-stimulating hormone, which enhances iodine uptake by the gland. Extensive destruction of thyroid tissue should be anticipated, and clinical manifestations of hypothyroidism may require replacement hormone therapy. Sore throat and transient swelling of the neck may develop. Antithyroid medications and recent administration of iodine in any form can suppress uptake of isotopic iodine. Allergy to iodine or seafood (which contains this element) mandates close observation of patients for anaphylactic or asthmatic reactions. Administration of high doses of this or other isotopes should be accompanied with radiation safety precautions to protect patients, visitors, and health-care personnel from inadvertent injury. Because of their carcinogenic and mutagenic potential, labeled iodine as well as other radioisotopes are usually contraindicated in pregnancy and during lactation.

Albumin with radiolabeled iodine is used to measure plasma volume, and iodohippurate tagged with this isotope can assess renal function.

^{32}P can suppress certain types of leukemia, and may alleviate polycythemia vera. Phosphorus concentrates in rapidly proliferating tissue such as bone marrow. Excessive myelosuppression can result in pancytopenia, and isotope-induced leukemias have been reported. Blood counts must be determined repeatedly before and after isotope therapy.

Radioactive gold (^{198}Au) can be instilled into body cavities (*e.g.,* pleural and peritoneal) to alleviate effusion and ascites that accompany malignancy. Open tumors or wounds contraindicate the use of this isotope. Labeled chromic phosphate can be used in a similar manner.

Additional uses of isotopes include measurement of cerebral and skeletal-muscle blood flow, body-water distribution, renal and hepatic function, utilization and storage of iron, and detection of pancreatic carcinoma, bone metastases, and ischemic heart disease.

Radiographic Diagnostic Contrast Media Agents

Radiopaque contrast media are used to visualize blood vessels and the biliary and urinary tracts. Because of their potential for inducing adverse reactions, these agents are administered only by personnel skilled in their use and in facilities equipped to manage life-threatening responses. Iodine atoms attached to a benzene ring confer radiopacity. Some of these agents, such as the diatrizoate salts, are negatively charged in solution. The addition of sodium or methylglucamine as a balancing cation results in a highly hypertonic preparation (2000 mOsm/kg compared to 300 mOsm/kg for blood). Intravenous administration of these agents induces pain, vomiting, and cardiovascular changes that may be related to their hypertonicity. Three agents, iohexol, iopamidol, and ioxaglate, with decreased ionic content (below 900 mOsm) produce a lower incidence of side effects, and may be safer for persons with cardiovascular or pulmonary disorders.

Hypersensitivity reactions are unrelated to osmolarity and can be lethal. The risk of cardiovascular collapse necessitates close observation of patients during and for at least 1 hour following diagnostic testing. Means for resuscitation must be immediately available. A small test dose of drug may be helpful, although a lack of adverse response does not always ensure safe administration of the full diagnostic dose. Severe myocardial depression and hypotension may occur by mechanisms other than anaphylaxis. Persons with a history of allergy (particularly to iodine) or of previous adverse response to contrast media appear to be at increased risk of shock and cardiac arrest. Pretreatment with antihistamines or corticosteroids may reduce the incidence of life-threatening reactions. Radiopaque media have induced renal toxicity in patients with multiple myeloma, especially if dehydration was coexistent. These agents can exacerbate symptoms of sickle cell anemia and may induce hypertension in the presence of pheochromocytoma. Renal impairment can hinder the excretion of radiopaque materials.

ANTIMICROBIALS

Antibacterials

Drugs that suppress bacterial growth are among the most widely prescribed in the United States. (The hazards of inappropriate use are discussed below.) Many of these agents are naturally occurring substances, synthesized by bacteria and fungi. Molecular modification of these antibiotics has yielded numerous semisynthetic substances, often with broader efficacy than the naturally occurring analogues. For example, acid-stable and penicillinase-resistant penicillins have increased the spectrum of activity of the parent drug, penicillin G (see discussion under ''Penicillins''). Some antibacterial agents such as the sulfonamides are totally synthetic anti-infectives.

The mechanism of action of the antibacterial drugs, indeed of all the antimicrobials, involves interference with some aspect of the physiological function of the microorganism, for example, suppression of cell wall or protein synthesis, or alteration of cellular metabolism. Bacterial cell function frequently differs sufficiently from mammalian cell function, so that some antibacterial agents are not markedly cytotoxic in humans. There is a range of antibacterial activity from bacteriostatic, which slows but does not irreversibly prevent bacterial growth, to bactericidal in which microbes are destroyed. Some agents are bacteriostatic at lower doses and bactericidal in larger amounts. Anti-infective drugs are most useful in persons with competent immune systems that assist in the removal of infectious agents.

Antibacterials vary widely in their spectrum of susceptible organisms. Some are active against a wide variety of pathogens (''broad spectrum'') while others are effective against a limited number of microorganisms (''narrow spectrum''). Viruses are generally impervious to these agents, which are appropriately administered to persons with viral infections *only* when secondary bacterial invasions are present. The sensitivity of specific pathogens to drugs should be determined so that the most appropriate antibacterials can be selected. Some conditions (*e.g.*, meningitis and bacteremia) require immediate institution of antibacterial treatment. The initial choice of agents is based on the probable infecting pathogen, and the drug regimen may be altered once the susceptibility of the specific organisms is identified. Body fluids for sensitivity testing should be obtained before drug therapy is begun.

Several *in vitro* susceptibility tests are available to aid in the identification of specific pathogens. Disk diffusion tests utilize paper filters impregnated with anti-infective drugs placed on the surface of agar inoculated with bacteria isolated from patients' body fluids or tissues. Following a period of incubation, the presence or absence of bacterial growth around each disk will indicate the effectiveness of the various drugs. Methods that test dilutions of antiinfectives against microbial cultures can provide information regarding minimal inhibitory concentrations (MIC) and minimal bactericidal concentrations (MBC), which are particularly important in the management of meningitis and endocarditis. The *in vivo* efficacy of a drug can be predicted by considering achievable serum or cerebrospinal fluid concentrations.

The inappropriate use of antibacterials has caused a number of serious consequences. Among these is the problem of acquired drug resistance: organisms once susceptible to a particular drug develop the ability to survive in the presence of that drug. Spontaneous mutations can occur among bacteria, and excessive administration of anti-infectives can suppress the growth of susceptible bacteria, therefore providing unopposed opportunity for survival of resistant cells. On the other hand, premature termination of antibacterial administration also fosters development of drug resistance, and it is important for patients to complete a full regimen of treatment even though the symptoms of infection have waned. Many nosocomial (hospital-acquired) infections are attributable to drug-resistant organisms.

Superinfections are secondary infections that arise from administration of antibacterials. The gastrointestinal, respiratory, and genitourinary tracts are normally inhabited by a variety of microorganisms that grow together and exert their own inhibitory influence to prevent overabundance of any one organism. Administration of drugs will suppress the growth of susceptible bacteria, and allow nonsusceptible organisms (with either acquired or natural resistance) to increase in numbers and induce infections. The risk of this response is increased when broad-spectrum agents are used, and when administration continues beyond 7 to 10 days. Elderly and seriously ill persons, in whom immune responsiveness may be less than optimal, are most susceptible to the development of superinfections. The best defense against this type of secondary infection is to administer antibacterials only when and as long as absolutely necessary, and to use agents known to be effective against the invading organism.

Prophylactic administration of antibacterials is appropriate in a limited number of clinical situations. Persons with a history of certain cardiovascular diseases, such as valvular heart disease, may be protected against bacterial endocarditis by brief regimens of penicillin or other antibiotics at times of dental or surgical procedures. Routine perioperative administration of antibacterials appears to reduce the occurrence of infection following some types of surgery, such as open heart surgery.

A frequent manifestation of superinfection is coli-

tis. Pseudomembranous colitis induced by *Clostridium difficile* causes severe diarrhea and dehydration that can be lethal. Many antimicrobials cause diarrhea, which if severe may require that drug therapy be terminated.

Allergic reactions are another frequent adverse response to anti-infective drugs. Symptoms can range from skin rashes to asthma and anaphylactic shock. Penicillin-responsive infections that occur in persons with penicillin hypersensitivity have been treated with the antibiotic after desensitization. Very low initial "desensitizing" doses are gradually increased until a favorable antibacterial response is obtained. However, persons thus treated must be closely observed for signs of anaphylaxis and supportive measures must be immediately available. Pretreatment with antihistamines may circumvent possible severe reactions.

Decreases in renal function, including those normally observed in older persons, require a reduction in dosage of antibacterial drugs inactivated by renal excretion. Plasma concentrations of anti-infectives should be monitored to ensure that toxic levels are avoided and therapeutic levels are achieved. Renal capacity should be determined before administration of drug to persons in whom inadequate function is suspected, and periodically during prolonged therapy. Many antibiotics are themselves nephrotoxic; changes in renal function detected during treatment with these agents usually require that drug administration be terminated.

Many antibiotics are well absorbed from the oral route, while others are not and must, therefore, be administered parenterally for the treatment of systemic infections. Oral administration of the latter, however, can be used to eradicate bacteria from the intestinal tract. Most antibiotics do not readily cross the blood–brain barrier; thus large doses must be given to treat central nervous system infections. Inflammation of the meninges can increase the permeability of cerebral capillary walls to drugs.

Carefully selected combinations of antibacterial agents are appropriately utilized for a limited number of clinical indications. Penicillins plus aminoglycosides can facilitate each others' effects against some bacteria. In contrast, some drug combinations result in reduced efficacy. In general, bactericidal and bacteriostatic agents are not administered concurrently. Bactericidal drugs are most effective against microorganisms that are rapidly dividing; this advantage is lost when bacterial replication is slowed by a bacteriostatic drug.

Antibacterial activity may be enhanced by concomitant use of other types of drugs. Probenecid competes for renal tubular secretion, prolonging the plasma half-life of penicillins and cephalosporins. β-Lactamase inhibitors such as clavulanic acid will broaden the antimicrobial spectrum of activity of agents that are destroyed by these enzymes. The characteristics of microorganisms and their responses to antiinfective agents are further described in Chapter 5, "General Microbiology and Immunology."

PENICILLINS

Penicillin G, a naturally occurring product of the *Penicillium* mold, was the first significantly effective agent developed in this group of drugs. It is, however, quite acid-labile and its characteristic β-lactam structure is rapidly destroyed by β-lactamase ("penicillinase") produced by some types of bacteria (*e.g.,* staphylococci and gonococci). Numerous semisynthetic penicillins (Table 7-31) have been developed; some derivatives are less susceptible to gastric acid degradation (*e.g.,* **ampicillin** and **amoxicillin**) while others are penicillinase-resistant (*e.g.,* **methicillin, oxacillin,** and **nafcillin**). A particularly broad spectrum of antibacterial activity is obtained in **mezlocillin** and **azlocillin.**

Penicillins block the action of a transpeptidase that is required for cross-linkage of structural units

TABLE 7-31. Penicillins

GENERIC NAME	TRADE NAME
Naturally Occurring	
Penicillin G	Pentids, Pfizerpen
Penicillin V	Pen-Vee, V-Cillin
Semisynthetic	
Penicillinase-resistant	
Methicillin	Staphcillin
Nafcillin*	Unipen, Nafcil
Oxacillin*	Prostaphlin
Cloxacillin*	Tegopen
Dicloxacillin*	Dynapen
Amdinocillin	Coactin
Extended spectrum	
Ampicillin*	Omnipen, Polycillin
Amoxicillin*	Amoxil, Wymox
Carbenicillin	Geopen
Ticarcillin	Ticar
Mezlocillin	Mezlin
Azlocillin	Azlin
Piperacillin	Pipracil
Pro-ampicillins	
Bacampicillin	Spectrobid
Hetacillin	Versapen

* Acid-stable penicillins.

of the bacterial cell wall. Deprived of their protection against a lower extracellular osmotic pressure, susceptible bacteria are destroyed by the influx of fluid from their environment. Penicillins are bactericidal, and are most effective during phases of rapid pathogen division when cell wall construction is essential to ensure survival.

The penicillins have a considerable range of antibacterial efficacy, and are the drugs of choice for many infections. Penicillin G is especially effective by parenteral routes; oral activity can be enhanced by administering large doses spaced between meals, when gastric acid secretion is relatively low. Penicillin V is a natural derivative with greater acid stability. Penicillin G and V are most effective against facultative gram-positive cocci and rods. Those penicillins resistant to the β-lactamase enzyme will destroy penicillinase-producing staphylococci. Broad-spectrum derivatives have a range of activity that includes several gram-negative rods. Among the infections commonly treated with penicillin are gonorrhea, bacterial endocarditis, syphilis, *Haemophilis influenzae,* and streptococcal invasions, and some urinary tract infections. The acquired ability to synthesize β-lactamase has conferred resistance on many strains of staphylococci that now cause nosocomial infections that are difficult to eradicate. Tetanus, typhoid, and diphtheria, which can be avoided through proper immunization procedures, can be treated with penicillins. **Amdinocillin,** which is slightly different from the basic β-lactam structure, is especially effective against gram-negative bacteria.

Penicillin G is rapidly absorbed following IM administration and rapidly extracted from the plasma as unchanged drug by the renal tubules. Probenecid blocks this tubular secretion and can sustain significant plasma levels of drug. Repository forms of penicillin (*e.g.,* procaine and benzathine penicillin G, or **Bicillin**) provide IM depots that can provide detectable plasma levels of drug for up to 4 weeks. Large doses of penicillins contain significant amounts of sodium, which may result in electrolyte imbalances. Intermittent rather than sustained therapeutic concentrations of penicillins are considered to be effective since microorganisms are sensitive only when replicating. In addition, drug levels are more uniformly maintained in body tissues and lymph, where bacteria are most abundant.

Penicillin allergy, occurring in up to 5% of patients, is one of the most frequent adverse effects of this group of antibiotics. Reactions range from mild transitory rhinitis and urticaria to angioneurotic edema, periarteritis nodosa, fever, and anaphylactic shock. The more severe reactions occur particularly following parenteral administration. Ampicillin has a marked propensity to cause skin rashes. Predetermination of sensitivity may be obtained through intradermal testing with a penicillin–polylysine conjugate. The previously used intradermal testing with penicillin G is no longer recommended, since sensitive persons can respond with a severe anaphylactoid reaction. Persons allergic to one form of penicillin are usually hypersensitive to all others, and may also be allergic to the cephalosporin antibiotics, which have a similar molecular structure. More slowly developing reactions ("accelerated reactions") may occur 1 to 72 hours following use of penicillin: urticaria is the most common of these. Delayed reactions may develop up to several weeks after administration; skin rashes, hemolytic anemia, and serum sickness characterize these late responses.

Oral administration of penicillins can cause nausea and diarrhea. Superinfections may develop, particularly with prolonged therapy using extended-spectrum drugs. Large doses of penicillins, especially when given IV to persons with meningeal infection or seizure susceptibility, may reach sufficient central nervous system concentrations to induce convulsions. Parenteral injection sites should avoid arteries or nerves. Thrombophlebitis may accompany IV administration, and pain often occurs at the IM site. Nephrotoxicity that can lead to acute renal failure is most characteristic of methicillin. Renal impairment necessitates reduction in dosage of all penicillins except nafcillin, which can be shunted to a hepatic route of inactivation. Penicillinase-resistant penicillins in particular have been linked to myelosuppression, and some penicillins interfere with platelet function.

Additional possible drug interactions include a reported reduced efficacy of oral contraceptives when penicillin V or ampicillin is concurrently administered, and an increased risk of dermatological reactions when ampicillin and allopurinol are present concomitantly. Penicillins should not be combined in solution with aminoglycosides because the latter drugs may be rendered inactive. Sulbactam and clavulanic acid are penicillinase inhibitors that are combined with penicillins to enhance their activity.

CEPHALOSPORINS

The cephalosporins, derived from the *Cephalosporium* mold, (Table 7-32) are similar to the penicillins in both structure (they possess a β-lactam nucleus) and mechanism of antibacterial action. A rapidly

TABLE 7-32. Cephalosporins

GENERIC NAME	TRADE NAME
First Generation	
Cephaloridine	Loridine
Cephalothin	Keflin
Cefazolin	Ancef, Kefzol
Cephapirin	Cefadyl
Cephalexin*	Keflex
Cephradine*	Velocef, Anspor
Cefadroxil*	Duricef, Ultracef
Second Generation	
Cefamandole	Mandol
Cefonicid	Monocid
Cefoxitin	Mefoxin
Cefuroxime	Zinacef
Ceforanide	Precef
Cefaclor*	Ceclor
Third Generation	
Cefotaxime	Claforan
Cefotetan	Cefotan
Ceftizoxime	Catizox
Ceftriaxone	Rocephin
Ceftazidime	Fortaz, Tazidime
Cefoperazone	Cefobid
Moxalactam	Moxam

* Available in oral formulations.

expanding and widely utilized group of drugs, the cephalosporins are classified into "generations" based upon their spectrum of activity. "First-generation" agents are particularly effective against gram-positive organisms that are also susceptible to penicillin. The "second-generation" agents are active against many anaerobic organisms, while the "third generation" includes gram-negative strains in its extended spectrum.

Many of the cephalosporins are β-lactamase resistant, and are useful in the eradication of penicillinase-producing bacteria including staphylococci, *Neisseria*, and *Haemophilus influenzae*. Most of the cephalosporins have a relatively short plasma half-life, although *cefonocid* is reported effective with once-daily dosing. The first-generation agents *cephalexin, cephradine,* and *cefadroxil,* plus second-generation *cefaclor,* are resistant to acid degradation, thus are orally active; other cephalosporins are administered parenterally. Since they are quite water soluble, these drugs are for the most part renally excreted (both by filtration and secretion) and do not cross the blood–brain barrier in appreciable amounts. However, some second- and third-generation agents are effective in bacterial meningitis; their entry into the central nervous system is enhanced by meningeal inflammation. Some cephalosporins bind extensively to plasma proteins. *Cefo-*

perazone is hepatically deacylated and secreted into bile.

Although often considered alternative rather than first-line drugs, the cephalosporins are highly effective against many bacterial invasions. Upper and lower respiratory tract as well as urinary tract pathogens are responsive. Second- and third-generation agents will destroy *H. influenzae, Pseudomonas aeruginosa, Serratia, Proteus,* and *Enterobacter.* Intraabdominal and gastrointestinal infections are often ameliorated by cephalosporins. Their use, however, is occasionally limited by cross-allergenicity with penicillins; extreme caution is necessary if cephalosporins are administered to persons reporting penicillin hypersensitivity.

The cephalosporins have a favorable therapeutic index. However, such adverse reactions as renal tubular damage (enhanced by concomitant administration of other nephrotoxic drugs) and superinfections (particularly with extended spectrum agents) can occur. Pain following IM injection and thrombophlebitis after use of the IV route are not uncommon. Several cephalosporins, most notably *cefamandole, cefoperazone,* and *moxalactam,* disrupt vitamin K metabolism and lead to deficiencies in clotting factors. Severe bleeding that may require transfusion of blood products can develop, especially in persons with renal impairment or poor nutritional status. Vitamin K supplementation can minimize the risk of coagulopathy.

Aztreonam (Azactam) is a monobactam antibiotic especially effective against specific gram-negative bacteria and *P. aeruginosa.* It is not susceptible to β-lactamase degradation and is active by oral and parenteral routes.

AMINOGLYCOSIDES

The aminoglycosides (Table 7-33), derived from *Streptomyces* strains of bacteria, are especially ef-

TABLE 7-33. Aminoglycosides

GENERIC NAME	TRADE NAME
Parenteral	
Streptomycin	Generic
Kanamycin	Kantrex
Gentamicin	Gentamycin
Tobramycin	Nebcin
Amikacin	Amikin
Netilmicin	Netromycin
Oral	
Neomycin	Mycifradin
Paromomycin	Humatin
Spectinomycin	Trobicin

fective against gram-negative infections. These bactericidal antibiotics bind intracellularly to the 30 S and 50 S subunits of the microsomes, disrupting protein synthesis. The aminoglycosides are not well absorbed from the gastrointestinal tract; oral administration is used to eradicate microorganisms from the intestinal lumen. Treatment of infections elsewhere in the body requires parenteral administration. Because of their marked water solubility, these agents are generally restricted to extracellular fluid compartments. Penetration into ocular and cerebrospinal fluids is poor, and the presence of ascites can draw large amounts of these drugs out of the circulatory system. Inactivation is by glomerular filtration, with large amounts of drug concentrating in renal tissue. Because of the narrow therapeutic index of these antibiotics, impairment of kidney function requires that dosages be reduced.

The major adverse effects of the aminoglycosides are ototoxicity (deafness and vestibular disturbance) and nephrotoxicity. The risk of toxicity is greatest in persons with renal impairment, in the elderly, and in the presence of dehydration. Tinnitus and ataxia are symptoms of auditory damage that may become irreversible. Audiometric testing before and throughout drug therapy can assist in the early detection of ototoxicity; high-frequency hearing is usually lost earliest. Preexisting hearing deficits preclude the use of these drugs, and concomitant administration of other ototoxic agents (*e.g.,* furosemide) should be avoided. Diuretics can also induce dehydration, which will enhance toxicity. Streptomycin and gentamicin have a greater propensity to affect vestibular function, while the other aminoglycosides most frequently cause hearing loss. Tobramycin affects both of these functions of the cranial nerve VIII.

Adequacy of renal function should be determined before initiation of aminoglycoside therapy. Impairment suggests that alternative drugs be considered. Periodic testing throughout therapy can detect deterioration of function that may require termination of the aminoglycoside. Maintenance of adequate hydration and avoidance of concomitant nephrotoxic agents (*e.g.,* furosemide and cisplatin) decreases the incidence of renal damage.

An additional adverse effect of these antibiotics is suppression of neuromuscular transmission that can be manifested in respiratory depression and muscular weakness. These become most evident in persons with preexisting disorders of transmission, such as myasthenia gravis. Calcium depletion, or concurrent administration of other neuromuscular junction blocking agents, can potentiate this action.

Aminoglycosides are therefore hazardous in persons undergoing surgery who may require administration of such drugs as curare and succinylcholine.

The aminoglycosides are reported to cause occasional changes in hepatic and bone marrow activity. Allergic reactions, skin rashes in particular, occur. Many bacterial strains rapidly acquire resistance to these drugs.

The use of **streptomycin,** the earliest of the aminoglycosides, has been largely replaced by the newer drugs in this class. Tularemia, brucellosis, and plague are special indications for the use of streptomycin. Gram-negative bacillary infections of the urinary tract can be treated with streptomycin as long as renal function is adequate and the microorganisms have not developed resistance. The use of streptomycin in the management of tuberculosis has declined; isoniazid and other antitubercular agents are discussed under that topic.

Gentamicin has a wide range of activity, including *Enterobacter, Serratia,* and *Staphylococcus aureus.* It can be effective against strains that have acquired resistance to other aminoglycosides. The combination of carbenicillin or ticarcillin plus gentamicin is especially useful in the eradication of *Pseudomonas.* Disruption of cell wall synthesis effected by the penicillin facilitates the action of the aminoglycoside at the intracellular ribosomes. As noted earlier, these drugs should not be combined in the same solution.

A penicillin plus gentamicin or streptomycin can be administered to persons with cardiac valvular abnormalities undergoing surgery or invasive diagnostic procedures. Such patients are particularly at risk of developing bacterial endocarditis. Gentamicin is frequently used in the initial therapy of bacteremia. Intrathecal and subconjunctival routes for gentamicin can make this drug useful in meningeal and ocular infections.

Amikacin, netilmicin, and *tobramycin* are used in much the same manner as gentamicin. Netilmicin and tobramycin are reported less ototoxic and nephrotoxic. Tobramycin is more active against *Pseudomonas.* Neomycin is no longer administered systemically.

TETRACYCLINES

The tetracyclines (Table 7-34) are broad-spectrum bacteriostatic antibiotics derived from *Streptomyces* bacterial strains. Semisynthetic analogues have been produced by molecular modification of the tetracycline structure. These agents inhibit protein synthesis by preventing attachment of transfer RNA to the 50 S ribosomal subunit. Gram-positive

TABLE 7-34. Tetracyclines

GENERIC NAME	TRADE NAME
Tetracycline	Achromycin
Chlortetracycline	Aureomycin
Oxytetracycline	Terramycin
Demeclocycline	Declomycin
Methacycline	Rondomycin
Doxycycline	Vibramycin
Minocycline	Minocin

and gram-negative facultative and obligatory anaerobes are susceptible to the tetracyclines, although many microorganisms have acquired resistance to these antibiotics. Brucellosis, syphilis, gonorrhea, cholera, pelvic inflammatory disease, chlamydia, rickettsia (typhus, Lyme disease, and Rocky Mountain spotted fever), and urinary tract infections are among the many clinical indications for tetracyclines, which can be used as alternative antibiotics in persons allergic to the β-lactam agents. Protozoal infections (*e.g., Entamoeba histolytica* and malaria due to *Plasmodium falciparium*) are frequently responsive to this group of drugs. **Minocycline** can be effective against *Staphylococci* and *Nocardia* that are resistant to other tetracyclines. Acne may be treated with chronic tetracycline therapy.

The tetracyclines can be administered orally or parenterally. Gastrointestinal absorption is inhibited by the presence of food, and particularly by ions such as calcium, iron, and magnesium. Dairy products and antacids should be ingested not less than 1 hour before or 2 hours after tetracycline dosages. Exceptions to this are **doxycycline** and **minocycline.** Tetracyclines vary in solubility. Doxycycline and minocycline are lipid soluble and will cross the blood–brain barrier. These two drugs have a longer plasma half-life than other tetracyclines. They are metabolized hepatically and excreted in bile and feces, being somewhat safer than many other antibiotics in persons with renal impairment. The less lipid-soluble tetracyclines are excreted by glomerular filtration, giving them greater efficacy in urinary tract infections.

Tetracyclines can induce renal dysfunction, and nephrogenic diabetes insipidus is reported to occur with demeclocycline. Hepatotoxicity may develop, in particular following large IV doses. Pregnancy or kidney impairment increases the risk of hepatic damage. Tetracyclines are antianabolic, causing elevated blood urea nitrogen levels. Fanconi's syndrome, consisting of acidosis, proteinuria, glycosuria, and aminoaciduria, is caused by degradation products in outdated tetracycline preparations. Because tetracyclines chelate with calcium ion, they are incorporated into dental enamel and bone. The risk of subsequent staining of teeth and suppression of skeletal development contraindicates the use of these drugs during pregnancy or in children younger than 8 years. Photosensitivity can be especially severe with demeclocycline; minocycline produces a high incidence of vertigo. Chronic administration of tetracyclines frequently induces secondary infection due to nonsusceptible organisms. Nausea and diarrhea can accompany oral administration and allergic reactions can occur. Tetracyclines enhance the actions of digoxin and anticoagulants, and reduce the efficacy of oral contraceptives.

CHLORAMPHENICOL

Chloramphenicol (Chloromycetin) is a broad-spectrum antibiotic with a range of activity similar to that of the tetracyclines. Typhoid fever, typhus, and other rickettsial infections are especially responsive. Chloramphenicol penetrates the blood-brain barrier, making it a useful agent in *Haemophilus influenzae* infections in the central nervous system. The mechanism of action of this antibiotic involves inhibition of protein synthesis by disruption of peptide bond formation at the 50 S ribosomal subunit level.

Chloramphenicol is well absorbed from the gastrointestinal tract, thus the oral route of administration is used most frequently. Inactivation is by hepatic glucuronidation and renal clearance by both filtration and secretion.

Myelosuppression is the major toxic effect of chloramphenicol. The risk of potentially lethal anemia, thrombocytopenia, and agranulocytosis limits the use of this drug to serious infections unresponsive to other forms of treatment. Chloramphenicol is hazardous in children, especially neonates, who appear to lack sufficient capacity to metabolize the drug. A cyanotic or "gray baby" syndrome that includes vomiting, abdominal distention, hypothermia, and respiratory and circulatory collapse is often fatal. Slowly developing hematological abnormalities, including leukemia, have been attributed to this antibiotic. Frequent monitoring of bone marrow function can assist in detecting early changes that may be reversed by immediate discontinuation of the drug. Renal and hepatic impairment increase the risk of chloramphenicol toxicity. The effects of dicumarol and the oral hypoglycemics can be increased during concomitant chloramphenicol administration. The efficacy of penicillins and the hematopoietic actions of iron and vitamin B_{12} may be reduced.

ERYTHROMYCIN

Erythromycin is a macrolide antibiotic available in several forms for oral, topical, and parenteral administration. The mechanism of its inhibition of protein synthesis is not clear. The spectrum of activity is similar to that of the penicillins but, like that of the tetracyclines, it also includes the psittacosis–lymphogranuloma venereum group of large viruses. Erythromycin is destroyed by gastric acid; the stearate and oleate salts are relatively acid-stable and are preferred for oral administration. Enteric coated forms of this drug also are available. Erythromycin is usually utilized as an alternative to penicillin.

Cholestatic hepatitis can develop over 2 to 3 weeks of therapy with the estolate salt, or may appear rapidly in persons who have previously experienced this reaction. Hepatic impairment precludes administration of this form of erythromycin. Nausea and diarrhea can follow oral administration.

Troleandomycin is a seldom-used orally administered macrolide antibiotic.

SULFONAMIDES

Once widely used, the sulfonamides have been largely replaced with newer antibiotic agents. The action of these synthetic anti-infective drugs involves interference with bacterial utilization of para-aminobenzoic acid (PABA) in the synthesis of folic acid. Since mammalian cells derive folic acid from dietary constituents, their growth is not affected by this action. The efficacy of the sulfonamides will be suppressed by pus or other sources of para-aminobenzoic acid. Low doses of the sulfonamides are bacteriostatic, while larger amounts are bactericidal. Bacteria, in particular gonococci, pneumococci, and streptococci, can acquire resistance to these drugs apparently by developing increased production of PABA or alternative enzymes that incorporate PABA into folic acid. Reduction in bacterial cell wall permeability to sulfonamides may also occur. Many of the organisms that have acquired sulfonamide resistance are susceptible to penicillins.

Sulfonamides can be administered orally or parenterally, according to their water solubility and intended site of action. Biotransformation of systemic sulfonamides is by enzymatic acetylation in the liver. Metabolites as well as unchanged drugs are excreted by the kidney. Crystallization of some sulfonamides in the nephrons can cause renal damage. ***Sulfisoxazole, sulfadimetine,*** and ***sulfacetamide*** are highly soluble in urine at low pH, making these drugs useful in the treatment of urinary tract infections.

Topical sulfonamide preparations are available for ocular and vaginal infections. Sulfonamides that are poorly absorbed following oral administration can be used to eliminate intestinal bacteria. *Sulfasalazine* is used in the management of ulcerative colitis; the 5-amino salicylate metabolite may account in part for its beneficial effects. *Silver sulfadiazine cream* (Silvadene) and *mafenide* (Sulfamylon) are used to control infection in burn patients. Absorbed systemically, mafenide can induce metabolic acidosis, particularly when renal excretion of the drug and its metabolites is hampered. Application of these preparations can be severely painful and is often preceded by administration of an analgesic.

Trimethoprim is an antifolate frequently combined with *sulfamethoxazole* (Bactrim, Septra). Synergistic antibacterial action occurs since the drugs inhibit different steps in the synthesis of folic acid. This combination is used especially in urinary tract infections, and may help to control *Pneumocystis carinii* in persons with acquired immune deficiency syndrome (AIDS).

Hypersensitivity reactions to the sulfonamides can include severe dermatological responses such as Stevens-Johnson syndrome. Hematological abnormalities can develop; persons deficient in glucose-6-phosphate-dehydrogenase (G6PD) are at significant risk of hemolytic anemia. Photosensitivity can occur. Precipitation of drugs in the kidneys can be nephrotoxic; adequate hydration and urinary alkalinization can help to prevent this adverse effect. Sulfonamides should not be administered in late pregnancy or to neonates since the competition of these agents with bilirubin for plasma protein binding sites can result in hyperbilirubinemia. Megaloblastic anemia due to folic acid deficiency may develop in pregnant or malnourished patients, particularly when trimethoprim is administered concurrently.

Systemic sulfonamides compete with other drugs for plasma protein binding sites. In bacteriostatic doses, these broad-spectrum agents reduce the efficacy of bactericidal antibiotics. Sulfonamides can prolong the plasma half-life of methotrexate, phenytoin, and the oral hypoglycemic agents.

ADDITIONAL AGENTS

Polymixins (colistin and polymixin B), which appear to increase bacterial cell wall permeability, have their greatest efficacy against *P. aeruginosa*. Nephrotoxicity limits the systemic use of these agents. Renal impairment delays the clearance of polymixins, which are extensively bound in many tissues and are slowly eliminated by glomerular filtration. Because they are poorly absorbed after oral administration, these drugs can be used to eradicate susceptible bacteria from the gastrointestinal tract. Several preparations for topical use (dermatological and ophthalmological) contain polymixin B. These drugs can induce respiratory failure in combination with neuromuscular blocking agents or in persons with myasthenia gravis.

Bacitracin interferes with bacterial cell wall formation, and has a spectrum of activity similar to that of the penicillins. It is reserved for topical use, since systemic administration presents a marked risk of renal damage. Ophthalmic and dermatological invasions of streptococci and staphylococci often respond to this agent. However, significant amounts of drug may enter the systemic circulation following application to infected or denuded skin.

Vancomycin, an inhibitor of bacterial cell wall synthesis, is derived from *Streptomyces orientalis*. Its action is directed mainly against streptococci and staphylococci, making it useful in treating methicillin-resistant infections. Parenteral administration is required for systemic efficacy. The oral route is used to eradicate infections, such as those caused by overgrowth of *Clostridium difficile*, within the lumen of the gastrointestinal tract. Vancomycin is ototoxic; hearing deficits contraindicate its use. Like most antibiotics, this drug is inactivated by renal excretion.

Lincomycin and *clindamycin* are closely related broad-spectrum antibiotics especially useful in alleviating anaerobic (*Bacteroides*) infections. Both are available as oral and parenteral preparations. These agents bind extensively to plasma proteins and penetrate most tissues except the central nervous system. Since these drugs are inactivated hepatically, impairment of renal function does not appear to enhance their toxicity. The potentially life-threatening pseudomembranous enterocolitis associated with these drugs (as well as occasionally with ampicillin, tetracyclines, and chloramphenicol) appears to be caused by a toxin elaborated by a resistant strain of *C. difficile*, which proliferates inordinately when other gastrointestinal flora are suppressed. Vancomycin administered orally ameliorates this superinfection. Unfortunately, lincomycin and clindamycin also cause a diarrhea that can be difficult to differentiate from colitis.

Nitrofurantoin is active against a variety of urinary infections. It is well absorbed following oral administration (delayed gastric emptying enhances absorption) and is rapidly concentrated in urine by both glomerular filtration and tubular secretion. Additional rapid metabolism of this drug by various tissues contributes to its brief (20 to 30 minute) plasma half-life. Renal impairment markedly prolongs this time interval, and decreases the drug's efficacy within the urinary tract. Low urinary pH promotes reabsorption and elevated drug concentrations in renal parenchyma; alkalinization of the urine enhances renal excretion. Persons with G6PD deficiency are at considerable risk of drug-induced hemolytic anemia. Late pregnancy and age of less than 1 month contraindicate the use of this drug. Pulmonary toxicity, occasionally due to hypersensitivity, is reported with nitrofurantoin. Chest pain, pleural effusion and interstitial fibrosis occur. Patients must be observed for dyspnea, cough, and other indications of respiratory changes since pulmonary damage may become irreversible.

Nitrofurazone, a topical agent related to nitrofurantoin, helps to control infection following severe burns or skin graft. The polyethylene glycol vehicle can be absorbed through damaged skin and attain toxic serum levels in persons with impaired renal function.

Nalidixic acid and *oxalinic acid* have been particularly effective in inhibiting growth of gram-negative bacteria in the urinary tract. They appear to act by inhibition of DNA synthesis. Administered orally, these agents are hepatically biotransformed (nalidixic acid to an active metabolite) and renally excreted. Adverse effects include photosensitivity, hypersensitivity, gastrointestinal and visual disturbances, and central nervous system and hematological abnormalities.

Norfloxacin (Noroxin) is highly effective against most urinary tract pathogens. Structurally similar to nalidixic acid, this orally administered fluroquinolone is hepatically biotransformed and excreted in bile as well as by glomular filtration and tubular secretion. Probenecid delays its appearance in the urine. In contrast to many urinary tract antibiotics, prolonged elevation of renal tubular concentrations of norfloxacin is attained even in the presence of marked kidney function impairment. Antacids and food in the gastrointestinal tract suppress drug absorption. Side effects, which are relatively mild and infrequent, include gastrointestinal disturbances, fatigue, headache, rash, joint inflammation, and hepatic and hematological changes. Maintaining adequate hydration reduces the risk of drug precipitation in the nephrons. Norfloxacin can inhibit hepatic biotransformation of coumadin and theophylline. Bacterial resistance does not readily develop to this bactericidal drug. Ciprofloxacin, also a fluoroquinolone, is administered in a variety of infections.

Methenamine (Urotropin) in an acid urine is converted to formaldehyde, which is bactericidal, particularly to gram-negative organisms. The drug is administered orally and is partially destroyed in the stomach. Enteric-coated formulations are available. Mandelic or hippuric acid, ammonium chloride, or acid-sodium phosphate often is administered simultaneously to attain a urinary pH below 5.5. Irritation of the urinary bladder can occur. Dehydration and renal impairment contraindicate the use of methenamine and its salts.

Phenazopyridine (Pyridium) imparts a local anesthetic action in the urinary tract to relieve pain and discomfort accompanying infections, injury, or diagnostic procedures. Administration by the oral route is usually limited to brief periods of time. Methemoglobinemia, hemolytic anemia, and hepatic and renal failure can occur. Renal dysfunction increases the risk of toxicity. Urine may become discolored; yellow discoloration of the skin or sclera can indicate dangerously elevated plasma levels of phenazopyridine.

Antitubercular Agents

Pulmonary *Mycobacterium* infections are usually treated with a combination of drugs administered for 6 to 9 months or longer. Isoniazid (INH) together with rifampin (Rifadin) is effective in uncomplicated tuberculosis unless the microorganism has developed resistance to this drug. Ethambutol (Myambutol), pyrazinamide (Aldinamide), or streptomycin can be added as a third drug in this regimen, particularly for the treatment of tuberculous invasions of other tissues including the meninges. Isoniazid-resistant strains of *Mycobacterium* are usually responsive to other antitubercular drugs; treatment with drug combinations suppresses the development of resistant microorganisms. *In vitro* drug susceptibility tests can assist in the selection of effective agents.

Isoniazid, a highly specific inhibitor of mycobacterial cell wall formation, is used in both the prevention and treatment of tuberculosis. It is most effective against actively replicating bacteria. Isoniazid is hepatically acetylated at varying rates dependent upon genetically determined enzyme capacities. Renal impairment slows excretion of the acetylated metabolite.

The major toxicity of isoniazid is potentially fatal hepatitis. Liver function must be monitored when this drug is administered. Up to 20% of patients receiving isoniazid will initially develop elevations in serum aminotransferase levels, although this frequently reverts to normal levels without drug termination. Persistent marked elevations of aminotransferase, a concomitant rise in serum alkaline phosphatase or bilirubin, or other indications of hepatic deterioration require that drug administration be interrupted. Persons between the ages of 35 and 65 appear to be at greatest risk of hepatic impairment. Chronic consumption of alcohol increases the incidence of this adverse reaction, and the presence of hepatic disease often precludes the use of isoniazid. Persons who have recovered from drug-induced hepatitis may be given a carefully controlled second trial of the drug. Recurrence of hepatic symptoms, however, requires abandonment of therapy with this agent.

Peripheral neuropathy and convulsions can be induced by isoniazid, particularly in malnourished persons. Pyridoxine (vitamin B_6) reduces this risk. Hematological aberrations and allergic reactions are additional adverse effects. Isoniazid slows the biotransformation of phenytoin, benzodiazepines, and carbamazepine, and can act as an MAO inhibitor. Overdoses of isoniazid can result in fatal central nervous system depression and respiratory failure. Convulsions may occur, and can be alleviated with IV barbiturates and pyridoxine. Concomitant metabolic acidosis may require sodium bicarbonate administration.

Prophylaxis with isoniazid may be indicated for close contacts of persons with active tuberculosis and for positive tuberculin reactors, particularly persons under age 35. Immunosuppressive therapy as well as disorders such as diabetes, leukemia, Hodgkin's disease, and AIDS increase the risk of tuberculosis and may justify preventive treatment with isoniazid. Although pregnancy is a relative contraindication, women at significant risk of disease can receive isoniazid.

Rifampin, usually coadministered with isoniazid, is active against tuberculosis, leprosy, and a number of other bacterial infections. This drug inhibits RNA synthesis by interacting with DNA-dependent RNA polymerase. Like isoniazid, rifampin enters cerebrospinal fluid and is effective in meningeal disease. Hepatic biotransformation produces an active metabolite. The parent drug is partially secreted into bile and is subject to enterohepatic circulation. Drug should be administered 1 hour before or 2 hours following meals, since food hinders gastrointestinal absorption.

Rifampin induces hepatic enzymes, lowering the efficacy of many drugs. Hepatitis can occur in persons receiving rifampin, particularly in the presence of liver dysfunction or other hepatotoxic drugs. Although synergistic hepatotoxicity from isoniazid combined with rifampin does not seem to occur, persons receiving both drugs must be closely observed. Since microorganisms can develop resistance to rifampin, drug sensitivity should be determined before therapy is begun. The most common adverse reactions include gastrointestinal symptoms, headache, ataxia, and hematological aberrations. Intermittent administration induces a flulike syndrome. Renal failure has been reported. Urine and other body fluids can acquire a red discoloration in persons receiving rifampin.

Ethambutol is not effective against all strains of *Mycobacterium,* and is administered only as an adjunct to other drugs. Unmetabolized drug is excreted in feces and urine; renal impairment may necessitate dosage adjustment. Optic neuritis is the unique toxicity of this drug, although it rarely occurs if daily doses do not exceed 15 mg/kg. A complete ophthalmological evaluation of the patient should precede institution of drug therapy, and vision should be tested periodically thereafter. Changes in acuity of red–green color discrimination mandate that ethambutol be terminated. Other reactions to this drug include hepatic dysfunction, hyperuricemia, allergy, and gastrointestinal and central nervous system symptoms.

Pyrazinamide combined with other antitubercular drugs can shorten the time required for successful eradication of mycobacterial infections. The drug and its metabolites are excreted renally. Hyperuricemia and hepatotoxicity occur. In contrast to that induced by ethambutol, elevation of serum uric acid levels induced by pyrazinamide is not alleviated by probenecid.

The aminoglycoside antibiotics streptomycin and kanamycin are effective agents for the management of tuberculosis. Because of their ototoxicity and nephrotoxicity, these drugs require caution in the elderly and in persons with auditory or renal impairment. Streptomycin-resistant mycobacteria frequently respond to kanamycin. Microorganism strains that are resistant to both of these drugs may be affected by *viomycin,* although the use of this drug is limited by its great incidence of toxicity. These drugs must be administered IM since they are not absorbed from the gastrointestinal tract.

Ethionamide (Trecator) and *cycloserine* (Seromycin) are less potent antitubercular agents occasionally used as second-line adjunctive agents. Magnesium depletion induced by the latter drug leads to neurological symptoms such as confusion, depression, convulsions, and psychosis. Para-aminosalicylic acid (PAS) frequently causes gastrointestinal ulceration and has been largely replaced by other drugs. This agent is bacteriostatic, and some myco-bacteria are not at all affected by it. However, PAS given concomitantly with other agents appears to suppress the development of drug-resistant strains. Serum levels of isoniazid are elevated by PAS. Hepatotoxicity and hypersensitivity reactions can occur.

Leprosy (Hansen's disease) is relatively rare in the United States and is optimally treated by specialists associated with the Public Health Service. The sulfone *dapsone* (Avlosulfon) is the drug of choice for this mycobacterial infection; rifampin may be coadministered. Several years of therapy are usually required to achieve complete eradication of the causative microorganism. Adverse reactions such as nausea, tachycardia, and hematological disturbances occur with relative infrequency and are generally mild. Hemolytic anemia may develop in persons deficient in G6PD. Dapsone-resistant strains of *M. leprae* have appeared.

Clofazimine (Lamprene) is effective against dapsone-resistant organisms. Combined with dapsone, it can hinder the development of drug resistance; rifampin can be added to this regimen. Clofazimine is slowly absorbed following oral administration. It accumulates in adipose tissue and leukocytes and has an elimination half-life of 2 months. An anti-inflammatory action, beneficial in erythema nodosum leprosum, has been reported for this drug. Clofazimine can cause reddish brown discoloration of skin, conjunctivae, and lepromatous lesions. Perspiration and lacrimation may be suppressed by anticholinergic action of clofazimine, and gastrointestinal disturbances are reported, particularly when large doses are given.

Antifungals

Fungal (mycotic) infections can be superficial or internal, thus both topical and systemic forms of antifungal agents are utilized. Microorganisms most commonly invading the human host include *Candida*, *Blastomyces*, *Cryptococcus*, *Histoplasma*, *Coccidioides*, and *Aspergillus*.

Since it has activity against all mycotic organisms, *amphotericin B* (Fungizone) is usually the drug of choice for systemic fungal infections. By combining with sterols in the fungal membrane, amphotericin B disrupts the selective permeability of the cell. Since it is poorly absorbed, this drug is usually administered IV. Intraventricular or intrathecal routes can be used for meningeal involve-ment, and topical forms are available for superficial infections (see below). Once-daily or alternate-day therapy may extend for several months. Amphotericin B is extensively bound within the body, and gradually excreted in the urine.

Amphotericin B has severe adverse effects. Suppression of renal function may persist for months following therapy; irreversible renal damage can occur. Renal function should be monitored; indications of significant renal failure require dosage reduction or termination of drug therapy. When serum creatinine levels are used to determine function, it must be remembered that in elderly patients this parameter may be low due to a decreased muscle mass. Thrombophlebitis (due to intravenous administration), hypokalemia and bone marrow suppression are additional reactions that can have serious sequelae.

The initial infusion of amphotericin B characteristically provokes wheezing, hypotension, hypoxemia, fever, and shaking chills. These symptoms may be ameliorated by concurrent administration of steroids, antipyretics, or antihistamines. Although hypersensitivity is uncommon, amphotericin B therapy is often initiated with a test dose of 1 mg in a small volume of 5% dextrose administered over 20 to 30 minutes.

Flucytosine (Ancobon) administered orally can be combined with amphotericin B in the treatment of systemic candidiasis or cryptococcosis. This drug interferes with nucleic acid synthesis; it is fungistatic and microorganisms can develop resistance. Inactivation is by renal excretion, and dosage reduction is required in persons with impaired kidney function. Adverse effects of flucytosine, which include hepatitis, myelosuppression, and diarrhea, can be severe. Blood counts, renal function, and serum levels of drug should be monitored. Amphotericin B may hinder the elimination of flucytosine, thus potentiating its toxicity.

Griseofulvin (Fulvicin), administered orally, is concentrated in the keratin layer of the skin. It is utilized in dermatophytoses that do not respond adequately to topical antifungal drugs. Concomitant ingestion of foods with high fat content promotes gastrointestinal absorption of this drug. Griseofulvin is metabolized hepatically and is excreted in bile. Headache, mental aberrations, gastrointestinal upset, and skin rashes can develop.

Ketoconazole (Nizoral) is effective in the treatment of a variety of fungal invasions. Oral absorption is substantial, although the therapeutic response may be gradual and courses of treatment may extend 6 to 12 months. Ketoconazole is inactivated hepatically and binds extensively to plasma proteins. Gastrointestinal side effects are most common, and may be alleviated by giving the drug with food. Drug-induced hepatic changes on rare occasions progress to potentially lethal hepatic necrosis. Ketoconazole suppresses testosterone synthesis and may be of benefit in prostatic cancer. Inhibition of corticosteroid synthesis has also been reported.

Miconazole (Monistat) administered IV can elicit cardiorespiratory arrest following the initial dose. Close observation and immediately available means for resuscitation are required. A variety of systemic fungal invasions are susceptible to this drug, which disrupts cell wall synthesis. Administration into the urinary bladder or the spinal column is suitable for treatment of refractory localized infections. Thrombophlebitis can occur with IV infusion; thrombocytosis and severe pruritus also may develop. Renal impairment usually does not enhance toxicity. Topical preparations of miconazole are also available.

Several additional agents are applied topically in the treatment of superficial fungal infections. *Tolnaftate, tioconazole,* and *undecylenic acid* and its salts are included in over-the-counter creams, ointments, and powders. *Clotrimazole* and *econazole,* analogues of miconazole, have a broad spectrum of antifungal activity. *Ciclopirox* (Loprox), which disrupts fungal cell energy metabolism, is active against several types of mycotic infections. *Nystatin* (Mycostatin), clotrimazole, and *miconazole* are used topically in the management of vaginal candidiasis. Localized burning and irritation can develop following the application of many of these drug forms.

Amebicides

Infection with *Entamoeba histolytica* is characterized by fatigue, fever, myalgia, arthralgia, intestinal bleeding, and severe diarrhea. Trophozoites in the lower bowel lumen can enter the circulatory system and infect extraintestinal tissues including lung and liver. Drug therapy for amebiasis is divided broadly into treatment of acute symptoms; treatment of tissue invasion such as intestinal ulceration, hepatitis, and liver, lung, and brain abscesses; prevention of relapse by eradicating all cysts from the gastrointestinal lumen; and elimination of cysts in asymptomatic carriers. Because of differing body locations and chemical susceptibilities of active motile trophozoites as contrasted with encysted microorganisms, no single drug has proved to be curative for both gastrointestinal lumen and tissue infections.

Metronidazole (Flagyl), the best single agent for treatment of amebiasis, is amebicidal at both intestinal and extraintestinal sites, but relapses of luminal infections occur. This drug, which inhibits DNA replication, is active against a broad spectrum of microorganisms. Metronidazole can be administered IV or orally, with good absorption from the gastrointestinal tract. It is inactivated hepatically and excreted via the kidney. Renal impairment does not prolong its usual half-life of approximately 8 hours. Hepatic dysfunction may necessitate dosage reduction. Treatment for 5 to 10 days is required to ameliorate amebiasis. To avoid drug decomposition, reconstitution and use of parenteral metronidazole must follow manufacturers' instructions precisely.

Gastrointestinal distress is the most frequently reported adverse response to metronidazole. Because the drug enters cerebrospinal fluid, central nervous system symptoms such as convulsions, vertigo, insomnia, and mental deterioration can occur. Peripheral neuropathy, leukopenia, changes in renal function, hypersensitivity reactions, and thrombophlebitis (the latter following IV infusion) can develop. Candidiasis may be exacerbated during administration of this drug. Metronidazole in therapeutic doses is carcinogenic for mice and rats but it has not been shown to be mutagenic for cells of other mammalian species. However, concentrations of metronidazole equivalent to those in body fluids of humans receiving therapeutic doses produce mutations in Ames' test salmonella (an *in vitro* mutagen assay system). This drug crosses the placenta and is secreted in breast milk. Teratogenicity and adverse effects in nursing infants have not been demonstrated to date but additional years of follow-up are necessary to rule out such actions. Use of metronidazole during late pregnancy and lactation is warranted only when risks of withholding metronidazole (hepatic amebiasis may be fatal) are greater than the risks of administering this drug.

The efficacy of metronidazole may be reduced by drugs that induce activity of hepatic enzymes. Metronidazole can potentiate the anticoagulant action of coumarin-type drugs, and concurrent alcohol consumption may provoke a disulfiram-like reaction.

Oral metronidazole is used frequently to eradicate vaginal trichomoniasis, as either a single dose or a 7-day course of treatment. Sexual partners, even when asymptomatic, should receive similar treatment to avoid reinfection. In research studies, metronidazole appears to enhance tumor responsiveness to radiation therapy. *Amacrine* in topical preparations can help to control this infectious agent.

The antimalarial *chloroquine* (Aralen), administered for 2 to 3 weeks, is amebicidal for extraintestinal infections but has little efficacy in alleviating acute symptoms of dysentery or in removing intraintestinal cysts, since it is almost completely absorbed from the upper gastrointestinal tract, and is present in low concentrations in the lower bowel lumen. The hydrochloride is available for IM administration when the oral route is inappropriate. Renal excretion of chloroquine is promoted by an acid urine.

Adverse reactions to chloroquine include alterations in ophthalmic and cardiovascular functions, gastrointestinal distress, headache, and occasional central nervous system stimulation manifested as convulsions or psychotic symptoms. Chronic administration (as in the management of malaria) can induce muscular weakness and exacerbation of psoriasis and porphyria. The occasional hepatotoxicity of chloroquine can be intensified by other hepatotoxic drugs. Chloroquine binds extensively to tissue proteins, particularly in the eye. Daily long-term use (years) for treatment of collagen diseases has caused irreversible retinal damage.

Emetine and *dehydroemetine* are toxic alkaloids derived from ipecac. They inhibit protein synthesis and eradicate trophozoites from extraintestinal sites such as liver. Prompt alleviation of symptoms including fever, arthralgia, and myalgia, and reduction in size, tenderness, and abscess of the liver have been obtained. In the past, these agents were usually combined with chloroquine to treat amebic hepatitis. Administered parenterally (IM or SC but not IV) emetine alkaloids are gradually excreted in the urine and may be detected in body tissues for long periods of time. The recommended 10-day course of therapy should not exceed a 650 mg total dose of drug, and a rest period of several weeks (6 or more) should elapse before a second course of treatment is given. Today, metronidazole is the drug of choice for treatment of extraintestinal amebiasis, and has replaced chloroquine and highly cardiotoxic emetine alkaloids for this purpose.

Iodoquinol (diiodohydroxyquin, Yodoxin) is an 8-hydroxyquinoline that will alleviate intestinal amebiasis. Intraluminal trophozoites and cysts are eradicated, but insufficient drug is absorbed for extraintestinal activity. Asymptomatic carriers of *E. histolytica* can be treated with iodoquinol. The usual course of therapy is 20 days; chronic therapy with hydroxyquinolines, particularly clioquinol, can elicit subacute myelo-optic neuropathy (SMON). More common adverse reactions are gastrointestinal and dermatological disturbances. Diarrhea or emesis with subsequent dehydration and electrolyte imbalance can occur, and thyroid function tests may be altered by iodoquinol (because of absorption of released iodine).

Diloxanide (Furamide), available from the Centers for Disease Control, is the drug of choice for treatment of asymptomatic cyst passers. The aminoglycoside *paromomycin* (Humatin) administered orally remains within the intestinal lumen where it destroys *E. histolytica*. Although a direct amebicidal action cannot be ruled out, the antiamebic efficacy of erythromycin and the tetracyclines is probably accomplished by their suppression of lower bowel flora that synergistically support growth and colonization of *E. histolytica*.

CHEMOTHERAPY OF OTHER PROTOZOAL INFECTIONS

Schistosomiasis is caused by trematodes (blood flukes) that enter the body through the skin or gastrointestinal mucosa and invade the vascular compartment. Malaise, fever, anemia, and hepatic and gastrointestinal symptoms appear within 2 to 3 weeks of exposure to the microorganism, several species of which can induce illness. *Schistosoma japonicum* and *mansoni* produce intestinal disturbance, while *S. haematobium* causes urinary tract symptoms.

Praziquantel (Biltricide) is active against the three species of schistosoma and other helmintic infestations as well. It is well absorbed following oral administration, and is rapidly excreted in the urine. Gastrointestinal disturbances are the most common adverse reactions to praziquantel.

Niridazole (Ambilhar, available from the Centers for Disease Control) also eradicates the three major species of schistosoma. Alteration of glucose utilization by microorganisms accounts for its efficacy. Given orally for 5 to 10 days, this drug will cause gastrointestinal disturbances and suppression of immune responsiveness. Niridazole is inactivated hepatically; liver dysfunction enhances its toxicity and contraindicates its use. Persons with G6PD-deficient red cells may develop hemolytic anemia. Pregnancy and seizure disorders also preclude administration of this drug.

Stibophen (Fuadin), administered IM, elicits gastrointestinal and cardiovascular symptoms, thrombocytopenia, anemia, and hepatotoxicity. *Oxamniquine* (Vansil), active against *S. mansoni* infections, can induce convulsions or central nervous system depression. The antischistosomal *hycanthone* (Etrenol) is contraindicated in hepatic disease, and may be teratogenic and carcinogenic. Single IM doses can be repeated at 3-month intervals.

Antimalarials

Malaria, caused by four species of plasmodia transmitted by the *Anopheles* mosquito, is endemic in many underdeveloped areas of the world. *Plasmodium falciparum* induces a potentially lethal tertian infection. Early treatment can be effective, although inadequate therapy often results in recurrence of symptoms caused by persistence of parasites in the circulatory system. *Plasmodium vivax* is a much milder malaria of tertian occurrence, although relapses may occur up to 2 years following the initial infection. Much rarer is infection with *Plasmodium ovale;* the course of this malaria is similar to that caused by *P. vivax. Plasmodium malariae* is quartan in nature; rarely, relapses can occur for several years. The malarial parasite, which gains entry to the human circulation via the bite of female *Anopheles,* localizes in hepatic cells. During this exoerythrocytic stage of 5 to 16 days' duration, tissue schizonts (primary tissue forms) develop and eventually rupture to release merozoites into the circulatory system. In the subsequent erythrocytic stage of malarial infections, the red blood cell is the site of development of trophozoites that mature into schizonts and cause the disruption of the erythrocyte and the classic malarial symptoms (nausea, headache, chills, and fever that may approach 105°F). Merozoites released in erythrocyte rupture will infect other red blood cells to propagate the cyclical nature (tertian or quartan) of clinical malarial attacks. *P. falciparum* and *P. malariae* leave no residual parasites in hepatic cells, while *P. vivax* and *P. ovale* may persist in dormant forms (secondary tissue forms) that can yield periodic recurrence of symptoms for several months or years. Plasmodial gametocytes also evolve during the erythrocytic stage but develop further only when transmitted back into the female *Anopheles.*

Drugs used in the treatment of malaria act at various points in the life cycle of the parasite. Agents that suppress primary tissue forms of plasmodia will prevent initial malarial attacks; those effective against secondary tissue forms can prevent recurrence of disease. Complete eradication of parasites from the body is referred to as a radical cure. Drugs that affect erythrocytic stages of malaria will achieve a clinical cure, that is, will terminate acute symptoms of disease.

Chloroquine (Aralen) is usually the drug of choice to alleviate symptoms and suppress recurrence of acute malarial attacks. The usual route is oral, although the hydrochloride salt is available for IM injection in patients with severe disease. Chloroquine is concentrated in infected erythrocytes where it destroys the parasite. *P. falciparum* has no secondary exoerythrocytic phase and can be completely eradicated by chloroquine unless the invading organism has acquired resistance to this drug. (Primaquine must be administered to effect radical cure in other forms of malaria, *i.e.,* to eradicate the secondary exoerythrocytic foci of reinfection.) Chloroquine taken once weekly prevents nonresistant malaria attacks in persons travelling to or residing in endemic areas. Administration is begun 2 weeks before exposure, and one daily dose of primaquine is added during the final 2 weeks of chloroquine prophylaxis to prevent reinfection and obtain a radical cure for *P. vivax* infections. The pharmacology of chloroquine is discussed under "Amebicides."

Quinine, an alkaloid derived from cinchona, is currently used mainly to eradicate chloroquine-resistant strains of *P. falciparum.* **Pyrimethamine,** sulfadiazine, and tetracycline may be concomitantly administered. Quinine is well absorbed from the gastrointestinal tract, metabolized in the liver, and rapidly excreted in urine. Urinary alkalinization decreases the ionization and promotes reabsorption of this weak base.

Cinchonism often develops with therapeutic doses of quinine; symptoms include tinnitus, vertigo, gastrointestinal disturbances, and visual changes that usually remit if the drug is promptly discontinued. Hematological deficits and hypersensitivity reactions, particularly skin rashes, occur. Hemolyic anemia of an allergic or idiosyncratic nature can develop. Quinine can potentiate the actions of oral anticoagulants, digitalis glycosides, and neuromuscular blocking drugs.

Quinacrine (Atabrine), which acts by suppressing DNA synthesis, is seldom used for malaria although it is still available as an anthelmintic. This drug binds extensively to plasma and tissue proteins and is slowly excreted in the urine. Common adverse effects include headache, vertigo, nausea, and diarrhea. Psychiatric symptoms, visual changes, severe skin rashes, and anemia can develop, and skin and urine may acquire a yellow discoloration.

Amodiaquin (Camoquin) is a congener of chloroquine and has similar antimalarial actions.

Primaquine is used to prevent relapses by eradicating secondary exoerythrocytic foci of reinfection in liver. It has little direct effect on erythrocytic infection, and other antimalarials such as chloroquine are used to prevent acute attacks or to produce a radical cure of falciparum malaria after the patient leaves the endemic area. Methemoglobinemia and potentially fatal hemolytic anemia can appear in persons whose red cells are deficient in G6PD or other enzymes involved in the reduction of methemoglobin to hemoglobin. Myelosuppressant drugs may exacerbate the hematological disturbances, including leukopenia, induced by primaquine. This is most common in black persons and certain residents of the Mediterranean basin.

Pyrimethamine (Daraprim) and *trithioprim* (Proloprim) block dihydrofolate reductase synthesis of tetrahydrofolate and inhibit the vital capacity of plasmodia to synthesize folic acid. Sulfonamides are PABA antagonists and are usually administered simultaneously with dihydrofolate reductase inhibitors to suppress further folate formation and to reduce development of resistant microorganisms. The slow antimalarial action of both types of antifolates makes them unsuitable for treatment of acute attacks. A single formulation, Fansidar, combines pyrimethamine with sulfadiazine. The considerable toxicity of these drugs limits their use to prophylaxis of chloroquine-resistant *P. falciparum*. Combining a sulfonamide with pyrimethamine increases the risk of severe dermatological reactions such as Stevens-Johnson syndrome. The appearance of a rash requires that drug administration be terminated. Pyrimethamine has a long duration of action, due in part to its ability to bind to tissue protein. Hematological disturbances induced by folic acid deficiency may develop; leucovorin (folinic acid, citrovorum factor) can reverse folate depletion in the human host but not the plasmodial parasite.

Anthelmintics

Anthelmintics are used to eradicate worm infestations. A variety of helminths can reside in the human gastrointestinal tract and induce debilitating, even life-threatening disease (*e.g.*, malnutrition, anemia). Some infections involve migration of microorganisms to additional sites in the body. Anthelmintic drugs take advantage of differing metabolic sensitivities of helminths compared to human cells.

Piperazine (Antepar) is effective against enterobiasis (pinworm) and ascariasis (roundworm) infestations, producing a flaccid paralysis that allows evacuation of worms from the intestine. The drug is available as tablets or syrup, administered for 2 days for roundworm (feces should be examined for expulsion of worm) and 7 days for pinworm. Adverse effects are relatively few, although piperazine is absorbed from the gastrointestinal tract. Gastro-

intestinal upset and allergic reactions can develop. Central nervous system toxicity, occurring particularly in persons with renal impairment, can include dizziness, tremors, visual disturbances, and seizures. Convulsive disorders contraindicate the use of this drug. Pinworms are easily transmitted; thus family members may also be infected and require drug therapy.

Pyrvinium (Povan) is administered in a single dose to eradicate pinworms; if required, a second dose can be given after 14 to 21 days. Administration with food reduces the incidence of gastrointestinal disturbance. Although this drug is poorly absorbed from the gastrointestinal tract, hypersensitivity reactions and Stevens-Johnson syndrome may occur. Pyrvinium kills worms by inhibition of oxygen and glucose uptake. The drug will color feces and vomitus a bright red; to avoid staining of dental enamel, drug tablets should not be chewed.

Thiabendazole (Mintezol) is useful in a variety of infestations including ascariasis, enterobiasis, strongyloidiasis (threadworm), trichinosis, cutaneous larva migrans, and uncinariasis (hookworm). Absorbed systemically, this drug can cause headache, drowsiness, hepatic changes, cardiovascular and visual symptoms, and hypersensitivity that can include severe dermatological reactions. Gastrointestinal disturbances are the most frequently reported adverse effects, and may be reduced by administering the drug with food. Courses of treatment vary depending upon the type of invading organism. Corticosteroids may be given concurrently to alleviate symptoms of trichinosis.

Mebendazole (Vermox) is effective against several species of helminth. Its mechanism of action—inhibition of glucose uptake—is similar to that of thiabendazole. Fever, hypersensitivity, and gastrointestinal disturbances (particularly when large numbers of worms are expelled) can occur. Little of the drug is absorbed systemically.

The antimalarial quinacrine (Atabrine) in large doses will eradicate several species of tapeworm. Interference in protein synthesis appears to be the mechanism of action. Sodium sulfate or saline is used to purge the gastrointestinal tract before and following drug administration. Feces should be examined for expulsion of worms. Brief courses of drug therapy can induce headache and gastrointestinal disturbances. Seizures and cardiovascular collapse may occur following ingestion of large drug doses.

Pyrantel (Antiminth) in a single oral dose is highly effective in the treatment of enterobiasis and ascariasis, while three consecutive daily doses are administered to remove hookworm. The drug is poorly absorbed from the gastrointestinal tract, although systemic amounts can become sufficient to cause headache, dizziness, and drowsiness. Gastrointestinal disturbances are the most frequently reported adverse effects. Depolarizing neuromuscular paralysis induced in worms accounts for the action of this drug.

Tapeworm infestations can be responsive to *niclosamide* (Niclocide), which inhibits mitochondrial oxidative phosphorylation. The dorsal part of the worm is killed, and may be digested in the gastrointestinal tract. *Taenia solium* (pork tapeworm) may release viable eggs that are not affected by niclosamide. Cysticercosis may be prevented by purging the intestine. Patients should be examined for 3 months to ensure the helminth eradication is complete. Little of this drug is absorbed, and gastrointestinal upset is the most frequent adverse reaction.

Diethylcarbamazine (Hetrazan) is effective in filariasis, apparently by promoting hepatic destruction of microorganisms. Fever, lymphadenopathy, leukocytosis, and tachycardia may occur as large numbers of filariae are killed. Drug treatment continues for 2 to 3 weeks.

The aminoglycoside *paromomycin* (Humatin), used primarily in intestinal amebiasis, will induce removal of tapeworms. Sufficient drug can be absorbed to cause nephrotoxicity. Paromomycin can decrease the intestinal absorption of methotrexate, and may interfere with vitamin K metabolism to potentiate the action of the oral anticoagulants.

Antiviral Agents

Because viruses invade and replicate within host cells, this type of infection is particularly resistant to drug treatment. Management of viral diseases often consists solely of supportive measures until the natural cycle of the pathogen is over. Anti-infective agents may be used to ameliorate secondary bacterial or other invasions. These drugs generally are not effective against viruses, although they have often been administered inappropriately to persons with "colds" or influenza. This use fosters the development of superinfections and resistant strains of microorganisms, as discussed under "Antibacterials." Certain viral diseases (*e.g.*, poliomyelitis, influenza, measles, mumps, hepatitis B) can be prevented by administration of immunostimulant substances. A few virucidal agents, with limited spectra of activity, are available.

Amantadine (Symmetrel) appears to block the entry of the influenza A virus into host cells. Although annual inoculation with influenza vaccine is the preferred prophylactic measure, persons at risk of developing this infection can be given amantadine in daily oral doses for several weeks. Following known or suspected exposure, vaccine and amantadine may both be utilized, the latter to prevent infection while an immune response is emerging. Amantadine is especially useful for persons in whom vaccine is contraindicated. Adverse effects of this drug include depression, dizziness, orthostatic hypotension, and congestive heart failure. Convulsions may occur, particularly in persons with seizure disorders. Renal impairment necessitates reduced dosage of this drug, which has an average plasma half-life of 20 hours.

Vidarabine (Vira-A) disrupts viral DNA replication, and has shown activity against herpes simplex types 1 and 2, varicella zoster, and cytomegalovirus. An analogue of adenosine, this drug is utilized locally (ophthalmically) and systemically (IV). Its passage across the blood–brain barrier makes it useful in treatment of herpes simplex encephalitis. Hepatic and hematological changes, nausea, vomiting, dizziness, and psychosis are possible adverse effects. Topical application can elicit lacrimation and localized irritation.

Acyclovir (Zovirax) is used in the management of shingles (herpes zoster), herpes encephalitis, and genital herpes infections. Initial episodes of the latter are most responsive, with a significant reduction in duration of pain and viral shedding. The occurrence and duration of viral reactivation may also be reduced. Oral, IV, and topical routes of administration can be used. Acyclovir can protect immunocompromised patients against local or systemic herpes infections, although viral activity frequently resumes when drug therapy is terminated.

Acyclovir, itself not active, is phosphorylated by viral thymidine kinase to a substance that inhibits DNA synthesis. Glomerular filtration and tubular secretion inactivate this drug. Frequent dosing, renal impairment, and dehydration enhance the risk of nephrotoxicity attributable to drug precipitation in the renal tubules. Bone marrow and hepatic changes may occur, and PO administration can elicit gastrointestinal disturbances. Appearance of drug-resistant strains has been detected.

Idoxuridine, which disrupts viral DNA synthesis, is available in topical ophthalmic preparations for the alleviation of herpes simplex infections of the cornea.

Ribavirin (Virazole) can inhibit both RNA and DNA replication. Administered as an aerosol, it will control lower respiratory syncytial virus infections in infants and young children. Such infections are frequently lethal in children who have cardiac disorders. A small particle aerosol generator intended specifically for drug administration is utilized, and high concentrations of drug are achieved in the respiratory tract. Persons requiring assistance in respiration are not good candidates for this therapy, because drug precipitation in respirator valves and tubing causes mechanical failure. Filters can reduce this danger.

The virulence of the human immunodeficiency virus (HIV, which induces AIDS) has stimulated a search for virucidal agents. *Zidovudine* (Retrovir, originally named azidothymidine [AZT]) inhibits the reverse transcriptase enzyme required for retroviral replication. Approved for use in certain AIDS patients, this drug can severely suppress bone marrow function. Anemia that necessitates blood transfusion can develop. Some studies have indicated that zidovudine ameliorates symptoms and can prolong survival. Zidovudine may interact unfavorably with many drugs including acetaminophen, ribavirin, and acyclovir. Zidovudine appears to be most effective when it is administered precisely every 4 hours throughout the day and night.

Numerous additional agents are under study for potential benefit in AIDS. α Interferon and interleukin-2, naturally occurring components of the immune system, may also be effective in the treatment of neoplasia. Dideoxycitidine, HPA-23, ribavirin, and others are potentially useful virucidal agents. Considerable effort is being expended in the development of an AIDS vaccine.

Many antimicrobial agents are utilized for the amelioration of opportunistic infections that develop in AIDS patients. The antiprotozoal drug *pentamidine* (Pentam 300) may be especially useful in *Pneumocystis carinii* pneumonia. Trimethoprim–sulfamethoxazole, usually the treatment of choice for this infection, appears to provoke severe reactions in the presence of AIDS. Among the numerous adverse effects reported for pentamidine are nephrotoxicity, hepatic changes, pancreatic damage, and cardiac and hematological abnormalities. A promising investigational treatment of *Pneumocystis carinii* pneumonia in AIDS patients involves simultaneous administration of a dihydrofolate reductase inhibitor (trimetrexate) and leucovorin (folinic acid).

Antiseptics

Several chemical preparations are used topically to remove microorganisms from body surfaces. Their actions involve alteration of pathogen protein and cell membrane integrity. Application of these substances to injured skin requires great caution, because toxic quantities may enter the systemic circulation.

Benzalkonium chloride (Zephiran) can be safely applied to skin, body cavities, the eyes (in concentrations less than 1:3000 or 0.03%) and mucous membranes (concentrations less than 1:5000 or 0.02%). Many vaginal infections respond to this antiseptic. Benzalkonium can be bacteriostatic or bactericidal, depending upon the concentration used. To avoid inactivation of this cationic antiseptic, substances such as soaps and detergents that are anionic must be completely removed from surfaces to be treated. Ingestion of benzalkonium can induce gastrointestinal irritation; systemic absorption elicits central nervous toxicity such as anxiety, weakness, convulsions, respiratory difficulty, and paralysis. Supportive care and evacuation of gastric contents may be necessary to prevent fatalities.

Hexachlorophene (pHisoHex) is used only on intact skin. Systemic absorption can induce hypotension and neurological symptoms including convulsions. Routine bathing of neonates with this detergent was discontinued following several deaths attributed to transdermal absorption. Application to injured skin or mucous membranes, or use with occlusive dressings, is contraindicated. Eyes should be protected from contact with hexachlorophene. This antiseptic leaves a surface film that is especially effective against many gram-positive bacteria. Irritation, photosensitivity, and dermatitis may develop in areas treated with hexachlorophene.

Chlorhexidine (Hibiclens), applied only to the skin, can be bactericidal to gram-positive and gram-negative bacteria. Eyes and ears should be protected from contact with antiseptic preparations. Adverse effects occur with less frequency than with hexachlorophene.

Iodine preparations including iodophors (water-soluble complexes such as povidone–iodine) release free iodine, which will destroy a broad spectrum of microorganisms. Of the iodine preparations, iodophors are reported to be the least irritating to skin. The most frequent adverse responses are allergic rashes that may be severe.

Mercury, in the form of *merbromin* (Mercurochrome) or *thiomerosal* (Merthiolate) may provide some antiseptic action when applied to skin or mucous membranes. It appears to act by inhibiting sulfhydryl enzymes and precipitating proteins.

Silver nitrate 1% may be used to prevent neonatal ophthalmic gonorrheal infections. More concentrated solutions treat dermatological disorders; 50% solutions are used in podiatry to remove plantar warts. Irritation of skin and conjunctivae can occur; application to injured skin is hazardous. Prolonged use can result in hyponatremia and hypochloremia as these ions are attracted to silver nitrate dressings. Ingestion of this antiseptic can induce severe gastrointestinal irritation and inflammation that can be lethal. Administration of 1% sodium chloride will precipitate inactive silver chloride. Nitrate ions in the circulatory system can elicit methemoglobinemia.

Ethylene oxide is a flammable gas used for the sterilization of instruments. Four hours of gas exposure at room temperature will effectively eradicate bacteria and viruses. Ten to 12 hours must then be allowed for dissipation of gas, since irritation and burns can result from minute amounts that remain on equipment. Exposure to this gas can cause nausea and neurotoxicity; appropriate safety precautions must be followed.

IMMUNOMODULATORS

Immunostimulants

Protection against many infectious diseases can be gained by exposure to naturally occurring pathogens or by administration of vaccines, toxoids, or immune sera. Vaccines and toxoids contain modified antigens that provoke an active immune response; the resulting production of antibodies and "memory" cells maintains prolonged resistance to infection. Immune sera contain antibodies (globulins) derived from humans or other animals and provide passive immunity that is immediate but transient. Both active and passive agents are administered following exposure to such diseases as hepatitis B or rabies; the passive agent provides immediate protection while the active agent stimulates an immune response. Otherwise, administration of these agents is separated by 3 months since antibodies present in passive agents may suppress the response to active agents. Agents for active immunity are most effective in persons with a responsive immune system.

All of the immunostimulants are biological preparations, derived from natural sources. Allergic reactions, especially to products from nonhuman species, must be anticipated with the availability of adequate means for resuscitation. To avoid drug decomposition, use and storage must comply with manufacturers' instructions.

Many vaccines and toxoids are routinely administered (*e.g.*, DPT, poliovirus vaccine), at an early age when possible, to establish life-long immunity. Other preparations are administered only to persons at risk of or following exposure to infectious materials (*e.g.*, hepatitis B or rabies). These agents are generally safe in most persons, and the benefit of avoiding potentially serious infections usually outweighs the risks incurred. Awareness of these risks can help to reduce the incidence and severity of occasional adverse reactions.

The DPT triple antigen contains pertussis bacteria and diphtheria and tetanus toxoids. Usually administered at age 2, 4, 6, and 18 months, a course of treatment can be given at similar time intervals later in life. Pertussis, however, should not be administered to children over 6 years of age because of an increased risk of adverse reactions. Preparations omitting this component are available. Pertussis has been implicated in rare but serious neurological responses in young children, and is contraindicated by the presence or familial history of neurological disorders or by severe reactions to previous doses of antigen. Diphtheria and tetanus immunity should be reinforced every 10 years. Localized reactions are the most frequent adverse effects, although allergic responses including anaphylaxis can occur. The latter contraindicate further administration of any component of the vaccine. DPT, like most agents of active immunity, is withheld in the presence of acute illness or immunosuppression.

Poliovirus vaccine is available in both oral and parenteral forms. Oral vaccine (TOPV, Orimune), which confers prolonged immunity, is administered in four doses to children as young as 2 months or as old as 18 years, or to adults at significant risk of exposure to the virus. Immunodeficiency in the candidate for vaccination or in others who reside in the same household will contraindicate oral polio vaccine. Viruses are present transiently in the gastrointestinal and upper respiratory tract, and rare cases of paralytic poliomyelitis have occurred. Immunosuppressed persons are at increased risk of infection, and parenteral vaccine is more appropriate in such circumstances.

Measles, mumps, and rubella vaccines are routinely administered to children at 15 months of age. Some of these preparations are produced in chick embryo cell cultures and are contraindicated by previous severe reaction to ingestion of eggs. Rubella vaccine is absolutely contraindicated in pregnancy because of the fetotoxic nature of this viral infection. (Most vaccines are best avoided during pregnancy, unless the risk of severe disease, *e.g.*, hepatitis B, poliomyelitis, or rabies, is present.)

Hepatitis B vaccines derived from human plasma

(Heptavax-B) and from DNA replication (Recombivax) are recommended for persons, including health-care professionals, who are at risk of exposure to this infection. If exposure has occurred, vaccine and hepatitis immune globulin (H-BIG) can be administered simultaneously. Infants born to carriers of this virus should receive immediate inoculation to prevent infection.

Annual administration of influenza vaccine is recommended for children with inflammatory disorders that require chronic aspirin therapy (due to the possible relationship between aspirin administration during influenza infection in children and the subsequent development of Reye's syndrome), for elderly persons, and for those with chronic debilitating disorders or immunodeficiency. The antigen content of this vaccine is varied yearly to include prevalent strains or mutations of virus. Localized reactions are the most frequent adverse response; neurological disorders such as Guillain-Barré syndrome are occasionally reported. Anaphylactic hypersensitivity to eggs contraindicates this preparation. Amantadine (Symmetrel) can be administered to prevent or ameliorate influenza (see ''Antiviral Agents''). *Haemophilus* influenza type B can be prevented by vaccination of children 2 to 5 years of age. The efficacy of a pneumococcal vaccine has continued to be controversial.

Rabies infections develop slowly and are generally fatal. Vaccines are available for both pre-exposure administration to persons at risk, and for postexposure administration together with rabies immune globulin, which imparts immediate passive protection. Because of the lethal nature of this disease, there are no contraindications to postexposure inoculation, which should be initiated as soon as possible after contact with the virus.

In addition to hepatitis and rabies immune globulins, several other agents of passive immunity are utilized. Immune serum globulin (gamma globulin) can forestall the development or reduce the intensity of measles, chickenpox, poliomyelitis, and hepatitis A and B. Although most immunostimulants are not administered IV, gamma globulin may be given intermittently by this route to immunodeficient persons. Headache, a flulike syndrome, and severe prolonged pain at IM injection sites are common reactions. Agents of active immunity usually are not administered within 3 months of immune globulins.

Rho(D) immune globulin (RhoGam), derived from human plasma, will prevent sensitization to the Rh blood factor. Rh-negative persons are at risk following transfusion of mismatched blood, or pregnancy with an Rh-positive fetus.

Antitoxins to botulism, diphtheria, and tetanus are derived from the blood of horses inoculated with these bacterial toxins. Hypersensitivity to equine proteins can result in anaphylactic shock or serum sickness. However, persons desperately in need of the life-preserving actions of these agents can be administered desensitizing doses accompanied by close observation and immediate availability of means of resuscitation.

Immunosuppressants

Immune responsiveness, beneficial when it protects the human body against potentially lethal infections, can be undesirable when it threatens the survival of grafted tissues, or when it aberrantly destroys normal host cells. The development of drugs that suppress the immune system has markedly enhanced the success of organ transplant surgery and may aid in the identification and alleviation of autoimmune diseases. However, the nature of these drugs' beneficial action leaves the recipient at significant risk of developing infections and neoplasms that are themselves a threat to survival. Therefore, these drugs are administered only by personnel well-skilled in their use, and in facilities that are adept at managing the special pharmacotherapeutic problems encountered. In the treatment of autoimmune disorders, which generally are not life-threatening, careful consideration must be given to the risk of potentially lethal consequences of immunosuppressant therapy. Severe disabling disease that is refractory to all other forms of treatment is the only acceptable indication for these drugs.

Cyclosporine (Sandimmune), a fungal derivative, has proven to be a valuable adjunct in kidney, heart, and liver transplantation and can suppress graft-versus-host disease in bone marrow recipients. Since this drug is water insoluble, it is prepared in alcohol and oil (olive oil for oral administration, castor oil for the IV route). Therapy is begun 4 to 12 hours before surgery, and must be maintained daily thereafter to prevent tissue rejection. Although gastrointestinal absorption is slow and incomplete, this is the preferred route; IV administration is utilized only when the oral route cannot be tolerated. The average plasma half-life of cyclosporine is 19 hours; it is metabolized hepatically and excreted in bile. Extensive binding to plasma proteins occurs, and the drug is sequestered in erythrocytes. Measurement of circulating levels will yield substantially higher values for whole blood than plasma.

Cyclosporine has a more selective action on the immune system than most previously available agents. The proliferation of T lymphocytes, in particular T helper cells, which are important to the mobilization of the immune response, is suppressed by this drug. Thus the risk of opportunistic infections is reduced but not completely abolished. Viral diseases such as Epstein-Barr infection and infectious mononucleosis have been troublesome in persons receiving cyclosporine.

Nephrotoxicity is a major adverse response to cyclosporine. In renal transplant recipients, deterioration of kidney function induced by drug toxicity is difficult to differentiate from that arising from graft rejection. Symptoms occurring soon after surgery suggest the latter, while more slowly developing impairment is characteristic of drug-induced damage. Cyclosporine can also produce hypertension and fluid retention, of particular concern following heart transplant. Neurotoxicity, hepatotoxicity, and hypersensitivity can occur. Embryotoxicity has been found in animal studies.

A corticosteroid such as prednisone is usually coadministered to enhance cyclosporine's effectiveness. Most other immunosuppressants, as well as other nephrotoxic agents, are avoided. Hepatic enzyme inducers can increase the rate of cyclosporine metabolism, while cimetidine and some antimycotic agents prolong drug action. To control secondary infections, concomitant use of antibiotics is often necessary during immunosuppressant therapy.

Azothioprine (Imuran), a derivative of the antineoplastic 6-mercaptopurine, suppresses bone marrow synthesis of the cells involved in immune responsiveness. This drug can be administered PO or IV. Xanthine oxidase is important for drug inactivation, thus the enzyme inhibitor, allopurinol, will markedly prolong the plasma half-life of azathioprine. Low doses of this drug are occasionally administered in severe degenerative rheumatoid arthritis refractory to other treatment. Adverse effects resemble those of antineoplastic agents: myelosuppression, nausea and vomiting, alopecia, hypersensitivity, hepatotoxicity, and carcinogenesis. Pregnancy is a contraindication. Azathioprine may be combined with other immunosuppressants, which increases the risk of infections. Nonsteroidal anti-inflammatory drugs can be added in the management of arthritis.

Methotrexate also may be administered to alleviate severe autoimmune disease, although this drug is highly toxic and fatalities have occurred. Myelosuppression, hepatic and pulmonary toxicity, nausea, and gastrointestinal ulceration are among the adverse reactions. Salicylates and other nonsteroidal anti-inflammatory drugs must be avoided, since these can inhibit renal excretion of methotrexate. Renal function must be monitored. Pregnancy contraindicates this drug, which is both teratogenic and abortifacient. Concomitant use of nephrotoxic drugs, or alcohol and other hepatotoxic agents, can increase the risk of organ damage. Corticosteroids may be concurrently administered to enhance anti-inflammatory action.

The antineoplastic cyclophosphamide (Cytoxan) can be used clinically for its immunosuppressant action. Hemorrhagic cystitis is of special concern with this drug (see "Antineoplastic Agents").

Antithymocyte globulin (Atgam), extracted from blood of horses sensitized to human T lymphocytes, blocks the immune reactivity of T cells. It is administered IV in combination with other agents to suppress transplant rejection. Aplastic anemia can also be ameliorated by this drug. Thrombophlebitis, chills and fever, arthralgia, diarrhea, and hypersensitivity (particularly to equine protein) are possible adverse reactions.

A recent addition to the available immunosuppressants is *muromonab CD-3* (Orthoclone OKT3), a monoclonal antibody that suppresses T-cell activity. Patients must be carefully screened for fever, fluid overload, or allergy to murine substances before this drug is administered. Fever and pulmonary edema are among the adverse effects. Therapy is usually limited to less than 14 days; during this time severe infections can develop.

High doses of corticosteroids such as prednisone and prednisolone continue to be useful when immunosuppression is required. The actions of these drugs are discussed under "Endocrine Pharmacology."

VITAMINS

Vitamins may be considered a special category of drug. Not only do they influence the actions of many types of cells, but they are also essential to proper physiological function. Vitamin deficiencies occur infrequently in the United States, except among persons who lack access to a well-balanced diet. Deficiencies may also be induced by malabsorption syndromes, extensive surgery, and the use of certain drugs, for example, inadequacy of fat-soluble vitamins when bile sequestrants are administered. Vitamin replacement therapy is highly effective in restoring proper nutrition. Widespread use of vitamins prophylactically and as therapy for actual or presumed subclinical deficiencies has occasionally resulted in ingestion of toxic amounts of these substances. Vitamin deficiency can often be alleviated by improved dietary intake.

Vitamin A is essential for retinal function, bone growth, and skin integrity. This fat-soluble vitamin is available as fish-liver oil with high content of the vitamin, as concentrates from such natural sources, and as manufactured synthetic products. Water-miscible forms can be administered by slow IV infusion; rapid injection can cause fatal anaphylactoid reactions. The recommended daily allowance of this vitamin for adults in 5,000 units. Hypervitaminosis A has occurred in numerous instances of excessive self-medication, causing symptoms such as irritability, headache, arthralgia, drying and cracking of the skin, and hematological deficits. Jaundice and enlargement of the liver may develop, since vitamin A is stored tenaciously in this organ. New bone formation and premature closure of the epiphyses have occurred, with serious alterations of skeletal development. Bone decalcification is also reported.

Vitamin D affects calcium and phosphate metabolism, influencing the development and function of tissues that use these essential ions. Endogenous vitamin D formation in the skin is induced by exposure to sunlight. This substance occurs in several forms: vitamin D_2 *(calciferol)* and D_3 *(cholecalciferol)* appear to have similar activity. Dihydrotachysterol (Hytakerol) is hepatically transformed to active vitamin; it is used particularly in amelioration of hypoparathyroidism. *Calcitriol* (Rocaltrol) has special application in alleviating hypocalcemia in renal dialysis patients. Bile is essential for the absorption of vitamin D from the gastrointestinal tract; persons with inadequate amounts of this digestive secretion often benefit from administration of bile acids.

The recommended daily intake of vitamin D is 400 units. Replacement dosages must be highly individualized. Symptoms of overdose include nausea, constipation, weakness, convulsions, polyuria, and metallic taste. Hypercalcemia can induce calcification of blood vessels, renal tubules, and other soft tissues. Serum calcium and phosphatase levels should be monitored; a reduction in the latter can warn of developing calcium excess. Vitamin D is lipid soluble and may be stored in large amounts in body tissues. Hypercalcemia in infants is occasionally reported to be induced by vitamin D administration. Persons receiving digitalis must avoid hypercalcemia, because this electrolyte may elicit cardiac arrhythmias. Hepatic enzyme induction decreases the efficacy of vitamin D.

Vitamin E occurs in several forms known collectively as the tocopherols. The functions of this fat-soluble vitamin appear to include antioxidant and enzyme cofactor. Deficiency seldom occurs, although malnourished infants may exhibit the characteristic hemolysis, muscle necrosis, and creatinuria. Premature infants maintained on formulas high in iron and polyunsaturated fatty acids also are at risk of vitamin E deficiency. Anemia in these patients is corrected by administration of vitamin E. Recommended adult daily intake ranges from 12 to 15 units.

Vitamin K is essential for the hepatic synthesis of several clotting factors including prothrombin. Intestinal bacteria are an important source for this vitamin; administration of certain antiinfective drugs can eradicate these microorganisms and induce coagulation deficits. Absorption of this fat-soluble vitamin is dependent upon the presence of bile in the intestine. Administration of vitamin K will correct vitamin-dependent coagulopathies only if hepatocytes retain their ability to synthesize clotting factors. Oral anticoagulants such as warfarin suppress formation of K-dependent factors; overdose or overresponsiveness to these drugs can be ameliorated by administration of the vitamin. The onset of improved coagulation requires several hours. Emergency measures such as transfusion of blood products may be necessary in severe hemorrhagic episodes.

Several synthetic analogues of vitamin K are available. *Phytonadione* (Mephyton) can be administered orally or parenterally, although the IV route is used only with extreme caution since anaphylactic reactions may occur. The efficacy and potency of this substance are nearly identical to those of the naturally occurring vitamin. Phytonadione has a more rapid onset and longer duration of action than other analogues, and appears to be safer and more effective in ameliorating responsive neonatal coagulopathies. *Menadione* and *menadiol* (Synkavite) do not require the presence of bile for gastrointestinal absorption. These analogues can provoke hemolytic anemia in G6PD-deficient persons or in neonates, and are contraindicated in late pregnancy. Newborn infants also are at risk of vitamin K analogue-induced hyperbilirubinemia. Administration of vitamin K can transiently suppress responsiveness to oral anticoagulants. There is no interaction between this vitamin and heparin.

Vitamin B complex includes several water-soluble substances that are essential for many physiological functions. Since these vitamins are not stored in body tissues to any appreciable extent, deficiencies readily occur if daily intake is inadequate. Usually more than one vitamin in this group will be lacking.

Thiamine (vitamin B_1) is a coenzyme in carbohydrate metabolism. Requirements for this vitamin are increased during pregnancy, febrile diseases, and by high dietary intake of carbohydrates. Thiamine deficiency (beriberi) leads to malfunction of the gastrointestinal, cardiovascular, and nervous systems. Korsakoff syndrome, characteristic of chronic alcohol abuse, is caused by inadequate amounts of this vitamin. Replacement can be given by oral or parenteral routes. Intramuscular injection can be painful; IV administration is hazardous and should be used only when other routes are unacceptable. Intradermal pretesting can help to identify hypersensitive persons.

Riboflavin (vitamin B_2) is an essential component of coenzymes involved in the transfer of hydrogen ions in tissue respiratory systems. Symptoms of riboflavin deficiency include corneal and dermatological changes. Oral and IM routes are used for replenishment of this vitamin.

Pantothenic acid (vitamin B_5) is a component of coenzyme A that takes part in many energy-releasing reactions. Synthesis and utilization of fatty acids and steroid hormones are dependent upon this vitamin. Deficiencies have not been reported, except when induced by administration of an antagonist of pantothenic acid.

Pyridoxine (vitamin B_6) interacts with carbohydrate, protein, and lipid metabolism. Deficiencies may occur in persons receiving isoniazid, oral contraceptives, hydralazine, or penicillamine. Chronic alcoholism, malnutrition, diabetes, and seizure disorders increase the risk of deficiency. Infants also may exhibit deficiency. Abdominal disturbances, convulsions, and peripheral neuritis are prominent symptoms. A genetic pyridoxine-dependent seizure disorder and pyridoxine-responsive anemia are occasionally reported. Pyridoxine reverses the antiparkinsonian efficacy of levodopa, unless a peripheral decarboxylase inhibitor is given simultaneously.

Cyanocobalamin (vitamin B_{12}) is required for cell replication, hematopoiesis and myelin synthesis. Deficits elicit neuropathies such as weakness, paresthesias, ataxia, and loss of bladder and bowel control. Erythrocytes fail to mature, resulting in megaloblastic anemia. Primary vitamin deficiency may respond to oral replacement therapy, although treatment in the presence of abnormal gastrointestinal absorption often requires parenteral forms of vitamin B_{12}. In pernicious anemia, oral administration of vitamin must be accompanied by intrinsic factor in order to effect absorption. Intramuscular and SC injections provide for rapid vitamin replacement. Since this is a water-soluble substance, excess amounts are not retained in body tissues. Adequate amounts of iron, potassium, and folic acid are also needed for the production of erythrocytes. Chloramphenicol and other drugs that suppress bone marrow function can reduce the hematopoietic efficacy of vitamin B_{12}.

Adverse responses to vitamin B_{12} administration include pain at the injection site, diarrhea, thrombosis, pulmonary edema, congestive heart failure, and allergic reactions. An initial intradermal test dose can help to avoid anaphylaxis. Preparations should not be administered IV. Large amounts of vitamin may be required to correct deficiencies, with smaller doses continued at monthly intervals.

Folic acid deficiency usually accompanies states of inadequate vitamin B_{12} and appears to contribute to the incidence of megaloblastic anemia. Both vitamins participate in synthesis of DNA. Folic acid is usually well absorbed following oral administration, and may also be given SC, IM, or IV. Few adverse reactions other than allergy have been reported. Folic acid can reduce the efficacy of phenytoin, leading to loss of seizure control. Phenytoin, primidone, and phenobarbital can accelerate folate metabolism. Several antineoplastic agents (*e.g.,* methotrexate) and antibiotics (*e.g.,* sulfonamides) are also folate antagonists. Oral contraceptives can induce mild folate deficiency.

Nicotinic acid (niacin) and *nicotinamide* are utilized in the prevention and treatment of pellagra. Administration of isoniazid may induce deficiency of nicotinamide, which is essential for lipid and carbohydrate metabolism. Nicotinic acid is a component of nicotinamide adenine dinucleotide (coenzyme II). This drug has some value in hyperlipidemia and is discussed under that topic. Peptic ulcer, hepatic impairment, and severe hypotention contraindicate its administration.

Vitamin C (ascorbic acid) is essential for many physiological functions. Deficiency leads to collagen changes (scurvy) and loss of integrity of bone, capillaries, and connective tissue, and inadequate healing of wounds. Fever, infections, extensive burns, chronic illness, and cigarette smoking will increase the daily requirement for vitamin C. This water-soluble substance is not stored in body tissues; its renal excretion can produce significant lowering of urinary pH. Formation of oxalate or urate stones in kidneys has occurred with large doses. Excessive amounts of vitamin C can cause diarrhea, and are contraindicated during pregnancy since an increased need for the vitamin may be induced in the neonate.

A variety of drug interactions has been attributed to vitamin C. Alterations in the actions of oral anticoagulants and interference with oral contraception may occur. Urinary acidification can enhance reabsorption of acidic drugs and reduce that of alkaline drugs. The action of disulfiram may be impeded. Vitamin C facilitates intestinal absorption of iron.

TOXICOLOGY

Exposure to **carbon monoxide,** a product of most forms of combustion as well as a constituent of artificial fuel gases, is exceptionally common. This gas combines with hemoglobin to form carboxyhemoglobin, which is incapable of transporting oxygen. When approximately 20% of the blood pigment is thus combined, the subject experiences headache and "dizziness"; with 40% combined, there is collapse; with 60%, coma; higher proportions of carboxyhemoglobin are usually lethal. The dissociation pressures of the remaining oxyhemoglobin are less than normal under these conditions. Carboxyhemoglobin is a red pigment, and cherry-red flushing of the skin can be diagnostic. Large skin blisters may occur. The combination of monoxide and hemoglobin dissociates slowly, since the affinity of monoxide for hemoglobin is 200 to 300 times greater than the affinity of oxygen for hemoglobin. Continuous exposure to a carbon monoxide concentration of 0.1% can be fatal in about 2 hours. Administration of oxygen, occasionally under hyperbaric pressure, promotes dissociation and restoration of hemoglobin; respiratory assistance may be required concomitantly.

Cyanides and **hydrocyanic acid** represent a special danger because of their use in industries and fumigation procedures. They are also encountered as poisons used in suicide attempts. Cyanides rapidly and directly inhibit the respiratory mechanism of cells by a highly sensitive inactivation of the cytochrome oxidase system. Histotoxic anoxia in the thoracic chemoreceptors induces pronounced hyperpnea. Convulsions, probably anoxic in character, are followed by respiratory failure. Rapid IV administration of amyl or sodium nitrite and sodium thiosulfate to inactive cyanide ion can be life-saving. Although less effective, methylene blue may be more readily available in an emergency.

Methemoglobin is formed by the action of certain inorganic substances (chlorates, nitrites), aniline dyes, and drugs such as acetaminophen and sulfanilamide that are aniline derivatives. (The use of acetanilid was discontinued because of its propensity to oxidize hemoglobin.) Methemoglobin, like carboxyhemoglobin, is incapable of transporting oxygen, since the ferrous ionic form is converted to the ferric state. Cyanosis, headache, and respiratory difficulty are symptomatic of methemoglobinemia.

Neonates, particularly premature infants, are at risk of methemoglobinemia. In adults, susceptibility follows genetic trends and is associated with deficiency of enzymes such as G6PD.

Methemoglobin is partially eliminated in the urine and partially reconverted to normal hemoglobin over the course of several hours. Erythrocytes are hemolyzed, and chronic methemoglobinemia will results in anemia. Treatment of the acute poisoning consists of oxygen administration and methylene blue (1 to 4 mg/kg intravenously or orally). Identification and elimination of the causative agent are necessary to prevent recurrence.

Kerosene ingestion often causes pneumonitis due to aspiration. Vomiting should not be induced, and gastric lavage must be carried out with extreme caution. There is evidence also that kerosene produces pulmonary inflammation due to transport through the bloodstream from the alimentary canal. **Turpentine** has about the same effects, with a more conspicuous degree of renal inflammation.

Methyl alcohol (methanol) is similar to **ethyl alcohol** (ethanol) in its central nervous system depressant action. This organic solvent is especially toxic to retinal cells and the optic nerve; its ingestion can lead to blindness. Methanol is metabolized to formate, which can induce metabolic acidosis. Sodium bicarbonate administered PO or IV will neutralize excess H^+ ions in plasma. Since ethanol slows the oxidation of methanol, its administration may minimize toxic effects.

Isopropyl alcohol is used extensively as a substitute for ethyl alcohol in external medicinal preparations, such as rubbing and disinfecting alcohols. Ingestion can cause marked renal impairment; large amounts of isopropyl alcohol can be lethal.

Boron hydrides such as pentaborane and decaborane have been responsible for acute and chronic toxicities. Mild symptoms resemble those of common respiratory infections and allergies. In more severe cases, muscle spasms, convulsions, disorientation, and coma develop, frequently after a latent period of several hours. Liver tenderness and abnormal liver function tests may continue for some time.

Lead is a commonly used element, found in paints, pottery, and other household items. Toxic effects can develop after ingestion of a few milligrams daily over several weeks. The most rapidly dangerous route of entry is through the respiratory tract (inhalation of dusts and of the volatile tetraethyl lead), although poisoning also results from oral ingestion and through absorption of organic compounds through the skin. Signs and symptoms of lead poisoning include stippling of red cells, reticulocytosis, anemia, pallor, lead line on the margin of teeth and gums, muscle weakness, and gastrointestinal distress. Encephalopathy, which induces convulsions and coma, can be fatal.

X-ray density at the epiphyseal line is diagnostic in infants who more commonly exhibit cerebral and meningeal symptoms.

The elimination of stored lead is promoted by IV administration of the chelating agent calcium disodium ethylenediamine tetraacetic acid (EDTA, Versene, Sequestrene). This substance complexes with lead to form a soluble compound that is readily excreted in the urine. Dimercaprol (BAL) may be administered concurrently to enhance excretion. The source of lead intake must be identified and eliminated.

Another effective chelating agent is penicillamine, which is capable of removing copper as well as lead. This drug is used in the management of copper excess such as Wilson's disease. It must be remembered, however, that the administration of an antidote carries the risk of drug side effects.

Mercury in soluble ionized form is intensely corrosive, and after absorption it has conspicuous toxic effects in the kidney tubules. Mercuric chloride (corrosive sublimate), metallic mercury (*e.g.*, in thermometers and manometers), and mercury contamination of fish are sources of this poisoning. Toxicity develops in two stages. The first, chemical trauma due to corrosive action, is characterized by immediate burning in the upper gastrointestinal tract, followed by severe vomiting and diarrhea. The second stage, systemic toxicity, becomes apparent within a few days as renal tubular necrosis and azotemia develop.

Treatment consists of stomach lavage, proteins from egg whites and milk to provide local protection, and parenteral fluids. The chelating agents dimercaprol and penicillamine assist in the removal of mercury ion but do not reverse renal damage, which can be lethal.

Arsenic, utilized in pesticides and weed killers, has been a frequent cause of accidental and suicidal poisonings. Acute poisoning may result from ingestion of as little as 100 mg arsenic trioxide (white arsenic). It is characterized by gastrointestinal disturbances, usually with severe vomiting and diarrhea. Arsenic can gain entry into the central nervous system, and will cause convulsions and coma. The chief systemic action is capillary dilation, most marked in the splanchnic area.

Replacement of fluids and electrolytes can be lifesaving. Gastric lavage followed by administration of ferric hydroxide or sodium thiosulfate and a sodium sulfate cathartic will evacuate metal from the gastrointestinal tract. Dimercaprol may prevent further systemic action of the arsenic.

Chronic **beryllium** poisoning was once of special interest, largely because of its incidence in the early days of the fluorescent-lamp industry. Presently it is used in alloys, atomic energy technology, and in ceramics. Skin granulomas may develop following direct contact. Small amounts of inhaled beryllium produce nodular and diffuse granulomas, replacing lung parenchyma. Symptoms of weakness, dyspnea, cough, and weight loss may develop at varying intervals following exposure. Polycythemia has been reported. Administration of prednisone may reduce the toxic effects of beryllium.

Cigarette smoking exposes the smoker to many toxic substances, particularly nicotine, carbon monoxide, tars containing known carcinogenic hydrocarbons, pesticides, and polonium 210 (^{210}Po). Concern over health hazards posed by these toxins has been emphasized by the report of the advisory committee to the Surgeon General of the Public Health Service. Conclusions were that cigarette smoking is causally related to lung cancer, is a significant factor in the incidence of cancer of the larynx, and may be related to cancer of the mouth, esophagus, and urinary bladder. It is considered to be the most frequent cause of chronic bronchitis in the United States and to have a causative relationship to pulmonary emphysema. Deaths attributable to these nonneoplastic conditions are significantly more frequent among cigarette smokers than among nonsmokers. Graded epithelial changes have been observed in the tracheobronchial tree in approximate dose–response relationships to cigarette smoking. These changes include loss of cilia, basal cell hyperplasia, and appearance of atypical cells with hyperchromatic nuclei; bronchial glands also exhibit hyperplastic changes. Smoking during pregnancy increases the risk of abortion, stillbirth, and low birthweight infants. Smoking is also associated with an increased incidence of myocardial infarction, hypertension, and peptic ulcer.

Radiation exposures to doses of the order of 50,000 rads at high dose rates are followed by immediate injury and death, presumably as the result of damage to the central nervous system; exposure to about 1,000 rad leads to death in several days as gastrointestinal epithelium is lost, total body irradiation with several hundred rads is followed by profound myelosuppression with death in 2 to 4 weeks;

smaller doses of 100 rad or less may produce only equivocal acute symptoms followed by slowly developing sequelae such as cataracts, development of degenerative disease, and neoplasia, long after the initial radiation insult.

The testing of nuclear weapons and more recently the construction of nuclear power plants has fastened interest on radiation effects in exposed populations, with intensive monitoring in various parts of the world. The predominant long-lived nuclide from fusion reactions is tritium; from fission reactions, ^{90}Sr. ^{90}Sr and ^{137}Cs appear in plants through uptake from soil. The fallout behavior of ^{131}I differs because of its short half-life and usually is related to rain and the surface area of plants; transfer of ^{131}I to humans occurs principally through milk.

Rodenticides and *insecticides* have been made increasingly effective, and their consequent greater use has increased the hazards of public exposure to these agents.

Red Squill is one of the oldest and most common rodenticides. It contains cardiac glycosides (scillaren) and other glycosides. It produces alternating convulsions and paralysis in rats. Household pets and humans usually vomit the poison before a lethal dose is absorbed.

Sodium fluoroacetate (1080) is volatile and stable and can be absorbed through the skin in toxic amounts. It is used only by specially trained commercial exterminators. The mechanism of death is by ventricular fibrillation.

Alpha-naphthol-thiourea (ANTU) stimulates powerfully the flow of lymph and kills by massive pulmonary edema and pleural effusion.

The anticoagulant *warfarin* is an effective rodenticide. Vitamin K can reverse the hemorrhagic effects of this drug, although several hours are required for the resynthesis of clotting factors.

Pyrethrum, a mixture of plant esters used as an insecticide, is a central nervous system stimulant. Oral ingestion by humans results in hydrolysis of the esters to inactive compounds, which gives it a wide margin of safety. However, its allergenic properties are marked in comparison with other insecticides.

Rotenone is a neutral crystalline derivative of derris root. It causes death in mammals through convulsions and respiratory depression.

Some chlorinated hydrocarbons are unusually effective against a considerable variety of infestations. Usually they are applied in kerosene solution and, when ingested accidentally, the symptoms of poisoning may be those of kerosene. *Chlorophenothane* (DDT) is a central nervous system stimulant and sensitizes the heart to fibrillation. Chronic poisoning is characterized by nervous system symptoms and severe liver damage. DDD, TDE, and methoxychlor are similar. Some isomers of benzene hexachloride, particularly gammexane or *lindane,* are extremely potent central nervous system stimulants, while others are depressant. Chlorinated *camphene* (Toxaphene) produces reflex excitability and convulsions that can be ameliorated by barbiturates. *Chlordane,* a chlorinated indane derivative, has action similar to DDT; it is more readily absorbed through skin thus has a greater incidence of toxicity. *Dieldrin* and *aldrin* also are chlorinated hydrocarbons related in action and uses to chlordane and camphene. The chlorinated hydrocarbons accumulate tenaciously in body fat, but their excretion rate increases in proportion to accumulated amounts. The organophosphate insecticides, which are inhibitors of cholinesterase, are discussed under "Autonomic Drugs."

DRUG ABUSE

Many drugs are misused or abused for a variety of purposes. This section will focus on those drugs that are used in a nonmedical or "recreational" manner based upon their central nervous system actions. Both stimulants and depressants of central nervous system function are included. The abuse of such drugs can lead to drug dependence that may be psychological or physiological. Psychological dependence, characterized by intense craving for drug, or by feelings of inability to function without drug use, fosters repetitious drug use that in many instances can lead to physiological (or physical) dependence. In the latter, the persistent presence of drug appears to induce poorly understood physiological changes; when the drug is not present, physical symptoms called an abstinence or withdrawal syndrome develop.

Persons dependent upon (or "addicted to") drugs often become totally preoccupied with obtaining drugs, first for their pleasurable aspects then as physiological dependence develops, for their ability to stave off the discomforts of withdrawal. Drug abuse has become a problem of major proportions in the United States, having economic, social, and moral as well as medical ramifications. Only the latter will be outlined here. However, the physician must be mindful that psychological and social assistance must be offered and encouraged along with medical care if the patient is to overcome his or her dependency.

Alcohol Abuse

Alcohol is a central nervous system depressant that sedates and induces a calm euphoric response in most persons. Chronic consumption of ethyl alcohol severely damages many body tissues. Hepatotoxicity, cardiomyopathy, esophageal varices, gastritis, central nervous system atrophy, nephrotoxicity, and teratogenicity are among the adverse responses attributed to the use of this drug. Large quantities of alcohol can severely, even fatally, depress respiration. Perhaps the greatest toxicity of alcohol is the number of persons killed and injured annually in accidents, automobile and other, caused by people under the influence of this drug.

Alcohol is metabolized hepatically, first to acetaldehyde through the action of alcohol dehydrogenase, then to acetate by aldehyde dehydrogenase. Acetate enters the tricarboxylic acid cycle to be transformed finally to carbon dioxide and water. The early steps of this pathway tend to follow zero-order kinetics, so that the rate of metabolism is not affected by the quantity of alcohol present. Blood levels of alcohol in most persons closely parallel the degree of intoxication, and in most states are accepted as medicolegal evidence of impairment. Emotional instability and motor incoordination occur with 80 to 100 mg/100 ml plasma (0.08 to 0.1%); "legal" drunkenness begins at 100 to 150 mg/100 ml; marked central nervous system depression appears at 200 to 400 mg/100 ml; loss of consciousness at 500 mg/100 ml; concentrations above this level can be lethal.

Alcohol provides substantial amounts of calories but virtually no nutritional components. In addition, alcohol appears to impair intestinal absorption of foodstuffs and nutrients. Thus persons who chronically consume quantities of alcohol frequently suffer from malnutrition. Mental aberrations such as Wernicke's encephalitis and Korsakoff's syndrome, frequent among alcoholics, are at least in part amenable to administration of thiamine (vitamin B_1).

Withdrawal from physiological dependence upon alcohol can be especially severe. Nausea, tremors, hyperreflexia, and hallucinations progress to seizures, delirium tremens, and disorientation. In extreme uncontrolled withdrawal, cardiovascular and respiratory failure can occur. Dehydration, electrolyte imbalance, and hypoglycemia can be present. Controlled detoxification from alcohol dependence can be accomplished in-hospital, with the administration of small, gradually reduced doses of a long-acting central nervous system depressant such as chlordiazepoxide, paraldehyde, or phenobarbital to suppress withdrawal symptoms. A marked craving for alcohol usually persists after detoxification, and patients will need a period of psychological support and assistance to avoid relapse into alcoholism.

Disulfiram (Antabuse) can occasionally be of assistance in maintaining abstinence from alcohol use. Disulfiram interferes with inactivation of alcohol, inducing accumulation of a toxic metabolite that is probably acetaldehyde. Alcohol ingestion in the presence of disulfiram elicits an unpleasant and at times hazardous reaction. Nausea, headache, dizziness, cutaneous vasodilation, hypertension, and tachycardia are characteristic. The rationale for such therapy is to provide negative conditioning or a perception that the results of alcohol consumption are not pleasant. Unfortunately, the disulfiram–alcohol interaction can also induce hypotension, coma, and death. Cardiovascular disease and psychiatric disorders contraindicate the use of disulfiram. This drug must be administered only to persons who willingly accept its use and have full knowledge of the potential severity of the consequences of concomitant alcohol consumption.

Opiate Abuse

The pharmacology of the opiates is discussed under "Narcotic Analgesics."

Because these drugs induce an intense euphoria, they are subject to abuse. Tolerance to the pleasurable responses, as well as physiological drug dependence, rapidly develop to drugs such as heroin, morphine, methadone, hydromorphone, meperidine, and other opiates. "Designer drugs," similar in structure to the potent narcotic fentanyl, have the curious situation of being "legal" substances simply because their chemical structure is not specified as "illegal." In addition to the usual dangers inherent in substance abuse, these drugs may contain contaminants such as 1-methyl-4-phenyl-1,2,3,6-tetrahydropyridine (MPTP), which has induced parkinsonian destruction of dopaminergic neurons.

Withdrawal from opiate dependence can be unpleasant but is rarely as severe as that from alcohol. Fatigue, anxiety, nausea, drug craving, chills, and fever are characteristic. Detoxification is often accomplished by substituting methadone, which is orally effective and has a long duration of action, for the abused opiate. Stepwise reduction in methadone dosages keeps abstinence symptoms under control while allowing physiological mechanisms to readjust to a drug-free existence. Clonidine also has been used to manage opiate withdrawal symptoms. Clonidine is a centrally active antihypertensive agent whose site of action is at the presynaptic, α-2 adrenoceptor. It suppresses the autonomic symptoms of withdrawal.

Detoxification does not abolish the patient's craving for opiates, and the rate of recidivism among abusers is high. For some persons, methadone maintenance programs offer a more stable life-style. Methadone, itself an opiate, suppresses (or satisfies) drug craving and also blocks the euphoriant action of other opiates. Naltrexone (Trexan), an orally active opiate antagonist, also can be used to block the pleasurable aspects of opiate use.

Sedative–Hypnotic Abuse

Dependence upon barbiturates and other sedatives often begins with legitimate use of these agents (see discussion under "Sedative–Hypnotic Drugs"). Psychological dependence on the calming or sleep-inducing effects fosters prolonged use and the development of physiological dependence. Overdose of hypnotics, not uncommonly with suicidal intent, can result in respiratory depression and failure. Withdrawal from dependence upon these drugs is similar to that from alcohol. Symptoms can be severe, and can be suppressed by gradual withdrawal of central nervous system depressant substances.

Antianxiety Drug Abuse

Benzodiazepines and related antianxiety agents produce both psychological and physiological dependence. In contrast to other central nervous system depressants, overdose of these drugs is not lethal unless other central nervous system depressants are ingested concurrently. Withdrawal symptoms from benzodiazepines such as diazepam and chlordiazepoxide may develop slowly, since these drugs have a long duration of action. Tremor and restlessness, often mistaken for return of anxiety, progress to seizures and delirium. As with other central nervous system depressants, dependence upon benzodiazepines is best managed by gradual reduction in drug dosage.

Psychostimulant Abuse

Central nervous system stimulants induce less pronounced physiological dependence than do the depressants. However, the intense euphoriant and energizing effects of drugs such as the amphetamines and cocaine promote marked and persistent drug craving. Termination of drug use can elicit depression, fatigue, and other subjective symptoms that may constitute a physiological withdrawal syndrome.

Amphetamines are used either orally or intravenously, and have a relatively prolonged duration of action. Intravenous abusers may carry out successive bouts of injection for several days without sleep or food. Restlessness, hyperthermia, increases in blood pressure and heart rate, psychotic episodes, cerebral hemorrhage, and convulsions can occur. Treatment of acute reactions involves supportive measures aimed at normalization of vital signs. An antipsychotic agent such as haloperidol can reduce agitation; urinary acidification promotes excretion of the weakly basic amphetamines.

Cocaine, in particular the free base ("crack"), has become a widely abused drug. The free base can be smoked to produce a rapid and intense but short-lived response that leaves the user craving additional drug. Physiological effects are similar to those of amphetamines: lethal arrhythmias, myocardial infarction, and seizures can occur. Haloperidol (to control agitation), diazepam (to alleviate seizures), and antiarrhythmics all can be used in the management of cocaine reactions.

Psychotomimetic Abuse

Tetrahydrocannabinol (cannabis, contained in marijuana and hashish) is rapidly absorbed from pulmonary alveoli. Euphoria; intoxication; drowsiness; alterations in auditory, visual, and time perception; failure of short-term memory; impairment of skilled behavior; hallucinations; and panic reactions are prominent central nervous system responses. Vasodilation, changes in blood pressure, and tachycardia occur. "Bloodshot" eyes are a hallmark of marijuana use. An "amotivational syndrome," characterized by apathy and personality changes, has been attributed to this drug. Physiological dependence does not seem to develop, and little tolerance occurs. Controversy has long centered on the relative "safety" of marijuana abuse. Possible therapeutic usefulness of tetrahydrocannabinol has fostered development of a synthetic analog, nabilone (Cesamet), for bronchodilation, antiemesis in antineoplastic therapy, and to decrease intraocular pressure in glaucoma. Tetrahydrocannabinol is available as Dronabinol.

Mescaline, an alkaloid derived from peyote, induces anxiety, tremors, nausea, and disturbed auditory and visual sensations.

Lysergic acid diethylamide (LSD) and an "alphabet soup" of related substances (DOM-STP, DMT, DET, MDA, MDMA, as well as psilocin and psilocybin) produce distortions in sensory awareness, hallucinations, euphoria or dysphoria, and panic, the latter often referred to as a "bad trip." These substances are active in extremely small (microgram) amounts. Flashbacks to previous drug experiences commonly occur. Schizophreniform psychoses, transient and more prolonged, can be induced by these hallucinogens. Tolerance to drug effects is rapidly developed and rapidly lost. Physiological dependence does not occur; time intervals between drug experiences may be extensive. Panic and psychotic reactions can be subdued with phenothiazine administration.

Phencyclidine (PCP, angel dust) has been a widely abused drug despite its tendency to produce personality changes and severe toxic psychoses. This substance appears to interact with several central nervous system neurotransmitter systems. Characteristic reactions range from a comatose state to agitated, violent behavior. Convulsions, hyperthermia, anxiety, suicidal ideation, stereotyped activity, hallucinations, and mood alterations are a few of the unpredictable responses elicited by phencyclidine. Irrational behavior may put the drug user or those around him or her in imminent danger of harm. The most appropriate management of severe adverse reactions usually consists of supportive measures administered in an environment relatively free of sensory stimuli. Diazepam can alleviate agitation or seizures. Neuroleptic drugs may suppress psychotic behavior but can also induce marked hypertension. Barbiturates can cause extreme central nervous system depression, and thus should be avoided.

The nutmeg spice contains a hallucinogen thought to be myristicin. Ingestion of large amounts produces euphoria, hallucinations, and psychosis as well as anticholinergic responses such as tachycardia, dry mouth, and apprehension.

Anticholinergics have become drugs of abuse. Excessive ingestion of tricyclic antidepressants and antiparkinson cholinolytics, as well as of belladonna and related plant alkaloids, induces central nervous system responses of disorientation, confusion, and hallucinations. Coma, convulsions, arrhythmias, and death may ensue. Physostigmine, discussed under "Autonomic Drugs," can be used cautiously to reverse anticholinergic overdose.

Numerous volatile substances and gases have been inhaled for their euphoriant actions. Industrial solvents in a variety of preparations ranging from glues to typewriter correction fluid and lighter fluid are often toxic to bone marrow, renal, hepatic, brain, and myocardial cells. Fatal reactions are not uncommon.

In addition to the adverse reactions that can be elicited by abused drugs, further physiological detriment can arise from contaminants that are used to "cut" street drugs. Polydrug abuse is often present, together with infections induced by sharing of needles among IV drug users. This latter practice places persons at extreme risk for development of the acquired immune deficiency syndrome (AIDS).

QUESTIONS IN PHARMACOLOGY

Multiple Choice Questions

ONE-ANSWER TYPE

1. Which of the following symptoms are alleviated by anticholinergic drugs?
   (a) Tardive dyskinesia
   (b) Parkinsonism symptoms
   (c) Both
   (d) Neither
2. Which of the following is (are) used only as a diagnostic agent in myasthenia gravis?
   (a) Edrophonium
   (b) Pyridostigmine
   (c) Both
   (d) Neither
3. Therapeutic doses of which of the following are associated with decreased heart rate at rest?
   (a) Propranolol
   (b) Pindolol
   (c) Both
   (d) Neither
4. The principal route for succinylcholine inactivation is a:
   (a) Mitochondrial enzyme
   (b) Microsomal enzyme
   (c) Plasma enzyme
   (d) Cytosolic enzyme
   (e) None of the above
5. The principal route for epinephrine methylation is a:
   (a) Mitochondrial enzyme
   (b) Microsomal enzyme
   (c) Plasma enzyme
   (d) Cytosolic enzyme
   (e) None of the above
6. The principal route for diazepam glucuronidation is a:
   (a) Mitochondrial enzyme
   (b) Microsomal enzyme
   (c) Plasma enzyme
   (d) Cytosolic enzyme
   (e) None of the above
7. Which of the following is associated with chronic alcohol consumption?
   (a) Depressed platelet function

(b) Hypertension
(c) Both
(d) Neither

8. Which of the following is the most serious and dose-limiting adverse effect of morphine?
   (a) Extreme sedation
   (b) Increased intracranial pressure
   (c) Decreased respiration
   (d) Decreased myocardial conductivity
   (e) Decreased blood pressure

9. Which of the following statements about enflurane is *not* true?
   (a) It is a halogenated compound.
   (b) It sensitizes the myocardium to catecholamines less than halothane does.
   (c) It undergoes more hepatic metabolism than halothane does.
   (d) It potentiates nondepolarizing muscle relaxants.

10. Which property of β blockers is unlikely to increase peripheral resistance?
    (a) Selectivity towards β_1-adrenoceptor
    (b) Intrinsic β-adrenoceptor stimulating activity
    (c) Both
    (d) Neither

11. Which property of β blockers is unlikely to produce respiratory distress?
    (a) Selectivity towards β_1-adrenoceptor
    (b) Intrinsic β-adrenoceptor stimulating activity
    (c) Both
    (d) Neither

12. The most commonly used hypnotic agents are from which following class of drugs?
    (a) Tricyclic antidepressants
    (b) Monoamine oxidase inhibitors
    (c) Phenothiazines
    (d) Benzodiazepines
    (e) Butyrophenones

13. An ideal general anesthetic would have all of the following properties *except:*
    (a) Low blood gas solubility
    (b) Nonflammable
    (c) Primary hepatic elimination
    (d) Muscle relaxation

14. Side effects of which of the following may include salivation and sweating?
    (a) Physostigmine
    (b) Pyridostigmine
    (c) Both
    (d) Neither

15. Which of the following is used as an antidote in tricyclic antidepressant overdose?

(a) Physostigmine
(b) Pyridostigmine
(c) Both
(d) Neither

16. Select the correct statement about nitrous oxide:
    (a) It is an adequate surgical anesthetic by itself.
    (b) It does not undergo biotransformation.
    (c) It has no analgesic properties.
    (d) It is rarely used in modern anesthesia techniques.

17. Injection of a drug X into an anesthetized dog increased blood pressure and decreased heart rate. Following bilateral vagotomy drug X elicited a pressor response without changes in heart rate. Drug X is probably:
    (a) A ganglionic stimulant
    (b) A sympathomimetic amine acting on α- and β-adrenoceptors
    (c) A sympathomimetic amine acting only on α-adrenoceptors
    (d) An indirect acting sympathomimetic amine

18. Which of the following is a veterinary anesthetic with hallucinogenic effects?
    (a) Cannabis
    (b) Cocaine
    (c) Phencyclidine
    (d) Mescaline
    (e) MPTP (methylphenyltetrahydropyridine)

19. Which of the following is a psychedelic phenylethylamine derived from a mushroom?
    (a) Cannabis
    (b) Cocaine
    (c) Phencyclidine
    (d) Mescaline
    (e) MPTP (methylphenyltetrahydropyridine)

20. Which of the following produces reddening of the conjunctiva and aggravation of angina pectoris?
    (a) Cannabis
    (b) Cocaine
    (c) Phencyclidine
    (d) Mescaline
    (e) MPTP (methylphenyltetrahydropyridine)

21. Each of the following is an effective antidepressant drug *except:*
    (a) Lithium
    (b) Imipramine
    (c) Phenelzine
    (d) Desipramine
    (e) Chlorpromazine

22. Which of the following drugs would have the shortest onset of action for its recommended indication?
    (a) Diazepam
    (b) Imipramine
    (c) Amitriptyline
    (d) Phenelzine
    (e) Desipramine

23. Which of the following causes muscle paralysis by sustained depolarization of the postjunctional membrane?
    (a) Pancuronium
    (b) Atracurium
    (c) Both
    (d) Neither

24. Dosage adjustment is not required for the patient with renal dysfunction for which of the following?
    (a) Pancuronium
    (b) Atracurium
    (c) Both
    (d) Neither

25. For which of the following drugs are blood levels *routinely* determined for therapeutic purposes?
    (a) Phenelzine
    (b) Lithium
    (c) Chlorpromazine
    (d) Diazepam
    (e) Flurazepam

26. Which of the following drugs has a short elimination half-life?
    (a) Diazepam
    (b) Oxazepam
    (c) Both
    (d) Neither

27. Dosage of which of the following drugs may have to be reduced during concomitant administration of cimetidine?
    (a) Diazepam
    (b) Oxazepam
    (c) Both
    (d) Neither

28. Which of the following has a low therapeutic index?
    (a) Diazepam
    (b) Oxazepam
    (c) Both
    (d) Neither

29. There is a high incidence of seizures during withdrawal from:
    (a) Heroin
    (b) Phenobarbital
    (c) Both
    (d) Neither

30. Tolerance and dependence develop with repeated use of:
    (a) Heroin
    (b) Phenobarbital
    (c) Both
    (d) Neither

31. Which of the following drugs has reduced effects in patients who chronically consume alcohol?
    (a) Barbiturates
    (b) Warfarin
    (c) Both
    (d) Neither

32. In an emergency room setting, which of the compounds listed below would probably be most useful in treating a drug overdose in a patient exhibiting coma, decreased respiration, and pinpoint pupils but no other remarkable signs?
    (a) Amphetamine
    (b) Diazepam
    (c) Haloperidol
    (d) Naloxone
    (e) Atropine

33. Which of the following statements about pentazocine is *false?*
    (a) It will not precipitate withdrawal in heroin addicts.
    (b) It has fair oral bioavailability.
    (c) It can cause dysphoria.
    (d) It can cause respiratory depression.
    (e) It possesses moderate analgesic activity.

34. Which of the following is *not* usually a therapeutic indication for the use of a strong narcotic agonist?
    (a) Obstetrical pain
    (b) Chronic "low-back" pain
    (c) Dyspnea of pulmonary edema
    (d) Myocardial infarction
    (e) Cardiac surgery

35. Cardiac arrhythmias caused by exogenous catecholamines are most commonly seen during anesthesia with:
    (a) Enflurane
    (b) Isoflurane
    (c) Halothane
    (d) Methoxyflurane
    (e) Nitrous oxide

36. Diminution or prevention of reflex tachycardia is caused by:
    (a) Ganglionic blockade
    (b) β-Adrenoceptor blockade
    (c) Both
    (d) Neither

37. Diminution or prevention of reflex bradycardia is caused by:
    (a) Ganglionic blockade
    (b) β-Adrenoceptor blockade
    (c) Both
    (d) Neither
38. Diminution or prevention of norepinephrine pressor response is caused by:
    (a) Ganglionic blockade
    (b) β-Adrenoceptor blockade
    (c) Both
    (d) Neither
39. Cardiotoxic side effects are particularly associated with:
    (a) Tricyclic antidepressants
    (b) Lithium salts
    (c) Both
    (d) Neither
40. Drugs reaching plasma via which route of administration may first undergo extensive hepatic degradation?
    (a) Intravenous
    (b) Intramuscular
    (c) Sublingual
    (d) Oral
    (e) Subcutaneous
41. Which of the following is associated with supersensitivity of dopamine receptors in the basal ganglia?
    (a) Tardive dyskinesia
    (b) Parkinsonlike syndrome
    (c) Both
    (d) Neither
42. Which of the following is managed with anticholinergic drugs?
    (a) Tardive dyskinesia
    (b) Parkinsonlike syndrome
    (c) Both
    (d) Neither
43. Which of the following is useful in treating nausea of cancer chemotherapy?
    (a) Dronabinol
    (b) Nabilone
    (c) Both
    (d) Neither
44. Antipsychotics such as haloperidol are useful in treating toxic psychoses produced by:
    (a) Amphetamine
    (b) Cocaine
    (c) Both
    (d) Neither
45. Which drugs are effective in the absence of a functioning adrenal gland?
    (a) Cortisone
    (b) Dexamethasone
    (c) Both
    (d) Neither
46. Which of the following drugs acts through the release of formaldehyde in the urinary tract?
    (a) Nitrofurantoin
    (b) Ammonium chloride
    (c) Methenamine
    (d) Nalidixic acid
    (e) None of the above
47. Which of the following is used to diminish heroin withdrawal symptoms?
    (a) Clonidine
    (b) Naloxone
    (c) Both
    (d) Neither
48. Which of the following causes decreased release of arachidonic acid from phospholipids?
    (a) Glucocorticoids
    (b) Aspirin
    (c) Both
    (d) Neither
49. Which of the following causes depressed formation of leukotrienes?
    (a) Glucocorticoids
    (b) Aspirin
    (c) Both
    (d) Neither
50. Which of the following causes depressed formation of prostaglandins?
    (a) Glucocorticoids
    (b) Aspirin
    (c) Both
    (d) Neither
51. Which of the following drugs is most likely to produce cardiac failure?
    (a) Quinidine
    (b) Diltiazem
    (c) Procainamide
    (d) Digoxin
    (e) Phenytoin
52. Which of the following drugs may produce "paradoxical tachycardia"?
    (a) Quinidine
    (b) Diltiazem
    (c) Procainamide
    (d) Digoxin
    (e) Phenytoin
53. Which of the following may result in a drug-induced lupus-erythematosus-like syndrome?
    (a) Quinidine
    (b) Diltiazem
    (c) Procainamide

(d) Digoxin
(e) Phenytoin

54. Which of the following drugs exerts an inotropic effect via inhibition of phosphodiesterase?
    (a) Aminophylline
    (b) Amrinone
    (c) Both
    (d) Neither

55. Propranolol antagonizes the cardiac inotropic effect of which of the following drugs?
    (a) Aminophylline
    (b) Amrinone
    (c) Both
    (d) Neither

56. Which of the following may induce methemoglobinemia and hemolysis when administered to a subject with glucose-6-phosphate-dehydrogenase-deficient erythrocytes?
    (a) Primaquine
    (b) Sulfonamides
    (c) Both
    (d) Neither

57. Fat-soluble vitamins:
    (a) Cause overdosage toxicity
    (b) Are stored in liver
    (c) Both
    (d) Neither

58. Deficiency of which of the following substances causes the disease beriberi?
    (a) Vitamin E
    (b) Vitamin A
    (c) Thiamine
    (d) Nicotinic acid
    (e) None of the above

59. Dose-limiting toxicity of anthracycline antitumor agents such as doxorubicin (Adriamycin) may be manifested as:
    (a) Myelosuppression
    (b) Congestive heart failure
    (c) Nausea, vomiting
    (d) Rashes
    (e) Anaphylaxis

60. The increased usefulness of amoxicillin and clavulanic acid combinations is due to the fact that they:
    (a) May be used safely in patients allergic to other penicillins
    (b) Are better absorbed when taken orally
    (c) Are effective against *Pseudomonas aeruginosa* infections
    (d) Are effective against penicillinase-producing microorganisms
    (e) None of the above

61. Prior to sensitivity studies, the most reasonable choice of an antibiotic to treat a *Staphylococcus aureus* infection acquired outside of the hospital would be:
    (a) Oxacillin
    (b) Penicillin G
    (c) Ampicillin
    (d) Carbenicillin
    (e) Amoxicillin

62. The treatment of choice for a patient with Legionnaire's disease is:
    (a) Penicillin G
    (b) Cefotaxime
    (c) Chloramphenicol
    (d) Erythromycin
    (e) Amikacin

63. Which of the following reduces blood pressure via suppression of angiotensin II formation?
    (a) Captopril
    (b) Propranolol
    (c) Clonidine
    (d) Guanethidine
    (e) None of the above

64. Which of the following has antihypertensive effects associated with blockade of α-adrenoceptors?
    (a) Captopril
    (b) Propranolol
    (c) Clonidine
    (d) Guanethidine
    (e) None of the above

65. Abrupt withdrawal of which of the following drugs may be accompanied by severe blood pressure elevation?
    (a) Captopril
    (b) Hydralazine
    (c) Clonidine
    (d) Hydrochlorothiazide
    (e) None of the above

66. A patient receiving timolol and epinephrine instillation into the eye for glaucoma experienced dizziness associated with hypertension. The most likely explanation for this event is that timolol:
    (a) Increased the release of norepinephrine
    (b) Unmasked epinephrine's pressor response
    (c) Prevented the urinary excretion of epinephrine
    (d) Increased the activity of the enzymes monoamine oxidase and catechol-o-methyl transferase
    (e) None of the above.

67. Pseudomembranous colitis is believed to be due to a toxin produced by *Clostridium difficile*. Appropriate treatment of this condition would be:
    (a) Intravenous vancomycin
    (b) Intramuscular vancomycin
    (c) Oral vancomycin
    (d) Intravenous clindamycin
    (e) Oral clindamycin
68. Which of the following statements about therapeutic doses of verapamil is *not* correct?
    (a) Verapamil diminishes conduction velocity through the AV node.
    (b) Verapamil is used in the management of supraventricular tachycardia.
    (c) Verapamil increases coronary blood flow by dilating coronary arteries.
    (d) Verapamil has a positive inotropic effect.

    (e) Verapamil has a negative chronotropic effect.
69. Neurotoxicity may be dose limiting for:
    (a) 5-Fluorouracil
    (b) Vincristine
    (c) Doxorubicin (Adriamycin)
    (d) Methotrexate
    (e) Bleomycin
70. Which pharmacological action of hydralazine causes reduction of blood pressure in hypertensive patients?
    (a) Increased renin release
    (b) Enhanced inotropism
    (c) Direct vasodilation
    (d) Blockade of α-adrenoceptors
    (e) Diminished sympathetic activity
71. Which of the following is one of the earliest dose-related signs or symptoms of aspirin toxicity in the adult?
    (a) Respiratory depression
    (b) Reye's syndrome
    (c) Metabolic acidosis
    (d) Tinnitus
72. Which of the following acts in the CNS?
    (a) Clonidine
    (b) Prazosin
    (c) Both
    (d) Neither
73. Which of the following promotes salt and water excretion?
    (a) Clonidine
    (b) Prazosin
    (c) Both
    (d) Neither

74. Which of the following inhibits norepinephrine release?
    (a) Clonidine
    (b) Prazosin
    (c) Both
    (d) Neither
75. Which of the following causes an initial syncopal reaction?
    (a) Clonidine
    (b) Prazosin
    (c) Both
    (d) Neither
76. Which of the following promotes uric acid excretion?
    (a) Chlorothiazide
    (b) Probenecid
    (c) Allopurinol
    (d) Furosemide
    (e) None of the above
77. The drug of choice for type II hyperlipoproteinemia is:
    (a) Nicotinic acid
    (b) Gemfibrozil
    (c) Cholestryramine
    (d) D-Thyroxine
78. N-Acetylcysteine would be indicated for treatment of an overdose of which of the following?
    (a) Aspirin
    (b) Ibuprofen
    (c) Acetaminophen
    (d) Diflunisal
    (e) Naproxen

MULTIPLE TRUE–FALSE

From the list following the question, select all of the correct items and match them to the answer according to the following list:

A. If *only 1, 2, and 3* are correct
B. If *only 1 and 3* are correct
C. If *only 2 and 4* are correct
D. If *only 4* is correct
E. If *all* are correct

79. In which of the following conditions should narcotics be used with extreme caution or not at all?
    1. Head injury
    2. Pulmonary edema of left ventricular failure
    3. Emphysema
    4. Myocardial infarction
80. Sublingual administration of drugs:

1. Results in the rapid achievement of therapeutic blood levels
2. Is limited only to drugs that are not lipid soluble
3. Is useful for drugs that are metabolized in the gastrointestinal tract
4. Results primarily in effects to the brain

81. Benzodiazepines:
    1. Enhance the inhibitory actions of GABA, one of the brain's major inhibitory neurotransmitters
    2. Show cross-tolerance and cross-dependence with alcohol
    3. Are the most widely prescribed psychotherapeutic drugs
    4. Are effective in the treatment of most forms of depression.

82. Opiates produce their analgesic effects by:
    1. Inhibiting CNS pathways transmitting pain stimuli
    2. Inhibiting the sensitivity of peripheral pain receptors to chemical and physical stimuli
    3. Blunting the emotional reaction to pain stimuli
    4. Nonspecific inhibition of sensory pathways

83. These drugs may produce urinary retention.
    1. Belladonna alkaloids
    2. Tricyclic antidepressants
    3. Antihistamines
    4. Antipsychotic drugs

84. These drugs are useful in treating motion sickness.
    1. Belladonna alkaloids
    2. Tricyclic antidepressants
    3. Antihistamines
    4. Antipsychotic drugs

85. Carbamazepine is effective in the therapy of:
    1. Tonic–clonic convulsions
    2. Trigeminal neuralgia
    3. Manic depressive disorder
    4. Absence seizures

86. The adrenergic–neuronal blocking agent, guanethidine, should not be administered to patients receiving MAO inhibitors because:
    1. Central effects of guanethidine antagonize MAO action.
    2. Guanethidine will prevent the storage of MAO inhibitors.
    3. Guanethidine will prevent the metabolism of MAO inhibitors.
    4. Guanethidine may elicit a pressor response.

87. Patients with myasthenia gravis frequently exhibit:
    1. Improved muscle tone following the edrophonium (Tensilon) test
    2. Decremental muscle response to repetitive nerve stimulation
    3. Antibodies to acetylcholine receptors
    4. High levels of plasma cholinesterase

88. Tardive dyskinesia is:
    1. Effectively controlled with benztropine (Cogentin)
    2. A consequence of blocking the reuptake of dopamine by neurons in the basal ganglia
    3. Rapidly produced by all antipsychotic drugs
    4. Rarely reversible

89. Treatment for major depression includes:
    1. Electroconvulsive therapy (ECT)
    2. Methylphenidate
    3. Tranylcypromine
    4. Amphetamine

90. Lithium's side effects include:
    1. Constipation
    2. Tremor
    3. Weight loss
    4. Polyuria

91. Less muscle relaxant is required during anesthesia with:
    1. Nitrous oxide–narcotic
    2. Enflurane
    3. Halothane
    4. Isoflurane

92. Drug combinations expected to have synergistic antibacterial actions include:
    1. Penicillin G and streptomycin
    2. Carbenecillin and gentamycin
    3. Trimethoprim and sulfamethoxazole
    4. Penicillin G and tetracycline

93. Overdose with which of the following analgesics is likely to produce coma, pinpoint pupils, and respiratory depression?
    1. Ibuprofen
    2. Meperidine
    3. Acetaminophen
    4. Morphine

94. Warfarinlike drugs:
    1. Are highly bound to plasma protein
    2. Reduce antithrombin III levels
    3. Interfere with the action of vitamin K
    4. Block the synthesis of thromboxane A_2

95. Which of the following is used in the treatment of supraventricular tachyarrhythmias?
    1. Digoxin

2. Phenytoin
3. Quinidine
4. Lidocaine
96. Which of the following is used as a prophylactic against the occurrence of severe ventricular arrhythmias following a myocardial infarction?
1. Digoxin
2. Phenytoin
3. Quinidine
4. Lidocaine
97. Which of the following drugs has (have) a high addiction liability?
1. Barbiturates
2. LSD (lysergic acid diethylamide)
3. Meperidine
4. PCP (phencyclidine)
98. Valproic acid:
1. May produce hepatotoxicity
2. Is used in the treatment of status epilepticus
3. May raise plasma phenobarbital levels if chronically coadministered
4. Is linked to a high incidence of gingival hyperplasia.
99. The signs and symptoms of withdrawal from physiological dependence on opiates include:
1. Runny nose
2. Hyperthermia
3. Diarrhea
4. Pupillary constriction
100. Chronic administration of which of the following may result in psychological dependence?
1. Temazepam
2. Lorazepam
3. Oxazepam
4. Chlordiazepoxide
101. Basic mechanisms of antimicrobial action include:
1. Inhibition of bacterial cell wall synthesis
2. Inhibition of bacterial protein synthesis
3. Disruption of bacterial cell membranes
4. Inhibition of nucleic acid synthesis
102. Which of the following is effective in reducing systemic heavy metal intoxication?
1. Deferoxamine
2. Calcium disodium edetate
3. Dimercaprol
4. Penicillamine
103. Which drug is useful in the treatment of Wilson's disease?
1. Deferoxamine

2. Calcium disodium edetate
3. Dimercaprol
4. Penicillamine
104. Which of the following could be expected in a case of severe aspirin overdose in a child?
1. Metabolic acidosis
2. Decreased respiration
3. Delirium, convulsions
4. Respiratory acidosis
105. Which of the following produces salt and water retention?
1. Clonidine
2. Hydralazine
3. Guanethidine
4. Minoxidil

Identification Questions

Identify the item listed in questions 106–111 according to the following list:

A. If *only 1, 2, and 3* are correct
B. If *only 1 and 3* are correct
C. If *only 2 and 4* are correct
D. If *only 4* is correct
E. If *all* are correct

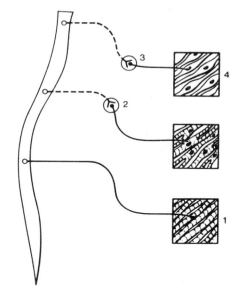

106. Acetylcholine release
107. Muscarinic receptors
108. Nicotinic receptors
109. Atropine inhibition

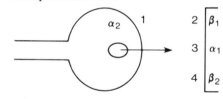

110. Epinephrine
111. Isoproterenol

Select the most appropriate choice for each question.

The following diagram presents the relationship between the recorded contraction of bronchial smooth muscle and the dose of injected acetylcholine (ACh). Identify drugs I and II from the list of choices.

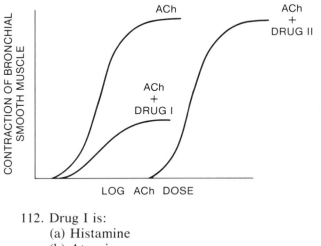

112. Drug I is:
    (a) Histamine
    (b) Atropine
    (c) Pilocarpine
    (d) Epinephrine
    (e) D-Tubocurarine
113. Drug II is:
    (a) Histamine
    (b) Atropine
    (c) Pilocarpine
    (d) Epinephrine
    (e) D-Tubocurarine

The following figure presents the relationship between heart rate and drug concentration in a vagotomized dog. Drug I is epinephrine. Identify drugs II, III, and IV from the list of choices.

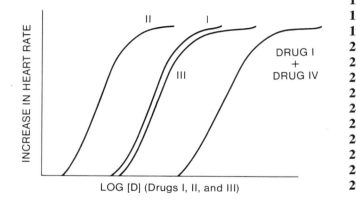

114. Drug II is:
    (a) Norepinephrine
    (b) Phenylephrine
    (c) Isoproterenol
    (d) Propranolol
    (e) None of the above
115. Drug III is:
    (a) Norepinephrine
    (b) Phenylephrine
    (c) Isoproterenol
    (d) Propranolol
    (e) None of the above
116. Drug IV is:
    (a) Norepinephrine
    (b) Phenylephrine
    (c) Isoproterenol
    (d) Propranolol
    (e) None of the above

ANSWERS TO PHARMACOLOGY REVIEW QUESTIONS

1. b	30. c	59. b	88. D
2. a	31. c	60. d	89. B
3. a	32. d	61. a	90. C
4. c	33. a	62. d	91. C
5. d	34. b	63. a	92. A
6. b	35. c	64. e	93. C
7. c	36. c	65. c	94. B
8. c	37. a	66. b	95. B
9. c	38. d	67. c	96. D
10. c	39. c	68. d	97. B
11. c	40. d	69. b	98. B
12. d	41. a	70. c	99. A
13. c	42. b	71. d	100. E
14. c	43. c	72. a	101. E
15. a	44. c	73. d	102. E
16. b	45. c	74. a	103. D
17. c	46. c	75. b	104. E
18. c	47. a	76. b	105. E
19. d	48. a	77. c	106. E
20. a	49. a	78. c	107. D
21. e	50. c	79. B	108. A
22. a	51. b	80. B	109. D
23. d	52. a	81. A	110. E
24. b	53. c	82. B	111. C
25. b	54. c	83. E	112. d
26. b	55. d	84. B	113. b
27. c	56. c	85. A	114. c
28. d	57. c	86. D	115. a
29. b	58. c	87. A	116. d

Behavioral Sciences

Ronald S. Krug, Ph.D.
David Ross Boyd Professor, Vice Chairman for
Education, Department of Psychiatry and
Behavioral Sciences, University of Oklahoma at
Oklahoma City—Health Sciences Center,
Oklahoma City, Oklahoma

Gordon H. Deckert, M.D.
David Ross Boyd Professor, Department of
Psychiatry and Behavioral Sciences, University of
Oklahoma at Oklahoma City—Health Sciences
Center, Oklahoma City, Oklahoma

INTRODUCTION

Behavioral Sciences Defined

Behavioral sciences is defined as the science of behavior. Because it is not the "art" of behavior, this topic belongs in the basic sciences section of medical education preparatory to the study of the clinical art of medicine.

It shares with other sciences use of the *scientific method,* or the generation of hypotheses about its content and the methodology for testing those hypotheses. The scientific method is a self-correcting style of thinking and inquiry. That is, from curiosity about and observation of the world, a general theory of how an event occurs is formulated. Hypotheses are then generated to test aspects of the theory, and, using appropriate controlled research design, the hypotheses are tested for their reliability and validity. Results are used to refine the theory, with the goal of replacing theoretical formulation with established fact.

The "behavioral" portion of behavioral sciences does *not* reflect the influence from the *behaviorism* school of psychology, which posited, "if you can't

see it or measure it, it doesn't exist." The basic parameters of mental behavior, particularly as they contribute to the practice of medicine, are legitimate concerns for scientific study. These include thought processes, thought content, subjective emotional state, and perceptual phenomena. The static personality structure of individuals (their traits) as well as varying adaptations to fluctuating internal and external states (the *dynamic* aspects of human behavior) are also valid foci of scientific investigation. Also included are those phenomena that are expressions of the "collective man," such as society, culture, subculture, and mores.

Behavioral sciences in medical education is a body of knowledge that is continually argued and refined. A consensus of content is found in the publications of the Association of Behavioral Sciences in Medical Education (ABSAME) and in the constituency of the Behavioral Sciences committees of the National Board of Medical Examiners. Both have representation from throughout the United States and operate from the studied and organized conglomeration of data supplied by its changing membership. The academic discipline sources are varied. From the basic sciences of biochemistry, genetics, pharmacology, and physiology come data loosely termed behavioral biology, which is the relationship between molecular events and human behavior. From the social sciences of anthropology and sociology come cultural, group, and social system influences, and from psychology comes the information about abnormal behavior, assessment of behavior, developmental processes, personality, psycholinguistics, and psychophysiology.

The behavioral sciences has wide application to all of the subdivisions of medicine. Sabshin indicated, "Patients with psychiatric problems constitute a major portion of the work load for those . . . in general medical practice. . . . more patients with mental illness are treated by health professionals than by mental health professionals. . . ." Rakel reported psychofamilial patient problems as the third most common difficulty encountered in a family physician's office. Large-scale studies have validated the finding that 50% to 60% of adults randomly sampled report psychophysiologic symptomatology. Obviously, it would be erroneous and perhaps dangerous to misconstrue behavioral sciences as simply, and only, an introduction to psychiatry.

Integration of Behavioral Sciences and Psychiatry

While we have noted that behavioral sciences is not simply an introduction to psychiatry, there are two practical ties between these fields. The first is academic history. For the most part, behavioral sciences was introduced through departments of psychiatry in medical schools. The second is an apparent similarity of content. Within behavioral sciences is a subsection of "abnormal behavior." Obviously, the diagnosis, intervention, and follow-up of many of these conditions are within the purview of psychiatry, not behavioral sciences. It should be remembered that the predisposers, precipitators, and maintainers of abnormal behavior may be orthogonal phenomena that call for different strategies. For example, a person may be genetically predisposed to alcoholism; however, that individual may begin to drink only because of the death of a child and continue to drink because of biochemical addiction to the drug. The genetic predisposition would have required genetic counseling, the precipitating stress would have required grief and bereavement work that provided more available and attractive alternatives than alcohol, and the biochemical addiction would demand medical detoxification from this class of depressant compounds.

Some of these activities are the legitimate domain of behavioral scientists, and all are within the scope of the practicing physician regardless of medical specialty. It is only through applied research that the issues and answers surrounding predisposers, precipitators, and maintainers can be addressed.

PHENOMENOLOGY OF MENTAL PROCESS

Mental processes are those functions that constitute the concept of "mind"; they are dimensions of behavior to which physicians attend as they evaluate the total person. These are the basic elements of mental functioning upon which the more complex and protean forms of human behavior are constructed. It is assumed that many are unique to man. Mental processes are not static events. They wax and wane, and they are in dynamic interchange with the person's internal and external environment.

Basic Concepts

MOTIVATION

Motivation is a concept that represents the energy that moves an individual to actively satisfy physical, psychological, and social needs. It is the *drives* or *tension states* created by "survival" needs as well as the *impulses,* or unexpected urges, over which the individual has little control. Other terms from various theories are *libido* and *will. Primary needs* are basically physiologic in origin, but through humans' symbolic and communication ability, psychological or social needs *(secondary needs)* also develop.

GRADIENT

Gradient refers to the relationship between two elements as depicted by the slope of a line on a graph. For example, in Figure 8-1, as one progresses on the x-axis, the value of y increases. For example, if x represents a patient's distance from the hospital's

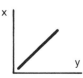

Fig. 8-1. Gradient. The graphic description of the relation between two variables.

surgical suite and *y* represents his anxiety levels, then this gradient would state that the closer the patient is to the surgical suite, the more anxious he feels.

STRESS

Stress involves the disruption of a person's internal homeostatic state. If one's homeostatic balance is disrupted, the individual is understood to be stressed. **Walter Cannon,** writing in the 1940s, characterized the attempt to correct this lack of homeostasis as the ***fight or flight*** syndrome—demonstrated by increased blood sugar, dilated pupils, increased blood pressure, and increased muscle tone—to prepare the person for battle or rapid retreat. **Hans Selye** (1956) posited the ***general adaptation syndrome,*** which ultimately implicated activation of the entire endocrine system in response to somatic, psychological or social stress. Arthur stated, ''Constant activation of the endocrine system can lead to adrenal exhaustion and deleterious bodily effects elsewhere from secondary processes such as elevated blood sugar.'' Selye's work is perhaps most applicable in those conditions where the stress emanates from an internal condition of the person from which it is not possible for the person to ''flee'' or that the individual cannot ''fight.'' Three conditions seem to be most important in internal psychologically based stress: loss of significant objects (*e.g.,* a body part, loved one, occupation), injury or threat of injury (*e.g.,* surgery, illness, terminal disease, a robber with a gun), and frustration (*e.g.,* rejected lover, crowded living space, sitting in a waiting room). These three will be elucidated below.

CONFLICT

Conflict is present when two or more drives arise simultaneously (*e.g.,* to study for specialty board exams or to attend a desirable social event), or when two or more incompatible responses, including feelings, are aroused simultaneously (*e.g.,* love and hate toward one's parents). By definition, conflict is within the individual. Conflict can be classi-

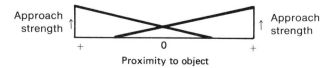

Fig. 8-2. Approach–approach conflict. Conflict generated by two equally positive objects.

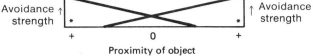

Fig. 8-3. Avoidance–avoidance conflict. Conflict generated by two equally negative objects.

fied into three types: ***approach–approach, avoidance–avoidance,*** and ***approach–avoidance.*** Figure 8-2 displays the schema for approach–approach conflicts. The conflict is maximal where the two gradients cross (*e.g.,* deciding whether to take a vacation in Tahiti or Hawaii). Once the individual has moved past the conflict point on either gradient (*e.g.,* once he has made a decision), no consequent difficulty arises because the level of the nonchosen gradient decreases as the individual approaches the chosen object.

Figure 8-3 displays the schema for avoidance–avoidance conflict. Again, conflict is maximal where the gradients intersect. For example, the point where one decides to stop smoking in order to avoid lung cancer is the crisis point in the conflict of avoidance of health problems vs. avoidance of stopping to smoke (avoidance of pleasure). However, in avoidance–avoidance conflict, once the individual makes a decision and moves towards an object, the avoidance gradient increases and pushes the individual back into the conflict again.

Figure 8-4 demonstrates approach–avoidance conflicts. Here the same object, for example, marriage, has both approach (gradient *a*) and avoidance (gradient *b*) attributes. The person begins the approach gradient, making wedding plans, before encountering the avoidance gradient, awareness of losing freedom; again, the conflict is maximal where the two gradients cross. If the individual proceeds on the approach gradient, the avoidance increases; if the person retreats, the approach becomes more attractive once again. The resolution is either to increase the positive value or to decrease the negative value of the object so the gradients never cross.

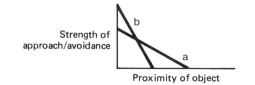

Fig. 8-4. Approach–avoidance conflict. Conflict generated by both positive and negative attributes residing within the same object.

ORGANIC–FUNCTIONAL

Organic–functional is a distinction that refers to the etiology of a given, usually "pathologic," human condition. *Organic* means the etiology is known, usually, in pathologic states, on the basis of one or more of the following conditions, which affect the central nervous system (CNS) either directly or indirectly: metabolic, inflammatory, traumatic, toxic, infectious, neoplastic, congenital, degenerative or vascular. (A handy memory aid, or mnemonic, is "MITTEN-CDV.") Behaviors that are organic in etiology can present to the physician as any of a number of psychiatric syndromes. However, organic brain syndromes can usually be distinguished by a disordered sensorium or unique types of perceptual experiences discussed below. The term *functional* historically is derived from the fact that pathology could not be seen by using a light microscope. Today it implies that there is no known organic pathological condition that is responsible for the observed behavior pattern. Functional pain, while sometimes inappropriately dismissed as "all in the head," does not make the experience of the pain any less for the patient who has it. Functional etiology can also imply a psychological or learned base to the behavior pattern observed by the physician.

ACUTE–CHRONIC

The acute–chronic dimension used in behavioral sciences, specifically the pathologic conditions of behavior, is applied differently than in medicine as a whole. In psychiatry and behavioral sciences, *acute* implies that the condition is reversible and *chronic* means that it is not reversible. In certain situations, multiple acute episodes can produce a chronic–organic condition (*e.g.,* multiple acute alcohol intoxications can produce Korsakoff's psychosis).

"The Mind"

EMOTIONS

For this discussion, the words *emotions* and *affect* will be considered synonymous. Emotions accompany the alteration of the homeostatic state of the human organism. The alterations may be small and are often ignored by the person, or they may be large and overwhelming. The accompanying emotion can vary accordingly. Both large and small perturbations and their emotional concomitants are important because small, unnoticed changes can accumulate into a large, overwhelming situation.

Emotions can be judged positive (*e.g.,* happy) or negative (*e.g.,* sad). However, because people usually do not seek help from the physician when they are happy, the following discussion will focus on the more disruptive emotions of anxiety–fear, anger–hostility and sadness.

Anxiety–fear is the typical emotional response to some type of real or imagined injury or threat of injury. However, a distinction between fear and anxiety can be made. *Fear* as an emotion is related to a real thing that the frightened person recognizes and usually understands, and against which the person can make protective behavioral responses. *Anxiety* as an emotion is best understood as fear of something that the anxious person cannot identify. The symptoms of anxiety are experienced subjectively but are not linked to an object in the anxious person's awareness. The event responsible for the anxiety is said to be repressed. It is not that the anxious person will not tell the physician the source of experienced anxiety, but rather that he cannot because he has no awareness of the threatening object.

The subjective evidence of anxiety (*i.e.,* what the patient reports) includes statements like, "I'm nervous," "I have butterflies in my stomach," or "My knees are shaky." The objective evidence (*i.e.,* what the physician sees) includes the following: excessive perspiration, fine motor tremor, speaking at the height of inspiration, head pulled back as if avoiding a blow to the face, eyes open wide so sclera is visible above and below the iris, eyebrows elevated leading to a wrinkled brow, frequent and rapid changes in body posture, fidgeting of the hands and feet, and, if the patient is sitting, the feet and lower legs positioned with one in front of the other as if to enable a "fast getaway."

The physiological correlates of anxiety include an epinephrine-like response peripherally. Overactivity of the sympathetic nervous system may result. Centrally, the locus ceruleus and the diencephalic limbic systems are implicated. These include excessive perspiration, skeletal muscle tension (*e.g.,* tension headaches, constriction of the back of the neck or chest, quivering voice, lower back pain), cardiovascular irritability (*e.g.,* transient dystolic hypertension, premature contractions, tachycardia, hypotension), genitourinary dysfunction (*e.g.,* urinary frequency, dysuria, erectile dysfunction in men, decreased vaginal lubrication in women), functional gastrointestinal disorders (*e.g.,* abdominal pain, anorexia, nausea, diarrhea, constipation), and respiratory difficulties. The extreme instance of the latter is known as the *hyperventilation syndrome,* which includes dyspnea; dizziness; paresthesias of the fingers, toes, and perioral area; and, in extreme cases, carpopedal spasm. Generally, hyperventilating patients subjectively report that they are oxygen deficient, but in fact their oxygen blood level is above normal.

Besides anxiety's role either as etiologic or, at least, an accompaniment of pathological behavior syndromes, there is a clear relationship between anxiety and performance, as expressed in Figure 8-5. To a certain degree, anxiety can enhance performance by making the person alert, active, and motivated. However, too much anxiety causes a decrease in performance.

The most common situations that provoke anxiety are as follows: *anticipatory anxiety,* where individuals frighten themselves with the unknown in advance of a given event (*e.g.,* stage fright), *castration anxiety,* which originated from psychoanalytic theory, meaning the anxiety/fear associated with the son's fear that the father will "cut off his penis" for "loving" the mother (today the concept is expanded to any situation where the person encounters threat from an authority figure such as a supervisor), *separation anxiety,* which is experienced when one is separated from another person who is needed (*e.g.,* the first day of school, frequently for both the child and the parents), *stranger anxiety,* which is a normal developmental event occurring in an infant between six and 12 months when the infant is confronted with anyone who is "nonmother." This is frequently distressing (*i.e.,* anxiety provoking) for the nonmother figure, usually the father; however, stranger anxiety simply indicates that the child has begun to discriminate between objects.

These specific examples demonstrate the signal–alerting function of anxiety/fear. The anxiety/fear signals the individual that danger is present. It is frequently difficult for a person to "unlearn" anxiety/fear attached to a specific event that is no longer dangerous because the symptoms are so uncomfortable that the frightened/anxious person automatically avoids the source of the distress whenever the alerting signals are perceived.

Anger as an emotional response usually has *frustration* as its stimulus. Frustration occurs when motivated (*i.e.,* goal directed) behavior either is blocked or there is a challenge to obtaining the goal. The goal may be a real or symbolic object that will satisfy a given primary or secondary need (*e.g.,* pulling into a parking space and someone else blocks the entry). The aim of the resultant anger is to remove the blocking agent and allow the accomplishment of the drive. Anger is a drive discharge emotion in that the emotion, appropriately directed, allows for satisfaction of the frustrated drive/need state.

Anger is also related to *hostility.* The major distinction between anger and hostility is that anger is relatively short-lived if the frustrating stimulus is removed. Some authors suggest anger should not last longer than 20 minutes. Also, anger is not necessarily destructive, but is more aggressive. Hostility, however, is an emotional condition that pervades the person's entire behavioral repertoire, is present over extended periods of time (*e.g.,* years) and is physically or psychosocially destructive. Hostility may or may not be related to a specific frustrating stimulus or condition.

Subjective reports from the angry patient include statements like, "I'm mad," "I'm angry," or "I'm pissed off." Objective signs the physician can observe include narrowed eyelids, "knitted" eyebrows, flared nares, clenched teeth (*i.e.,* protruding masseter muscles), lips thin and tightly pursed, head and neck jutted forward, protruding and throbbing temporal and neck blood vessels, rigid back, arms crossed tightly across the chest, and feet planted flatly and firmly on the floor.

The psychophysiologic concomitants of anger are peripherally epinephrine (and possibly norepinephrine) in nature. These include increased heart rate and blood pressure, dilated pupils, increased muscle tension, increased energy, constriction of peripheral vessels, and increased metabolic rate.

Primate studies have implicated the diencephalic–limbic system in anger. *Rage* reactions have been observed after intercollicular section and nociceptive stimulation in the posterior and lateral portions of the hypothalamus as well as other areas of the limbic system. Also, there appear to be modifying influences from the forebrain and rostral thalamic nuclei. Important considerations are the "forced activity" observed in *temporal lobe epilepsy* (also called partial complex seizures), and the absence of fear and aggression responses as well as

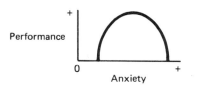

Fig. 8-5. Anxiety and performance. Mild to moderate anxiety enhances performance; however, higher levels of anxiety interfere with performance.

the hypersexuality of the *Kluver–Bucy syndrome* associated with bilateral lesions of the amygdala and hippocampus.

Sadness as an emotional response usually has *loss* of a significant object as the etiologic event. The lost object may be a person, job, health, youth, or anything to which the individual is strongly attached. The subjective evidence for sadness is the patient's report that "I feel down," "I feel blue," or "I am sad." The objective evidence the physician can observe includes flaccid face, downcast gaze, sighing respiration, speaking at the end of expiration, head tilted down, shoulders slumped, decreased associative arm movement in walking, hands held loosely in the lap, legs crossed at the ankles, and general decreased amounts of body movements.

Sadness as an accompaniment of the *mourning* process is expected and must be distinguished from the *depressive syndrome,* which is characterized by dysphoria accompanied by dysfunctions in sleep, appetite and weight, "libido," concentration, and psychomotor activity, with feelings of guilt and worthlessness and suicidal ideation/impulses. Mourning should be completed in 6 to 12 months after major loss. If mourning extends into the second year, the physician should suspect that the patient is no longer mourning, but is depressed and should be treated accordingly.

There are two important variations of sadness. The first is *guilt,* which can be conceptualized as a mixture of sadness plus anger turned back upon the self. The individual angrily blames the self for some event. For example, a mother whose child is born retarded may be sad over the "loss" of a "normal" child and may inappropriately assume the responsibility for the retardation with a statement such as, "If only I had (not) done. . . ." *Shame,* on the other hand, can be conceptualized as sadness in the face of external environment disapproval. For example, with the same mother noted above, the immediate family might say, "If only you had (not) done. . . ." Shame can also be viewed as the feeling one experiences in the presence of another's disgust.

There are five major descriptions that characterize emotions. First, they are *bipolar:* anxious–calm, angry/hostile–warm (similar to hate–love continuum), and sad–happy. Next, an emotion can be *ambivalent* in that an individual simultaneously experiences both ends of the bipolar continuum toward the same object. This is similar to the approach–avoidance conflict noted above (*e.g.,* loving and hating an individual at the same time). Third is the ability to express emotions either subjectively with

words or objectively by facial expression, or both. Some persons have decreased or constricted expression, some have increased expression, and some demonstrate no emotional response. The absence of emotional expression is termed *flat affect.* Fourth is the *appropriateness* of an expressed emotion relative to the content to which it is attached. (*e.g.,* It is generally appropriate to cry at the loss of a loved one, but not to laugh.) Last, it is the rapidity of emotional change. All persons experience fluctuations in their emotional state; however, some individuals' emotions change markedly quite frequently (*e.g.,* every 30 seconds). This is termed *lability* of affect.

Disgust may also deserve attention. It is often a clue to the values held by a given individual. Its somatic expression may be significant in the evolution of certain symptoms (*i.e.,* nausea and vomiting). There is increasing evidence of its involvement in the development of compulsive behavior in some individuals.

THOUGHT

Thinking is "mental" manipulation of symbolic processes usually for creative or problem-solving purposes. Since thoughts are intangible, thinking can only be judged objectively by verbal, written, or other products. For discussion purposes, thought will be divided into two separate portions: the process and the content.

Thought process, the first major division, describes *how* a person thinks. There is a given production rate, which may be inferred from the rapidity with which a person speaks, but geographic and cultural variations may be misleading. It is clearer to conceptualize production rate of thoughts as a person walking. *Accelerated thought* process is similar to a person descending a steep hill and about to lose balance. That person takes short rapid steps to prevent stumbling. The physician may try to intervene, but the person cannot help but continue rapidly downhill. *Retarded thought process* is similar to a person ascending a steep hill. The progress is slow and labored and, regardless of the physician's attempt to assist, the person maintains a slow pace. *Blocking* is exemplified by the person who, while walking, encounters sudden darkness in which the appropriate direction cannot be ascertained. This individual is confused, doesn't understand why the darkness occurred and can't extract himself from the darkness. Accelerated and retarded production rates generally accompany major affective disorders and certain organic conditions. Blocking is usually psychologically determined and precipitated by content issues that are in conflict; it is most common in major thought disorders.

When examining how a person thinks, besides rate there should be consideration of the *continuity* with which thoughts are connected. Most formal thought process is characterized by Aristotelian logic (*i.e.,* A → B → C → D . . . → Z). The term *looseness of association* refers to thought process that is non-Aristotelian, where associations between thoughts are formed on unique bases that have very loose connections. Sometimes this is called *predicate logic* (*e.g.,* von Damerus' Principle), where the association is based on the objects of sentences (*i.e.,* "The Virgin Mary was a woman, I am a woman, I am the Virgin Mary.") In other forms, the associations between thoughts are on the basis of sounds and are called *clang associations,* like bang, rang, dang, sang, and clang. Another disorder of continuity is *circumstantial* thinking, in which the person produces every detail or circumstance surrounding a given event. For example, when asked, "What did you do this morning?" the person might respond, "I heard the alarm, opened my left eye, then my right eye, opened my mouth, yawned, stretched my right arm, then my left. . . . (*three hours later*) and then stood up at the side of the bed." These persons will eventually arrive at the end goal; however, the physician hardly has time to wait. *Tangential* thinking is that process characterized by the person slightly missing the goal. For instance, "Are you a good tennis player?" may elicit the answer, "I like to play tennis." While the questioner has some data relative to the inquiry, an "on-target" response was not made. The thought process known as *perseveration* is when persons repeat the same response regardless of the context of the question. (Q: "How old are you?" A: "30." Q: "How many children do you have?" A: "30." Q: "How tall are you?" A: "30.")

Thought content, the second major division, is concerned with the message or meaning of the thoughts. The first consideration is the thought's *relationship to reality,* which is identified by three components: *sense of reality* (*e.g.,* knowing that the four-legged object on which one is sitting is a chair), *testing reality* (*e.g.,* validation with someone else or through functional experimentation that the object is, indeed, a chair), and *adapting to reality* (*e.g.,* using the chair to sit comfortably at a table to eat when the table is too high or low without it). The most significant aspect of relationship to reality is whether the individual is either realistic or *autistic* in thought content. Autistic means the individual has a private understanding of the world or external events which is not shared by others; for instance,

Einstein's theory of relativity when initially proposed. If the autistic thinking becomes fixed in the face of contrary, overwhelming evidence and takes on a maladaptive or malevolent quality, the thought content is called delusional. *Delusions* are defined as false–fixed belief systems. Autistic thinking is characteristic of major thought disorders like schizophrenia.

The second aspect of thought content is the relative level of *abstraction* that an individual can attain. For example, upon request, can the individual abstract the common essence from examples of a general category (*e.g.,* an orange and banana are both fruit) and distill a general principle from a concrete example (*e.g.,* "A stitch in time saves nine" means prevention is cost effective)? If abstractability is impaired, the person can only identify superficial *concrete* qualities of diverse objects of a general class (*e.g.,* an orange and banana both have peelings) or can only repeat the example or give literal interpretation of the example (*e.g.,* "Sew a tear when it starts and it won't take as many stitches to fix"). While poor abstractability is found in functional and organic thought disorders, it is also characteristic of mental retardation and the thought processes of young children.

The next characteristic of thought content is whether the individual can develop *insight.* Can the person interdigitate relations between events in a cause–effect manner, or can the individual recognize stress events or internal conflicts and their subsequent emotional effects? Related to insight is *judgment.* Given insight, how does the person relate in social situations, generally exercise control over life, and judge the consequences of given situations and adjust to them?

Another significant element of thought content is the relative *obsessional* nature. That is, whether the same thought content characteristically intrudes uncontrollably into the person's awareness or whether characteristic thoughts are varied and rich in content.

It is useful to consider the major topics, themes or issues that appear in a given patient. The physician stands back, so to speak, examines the patient's verbal landscape, and notes a title: "I constantly suffer at the hands of people who don't understand me," for example.

ORIENTATION

Orientation is knowing who and where one is at the present time. There are four dimensions of orientation that are considered: person, place, time, and situation.

Orientation to person means the individual knows who he is (*i.e.,* name, birthdate, can identify parts of the body or knows that the body belongs to himself). The phenomenon of *depersonalization* is a disorientation to person in which the body as a whole or parts of it seem dissociated from the "mind" (*e.g.,* the mind drifts from the body and observes events from the corner of the room). Two other disruptions in orientation to person are *anosognosia,* not knowing that one is ill, and *autotopagnosia,* not being able to correctly locate one's own body parts.

Orientation to place means the individual can locate himself geographically and spatially. If orientation to place is disrupted, the most common forms are *derealization,* a sensation of distortion of spatial relations and unreality, *deja vu,* a feeling when in a strange environment that "I've been here before," and *jamais vu,* the reverse of deja vu, where the individual is in a familiar environment and suddenly wonders, "Where am I?"

Orientation to time is the individual's ability to know present position in linear time; for example, day or night, morning or evening, day of the week, month, and year. The latter is emphasized because of the common assumption that if a person knows the date and month, that person automatically knows the year. This is frequently untrue, particularly in the various forms of organic brain disorders and syndromes.

Orientation to situation is a synthesis of the above three. That is, to repeat the definition of orientation, does this person know who he is, where he is, when it is, and the present contextual situation that relates these three together?

CONSCIOUSNESS

Within behavioral sciences, the concept of conscious mental processes has three distinct definitions. First, consciousness is used to refer to the relative level of physiologic arousal. Second, it can mean that the person is physiologically alert, but there is a psychodynamic condition present that may grossly affect mental processes. Third, it is used to define whether a piece of data is in a person's awareness at the present time, with the assumption that the individual's physiological arousal level is normal and alert.

The first point (relative physiologic arousal) refers to the level of activation of the CNS and the associated nonfluctuating nature of consciousness. This aroused condition of the organism is intimately tied to the integrity and functioning of the *reticular activating system (RAS).* Apparently the RAS is also central to the behavioral *alerting* or *orienting response* which is the primary determinant of *attention.* If the RAS is functioning in an activating manner, it is transmitting signals to other portions of the brain and the person is alert and attending or orienting to incoming stimuli. However, if the RAS is compromised in function, the individual experiences a condition ranging from mental confusion, through clouding of consciousness, stupor (*i.e.,* the individual's senses are dulled and the person is capable of very little environmental interchange), to coma, where there is no awareness of the environment. These alterations in physiologic alertness are common sequelae of CNS dysfunction and particularly *traumatic head injury.* In addition to the characteristic level of consciousness, fluctuating levels of consciousness (or attention) frequently accompany pathologic CNS conditions as well as psychologically based disorders. Organic conditions should be suspected if the person is well rested and is attempting to focus attention or concentrate, and cannot.

The second definition of consciousness implies that the person is physiologically alert; however, some psychologically based conflict has precipitated a condition in which the person seemingly functions in a "normal" manner but is unaware of massive amounts of personal experience. The most common of these conditions are *fugue states,* which are characterized by the assumption of a totally "new life" without being aware of a different earlier life (upon recovery of the earlier memory, the fugue life is forgotten) and *dream* or *twilight states* in which the physiologically alert person seems to focus all attention on an inner or far-off event. During the latter condition the person is relatively immobile and markedly unresponsive to environmental stimuli; amnesia for the event is expected. *Somnambulism* (*i.e.,* sleepwalking) is the third major type of psychologically based alteration in consciousness. It is similar to a short-lived fugue state, except that it begins while the person is asleep. Upon awakening, the individual has no recollection of the events that transpired during the sleepwalking episode.

The third definition of consciousness historically is derived from psychoanalytic theory, and recently from studies that focus on how the brain processes information, and it refers to whether given material is in the awareness of the person. Freud spoke of three levels: first, conscious material, which is in full awareness; second, preconscious material, which is not in awareness but can be readily recalled at will (*e.g.,* one's own telephone number); and third, unconscious material, which is not in awareness and cannot be brought into awareness without special techniques like hypnosis or free association.

SENSATION

Sensation is defined as the experience that results from stimulation of sensory nerve endings of any of the five senses: sight, sound, touch, smell/taste, and kinesthesia.

Primary sensation tends to provoke anxiety because of its "unknown" quality. This unknown disrupts the homeostatic condition of the person, which the person attempts to correct through understanding or perception as discussed below. Toxic conditions (*e.g.,* various drugs) and other neuropathologic conditions, such as irritating lesions of the visual cortex or migraine headache, can produce sensory phenomena. It is emphasized that primary sensations without environmental stimuli (*e.g.,* visual scotoma and "sparklers," tinnitus, foul odors) usually imply organic conditions. The primary sensory pathways, their projection sites in the brain, and behavioral correlates will be included in the discussion of the physiologic contributions to the determinants of behavior.

Psychogenically based disorders of sensation are best represented by the phenomenon of chronic, psychogenic pain.

PERCEPTION

The understanding of sensory stimuli referred to above is the operational definition of perception. As stimuli enter the brain, in addition to the specific sensory nerve tracts that pass to the sensory cortical areas, there are collateral sensory inputs to the reticular formation which apparently activate the RAS. This activation results in *attention* to the stimulus and is called an *orienting response.* With attention and *concentration* on the nature of stimuli and past experience or frames of reference, the person "understands" or perceives the stimuli. For example, one is awakened in the night by a noise. Until the cause of the noise is perceived, arousal (*i.e.,* orienting response or attention) and anxiety remain at high levels. With perception, anxiety may change to fear or disappear depending upon the cause. The arousal may turn to concerted effort to deal with the perceived stimulus. Sometimes, for either organic or functional reasons, misperceptions of environmental stimuli occur. For example, a

drape blown by a draft is perceived as someone entering a window, or the shadow of a leaf on a wall at night is perceived as a tarantula spider. These are *illusions,* defined as misinterpretations or misperceptions of real environmental events.

However, exteroceptive stimuli are not always necessary for perception to occur, as in imagination or dreaming. On occasion, internal stimuli like thoughts can become so intense that they are projected as perceptions onto the external world in the form of *hallucinations.* That is, the person perceives as imaginary or interoceptive event as an exteroceptive reality. While hallucinations are usually considered pathologic (auditory being more functionally based, and visual, tactile, olfactory/taste, and kinesthetic more organic) there are two forms of hallucinations that seem to be unrelated to significant pathologic conditions. In stages of sleep when control over "conscious" processes is marginal, hallucinations—particularly auditory types—are frequently reported. If a hallucination occurs as one enters sleep it is called a hypnagogic hallucination and if it occurs as one is gaining wakefulness it is called hypnopompic hallucination.

Advances in neuroscience confirm the statement that perception is a constructional process; it is not veridical. All of us literally see and hear the world differently. In that sense illusions are universal.

MEMORY AND FORGETTING

Memory (*mnesis*) is the ability upon demand to bring into awareness past events and experiences. It is customary to divide the concept of memory into three arbitrary types based on how much time has elapsed since the original event occurred. *Immediate memory* or recall is the ability to reproduce data to which one has just been exposed; for example, finding a telephone number in a telephone book and having the number available for a few seconds, or the repetition of a serial set of numbers. This ability is apparently limited to seven "bits" or "chunks" of data. *Recent* or *short-term memory* is the ability to remember information after at least a ten-minute interval between exposure to and recollection of the data (*e.g.,* recollection of three independent items presented by an interviewer at the beginning of an interview, or notable news events that occurred within the last two weeks). *Remote* or *long-term memory* refers to the availability of information learned by the individual a considerable time before (*e.g.,* when was Pearl Harbor bombed, or when was John F. Kennedy assassinated?).

Research has established that both neuroanatomical sites and neurochemical processes are important in the mnestic process. Apparently the mesencephalic reticular systems is important early in the memory process, and activation of the thalamic reticular system with attendant inhibition of the mesencephalic reticular system is crucial later in the memory process. The hippocampus appears to be particularly central to the transfer of information from short-term to long-term memory. Synthesis of ribonucleic acid (RNA) and protein is important, particularly in the formation and storage of long-term data. Recent work specifically involving research into *Alzheimer's disease* has documented the contribution of the CNS acetylcholine (ACh) neurotransmitter system in memory process. In the CNS, ACh is concentrated in the basal ganglia and the basal forebrain cholinergic complex. This concentration in these two areas is thought to play a pivotal part in memory processes.

Special states of memory include *hypermnesia,* which is unusual memory for detail of a specific or selected situation, *iconic* memory, which is the brief, detailed retention of visual stimuli, and *eidetic* ("photographic") memory, which is the unusual ability to glance at an object like a book page, look away, and recite it without error as if reading the page.

Forgetting *(amnesia)* is the inability to recall material to which one has been previously exposed. It is assumed that the forgetting of material has either a "dynamic" or functional base (*i.e.,* the information is "blocked" from awareness by psychological processes), or is organic. The most common types of amnesia are as follows. In *patchy* or *lacunar* amnesia, the person has intact memory around a given amnesic "hole;" for example, the grandparents who can remember all grandchildren's names and birthdates except the one whose mother died at its birth. In *anterograde* amnesia, the person forgets all information following a given significant life event (*e.g.,* memory loss for 24 hours after being raped). *Retrograde* amnesia is the loss of memory for events preceding a significant life event (*e.g.,* 24 hours prior to being knocked unconscious from an automobile accident). *Paramnesia* (*i.e.,* retrospective falsification) is the distortion of remembered data. The person who experiences this is firmly convinced of the validity of the recollection. One specific instance of this phenomenon is called *confabulation,* characteristic of the organically based Korsakoff's disease, which is now called alcohol amnestic disorder. In confabulation, the individual weaves data from the here-and-now into the recalled experience. Sometimes the interwoven data

is suggested by the physician as a way to test for confabulation.

In general, a memory defect is considered to be of psychogenic origin if the individual has no disturbed level of consciousness and there is no intellectual impairment. If recovery of lost memory is abrupt, a psychogenic etiology is implied. Organically based memory disorders have the following associations. Bilateral lesions of the hippocampus or mamillary bodies produce profound deficits, particularly in short-term memory. Long-term memory is usually unaffected by organic conditions unless accompanied by psychosis. If organic memory loss occurs, recovery is typically gradual and is regained from the extremes to the precipitating event (see Fig. 8-6).

INTELLIGENCE

The concept of intelligence is defined as the aggregate or global capacity of the individual to act purposely, to think rationally, and to deal effectively with his environment.

Intelligence is usually subdivided into two types: verbal and performance. These can be related to CNS lateralization of higher mental or cognitive processes in the brain with verbal abilities under greater executive control of the left hemisphere and nonverbal visual–spatial skills associated more predominantly with right-hemisphere functioning for most people, regardless of hand dominance.

A central issue in the discussion of intelligence involves the *nature–nurture* controversy: whether intelligence is determined by heredity or environment. Evidence in favor of the nature position includes twin studies, which have consistently shown a concordance rate between monozygotic twins that is higher than the rate for dyzogotic twins, which, in turn, is higher than that of natural siblings. Also, an adopted child's IQ correlates higher with that of biological parents than with the IQ of adoptive parents.

For the nurture position, there is favorable evidence as well. Social, cultural, and interpersonal

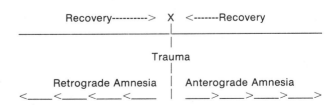

Fig. 8-6. Diagram of traumatic memory loss and its characteristic pattern of recovery.

deprivation are correlated with low IQ scores. Rural, isolated, and mistreated children have lower IQ scores than matched urban, stimulated, and well-treated peers; minority children taught in inferior school systems who are moved to enriched schools have positive correlations between IQ scores and length of time in the enriched school system.

The ***intelligence quotient (IQ)*** is a mathematical expression of the relation between mental ability and age. IQ will be discussed in detail below under psychological assessment; however, dependent upon the particular IQ test administered, an average IQ is 100 with 10 to 15 points of variation on either side.

The distribution of intelligence is assumed to follow a normal, or "bell-shaped," curve; however, due to early trauma, infections, or poor maternal prenatal health care, there is a higher than expected number of persons with lower intelligence in the population. Generally intelligence scores are grossly classified as below normal, normal, and above normal.

In the below-normal range are those persons diagnosed as having primary ***mental retardation.*** Primary mental retardation is a syndrome defined by low intelligence, poor social adaptation, and developmental problems. This definition excludes those persons whose intellectual ability is compromised by acquired brain dysfunction and related disorders. These are classified as having secondary mental retardation. The IQ distribution and functional classification according to the Diagnostic and Statistical Manual of Mental Disorders III-R (American Psychiatric Association, 1987) is as follows:

IQ = below 20 or 25: ***profound*** mental retardation
IQ = 20–25 to 35–40: ***severe*** mental retardation
IQ = 35–40 to 50–55: ***moderate*** mental retardation
IQ = 50–55 to approximately 70: ***mild*** mental retardation
IQ = 70 to 89: ***borderline*** mental retardation

Another classification that is sometimes more useful is based on prognosis in self care (Pardes, 1985). This divides retarded individuals into the following classifications:

IQ = below 30: ***custodial*** (These persons cannot distinguish between safety and danger and, therefore, must live in a protected custodial environment.)
IQ = 30–50: ***trainable*** (Persons classified here can distinguish safety from danger; however, they cannot learn the essentials of symbolic communication, that is, reading, writing, and arithmetic.)

IQ = 50–70: ***educable*** (These individuals can learn the basics of symbolic communication but encounter difficulty in abstract thinking and complex judgment.)

The IQ range of 70 to 90 does not have a specific "label"; however, these persons usually can be self-supporting financially and can care for their own personal needs. They can do minimal abstracting and can complete the basics of education.

Normal intelligence, then, is bordered by IQ scores of 90 and 109. The majority of persons fall within this range of IQ scores.

The person of above-average intelligence has an IQ score greater than 109. The classification according to Wechsler is as follows:

IQ = 110–119: ***bright*** normal
IQ = 120–129: ***superior***
IQ = 130 and above: ***very superior***

In addition to intelligence, there are persons with unique abilities. On the low-IQ end of this continuum, some persons have IQs in the range of "retarded," but show some dramatic, singular talent. These individuals are called ***idiot savants.*** Some have spectacular achievement in arithmetic calculation, playing musical instruments, and calendar calculation for the remote past and distant future. On the high end of the continuum are persons with IQs in the range of ***genius*** but who have some singular, outstanding deficit. For example, Albert Einstein, for all practical purposes, had an IQ that was so high as to be untestable. However, at age 15 his grades in history, geography, and language were poor and he left school with no diploma.

These aspects of the "mind" constitute what can be conceptualized as the phenomenology of mental process. The focus has been on delineating mental activity, which is the basis of an individual's interaction with the external environment. These parameters are conceptualized as biological "givens," which must function in a "normal" manner for the individual to be maximally adaptive in the world.

Frequently the physician must determine if a given individual's "mind" is functioning correctly. To do this in a valid manner, the physician must use a standard procedure that reflects the important dimensions of mental processes. This procedure is called the ***mental status examination.***

DETERMINANTS OF BEHAVIOR

The preceding section addressed the mental process of behavior. This section summarizes how behavior is influenced, beginning with genetic events and proceeding through biochemical influences, psychophysiologic parameters, learning, growth and development, sociocultural considerations, and psychosocial issues in current American society.

Genetic Influence on Human Behavior

Genetic factors are responsible for unique human conditions. Basic genetic concepts are as follows:

Genes: The elemental unit of heredity composed of biochemical substance called deoxyribonucleic acid (DNA) provides hereditary information and controls.

Chromosomes: The 23 pairs of "strands of genes" are present in virtually all cells of the body. The exception are sex cells, which are unpaired and have only 22 chromosomes.

Genotype: the genetic makeup of the person

Phenotype: the expression of the genotype; unless special conditions are present, the genotype may not be observable or manifested as a phenotype.

X chromosome: "female" chromosome (XX); can be provided by either the male or the female

Y chromosome: "male" chromosome (XY); can only be provided by the male

Karyotype: the chromosome composition of the somatic or body cells

Mutations: alterations in the chemical composition of genes so new cells produce substances different from those produced by the cells that preceded the mutation; some are "spontaneous" (*i.e.,* unknown etiology), which are rare, and some are due to exposure to x-rays, chemical actions, and so forth

Centromere: the pale-staining primary constriction on each chromosome which divides the chromosome into two arm lengths

Sex chromatin, or *Barr body:* a chromatin mass present in the somatic nuclei of normal females during interphase; Normal males have no Barr bodies; thought to be inactivated by X chromosomes; number of Barr bodies is always fewer than the number of X chromosomes.

Autosome: the 22 homologous pairs of nonsex chromosomes formed at the union of the sperm and the egg; because each complement of chromosomes from each parent is a chance assortment of half of each parent's chromosomes, every human is a unique genetic entity; also leads to an equal or random distribution of an autosomal trait between sexes

Sex-linked: gene responsible for a trait is located on an X or Y sex chromosome; results in an unequal distribution of the given trait between the sexes

Homozygous: both corresponding genes of sperm–egg chromosome pair carry a given trait

Heterozygous: only one gene of sperm–egg chromosome pair carries a given trait

Dominant single-gene inheritance: when the genetic effect (*i.e.,* phenotypic expression) requires only one gene of a sperm–egg chromosome pair to carry a trait

CHROMOSOMAL DISORDERS

Those behavioral disorders that have been established to be genetic in etiology can be divided into three major subgroups: Sex chromosome disorders, inborn errors of metabolism, and translocation/nondisjunction errors.

Sex Chromosome Disorders. *Turner's syndrome* occurs in one per 3000 to 5000 girls and is characterized by underdeveloped external female genitalia, a small uterus, short stature, webbed neck, and usually a lack of ovaries. Often these girls show intellectual impairment but not usually severe mental retardation. The karyotype of these women shows 45 chromosomes with a sex chromosome constitution of XO, and there is no Barr body observed. Presumably this is due to nondisjunction of an X chromosome of one parent during gametogenesis.

Klinefelter's syndrome is an anomaly of males and is characterized by external male genitalia with small atrophic testes. These men are usually sterile, and they often have gynecomastia, sparse body hair, long legs, and an increased excretion of gonadotrophin. The syndrome occurs at a rate of one per 340 to 500 male births. Mental retardation is usually, but not invariably, present. The etiology is presumed to be nondisjunction of an X chromosome, leading to a karyotype of 47 chromosomes with an XXY sex chromosome constitution. There is a Barr body present, which is unusual for males.

XYY karyotype has led to a great deal of controversy because of a suggested link between this karyotype and criminality. These men—"supermales"—have been characterized as tall, displaying poor impulse control, and having disrupted interpersonal contacts and a greater than average sexual drive. If they have criminal histories, the criminality tends toward crimes of violence. The *XYY* karyotype has been demonstrated to have a higher prevalence rate in incarcerated men. Further research, however, has also demonstrated a high frequency of the karyotype among nonincarcerated males.

XXY karyotypes are females—"superfemales"—who are sexually infantile, sterile, and amenorrheic. These women have two Barr bodies.

Inborn Errors of Metabolism.
Phenylketonuria (PKU) results from insufficient amounts or absence of the enzyme phenylalanine hydroxylase, which oxidizes phenylalanine to tyrosine. As a consequence, phenylalanine is metabolized by alternate pathways, and either the excessive unmetabolized phenylalanine or the alternative metabolites alter brain metabolism. The disease can be diagnosed in the infant by detection of phenylpyruvic acid in the urine. Through dietary control (*i.e.*, low phenylalanine content), mental retardation can be prevented. Most states in the United States require urine testing of newborns for PKU. The incidence of the disease is about 1 per 16,000 births. If untreated, mental retardation appears at about six months. The ultimate result is severe retardation. This has an autosomal recessive transmission, and persons who are carriers have no clinical manifestations. However, carriers can be detected by their inability to rapidly metabolize test loads of phenylalanine.

Tay-Sachs disease is a disorder caused by a specific enzymatic deficiency. It has an autosomal recessive transmission, most prevalent in—but not confined to—Ashkenazi Jews. The disease is characterized by progressive mental deterioration, loss of visual function, cerebromacular degeneration, and accumulation of lipid substances throughout the CNS. The usual onset is from 4 to 8 months of age, with death by 3 years. The infants become hypotonic, display slow developmental progression, and are weak and apathetic. They become spastic with primitive postural reflexes, frequently have convulsions, and display progressive mental and physical deterioration. A cherry-red spot in the macula lutea of each retina can be discerned upon examination.

Translocation/Nondisjunction Errors.
Down syndrome (*i.e.*, "mongolism") is characterized by a prominence of the median folds of the eyelids, short stature, stubby hands and feet, and peculiarity of palm prints. Other congenital malformations, (*e.g.*, cardiovascular) may be present. Mental retardation is present. This condition represents the single most definable clinical entity causing severe mental retardation. There are two causes of Down syndrome, which are phenotypically identical. The first type,

trisomy 21, has chromosome 21 represented three times instead of two. This produces a karyotype with 47 chromosomes. Apparently this is due to nondisjunction of chromosome 21. The second type apparently is due to translocation of chromosomes 21 and 15. There are 46 chromosomes: the 21s are normal, one of the 15s is normal, and there is one large, unpaired chromosome that is interpreted as a fusion of 15 and 21. While it is not known *why* these alterations occur, it is known that they have a higher prevalence in offspring of older mothers, and there is some relationship to the mother's having been exposed recently to x-rays.

The Inheritability of Emotional Disorders.
Schizophrenia, as with intelligence, has a concordance rate among family members that varies with the degree of genetic similarity. Franz Kallman's early work (1953) demonstrated that monozygotic twins raised together have a concordance rate of 86%, and monozygotics raised apart have a somewhat lower concordance rate; however, monozygotics reared apart have a higher rate than fraternals reared together, which is 15%. Other studies suggest concordance figures for monozygotics that range from 50% to 88%. Children of schizophrenic mothers who were raised away from the mother since day three were studied and found to experience significantly more difficulty on a number of relevant variables than did the controls (*e.g.*, total years incarcerated in mental institutions was 112 for children of schizophrenics versus 15 for children of nonschizophrenics). The degree of familial relationship to a schizophrenic yields an expectancy rate for becoming schizophrenic as follow: general population, 0.85%; half sibs, 7% to 8%; full sibs, 5% to 15%; parents, 5% to 10%; children of one index case, 8% to 16%; and children of two index cases, 53% to 68%.

Bipolar disorder (*i.e.*, manic–depressive illness) appears to be the major affective disorder that has a hereditary component. Some authors have suggested a 100% concordance rate in monozygotic twins and postulate evidence for an X-linked, dominant mode of transmission. Reported expectancy rates are as follows: half sibs, 16.7%; parents of an index case, 23.4%; siblings, 22.7%; fraternal twins, 25.5%; and monozygotic twins, 100%.

Other behavioral complexes for which there has been support for a genetic base include various neurotic and personality disorder symptom complexes as well as identifiable nonpsychiatric behavioral patterns, *e.g.*, dysthymia, obsessive–compulsive disorder, some forms of homosexuality, criminality (discussed under XYY genotypes), antisocial personality disorder, and alcoholism and other forms of substance abuse (*e.g.,* narcotic and nicotine addiction).

In some of these, other factors appear to exert a stronger influence than the suggested genetic substrate.

Biochemical Determinants of Behavior (Neurotransmitters)

Neurotransmitters are biochemical substances that facilitate transmission of information from one neuron across the synapse to the next neuron, or from neuron to muscle fibers at the myoneural junction. Over 100 such substances have been identified to date. They are released from the presynaptic neuron into the synaptic cleft, where they attach to highly specific receptors at the postsynaptic site. They may be eliminated from the body through metabolism or reabsorbed by the presynaptic neuron. Their duration of action is very short. Different types of neurotransmitters are found in different areas of the nervous system. Recent studies suggest that some neurons may contain more than one transmitter substance.

There are four general neurotransmitter systems that today appear to be the most important in the understanding of human behavior: *monoamines,* which are the catecholamines, dopamine (DA), norepinephrine (NE), and epinephrine (E), and the indolamine, serotonin (5-HT); *acetylcholine* (ACh); *amino acids* (*i.e.,* gamma-aminobutyric acid or GABA); and *peptides* (*i.e.,* endorphans, cholecystokinin, and neurotensin).

MONOAMINES

The *catecholamines* are formed by the breakdown of phenylalanine to tyrosine, tyrosine to 3,4-Dihydroxyphenylalanine (DOPA), DOPA to dopamine, and dopamine to norepinephrine and then epinephrine.

In general, it appears that *dopamine* neurons selectively inhibit transmission of sensory information to enhance the signal-to-noise ratio. Dopamine has been most associated clinically with the psychiatric disorder, schizophrenia.

There is strong evidence that the *antipsychotic (neuroleptic) compounds* have antidopamineric effects, and that all antidopamineric agents possess antipsychotic activity. This led to the *dopamine hypothesis* of the schizophrenias.'' It has been established there are two DA receptors, D1 and D2. The role of D1 receptors is unclear. There has been

demonstrated an increase in the number of D2 receptors in the caudate, putamen, and nucleus accumbens of schizophrenic patients. The clinical effects of antipsychotic drugs are related to their relative ability to block the D2 receptors. Other neurotransmitter systems are certainly involved in the schizophrenias since these disorders are extremely complex behavioral expressions.

The other most important behavioral correlate of the DA systems is the appearance of *Parkinsonism* in persons who have deterioration in the nigrostriatal tract of the DA system. This may also be the system involved in *tardive dyskinesia,* a movement disorder secondary to relatively long-term maintenance on antipsychotic medications.

The *norepinephrine* (NE) cell bodies are found in the gigantocellular nucleus and, especially, in the *locus ceruleus,* but their highly branched axons project to all parts of the CNS. NE has been found to have inhibitory influences on some postsynaptic neurons and exciting effects on others. There are some reports for increased levels of NE in the schizophrenias.

There is very strong evidence that this catecholamine plays an important role in the mood disorders such as the depressive syndrome noted above. First, rauwolfia drugs, whose action reduces catecholamines, produce depression in some patients. Second, the mode of action of drugs that are most effective in the clinical management of depression all increase the available NE (and 5-HT; see below) at the receptor sites, probably by decreasing reabsorption. More recent evidence suggests that certain depressions may be associated with low NE synthesis and release, and others with low 5-HT. The *catecholamine hypothesis* of affective disorders suggests that depressions are associated with low levels of NE, and the manic syndrome is associated with excessive levels.

Other behavioral correlates of NE include anxiety, arousal, pain, and possibly components of the sleep cycle.

The role of *epinephrine* in stress is well recognized; however, little is known about epinephrine as a central neurotransmitter except in the locus ceruleus, where it inhibits firing of the neurons.

The neurotransmitter *serotonin* (5-HT), an *indolamine,* is synthesized from tryptophan. The majority of neurons that produce this substance are in the *raphe nuclei.* Its role in complex human behaviors is still poorly understood; however, 5-HT does play a role in pain, aggression, cardiovascular components, and respiration.

The suspected role of 5-HT in affective disorders has been noted above, but the definition of that role is unclear. Recent data implicate 5-HT in obsessive compulsive behavior. 5-HT's role in the major thought disorders is unclear.

ACETYLCHOLINE

Today the most important role of ACh is in its link to Alzheimer's disease and, therefore, to memory and cognition. Present research into this disorder demonstrates reductions in choline acetyltransferase activity and the inability of brain tissue from Alzheimer's patients to synthesize acetylcholine.

The other behavioral role of ACh is in movement. When there is an imbalance between CNS levels of DA and ACh, Parkinson-like movements appear.

AMINO ACIDS

GABA is probably the major inhibitory neurotransmitter in the CNS. Apparently, within the CNS its role is to modulate the activity of the other neurotransmitter systems.

A dysfunction in this modulation may be central to the psychiatric syndrome called *generalized anxiety disorder* and, especially, in other syndromes involving panic.

PEPTIDES

The opioid peptide neurotransmitters emanate from one of three precursors: the beta-endorphin/ACTH (adrenocorticotropic hormone) precursor, the enkephalin precursor, and the dynorphin/neo-endorphin precursor. The receptors of these neurotransmitter systems are distributed in the CNS close to the dopaminergic systems that have been implicated in the schizophrenias. All of these neurotransmitters seem to be important in the CNS systems that are responsive to stress.

Because of the location of peptide neurotransmitter systems in relation to dopaminergic systems, a great deal of research has been conducted relative to the role of peptides in the schizophrenias. Clinical studies provide no convincing support for an excess or deficiency of endorphin activity in schizophrenia. However, there may be an interactive effect between the peptide and dopamine systems. Because of the proximity of the two systems and the fact that neurotensin (NT) and cholecystokinin (CCK) coexist with dopamine in certain dopaminergic neurons, research in this important area is ongoing. Neuropeptides appear to coexist in all of the major neurotransmitter systems. In discussing peptides, increasingly a distinction is being made by

investigators between neurotransmitters and neuromodulators.

Current speculation regarding *narcotic addiction* and the endorphin system involves the hypothesis that a constant external supply of morphine substances suppresses the natural production of endorphins. Withdrawal, then, would be defined as an endorphin deficiency with an extended period of time to return to normal functioning level. This would, in part, account for the long-lasting depression and *protracted abstinence syndrome* common in narcotic withdrawal. A second hypothesis concerns congenital endorphin deficiency. Since congenital endorphin excess can be postulated from case studies of insensitivity to pain, such insensitivity being reversed by administration of a narcotic antagonist, it is logical the converse may occur. Such a finding would assist in understanding how some persons use narcotic substances without becoming addicted, and others report addiction-like "craving" behavior from first exposure.

Physiologic Determinants of Behavior

LIMBIC SYSTEM

The limbic system primarily is composed of the phylogenetically older cortex and associated structures: the *hippocampus, fornix, mammillary bodies, anterior thalamic nuclei, cingulate gyrus, septal nuclei* and *amygdala*. This system is arranged in circuits and influences behavioral expression regulated by the hypothalamus. Activities of the limbic system include modulation and coordination of the central processes of emotional elaboration, motivation, establishment of conditioned reflexes and memory storage. The major behavioral correlates of limbic system dysfunction are:

Bilateral lesions of the hippocampus produce profound deficits of short-term memory storage and retrieval.

Patients with irrepressible rage reactions demonstrate spiking on EEG tracings originating from the amygdala.

The Kluver–Bucy syndrome of submissive behavior, hypersexuality, visual agnosia, and oral exploration of objects—first noted in vicious monkeys after removal of the temporal lobes, uncus, amygdala, hippocampus and the tail of the caudate—has been demonstrated in humans with lesions to the amygdala.

Electrical stimulation of the septal region produces intense pleasure responses and pain/seizure blockade.

Electrical discharges from the uncus (*i.e.,* uncinate fits) are correlated with olfactory hallucinations of foul odors, such as feces or burning rubber, anxiety–fear (*e.g.,* "empty feeling in the stomach"), jamais vu, or déjà vu.

RETICULAR ACTIVATING SYSTEM

The RAS and its thalamic projections is one of the phylogenetically oldest parts of the brain involved with determining behavior. As noted in the section on consciousness, the RAS is intimately involved in *arousal* and *attention.* Most sensory and motor impulses pass through the RAS as they enter and exit the brain. Functionally, the RAS can, through diffuse activation, "prime" the entire brain to process stimuli; facilitate or inhibit sensory or motor stimuli; "filter" incoming information; and facilitate the active process of sleep through inhibition of the midbrain reticular system.

Based on evidence that all antipsychotic preparations have their effect in the RAS and limbic system, some theorists have postulated RAS dysfunction in the schizophrenias. In this framework, schizophrenia would be seen as the behavioral expression of improper filtration of environmental stimuli. The resultant stimulus influx overwhelms the schizophrenic's cortical function, reflected in the schizophrenic's inability to cope appropriately with the world.

CORTICAL SITES

Cortical sites are in executive control of much of human behavior. The left cerebral hemisphere is responsible for verbal abilities—with the exception of a very few right-hemisphere-dominant persons. Prerolandic areas are correlated with the motor act of speech. Dysfunction here results in *motor* or *Broca's* or *expressive aphasia*—synonymous terms. Persons with such an aphasia usually are able to understand symbolic communication, but have difficulty expressing themselves freely in good grammatical form. Postrolandic areas (i.e., temporal and parietal) appear to be in executive control of the comprehension of symbolic communication. Lesions here produce *sensory* or *Wernicke's* or *receptive aphasia* (also synonymous).

Damage to the right cerebral hemisphere in postrolandic areas is correlated with *visual–spatial dysfunctions* (*e.g.,* inability to follow a blueprint or road map) and *construction dyspraxias,* the inability to motorically reproduce a visual stimulus. Sensorimotor abilities tend to be under control of the contralateral sensory/motor gyri of the cortex. Audi-

tion is primarily contralateral in executive control, although there is an 80% to 20% split of fibers from the cochlea to the temporal lobes, with the 20% represented on the ipsilateral temporal cortex.

Vision is somewhat more complex. *Visual fields* are divided into quadrants. The right half of each retina and, therefore, the left visual field, is represented on the right occipital cortex. Conversely, the left half of each retina (the right visual field) is represented on the left occipital cortex. Fibers from the upper quadrants sweep through the temporal lobes, and fibers from the lower quadrants course through the parietal region. When corresponding fields in each eye are defective, it is called a *homonymous hemianopsia* if both upper and lower quadrants are defective. A homonymous hemianopsia implies either occipital lobe dysfunction or temporal and parietal dysfunction in the brain hemisphere contralateral to the field defect. Bilateral upper and lower outer field cuts imply dysfunction at the optic chiasm, usually tumors of the pituitary gland. Single-eye impairment suggests dysfunction anterior to the optic chiasm.

Stereognosis is the ability to perceive spatial configuration of objects from tactile sense alone. This is characteristically under executive control of the contralateral postrolandic area. Dysfunction is called *astereognosis.*

SENSORY DEPRIVATION

Sensory deprivation is a physiologic condition presumably tied to activity of the RAS. Sensory deprivation in the laboratory is attained through constant control of visual, auditory, olfactory, kinesthetic, thermal, tactile, and gustatory stimuli. When environmental sensory stimuli are decreased or removed, the RAS apparently can no longer maintain a homeostatic balance between internal and external reality. In perceptual terms, all external frames of reference to interpret cues are absent. The major correlates of sensory deprivation are profound anxiety; depression or hostility (*i.e.,* irritability); auditory, visual, and tactile hallucinations; depressed level of consciousness and alertness; and extreme stimulus hunger. The basic similarity between monotonous night driving, isolation for "brainwashing" or suggestability effects, and sensory deprivation is apparent.

SLEEP

Sleep behavior is an active physiologic process. Apparently, structures in the lower pons and medulla are responsible for initiating and/or maintaining sleep through synchronization of cerebral cortical rhythms. Presumably these mechanisms act through inhibition of the midbrain reticular system. Sleep is divided into stages reflected by electroencephalogram (EEG) activity.

Stage 1: The EEG is characterized by low-voltage mixed frequency, but most predominant is theta activity (5 to 7 per second). This is the same wave form demonstrated by experienced meditators.

Stage 2: The EEG shows waxing and waning bursts of regular waves called sleep spindles. Sleep spindles are 12 to 14 per second and each spindle lasts 1 to 2 seconds. These are present against a background of low-voltage irregular rhythms.

Stage 3: High-voltage slow EEG activity is observed.

Stage 4: Continuous high-voltage slow EEG activity at about 1 per second is seen. *Night terrors* in children, *enuresis* and *sleepwalking* apparently all arise from stages 2, 3, and 4.

During *rapid eye movement (REM),* the background EEG is indistinguishable from Stage 1, except that bursts of REM are recorded. Accompaniments of REM sleep include vivid visual dreams, penile tumescence in males from infancy through old age and vaginal lubrication in females, disappearance of torso EMG, and the greatest variability in activity of the autonomic nervous system (ANS). *Nightmares* arise here. *Sedative–hypnotic medications* reduce REM, and withdrawal of these medications results in *REM rebound.* REM deprivation is correlated with subsequent neural hyperexcitability and decreased electroconvulsive seizure threshold. Nonvisual dreams, similar to thoughts running through the mind, occur in other sleep stages.

Apparently, REM sleep interrupts non-REM sleep an average of every 90 minutes, with the amount of REM sleep increasing during the total sleep period. Over a lifetime, progressively less REM, and less sleep overall, is obtained. During a single, normal sleep period, individuals proceed regularly through consecutive stages of sleep, with few or no fully awake episodes during the period. Also with increased age, the trend is toward lighter sleep patterns and, therefore, more awakenings are to be expected. CNS–depressant drugs like alcohol produce similar effects at any age.

Sleep deprivation results in errors of omission (as opposed to errors of commission). When prolonged for more than 72 to 96 hours, the effects can be profound, resulting in a delerium-like organic brain syndrome.

Disorders of sleep other than those noted above include *narcolepsy,* which is characterized by four symptoms. Sudden onset of REM sleep resulting in excessive daytime sleepiness, *cataplexy* (a sudden loss of muscle control and tone) precipitated by strong emotion or excitement, sleep paralysis, and hypnagogic hallucinations. There is evidence for a recessive genetic component in narcolepsy. *Sleep apnea* syndromes, or sleep-induced respiratory impairment, are another group of disorders, characterized by three types: those associated with REM and non-REM (type A), those associated with non-REM only (type B), and those associated with REM and the transitions from wakefulness to stage 1, and transition to REM (type C). *Drug dependency insomnia* results from habitual use of hypnotics and tranquilizers. *Nocturnal myoclonus* is another sleep disorder which sometimes occurs with the "restless leg syndrome." *Circadian rhythm disturbance,* or "jet-lag," is a dissonance between the internal body clock and external time zone. In phase–lag syndrome, the individual has difficulty falling asleep; in phase–lead syndrome, the patient falls asleep and awakens too early. *Pseudoinsomnia* is a condition in which the patient sleeps six or more hours but believes (perhaps dreams) he is not sleeping. However, most insomnias relate to anxiety or depression.

CIRCADIAN RHYTHMS

Circadian rhythms are cyclic physiologic activities of the body which may have significant influence on behavior. The different rhythms have regulators of two origins. The first are *endogenous regulators,* which arise from within the person. With total isolation from atmospheric and/or other relevant influences, these will continue in a more or less regular fashion. The second are *exogenous regulators,* which originate outside the person. The major exogenous regulators that have been studied are the 24-hour light–dark cycle, the disruption of which is responsible for jet-lag; chemicals like alcohol, amphetamines and other drugs that can produce a new pattern in the circadian rhythms; and stress, emotional or physical, that can disrupt the normative rhythm.

The major circadian rhythms are the sleep–wakefulness period of the 24-hour day, menstrual cycle in women, adrenal steroid secretion, liver enzymes for metabolism, REM–non-REM variations in sleep, body temperature, heart rate, blood pressure, and cell reproduction and sensitivity. The latter rhythm has clinical significance for conventional radiation therapy, in that radiation of some tumors may kill more cancerous cells in the morning than at other times.

Acquisition of Behavior (Learning)

Genetic, biochemical, and physiologic determinants of behavior address "inborn" or "natural" events over which the individual has little control. The following discusses behaviors that either are acquired or strongly influenced by learning.

Learning is defined as the relatively permanent change in a behavioral tendency that occurs as a result of reinforced practice. This definition involves a number of assumptions. First, "change" implies that one can learn to do or learn not to do. Second, "behavioral tendency" implies that learning is inferred from behavior. Third, practice accompanied by reinforcement is the "cause" of acquisition and maintenance of a change in behavioral tendency. The neurophysiology of learning is a very exciting field of research by neurobiologists of various disciplines.

REINFORCEMENT

Reinforcement has a central role in acquisition of most behavior. Reinforcement is a "payoff" and is commonly conceptualized as *positive* when the person is *given* something that strengthens the response tendency, like food or money, or *negative* when something is *withdrawn,* which strengthens the response tendency (*e.g.,* pain, nagging, or other discomfort is removed). *Punishment* is classified as *aversive* stimulation and is usually only effective in suppressing behavior for a short while, or teaching the person who is punished to stay away from the punishing individual.

Also of considerable significance is the *schedule of reinforcement.* The person may be placed on an absolute reinforcement schedule, either reinforced every time the behavior occurs (which results in the reinforcement losing its effectiveness) or never reinforced for the behavior (which results in *extinguishing* a given behavior). Periodically the extinguished behavior will reoccur, "just to see if maybe it will work this time." This is called *spontaneous recovery.* Or the person may be placed on a *partial reinforcement* schedule. Partial reinforcement schedules produce the most stable behavior patterns and behavior resistant to extinction. The major schedules can be diagrammed as follows:

	Fixed	Variable
Interval		
Ratio		

Fixed-interval means reinforcement is available only after a given, consistent period of time has elapsed. This produces "bursts" of behavior immediately prior to the time reinforcement is available (*e.g.,* "cramming" for scheduled exams). This yields the fewest responses per unit of time and the least consistent rate of response (4th place).

Variable-interval means reinforcement again is available after a period of time; however, the time period changes (*e.g.,* an instructor gives random "pop quizzes.") This improves response and consistency rates to 3rd place.

Fixed-ratio improves response and consistency rates to 2nd place. In this mode reward is available after a given constant amount of responding (*e.g.,* being reimbursed $5.00 per 100 stitches sewn).

Variable-ratio schedules produce the highest response and consistency rates. Again, reinforcement is available after the person produces a given number of responses; however, the response rate for "payoff" varies (*e.g.,* playing slot machines). This partial reinforcement schedule produces high rates of behavior because the person knows it's a variable-ratio reward system; therefore, the more responses, the sooner the reinforcement will appear—and maybe the ratio will be small "next time."

Two general types of reinforcement have been demonstrated. *Primary reinforcements* are those that address some type of primary need the organism has, such as food, sleep, or water. *Secondary reinforcements* are learned, such as money, a smile, verbal approval, or job promotion.

As a rule, the acquisition of behavior is maximal if practice is distributed over a series of trials rather than the same number of responses massed into fewer numbers of episodes.

TYPES OF LEARNING

Different types of learning are discussed below. These are ordered in terms of increasing complexity as well as chronological appearance:

Instincts. Instincts are defined as inborn predispositions to behave in a specific manner when appropriate stimulation is experienced. Today most writers refer to instincts as "primary drives" or "primary needs." While inborn and, therefore, not learned, their expression in humans is strongly modified by the milieu. Those instincts central to modern psychodynamic theories are sexuality, aggression, and dependence. Other writers include curiosity, mastery, nutrition, oxygen, and other vegetative functions. Whether called instincts, primary drives, or needs, they presumably originate from genetic, biochemical, or physiologic substrates; therefore, while they can be modified in expression (and actually, in some instances, suppressed for extended periods of time) they will recur given appropriate stimulation or through circadian fluctuation.

Imprinting. Imprinting was considered by **Konrad Lorenz** to be an innate mechanism which precipitated attachment to a significant parenting object, released by a set of stimuli at a critical time in neonates, and in which the role of reward was minimal. Lorenz adequately demonstrated the phenomenon in neonatal ducks and geese as they "imprinted" him as their "mother." Subsequent theoreticians have linked imprinting in lower animals to **bonding** or **attachment** in human infants. While the analogy is obvious, whether the mechanisms are truly similar have not been established.

Classical Conditioning. Classical conditioning is the form of learning popularized by **Pavlov,** which is described as **stimulus substitution.** An event that does not produce a given effect is presented immediately prior to an event that will reliably produce a given effect, that is, the first stimulus (event) has been substituted for the second. A clarifying example is a child who is only brought to the physician for immunizations. The child walks in the door, sees the doctor, is stuck with a needle, and begins to cry. With repetition, the child begins to cry when the doctor is first encountered. In classical conditioning terms the needle stick is the **unconditioned stimulus (UCS)** that produces the cry, or **unconditioned response (UCR).** The physician is the **conditioned stimulus (CS)** and the cry on seeing the physician is the **conditioned response (CR).** The conditioning is the new link between the physician and the cry. Sometimes not only the physician, but also the waiting room, the nurse, the word "doctor," the front door of the office, and all things associated with the needle stick begin to elicit the same conditioned response of crying. This is called **stimulus generalization** or **stimulus gradient** and is probably the factor responsible for the observation that

hypertensive patients produce more hypertensive readings in the physician's office than in their home environment (so-called "white coat" hypertension).

Classical conditioning has been demonstrated in all animal life forms from unicellular animals through humans, both before and after birth. Classical conditioning is associated with sympathetic and parasympathetic responses of the ANS and, therefore, is not ordinarily under much cognitive control. There is an optimal time interval of 0.5 seconds separation between the CS and the UCS for the stimulus substitution to occur. Also, the UCS must occur regularly for the behavior to remain stable. If it does not, then extinction occurs (*i.e.*, weakening, and eventual disappearance of the CR). If the child does not experience the prick of the needle each time the physician is seen, soon the child will no longer cry when the physician enters the room. Heart rate, galvanic skin response, insulin shock, and immune reactions are a few of the responses that have been classically conditioned to neutral stimuli like a word or picture.

Classical conditioning may be the basic process by which certain early fears and emotional responses are acquired. Many authors feel the foundations of so-called **psychosomatic illnesses** are laid down in the infant through this process. There is some evidence that the **placebo reaction** alleviating pain may be a classically conditioned endorphin response.

Operant Conditioning. Operant, or instrumental, conditioning if frequently linked to the work of **B. F. Skinner.** It is the production of a given response through environmental reinforcement. For instance, the child stops crying and the physician gives the child a piece of candy, or the medical student diligently studies and receives an "F." Later the same student doesn't study and receives an "A." The student learns to **discriminate** which response the environment will differentially reinforce and thereafter does not study.

Operant conditioning is the general case of learning, and it affects all behavior including activity of the ANS. **Biofeedback** is a direct outgrowth of operant conditioning. In biofeedback, a person receives positive secondary reinforcement (*e.g.*, a light or buzzer is activated for increasing periods of time, or a smile or approval from the experimenter) for controlling a body function, be the function under ANS control or not. The body function that is trained to appear is one that is incompatible with distress. For example, tension headache sufferers are trained to decrease frontalis muscle EMG. Biofeedback has been applied experimentally to a wide variety of medical problems including migraine and tension headaches, hypertension, and peripheral circulatory disorders. The technique, however, is still controversial as a therapeutic modality.

In direct opposition to classical conditioning, where the UCS (*i.e.,* the reinforcement) must always be present to insure stable response patterns, in operant conditioning the reinforcement is present 100% of the time *only* during the response acquisition phase. After acquisition, a schedule of partial reinforcement (explained above) is instituted to maintain a stable response pattern. For example, parents who want to guarantee that children are disruptive should inconsistently provide either approval of the behavior or disapproval. Such partial reinforcement produces behaviors that are resistant to extinction.

A variant of operant conditioning is **shaping.** In this procedure, successive approximations of a complete behavior are developed through 100% reinforcement, and then a more complex form is developed and stabilized. For example, an elective mute child first would have *sounds* developed through 100% reinforcement and stabilized by partial reinforcement—then syllables, then words, then phrases, then sentences, and so forth. Shaping can also be used to decrease unwanted behaviors like toewalking: the child first is reinforced for partial toewalking, then for partial sole walking, and then for flat foot walking.

Cognitive Learning. Cognitive learning, as opposed to conditioning, emphasizes the role of understanding. It assumes the individual is fully aware and attention is focused. (Data acquired by classical and operant conditioning may be employed to acquire material through this process.)

Piaget and associates have contributed significantly to our understanding of cognitive learning. Piaget emphasized that the cognitive apparatus to understand the world changes dramatically as a person matures. The child is not a miniature adult. Rather, the child at different ages and stages has different capacities to comprehend. The child is moved into more mature ways of understanding through the equilibration process, which has two components. First, **assimilation** means that the child, through active interchange with the environment, incorporates data from the external world. The child assimilates data until the extant mental structure can't manage the mass of assimilated data. At this point, **accommodation** takes place and the mental apparatus changes to the next more complex structure of cognitive processing and understanding. With this new structure the child assimilates more data until forced to accommodate the mass of assimilated data to an even more complex cognitive structure.

In addition to the equilibration process, Piaget posited that physical maturation, active experience with environment, and social transmission of information were the essential elements for changing cognitive structure. Deprivation of any or all of these was believed to result in less than maximal cognitive functioning.

Piaget posited four stages of cognitive development:

Sensorimotor stage. During this stage, from birth to roughly 18 months, the infant employs senses and motor activity to interact with the environment. The focus is coordination of senses and movement. Pure sensations are relied upon; therefore, the infant operates on the principle, "out of sight out of mind," which explains why "peek-a-boo" can be a never-ending source of distraction and pleasure for the infant. During this stage, the infant moves beyond its body to interaction with the world. Continued practice produces more systematic and well-organized interaction. This sensorimotor period ends with the infant having an active interest in new behaviors and novel events. The infant has shifted from reflex activity to intentional means–ends action sequences, with independent motor systems purposely coordinated.

Preoperational stage. In this stage, roughly from 18 months to 7 years of age, the child relies specifically on perception and "intuition" in thought processes to comprehend the world. However, the conservation of identity of objects is not yet possible. For example, if one of two same-sized pieces of clay is elongated, it is reported to be "more" or "bigger" than the one that was not altered. The child at this stage can only focus cognitive processes on one dimension at a time.

Concrete operations stage. At this time, roughly from age 7 to 11–13 years, the child begins to abstract commonalities from tangible objects. When the child can see, touch, or gain images from objects, similarities between them can be extracted. This child can add and subtract elements to or from each other and yet conserve the essence of separate elements. Totally abstract discussions are not possible yet and "reversibility" in thought processes is difficult.

Formal operations stage. This last stage, beginning

at about 11 to 13 years of age, is characterized by the ability to indulge in abstract, conceptual thinking where tangible objects are not necessary for the conceptualization to occur. This individual can think in terms of relations and reversibility. Reflective conceptual cognitive reasoning and understanding is a reliable process at this stage.

Social Learning. Social learning theories focus on reciprocal *interpersonal relations* and those behaviors acquired as a result of *modeling.* The learner observes another person perform an act and models behavior after the observed person. The observer learns without the reinforcement necessary for conditioning-type learning. Indeed, vicarious reinforcement and vicarious extinction have been observed in children. If a child sees another rewarded for a behavior, the observing child will produce the same behavior—and vice versa with vicarious extinction. It is assumed that the intergrated, conforming, social behavior which children acquire is based on observation either of peers being reinforced for producing a behavior or through imitation of parental behavior. Some of the most current controversial issues in social learning are those that involve the influence of media on children's behaviors (specifically sexuality, aggression, and violence observed on television) and peer influence in substance abuse.

While reinforcement—especially primary reinforcement—does not play a truly central role in social learning theories, it is important. Models may provide behavioral roles for others to follow; however, if primary or secondary reinforcement of the newly acquired behavior does not occur, it will soon extinguish.

Growth and Development

In addition to biochemical, physiologic, genetic, and learned influences on behavior, there is impact from the natural unfolding growth and development process. This process will be presented in two parts: the theories and the phenomenal observations.

THEORIES

Psychoanalytic. *Psychoanalytic theory,* associated most with Sigmund Freud and his cohorts, focuses on the *intrapsychic* aspects of the mind. Central to early psychoanalytic theory was the concept of *libido,* defined as "psychic" energy (*i.e.,* motiva-

tion) and presumed to emanate from tissue metabolism. During "psychosexual" development, this psychic energy, or libido, is invested (concentrated or "collected") in different somatic areas at different stages of maturation. There are five stages:

1. *The oral sensory stage:* Approximately from birth to 18 months, the child's major source of interest and gratification is the mouth, which serves as the major focus for exploration of the environment. "Oral receptivity" (*i.e.,* sucking) is characteristic of the early portion and "oral aggression" (*i.e.,* biting) is characteristic of the latter portion of this stage. The central psychological "personality" issues involve trusting others, the relative safety of the world, and dependency needs. "Separation anxiety" often has its roots in this period.

2. *The anal musculoskeletal stage:* Approximately from 18 months to 3 years of age, the anus and the musculoskeletal system are the major repository of libidinal energy and the primary source of gratification or pleasure. Personality issues of control (including excretory functions), mastery, attitudes about authority's rules, savings (holding on), and spending (letting go) are considered to emanate from this stage. The emotions of disgust and anger, from and toward others, have considerable influence in this period.

3. *The phallic/urethral stage:* From about 3 years to 6–7 years of age, libidinal energy is primarily invested in the sexual organs and sensual experience. Activity is concentrated in extension to others and awareness of sex differences. It is at this stage that the Oedipal/Electra complex develops and is, one hopes, resolved.

    Oedipal/Electra complex is a normal phase through which all persons pass. It encompasses the child's developing a "love" attachment to the parent of the opposite sex and a conflicting desire to "get rid of," as well as maintain a relationship with, the parent of the same sex so the son–mother or daughter–father love can be consummated. Characteristic of this phase is the child's saying to the loved parent, "I want to marry you when I grow up." Successful resolution of this conflict is through the child realizing the same-sexed parent is more powerful; therefore, attempts to "get rid of" that parent may precipitate dire consequences including removal or envy of the penis and loss of love, that is, *castration anxi-*

ety. To resolve this, the child identifies with the same-sexed parent, gives up the opposite sexed parent as a primary love object, and says, ''When I grow up I want to be like my (daddy/mommy) and marry a (woman/man) like you.''

4. *The latency stage:* From approximately 7 to 12 years of age, libidinal energy is not concentrated in any specific body zone. It is characterized by same-sex peer relations and avoidance of opposite-sex interactions, although girls seem to be more interested in relations with boys than are boys to girls. Socialization, acquisition of social customs, and companionship are major issues.

5. *The genital stage:* From about 12 years of age to death, fully integrated, aware activities involve persons of the opposite sex and include romantic love. Fully established sexual identification, independence from parents, selecting a spouse, and vocational goals should be established during the early portions of this stage.

Throughout this maturational process, difficulty can be encountered through several mechanisms. First, *fixation* can occur at a particular stage of development, and little progress is made toward increasingly adaptive or mature levels of functioning. Second, normal progression through various stages occurs but during periods of stress, *regression* to an earlier stage of maturity can be observed. This is particularly true if a significant trauma occurred at an earlier stage producing a ''weakness'' or vulnerability. In this case, normal development may continue but later, under stress that is either literally or symbolically similar to the original trauma, the individual regresses to the stage at which the original trauma occurred. Because the content of the original trauma was *repressed* (*i.e.,* forgotten), the individual experiences the anxiety from the original threat without cognitive awareness of the frightening stimulus.

The concepts of conscious, preconscious, and unconscious as nonphysiologic referents stem from psychoanalytic theory. As noted above, *conscious* means material that is in present awareness of the person (*e.g.,* what is being read at this time), *preconscious* refers to material not presently in awareness (*e.g.,* one's phone number), and *unconscious* refers to material that is not in the person's awareness and cannot be brought into awareness without special techniques.

In addition to stages of development and levels of consciousness, Freud also posited the *pleasure principle,* meaning that people seek pleasure and avoid pain. The pleasure principle, modified by experience, is the *reality principle,* which allows for the delayed gratification of needs until an appropriate time.

Freud divided intrapsychic life—''mind''—or personality into three conceptual subdivisions: the ego, superego, and id. The *ego* is the portion that interfaces internal needs with the external reality. It has the most conscious awareness and operates predominantly by the reality principle. The functions that are characteristically assigned to the Ego are as follows:

Reality is the relationship to, testing, and sense of whether one is operating in the real world or in delusion.

Object relations refers to whether one can establish and maintain long-term close, interpersonal relations with at least one other person.

Autonomous functioning is the ability to care for oneself and meet the ordinary demands of living. This includes those ''conflict-free'' mental functions such as memory, mobility, and vocabulary.

Defense is protection of the ego from being overwhelmed by demands from the other sectors of the ''mind'' (A partial list of ego defense mechanisms is presented below.)

Synthesis is the ability to integrate data about the self and portions of behavior into a meaningful integrated whole (*e.g.,* ''I am a physician.'').

Identity usually refers to sexual identity (*i.e.,* maleness/femaleness) or, more broadly, to a sense of ''who am I?''

Thinking refers to those elements discussed above under the process of thought.

(A helpful mnemonic for ego functions is ''ROADSIT,'' comprised of the first letters of each word.)

The *id* is the repository of basically unconscious instinctual drives (*i.e.,* needs) and impulses. It operates on the pleasure principle and, therefore, constantly seeks immediate gratification of needs—which is unrealistic.

The *superego* is the ''conscience'' or value system that was acquired at a very young age from parents through introjection and identification. Because it is acquired at an early age, it is in pure form, usually irrational, punitive, and rigidly understood. Its function is control of instinctual needs (*i.e.,* id): ''Thou shalt not!''

The unconscious instincts of the id constantly seek gratification and are controlled by ego reality functioning and superego restrictiveness. In order for the ego to function in reality and not be overwhelmed by demands from the id, protective mental devices develop called ego defense mechanisms. These allow at least partial gratification of instinctual needs. All people have defense mechanisms, but some defense mechanisms are more healthy than others. The major ego defense mechanisms are as follows:

Repression is involuntary exclusion of material, particularly conflicted data, from conscious awareness. (Repression is considered to be the basic defense mechanism, operating in conjunction with one or more of the following.)

Suppression is the intentional exclusion of material from consciousness.

Introjection is the total assimilation of the values, attitudes, and prejudices from parents into one's own ego and, especially, the superego.

Identification, while similar to introjection, is less total or complete. It is modeling oneself after a significant other. It can also be the conforming to the values and attitudes of a group.

Displacement is employed when the object that will satisfy an instinctual need is changed. For example, a resident physician on the house staff may strike his spouse instead of the attending physician at whom the resident feels rage.

Projection is the attribution of one's own impulse and/or thoughts (particularly if they are unacceptable) to another person. This is the mechanism underlying scapegoating, the central core of prejudice.

Reaction formation is turning an impulse, feeling, or thought into its opposite (*e.g.,* persons who cannot accept their own sexual impulses may work as a censor of pornographic movies, thereby partially gratifying their sexual needs).

Sublimation is turning "unacceptable" impulses, thoughts, or feelings into socially acceptable ones (*e.g.,* an individual may have murderous rage as a characteristic feeling state, but become a butcher). Sublimation is one of the healthiest defense mechanisms because of constructive end products and elements of conscious decision-making involved.

Compensation is employed when one encounters failure or frustration in one activity or arena, and overemphasizes another (*e.g.,* an uncoordinated child may overstress intellectual pursuits).

Denial is the failure to recognize or be aware of obvious and logical consequences of a thought, act, or situation. (*e.g.,* the student who blatantly cheats on an exam while a proctor is observing the student). This is a rather primitive defense mechanism and is almost always pathologic in the adult.

Conversion is the somatic representation of conflicting impulses, feelings, or thoughts. The representation is in body functions under executive control of sensory nerves or the voluntary nervous system. The *primary gain* from a conversion reaction is neutralizing painful affect with the symptom symbol of the conflict; for instance, a student fearful of failing an exam may experience paralysis of the dominant hand. The student may gain a great deal of attention and sympathy from others—this is the *secondary gain.* This defense mechanism is always pathologic because it doesn't facilitate free function of the individual.

Somatization, in contrast to conversion, is the physical expression of conflicts through body parts under executive control of the ANS, both the sympathetic and parasympathetic branches (*e.g.,* peptic ulcer).

Regression is the return to an earlier level of maturation or personality development. As noted above, this usually occurs under periods of stress and can be expected to appear in certain specific situations. For example, at the birth of a sibling, an older sib may begin to behave below the achieved maturation level. Patients admitted to hospital characteristically become whining, demanding, and dependent. Elements of regression may be a normal, expected response to severe illness.

Dissociation is the responsible defense mechanism in "multiple personalities." A group of thoughts, feelings, and actions is split off from the main portion of consciousness, that is, they are compartmentalized. One personality is "good," the other is "bad." More commonly, amnesia, fugue states, or feelings of unreality become manifest.

Rationalization is offering a socially acceptable and more-or-less logical reason for an act usually produced by unconscious or nonverbalized impulses (*e.g.,* "I was drunk; therefore, I sexually approached my attending's spouse." The person misleads the self as well as others.

Since psychoanalytic theory emanated from observations of and attempts to intervene in pathology, some concepts unique to management of patients are important. *Transference* refers to a situation in which the patient begins to inappropriately project thoughts, feelings, and impulses onto the health care provider which are derived from unconscious internal states of the patient, often those he holds toward other significant persons (*e.g.,* mother). Presumably these are from unmet needs that the patient is experiencing. Somewhat similar to transference is the behavior complex called "acting out." Instead of dealing maturely with the transference the patient behaviorally expresses (*i.e.,* displaces) the impulses outside the treatment setting. In *countertransference,* the health care provider projects personal unmet needs, feelings, and impulses from unconscious processes onto the patient. "Acting out" by the professional may end in a malpractice suit or "divorce."

Psychosocial Model. The *psychosocial model* or theory also has psychoanalytic origins but emphasizes the person in interaction with the environment. *Eric Erikson* postulated eight stages in the psychosocial development of man. Each stage has a "task" for resolution before the next stage can be entered successfully. Defective resolution of a stage forms an inadequate foundation upon which subsequent stages are constructed. The stages and tasks follow:

1. *Trust versus mistrust* (from birth to age 18 months): To know and feel that the world is intrinsically safe and trustworthy, the developing infant must have basic needs met appropriately (*e.g.,* the hungry infant must be able to trust that when it cries, it will be fed). There must be continuity between the infant's action and the world's reaction.

2. *Autonomy versus shame and doubt* (from age 18 months to 3 years): In this stage, the young child must attain confidence in his ability to operate in the world somewhat autonomously of parents or significant others. He must not end this period doubting "he can stand on his own two feet" or ashamed of attempts to differentiate from significant others. Issues of self-control (including bodily functions) are primary at this stage, exemplified by toilet training and the automatic "no" of the "terrible twos." Usually this is not obstructionism or rebellion, but rather the child's way of saying, "I'm not you."

3. *Initiative versus guilt* (from age 4 to 6 years): At this stage, the child must achieve the ability to initiate independent activities in the world, and to effectively carry these activities to fruition without others overwhelming the plans through guilt induction. Disproportionate fear (*i.e.,* inadequate resolution of the Oedipal/ Electra complex) and superego anger can combine to form guilt as an inadequate resolution of this stage.

4. *Industry versus inferiority* (from age 6 to 13 years): Industry refers to the child's accomplishments of goals without parental support. The child attends school with peers who are relative equals in ability to produce. If the child does not successfully compete in interaction with these peers without the support of the parents, then a sense of inferiority develops that can color the remaining stages of development. This frequently produces in children the overwhelming impression of having nothing to offer others.

5. *Identity versus role confusion* (from age 13 to 18 years): During this phase, the young adult experiences extremely rapid physical/endocrine changes and simultaneously feels the impact of numerous new environmental influences. The major task is to develop fully a sense of personal identity, which includes the establishment of a solid sexual role. The adequate resolution must be, "I know myself, and I can make it as an adult." If, in the face of these extreme pressures, the young adult can't establish this sense, then adult role confusion develops.

6. *Intimacy versus isolation* (from age 18 to 25 years): With foregoing stages mastered, the adult has the task of developing an intimate, trusting, and committed relationship with at least one other person. If, by the end of this stage, an individual has not established that intimate relationship, a pervasive state of singular isolation is experienced in which a person feels he can neither share his life with nor gain support from others.

7. *Generativity versus stagnation* (from age 25 to 40 years): Generativity refers both to establishment of offspring and the guidance of those children's development, and entrance into an occupational arena where accomplishment and continued growth are feasible. Without developing children as personal extensions of the self or developing opportunities for occupational advancement, individuals find little meaning in life and become stagnant. By the end of this stage, an individual must take active responsibility for himself. That is, if at age 40 the person still attributes all responsibility for present conditions to parents and early childhood experiences, serious difficulty in adaptation usually occurs.

8. *Integrity versus despair* (age 40+): During this time, a person develops emotional integration, examines his life and begins to evaluate per-

sonal status. Hopefully the individual looks at the past, present, and future and perceives a continuity of which that person is proud. That is, the individual looks at his past life and says, "Given the various influences that were ongoing, I lived my life well and I'm happy with it." If this examination results in unrectifiable disapproval, despair is the consequence.

In summation, these theories—psychoanalytic and psychosocial—and the concepts that Piaget developed should not be regarded as adversarial. Instead they are different, but complementary, dimensions of human development. Freudian theory focuses on psychodynamic and psychosexual internal processes, Erikson examines interpersonal or psychosocial issues, and Piaget attends to development of cognition. There are other theories, but these are the most commonly encountered.

THE LIFE CYCLE OF GROWTH AND DEVELOPMENT

Pregnancy and Birth. From conception to birth, a number of variables have an impact on the fetus. High maternal emotional levels have been reported to result in high levels of ACTH, NE, and epinephrine substances in the fetal bloodstream, and concomitant irritability of the fetus has been observed. Maternal attitudes toward the pregnancy and the number of siblings predict postpartum childrearing practices (*e.g.,* Warm–Cold and Permissive–Restrictive).

An area of recent concern is maternal psychoactive drug use during pregnancy. A *general withdrawal syndrome* in neonates born to mothers who consistently use psychoactive drugs during pregnancy has been documented and a rating scale of severity established. This syndrome can be fatal to neonates if not appropriately managed, with fatality apparently due to pervasive CNS and behavioral hyperactivity resulting in dehydration and consequent febrile seizure activity. Long-term effects of neonatal addiction and the general withdrawal syndrome have not been fully established. *Fetal alcohol effects* have resurfaced as a primary concern. These effects have been associated with maternal alcohol consumption during pregnancy. In severe cases, the syndrome can include microcephaly, mental retardation, various system abnormalities, and stigmata suggestive of Down syndrome. Low birth weights are common. In mild cases, only behavioral hyperactivity may be seen. No exclusive causal relationship between alcohol, or its metabolites alone, and the described syndrome has been

definitely established in humans, suggesting interaction between alcohol and other idiosyncratic factors. There appears to be a dose-dependent relationship.

The utilization of CNS-depressant medications and anesthesias to assist the birth process is being scrutinized. The most common include inhalation anesthetics, barbituates, meperidine, "major tranquilizers," and local anesthetics. Most of these drugs may affect maternal physiology and labor, changing the intrauterine environment, the newborn directly by altering activation of functions that have been dormant, or the neonate's behavior by altering EEG activity level and its behavioral correlates.

Due to these medication issues and suggested "dehumanization" of hospital births, natural or *prepared childbirth* is being reexamined. *Lamaze* and Dick–Reed have been major proponents of unmedicated labor and birth, with the father present and providing support for the delivering mother.

At birth, neonatal function can be assessed by using the *Apgar* rating system. Assessment is done at one minute and five minutes using five indicators: heart rate, respiratory effort, muscle tone, reflex irritability, and color tone. Each indicator is rated on a three-point scale: 0 = no function; 1 = function present, but poor; 2 = function perfect. The five-minute score, in combination with birth weight, has the best predictability. The following correlates have been suggested: 0 to 3 = likely death; 4 to 6 = serious subsequent problems; 7 to 9 = later attentional defects and possible learning disability; 10 = perfect functioning.

Infancy. The major abilities with which neonates can interact with the world are *reflexes*. The main primitive reflexes are as follows:

Babinski: When scratched on the lateral aspect of the sole of the foot, heel to toes, the infant responds with dorsiflexion of the big toe and fanning of the others. This response continues from birth to between 12 to 18 months of age, when it disappears in normal children.

Moro: Any sudden movement of the infant's head and neck stimulates a rapid abduction, extension and supination of the arms with opening of the hands. The fingers of the hands adopt a distinctive "C" formation of the thumb and index finger and other digits of the hand are extended. In normal infants, the reflex persists until 4 to 6 months of age. The reflex is absent in newborns with diffuse CNS depression and other brain stem disorders. Its persistence beyond 4 to 6 months of age has been associated with mental retardation and brain damage.

Eye blink: Tactile stimulation of eyelashes, tapping the bridge of the nose, a bright light, or a loud noise provokes the blink response.

Grasp: Palmar pressure causes a grasp response in infants from one month to 5 to 6 months of age. A similar response of plantar flexion can be elicited up to between 9 to 12 months of age by pressing an object on the sole of the foot behind the toes.

Crossed extensor: If the leg of a supine infant is extended by pressure exerted on the knee and the sole of the extended foot stimulated with a sharp object, the result is extension and slight abduction of the unstimulated limb. This reflex normally disappears by 2 months of age.

Deep tendon reflexes: The response of striated muscles to sudden stretching is termed a deep tendon reflex. Those characteristically tested in infants are: jaw jerk (C5), biceps (C5-6), radical periosteal (C5-6), triceps (C6-8), knee (L2-4), and ankle (S1-2).

Suck: Stimulation of the perioral and oral area results in orientation to the stimulus and sucking behavior if the stimulus is encountered.

Normative motor control in the infant is always individually different and no developing infant is "normal" at all milestones of development. The following are presented as general guides (at ages in months):

1 month:	Can lift head briefly
2 months:	Can raise chest for brief periods
3 months:	Makes stepping motions, can lift the head and hold it above the body plane, and can retain a hold on objects
4 months:	Can sit on a lap, look around, and display some lumbar back curvature; the hands can be grasped together, played with, and unilateral open-handed approach to objects can be observed
5 months:	Can sit alone briefly and grasp objects in a one-hand directional motion
6 months:	Can do knee push or swimmer movements and can get up on hands
7 months:	Can roll over unassisted
8 months:	Can stand with help
9 months:	Can sit alone unassisted and make some progress on the stomach
10 months:	Can scoot backwards and is able to crawl
11 months:	Can stand holding on to furniture; can grasp an object in each hand and bring them together, and can use the thumb

and opposing forefinger to pick up small objects

12 months:	At the end of the first year can pull to a stand, walk when led, take and release small objects, and place them in containers
15 months:	Can stand and walk alone
18 months:	Can walk forward and backward, throw a ball, feed self and use a cup
24 months:	Can hold a pencil and draw with it

Social behavior development in the infant is characterized by appearance of selected behaviors. Appropriate *social smiling* appears at about two months. *Stranger anxiety* (*i.e.*, fear response to "nonmother" persons) normally appears between 6 to 12 months of age. (This indicates the capability of Piagetian object constancy has developed). During infancy, play activity is singular and concentrated in sensorimotor exercise. This moves the infant from reflexive–respondent behavior into controlled–purposive, externally directed activity.

Verbalizations by the end of the first two years have reached an average frequency of 200 words. The acquisition of language is from early reflexive laughing and crying to self-motivated babbling, which appears at about 6 to 8 months of age. Words as meaningful symbols first appear at about the age of 12 months; however, a range of between 1 to 3 years is normal.

Toilet training is not feasible until sphincter control has developed at between 1.5 and 2.5 years of age. This is contrary to data that many American parents "toilet train" their children between 9 and 14 months. If a child is toilet trained prior to 18 months of age, it is the "mothering person" who has been trained to observe when elimination is imminent and, consequently, rushes the child to the "potty." In the latter stages of infancy, the *terrible twos* appear, in which the child responds with "No!" to any request. This behavior is the reflection of the infant's initial attempts to establish autonomy and reflects entrance into Erikson's second stage.

During the latter stages of infancy and extending into the first preschool year, the *gender identity* is established. Dependent upon how parents and significant others interact with the child, he or she establishes the basic feeling of being male or female. This feeling is learned and set by the age of 3 years. It is the private experience of the child's sexuality.

Major problem areas for infants include maternal deprivation, which may precipitate the infant's withdrawal from all social interaction. If no mothering substitute is provided, the infant can enter an extremely withdrawn condition known as **anaclitic depression,** proceed to **marasmus,** and even die. Institutionally raised children display milder, but similar, withdrawn characteristics. Although they may not die, their ability to form close interpersonal relations in later life is seriously compromised. They are unresponsive and demonstrate retardation in cognitive, language, and motor development. In addition to maternal deprivation, highly nervous mothers have a higher prevalence of infants who demonstrate behavioral dysfunctions, such as sleep disorders, irritability, hyperactivity, and feeding disorders, and also prematurity.

Preschool. During the **preschool age** (2 to 5 years) psychomotor maturation involves development of gross and fine motor skills, and handedness is typically established.

Parental childrearing attributes seem to be most influential here. The Warm–Cold and Restrictive–Permissive dimensions in parental childrearing practices are correlated with characteristic behavior patterns in children. This relationship is characterized by Fig. 8-7.

Play activities progress from individual play to **parallel play,** in which two children are in physical proximity; however, each is playing alone with his own toys and games. The only reliable interaction is one child taking a toy from the other, precipitating a relatively violent interchange.

During preschool years, the child is extremely **egocentric;** all understanding of events in the external world are referred to the self for causal relations (*e.g.,* "The sun came up because it's time for me to get up.") Serious problems often arise from this egocentricity. If parents argue or divorce during this stage, the child may assume personal responsi-

bility for that event (*e.g.,* "My daddy left because he doesn't like me.")

In these five five years, language has fully developed and that progression is presented here as a cohesive whole process. The structure of language is roughly divided into **phonemes, morphemes, syntax,** and **semantics.** A phoneme is the smallest possible unit of language identifiable as a discrete sound. For example, in the word "pot," the "p" (written p) is a phoneme; the "k" sound of both words "cow" and "keep" is the same phoneme (K) even though the two words are spelled differently. A morpheme is comprised of several phonemes and is the smallest linguistic unit that can have independent meaning. The word "apples" has two morphemes: (1) "apple," and (2) the "s" that makes it plural. Syntax is defined as the rules by which people speak and understand a language. Syntax or grammar rules specify how morphemes are connected to produce meaningful units like phrases and sentences. Semantics is the inherent meaning, frequently involving emotional attachment, that is assigned to a particular piece of syntax. It is in this portion of language that major communication difficulty arises between persons, particularly if they are from different backgrounds. For example, the meaning of the word "white" is different depending upon one's skin color (*e.g.,* black, red, white, or yellow), occupation (artist versus bleach manufacturer) and so forth.

Acquisition of language is interpersonal and represents an interplay between developmental process and the milieu within which a child is raised. Developmentally, prior to age six months, infants produce random sounds that are used in every known language. These sounds are identical, regardless of the infant's nationality, and are probably

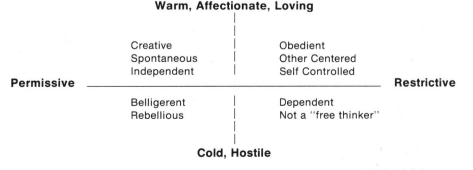

Fig. 8-7. Parental childrearing dimensions and correlated child behavior.

due to neuromuscular development of the throat and mouth. During the sixth to twelfth month, when self-motivated babbling appears, apparently selective reinforcement by significant others shapes the infant's babbling into characteristic national language. The first words to appear are nouns, next are verbs, third are adjectives, and finally pronouns. Between 1 and 2 years of age, the phrases and sentences are simple and may be only one word (*e.g.,* "water"). Between 18 months and 2 years of age, the utterances become longer, with brief phrases and rudimentary sentences being assembled. By age 5, adult syntax (including past tenses, plurals and active as well as passive sentences) is established. Severely retarded persons are very slow to develop speech; however, for persons of normal and higher intellect, there is no correlation between the rapidity with which children talk and intelligence.

Issues in language development as influences on behavior include, especially, minority–majority issues. The majority of social institutions in America are white, Anglo–Saxon, and Protestant ("WASP"). Children who are not from a WASP background have been raised in a cultural milieu that has a different syntax than WASP, or that may assign a semantic meaning to the WASP language. The result is that a minority child entering a majority school must become semantically bilingual and live in two different semantic worlds (the one of school and the one of home) in order to progress in WASP educational structure. Majority instructors frequently do not recognize this variance; therefore, when using a specific WASP word or phrase in the presence of a minority student, two things may occur: the student translates the word to and from minority semantics which gives the appearance of the student being slow, or the student may display a different emotional reaction to the word than the instructor expects, and, therefore, seem "strange" or "crazy."

School Age.   By the time the child has reached *school age* (6 to 12 years of age), psychomotor development is complete and play activities have developed to a phase of *cooperative* interactional activity. In Erikson's framework, industry and adequacy in peer relations are of foremost importance. The beginning school years are when the child leaves the primary influence of parents and enters the control sphere of other adults—teachers—and peers. Typically, there is eager anticipation of school, which lasts for the first two years. The relationship children develop with teachers can be predicted by the child's relation to parents, that is, there is generalization between parents and teachers. Physical handicaps, eye–hand motor coordination difficulties, learning disabilities, percep-

tual problems, and hyperactivity can become barriers to adequate school performance which, in turn, will have an impact on the child's feeling of adequacy. Research suggests that males, children from lower classes, and children from minority groups—particularly if they also form a minority in the school—have a more difficult time adjusting to the WASP, sexist school situation characteristic of American public education.

During this stage, increased sexual exploration of self (*i.e.,* masturbatory activity) and others is normal. Because this age group is also characterized by same-sex interpersonal relations, same-sex sexual activity is also normally expected.

Sex role differences that began to appear in the previous stage are further defined and refined. Children learn at this time to regulate and sometimes to totally inhibit natural emotions. For instance, male children are taught not to cry (*i.e.,* not to demonstrate sad feelings: "big boys don't cry"); however, they are groomed to display aggressive, angry, hostile emotions. Conversely, female children learn that crying is perfectly permissible but that "nice girls never say damn." As a consequence of this sex role training, males often display anger when they are sad, and females often cry when angry. Fortunately, several of the issues described above relating to language development, physical handicaps, physical orientation, and sex role differences are being perceived by educators and are being corrected.

Child abuse sometimes occurs during infancy, preschool, and subsequent school-age phases. Child abuse encompasses neglect, active physical trauma, and sexual abuse. Each state in the United States has laws against child abuse, which require physicians to report suspected child abuse and protect the physician from retaliatory acts. According to the National Center on Child Abuse and Neglect and researchers, parents reported for abuse of their children themselves were abused children, the parent seldom looks at or touches the child, the family is isolated (*e.g.,* unlisted phone number, no social club memberships, cannot be located, seems to trust no one, does not participate in school activities or events), the parents expect or demand behavior beyond the child's years or abilities, they don't care for the physical hygiene of the child, the parents over or under-react to the child's condition, they appear to be misusing alcohol or other drugs, and they are overcritical of the child. These parents perceive the child's expression of needs as being purposeful acts of frustration and irritation to the parent (*e.g.,* a hungry child cries at night and the parents say, "That child won't let me sleep.").

They are reluctant to give information about the child's injury or condition and are either unable to explain injuries or offer illogical or contradictory information. They appear to lack control or, at least, they fear losing control, and they generally know no other disciplinary techniques except physical punishment.

Characteristics of the **abused** or **neglected** child include obvious welts or skin injuries, inappropriate clothes for the weather, severely abnormal eating habits (*e.g.,* eating from garbage pails and drinking from toilet bowls) and begging or stealing food, and exhibiting extremes of behavior from aggression to extreme passivity/withdrawal. While these children appear overly mature, they also seem unduly afraid of parents and other adults. They generally cause trouble with peers, are wary of any physical contact, and are apprehensive around other children who are crying. They frequently engage in vandalism, sexual misconduct, and use alcohol and other drugs. Often these children need glasses or other medical attention, show severely retarded physical growth, and are often tired and without energy. Usually there is only one child in the family who is abused, and most research indicates that the abused child is either different in some way (*e.g.,* has a higher or lower IQ than others in the family or is physically handicapped) or is perceived by the family as "ugly."

In general, child abuse occurs in a constellation of a **culture/community** that offers little support for the family unit and perceives children as having few rights, in a family with limited disciplinary knowledge except physical punishment, and with a child who is perceived as "different." Viewing child abuse simply as a function of parental pathology is naive.

Puberty and Adolescence. The onset of **adolescence** (from 12 to 17 years of age) is introduced by **puberty:** menstruation for females and seminal emissions for males. At puberty there is a physical growth spurt accompanied by radical endocrine shifts that control the onset of secondary sex characteristics (*i.e.,* distribution of body fat, pubic hair, voice changes, and facial hair in males). This endocrine shift also provides the overwhelming sexual drive observed in this phase. Females have an earlier onset of puberty than males, and there is evidence that onset of menses is occurring at younger ages, with the average age at 12.5 years and a normal range of 10.5 to 15 years of age. The onset of menses is apparently controlled in part by body size. Sperm production in males begins at about 14.5 years with a range of 12.5 to 16.5 years of age. Both masturbatory and interpersonal sexual activity heightens during this phase. Each year in America, there are approximately 30,000 pregnancies to females under the age of 15 years, and 1,000,000 to females between 15 and 19 years of age. As a result, teenage marriages frequently occur, 50% of which are because of pregnancy. While some of these are extremely stable and endure, one third end in divorce within four years.

During adolescence, a major achievement/milestone is for the young person to separate from the dependent role with parents. Cognitively, adolescents can meaningfully ask the question, "Why are things like they are?" but, because they have not fully developed delay of gratification, they want changes in perceived inequities now! In this constellation, the adolescent is faced with the necessity of separating from the parents, requiring affectional and emotional support needs, being associated with peers who share the perceived inequities and can supply the support system. This configuration, in combination with the adolescent perception of personal invulnerability, contributes to high levels of illicit substance abuse, accidents being the leading cause of death among white teenagers, suicide being the second-leading cause of death, crimes of violence beginning to peak at about 15 years of age, and homicide being the leading cause of death of black youth.

Throughout the above stages, **moral development** has also been maturing along with other psychosexual, psychosocial, and cognitive abilities. Depending upon social model transmission, cognitive ability development, and other issues, the individual should have reached a high level of moral sophistication by the end of adolescence and entering into young adulthood. As with all developmental phases, persons may become fixated at one level or regress under special conditions of internal or external stress. **Kohlberg** provided the following framework for understanding moral development:

Stage 1: Punishment and obedience orientation. The physical consequences determine "goodness" or "badness." (*e.g.,* "It was bad because I got punished.")
Stage 2: Instrumental relativist position. An action is right because it satisfied one's needs.
Stage 3: Interpersonal concordance. Good behavior is that which pleases or helps others and is approved by them.
Stage 4: Orientation to authority. Respect for law, authority and order for its own sake.
Stage 5: Social contract orientation. Laws are agreements or contracts, and the contracts

are what define right and wrong. Contracts are changeable.

Stage 6: Universal ethical principle orientation. Universal principles of justice prevail (*e.g.,* taking another's life is wrong).

Young Adulthood. In Erikson's framework, the major tasks during the young adult period (18 to 35 or 40 years of age) are developing an intimate relationship and establishing oneself in an occupational position. An intimate relationship in the United States usually implies love; according to Maslow, this is either **B love** or **D love.** "B" love is that which is based on each individual feeling personally secure—a full "genital" character in a psychodynamic framework. These persons like themselves, feel complete individually and have an appreciation for "being." From this security and well being, two persons choose each other to share their lives and create children from the union. Within this nuclear family, there is a maximum of respect for individuality with no ulterior motive to change the other person. Children in these families are guided, through warmth, permissiveness, and limit-setting, toward self-discovery and maximizing individual potential. "D" love is deficient love. In this framework, each person comes to the relationship out of perceived personal deficit and selects the other to fill the missing characteristic in the self. Such marriages frequently have an ulterior motive to alter the other person after the marriage is established. Children in these nuclear families are acquired to fulfill needs the parents have (*e.g.,* to be an "average" family, to hold the marriage together, so the mother has "something to do," and so forth). Such arrangements/dynamics predispose a nuclear family to later difficulties when the marriage partners can't or won't meet each other's needs, or the children leave the home.

The resolution to the second part of this Eriksonian phase, occupational choice—and particularly professional choice—is frequently based on irrational decisions. Early childhood or adolescent experiences often shape a premature decision, which is retained as an irrevocable law. Sometimes persons enter a particular field owing to familial or other social pressures (*e.g.,* "All the women in this family have always been nurses.") and maintain in their training "until. . . ." Unfortunately, "until" never comes and these persons frequently shift jobs at middle age. Terkel (1974) described four aspects of *work:* it influences the conception a person has about self and the surrounding world, it is used as a social locator, it can provide a source of power and

autonomy, and it can be a source of major frustration and devaluation. In the United States, there is a work ethic that values and promotes productivity. While this orientation provides solid base to the economy, it creates considerable difficulty for youth who can't produce and the elderly who are forced into idleness at retirement age, particularly with regard to the first three of Terkel's items. Since *socioeconomic status* is based on income, education, and occupation, the young and old clearly wear a "label" of nonvalued lower socioeconomic status.

A major complicating factor, which develops for young adults, is forced incompatibility between marriage partners in Erikson's psychosocial context. Because extended family structure in the United States is no longer the rule, each new nuclear family must quickly establish its own independent existence. This forces the husband to be preoccupied with work (*i.e.,* generativity), leaving the wife to raise the children and be the major source of warmth and intimacy. By the latter part of this stage, the husband frequently has established himself occupationally and wants to return to the family for the intimacy he has foregone while "becoming a success." However, the wife has "run out" of intimacy and wants to begin her generativity. This decrease in extended family dependence and psychosocial incompatibility certainly contributes to the observed increase in American divorce rates (40% in 1977 and the rate has been increasing at about 5% a year). About 1.5 million families in the United States have a separated or divorced person as head of the family, and those families involve more than 2.4 million children, 90% of whom live with their mothers. This condition, coupled with data presented earlier regarding sex role acquisition, egocentricity of youth, and so forth, provides a situation in which youth can become confused in identity, assume responsibility for the divorce of parents and, in frustration, act out maladaptively. Whether the increase in the number of wives entering into the workforce over the past few decades will alter these astounding data remains to be seen.

Middle Age. As individuals enter the middle years (from 40 to 60 or 65 years of age), regardless of their previous occupational role—housewife or financial provider—they encounter the **career clock** phenomenon. They critically review accomplishments to date, reexamine the reasons for entering the role, and evaluate whether things should remain as they are. Frequently, the occupational, marital, social, and geographic status changes at this point because of no wish to carry through previous decisions that are inappropriate at this time. Others evaluate their present situations and find them unacceptable, yet do nothing to alter them, resulting in a subsequent life of desperation. Others evaluate, are happy with their present state, and continue with an integrity between previous, present, and anticipated future life-style. During this time, sex role stereotypes are better modulated, prejudices are relaxed, and overall tension levels are reduced. The issue of personal mortality is also confronted and, in the main, resolved. (This is often difficult for physicians.) Consistently, this age range is reported as the most gratifying for the majority of persons.

On the negative side, women who have overinvested in their children sometimes develop the **empty nest syndrome** and frequently experience a rather severe depressive episode when the last child is gone. Men at 45 to 54 years of age are at the peak of their earning power and careers; consequently, stress syndromes (*e.g.,* gastrointestinal distress, myocardial infarctions) may become manifest. Divorce also may occur due to waiting ''until the children are grown'' or to both persons being required to deal with each other rather than through the children.

Old Age.   The technocracy in the United States has provided a socioeconomic climate which has drawn attention to the elderly of America. In this focus on the elderly, a number of myths have been generated. The most popular are as follows:

The elderly live alone in nursing homes. The reality is that 5% of elderly live in residential institutions, 60% own their own homes, and between 65% and 80% live with someone else. However, the percentage of elderly in nursing homes dramatically increases in the 75 to 85-year age group and increases more in the 85 to 95-year group.

The elderly are asexual. Realistically, 70% of elderly males and 20% of females report active sexuality. The disparity between males and females probably reflects the fact that males marry younger females and have a shorter life expectancy; therefore, more females are left without a sexual partner in later life.

The elderly are senile. While senility does have some correlation with plaque formation in the CNS, other determinants of senility are social isolation, forced inactivity, and lack of significant interpersonal involvement. One need only consider Albert Einstein to realize age per se has little to do with senility.

The realistic issues with which the elderly are confronted are multiple:

Mental processes: As persons age, two significant changes occur. First, reaction time slows. As a consequence, because quick sensorimotor reactions are the basis for performance items on most intelligence tests, there is an apparent but illusionary decrease in IQ as persons age. Second, immediate and recent memory are attenuated while remote memory is unimpaired. This results in older persons ''boring'' younger adults with repetition of remote data. However, young children are as fascinated with these recollections as they are with the retelling of fairy tales. While these acquisitional problems are relative and not absolute—older persons can and do learn—it does take longer for them to acquire new data.

Fixed income: 15% of American elderly are living on poverty level, fixed incomes that make them most vulnerable to fluctuations in national economics.

Chronic health conditions: About 85% of the elderly have at least one chronic health problem, twice as many are likely to be hospitalized, Medicare meets about 50% of total health care costs, 14% need assistance in their homes, 50% of the blind are 50 years of age or older, 25% of all prescribed drugs are consumed by the elderly, and 15% of the elderly make serious errors in the consumption of prescribed medication, mainly due to the recent memory problems (forgetting if and when they took medications).

Nutrition: Nutritional deficiencies affect about 10% of the elderly due to fixed income and rising food costs, loss of interest in preparing food and eating if they live alone, and compromised access to food based on transportation problems.

Transportation: The breakdown of extended families has led to the elderly being excluded from regular travel previously provided by their children. Health problems may limit the ability of the elderly to drive, and inadequate or expensive public transportation further limits mobility. In some studies, this is reported by the elderly as their major problem.

Inactivity: Enforced idleness is due to mandatory retirement with financial penalties for earning extra money, lack of mobility, and decreased social contacts as friends and relatives of the same age die.

The people who successfully age are those who actively planned for retirement, continue activities of the middle years, maintain an active social involvement and provide themselves with continued growth experiences. The best predictors of successful aging are a good IQ, higher education, financial security, how active and integrated the individual was prior to onset of the rapid aging process, and the presence of an intimate relationship.

Interpersonal and Small Group Determinants of Behavior

GROUP DYNAMICS

When an individual interacts with one or more persons, the needs of the single individual are placed in a context of the needs of the other. Usually, in such a setting, no single individual's needs are completely met. Group size dictates some basic influences on human behavior. Two interacting people—a *dyad*—have an opportunity to develop intimacy and resolve differences when lack of consensus develops. Three people—a *triad*—are involved in a more complex issue in that relations must be maintained at less than an intimate or dyadic level to avoid exclusion of one person. If dyadic intimacy does develop between persons in groups larger than two, priorities must be clearly established; for example, children in a family must understand they cannot destroy the marital bond and be the primary intimate object for one of the two parents. Likewise, parents must align solidly together for the child to mature appropriately. Triads always have the potential to move into the "drama triangle," where the roles of persecutor, victim, and rescuer are stable, but persons in the triangle assume different roles at different times. When more than three people interact, members tend to subdivide and form relationships with at least one other person in the group that are *affiliative* (*i.e.,* attraction) and *differentiating* (*i.e.,* repulsion). The affiliations and differentiations occur along multiple dimensions, such as sex, age, race, ethnicity, occupation, and socioeconomic status, as well as various combinations. These dimensions of affiliation and differentiation within a group frequently get superimposed upon the nature of the group.

The nature of the group is defined as whether the group has an end product, task, or goal—*task-oriented group*—or whether it assembles to support a given identity—*sentient group*—with no task or goal product expected.

Related to these affiliation–differentiation and task–sentient dimensions is the focus of the group; that is, does the group focus on the *content–decision* issue of a topic (more characteristic of task groups) or does the group focus on the *process* of how things are occurring? Typically, these content–process issues are always ongoing but difficult to attend to simultaneously. A neurosurgical team doing surgery is a task group focused on content–decision outcome issues. The outcome may be less acceptable if all team members are in the process of undercutting other members' effectiveness. That same team later in an informal setting discussing the outcome of the surgery, "rehashing" how well everyone performed and sharing personal feelings with each other, transforms to a sentient group, which is process oriented and no tangible product is expected.

LEADERSHIP

Leadership is tied to the nature, focus and needs of the group. Leaders are typically polemically divided into authoritarian or democratic styles. *Democratic leaders* provide a setting in which group members are true contributors to decision-making. Their groups perform consistently, display high morale, and produce when the leader is absent. They perceive themselves as an integral part of a whole. *Authoritarian leaders* have groups that have sporadic high performance when the leader is present, but noticeably diminished production when the leader is absent. Typically, in a group that is product-oriented but led by an authoritarian person who makes all meaningful decisions, the group concerns itself with irrelevant process issues or incidental content items. This group is not productive either in a task-oriented or a sentient sense.

Group needs and the consequent *expectation* by the group of the leader interact with the relative maturity of the group. Rioch has defined these issues as outlined in Table 8-1. Leaders who attempt to fulfill the fantasy demands of an immature group or who approach leadership from the fantasy/immature posture generally fail and the group either ostracizes the leader or deteriorates in functioning.

DESTRUCTIVE ISSUES

Other destructive variables to internal group structure are excessive competition and inappropriate aggression. Both of these variables not only inter-

TABLE 8-1. Group Expectations

GROUP NEED	GROUP EXPECTATIONS OF LEADER	
	Fantasy–Immature	Mature
Dependency	Omnipotence	Dependable
Fight–Flight	Unbeatable	Courageous
Pairing/Affiliation	"Marvelous unborn"	Creative

fere with group performance but, in some instances, also dissolve the extant group. The group, however, can extrude the offending member, close the group to the extruded person, and gain solidarity by closed-rank resistance to attempts from the extruded person either to rejoin or further destroy the group structure.

GROUP AS A SYSTEM

A basic assumption underlying large and small groups is that a group is a relatively rigid, closed system that is tightly interdependent. Any alteration in the system, such as a person entering, exiting, or changing, requires compensatory alteration in another person in the system to maintain stability.

Families can be viewed as such systems in which there are extremely stable roles that are resistant to change; however, the individual who fills a role can be variable (*e.g.*, the mothering role can be assumed by any family member). This role stability and resistance to change exists regardless of the relative functional adaptability or health of the family. Attempts to enter or alter the structure either are resisted or the system structure of the family group must change.

Family systems characterized by inclusion factors have changed considerably in the recent past. A **nuclear family** is a unit of procreation: mother, father, and children. **Extended families** are those in which there is inclusion of more than one unit of procreation, such as grandparents, parents, grandchildren, great grandchildren, aunts, and uncles. As a general rule, in America today most families are nuclear with only loose ties to other familial, procreative units. This weakening of bonds in extended family units has serious implications for a support system for orphaned, single, older, or new family members. Previously, new marriages in an extended family could rely on that system to provide support while the new family stabilized. Now new marriages must establish a stable nuclear family in an extremely short period of time.

Assessment of Behavior

Observation of specific aspects of human behavior has been standardized by psychological tests. Because these are formal and consistent observations, normative data have been collected about performance of people. Consequently, any person's performance can be compared to the norms, and statements about that person's relative standing on a particular variable can be made. Normative data comprising the sample against which an individual's score is compared can be collected by selecting people **randomly,** when everyone in a given population has an equal opportunity to be selected for the sample, or through **stratification** of the sample, when the sample is constituted to reflect relevant variables in the overall population at the rate the variables occur in the overall population (*e.g.,* including the percentage of Eskimos in the sample that reflects the incidence of Eskimos in the population).

The major types of psychological tests are described below. While some are administered in a group, individualized assessment is always more valid.

DEVELOPMENTAL SCALES

These are standard observations of the psychomotor/social development of infants and children. For example, the **Denver Developmental Scale** is applicable from birth to the age of six years, and provides data on gross developmental progress in personal–social, fine motor, language, and gross motor areas. The **Vineland Social Maturity Scale** is a standard interview, usually with the parent, about a child's socialization level that can be applied from birth to maturity.

INTELLIGENCE TESTS

These are psychological tests that presumably reflect the concept of intelligence presented earlier. An IQ is derived by one of two methods. The first is the **mental age concept,** where a mental age (MA) score is derived from a standard test. That MA is divided by the person's chronological age (CA) and multiplied by 100 to yield the IQ. The formula is $MA/CA \times 100 = IQ$. The **Stanford–Binet Intelligence Test** is an example of this process.

The second method of IQ derivation, called the **deviation IQ,** is exemplified by the Wechsler scales: **Wechsler Adult Intelligence Scale (WAIS)** for those 16 years of age and older and the **Wechsler Intelligence Scale for Children (WISC)** for those under the age of 16. The IQ is derived from age subgroup norm tables; therefore, age-related factors that might contaminate scores are controlled. The Wechsler tests provide a **verbal IQ (VIQ),** a **performance IQ (PIQ),** and a **full-scale IQ (FSIQ).** The separate verbal scales that are combined to obtain the VIQ are **Information,** general fund of knowledge; **Comprehension,** social judgment; **Arithmetic,** mathematical ability; **Similarities,** ability to abstract commonalities from objects of a class; **Digit Span,** rote recall forward and backward; and **Vocabulary,** general vocabulary level. The timed performance scales that are combined to obtain the PIQ are **Digit Symbol,** a coding task; **Picture Completion,** visual recognition of incomplete pictures; **Block Design,** psychomotor reproduction of progressively more complex visual geometric designs; **Picture Arrangement,** visual appreciation of nonverbal social judgement situations; and **Object Assembly,** recognition of a gestalt from diverse parts of an object. The Verbal and Performance scales are combined through norm tables to provide the FSIQ. The IQ tests tend to be highly correlated with adequate education. The norms on IQ tests also tend to be nonhandicapped and "WASP"-biased; therefore, one must carefully interpret test results if the person examined is non-WASP, is poorly educated or has a physical or mental handicap.

ACHIEVEMENT TESTS

These are norm-based assessments which usually have been established on stratified representative national samples. They purport to reflect the amount an individual has "learned" or accomplished. The **National Board of Medical Examiners** tests are examples, as is the **Wide Range Achievement Test (WRAT).** The WRAT has subdivisions of reading, spelling, and arithmetic, with national norms applied from preschool through high school years.

APTITUDE SCALES

Ability or aptitude tests are those attempts to assess "native" endowment in areas like creativity, musical and artistic aptitude, and psychomotor coordination and speed.

INTEREST TESTS

Scales like the **Strong Vocational Interest Inventory** were empirically derived by administering many diverse items to persons who were successful and satisfied in different occupations. Those items to which persons in a given vocation responded uniquely were combined into a scale. Persons who answer items in a similar manner are presumed to be good candidates for that vocation. In such empirical derivation, it is not necessary that item content have "face validity," or make sense.

PERSONALITY SCALES

These tests presume to assess dimensions of stable intra- and interpersonal interaction patterns. They are typically subdivided into objective (*i.e.*, empirical) versus subjective (*i.e.*, projective) tests:

The Minnesota Multiphasic Personality Inventory (MMPI) is the best known objective test. It is objective in that it was derived from empirical analysis and not theory. The MMPI has hundreds of true–false, psychiatric symptom-related questions, which are scored on ten clinical scales and three validity scales. It is not a true personality inventory because the clinical scales presumably reflect the relative absence or presence of psychopathology but not underlying personality dimensions.

The Meyers–Briggs Inventory is an objective personality scale based on Jungian theory. The major dimensions reflected by this test are: Extroversion–Introversion, Sensation–Intuition, and Feeling–Thinking.

These dimensions in combination, yield eight "types," which are personality descriptions, not degrees of psychopathology as with the MMPI. Norms are available for an individual's type as well as type compatibility in some special professions.

The **projective** or **subjective personality tests** are those derived from personality theories and based on the **projective hypothesis.** The projective hypothesis states that given an ambiguous stimulus, people will structure the ambiguity according to their own needs and underlying dynamics. The clinician analyzes responses to the ambiguous stimuli and infers internal needs and underlying dynamics. The major projective tests are the **Rorschach** (known as the "ink blot test"), which is associated more with unconscious intrapersonal dynamics, and the **Thematic Appreciation Test (TAT),** which consists of ambiguous pictures of different persons and objects in vague settings about which the person creates a story. Again, the examiner infers from the stories the underlying personality needs and dimensions. The TAT reflects more interpersonal dynamics although some intrapersonal data can be obtained. There is a **Children's Appreciation Test (CAT),** similar to the TAT, which involves animals instead of humans in the vaguely structured pictures. Other projective tests are the **Draw-a-Person (DAP)** and the **Sentence Completion Test** (*e.g.*, "Right now I feel. . . .").

NEUROPSYCHOLOGICAL TESTS

These are psychological instruments sensitive to cerebral (specifically, cortical) dysfunction. The *Bender–Gestalt,* a test of graphic reproduction of nine rather simple geometric designs, has been used for this purpose. The *Halstead–Reitan battery,* a combination of many different tests, has a long research and clinical history of proven utility in reflecting specific brain-behavior relationships. The *Luria* scales currently show promise in this regard. With biomedical advances (*e.g.,* CAT scans), the utility of these as primary differential diagnostic tools has decreased; however, they are helpful as noninvasive techniques for documenting relative progression of dysfunction or relative recovery of function after cerebral trauma. They are particularly meaningful in those situations where structural lesions are not present and other biomedical procedures cannot detect disease progression, for example, posttraumatic syndrome and its legal sequelae.

PSYCHOSOCIAL ISSUES IN HEALTH CARE DELIVERY

The following section addresses generic topics that have surfaced as major areas of concern in delivery of health care. They represent the interface between internal psychological/biological processes and social efforts to control them. For clarity, they have been divided into those issues associated with the patient versus those associated with the health care delivery system. However, in reality the issues are present for both the patient and the physician at all times in an interactive process.

Sociocultural Influences

The sociocultural milieu in which the patient is immersed defines for the patient what is "normal," allowed or sanctioned, how expression of allowed behavior is permitted, and how the patient can attend to illness. The cultural subgroup to which the patient belongs establishes the rewards and, through application of those rewards, controls behavior. While the term *minority* means a group that has less representation in the United States population, in the past it has been used to connote a value judgement of "weak" and "inferior" or "bad." It has been specifically applied to ethnic subgroups and has provided a basis for prejudice and negative discrimination. In health care this is exemplified by

at least two classes of health care delivery: that applied to the majority (*i.e.,* private fee for service, private health insurance, Preferred Provider Options, Health Maintenance Organizations), and that delivered to the minority through a public health service model, which is government-subsidized and usually not considered to be as adequate or "caring" about the patient. In this instance, economic status plays a major role in defining "minority" or "majority."

Beliefs, attitudes, prejudice, and values are core psychosocial issues in health care delivery:

Beliefs are the cognitive information an individual accepts about an object. The belief may or may not be based in fact and varies in strength from an opinion, which is a lightly held belief, to a strong belief for which a person may die (*e.g.,* "women and children first").

Attitudes encompass the evaluative (*i.e.,* good–bad) and affective aspects of responses toward a given object or situation. There are two basic components to an attitude: a belief portion and an affective part. For example, not only must a physician believe that the medical profession is worthwhile, but that physician also must derive a positive feeling from the practice of medicine.

Prejudice is an attitude that is harmful and based upon the distortion of some small element of truth and frequently is directed towards a subgroup—usually a minority subgroup—of people. Within any group, prejudice toward those not in the group is common whether majority toward minority or vice versa. The distortion involves overgeneralization, oversimplification, and alteration of reality, and at times employs the phenomenon of *scapegoating.* In scapegoating (and prejudice), the defense mechanism of projection is used to project onto the victim qualities that persons are unconsciously ashamed or afraid of in themselves. The case against the scapegoat is justified by vices attributed (correctly or incorrectly) to the scapegoat. Usually the scapegoat is weak enough not to retaliate effectively but strong enough not to be easily victimized, easily accessible, and identifiable. It has been reported that persons who are subjected to scapegoating for protracted periods of time take on the attributes of the scapegoat role.

Typically, prejudice begins to appear at about the preschool age and is often conveyed by the parenting persons in the child's life. While influenced by cultural norms and the significant group to which the person belongs, prejudices also vary with socioeconomic status, education, and religious affiliation. Persons who are strongly prejudiced tend to have *aggressive, authoritarian personalities* that do not allow them to consider alternative views of the scapegoated object.

The alteration of prejudice, and other attitudes, is a complex process, which involves variations on the basic theme of extended exposure to the prejudiced object over time. Distorted facts are recognized and negative affects extinguished, and these are replaced with affiliative bonds. Other factors in attitude change include the creditability and prestige of the source, whether the source displays disinterest in changing the attitudes (*e.g.,* "overheard" conversations), whether the source argues a position against his own self-interest, the arousal of emotions other than fear or anger, and the intensity with which the prejudice is held.

Values are the personal guide an individual develops that give direction to life. They help the person relate to the world and take decisive personal action. Values are usually developed later in life as the result of considerations of various alternatives, and they usually have three aspects: choosing them consciously, prizing or feeling good about them, and acting on them.

The *sick role* significantly affects human behavior. People from different professional, socioeconomic, sexual, and ethnic backgrounds display illness differently. For example, health professionals frequently resist recognition of illness in themselves because of the "omnipotent" role forced on them by the culture and accepted by their own fear of disease. There is no more confining prison than being placed on or placing oneself on a pedestal. Women tend to seek more health care than men, even when the effects of pregnancy are controlled. Persons of lower socioeconomic levels do not seek as much preventive care as do those from the middle and upper classes. Consequently, hospital stays for poorer persons tend to be longer because illness progresses further in its course before care is sought. Basically, persons of lower socioeconomic status define illness when, in the course of dysfunction, there is impairment of earning power.

Ethnicity helps shape how individuals display their illness. Cultures that encourage open display of emotions (*e.g.,* Italians), will be volatile in expression, while less emotionally apparent cultures (*e.g.,* Chinese), will endure in quiet reservation. Ethnicity also determines what health care person is sought—medicine man, priest, chiropractor, physician, midwife, and so forth.

The psychosocial environment provides at least four additional considerations: *Hollingshead and Redlick* (1958) demonstrated that some types of mental illness are more likely to receive medical treatment at earlier stages among the rich as compared to the poor and in cities compared with rural areas. There is a positive correlation between low socioeconomic status and severe symptom impairment, particularly schizophrenia. There does not seem to be a relationship between rural versus urban setting with regard to overall rates of mental disturbance. Rates for all functional psychosis tend to be higher in rural settings, and rates for neuroses and personality disorders appear higher for urban areas.

Holmes and Rahe (1967) established a strong relationship between *life change events and illness.* Their Social Readjustment Scale has proven effective in predicting relative mental and physical illness from cumulative social events such as divorce, Christmas holidays, and so forth.

Human Sexuality

Gender refers to sexual anatomy. The *gender identity* refers to the sexual role of the child in which it feels it belongs—either that of a man or woman. It is the private experience of sexuality. *Gender identification* means how the child, through modeling (*i.e.,* social learning), is taught to act, whether masculine or feminine. It is the public expression of the person's sexuality. These three can be independent of each other.

Sexual behavior that is considered normal in America includes sexual excitement from birth until death, masturbation from early adolescence until death, and same-sex exploration from late childhood/early adolescence until opposite sex attachments form in middle to late teens.

Masters and Johnson (1966) pioneered modern medicine's objective knowledge about adult human sexuality. Their work separates the human sexual response cycle into four phases. Table 8-2 summarizes their data, the work of Sherfey (1972), and Sadock (1982).

In addition to these states, a *refractory period* after orgasm occurs for the male, during which time he cannot become erect or have additional orgasms. Females can be multiorgasmic. There are data in the literature that suggest some females may also have ejaculate at orgasm. These data are associated with the discussion of the *"g" spot* (for Graffenberg) in females.

The normal effects of *aging* on the human sexual response are shown in Table 8-3. In the man over 60 years of age, it has been observed that the refrac-

TABLE 8-2. Sexual Stages

STAGE	FEMALE	MALE
Excitement	Vaginal ballooning Vaginal lubrication Nipple erection Clitoral erection	Penile erection Nipple erection
Plateau	Clitoral retraction Further vaginal ballooning HR, BP, Resp. increase	Testes increase in size Additional penile engorgement HR, BP, Resp. increase
Orgasm	Vagina and uterus contract at about ¾-sec. intervals for 3–15 contractions. HR, BP, Resp. may increase further	Ejaculation of seminal fluid: Marked penile and prostate contraction at .8 sec. for 3–4 major contractions. HR, BP, Resp. may increase further
Resolution	All changes return to unstimulated state within 30 min.	All changes return to unstimulated state within 30 min.

tory period is quite extended—to perhaps days—before the male can become erect again.

The human sexual response cycle is biologically stable and apparently correlated with normal biochemical/physiologic functioning. In the physiologically intact person, what is necessary is "friction and a frame of mind." Dysfunction can occur at any or all of the stages of the cycle for both males and females. These dysfunctions are noted in Table 8-4. Generally, if there is no underlying organic pathology, the etiology of these dysfunctions can be traced to inadequate education and social programming, getting out of the "here and now pleasure"

TABLE 8-3. Sex and the Elderly

STAGE	FEMALE	MALE
Excitement	Decreased vasocongestion Delayed vaginal lubrication	Decreased vasocongestion Increased time to erect
Plateau	Vaginal expansion is reduced	Increased duration of erection and activity without orgasm Full erection not until entering orgasmic phase
Orgasm	Contractile phase reduced in duration	Slower ejaculatory experience with decreased contractions Prostatic contractions are absent
Resolution	Very rapid return to unstimulated state	Very rapid detumescence of the penis

TABLE 8-4. Sexual Dysfunction

STAGE	FEMALE	MALE
Excitement	General sexual dysfunction ("frigidity") Vaginismus (strong vaginal contractions) Dyspareunia (painful intercourse)—usually organic base	Erectile dysfunction ("impotence") Dyspareunia (painful intercourse)—usually organic base
Orgasm	Inorgasmia (usually due to low trust level of partner)	Inorgasmia (performance anxiety) Premature ejaculation (inadequate learning or control).

and anxiously going into remembered past or projected future, or assuming a critical spectator role during sexual activity. It should also be noted that a number of primary physiologic illnesses (*e.g.*, diabetes melitis), aging, and drug use (prescription and otherwise) can produce identical sexual dysfunctions.

Through the utilization of behavioral modification techniques, resolution of physical abnormalities, and counseling toward improved communication between sexual partners (oriented to trust and taking personal responsibility for one's own pleasure), has resulted in high rates of resolution for many of these dysfunctions.

Besides the predominant heterosexual pattern, there are different sexual preferences, which form large subgroups within the population. Although there is some evidence that some of these preferences occur on a genetic basis, most are viewed as being the result of early learning experiences based in either the gender identity formation prior to 3 years of age or role identification issues later in childhood. Some authors view the acquisition of sexual preference as similar to the acquisition of language. There is a biologic readiness upon which the preference (like the primary language) is acquired. Regardless of later preferences (or languages), there is the first acquisition, which is always present. Some data also suggest there may be biologic substrates to some different sexual preferences. As with language acquisition, the longer one stays with a sexual preference (or primary language), the more difficult it is to acquire a different one. Likewise, if one continues to practice the primary preference (language) while acquiring a different one, the new one is less well acquired.

Kinsey reported that 4% of adult, white males

live an exclusive homosexual existence, and about 10% are "more or less" exclusively homosexual for at least three years between the ages of 16 and 65; 48% of male adolescents report same-sex genital play. According to Kinsey, there are a third to a quarter as many female (lesbians) as male homosexuals. Apparently, the discrepancy is correlated with relative definitions and differentially allowed or accepted behaviors between males and females in American society. Overall, the best estimate of adult homosexuality is that 10% of adults are homosexual. Of that 10%, 60% are males and 40% are females.

There are no valid data with regard to the number of practicing bisexual persons. However, the present AIDS epidemic strongly suggests this is a more prevalent behavior pattern than previously suspected.

The major medical concern regarding homosexuality is the prevalence of **sexually transmitted diseases** (STDs) among a subgroup of homosexual males who tend to be quite promiscuous and have a high STD rate. The advent of Human Immunodeficiency Virus (HIV) and Acquired Immuno Deficiency Syndrome (AIDS) has led to concern regarding the sexual practices of some homosexual and bisexual males.

Transvestism is defined as intermittent, but regular, dressing in clothes of the opposite sex (*i.e.,* crossdressing), which is experienced as sexually pleasurable. In the United States, this syndrome is confined to males since females are allowed to crossdress with no social proscriptions.

In the above three conditions—heterosexuality, homosexuality, and transvestism—the gender identity is consistent with the gender (*i.e.,* biologic sex) and the major etiologic issue is gender identification.

Transsexuality apparently is due to gender **identity inversion:** the gender identity is opposite of the biologic sex. Since first memories, these persons feel as if they are the opposite-sexed person trapped in the body of the biologic sex of birth. They crossdress frequently from early childhood; it is not for sexual pleasure, but for role fulfillment. They usually are married with a family and, in middle years (30 to 50 years of age), seek cosmetic surgical intervention to align the external genitalia with internal feelings. These surgeries have been very successful from the patient's point of view.

Other sexual variations include organic-based differences, such as Turner's syndrome and Klinefelter's syndrome, noted above.

Functionally based differences include **pedophilia,** which is defined as sexual interest in young children. This syndrome is predominantly heterosexual (95%) and is illegal in all states. **Voyeurism** is sexual gratification from watching sexual acts or looking at sexual organs. This is believed to be confined to males; however, differentially allowed (*i.e.,* prosecuted) behavior between males and females must be considered. **Exhibitionism** is the compulsive need to expose one's genitals, and it is usually only prosecuted in males. The act of exposure does not provide release of sexual tension, but the reaction from the female to the exposure does. Exacerbation of these syndromes apparently occurs when the male is faced with defeat, ego deflation, or other threat to adult functioning. Theoretically, these alternatives are taken because approaching a mature female in a situation where rejection is possible is too threatening.

While **incest** is verbalized as a universal taboo, high prevalence rates are reported. Incest is defined as sexual activity between close members of a family. Father (or stepfather) and daughter is most common by report, although mother–son and sibling (heterosexual and homosexual) are not infrequent patterns. Typically, parent–child incest is correlated with a family constellation in which the same-sex parent as the child involved is an extremely poor and incompetent marriage partner who, at least passively, encourages and condones the relationship because it relieves that parent of unwanted and overwhelming responsibilities. Alcohol consumption is frequently involved in incest. While general statistics imply this is a phenomenon of persons of lower socioeconomic status, clinical experience suggests a differential legal prosecution and detection rate among the social classes.

Death and Dying

Death and the process of dying in the United States has become a hospital-focused issue because today few Americans die in their homes. **Elizabeth Kubler-Ross** pioneered the therapeutic work in death and dying. Since that time, the process stages identified by her (listed below) have been recognized to accompany any serious health loss of which the patient is informed. That is, if the patient is informed of a serious, though not fatal, illness, these stages can be observed, and until the patient works through the stages, compliance with proper medical regimens is not good.

THE ADULT

The stages of dealing with death in an adult are as follows:

Denial: The patient firmly insists there is a diagnostic error. Frequently, requests for independent validation are made or the patient disappears from the physician's practice. If the physician recognizes this stage and facilitates further evaluation, the patient usually will stay with the physician.

Anger: In this phase, the patient moves out of the denial stage and enters a phase of angrily asking the question, "Why me?"

Bargaining: As the anger is dissipated, the patient attempts to strike compromises with the physician, self, or a diety. These frequently take the form of "If I can live until (a given time or event), then I won't ask for more," or "I'll do (usually a sacrifice)." Temporary remissions during this phase frequently are interpreted by the patient as fulfillment of the bargain. These should be anticipated by medical personnel and carefully discussed with the patient to prevent over-interpretation.

Sadness or depression: During this stage, the patient becomes fully cognizant of the terminal nature of the condition and emotionally experiences the finality of the diagnosis. The anger and bargaining of previous stages is replaced with appropriate sadness, which accompanies any significant loss.

Acceptance: This is not a euphoric happiness, rather a condition in which the patient resolutely foregoes the sadness and depression, puts his life in order, and makes plans to live out the remainder of his life with the given situation. It is during this time that the dying person can truly say "goodbye" to surviving significant others.

While these stages are listed as discrete entities, in reality they are fluid, and they overlap each other. The individual moves in and out of a given stage in a progression–regression pattern; however, there is usually predominance of one stage over the others. The issue for the physician is *how* to tell the patient of a serious condition, not *whether* to tell the patient. Collusion among health care personnel and relatives not to inform the patient of the true nature of the condition is ill-advised. It should be the patient's choice not to hear (*i.e.,* denial), not the physician's preference to withhold the information. Dying patients have also pointed up the serious error of the physician announcing to the patient what stage he is in as a way of circumventing dealing with the patient as a dying person; for example, "Oh, you're in the stage of anger, you'll be out of it soon and start bargaining with me."

THE CHILD

The dying child poses special issues. Because the child is in preoperational or concrete-operations stage, the full, cognitive understanding of imminent death is not a true reality. The child comprehends it as going to sleep from which the child believes he will awaken. Dying children tend not to fear death, but rather they are most disturbed by separation from parents and mutilation that will make them different or which they may misperceive as punishment.

MANAGEMENT ISSUES

Commonly, physicians and other health care providers have avoided dealing with the dying patient by giving the patient no entree for discussion (busily making rounds and moving in and out of the patient's room quickly), geographically isolating the patient in a single room at the end of the hall or keeping the room door closed, making a contract with significant others not to inform the patient of the nature of the condition, extending unrealistic hope (*e.g.,* "We're expecting a breakthrough any day." or automatically saying, "You're going to be just fine."), and maintaining a clouded sensorium in the patient through medication. Appropriate management of the dying patient tends to emphasize the opposite of these.

These realities, coupled with the American penchant for keeping dying relatives isolated in social institutions, has led to the *hospice* movement, where persons with terminal illnesses are assisted in their dying process by involving the whole family as much as possible, allowing the patient to be afraid and discuss the fear, providing physical contact in a warm and supportive atmosphere, allowing the patient to talk and cry about the loss, managing temporary remissions without building unrealistic hope, providing as much dignity in the health care as is feasible, and using medications that provide pain relief without clouding the sensorium (*e.g.,* Brompton's mixture, a combination of narcotics and stimulants).

Grief and Bereavement

The persons remaining after the loss of a loved one through death or permanent separation (and, some authors report, after the loss of a body part like a limb, breast, or testicle) undergo predictable reactions. The grief and bereavement process reflects significant loss; therefore, it is related to the emotion sadness. The expression of these reactions is culturally determined and varies by ethnic subgroup. It is expected that the normal process of mourning should be completed within 6 to 12 months after loss. Grieving/mourning is a process—not a condition—and, as such, changes with time like a contusion that is in the process of resolution.

THE ADULT

The stages of the grief process for adults are as follows:

Acute disbelief or phase of protest: This may last for minutes, hours, or days, during which the individual is not fully aware the object is gone. It is a state of mental "shock" during which the person may intellectually know the loss has occurred but not affectively experience it. Anger is often projected toward the physician, relatives, and friends because these support people allowed the loved one to die or will not help the grieving person recover the loved one.

Grief work or phase of disorganization: In this second phase, the grieving person develops an emotional sense of loss. The world is experienced as empty, meaningless, and barren. The grieving person tends to withdraw from social contacts and isolates himself. Initially, mental activity is almost exclusively involved with memories of the lost object. Frequently, the mourner will report feeling the "presence" of the individual in the room or close by. Waves of grief which seem to "come from nowhere" tend to overwhelm the grieving person. As this stage continues, the mental preoccupation with the lost one, the withdrawal/isolation, and the waves of grief diminish.

Resolution or phase of reorganization: Through the first two phases, the mourner emerges with an acceptance that the loss is real. He has formed a new relationship with the loss object in terms of realistic memories, not vows to preserve the world as it was the day the loss occurred. This phase signals that the grieving individual is ready to return to the world and form relationships without experiencing guilt over fantasized unfaithfulness or what might have been.

AGE-RELATED GRIEVING

Humans react differently to the loss of another depending upon their age and ability to comprehend the loss. The conditions listed below are common and normal accompaniments of mourning.

Infants may withdraw from social contact, refuse to eat, and die if a mother figure is lost and not replaced. This condition, known as marasmus, was discussed previously.

Children will frequently react with hyperactivity and assume a jocular attitude.

Adolescents and young adults will frequently react with hypersexuality, delinquent activity, and significant substance abuse.

Adults often develop psychosomatic illnesses or an exacerbation of a previous pathologic condition and are highly vulnerable to physical disease. Substance abuse is a potential problem.

Elderly adults, like infants, frequently withdraw from social contact and often die within the one year of mourning unless supportive steps are taken to involve them in the life process.

NORMAL VARIANTS

Anticipatory grief sometimes accompanies the death of someone who has had protracted illness. The grieving person has worked through the loss prior to the actual death and, frequently at the time of loss, is ready to begin establishing new, guilt-free relationships immediately. The major problems observed from this pattern are that the person may feel guilty because he is relieved at the death, and he is not reacting as others expect. *Delayed grief* is the maintaining of the affectless shock from stage I until a protracted period of time after the death. Often delayed grief is triggered by accidentally finding a possession of the dead person. It is as if the possession or event has "slipped through" a defense mechanism and triggered the grief. Delayed grief reactions frequently appear in the person who was strong for the other grieving persons, made all funeral arrangements, and postponed the mourning. Similarly, persons who have been separated from a parent at a young age and subsequently learn of that parent's death may experience a variant of a delayed grief reaction. They mourned the loss with the original separation and, with the final one, they experience the old grief—and also the anger that the parent died before a reuniting and resolution of desertion issues were managed. These delayed grief reactions can precipitate profound, acute clinical depression with impulsive suicidal acts. ***Anniversary reactions*** are exacerbations of the pain, sadness, and loss triggered by birthdays, or the wedding or death anniversary of the dead person. Usually these decrease in intensity with years; however, when they serve as a trigger for a delayed grief reaction, the initial grieving may be of equal or greater intensity than would have been expected with an immediate grief reaction.

ABNORMAL GRIEF PATTERNS

Abnormal variants of the grief process are usually of two types. First, the individual may become fixated in one of the age-related reaction patterns noted above and not move beyond it. For example, an adolescent may react to the loss of a sibling, friend, or parent with substance (*i.e.,* drug) abuse. The substance abuse becomes a defense against addressing the loss. Consequently, when the loss begins to surface (or the patient develops tolerance to the drug), drug use is increased to manage the uncomfortable feelings. Obviously, physicians who chronically medicate a grieving patient are preventing the patient from appropriately working through the grief and sometimes create iatrogenic addiction. Second, the adult patient may become fixated in the second stage of the grief process and not move into resolution. If grieving extends more than 12 months, the patient should be assumed to be clinically depressed and be treated appropriately.

Substance Abuse

Substance or drug abuse involves use of psychoactive chemicals taken for nonmedical reasons in a nonprescriptive pattern which is harmful to the person or society. Basically these are alcohol, narcotics, sedative–hypnotics, psychedelics, and stimulants. Definitions for substance abuse are not clear because substance abuse is socially defined and subject to social subgroup variation regarding "normal" or "deviant."

ALCOHOLISM

This is best defined as that pattern of alcohol consumption which results in dysfunction in one or more of five areas: marital, social, legal, occupational, or physical, *and* the person cannot stop drinking, that is, the individual has lost control of

consumption. Problem drinking is defined as problems in any or all of the same five areas, but when the person is confronted with these as a result of alcohol consumption, the person can alter the drinking pattern so it no longer creates the problem.

ADDICTION

Addiction is defined as the nonprescriptive use of a drug harmful to society and/or self, that has the following properties: ***tolerance,*** increasing amounts of the drug are needed over time to achieve the same effect (a cellular, biochemical event), ***dependence,*** abrupt cessation of use of the drug precipitates a recognizable and characteristic withdrawal syndrome (a biochemical–physiologic condition), and ***habituation,*** the drug is taken for the psychological effect or it may be taken out of "habit."

PREVALENCE

Prevalence data for substances of abuse vary with time and the substance in question. However, the figures of 7% to 10% of adult Americans being alcoholics or having a drinking problem and 300,000–400,000 being narcotics addicts seem to be stable consensual estimates of these problems. Statistics on prevalence of other drugs of abuse, particularly marijuana, indicate increases in use; however, whether this reflects a higher rate of actual use or whether more use is now reported is not clear. What is true is that substance abuse is a significant health care problem and it is extending to younger populations as well as to all socioeconomic and ethnic groups.

ETIOLOGY

The etiologic theories of substance abuse (particularly alcoholism) fall into three major categories:

1. ***Physiologic*** and ***biologic*** models
    a. ***Genetotrophic*** issues include research on inherited metabolic defects that result in the need for greater than average consumption of certain foodstuffs such as alcohol.
    b. ***Endocrine*** research data emphasize a defect that leads to episodic hypoglycemia. This produces emotional symptoms that stimulate drug-taking to balance the system.
    c. ***Normalizing effect*** of drugs. Multiple studies have demonstrated physiologic, biochemical, and neurophysiologic differences between substance abusers and nonabusers that disap-

pear after acute drug ingestion. Unfortunately, no presubstance abuse measures have been available on these persons; therefore, it is not possible to know if observed differences are drug induced.

   d. *Genetic* marker variables (*i.e.,* inherited color blindness, primary depression in female family members of male alcoholics, alcoholism and antisocial behavior patterns in male family members of female primary depressed persons), genetic mice strains that drink alcoholically, and concordance rates between adopted children and biologic, alcoholic parents all suggest a genetic component to substance abuse *for some persons.*

   e. Recent research has documented **evoked potential** differences between seven-year-old male offspring of alcoholic men and matched controls.

   f. Beta-**endorphin** and salsolinol level differences between groups of alcoholic persons and matched controls suggest a self-medication of deficits in pain modulation systems of the body. All suggest a physiologic component to substance abuse for some persons.

2. ***Psychological models***

   a. The **psychodynamic model** focuses on unconscious conflicts and low self-esteem as stress variables. The reinforcer of substance abuse is the stress reduction induced by the drug consumption.

   b. **Personality trait** models have identified low stress tolerance, dependence, decreased self image, insecurity, impulsiveness and tolerance, or deviant behaviors as traits associated with substance abuse.

     Both the psychodynamic and personality trait models have only identified their core findings in persons who are substance dependent. They have neither examined the dependent persons prior to the substance dependence nor presented data on the number of persons who possess the traits and are not substance dependent.

     It is important to know that there has *never* been a substance abuse personality identified, that is, a personality that, once identified, will predict substance abuse in all persons with the personality. Each time such a personality has been suggested, a significant number of persons who have the personality but no substance abuse are identified.

   c. Behavioral **learning models** explain drug ingestion as a learned response which decreases felt stress. As a result of the chemical's properties and reported use, the body becomes physiologically dependent leading to continued drug use to avoid withdrawal.

   d. **Psychological dependence** is a concept that has found popularity in the recent past and is defined as that individual who is self-mediating a psychological/psychosocial problem.

3. ***Sociocultural models***

   a. Cultural and **socialization** issues focus on cultural norms that promote substance abuse.

   b. The **cultural stress** factors model relates substance abuse to the degree of stress and inner tension produced by the culture. It also explores the cultural drinking attitudes and the alternatives for stress management provided by the culture.

   c. **Familial** pattern research is focused on role modeling, with social learning providing the basis for the substance abuse.

   d. **Environmental instabilities** and crises produce changes in individual life situations or social roles that precipitates instability, confusion, and stress. In this model drugs are taken as a mechanism to decrease these conditions.

DRUG EFFECTS AND TREATMENT

The effects of various psychoactive substances of abuse, their toxicology and some aspects of treatment are presented in Table 8-5. Different levels of drug toxicity involving different chemicals of abuse are frequently misdiagnosed as functional emotional disturbances. Most notably, psychedelics and stimulants have produced conditions similar to acute manic or paranoid schizophrenic reactions; and phencyclidine (PCP) can present as a dissociated, catatonic (*i.e.,* agitated or depressed) schizophrenic reaction. These toxic conditions can be complicated by unusually long abstinence syndromes from some drugs (sometimes weeks) presumably on a basis of the lipophilic binding properties. Failure to obtain toxicologic studies on patients with distorted behavior patterns can result in improper medical regimens that exacerbate or prolong the episode rather than assist in its resolution. Sometimes inappropriate management due to inadequate diagnostic studies can be fatal.

Violence

Violence may be a special case of uncontrolled aggression or a separate entity that has independent etiologies. While aggression can be directed toward

TABLE 8-5. Drug Effects

	ALCOHOL	NARCOTICS	SEDATIVE HYPNOTICS	PSYCHEDELICS	PHENCYCLIDINE	STIMULANTS	MARIJUANA
Physiologic Aspects							
Tolerance	X	X	X	X	X	X	X
Dependence	X	X	X		?	X	X
Habituation	X	X	X	X	X	X	X
Fatal in:							
a. Overdose	X	X	X	?	X	X	
b. Withdrawal from							
addiction	X		X		?		
Discomfort on withdrawal							
from addiction	X	X	X		?	X	?
Physiological Effects							
Pain blockade	X	X	X	X	X	X	?
Euphoria	X	X	X	X	X	X	X
Energy level							
increase	?			?	?	X	
decrease	X	X	X	?	X		X
Anxiety decrease	X	X	X		X		X
Perceptual changes (e.g.,							
hallucinations)				X	X	X	X
Psychomotor impairment	X	X	X		X		X
Time sense changes	X	X	X	?	?	X	X
Toxicologic test available	X	X	X		X	X	X
Treatment							
Titrated withdrawal rec-							
ommended	X	?	X				
Chemical blockade							
available	X	X				?	
Antagonist available		X					

Adapted from the National Institute on Drug Abuse Medical Monograph Series (1976).

a single person, groups of people, or an inanimate object, violence usually denotes interpersonal acts. For both aggression and violence, it is important to distinguish the ***intentionality*** of the act. That is, while war and crime are aggressive and violent acts, they are usually not premeditated to do harm to an individual person.

In the United States, reported juvenile crime has increased dramatically over the last few decades; one out of every nine youths below the age of 18 years will be arrested and will go through the court system. United States data reported regarding violence and school-age children suggest the following annual figures involving teachers and peers: 100 murders, 12,000 armed robberies, 9,000 rapes, 204,000 aggravated assaults and 270,000 school burglaries. Most school violence is predictable and occurs during school hours, at midweek, in February, between classes, and to a victim who is a 7th-grade, minority male in the school who has been victimized before. The offender is usually the same age and sex and is known to the victim.

Toch reported that adult acts of violence fall into the following categories: preservation of self-image (41%), pressure-removing (12%), as a tool (26%), exploitation (10%), bullying (6%), self-defense (6%), self-indulgence (6%), norm-enforcing (4%), and cathartic (3%).

Specific data on the predictability of adult violence are not as clear as for youth. The major correlates are as follows. Most murders—about 25%—are a family affair in the heat of a quarrel. There is a strong correlation between alcohol consumption and violence/aggression; 50% of all arrests, 24% of violent deaths, 50% to 64% of all homicides (killer or victim), 34% of all forcible rapes, and 41% of all assaults. Repressive social conditions precipitate outbursts of violence.

Four special forms of violence are frequently seen by the physician: chemically induced (most frequently alcohol, amphetamines, or phencyclidine), child abuse, spouse beating, and rape.

Spouse abuse by men has been reported to occur in a three-stage cycle. In ***phase I,*** which may last from a few days to years, the husband becomes increasingly critical, verbally abusive, and perhaps destructive to things (*e.g.,* throws a plate of food on the floor). This phase I build-up reaches a peak, at which time he enters phase II. *Phase II* is the violent beating of the wife. This phase is similar to a child's temper tantrum in that nothing the wife can say or do will intervene in the behavior, which may last from minutes to days. *Phase III* follows, during which the husband is extremely repentant and attentive and offers convincing statements that he will "never do it again." This phase III behavior is the positive reinforcement that prevents the wife from pressing legal charges. Unless the wife does bring action at the first episode, the husband assumes her tacit agreement to participate in the activity. The great majority of wives do not obtain masochistic pleasure from the beating; rather, they usually stay in the relationship because of loneliness and financial considerations. The husbands are usually emotionally immature and insecure and the wives are the "emotional glue that holds them together." The wives will usually tolerate the behavior until it begins to occur with the children.

In *rape,* the act is a violent—not a sexual—one. Characteristics of the noninstitutional (*i.e.,* nonprison) *typical rapist* include the following: 15 to 19 years of age, of a lower socioeconomic status, and sexually abused as a child (75%). Usually these men are sexually conservative and naive. The most frequent scenario is that the rape occurs in the victim's home (50%) by someone with whom the woman has at least a minimal acquaintance. Psychologically, the rape is best understood as a displacement onto the victim of anger or revenge toward a mother or other woman perceived as hostile/castrating/rejecting.

Recommendations for *control of aggression* (and perhaps violence) include the following: eliminate sources of frustration, don't reinforce aggressive behavior, reinforce nonaggressive behavior, eliminate associated objects (*e.g.,* toy guns), provide alternatives to violence, confront aggression/violence with an equal-strength, nonaggressive reaction, and decrease the use of physical punishment because it serves as a model of aggression.

Suicide

If aggression can't be directed appropriately, displaced, or scapegoated, it may be turned upon the self, and suicide occurs. Four different definitions or descriptions of suicide can be applied: (1) anyone who takes his own life, (2) taking one's own life where a given set of circumstances (*e.g.,* physical health, environmental conditions) are so hopeless that a person actively "gives up," (3) taking one's own life where unexpressed hostility toward others is involved, for example, "I'll show you, you son-of-a-bitch, you'll miss me when I'm gone." (Menninger wrote about this anger/self-destruction as simultaneously containing the wish to kill, the wish to be killed, and the wish to die), and (4) taking one's own life as an accompaniment of a serious depressive syndrome or other mental disorder.

The latter three definitions all incorporate the feeling of hopelessness for change: "Things will never get any better and I don't want to continue like this." Hopelessness, helplessness, and loss of future orientation are the best predictors of active suicidal intent.

Statistically, approximately 26,000 to 30,000 persons in America are reported to commit suicide each year and about ten times that number attempt it. In adolescents and college students (15 to 24 years of age) suicide is the *second* leading cause of death and accidents are first. It is likely that many accidents, particularly single-person vehicle deaths, are actually suicides. Overall, suicide is one of the ten leading causes of death in America.

The demographics correlated with successful suicides are as follows. These are most significant; previous attempts, more males then females are successful (more females attempt it), single, widowed, or divorced, living alone, over 45 years of age, white, unemployed, a suicide note, poor health, early stages of recovery from depression (*i.e.,* energy and concentration levels have improved to where the individual can make plans and carry them through), and 25% to 36% are alcohol related. These are other correlates: eight out of ten have given a warning, hits all social classes (relative standing is difficult to ascertain due to differential recording), and it increases in incidence after a national crisis. It is commonly reported that physicians have a higher rate of suicide than the general population; however, if socioeconomic status is controlled, their rate is not significantly different.

Since suicidal persons usually are only actively suicidal for a short period of time, appropriate management of the suicidal person should entail close supervision. Preferably, this is done by a close support system (*i.e.,* family or friends) on an ambulatory basis—admission to a mental hospital presupposes subsequent release, and the rate for suicidal persons discharged from mental hospitals is 34 times that of the general population. However, if no adequate ambulatory support system is available, hospitalization is indicated.

The Doctor–Patient Relationship

A major factor in the care of patients is the ***rapport*** that develops between the physician and the patient. Rapport is not simply, or necessarily, that "I like you;" rather, it is the understanding each has of the other and the cooperative effort to cure or control the patient's condition. That is, both the patient and the physician must be involved in the treatment process and the patient must actively attempt to "get well." This is best accomplished by the physician talking with the patient, not at him.

The verbal and nonverbal messages that physicians convey must be congruent and of a particular nature. The physician must be a warm, "nurturant parent." That does not necessarily mean totally permissive or all-giving. It does mean caring enough to sometimes set very specific boundaries (*e.g.,* "I won't let you kill yourself.") and being honest (*e.g.,* "Your test results and examination suggest you have a malignancy"). The physician must maintain a mature adult reality with all patients. The physician must have an active, inventive mind to bring new solutions to patients' problems.

There are three major ***interviewing styles,*** which will predictably produce different outcomes with patients There is no one correct style; however, each can be used differentially for specific purposes.

Laundry List: The physician asks a series of preprogrammed, structured questions, which effectively communicates to the patient, "I will tell you when to talk and what to talk about." This interview style is probably the least efficient in gathering data meaningful to the care of patients and certainly does the least to promote doctor–patient rapport. It is useful to structure persons with thought disorders or affective disorders, particularly mania, and to intervene in obsessive–compulsive verbal detail. That is, it can assist some patients by structuring their internal state and maintaining effective communication patterns.

Associative: In this style, the physician listens to and observes the patient. Any communication from the physician is associated to what the patient is presenting. The physician inserts minimal structure into the interview. This is considered the most efficient method of relevant data collection, first, because more pertinent information is

elicited than by laundry list interviewing and, second, the best rapport is developed. Obviously, those conditions listed above for which a laundry list interview is indicated are those for which the associative interview is contraindicated.

Open-ended: This format is not truly appropriate for general medical interviewing because, it tends to focus on process rather than content issues. In true open-ended interviewing, whatever the patient wishes to verbalize is the topic at hand and no focus is necessary. This is useful in certain psychotherapeutic encounters, but not the majority of medical practice.

Some specific concepts for interviewing are as follows:

Support: any response, verbal or nonverbal, that demonstrates interest in, concern for, or understanding of the patient

Reassurance: a response that helps the patient feel good about himself, including feelings of merit and self-assurance

Empathy: a nonjudgemental response that shows the patient the doctor recognizes and accepts the patient's feelings, even though the doctor may personally disagree with them

Confrontation: a response that points out to the patient the patient's feelings or behavior; confrontation need not be a hostile or accusatory action

Reflection: a response that echos or mirrors a portion of what a patient has just said, which is generally intended to allow patients to become aware of what they have verbalized

Interpretation: a statement based on inference rather than on observation (*e.g.,* "Given those frustrating events, I assume you became angry.")

Silence: Different types can be communicated—interested silence, disinterested silence, and withdrawn silence—however, silence can be a very effective communication device.

Summation: a response that reviews information given by the patient

Adherence Issues

Adherence to medical treatment is a significant issue in health care delivery, because research indicates that only 30% to 35% of patients totally follow their physician's recommendations, and 30% to 35% do not comply at all. The following variables have been documented as contributing to this issue and are probably rooted in the values of both the physician and patient.

Patients who have chronic illnesses (*e.g.*, cardiovascular disease, mental disorder, arthritis) tend to adhere less. Often they require long-term medication maintenance or use preventive medications which, when discontinued, do not produce immediate or noticeable effects. Young, elderly, and disadvantaged patients adhere less, as do persons who are described as hostile risk-takers and/or hypochondriacal. Patients who follow medical instructions perceive their physicians as caring, have a positive relationship with their doctor, are satisfied with their management, and believe they are ill.

Medication variables that tend to decrease adherence include "lock top" dispensers. Adherence also decreases if more than three medications at a time are taken and if the medications are prescribed either more than four times per day or on an as-needed basis. Adherence can be enhanced by correlating medication taking with daily activities such as meals, using dispensers that have daily/hourly reminders, selecting medications with few side effects, and—most important—ensuring that the patient knows the name and action of the medication.

Treatment regimen variables that increase adherence include therapeutic recommendations that are easy to learn and carry out, take little time to complete, do not lead to social isolation, and do not increase fear.

Physicians who obtain good compliance talk with their patients regarding the patient's feelings about the treatment (*e.g.*, prescribing multiple drugs may mean to a patient that he is more ill). These physicians have a positive attitude toward both the drugs they prescribe and their patients, and they closely supervise the therapy prescribed. They give patients a specific appointment and keep the appointment on time, rather than having the patient "drop in" and keeping the patient waiting in the waiting room. Most important, the physician who has patients that adhere to therapy establishes a cooperative interpersonal working relationship where he and the patient take responsibility for the patient's health care.

Assuring that a patient follows through with a referral is increased by a short referral time, referring the patient to a specific clinician, and referring by letter, not telephone.

Legal and Ethical Considerations

The major, controversial ethical considerations today, as in the past, are those associated with life and death.

BIRTH CONTROL

A central issue of birth control is the physician's legal right to disseminate information or contraceptive devices to persons below the age of majority. While such information is available to adults in each state in the United States, some states maintain laws prohibiting the physician's dissemination of information to minors without parental consent.

ABORTION

The arguments about abortion are multifaceted but include these major points: public financing of abortion for indigent persons; the general ethics of performing elective abortions; whether a wife, without consent of her husband, should be able to receive an abortion; the physical or mental conditions under which abortions should be available.

THE PATIENT'S RIGHT TO DIE

These are central issues concerning a patient's right to die: first, if the patient is of sound mind, is in severe discomfort, or has a condition which, without medical support, will be fatal and the patient does not want the medical support, should it be withdrawn, particularly if the legal next-of-kin opposes the removal of life support system? Second, if the patient has only vital signs, which is clear indication that cortical death has occurred and that auxiliary life support systems are presumably maintaining basic physiologic functioning, by whose authority can the life support systems be withdrawn?

THE PATIENT'S RIGHT TO LIVE

While a patient's right to live is beginning to be a focal issue, as medical economics tighten it will become more critical. It encompasses the reality that as medical science advances, expensive technologies are developed. The available public health care dollar may not be able to subsidize these services for all persons who cannot personally afford them, and, if private, third-party health insurance carriers attempt to provide them, premium payments for all persons will increase dramatically. However, if a mechanism is not provided for the less affluent, then health care delivery for "rich people" and "poor people" will demonstrate more disparity than presently exists.

PARENTAL REFUSAL OF CHILD MEDICAL CARE

A life and death issue involves the emergent medical care of children whose parents reject medical intervention on religious or personal grounds. The basic legal maneuver to circumvent this difficulty has been to have the child declared a ward of the court and treatment effected. The aim is to provide care until the child is of legal and mental age to decide personally about medical intervention.

LEGAL ASPECTS

The legal issues that form a present, major focus are those that surround informed consent and the committed "mentally ill" person, although all patients are included.

Informed consent involves the patient knowing what a particular treatment regimen involves, including what specifically is being prescribed (*e.g.,* medicine, surgery), what options or alternative treatments are available, what the probable outcomes are, and what side effects are known to occur. The latter is particularly relevant both with antipsychotic medications and their association with tardive dyskinesia, as well as with the utilization of addictive drugs. If a patient is not physically or mentally able to comprehend the information, it is generally permissible to administer the least traumatic effective treatment if that treatment is responsible medical practice. As soon as the patient is able to comprehend the management, the patient must be fully informed. A better option, if available, is to discuss management with responsible family members and follow their wishes. In either case, documentation with time and date is essential.

Committed mentally ill adults legally are entitled to the following: they must have treatment available, they can refuse treatment, they can require a jury trial to determine sanity, and they retain their competence for conducting business transactions (*e.g.,* marriage, divorce, voting, driving). The words "sanity" and "competence" are legal, not psychiatric, terms. They refer to prediction of dangerousness, and most medical–psychological studies show that health care professionals cannot reliably and validly predict such dangerousness. The committed only lose the civil liberty to come and go. In most states, emergency detention can be effected by a physician or a law-enforcement person for 48 hours pending a hearing. A physician can detain only; a judge can commit.

With children, special rules exist: *physicians cannot detain.* Other than parents, only juvenile courts have authority over children. Children can be committed only if they are an imminent danger to self or others, they are unable to care for themselves in daily needs, or the parents have absolutely no control over the child and the child is a danger (*e.g.,* fire-setter).

RESEARCH METHODOLOGIES FOR THE STUDY OF HUMAN BEHAVIOR

Statistical Distributions

In research, a statement of significant difference is made based on statistical probabilities. The statement that the results are significant at the 0.05 level means that by chance alone the results are expected 5 times out of 100. The often-quoted statement should be remembered, "Statistics are like a light pole—they can be used for support as does the drunk or to illuminate a given area as does the sober person."

NORMAL DISTRIBUTION

The ***normal distribution*** is the "bell-shaped" curve, which has been used to describe human traits. The curve is presented below. The percentage figures given in this diagram reflect the proportion of events that fall within a given standard deviation of the curve. Abnormality is defined as the amount of deviation from the mean or statistical average, not by social agreement.

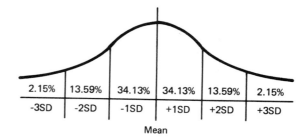

IRREGULAR DISTRIBUTIONS

Other distributions that do not have a "bell-shaped" or normal curve are:

Bimodal

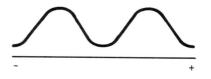

Skewed-negative

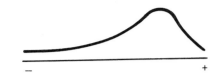

Skewed-positive

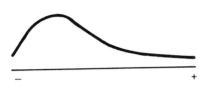

Skewed distributions are named in terms of their "tail."

DISTRIBUTION STATISTICS

There are various statistics that describe the distribution of events (*i.e.*, scores). The major ones are measures of central tendency and measures of variation. The measures of central tendency are the **mean** ($\overline{X}$), the arithmetic average of all individual scores; the **mode**, the most frequent score; and the **median**, the point above and below which 50% of scores occur. For normal distributions, these are all the same point. One of the measures of variation is **standard deviation** (SD), the mathematical expression of the variability of all scores around the mean. Usually plus-and-minus-1 SD is considered to be "normal variation;" for example, if the mean IQ score is 100 and the SD is 10, then "normal" scores would be 90 through 110. **Variance**, the standard deviation squared, and **range**, the highest to the lowest scores of a distribution, are two other measures of variation.

Research Concepts

CONTROL GROUPS

Control groups are the core of experimental designs. These are groups that are as identical as possible to the experimental group upon which experimentation is done and that only differ in the experimental treatment being applied. There are two major types of control groups.

No-treatment control groups are used, for example, with pathologic groups. In this design, the control group does not get an investigational treatment. After treatment is applied to the experimental group, the two groups are compared for improve-

ment in the treated group. Use of such a design helps examine treatment efficacy relative to spontaneous remission rates.

Same-subject control groups are those in which measurement on the criterion of change is taken before a treatment is applied and again after the treatment. Scores are examined for significance of change. This design helps control extraneous factors, which might arise from using a matched control design of totally independent persons.

INDEPENDENT AND DEPENDENT VARIABLES

Independent variables are those that are manipulated (*e.g.*, a given medication). *Dependent* variables are those that reflect the effects of the independent variable (*e.g.*, decrease in a febrile condition after a certain medicine is administered).

VALIDITY

Validity refers to the true accuracy of the observed experimental effect. Using the above illustration, if the febrile condition decreased, was it the effect of the medication or the differential time of day the temperature reading was taken? Generally, cross validation of an experimenter's results by independent researchers is required before a given conclusion is accepted as valid.

RELIABILITY

Reliability means the regularity with which the phenomenon can be reproduced. Using the example from above, does the medication reduce the febrile condition 100% of the time it is administered or 50% of the time?

TRUE AND FALSE POSITIVES AND NEGATIVES

The concepts of true and false positives and negatives refer to the issue of accuracy of test results and are tied to the issues of sensitivity and specificity (below).

True positive: pathology present and results positive

True negative: pathology absent and results negative

False positive: pathology absent and results positive

False negative: pathology present and results negative

SENSITIVITY

Sensitivity is applied to a test of a given entity. A test is sensitive if it correctly picks up the *presence* of pathology in persons who have the pathology. Sensitivity is expressed as a percentage. It is equal to the number of true positives divided by the number of true positives plus false negatives, multiplied by 100.

SPECIFICITY

Specificity is defined as the ability of a test to pick up the *absence* of pathology in a person who does not have the pathology. Specificity is also expressed as a percentage. It is equal to the number of true negatives divided by the number of true negatives plus false positives, multiplied by 100.

EPIDEMIOLOGICAL CONCEPTS

Special statistics related to rates of occurence of a phenomenon in a given population or sample from the entire population are important in behavioral sciences. There are four major epidemiologic statistics. *Incidence* is the rate of new cases of a phenomenon in a given group of persons. *Prevalence* is the rate of all cases of a phenomenon in a group. *Morbidity* is the ratio of the number of ill persons to the total population of a community. *Mortality* is the death rate in a given population.

Research Designs

The manner in which data are collected on a given research topic constitutes the research design.

LONGITUDINAL

Longitudinal studies track the same group of subjects over an extended time period. Periodic observations are made and changes in the group over time are tested for significance of change or are related through correlational statistics. This design can incorporate "no-treatment" or "same-subject" control groups and is employed when unpredictable extrapersonal events, like a world war, may confound results.

A special form of longitudinal study is the treatment follow-up design; for example, after patients have received a given treatment, does the treatment last or is it a temporary phenomenon? This is a particularly relevant research question when the treatment is expensive in physician's time, financial cost, or social–personal consequences.

CROSS SECTIONAL

Cross-sectional designs examine different groups at various levels of a given variable all at the same time and compare the different groups for a given effect. For example, groups at ages 10, 20, 30, 40, 50, 60, and 70 years are administered IQ tests all on one day and results compared to evaluate the hypothesis that IQ decreases with age. This design does not control for the extrapersonal events (such as the fact that, as time goes by, the tendency is for more persons to get more education), which are controlled through the longitudinal design. This design is most applicable when one wishes to examine the effects of a given treatment on various levels of a variable, such as the response of different-aged carcinomas to a given chemotherapeutic regimen.

DOUBLE BLIND

Double-blind designs are those in which neither the subject (S) nor the experimenter (E) knows if the treatment an S is receiving is true treatment or a "placebo." This design is useful to control the subjective bias of both the S and E which frequently, without awareness, influences the outcome of research.

CROSS-OVER

Cross-over designs are a combination of no-treatment and same-subject control groups. In order to prove the efficiency of a given treatment, midway through the experiment, the experimental group is subjected to the events applied to the control group and vice versa. If the experimental treatment is effective, the respective positions of the two groups relative to the dependent variable will shift; or if treatment is permanent, the control group should approximate the experimental group. This is a powerful design that assures treatment effect and addresses the ethical issue of withholding a treatment from a group of persons (*e.g.,* patients with carcinoma not receiving a given type of chemotherapy that proves to be effective).

Research Statistics

Research statistics in behavioral sciences essentially test how similar or how different groups of subjects are.

MEASURES OF DIFFERENCE

Central to probability statistics based on the normal curve, is testing if an observation is significant or if it is a common, "chance" variation within the normal range. Distribution data characterized by a mean and standard deviation can be tested to see if two groups (*e.g.*, experimental and control) differ significantly on the dependent variable. This is done with the *"t"* test. This statistic compares the difference between the means of two samples using the standard deviations of each sample to "pace off" the distance between the two means. If the distributions don't overlap a great deal, it is concluded that the two groups are "significantly different." The significance of the "t" value is determined by reference tables based on sample size and level of significance desired. The larger the sample and the lower the significance one is willing to accept, the smaller the "t" and vice versa.

The *"F"* statistic (*Analysis of Variance* or *ANOVA*) is similar to "t" except the "F" statistic can compare more than two means at a time (*e.g.*, different doses of a medication or the effects of different medications, time of day administered, and different doses of each on the dependent variable). The "F" statistic can reflect whether each of the independent variables is associated with the change in the dependent variable or whether it is an interaction among given variables that is significant.

MEASURES OF RELATIONSHIPS

In addition to statistics of central tendency and variation used to test differences between groups and to generally describe how a group of people present, there are also statistics of relationship between conditions.

The basic relationship statistic is the *correlation coefficient* ("r"). This statistic measures how two variables relate to or co-vary with each other. The "r" that is positive means, as one variable increases so does the other; the "r" that is negative means, as one variable increases the other decreases. The value of "r" can only range from 0.00 to 1.00; the higher the value, the stronger the relation. Therefore, "r" values can vary from -1.00 to $+1.00$. (An r = $-.85$ expresses a stronger relation than an r = $+.75$.) Correlational statistics can *never* be interpreted as cause–effect. There are three possible interpretations to all correlational data. If the "r" is between variables *a* and *b*, these are permissible interpretations: *a* leads to *b*, *b* leads to *a*, or *a* and *b* are related through a third variable, *c*. Corre-

lations can be tested for significance of the size of the correlation (*i.e.*, significantly different from r = 0). One can also establish correlations among multiple variables. Multivariate analyses (*e.g.*, *factor analysis*) are examples of this approach.

REFERENCES

Hollingshead AB, Redlich FC; Social Class and Mental Illness. New York, John Wiley & Sons, 1958

Holmes TH, Rahe RH: The social readjustment scale. J Psychosom Res 11:213, 1967

Kallman FJ: Heredity in Health and Mental Disorder. New York, Norton, 1953

Masters WH, Johnson VE: Human Sexual Response. Boston, Little, Brown & Co, 1966

Pardes H: The syndrome of mental retardation. In Simons R (ed): Understanding Human Behavior in Health and Illness, 3rd ed. New York, Williams & Wilkins, 1985

Sadock VA: Sexual anatomy and physiology. In Grinspoon L (ed): Psychiatry 1982: Annual Review. Washington, American Psychiatric Press, 1982

Selye H: *The Stress of Life*. New York, McGraw-Hill, 1956

Sherfey MJ: The Nature and Evolution of Female Sexuality. New York, Random House, 1972

Terkey S: Working: People Talk About What They Do All Day and How They Feel About What They Do. New York, Random House, 1974. Cited in Mumford E: The social significance of work and studies on the stress of life events. In Simons R (ed): Understanding Human Behavior in Health and Illness. New York, Williams & Wilkins, 1985

Walker L: Battered Women. New York, Springer Publishing, 1984

Wechsler D: Manual for the Wechsler Adult Intelligence Scale. New York, The Psychological Corporation, 1955

QUESTIONS IN THE BEHAVIORAL SCIENCES

Multiple Choice Questions

1. The latency phase of psychoanalytic theory occurs at the same time as which of Erikson's stages?

(a) Trust vs. mistrust
(b) Identity vs. role confusion
(c) Industry vs. inferiority
(d) Autonomy vs. shame & doubt
(e) Initiative vs. guilt

2. A 32-year-old housewife from an upper middle class background is married to an affluent junior executive who must travel a great deal. She does not work but pours herself into volunteer organizations, bridge club, working at the local orphanage, and visiting sick people in hospitals. In a social gathering she rather pointedly occupies the center of attention and generally gives the impression of "anything you can do, I can do better." She is also deathly afraid of riding on elevators. At which stage of Erikson's tasks of development is this woman fixated?
(a) Initiative vs. guilt
(b) Industry vs. inferiority
(c) Identity vs. role confusion
(d) Intimacy vs. isolation
(e) Generativity vs. stagnation

3. Which of the following defense mechanisms would you naturally expect to occur as a psychological concomitant of physical illness, where the person is placed in a hospital?
(a) Symbolization
(b) Regression
(c) Isolation
(d) Compensation
(e) Introjection

4. According to the *Diagnostic and Statistical Manual of Mental Disorders,* Edition III (DSM-III), an IQ of 65 classifies a person as:
(a) Borderline mental retardation
(b) Mild mental retardation
(c) Moderate mental retardation
(d) Severe mental retardation
(e) Profound mental retardation

5. Which of the following is *not* expected after one hour of sensory deprivation?
(a) Anxiety
(b) Depression
(c) Hostility
(d) Fugue
(e) Hallucinations

6. A 14-year-old male is brought into your office by his mother. They have had an argument over the length of his hair. The boy reacts to you in a hostile, argumentative fashion even though you have reasonably long hair, a beard, and have not provoked the reaction

from the young man. You would say that the phenomenon that is occurring is:
(a) Countertransference
(b) Transference
(c) Acting-out
(d) Regression
(e) Synthesis

7. With regard to children who have debilitating and terminal illness, their greatest fear is:
(a) Pain
(b) Death
(c) Separation from parents
(d) What will become of their pets
(e) Being anesthetized

8. In the prediction statistic, the correlation, the value that would have the most predictive power would be:
(a) +.95
(b) −.35
(c) 0
(d) −1.0
(e) +.65

9. Which of the following defense mechanisms is always pathologic?
(a) Rationalization
(b) Isolation
(c) Denial
(d) Disassociation
(e) Conversion

10. In a crisis management of persons who abuse drugs, there are certain drugs of abuse from which persons often die if they are abruptly withdrawn from the substance. Which of the following preparations constitutes a danger of death from abrupt withdrawal?
(a) Stimulants
(b) Sedative hypnotics
(c) Psychedelics
(d) Opiates
(e) Volatiles

11. In the grieving and mourning process we know that at different ages the mourning can take different forms. Which of the following is an *incorrect* statement?
(a) The infant might protest, deny, and detach himself.
(b) A child in the latency stage would probably be jocular and perhaps hypomanic.
(c) A child in the adolescent stage might turn to antisocial acting out.
(d) Middle-age persons quite frequently turn to hypochondriacal symptoms.
(e) Elderly persons typically are relieved and feel somewhat released.

12. The Thematic Apperception Test (TAT) is an example of what type of psychological test?
    (a) Intelligence
    (b) Achievement
    (c) Ability
    (d) Interest
    (e) Personality

13. In speaking of orientation, four spheres are usually examined. All of the following are included *except:*
    (a) Relationship of self to a place in time
    (b) Awareness of self as a person
    (c) Knowledge of geographic location
    (d) Awareness of internal affective state
    (e) Knowledge of present position in time

14. In terms of etiology, anxiety is usually viewed as repressed or forgotten:
    (a) Fear
    (b) Guilt
    (c) Sorrow
    (d) Grief
    (e) Anger

15. All of the following are true statements about the memory process *except* one:
    (a) Long-term memory is rarely defective in organicity unless accompanied by psychosis.
    (b) If memory loss occurs, recovery is typically from the extremes of loss to the precipitating event.
    (c) Memory is particularly disrupted with bilateral lesions of the hippocampus and/or mammillary bodies.
    (d) In general, memory defect is psychogenic if there is no disturbance of consciousness and no intellectual impairment.
    (e) If there is short-term memory loss and motivation and attention is good, it is suggestive of psychogenic involvement.

16. In Freudian theory, a child who has begun to be strongly attached to the parent of the opposite sex and display some "fear" of the parent of the same sex would be in which stage of psychosexual development?
    (a) Oral
    (b) Latent
    (c) Anal
    (d) Phallic/urethral
    (e) Genital

17. All of the following are considered to be functions of the ego *except:*
    (a) Personal values
    (b) Defense mechanisms
    (c) Object relations
    (d) Reality testing
    (e) Thought processes

18. In Erikson's theory of psychological tasks, which of the following is *not* a correct task?
    (a) Integrity vs. despair
    (b) Industry vs. inferiority
    (c) Intimacy vs. isolation
    (d) Generativity vs. stagnation
    (e) Identity vs. shame and doubt

19. The patient states: "I feel uptight about my new job." This is an example of:
    (a) Objective evidence of anxiety
    (b) Subjective evidence of anxiety
    (c) Inappropriate effect
    (d) Repression of affect
    (e) A drive discharge emotion

20. All of the following are examples of psychophysiologic responses to anxiety *except* one:
    (a) Excessive perspiration
    (b) Tension headaches, constriction in the chest, backache
    (c) Aphasia, apraxia, and a right homonymous hemianopsia
    (d) Dyspnea, dizziness, and paresthesias
    (e) Transient systolic hypertension, premature contractions and tachycardia

21. A student did poorly on an examination. The student is afraid he will fail the course. On the next occasion he walks into the room in which the examination was given he experiences fear. This is an example of:
    (a) Classical conditioning learning
    (b) Social learning
    (c) Cognitive learning
    (d) Inhibition learning
    (e) Fixed-schedule learning

22. In learning theory, grades in an academic course would be an example of:
    (a) Acquisition
    (b) Generalization
    (c) Primary reinforcers
    (d) Secondary reinforcers
    (e) Ratio reinforcement

23. All of the statements below regarding adolescence (ages 13 to 18) are true *except:*
    (a) In Erikson's framework the basic task to be resolved is to develop affiliation with others.
    (b) Fifty percent of teenage marriages occur because of pregnancy.

(c) One-third of teenage marriages end in divorce within four years.
(d) They are in Piaget's stage of formal operations.
(e) Adolescents must maintain a sense of identity in the face of rapid changes.

ANSWERS TO MULTIPLE CHOICE QUESTIONS

1. (c)	7. (c)	13. (d)	19. (b)
2. (a)	8. (d)	14. (a)	20. (c)
3. (b)	9. (e)	15. (e)	21. (a)
4. (b)	10. (b)	16. (d)	22. (d)
5. (d)	11. (e)	17. (a)	23. (a)
6. (b)	12. (e)	18. (e)	

Index

Page numbers followed by *f* indicate figures; numbers followed by *t* indicate tabular material.

797